CANADIAN BATES'

Guide to
Health
Assessment
FOR NURSES

Tracey C. Stephen, MN RN
Faculty Lecturer
Faculty of Nursing
University of Alberta
Edmonton, Alberta

Rene A. Day, PhD RN
Professor
Faculty of Nursing
University of Alberta
Edmonton, Alberta

D. Lynn Skillen, PhD RN
Professor Emerita
Faculty of Nursing
University of Alberta
Edmonton, Alberta

Lynn S. Bickley, MD
Clinical Professor of Medicine
School of Medicine
Texas Tech University Health
   Sciences Center
Lubbock, Texas

 Wolters Kluwer | Lippincott Williams & Wilkins
Health
Philadelphia · Baltimore · New York · London
Buenos Aires · Hong Kong · Sydney · Tokyo

Executive Acquisitions Editor: Elizabeth Nieginski
Product Director: Renee A. Gagliardi
Senior Marketing Manager: Jodi Bukowski
Designer: Joan Wendt
Compositor: Spearhead Global, Inc.

First Edition

351 West Camden Street   530 Walnut Street
Baltimore, MD 21201   Philadelphia, PA 19106

Printed in China

9 8 7 6 5 4 3 2 1

Library of Congress Cataloging-in-Publication Data

Canadian Bates' guide to health assessment for nurses / Tracey Stephen ... [et al.]. — 1st ed.
    p. ; cm.
  Includes bibliographical references.
  ISBN 978-0-7817-7867-1
  1. Nursing assessment. 2. Physical diagnosis. 3. Medical history taking. I. Stephen, Tracey. II. Title: Bates' guide to health assessment for nurses. III. Title: Guide to health assessment for nurses.
  [DNLM: 1. Nursing Assessment—methods. 2. Medical History Taking—methods. 3. Physical Examination—methods. WY 100.4 C212 2009]
  RT48.C35 2009
  616.07′5—dc22
      2009006615

Acknowledgments

The Beginning. The *Bates' Guide to Physical Examination and History Taking* has always been outstanding for its accuracy and comprehensiveness. The excellent examination techniques, clear images, and detailed history taking have contributed to learning among nursing students for more than a quarter century. We were thrilled to be asked to take this well-respected text and turn it into a Canadian textbook for nursing students and nurses in practice. This exciting opportunity allowed us to bring health promotion, interprofessional collaboration, and nursing concepts and documentation to the fore. We incorporated our philosophical views about the client as a concept, replaced "normal" with expected and unexpected findings, and highlighted the essence of nursing that includes dignity, respect, comfort, and safety. We are thankful for the opportunity to collaborate on this textbook. The experience of working together with our shared passion for health assessment has been a joy. Publication of this textbook is a culmination of the legacy initiated by Pauline Marie Kot who was a dear friend and mentor in the Faculty of Nursing, University of Alberta.

Barbara Bates demonstrated amazing foresight when she initiated the first edition of her textbook for medical students. **Lynn S. Bickley** has continued Bates' commitment to assist health professionals in developing excellence in assessment of clients and maximizing health outcomes.

Lippincott Williams & Wilkins (a Wolters Kluwer Company). Working with the talented and dedicated acquisitions and editorial teams has been a very positive experience. We appreciate their respect for our judgment about critical content to be added to the book, and their confidence in our ability to maintain high standards and bring this project to completion. **Peter Darcy**, publisher, supported the idea for the book, facilitated the process, and kept the momentum going. **Renee Gagliardi**, senior product manager, provided support, encouragement, willingness to understand different points of view, patience, and flexibility in the face of our individual pressures and demands. Her crazy ability to reword sentences while maintaining the essence of what we were trying to say contributed to the readability and overall quality of the work. Renee looked at our challenges creatively and presented us with viable options. We enjoyed our teleconferences with Renee because of her enthusiasm, respect, and empathy. Her professionalism was outstanding.

Recognition by **Corey Wolfe, Barry Wight,** and **Dan Renaud** of the need for a Canadian nursing assessment textbook provided the impetus for this project. They knew our passion for health assessment and our desire to have an outstanding Canadian resource for learners in nursing. Their openness to innovation, enthusiasm, knowledge of Canadian networks, and determination to keep the project moving forward were a constant support.

The Canadian Chapter Authors. Colleagues from British Columbia, Alberta, Saskatchewan, Manitoba, and Ontario willingly shared their expertise, made clinically relevant contributions, and brought the chapter templates to life. They, too, recognized the importance for students to have excellent materials for the Canadian context.

The University of Alberta Team. **Wayne Day**, our project director and Internet researcher *extraordinaire,* kept us organized, focused on details, caught things we missed, and ensured that we stayed sane. **Leona Laird** and **Alice DaSilva** efficiently handled the many courier packages to the publisher with smiles, and contributed to a timely flow of materials. Our **colleagues** supported, encouraged, empathized, and were excited about the product to come. **Students and graduates** over the years raised provocative questions, showed keen interest, and recognized that health assessment is critical in nursing. They applied their learning in practice and in their own personal and family health experiences. Many shared how health assessment education and skillful instruction have influenced their careers. They remember lab demonstrations and lab environments that were warm, respectful, fun, and exciting. **Simulated clients** made major contributions to student learning. Their patience, willingness to allow us to demonstrate approaches and skills, and their openness to having students practise on them contributed to positive learning experiences. In particular, they assisted students with pointers about how to approach and examine clients of the opposite sex. They always tried to help students relax during test situations, and they even allowed their photos to be taken for the book!

We dedicate this book to the memory of a dear colleague and friend, Pauline Marie Kot (1930–2008). Pauline was thrilled to hear that her favourite health assessment book was being recreated for nursing students and nurses in practice. A fine teacher and mentor, she was highly regarded by her students and colleagues, and was influential in helping each of us to further develop our health assessment skills.

Pauline was a caring individual; a woman of integrity who treated everyone with respect, fairness, and kindness. An expert in the field of health assessment, she paid attention to detail and pursued excellence. She provided a supportive, safe learning environment for students and had a wry sense of humour that she used in her teaching. Pauline was at the vanguard of introducing health assessment into nursing curricula. She showed leadership at the University of Alberta as a member of the nursing faculty, teaching health assessment for students and working nurses, embracing computer-managed learning, and developing a structured, comprehensive course syllabus for health assessment that is still in use today.

Tracey Stephen   S Lynn Skillen   Rene A. Day

About the Canadian Author Team

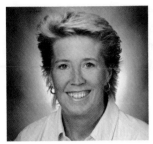

Tracey C. Stephen is a Faculty Lecturer in the Faculty of Nursing, University of Alberta. She has been teaching nursing students since 1991, teaching health assessment for the past 17 years, and currently teaches critical care nursing and health assessment. Tracey is passionate about working with nursing students, nurses, and clients and their families. She is committed to developing excellent learning resources for nursing students. Tracey appreciates her colleagues and students for all their support. She sends a very special thank you to FP for such unwavering support and friendship.

She thanks her wonderful husband, Andy, and three awesome children, Jenelle, Taylir, and Mackenna, for all that they are and for all that they do to make her life so fantastic. She thanks them for their love, cheering, and patience during this adventure and sends this message, "I love you as blue as the sky, as bright as the sun, and all the way to the moon and beyond."

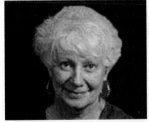

D. Lynn Skillen received a PhD in Sociology (Workplace Health and Safety) from the University of Alberta, and an MHSc (Health Care Practice) and BScN (Community Health) from McMaster University. Throughout her academic career at the Faculty of Nursing, University of Alberta she taught undergraduate and graduate health assessment, including advanced health assessment in Spanish to nurse educators in Mexico and Peru. A nurse clinician earlier in her career, she used health assessment skills in remote and urban Alberta. She values the opportunity to write with two dear, respected colleagues who share her passion for excellence in health assessment in nursing. Lynn is grateful to Bud, Sammy, and Sofie for their unconditional support. As a Professor Emerita, her lifelong interest in languages (Spanish, French, and Italian) guides her travel choices for hiking, biking, and skiing.

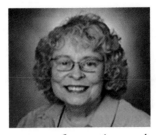

Rene Day is a Professor at the Faculty of Nursing, University of Alberta. She received her PhD from the University of Alberta, MS (nursing) from the University of Hawaii, and BScN from the University of Alberta. Since 1976, Rene has taught health assessment for nursing students, practising nurses in northern and central Alberta, and nurses working in correctional facilities in the Province of Alberta. Her lifetime approach to teaching has been about supporting students to be successful. Rene has been honoured with a Lifetime Achievement Award from the College and Association of Registered Nurses of Alberta, a Nursing Education Leadership Award from the Alberta Nursing Education Administrators, and a national award for Nursing Education Administration from the Canadian Association of University Schools of Nursing. Heartfelt thanks go to her husband Wayne for his patient, unwavering, and loving support and to Jason, Mary, Stephen, and Julia for their understanding about fewer family dinners when book chapters took over the dining room table.

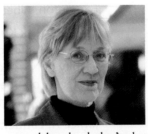

Lynn S. Bickley is the award-winning author of *Bates' Guide to Physical Examination and History Taking*, *Bates' Pocket Guide to Physical Examination and History Taking*, and *Bates' Visual Guide to Physical Examination and History Taking*. She earned her bachelor's degree from Smith College and her medical degree from the University of Rochester School of Medicine and Dentistry. This distinguished clinician and educator has specialized in programs involving student and physician training in geriatrics and patient-centered cultural competence. At Texas Tech University, she oversaw a comprehensive curriculum redesign for the School of Medicine. She serves on a national committee setting standards for teaching clinical skills.

Canadian Contributors

Joan Anderson, PhD
Professor Emerita
School of Nursing
University of British Columbia
Vancouver, British Columbia

Marjorie C. Anderson, PhD RN
Associate Professor (Retired)
Faculty of Nursing
University of Alberta
Edmonton, Alberta

Judy A. Bornais, MSc RN
Experiential Learning Specialist
Faculty of Nursing
University of Windsor
Windsor, Ontario

Angela Bowen, PhD RN
Assistant Professor
College of Nursing and Associate
    Member
College of Medicine Department
    of Psychiatry
University of Saskatchewan
Saskatoon, Saskatchewan

Annette Brown, Ph RN
Associate Professor
School of Nursing
University of British Columbia
Vancouver, British Columbia

Kim Brunet, MSc RD
Nutrition Service Manager
Alberta Health Services
Capital Region
Edmonton, Alberta

William L. Diehl-Jones, PhD RN
Associate Professor
Faculty of Nursing and Faculty
    of Science
University of Manitoba
Winnipeg, Manitoba

Dana S. Edge, PhD RN
Associate Professor
School of Nursing
Queen's University
Kingston, Ontario

Nicole Harder, MPA RN
Learning Labs Coordinator
Faculty of Nursing
University of Manitoba
Winnipeg, Manitoba

Kathleen Hunter, PhD RN
Assistant Professor
Faculty of Nursing
University of Alberta
Edmonton, Alberta

Kaysi Eastlick Kuschner, PhD RN
Associate Professor
Faculty of Nursing
University of Alberta
Edmonton, Alberta

Janice A. Lander, RN PhD
Professor
Faculty of Nursing
University of Alberta
Edmonton, Alberta

Gerri C. Lasiuk, RN PhD
Assistant Professor
Faculty of Nursing
University of Alberta
Edmonton, Alberta

Diana Mager, RD PhD
Assistant Professor
Clinical Nutrition
Alberta Institute for Human
    Nutrition
Department of Agricultural, Food,
    and Nutritional Science
Faculty of Agricultural, Life, and
    Environmental Sciences
University of Alberta
Program Manager, Research
Nutrition Services
Alberta Health Services
Capital Region
Edmonton, Alberta

Linda Reutter, PhD RN
Professor
Faculty of Nursing
University of Alberta
Edmonton, Alberta

Sheri Roach, BComm BJ BScN RN
MN/MHA Student
Dalhousie University
Halifax, Nova Scotia

Pat Roddick, MHS RN
Instructor
School of Nursing
MacEwan College
Edmonton, Alberta

Sarla Sethi, PhD RN
Associate Professor (Retired)
Faculty of Nursing
University of Calgary
Calgary, Alberta

Colleen Varcoe, PhD RN
Associate Professor
School of Nursing
University of British Columbia
Vancouver, British Columbia

Contents

CHAPTER 14

The Thorax and Lungs 381

CHAPTER 15

The Cardiovascular System 423

CHAPTER 16

The Breasts and Axillae 479

UNIT III

Special Populations 847

CHAPTER 24

Assessing the Woman Who Is Pregnant . . 849

CHAPTER 25

The Older Adult 887

Preface

Entering the realm of health assessment, nursing students begin to integrate the art and practice of nursing. Their experiences grow, expand, and trigger the required levels of critical thinking from the first moments of their encounters with clients. Working through the steps of the health history and physical examination reveals to them the multifaceted profile of the client. Students learn to identify concerning symptoms and signs, lifestyle practises, unexpected findings, and a nursing diagnosis that considers the client holistically. The skills that allow them to assess all clients also shape the image of the unique human allowing them to conduct an assessment and provide care. Collecting a comprehensive client history begins to reveal the individual as that unique human being. During the history interview, students and nurses in practice become aware of areas for health promotion, identify symptoms and signs that require scrutiny, differentiate expected and unexpected findings, and interpret all the data to determine a nursing diagnosis.

The techniques of physical examination and history taking embody time-honoured skills of healing and client care. The ability to gather a sensitive and nuanced history and to perform a thorough and accurate examination deepens the relationships with clients, focuses the assessment, and sets the direction for clinical thinking. The quality of the history and physical examination governs the next steps with the client and guides the choices for subsequent tests. These important relational and clinical skills contribute to the development of accomplished clinicians.

The *Canadian Bates' Guide to Health Assessment for Nurses* is designed for nursing students who are learning to talk with clients, collect subjective data, perform physical examinations, and apply clinical reasoning to understand and assess client concerns. Sections of this edition will also be useful to nurses in practice, including nurse practitioners. The book is divided into three units to facilitate learning: *Foundations of Health Assessment, Regional and System Examinations,* and *Special Populations.* Five original chapters in this first Canadian edition encompass health promotion, culture, pain, nutrition, and documentation. An original section on psychosocial assessment has been added.

The first two chapters on health promotion and culture provide critical concepts that cross-cut all subsequent chapters. Key features of Chapters 3 through 25 are:

- Collection of subjective data
- Key symptoms and signs reported by clients
- Symptom/sign analysis
- Important topics for health promotion (including risk factors and screening)
- Canadian guidelines and standards for assessing health and risks to health
- Canadian demographics
- Canadian statistics
- Techniques for obtaining objective data
- Recording and analyzing client findings
- Interprofessional collaboration
- Critical thinking
- Citations and additional references
- Alignment with evidence from the health care literature
- Relevant Canadian associations and Web sites
- Canadian research related to health assessment.

In Unit I, *Foundations of Health Assessment,* readers will find in Chapter 1, *The Broad Scope of Health Promotion in Health Assessment,* the foundation for the application of health promotion in health assessment by nurses. This chapter provides a comprehensive discussion of health promotion in the Canadian context, including a history of the different approaches to health in Canada and the characteristics of health promotion. Chapter 2, *Cultural Considerations in Health Assessment,* introduces the concept of cultural safety and describes how every clinical encounter is cross-cultural, involving differences between nurse and client. It provides learners with the current discussion on how culture is understood from different perspectives, the importance of cultural considerations, and how these are relevant for the Canadian context. Chapter 3, *The Health History: Subjective Data,* guides students through the techniques of skilled empathic interviewing, with a special focus on ethics, and encompasses the vital components of a health history that capture the client's subjective data. Chapter 4, *The Physical Examination: Objective Data,* introduces the essential elements for proceeding with the physical examination. It includes the principles of the four basic examination modes: inspection, palpation, percussion, and auscultation, and provides the beginner with an understanding of the anatomical position, anatomical terms, and terms for movement and comparison. The chapter also contains information about sequences for comprehensive and focused physical examinations. Chapter 5, *Documenting and Analyzing Findings,* details the fundamentals of documentation, including the principles and methods for developing the written record using subjective and objective data. It presents guidelines for documentation, types of documentation systems, and an actual written record. Chapter 6, *General Survey and Vital Signs,* provides guidance for the traditional vital signs and incorporates the new fifth and sixth vital signs. Chapter 7, *Pain Assessment,* presents the current theory for addressing pain, available assessment, and the subjective and objective aspects of pain. Chapter 8, *Nutritional Assessment,* considers the digestive process, Canadian guidelines, measurements, and approaches to assessing nutritional status, including food intake and activity. Chapter 9, *Psychosocial and Mental Status Assessment,* is foundational to every encounter with clients and includes genetic, physiologic, psychologic, developmental, emotional, and spiritual dimensions of individuals within the context of their physical and social environments.

Unit II, *Regional and System Examinations,* is devoted to the techniques of examination of each body region/system. These chapters are arranged in the "head-to-toe" sequence that is commonly used in a **comprehensive** physical examination. When conducting a **focused** physical examination, learners will consult appropriate chapters according to the regions/systems they plan to scrutinize. Each examination chapter begins with a review of relevant anatomy and physiology, followed by pertinent health history, common symptoms and signs reported by clients, important topics for health promotion, important information useful for health counselling, specific prevention for specific diseases, and emergency concerns. The chapters then continue with the techniques of examination, including expected and unexpected findings, and examples of documentation for the focus of the chapter. Each chapter closes with tables to help students recognize selected unexpected findings and their implications. Unit II contains:

- Chapter 10: *The Skin, Hair, and Nails*
- Chapter 11: *The Head and Neck*
- Chapter 12: *The Eyes*
- Chapter 13: *The Ears, Nose, Mouth, and Throat*
- Chapter 14: *The Thorax and Lungs*
- Chapter 15: *The Cardiovascular System*
- Chapter 16: *The Breasts and Axillae*
- Chapter 17: *The Abdomen*
- Chapter 18: *The Peripheral Vascular System*
- Chapter 19: *The Musculoskeletal System*
- Chapter 20: *The Nervous System*
- Chapter 21: *Male Genitalia and Hernias*
- Chapter 22: *Female Genitalia*
- Chapter 23: *The Anus, Rectum, and Prostate*

In Unit 3, *Special Populations,* learners will find chapters relating to two special stages of the life cycle: pregnancy and aging. Chapter 24, *Assessing the Woman Who Is Pregnant,* contains Canadian guidelines for nutrition, supplements, and weight gain; health-promoting activities; changes in anatomy and physiology related to pregnancy, and risks. The final chapter, *Assessing the Older Adult,* outlines the approach to the heterogeneous older adult population in Canada, and details techniques for promoting the special goals related to aging: maintaining health, social well-being and optimal levels of function, and delaying unnecessary depletion of physiologic and cognitive reserves.

Learners are expected to have had basic courses in human anatomy and physiology. The sections on these subjects in the chapters of Unit II are intended to help students apply this knowledge to interpretation of symptoms, client examination, and understanding of physical findings.

This first Canadian edition for nurses emphasizes health promotion, common health concerns, and important challenges to health. Occasionally, a physical sign of a rare condition is included when it occupies a solid niche in classic physical examination, or when recognizing the condition is especially important for the health or even the life of the client.

Most students develop their health assessment skills first by practising on each other. These skills can be used in any setting as most examination techniques and expected findings are common to both adults and children.

CANADIAN BATES' GUIDE TO HEALTH ASSESSMENT FOR NURSES

This first Canadian edition for nurses introduces new content and approaches that build on *Bates' Guide to Physical Examination and History Taking.* This content springs from the learning needs of nursing students and our approach as nurse experts teaching health assessment. Our goal is to capitalize on Bates' high quality content on physical examination and history taking, and tailor the book for nursing and the Canadian context.

The three units of the Canadian text bring a coherent and helpful organization to students who are learning to assess clients from Canada's diverse populations. The foundational chapters on health promotion, culture, health history, physical examination modes and anatomical vocabulary, documentation, current approaches to general survey and vital signs, pain assessment, nutritional assessment, and psychosocial and mental status assessment provide additional substantive content to the *Bates' Guide to Physical Examination and History Taking.* All chapters in Units II and III contain current and comprehensive information related to health promotion, risk assessment, and counselling. Each chapter reflects an *evidence-based perspective,* listing key Canadian citations and references where possible as well as relevant Canadian associations and Web sites. All tables are vertical so readers can page through the chapters easily.

Each chapter in Unit II contains sections on Anatomy and

Physiology, Health Promotion, Screening, Prevention, History, Techniques of Examination, Examples of Documentation, and a Case Study with Critical Thinking questions that address knowledge, comprehension, application, analysis, synthesis, and evaluation. Symptom information is incorporated in the regional/system chapter most relevant to the particular symptoms. For example, headache is presented in Chapter 11, *Head and Neck*, while diarrhea is addressed in Chapter 17, *The Abdomen*. The sections on Important Topics for Health Promotion in each chapter provide Canadian statistics, demographics, and guidelines, such as for obesity, classification of hypertension, and screening mammograms.

Colour demarcates chapter sections and tables clearly, leading students to insets of key material and special tips for challenging aspects of examination and considering comfort, dignity, and safety during the physical examination. Canadian photographs and drawings have been added to better illustrate key points.

The basic core organization of the text permits students to study or review the Anatomy and Physiology sections according to their individual needs. They can study the Canadian demographics and statistics, important topics for health promotion, common concerning symptoms and signs reported by clients, cultural considerations, and Canadian guidelines. They can review Techniques of Examination to learn how to perform the relevant examination, then practise it under faculty guidance, and review it again afterward. Students and faculty will also benefit from identifying common unexpected findings, which appear in two places. The right-hand column of the Techniques of Examination sections presents possible unexpected findings. These are highlighted in red and linked to the adjacent text. Distinguishing these findings from the expected findings improves learners' observations and clinical acumen. For further information on unexpected observations, readers also can turn to the Tables of Unexpected Findings at the end of each of the chapters in Unit II. These tables display or describe various unexpected conditions in a convenient format that allows students to compare and contrast related unexpected findings in a single table.

SUGGESTIONS FOR USING THIS BOOK

Although the health history and the physical examination are both essential for client assessment and care, students often learn them separately, sometimes even from different faculty members. Students becoming proficient at interviewing are advised to return to Chapter 3, *The Health History: Subjective Data*, as they gain experience talking with clients of different ages and emotional states. As learners begin developing a smooth sequence of examination, they may wish to review the sequence of examination outlined in each of the regional/system examination chapters.

It is essential that students learn to integrate the client's story and the client's physical findings. Students will benefit by studying the relevant portions of the Health History as they learn successive parts of the examination. In a few areas, symptoms may lead to examination of more than one body system. For example, chest pain prompts evaluation of the cardiovascular, musculoskeletal, and respiratory systems. The symptoms of the urinary tract are relevant to the chapters on the abdomen, the prostate, and the male and female genitalia.

As students progress through the body systems/regions, they need to study the documentation of findings of the client who is presented in Chapter 5, *Documenting and Analyzing Findings*. They also may refer frequently to the sections on Recording and Analyzing Findings that display selected examples related to the focus of each chapter. This cross-checking will help students learn how to describe and organize information from the interview and physical examination into an understandable written format. Further, studying Chapter 3, *The Health History: Objective Data*, will help students select and analyze the data they are learning to collect.

Skimming the Tables of Unexpected Findings makes students more familiar with what they should be looking for and the rationale for asking certain questions. Students should not try to memorize all the detail that is presented. The best time to learn about unexpected conditions and diseases is when a client, real or described, appears with a concern. Students could then use this tool to try to analyze the concern or finding, and make use of other clinical texts or journals to pursue the client's situation in as much depth as is necessary. Students can refer to the Citations, Additional References, and Canadian Associations and Web Sites at the end of each chapter for additional relevant sources.

RELATED LEARNING MATERIAL

Faculty and teachers can turn to resources available on Lippincott's ThePoint Web site.

EQUIPMENT

Equipment necessary for a physical examination includes the following:

- Ophthalmoscope and otoscope
- Penlight
- Glass of water
- Tongue depressors
- Ruler and flexible tape measure marked in centimetres
- Thermometer
- Watch with second hand
- Sphygmomanometer
- Stethoscope with the following characteristics:

- Ear tips that fit snugly and painlessly. To get this fit, choose ear tips of the proper size, align the ear pieces with the angle of your ear canals, and adjust the spring of the connecting metal band to a comfortable tightness.
- Thick-walled tubing as short as feasible to maximize the transmission of sound: about 30 cm if possible and no longer than 38 cm
- Bell and diaphragm with a functional changeover mechanism

■ Gloves (sterile and unsterile)
■ Lubricant for vaginal and rectal examinations

■ Vaginal specula
■ Equipment for cytologic and perhaps bacteriologic study
■ Reflex hammer
■ Tuning forks, one of 128 Hz and one of 512 Hz or 1024 Hz
■ Cotton balls for testing sense of light touch
■ Disposable tissues
■ Felt marking pen
■ Samples of pungent odours for testing sense of smell
■ Paper and pen or pencil
■ Sheet to use for draping

Foundations of Health Assessment

CHAPTER 8
Nutrition Assessment

CHAPTER 9
Psychosocial and Mental Status Assessment

The Broad Scope of Health Promotion in Health Assessment

Linda Reutter and Kaysi Eastlick Kuschner

Health promotion is a key concept in nursing and the other health sciences. Promoting health is at the heart of all nursing activities in every setting and is one of the four core metaparadigm concepts of nursing.

Health promotion is conceived of in many different ways. It is not easily defined, and setting, time, academic discipline, and societal factors influence how it is put into practice. In Canada and Canadian nursing, the understanding of health promotion has evolved over time. A brief history of the different approaches to health in Canada and a description of the characteristics of health promotion provide a foundation for the application of health promotion in health assessment by nurses.

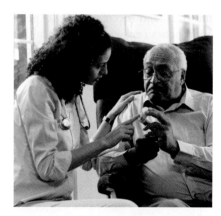

 ## HEALTH PROMOTION IN CANADA

Canadian nurses need to be aware of the degree of respect with which Canadian initiatives related to health promotion are viewed by the global community. The Canadian nursing perspective on primary health care (PHC) is consistent with many global initiatives for health. Conceptualizations of health and its determinants influence the scope of Canadian nursing practice.

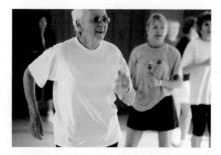

HISTORICAL APPROACHES TO HEALTH AND HEALTH PROMOTION

In Canada's recent past, there have been three major approaches to health: medical, behavioural, and socioenvironmental (Labonte, 1993). Each approach takes a different view of health and its determinants; all three are important.

Medical Approach. A *medical approach* usually is associated with a biomedical definition of health as the "absence of disease." The focus is on illness care, and the underlying assumption is that the major determinant of health is a good health care system. While a health care system is important, this approach does not emphasize a holistic view of health, nor does it focus on keeping Canadians well. Globally, it has become obvious that increasing the funding for curative care systems does not appreciably improve the health of populations as a whole.

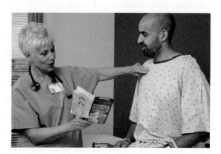

Nurses use the medical approach during the health history when they ask clients about their medications, how they take them, and what effect medications have. During the physical examination, nurses use this approach when they observe for expected and unexpected findings.

Behavioural/Lifestyle Approach.

In Canada, the *Lalonde Report* (1974) introduced the concept of four influences on health: biology, environment, lifestyle, and health care organization. This report was heralded as a major breakthrough in the analysis of determinants of health and is recognized as the beginning of "health promotion" in Canada. By 1978, the Canadian government had created a Health Promotion Directorate—the first of its kind in the world (Pinder, 2007). Directorate activities tended to focus on lifestyle issues, particularly choices regarding tobacco, alcohol, drugs, nutrition, and exercise, to the exclusion of other determinants, especially environments.

The *Lalonde Report* ushered in the *behavioural approach* to health, with an emphasis on personal health practices as major health determinants. Nurses subsequently directed their primary strategies for enhancing health toward promoting healthy lifestyles and decreasing risk behaviours. They emphasized health-education approaches (e.g., individual health counselling and education, social marketing, advocacy for policies that supported lifestyle change).

In health assessment, nurses assess many lifestyle practices while taking the comprehensive health history. For example, they inquire about exercise, breast or testicular self-examination, alcohol and drug use, skin protection, tobacco use, spirituality, dental care, use of protective devices in sports and recreation, and nutrient intake (see Chapter 3). When conducting physical examinations, nurses look for correlated subjective and objective data. These include taking height, weight, and vital sign measurements, and assessing for needle tracks, inspiratory wheezes, staining of fingers from nicotine, dental caries, skin lesions, and breast or testicular lumps (see Chapters 6, 10, 13, 14, 16, and 21).

Critics of the behavioural approach fault its lack of attention to the direct and indirect influence of social and environmental factors on health (through health practices). Although behavioural factors are influential, research findings suggest that individual risk behaviours explain only 25% to 30% of differences in mortality rates for chronic diseases (Adler et al., 1994). In addition, risk-reduction programs are most effective for clients with higher income (Lyons & Langille, 2000). Risk behaviours actually may serve as coping strategies for people who must manage the stress of unhealthy living and working conditions over which they have little control. For example, low-income women may use smoking as a coping strategy to manage the stresses associated with poverty (Stewart et al., 1996, 2004).

Socioenvironmental/Ecological Approach.

A *socioenvironmental* or *ecological approach* (a social view of health and health promotion) recognizes that the *root causes* of ill health reside in societal structures and environments. This approach emphasizes *psychosocial factors* (e.g., social support) and *socioenvironmental conditions* (e.g., income, workplace conditions, social inclusion, equitable distribution of resources) as key determinants of health (Labonte, 1993). The view of health is in positive, holistic terms rather than simply the absence of disease.

The *Ottawa Charter* introduced an ecological view of health. This watershed document was the outcome of the first international conference on health promotion, co-hosted by the Canadian government, World Health Organization (WHO), and Canadian Public Health Association (CPHA). The authors considered health to be the ability to satisfy needs, realize their aspirations, and deal with the environment. They labelled the determinants of health as "prerequisites for health" and defined health promotion as "a process of enabling people to increase control over, and to improve, their health" (WHO, 1986, p. 1).

Nurses apply the ecological approach during the health history when they inquire about occupational/workplace hazards, dangers in the home and community, family relationships, spoken, and cultural beliefs and practices related to health and illness. Following the physical examination, they record and analyze findings in the context of the client's socioenvironmental conditions.

Not all definitions of health promotion reflect a socioenvironmental or ecological approach to health. The following table contains three examples congruent with the socioenvironmental/ecological approach.

■ *Definitions of Health Promotion*

"The process of enabling people to increase control over, and improve, their health" (Most cited definition of health promotion) (WHO, 1986, p. 1)

"Health promotion represents a comprehensive social and political process, it not only embraces actions directed at strengthening the skills and capabilities of individuals, but also action directed towards changing social, environmental and economic conditions so as to alleviate their impact on public and individual health. Health promotion is the process of enabling people to increase control over the determinants of health and thereby improve their health. Participation is essential to sustain health promotion action" (Nutbeam, 1998, p. 351)

The "combination of concerted, integrated strategies of action on the broad determinants of health through the values-based process of enabling and empowering people to have control over these determinants" (Hills et al., 2007, p. 330)

In *Achieving Health for All: A Framework for Health Promotion* (Epp, 1986), the Canadian government identified three major challenges to achieving health: *reducing inequity, increasing prevention,* and *enhancing coping.* Nurses confronted these challenges and used the strategies proposed in the document in various settings. The government established Health Promotion Centres in six Canadian universities. Nevertheless, health promotion in Canada continued to concentrate on health education and lifestyle change (Pinder, 2007).

POPULATION HEALTH: A DETERMINANTS VIEW OF HEALTH

The greatest single new influence on national health promotion in Canada was likely the emergence of the population health paradigm in the 1990s (Pinder, 2007). In *Strategies for Population Health* (Advisory Committee on Population Health [ACPH], 1994), the federal, provincial, and territorial Ministers of Health endorsed the work of the Canadian Institute of Advanced Research. *In a population health approach, planning to improve health considers all known factors, conditions, and interactions that affect the health status of the population* (Health Canada, 1998). It emphasizes the use of *epidemiological data* to determine the causes of health and disease. In health assessments, nurses consider Canadian statistics on preventable disorders to identify risk factors relevant to their clients' health.

By 1996, Health Canada had profiled 12 determinants of population health, as shown in the accompanying table. These include *individual* factors (personal health practices, individual capacity, and coping skills) and *population-level* factors (social, economic, and physical environments, and health services, which are viewed as foundational to individual factors) (ACPH, 1994). By 1997, the Population Health Directorate had replaced Canada's Health Promotion Directorate and the population-health approach was guiding health policy in Canada (Pinder, 2007). The *Toronto Charter on the Social Determinants of Health* contains a somewhat different view of what determines health (Raphael et al., 2004). This conceptualization focuses on the influence of economic and social policies on the distribution of resources in society. The authors go beyond individual responsibility to societal responsibility for health and provide direction for policy advocacy by nurses.

■ *Conceptualizations of Health*

Prerequisites for Health	Population Health Determinants	Social Determinants of Health
Ottawa Charter (WHO, 1986) Jakarta Declaration (WHO, 1997)	*Public Health Agency of Canada (2002)*	*Toronto Charter on Social Determinants of Health (Raphael et al., 2004)*
■ Peace	■ Income and social status	■ Early childhood development
■ Shelter	■ Social support networks	■ Education
■ Education	■ Education	■ Employment and working conditions
■ Food	■ Employment and working conditions	■ Food security
■ Income	■ Physical environments	■ Health care services
■ Stable ecosystem	■ Biology and genetic endowment	■ Housing shortages
■ Sustainable resource use	■ Personal health practices and coping skills	■ Income and its equitable distribution
■ Social justice	■ Healthy child development	■ Social safety nets
■ Equity	■ Health services	■ Unemployment and employment security
■ Empowerment of women	■ Gender	■ Social exclusion
■ Social security	■ Culture	■ Aboriginal status
■ Respect for human rights	■ Social environments	
■ Social relations		

PRINCIPLES AND CORE VALUES OF HEALTH PROMOTION

Ecological definitions of health promotion that remain relevant reflect several principles articulated by the CPHA (1996) in its *Action Statement for Health Promotion.*

PRINCIPLES OF HEALTH PROMOTION

- Recognize the relationships among individual, social, and environmental factors.
- Support a holistic approach (physical, mental, social, ecological, cultural, and spiritual aspects of health).
- Take a long-term perspective.
- Use a multisectoral approach (i.e., health professionals must work with other sectors such as housing,

environment, labour, and employment to ensure that people have equitable access to health determinants).
- Use knowledge from various sources, including formal knowledge from diverse sciences and people's experiential knowledge, so that experiences, voices, and research contribute to what is known about health.

Health promotion embraces core values such as *empowerment*, *participation*, and *sense of control* by ordinary people. It gives primacy to *community action*, focusing on *capacity and capacity building* (Raeburn & Rootman, 2007). Health promotion emphasizes *equity*, *social justice*, and the *common good* (CPHA, 1996).

DETERMINANTS OF HEALTH

The table on p. 6 summarizes three major conceptualizations of what determines health. The *prerequisites for health* from the *Ottawa Charter* are very inclusive and convey a strong societal responsibility. The *population health determinants* from the Public Health Agency of Canada (PHAC) are fairly comprehensive and include both individual and societal factors. The PHAC Web site provides an excellent discussion of each and includes Canadian evidence for the effects on health (see also Reutter, 2006). The *social determinants of health* from the *Toronto Charter* are consistent with other formulations and evidence, as well as with lay understandings of what determines health. They align with existing Canadian government structures and policy frameworks, and are therefore relevant to Canadian decision makers and citizens. The social determinants make apparent those areas where there is either active governmental policy activity or inactivity (Raphael, 2004), informing nurses who are involved in political action.

HEALTH ASSESSMENT AND THE DETERMINANTS OF HEALTH

Nurses better understand the complexity of clients' health situations when they appreciate the interrelationships among health determinants and their influence on health. Understanding the relationships promotes more sensitive, nonjudgmental, and appropriate questioning and counselling during health assessment. Nurses consider how income, culture, education, age, gender, social support, working and living conditions, and environments influence personal health practices and coping skills. They also appreciate that such factors may be beyond the control of clients and instead are determined by government policies.

In health assessment, nurses use questioning to explore the influence of these broader social and physical environments on individual health. The health information or counselling they provide is relevant to the context of clients' daily lives, and recognizes physical and psychological barriers to client engagement in health practices. By understanding the *root causes* of health situations and the *role of contextual factors* on individual health, nurses strive to influence these determinants directly. The nursing scope of practice incorporates multiple strategies that go beyond individual client assessment to influence programs, services, and policies with effects on individual health. Nurses work collaboratively with other disciplines and sectors to change policies that inhibit health, and to ensure that supportive programs, services, and health policies are in place.

THE *OTTAWA CHARTER*: STRATEGIES FOR HEALTH PROMOTION

The five broad strategies in the *Ottawa Charter* for enhancing health provide an organizing framework that directs nurses' activities for health promotion in every practice setting (see the table on page 10). Every experience with individual health promotion creates a basis and stimulus for broader nursing action, whether at the organizational, municipal, provincial/territorial, or federal level. Nurses advocate for strategies that promote health locally in their organization, regionally in their political jurisdiction and health authority, provincially or territorially with their professional organizations, and nationally with nongovernmental organizations (NGOs) and federal bodies. All five strategies in the *Ottawa Charter* are within the scope of nursing practice.

Develop Personal Skills.   Nurses know this strategy very well. The focus is on helping clients to develop personal health practices and to enhance coping skills as a result of health education that emphasizes client knowledge for directing choices and actions. Health education to individuals and groups is the traditional health promotion strategy that nurses use. For example, they provide information in diverse areas such as nutrition, physical activity, and parenting. They help clients to acquire adequate resources and supports for carrying out health recommendations. On a broader scale, nurses use social marketing to influence health behaviours widely and often incorporate media messages. For example, British Columbia uses a Web site to increase awareness of all facets of smoking (http://www.tobaccofacts.org).

Create Supportive Environments.   Nurses work with others to ensure healthy and safe physical environments as well as stimulating and satisfying living and working conditions (WHO, 1986). Supportive environments can influence health and health practices directly, and nurses counsel clients to access and evaluate available programs.

Reorient Health Services.   Currently, health services in Canada and other high-income countries focus disproportionately on illness care. Many health professionals, including nurses, focus more on health promotion, illness prevention, and assisting clients living with chronic illness than on curative care. One example of reorienting health services is a PHC system that ensures more equitable access to health care and health promotion. More attention to the provision of health care services in the home is another example. In addition, local and regional health services in many areas of Canada support the establishment of primary care networks as reoriented services (Health Council of Canada, 2005). These interprofessional and multidisciplinary centres offer preventive, therapeutic, and emergent services at a single site.

Strengthen Community Action.   Health is created and sustained in community relationships (CPHA, 1996). Community development is a strategy for health promotion that emphasizes *empowerment*. Health professionals work with communities to increase their capacity to identify areas to enhance health. They work with other sectors to facilitate change. Involvement of communities in their own issues leads to more relevant and sustainable health programs, services, and policies. Neighbourhood Watch is one widely established initiative that enhances neighbourhood safety and is active in many cities and towns across Canada. This mechanism for reducing opportunities for crime enlists private citizens to work with local police (http://www.neighbourhoodwatchregistry.com/directorieschapters.html).

Build Healthy Public Policy. Policy advocacy is a legitimate nursing role increasingly incorporated in Canadian documents on nursing standards, competencies, and scopes of practice. Advocating healthy public policy is the broadest and most effective way to address the determinants of health. It has been identified as a priority strategy for health promotion (CPHA, 1996) and is at the foundation of all other strategies. Because policies in many nonhealth sectors (e.g., agriculture, education, transportation, social services, housing) influence health determinants, their decision makers need to ensure health-enhancing public policies. For example, by establishing a policy that bans the use of trans fat in industrially produced foods, the healthier choice becomes the easiest choice for individuals and their families.

The *Toronto Charter* determinants specifically focus on areas that policy advocacy can address. Policies that affect health include adequate and affordable housing, child care, living wages, adequate welfare incomes, and progressive taxation.

■ *Examples of Canadian Initiatives to Implement the Ottawa Charter Strategies for Health Promotion*

Strategy for Health Promotion	Examples
1. Develop Personal Skills	
■ *With seniors*	*Steady As You Go*, a widely disseminated Canadian program, has reduced falls effectively in community-dwelling seniors. Trained facilitators offer it to small groups of seniors with support from a health professional, usually a nurse. Seniors learn to identify their personal risk factors for falls and then to implement their own strategies to reduce their risks.
■ *With the general population*	The *Act Now BC campaign* promotes healthy living through partnerships with government and organizations in health, education, agriculture, and sports. Initiatives targeted to the general population range from social-marketing campaigns on lifestyle practices (e.g., nutrition, activity) to harm-reduction strategies on tobacco and alcohol use.
■ *With Northerners*	The 2006 *Drop the Pop Challenge* involved Northerners across the Yukon, Northwest Territories, and Nunavut in a project to support healthier drink choices. The Challenge was consistent with the Pan-Canadian Healthy Living Strategy. Interdisci-plinary collaboration from teachers, nutritionists, dental therapists, nurses, and community health representatives promoted the contest, which offered strong educational component.
2. Create Supportive Environments	
■ *In the workplace*	The *Innovative Workplace Health Initiatives* project, consistent with a workplace health-determinants approach to workplace wellness, was launched in diverse corporate, industrial, and health care organizations in British Columbia, Saskatchewan, Manitoba, Ontario, Nova Scotia, and New Brunswick. The emphasis is on healthy physical work environments, physically healthy employees, and healthy social environments that support employees at work and in work–life balance. This is highly relevant to nursing practice from the perspective of nurses in occupational settings, as well as nurses in health institutions (Sangster, 2002).
■ *In the hospital*	In 1992, the WHO established the *Baby Friendly Initiative* (BFI) to promote breast-feeding in hospitals. Only 1 of the 14,000 BFI-designated hospitals worldwide is Canadian (in Manitoba). The Provincial Coordinating Committee collaborates with the Breastfeeding Committee for Canada and aims to support the Regional Health Authorities in implementing the BFI in Manitoba's hospitals and communities.
■ *In the grocery store*	The Alberta Council on Aging administers the *Senior Friendly Program* in Canada. The program helps communities, businesses, and organizations provide services in a way that meets the needs of seniors and ultimately will improve their quality of life. The program has several components. For example, the *Senior Friendly Grocery Store Guide*, a

(continued)

Examples of Canadian Initiatives to Implement the Ottawa Charter Strategies for Health Promotion (Continued)

Strategy for Health Promotion	Examples
	collaborative project between the Dietitians of Canada and Alberta Council on Aging, provides guidance for groceries to ensure they meet the needs of seniors. Its steering committee reflects a wide range of sectors and disciplines, including a PHN specializing in health promotion of older adults (www.acaging.ca/sf.htm).
3. Reorient Health Services	
To address accessibility	Nurses are integrally involved in the expanding use of communication technology to ensure accessible health services, particularly for rural and remote communities. For example, the *National Telehealth Project* implemented and evaluated initiatives in First Nations communities in British Columbia, Alberta, Saskatchewan, Manitoba, and Quebec that enhanced health service delivery and shared health information and expertise. In several provinces, nurses are involved in telephone health information services such as *Health Link* in Alberta and *BC NurseLine* in British Columbia, which provide topical health information, identify relevant symptoms, and assist clients to make decisions about seeing a health care professional.
To promote health	*Community Health Centres* in Canada offer both primary health care (PHC) and social programs and services. They focus on health promotion in its widest sense, with an emphasis on meeting the prerequisites or determinants of health beyond illness care. The *Calgary Urban Project Society* (CUPS) in inner-city Calgary provides: • *Multidisciplinary-staffed health clinics* (e.g., prenatal and maternal child clinics, chiropractic care, dentistry, shared care mental health, eye care) • *Counselling and advocacy* • *Family resource centre* (e.g., life skills and parenting programs, breakfast and hot lunch, basic needs services, referrals, socialization) • *Community outreach* (e.g., home visits, referrals, emergency transportation) • *Educational and early intervention programs* • *Housing registry* (CUPS, 2006)
4. Strengthen Community Action	
For food security	Advocacy, networking, and coalition building are strategies used to address food-security issues, commonly leading to the development of collective kitchens and community gardens. In Québec, the collective kitchen strategy has flourished for more than 2 decades, and a provincial lobby coordinates activities. The *Calgary Health Region* provides training sessions for people to become collective kitchen coordinators. Community garden initiatives are supported in urban centres such as Toronto, Ontario, and Victoria, BC, contributing to food security for participants and opportunities for collective community action to address social concerns. Nurses can share information about these programs with their clients during health assessments. In public health services and nongovernmental organizations (NGOs), nurses work closely with communities to develop and sustain these programs.
For physical activity	The *"PEI Active" Campaign* began in 2007 to create friendly competition among 12 communities for physical activity. All types of physical activity (e.g., mini golf) were converted into kilometres for tracking by each community. In 2008, the campaign broadened to pair Prince Edward Island communities with those across Canada.
5. Build Healthy Public Policy	
To promote safety	The rural culture of Newfoundland and Labrador fosters widespread recreational use of all-terrain vehicles (ATVs) by children and adults, who often fail to wear helmets during use. Statistics on injuries and deaths related to ATVs are alarming. Nurses in this province actively participated in the lobby for legislation on safer use of ATVs, which the Department of Government Services passed in 2005. The legislation mandates use of helmets with ATVs, avoidance of public roads and highways, abstinence from alcohol while driving, and minimum age of 16 years for drivers of adult-size ATVs.

(continued)

■ *Examples of Canadian Initiatives to Implement the Ottawa Charter Strategies for Health Promotion (Continued)*

Strategy for Health Promotion	Examples
■ *To reduce childhood obesity*	On January 1, 2007, the Canada Revenue Agency implemented a policy established by the federal Financial Department in conjunction with Health Canada to confront the national epidemic of childhood obesity. The policy permits a parent to claim as a tax credit up to $500 per child for costs paid to enrol the child in eligible physical activities.
■ *To reduce homelessness*	Cathy Crowe, a Toronto Street Nurse, advocates tirelessly to reduce homelessness. She co-founded the Toronto Disaster Relief Committee (TDRC), which succeeded in declaring homelessness in Canada a national disaster, and advocates on numerous issues related to the health of homeless people. The main goal of the TDRC is to decrease homelessness, beginning with the "1% solution," whereby all levels of government spend an additional 1% of their budget on housing (www.tdrc.net/).

CANADIAN POPULATION HEALTH PROMOTION MODEL

In an effort to integrate the concepts of population health and health promotion, the Health Promotion Development Division of the Population Health Directorate of Health Canada developed the Population Health Promotion Model (Hamilton & Bhatti, 1996). Presented below is the original model that was subsequently augmented to include three additional determinants of health: culture, gender, and social environments.

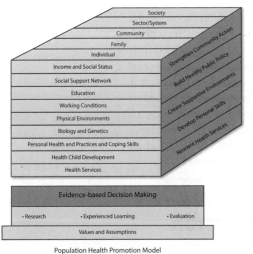

Population Health Promotion Model

The model explores four major questions:

■ On WHAT can we take action? (determinants of health)

■ HOW can we take action? (health promotion strategies)

■ On WHOM do we focus? (levels where action can be taken)

■ WHY should we take action? (best available evidence that is consistent with community needs, values, and resources)

This model aligns with nurses' understanding of what determines health and how they can influence health status. It informs a population health approach (see http://www.phac-aspc.gc.ca/ph-sp/index-eng.php).

A POPULATION HEALTH PROMOTION STRATEGY FOR SASKATCHEWAN

In 2001, Saskatchewan Health began creating a strategy for directing health promotion activities in the province. Recognizing that citizens are likely to be healthy when they live in healthy communities, the provincial government developed an action plan using a population-health approach. It defined 3-, 5-, and 10-year outcomes for four priority areas for action: mental well-being, accessible nutritious food, decreased substance use and abuse, and active communities.

GLOBAL FACTORS INFLUENCING HEALTH PROMOTION: BEYOND THE *OTTAWA CHARTER*

Since 1986, global changes have perhaps shifted priorities and led to alterations in earlier strategies, although the major strategies and principles of health promotion in the *Ottawa Charter* have been affirmed. Two influential documents are the *Jakarta Declaration* (WHO, 1997) and the *Bangkok Charter* (WHO, 2005).

JAKARTA DECLARATION ON LEADING HEALTH PROMOTION INTO THE TWENTY-FIRST CENTURY (1997)

The *Jakarta Declaration* evolved from the first international conference on health promotion held in a developing country and involving the private sector. Its writers affirmed the *Ottawa Charter* prerequisites for health (see pp. 8–11) and added four more: empowerment of women, social security, respect for human rights, and social relations. They declared poverty to be the greatest threat to health. Perhaps what is "new" in this document is its emphasis on the role of the *private sector* in health promotion. The *Declaration* presents several priorities for action: promotion of social responsibility for health in public *and* private sectors, increased investments for health in all sectors, consolidated and expanded partnerships for health at all levels of government and in the private sector, increased community capacity, individual empowerment, and adequate infrastructure for health promotion.

BANGKOK CHARTER FOR HEALTH PROMOTION IN A GLOBALIZED WORLD (2005)

This *Bangkok Charter* affirms that health promotion is grounded in health as a *human right*. Its authors recognize health as encompassing well-being, both mental and spiritual. The charter identifies several critical factors influencing health:

- Increased inequalities within and between countries

- New patterns of consumption and communication

- Commercialization

- Global environmental change

- Urbanization

The charter highlights the vulnerability of children and the exclusion of marginalized, ability-challenged, and indigenous peoples. The authors emphasize the need for strong political action, broad participation, and sustained advocacy. The countries that subscribed to the charter committed to making health promotion central to global development and a core responsibility for all governments for the purpose of capacity building and empowering communities with adequate resources. The charter emphasizes securing corporate sector commitment to maintain health-promoting workplaces and ethical business practices.

ADVANCING HEALTH PROMOTION IN CANADA

Many organizations advance health promotion in Canada. Among them are NGOs, government agencies, and professional organizations. The *Canadian Public Health Association* (CPHA) has played a pivotal role in the development of health promotion in Canada. Its mission is to advocate for individual and community health according to the public health principles of health promotion and protection, disease prevention, and healthy public policy (see www.cpha.ca). With the support of Health Canada and stakeholders across Canada, the CPHA produced the seminal document *Action Statement on Health Promotion* (1996), outlining important concepts and principles of health promotion and priority health promotion strategies from the *Ottawa Charter*.

The federal government's *Health Canada* is involved in the delivery of health promotion programs, which inform nurses who counsel individual clients regarding preventable disorders (www.hc-sc.gov.ca). Two prime examples are the Federal Tobacco Control Strategy and the Canadian Diabetes Strategy, which incorporate intersectoral collaboration.

CANADIAN DIABETES STRATEGY

In Nunavut, the Health Promotion Programs Unit (Health and Social Services) is taking a proactive approach and has introduced the Aboriginal Diabetes Initiative as a component of the Canadian Diabetes Strategy. The priorities are to identify people at risk, develop awareness and prevention programs, and provide training for caregivers.

Programs with strong government support include the *Canadian Health Network*; a bilingual Web-based information service that covers an extensive list of health topics to help Canadians make healthy choices (as of April 2008, this service is now incorporated into the PHAC Web site); and the *Pan-Canadian Healthy Living Strategy*, which addresses risk factors contributing to noncommunicable diseases. These resources help nurses to provide accurate and current information during individual health assessment. Raphael (2007) suggests that more support for policies that address the social determinants of health is needed to reduce health inequities in Canada today.

In response to catastrophic public health events (e.g., SARS), the *Public Health Agency of Canada* was created in 2003. Dr. David Butler-Jones was appointed as the first Chief Public Health Officer of Canada. The PHAC focuses on the five essential public health functions: health promotion, health protection, health surveillance, disease and injury prevention, and population health assessment. It created six *National Collaborating Centres for Public Health* across Canada, which focus on developing knowledge related to health promotion strategies and population health based on:

■ Determinants of health (Atlantic region)

■ Public policy and risk assessment (Québec)

■ Public health methodologies and tools development (Ontario)

■ Infectious diseases (Manitoba)

■ Environmental health (BC)

■ Aboriginal health (BC)

The PHAC also led the development of public health goals for Canada, reflecting a broad vision of health congruent with health promotion, and created the *Pan-Canadian Public Health Network*. This network facilitates collaboration and sharing of public health expertise among provincial and territorial jurisdictions. Six expert groups have been established to address public health issues, including health promotion (see www.phac-aspc.gc.ca).

Provincial and national nursing organizations are ideally positioned to advocate for healthy public policy and to reorient health systems in the direction of PHC. The *Canadian Nurses Association* (CNA) is a member of the *Canadian Coalition for Public Health in the 21st Century (CCPH)*, established in 2005. It is a national network (nonprofit organizations, professional organizations, health charities, and academic researchers) formed to influence public policy for sustaining the health of Canadians.

EXAMPLE OF THE REGISTERED NURSES ASSOCIATION OF ONTARIO (RNAO)

The RNAO has been particularly active in advocating for policies to reduce child and family poverty, including increasing social assistance rates and supporting the "1% solution" to reduce homelessness. The CNA has long advocated for a reformed primary health care (PHC) system.

The *WHO Commission on the Social Determinants of Health*, established in 2005, has the mandate to recommend interventions and policies that narrow health inequities through action on the social determinants of health. Dr. Monique Begin and Mr. Stephen Lewis represent Canada, which funds three of the nine knowledge networks: early child development, globalization, and health systems. The commission held its eighth meeting in 2007 in Vancouver, BC.

MANDATE OF CANADIAN NURSING: HEALTH PROMOTION WITHIN PRIMARY HEALTH CARE

Canadian national, provincial, and territorial nursing associations have long supported PHC, which the WHO introduced in 1978 as the most effective way to ensure accessible, appropriate, sustainable, and comprehensive health care (Ogilvie & Reutter, 2002). A PHC approach includes first-level primary care (basic medical and curative care), draws attention to the social determinants of health, and supports client and citizen decision making (CNA, 2005).

Nurses in all settings incorporate PHC principles into their practice (CNA, 2003). The principles most often associated with PHC are as follows:

- *Accessibility* to essential, comprehensive health care services for all people, with no unreasonable geographic, financial, or cultural barriers

- *Public participation* by individuals and communities in decision making about their health care and the health of their communities

- *Health promotion* involving activities related to health education, illness prevention, policy advocacy, and strong community participation

- *Appropriate technology* so that methods of care and service delivery are socially acceptable and affordable

- *Intersectoral and interdisciplinary cooperation* to address health determinants (CNA, 2005)

LEVELS OF PREVENTION

Primary health care incorporates the three levels of prevention recognized for more than half a century (Leavell & Clark, 1965): prevention activities before signs and symptoms of disease (primary); screening, early detection, and treatment (secondary); and rehabilitation to maximize health outcomes (tertiary).

Although *primary care* and *primary health care* are often used synonymously, traditionally, primary care has been provider-driven, institutionally oriented, and individually focused with an emphasis on clinical diagnosis and treatment (service provision). Under a PHC umbrella, primary care would incorporate health determinants, health promotion, preventive health care, clients as partners in care, and meaningful community agency relationships to facilitate accessibility and referrals (CNA, 2005).

Nurse scholars (Hills et al., 2007) contend that PHC is the approach needed to "reorient health systems" so that professional health practice incorporates health promotion. They suggest that health promotion and PHC could be integrated through interprofessional education and multidisciplinary teams in community health practice. These organizational structures are beginning to take hold in several Canadian provinces, primarily as a result of the federal government Primary Health Care Transition Fund (Health Council of Canada, 2005). The emerging role of nurse practitioners in reoriented health systems is promising, provided that they maintain a strong health promotion focus.

The nurses' value base aligns with that of health promotion: client participation, empowerment, and equity (Hills et al., 2007). The CNA envisions that future nurses will "provide the bulk of primary care, including assessment, diagnosis, treatment, prescribing, making referrals, and evaluating effectiveness of care" (Villeneuve & MacDonald, 2006, p. 99).

SETTINGS AND HEALTH ASSESSMENT

A "settings" approach (Green et al., 2000) acknowledges how context (environmental conditions) influences the development and maintenance of healthy behaviours and health itself. Settings represent health-influencing environments, based on the belief that individuals are in dynamic transaction with their sociophysical milieu (Kalnins, 2000). The resources available in the social settings where individuals act and live affect the potential for social systems, including health promotion programs, to promote health-enhancing behaviours in these same clients. By integrating settings in the health history, nurses consider each client not only as an individual but also as a member of groups or populations in different social and physical environments. This dual perspective increases awareness of the environmental conditions and broader determinants of health that shape clients' health experiences. It is consistent with a socioenvironmental or socioecological perspective of health promotion and avoids limiting individual-focused practice to biomedical intervention and behaviour change.

Five different settings that nurses need to consider in health assessments are schools, homes, workplaces, health care facilities, and communities. During the health history, nurses ask questions that capture the influence of the social and physical environments on client health in these settings (see Chapter 3). The *social* environment incorporates culture, income and social status, gender, social support and inclusion, empowerment, personal health practices, and coping skills. The *physical* environment includes the physical structure of the environment and health services.

SCHOOL SETTING

Healthy child development is a critical health determinant because of its implications for lifelong health (Hertzman, 2000). Children, adolescents, and young adults spend considerable time each day under the influence of schools or postsecondary institutions. School environments are influential on the quality of education, which is a highly significant determinant of health and well-being.

Worldwide, numerous programs and initiatives aim to provide supportive healthy educational settings. During the 1990s, the WHO, European Commission, and Council of Europe developed a health-promoting schools initiative. This multifactorial approach includes teaching health knowledge and skills, changing the social and physical environments of the school, and creating links to the wider community (Health Evidence Network, 2006). It is particularly effective in promoting mental health, healthy eating, and physical activity (Health Evidence Network, 2006). "Supportive school environments that foster resilience and focus on asset development, protective factors, and social connectedness reduce the risk of health-related problems and support the healthy growth and development of children and youth" (Canadian Consensus Statement, 2007, p. 1). In Canada, the Comprehensive School Health (CSH) initiative reflects the tenets and criteria set out by WHO (Health Evidence Network, 2006). It incorporates four main components:

- Formal and informal teaching and learning about health, health risks, and health issues

- Health and support services for early identification and treatment of problems that can influence learning (e.g., public health services, social and psychological assessments, mental health services, services for special needs)

- Supportive social environments (e.g., friends, peer support, teacher support, school discipline policies)

- Healthy, clean, and safe physical environments, including opportunities for physical activity and healthy nutrition (Canadian Consensus Statement, 2007)

The health promoting university initiative emerged in 1998. *The Edmonton Charter for Health-Promoting Universities and Institutions of Higher Education* (Health Promotion and Worklife Services, 2006) includes goals, principles, and priorities for educational institutions to be healthy learning and working environments. The focus is to help people develop personal health practices and coping skills through education and environmental conditions that are appropriate and safe for everyone.

During comprehensive health histories with youth or young adults, nurses consider social and physical factors in the learning environment that may influence health. In addition to the general setting questions, they also inquire about specific school setting topics. If clients have a chronic health condition or disability (e.g., asthma, allergies, physical or mental challenges), then nurses need to ensure that the school environment supports their needs.

SPECIFIC HEALTH HISTORY QUESTIONS FOR THE SCHOOL AS SETTING

- How is the client doing at school? Does he or she enjoy school?
- What friends does the client have at school? How included does he or she feel in school and extra curricular activities? This may be particularly important when considering the effects of income and culture.
- How healthy is peer support?
- How much support do teachers provide to the client?
- Do school discipline policies and effective management practices convey respect?

- How available are mental health services (e.g., counselling)?
- To what extent are there adequate and safe physical activity facilities and programs that provide opportunities for physical activity including sports and extra-curricular activities?
- To what extent are foods low in nutritive value restricted?
- What written policies exist for the administration of medications?

HOME SETTING

Home is a social and physical environment where most health-promoting behaviours are learned and maintained (Soubhi & Potvin, 2000). An integrated health assessment includes individual behaviours, interpersonal family relations, and physical home conditions. The family is the dynamic context for individual health experience (Soubhi & Potvin, 2000). Research has shown that characteristics of the family, socialization, and interactional processes are associated with health-related behaviours including nutrition, physical activity, risk taking, and coping responses. Assessment of the family context is relevant to enhancing individuals' social, emotional, spiritual, and physical well-being (Ford-Gilboe, 1997). Nurses may be guided by family assessment models, such as the McGill Model of Nursing (also called the Allen Model or the Developmental Health Model) (Gottlieb & Ezer, 1997), and the Calgary Family Assessment Model (Wright & Leahey, 2005).

In addition to consideration of the family as a social environment, the physical environment in which the family lives is important. Home safety is a major issue for health promotion. Injury statistics indicate that the home is not a particularly safe physical space. For example, injuries in the home are the most common reason for emergency department visits for children (Pless & Millar, 2000), and almost 62% of hospitalizations for injury in Canadian seniors are from falls in private dwellings (PHAC, 2005).

SPECIFIC HEALTH HISTORY QUESTIONS FOR THE HOME AS SETTING

- How does the client relate to family members in the home?
- To what extent are family members a source of social support for the client?
- Does the client feel safe and nurtured in the family?
- What are the health practices and beliefs, values, and social status in the home?

- What is the family working on or dealing with? What are the effects on the individual?
- What aspects of the broader context of family life might explain the present behaviour, situation, and concerns?
- Can the individual afford adequate housing?
- What are the exercise, nutrition, and hygiene practices of the family?

WORKPLACE SETTING

The workplace as a health promotion setting "holds a unique place, in that the health and well-being of workers in the workplace inevitably impacts the health of individual families, the local community and society at large" (Whitehead, 2006, p. 59). Employment and working conditions are recognized as a health determinant and as a setting in which other health determinants are influential. Healthy workplaces contribute to individual well-being by preventing occupational disease and injuries, promoting positive lifestyle behaviours, and enhancing workforce well-being and productivity. A healthy workplace promotes job satisfaction, retention, quality performance, and reduced costs related to injury, worker compensation claims, and health benefit claims (Lowe, 2004).

The workplace as a health promotion setting incorporates both the physical and the psychosocial environments (Polanyi et al., 2000). The physical environment includes the building or space in which work is conducted as well as the work processes and products. The psychosocial environment reflects the organizational, economic, legal, cultural, ethical, and political context of the workplace.

Elements of a healthy workplace include environmental and occupational health and safety programs, health and lifestyle practices, workplace culture, and supportive environments (National Quality Institute, 2007). Research suggests that health outcomes among workers are linked to the content, organization, and arrangements of paid work (Polanyi, 2004). Healthy workplaces provide job and employment security, safe physical conditions, a reasonable work pace, low stress, opportunities for self-expression and individual development, participation, and work–life balance (Jackson, 2004). In contrast, unhealthy work conditions include dirty and dangerous jobs (e.g., exposures to harmful substances or high noise levels) and jobs that are stressful because of the use of arbitrary power; failure to meet human developmental needs; conflict; and increased pace, demands, or repetitive content of the labour process (Jackson, 2004).

In recent years, Canada has given priority attention to working conditions in the *health care sector*. Nurses need to consider the workplace from four perspectives: (1) as providers of client care, (2) as employees, (3) as managers of personnel, and (4) as members of a professional organization. The leadership of the Office of Nursing Policy at Health Canada has examined several reports on the health care sector:

- Canadian Health Services Research Foundation (2001)
- Canadian Nurses Advisory Committee (2002)
- Standing Senate Committee on Social Affairs, Science and Technology (Kirby Report, 2002)
- Commission on the Future of Health Care in Canada (Romanow Report, 2002)

Job stress increases the risk of musculoskeletal injuries, accidents, physical and mental illness, substance abuse, and smoking (Shamian & El-Jardali, 2007). Federal, provincial, and territorial governments have committed to developing and implementing an action plan to promote healthy workplaces in the health care sector (Shamian & El-Jardali, 2007).

Three approaches to workplace health promotion have emerged in Canada. They provide a useful framework for nurses to determine areas for client assessment, because they exemplify how the social and physical environments of the workplace influence individual health:

- *Occupational health and safety* traditionally emphasizes health protection, safety, and reduction of biological, chemical, ergonomic, physical, and psychosocial hazards and risks in the workplace setting.

- *Workplace health promotion* initiatives broaden the individual worker focus to include healthy lifestyles, education, and resources in the workplace (e.g., smoking cessation, exercise facilities, weight reduction groups, stress management).

- Most recently, the *promoting workplace determinants* approach further extends initiatives to consider organizational factors (i.e., health-promoting organizations) (Polanyi et al., 2000). The focus is to reduce stress and improve employee wellness, including flexible work hours, worksite redesign, enhanced supervisor skills and practices, office communications, educational advancement opportunities, and family–work or work–life on-site provisions (e.g., child care, family leave). This approach considers individual job factors such as control and decision latitude, the nature and structure of work (includes psychological strain), physical demands, pace and volume of work, repetitiveness of tasks, and skill range used. Organizational factors at the unit or company level include remuneration and benefits, worker participation in decision making, management philosophy, and the structure of personnel relations (Polanyi et al., 2000).

SPECIFIC HEALTH HISTORY QUESTIONS FOR THE WORKPLACE AS SETTING

- What work–life policies exist in the workplace? Are they accessible to workers (e.g., are supervisors or decision-makers supportive of using available policies)?
- How well does the client relate to co-workers and managers? How are concerns addressed?
- What job factors influence individual sense of well-being (e.g., control and decision latitude, structure of work relationships, psychological strain, pace and volume of work expected)?
- What are the client's exposures to biological, chemical, ergonomic, and physical hazards in the workplace?
- What engineering controls (e.g., splatter guards), administrative controls (e.g., prohibition of eating and drinking in work areas), and personal protective equipment (e.g., puncture-proof footwear) are used to protect the worker/client?
- What physical demands are involved in the particular work performed? Is the pace, volume, or repetitiveness of tasks a concern?
- Are Material Safety Data Sheets available for hazardous chemicals?
- Are workers trained under the Canadian Workplace Hazard Management Information System (WHMIS) program?
- What policies are in place to reduce exposure to allergens and toxins?
- What health-promoting facilities are available to workers (e.g., fitness, food services)?

HEALTH CARE FACILITIES AS SETTING

Health care institutions have expanded their mandate beyond diagnosis and curative medical care. This was in response to social conditions such as changing morbidity and mortality patterns, the consumer movement for informed decision making, and political support for reorienting health services to be consistent with a determinants-of-health perspective and focus on health promotion (Johnson, 2000). Health care facilities often are assumed to be a positive influence on health, but a settings approach challenges this belief. Consumers and health professionals have increased awareness of the potential for health-compromising conditions as well. Although health care institutions are typically defined by their focus on providing acute care, long-term care, psychiatric care, and rehabilitation (Johnson, 2000), settings include community-based facilities, such as retirement residences that also deliver health care. Of particular interest is health promotion for clients who receive health services and residents who receive broader health services.

The WHO advocated for a health-promoting hospital framework in 1997. Such a framework focuses on client well-being, organizational practices to support inter-professional collaboration, and contributions to community and public health (Whitehead, 2005). It has implications for a more inclusive or holistic perspective of the health experience beyond acute episodes of care. This means that clients are provided with health education to assist them in coping with their health situation after discharge, enhancing self-care and health behaviours. A health-promoting hospital environment also enables clients to be involved in decision making about their care.

Long-term care or nursing home settings provide a unique opportunity for nurses to focus on health promotion. These settings are "home" for clients, in contrast to acute care institutions where discharge to the community is the goal. Typical goals of care include providing a safe and supportive environment, supporting functional independence, preserving individual autonomy, and managing chronic and acute medical problems (McElhone & Limb, 2005). The professional-centred work focus of this setting may contribute to social isolation for the resident, role ambiguity among family members, and stress for everyone (Logue, 2003). Promoting cooperative staff and family activities provides opportunities to integrate the family unit into resident care and enhance well-being. Activities to promote family stability and connectedness include encouraging continuity in family caregiving activities; providing opportunities to maintain emotional bonds; giving access to communication media, including computers for residents; and providing private areas for celebration of family events or meals. A family-centred nursing approach fosters family relationships in nursing homes; may prevent deterioration in family ties; and provides emotional, spiritual, and health benefits to both the family system and the older adult who is institutionalized (Logue, 2003).

Retirement communities are distinctive settings that integrate housing and programs to promote the health, well-being, and social functioning of residents. They provide independent and assisted-living programs for older adults, including a range of food, social, recreation, housekeeping, personal care, and wellness services (Young et al., 2006). Residents range from healthy older adults to frail older adults with complex health problems. The scope of services includes health care, as well as daily living issues related to meals, social engagement, and activity. Nurses' health assessment of residents should consider the social and physical environmental determinants of health.

In health-promoting health care facilities, outcomes should focus on assisting people to increase control over their health. This may include "situational control, self-efficacy, enhanced self-care, enhanced self-concept, improved pain control, enhanced social support, improved functioning with activities of daily living, and improved health status" (Johnson, 2000, p. 193, citing Berkman, 1995; Jenny, 1993, Kemper et al., 1993; Lincoln & Gladman, 1992). Comprehensive health assessment by nurses identifies institutionalized client and resident concerns and the potential for health promotion. Their assessment should consider selected, relevant aspects of the organization, the service providers, and the community of the clients or residents (Johnson, 2000).

SPECIFIC HEALTH HISTORY QUESTIONS FOR HEALTH CARE FACILITIES AS SETTING

Note: Nurses need to adapt specific questions to reflect the difference in focus between acute care settings (which aim to return clients to their homes and communities) and long-term care or residential settings (which represent the homes of clients).

- How does the client relate with care providers in the acute care, long-term care, or residential setting?
- What social support does the client have from family and friends?
- How is the client involved in care decisions? Is opportunity provided for involvement from family or support a network?
- What opportunities for social interaction does the client have?
- What recreational opportunities does the client engage in and how often? Are these satisfactory to the client?
- How adequate and comfortable is the functional space and layout of the facility?
- Is required assistance available when needed?
- Does the client have access to needed resources within or beyond the facility?
- What hygiene practices and policies are in place to protect residents?
- What strategies are implemented to prevent, detect, or treat health problems arising from the health facility (e.g., minimizing adverse drug events)?
- What supports would benefit the client on discharge from an acute care facility to promote successful return to the home, workplace, and community?

COMMUNITY SETTINGS

Community provides a "middle ground" between an individual perspective and a societal perspective in health promotion, and as such represents the "everyday living and working context. It is the setting in which we customarily act, associate with others, learn about life, and express our values. It is here that we most strongly interact with our culture and with others' cultures" (Raeburn, 2000, p. 281). Communities influence health. In particular, the quality and availability of services and resources, and the involvement and engagement patterns of the community are important factors influencing health (Beauvais & Jenson, 2003). For example, an increased sense of community belonging has been linked to self-rated health (Ross, 2002). One of the best examples of acknowledging the importance of communities to health and well-being was the Healthy Communities/Healthy Cities initiative prominent in the late 20th century (Manson-Singer, 1994).

The purpose of a focus on community in individual health assessment is to understand the community conditions (social and physical environments) that shape individuals' health experience, especially the resources available and risks that may be evident in the community environment. The Community Assessment Wheel is a useful framework for nurses to assess resources and risks (Vollman et al., 2008). It addresses aspects of the *physical* environment (e.g., available facilities or programs related to health and social services, safety, transportation, education, communication, recreation, and economic, including commerce to support daily life). Nurses also use this framework to explore the *social* environment of the community (e.g., communication networks, cultural or ethnic diversity and relations, community values and norms, and opportunities for community participation). Nurses adapt their health assessment according to the individual's health situation, age, and other characteristics.

SPECIFIC HEALTH HISTORY QUESTIONS FOR COMMUNITY AS SETTING

- How connected or included does the client feel in the community?
- What support networks does the client have in the community?
- What community issues are identified and how do they influence the individual's health experience?
- What opportunities exist for participation in community events, initiatives, and issues?
- How active is the client in community activities and issues?
- Is there a sense of community voice and action (empowerment)?

- How well does the client know and relate with neighbours and leaders in the community?
- What community conditions influence individual sense of well-being?
- How suitable is the physical layout of the community for the client?
- What services and resources are available to the client in the community, particularly in relation to individual need or preference (e.g., transportation, recreation, communication, education, health and social services)?

Critical Thinking Exercise

- Identify and describe the key components of the Population Health Promotion Model. (*Knowledge*)
- What factors in the workplace can influence the health status of a single-parent mother? (*Comprehension*)
- How would you incorporate a health-determinants perspective during a health assessment for an older adult living alone in her own home in the community? (*Application*)
- Compare and contrast the behavioural and socioenvironmental approaches to an individual health assessment. (*Analysis*)
- Identify the advantages and the challenges to incorporating a socioenvironmental or socioecological health promotion perspective in health assessment. (*Synthesis*)
- How will you evaluate the effectiveness of a health promotion perspective in your health assessment of a post-secondary student? (*Evaluation*)

Canadian Research

Jackson, A. (2004). The unhealthy Canadian workplace. In D. Raphael (Ed.), *Social determinants of health: Canadian perspectives* (pp. 79–84). Toronto, ON: Canadian Scholars Press.

Lowe, G. (2004). *Healthy workplace strategies: Creating change and achieving results.* Ottawa, ON: The Graham Lowe Group & Health Canada.

Stewart, M., Kushner, K., Spitzer, D., Letourneau, N., Greaves, L., & Boscoe, M. (1996). Smoking among disadvantaged women: Causes and cessation. *Canadian Journal of Nursing Research, 28*(1), 41–60.

Test Questions

1. To enhance personal health practices, the most fundamental and effective approach to individual client assessment would be:
   a. ascertaining past and current use of health care services.
   b. determining client stress levels related to lifestyle choices.
   c. using reputable health education strategies to reduce risk behaviours.
   d. understanding the environments in which clients experience everyday life.

2. During the initial stages of working with a group of single teenage mothers to improve their living circumstances, a community health nurse would begin by assessing the:
   a. availability of needed health education resources.
   b. physical health status of the teens and their infants.
   c. teens' identified lack of knowledge about birth control.
   d. social and physical conditions that influence the teens' health.

3. A few nursing students revealed to a faculty advisor that they were concerned about the effects of their program demands on their personal health practices. Follow-up with other students indicated that this was a common concern among the student group. Further assessment showed that the students expressed their belief in the importance of maintaining good health practices, but that most students had discontinued weekday efforts because

of their focus on school-related stress and limited economic resources. Faculty members supported the concept of integrated health programs and were prepared to develop a program as a project.

To assess the need for health promotion among the group of students, which of the following assessment methods would be most useful?

a. Physical assessment and health history
b. Individual student interview and questionnaire
c. Review of literature and consultation with faculty
d. Walk-through of education facility and faculty questionnaire

4. Program strategies consistent with a socioenvironmental approach to health and health promotion for the nursing students in Question 3 would include:

a. promoting personal health practices such as nutrition and fitness.

b. advocating policies that ensure adequate financial support for students.
c. screening for occupationally induced physiological risk factors of disease.
d. supporting lifestyle change to manage stress with exercise and time management.

5. From Question 3, the program planners work with the students and faculty to develop and implement a set of strategies that provide students with alternatives such as peer support, life skills counselling, fitness activity groups, and a social action student coalition. These strategies best reflect which of the *Ottawa Charter* strategies for health promotion?

a. Building healthy public policy
b. Creating supportive environments
c. Developing personal skills
d. Reorienting health services

Bibliography

CITATIONS

Adler, N., Boyce, T., Chesney, M., Cohen, S., Folkman, S., Kahn, R., et al. (1994). Socioeconomic status and health: The challenge of the gradient. *American Psychologist, 49,* 15–24.

Advisory Committee on Population Health. (1994). *Strategies for population health: Investing in the health of Canadians.* Ottawa, ON: Minister of Supply and Services Canada.

Beauvais, C., & Jenson, J. (2003). *The well-being of children: Are there "neighbourhood effects"? Discussion Paper F/31 Family Network.* Toronto, ON: Canadian Policy Research Networks.

Calgary Urban Project Society. (2006). *CUPS Annual Report 2006.* Calgary, AB: Author.

Canadian Consensus Statement. (2007). *Comprehensive school health.* Retrieved July 26, 2007, from www.safehealthyschools.org

Canadian Health Services Research Foundation. (2001). *Commitment and care: The benefits of a healthy workplace for nurses, their patients, and the system.* Ottawa, ON: Author.

Canadian Institute of Child Health. (1994). *The health of Canada's children: A CICH profile.* Ottawa, ON: Author.

Canadian Nursing Advisory Committee. (2002). *Our health, our future: Creating healthy workplaces for Canadian nurses.* Ottawa, ON: Author.

Canadian Nurses Association. (2003). Primary health care: The time has come. *Nursing Now, 16,* 1–4.

Canadian Nurses Association. (2005). *Primary health care: A summary of the issues. C.N.A Backgrounder.* Ottawa, ON: Author.

Canadian Public Health Association. (1996). *Action statement for health promotion in Canada.* Ottawa, ON: Author.

Commission on the Future of Health Care in Canada. (2002). *Building on values: The future of health care in Canada.* Ottawa, ON: Health Canada.

Epp, J. (1986). *Achieving health for all: A framework for health promotion.* Ottawa, ON: Health and Welfare Canada.

Ford-Gilboe, M. (1997). Family strengths, motivation, and resources as predictors of health promotion behaviour in single-parent and two-parent families. *Research in Nursing and Health, 20,* 205–217.

Gottlieb, L., & Ezer, H. (1997). Preface. In L. Gottlieb & H. Ezer (Eds.), *A perspective on health, family, learning, and collaborative nursing: A collection of writings on the McGill Model of Nursing* (pp. i–iii). Montreal, QC: McGill University School of Nursing.

Green, L., Poland, B., & Rootman, I. (2000). The settings approach to health promotion. In B. Poland, L. Green, & I. Rootman (Eds.), *Settings for health promotion: Linking theory and practice* (pp. 1–43). Thousand Oaks, CA: Sage.

Hamilton, H. & Bhatti, T. (1996). *Population health Promotion: An integrated model of population health and health promotion.* Ottawa: Health Promotion Development Division, Health Canada.

Health Canada. (1998). *Taking action on population health: A position paper for health promotion and programs branch staff.* Ottawa, ON: Author.

Health Council of Canada. (2005). *Primary health care.* Toronto, ON: Author.

Health Evidence Network. (2006). *What is the evidence on school health promotion in improving health or preventing disease, and specifically, what is the effectiveness of the health promoting schools approach?* Copenhagen, Denmark: WHO Regional office for Europe. Retrieved August 1, 2007, from www.euro.who.int/Document/E88185.pdf.

Health Promotion and *WorkLife* Services. (2006). *The Edmonton charter for health promoting universities and institutions of higher education.* Edmonton, Alberta: University of Alberta.

Hertzman, C. (2000). The case for an early childhood development strategy. *Isuma, Autumn,* 11–18.

Hills, M., Carroll, S., & Vollman, A. (2007). Health promotion and health professions in Canada: Toward a shared vision. In M. O'Neill, A. Pederson, S. Dupere, & I. Rootman (Eds.), *Health promotion in Canada* (2nd ed., pp. 330–346). Toronto, ON: Canadian Scholars' Press.

Jackson, A. (2004). The unhealthy Canadian workplace. In D. Raphael (Ed.), *Social determinants of health: Canadian perspectives* (pp. 79–94). Toronto, ON: Canadian Scholars Press.

Johnson, J. (2000). The health care institution as a setting for health promotion. In B. Poland, L. Green, & I. Rootman (Eds.), *Settings for health promotion: Linking theory and practice* (pp. 175–199). Thousand Oaks, CA: Sage.

Kalnins, I. (2000). Commentary: An environmental perspective on health promotion in the home setting. In B. Poland, L. Green, & I. Rootman (Eds.), *Settings for health promotion: Linking theory and practice* (pp. 76–85). Thousand Oaks, CA: Sage.

Labonte, R. (1993). *Health promotion and empowerment: Practice frameworks.* Issues in Health Promotion Series #3. Toronto, ON: Centre for Health Promotion, University of Toronto, & ParticipACTION.

Lalonde, M. (1974). *A new perspective on the health of Canadians.* Ottawa, ON: Government of Canada.

Leavell, H. R., & Clark, H. G. (1965). *Preventive medicine for the doctor in his community* (3rd ed.). New York: McGraw-Hill.

Logue, R. (2003). Maintaining family connectedness in long-term care: An advanced practice approach to family-centred nursing homes. *Journal of Gerontological Nursing, 29*(6), 24–31.

Lowe, G. (2004). *Healthy workplace strategies: Creating change and achieving results.* Ottawa, ON: Author.

Lyons, R., & Langille, L. (2000). *Healthy lifestyles: Strengthening the effectiveness of lifestyle approaches to improve health.* Halifax, NS: Atlantic Health Promotion Research Centre, Population and Public Health Branch, Health Canada.

Manson-Singer, S. (1994). The Canadian healthy communities project: Creating a social movement. In A. Pederson, M. O'Neill, & I. Rootman (Eds.), *Health promotion in Canada* (pp. 107–122). Toronto, ON: WB Saunders.

McElhone, A., & Limb, Y. (2005). Health promotion/disease prevention in older adults—an evidence-based update. Part III: Nursing home population. *Clinical Geriatrics, 13*(9), 24–31.

National Quality Institute. (2007). *Canadian healthy workplace criteria overview document.* Ottawa, ON: Author.

Nutbeam, D. (1998). Health promotion glossary. *Health Promotion International, 13*(4), 349–364.

Ogilvie, L., & Reutter, L. (2002). Primary health care: Complexities and possibilities from a nursing perspective. In J. Ross-Kerr & M. Wood (Eds.), *Canadian nursing: Issues and perspectives* (4th ed., pp. 441–465). Toronto, ON: Harcourt Canada.

Pinder, L. (2007). The federal role in health promotion. In M. O'Neill, A. Pederson, S. Dupere, & I. Rootman (Eds.), *Health promotion in Canada* (2nd ed., pp. 92–105). Toronto, ON: Canadian Scholars' Press.

Pless, B., & Millar, W. (2000). *Unintentional injuries in childhood: Results from Canadian health surveys.* Ottawa, ON: Health Canada.

Polanyi, M. (2004). Understanding and improving the health of work. In D. Raphael (Ed.), *Social determinants of health Canadian perspectives* (pp. 95–105). Toronto, ON: Canadian Scholars Press.

Polanyi, M., Frank, J., Shannon, H., Sullivan, T., & Lavis, J. (2000). Promoting the determinants of good health in the workplace. In B. Poland, L. Green, & I. Rootman (Eds.), *Settings for health promotion: Linking theory and practice* (pp. 138–166). Thousand Oaks, CA: Sage.

Public Health Agency of Canada. (2005). *Report on seniors' falls in Canada.* Ottawa, ON: Division of Aging and Seniors.

Raeburn, J. (2000). Commentary. In B. Poland, L. Green, & I. Rootman (Eds.), *Settings for health promotion: Linking theory and practice* (pp. 279–287). Thousand Oaks, CA: Sage.

Raeburn, J., & Rootman, J. (2007). A new appraisal of the concept of health. In M. O'Neill, A. Pederson, S. Dupere, & I. Rootman (Eds.), *Health promotion in Canada* (2nd ed., pp. 19–31). Toronto, ON: Canadian Scholars' Press.

Raphael, D. (2004). Introduction to the social determinants of health. In D. Raphael (Ed.), *Social determinants of health* (pp. 1–18). Toronto, ON: Canadian Scholars' Press.

Raphael, D. (2007). Addressing health inequalities in Canada: Little attention, inadequate action, limited success. In M. O'Neill, A. Pederson, S. Dupere, & I. Rootman (Eds.), *Health promotion in Canada* (2nd ed., pp. 106–122). Toronto, ON: Canadian Scholars' Press.

Raphael, D., Bryant, T., & Curry-Stevens, A. (2004). Toronto Charter outlines future health policy directions for Canada and elsewhere. *Health Promotion International, 19,* 269–273.

Reutter, L. (2006). Health and wellness. In P. Potter, A. Perry, J. Ross-Kerr, & M. Wood (Eds.), *Canadian fundamentals of nursing* (3rd ed., pp. 1–17). Toronto, ON: Elsevier Mosby.

Ross, N. (2002). Community belonging and health. *Health Reports, 13*(3), 33–39.

Sangster, D. (2002). *Twelve case studies of innovative workplace health initiatives: Summary of key conclusions.* Retrieved June 26, 2008, from http://www.cibc.ca/Research_and_Reports/Case_Studies.asp

Shamian, J., & El-Jardali, F. (2007). Healthy workplaces for health workers in Canada: Knowledge transfer and uptake in policy and practice. *Healthcare papers, 7*(Sp), 6–25.

Soubhi, H., & Potvin, L. (2000). Homes and families as health promotion settings. In B. Poland, L. Green, & I. Rootman (Eds.), *Settings for health promotion: Linking theory and practice* (pp. 44–67). Thousand Oaks, CA: Sage.

Standing Senate Committee on Social Affairs, Science and Technology. (2002). *The health of Canadians—The federal role.* Ottawa, ON: Author.

Stewart, M., Gillis, A., Brosky, G., Johnston, G., Kirkland, S., Leigh, G., et al. (1996). Smoking among disadvantaged women: Causes and cessation. *Canadian Journal of Nursing Research, 28*(1), 41–60.

Stewart, M., Kushner, K., Spitzer, D., Letourneau, N., Greaves, L., & Boscoe, M. (2004). *Support intervention for low income women smokers: Phase I Public Report.* Retrieved April 29, 2008, from http://www.ssrp.ualberta.ca/projects_women_smokers.html

Villeneuve, M., & MacDonald, J. (2006). *Toward 2020: Visions for nursing.* Ottawa, ON: Canadian Nurses Association.

Vollman, A., Anderson, E., & McFarlane, J. (2008). *Canadian community as partner* (2nd ed.). Philadelphia: Lippincott Williams & Wilkins.

Whitehead, D. (2005). Health promoting hospitals: The role and function of nursing. *Journal of Clinical Nursing, 14,* 20–27.

Whitehead, D. (2006). Workplace health promotion: The role and responsibility of health care managers. *Journal of Nursing Management, 14,* 59–68.

World Health Organization. (1986). *Ottawa Charter for health promotion.* Ottawa, ON: Canadian Public Health Association.

World Health Organization. (1997). *The Jakarta Declaration on health promotion into the 21st century.* Geneva, Switzerland: Author.

World Health Organization. (2005). *Bangkok Charter for health promotion.* Geneva, Switzerland: Author.

World Health Organization. (2006). *Commission on the social determinants of health.* Geneva, Switzerland: Author.

Wright, L. M., & Leahey, M. (2005). *Nurses and families: A guide to family assessment and intervention* (4th ed.). Philadelphia: F.A. Davis.

Young, H., Sikma, S., Trippett, L. J., Shannon, J., & Blackly, B. (2006). Linking theory and gerontological nursing practice in senior housing. *Geriatric Nursing, 27,* 346–354.

ADDITIONAL RESOURCES

Canadian Coalition for Public Health. (2005). *National public health coalition looks to government to build on public health momentum.* News release, Ottawa, February 23, 2005.

Mitchell, I., & Laforet-Fliesser, Y. (2003). Promoting healthy school communities. *Canadian Nurse, 99*(8), 21–24.

Public Health Agency of Canada. (2005). *Population health approach.* Retrieved February 8, 2009 from http://www.phac-aspc.gc.ca/ph-sp/index-eng.php

World Health Organization. (1984). *A discussion document on the concept and principles of health promotion.* Copenhagen, Denmark: European Office of the World Health Organization.

CANADIAN ASSOCIATIONS AND WEB SITES

- Public Health Agency of Canada: http://www.phac-aspc.gc.ca/

- Canadian Population Health Initiative: www.cihi.ca/cphi

- Health Canada Population Health Approach: www.phac-aspc.gc.ca/ph-sp/phdd/

- Canadian Public Health Association: www.cpha.ca

- Canadian Consortium for Health Promotion Research: www.utoronto.ca/chp/CCHPR

- WHO Commission on Social Determinants of Health: http://www.who.int/social_determinants/en/

- WHO Web site on Health Promotion Conferences and Charters: www.who.int/healthpromotion/conferences

- International Union of Health Promotion and Education (UHPE): www.iuhpe.org/

Relevant Web sites pertaining to school health programs and assessment and health promotion of children in schools:

- Comprehensive School Health (CSH) and Health Promoting Schools (HPS): www.safehealthyschools.org

- Quality School Health—Canadian Association for Health, Physical Education, Recreation and Dance: www.cahperd.ca/eng/health/about_qsh.cfm

- School Health Research Network: www.schoolhealthresearch.org

- Safe Kids Canada: www.safekidscanada.ca

- U.S. Centers of Disease Control self-assessment guide for healthy schools: The School Health Index-SHI: www.cdc.gov/HealthyYouth/SHI/

Relevant Web sites pertaining to workplace health programs and assessment:

- Workplace Health Strategies Bureau, Health Canada: http://www.hc-sc.gc.ca/ewh-semt/occup-travail/work-travail/wh-mat-strategies_e.html

- The Pan-Canadian Healthy Living Strategy: http://www.phac-aspc.gc.ca/hl-vs-strat/index.html

- Canadian Policy Research Networks (Job quality theme): http://www.cprn.org/theme.cfm?theme=81&l=en

- Canadian Health Services Research Foundation (Management of the Healthcare Workforce theme): http://www.hc-sc.gc.ca/hcs-sss/hhr-rhs/strateg/recru/init-work-travail/index_e.html

- Canadian Centre for Occupational Health and Safety: http://www.ccohs.ca

- National Quality Institute: http://www.nqi.ca/

Cultural Considerations in Health Assessment

COLLEEN VARCOE, ANNETTE BROWN, AND JOAN ANDERSON

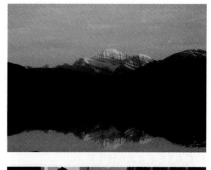

"OK, Mrs. Peter. Take off your clothes and put on this gown. I'll be right back." How often do health assessments begin this way? Does this seem routine and acceptable to you? Does this approach deter clients from accessing health care? How many clients leave without being seen (even if injured) or comply but avoid further health care encounters?

Every clinical encounter is cross-cultural and involves differences between nurse and client. Nurses bring their personal experiences, which are part of their culture; they are also bearers of the culture of health care. Clients bring their personal culture, which is always multifaceted and includes a culture or cultures of health. Similarities may exist between nurses and clients, but most often, there will be differences, even when both share a similar heritage.

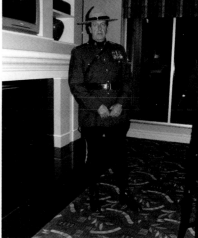

Cultural considerations are important to every health assessment for at least three interrelated reasons:

- To be *effective* and *efficient*: Nurses should understand clients as well as possible. Doing so requires nurses to consider how meanings are shaped culturally.

- To be *equitable*: Nurses need to provide the best possible care to all clients. This requires challenging stereotypes and discrimination.

- To be able to validly *draw on evidence* in relation to individuals: Nurses need to understand how social relations shape health and illness and to see clients within their social, economic, and citizenship contexts.

The focus of this chapter is how to consider culture in the health assessment of clients who come from backgrounds similar to and different from your own. This requires consideration of what culture means and how it is understood from different perspectives. A critical cultural perspective is used to consider the Canadian context, to explore how culture is understood and shaped in Canada, and to introduce an approach to integrating cultural considerations in your health assessments.

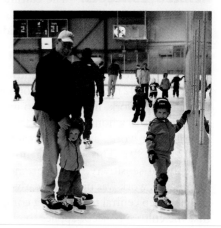

THEORIES RELATED TO CULTURE AND HEALTH

How nurses understand culture, and what they understand it to be, shapes their use of culture and related ideas in their health assessments. In Western societies, the way nurses perceive culture is primarily based on how they think about race. The idea has been that there are different races and that different races have different cultures. This is generally a *culturalist* approach.

CULTURALIST APPROACH

In a culturalist view, culture is the shared values, beliefs, and practices of groups of people—a "thing" that people have. Culture, frequently a euphemism for race, is used to explain people's practices, implying biological differences. Using race thinking, people grouped by race or ethnicities are seen as having certain traits.

Because the culturalist approach has been dominant in Western thinking, it has been the most common approach used in health care. For example, past health professionals believed that each group coming into Canada from a given country (e.g., Mexico) would have a specific culture. Nurses thought the best approach was to learn the "facts" about these cultures and tended toward formulating and applying "recipes" for cultural care. Working more closely with people from different parts of the world, researchers came to realize that the issues are far more complex. Although background knowledge about individuals' histories and predominant systems of meaning for given groups is useful, health care providers cannot just apply "cultural facts" to everyone. For example, all immigrants to Canada from India cannot be assumed to be vegetarian or want particular rituals observed when dying. Moreover, recipes for culture can lead to stereotyping—doing more harm than good in terms of client outcomes.

CASE EXAMPLE

An agitated and confused woman dressed in traditional ethnic clothing was brought to a large urban emergency unit by her husband and her brother-in-law, who were concerned that the client had "gone crazy." English was a second language for all three, although the husband, who did most of the talking for the family, was fluent in English. Hospital staff perceived the husband and brother-in-law as controlling, overly attentive, and protective. They worried that domestic violence was the key issue, saying "*It's in their culture to control women*" and "*Some level of physical abuse is acceptable in their culture.*" The staff quickly isolated the woman and called for intervention from a social worker. Unfortunately, this de-layed further assessment, which later revealed that the woman had a sig-nificant brain tumour. Not surprisingly, the family was upset and angry.

Related Concepts. The culturalist approach to health and health care has included two key concepts: *cultural sensitivity* and *cultural competence*. *Cultural sensitivity* means that health care providers should be sensitive to individuals' values, beliefs, and practices.

Over the past four decades, groundwork by nurse-anthropologist, Dr. Madeleine Leininger (2002), led to the development of a widely drawn on culture care theory. Based on her work, nurses tried to integrate the concept of culture into their care for individuals whom they saw as different from themselves. Leininger herself describes her work "as a great breakthrough in caring for the culturally different" (2002, p. 189). This implies a norm that defines others as different. Striving for cultural sensitivity, nurses attended to clients' values, beliefs, and attitudes. Leininger's work was pivotal in early conceptualizations of culture and health care, and has been central to providing compassionate care. Researchers have recognized that the culture concept applies to all clients, needs to examine the intersection of these factors with the broader social determinants of health, and considers how those determinants, along with power relations, shape peoples' lives.

Cultural competence, a more recent concept, emphasizes a more active role for nurses by encouraging them to go beyond sensitivity in their work with clients. The Canadian Nurses Association (2004) assigns responsibility for providing culturally competent care to various entities: individual nurses, professional and regulatory associations, educational institutions, accrediting bodies, governments, and health care institutions. Cultural competence has been used from different perspectives. Its meaning varies in the way culture and race are understood and the extent to which it includes attention to power and the broader social determinants of health:

- Srivastava (2007) built on Leininger's work using attention to power to consider culture in ways that directly address racism and inequity.

- Some understanding of cultural competence tends to focus on learning more about the culture of others to improve health care and generally do not challenge the basic premise of categorizing individuals by race.

- Other approaches to cultural competence are similar to the evolving concept of *cultural safety* (see pp. 38–39, 46).

As understanding of culture has evolved, so has understanding of race, which is far more complex than a fixed category. Henry et al. (2006) stated:

> Race is a socially constructed category used to classify humankind according to common ancestry and reliant on differentiation by such physical characteristics such as colour of skin, hair texture, stature, and facial characteristics. The concept of race has no basis in biological reality and, as such has no meaning independent of its social definitions. But as a social construction, race significantly affects the lives of people of colour. (p. 351)

In 1952, the United Nations Educational Scientific and Cultural Organization released its first statement on race, dispelling its validity as a biological category. Despite efforts to challenge the idea of race as biological, nurses often tend to confuse race with genetic characteristics. For example, sickle-cell anemia among African Canadians is genetically linked but often offered as evidence of race, even though it is similar to other genetic problems such as cystic fibrosis or Hodgkin's disease. Unfortunately, distinguishing individuals according to race is a common contemporary practise.

Ethnicity is often used as a substitute for race. Ethnicity refers to a group or "community maintained by a shared heritage, culture, language, or religion" (Henry et al., 2006, p. 350). This complex concept frequently implies geographic and national affiliation, but it can be ambiguous. It can encompass race, origin or ancestry, identity, language, and religion, and is dynamic, changing with new immigration flows and new identities (Statistics Canada, 2006a). *Statistics Canada* specifies three fundamental ways of measuring ethnicity: origin or ancestry, race, and identity. However, origin or ancestry is ambiguous because it does not usually specify a historical reference point (when do the ancestors of immigrants from England stop being "English"?). Race is ambiguous because the basis of racial categories continually shifts even as the tendency to treat race as biological persists despite all evidence to the contrary.

Identity depends on how individuals perceive themselves. It is "a subjective sense of coherence, consistency, and continuity of self, rooted in both personal and group history" (Henry et al., 2006, p. 350). People may interpret identity differently, basing it on origin, race, or citizenship. The same person may identify as Italian, Caucasian, and Canadian. It is important to distinguish between how people are categorized by others and how they self-identify. One's identity may be shaped by others' categorizations but be quite different from those imposed categories. Individuals and groups can use identity in powerful ways, both to suppress others (e.g., think "Aryan Nation") and resist suppression (e.g., think "Black Power").

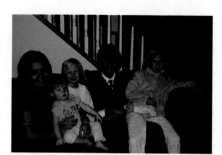

A CRITICAL CULTURAL PERSPECTIVE

A critical perspective of *culture* is based on understanding it as a dynamic, shifting process in which we all engage. Rather than seeing values and beliefs as determining people's behaviours and circumstances, a critical perspective sees them as being part of systems of meaning on which people draw. Health and illness meanings are understood as they intersect with factors such as economics, everyday-living conditions, racism, and racialization.

People create culture as they live in relation to one another. Culture is created, culture is lived, and culture is always in process. Culture is a relational process (Browne & Varcoe, 2006; Hartrick-Doane & Varcoe, 2005), that is, people create culture in relation to one another and their environments. Nurses need to understand how they are bearers of health care and other cultures and how they create culture even as they do health assessments.

A critical cultural perspective simultaneously draws attention to power and to historical, social, economic, and political relationships. The extent to which an ethnic group engages with wider Canadian society is partly a consequence of power relations between them and how that group has been treated socially, economically, and politically. Nurses need to understand how wider circumstances shape individuals' lives and to pay attention to their own power. For example, *the very act of instructing someone to take off his or her clothes enacts power and the culture of health care.*

Values, beliefs, and practices are powerful, not as *determining* factors in individuals' lives but as dynamic and interacting with multiple factors in their social contexts. For example, a cultural perspective helps nurses examine what people eat as shaped by the intersection of beliefs, values, and traditions with factors such as income and geography. When a nurse takes a health history from a client with diabetes, the nurse's understanding of the client's access to food, and the ability to afford and prepare food, is as important as understanding the client's preferences and traditions.

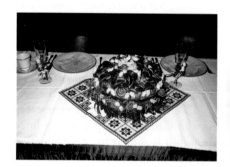

Viewing culture as a relational process with multiple factors draws attention to factors that affect health. These include clients' life circumstances and the *broader determinants of health*, such as poverty, education, migration, and citizenship status. Not least among these factors is how nurses interact with their clients—how they enact their power and the culture of health care and seek to listen to and understand clients.

From a critical perspective, nurses are not required to know discrete cultural facts about every group. Nurses do need a body of knowledge that focuses more sharply on the *varied systems of meaning on which people draw* (e.g., how people make sense of a particular illness, which might be quite different from the biomedical understanding). Nurses are not required to memorize different explanations that clients might have of an illness; they need to *listen* to different explanations so that they can best respond to individuals in *the context of their lives.*

A critical perspective also requires nurses to be more *aware of their own beliefs and values* and *to question their assumptions* about different groups. For example, to understand how poverty limits life choices, nurses need to confront their assumptions about people who are poor. They need to understand how systemic racism and other forms of discrimination keep some groups in poverty. If clients cannot get work because of discriminatory employment practices, or if the only jobs they can get are well below their capabilities, this may have profound effects on their health and ability to manage illness.

A *critical perspective* helps nurses build knowledge, frame the questions to ask clients during health assessments, and interpret what clients tell them.

SOCIOPOLITICAL, ECONOMIC, AND CULTURAL COMPLEXITY IN CANADA

Canada is a country of great diversity and complexity. Its original inhabitants were diverse indigenous peoples; over the past 500 years, the English and French first colonized Canada, which later became a destination for migrants from all over the world.

ABORIGINAL PEOPLES

Canada has always been home to diverse peoples. Its many indigenous groups experienced contact with Europeans differently in various locations and times, but the shared experience was one of colonization. *Colonization* is the "loss of lands, resources, and self-direction and . . . the severe disturbance of cultural ways and values" (LaRoque, 1993, p. 73).

Colonizing policies and practices in Canada include the following:

■ Creation of the Indian Act

■ Removal of entire communities onto reserves, often with insufficient resources to sustain them, and continued underfunding of these reserves

■ Historical and ongoing government appropriation of Aboriginal lands

■ Forced removal of children to residential schools; ongoing widespread state apprehension of Aboriginal children

■ Outlawing of cultural and spiritual practices

■ Widespread discriminatory attitudes toward Aboriginal peoples

The effects of colonization continue to influence the health and social and economic status of Aboriginal peoples. Colonizing practices continue as the wider society racializes Aboriginal people, governing them with different policies, including those related to land ownership, banking, and health care.

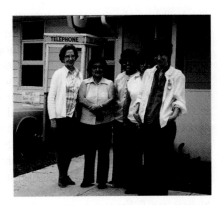

Although colonization decimated many groups, numerous indigenous peoples continue to reside in Canada. In 2001, 1.3 million people (4.4% of the total Canadian population) reported Aboriginal ancestry (Statistics Canada, 2003a). The term *Aboriginal peoples* generally refers to First Nations, Métis, and Inuit peoples (Indian and Northern Affairs Canada, 1996) These terms replace the inaccurate labels imposed during colonization: First Nation replaces Indian, Inuit replaces Eskimo, and Métis refers to people of mixed European and Aboriginal ancestry. Nevertheless, the earlier labels persist in the media, federal policy and legislation (e.g., the Indian Act still in effect), statistical reports, and wider public discussions.

Those belonging to the three political and cultural groupings of Aboriginal peoples use more than 50 languages: First Nations represent at least 10 language families, Inuit represent a separate language family, and Métis represent a unique mixed language (Cook & Howe, 2004). Various colonial processes, including residential schools where children were punished for speaking their own languages, eroded and even eradicated many indigenous languages. As of 1996, only 3 of 50 Aboriginal languages (Cree, Inuktitut, and Ojibway) had large enough populations to be considered truly secure against extinction (Statistics Canada, 1998, December 14).

Aboriginal people are generally younger than other Canadian groups as a result of higher mortality rates and shorter life spans. Increasingly, Aboriginal people are moving to cities from rural or northern communities in an effort to benefit from economic opportunities, jobs, and educational programs. Many who move to urban centres are families with young children. Canadian Aboriginal people are initiating significant cultural, economic, and political reclamation:

- A resurgence in community-level language programs

- Various entrepreneurial initiatives

- Legal actions regarding the extensive physical, emotional, and sexual abuse of children by state and church officials

- Widespread political activity supporting treaty negotiations and the settlement of land claims with the government of Canada

The complex history of colonial politics and contemporary policies and practices has detrimental effects on the overall health and social status of Aboriginal individuals, families, and communities. Recently, Canada's ranking dropped from first to eighth as the best country in the world to live, primarily because of the housing and health conditions in First Nations communities (Assembly of First Nations, 2007). On most health indicators, Aboriginal people fare more poorly than the rest of the population. In 2000, life expectancy at birth for the "Registered Indian" population was 68.9 years for males and 76.6 years for females, a difference of 7.4 years and 5.2 years, respectively, from the general Canadian population (Health Canada, 2007). Compared with the general population, Aboriginal peoples have higher proportions of births to teenaged mothers, higher rates of suicide in youth, almost twice as many high birth weights, and higher rates of smoking. Furthermore, heart disease is 1.5 times more common, tuberculosis infection rates are up to 10 times more frequent, and incidence of type 2 diabetes can be 5 times higher (Health Canada, 2007).

The health of Aboriginal people is often presented out of context, neglecting factors such as unemployment, poverty, geographical isolation, and conflict between levels of government (Roscelli, 2005; Stanhope et al., 2008). Late access to prenatal care, higher infant mortality rates, and worse birth weights than the general population are routinely cited problems. Historically, these indicators resulted in a focus on infants rather than on living conditions that shaped such outcomes and were used to justify interventions in Aboriginal people's lives. Examples include requiring women to go to urban centres to give birth or apprehending children to state care (Benoit et al., 2007; Kaufert & O'Neil, 1993). Health indicators that are not understood within their social, economic, and political contexts can be erroneously seen as cultural problems (a culturalist perspective).

Nurses can fail to see how social conditions, systemic racism, and discrimination shape suicide and substance use among Aboriginal people. They can overlook the consequences of policy and politically created social conditions. For example, judgemental racist attitudes from care providers, poverty, and limited resources in rural settings hamper prenatal care for Aboriginal women (Browne, 2007; Browne & Fiske, 2001), yet nurses may judge these same women for not accessing care.

EARLY SETTLERS, MIGRANTS, AND REFUGEES

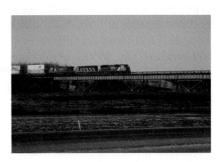

Canada has had immigrants since Aboriginal peoples witnessed the arrival of the first settlers, many of whom came from European countries as part of colonial expansion to meet the labour market needs of "settling the land." People of non-European descent experienced the colonizing process through discriminatory policies. For example, more than 10,000 men were temporarily brought from China to build the Canadian Pacific Railway in the 1880s, but their families were not allowed to accompany them. Similarly, women from the Caribbean were brought to Canada primarily as domestic labourers, and their families were barred (Arat-Koc, 1999).

Until the 1970s, the United States and Europe (e.g., United Kingdom, Italy, Germany, the Netherlands) were the primary sources of immigrants to Canada (Statistics Canada, 2007a). With changing Canadian immigration policies, the proportion of Europeans has declined steadily in each subsequent wave of immigrants. By 2006, 1 in 5 Canadians were born in another country, and no longer did Europe represent the primary source of immigration (Statistics Canada, 2007b, 2007c).

Reasons for migration are often complex and varied; they include relocation to explore new economic opportunities, escape from persecution or oppression, or reunion with family. Refugees usually come from war-torn countries or leave home during political unrest. Because of the global political and economic climate, changing immigration policies, and international events related to the movement of migrants and refugees, the numbers fluctuate; however, increasingly people come from various source countries.

As of 2001, approximately 1.8 million people (6.2% of total population) living in Canada were immigrants who had arrived within the past decade. The number of people coming to Canada annually since has fluctuated around 250,000 (e.g., in 2006, 251,511 new immigrants arrived in Canada).

Most newcomers to Canada settle in urban areas, but increasingly rural settings are seeking to attract them to bolster diminishing populations and meet labour needs. Between 2002 and 2004, the vast majority of immigrants (88% in 2004) settled in the three most populous provinces: Ontario, Quebec, and British Columbia (Statistics Canada, 2006c).

The terms used to refer to newcomers is important. Although the term *immigrant* applies to any person whom immigration authorities have granted the right to permanently live in Canada (Statistics Canada, 2006a), it is sometimes wrongly used synonymously with *people of colour*.

> Many people of colour are not immigrants and are from families who have lived in Canada for several generations. Nurses must not make assumptions about nation of birth or citizenship status based on appearance.

The term "visible minority" is sometimes confused with "immigrant" and "people of colour." *Statistics Canada* uses a racialized understanding to define "visible minority" as people who are non-Caucasian in race or nonwhite in colour and does not consider Aboriginal people as members of visible minority groups (Statistics Canada, 2006a). However, some Aboriginal people and many people with visible "differences" (e.g., physical disabilities, those who are very small or very large) may consider themselves as belonging to a visible minority.

Some people of colour view the term visible minority as demeaning, marginalizing, and discounting of individuals' different histories. Many prefer "people of colour" because it acknowledges differences while recognizing shared systemic discrimination in Canada (Carty, 1991). Immigrants and refugees are not a homogeneous cultural or socioeconomic group, even when originating from the same country. They have different levels of education, French- and English-language skills, and understandings of Western health services. Some highly educated middle-class immigrants and refugees from large cities are used to health care similar to that in Canada; those who are poor or from rural areas might not be.

The processes of migration and resettlement have effects on health. Recent data from large national databases (e.g., the National Population Health Survey) provide compelling evidence that although immigrants come to Canada healthy, their health, especially for non-European immigrants, deteriorates compared with Canadian-born residents and European immigrants (Pederson & Raphael, 2006). This decline is attributable to social determinants. Low income despite higher education levels, precarious employment, racism, discrimination, and low levels of social support constrain their access to resources and services required to maintain health.

RELEVANT CANADIAN LEGISLATION

Legislation, which is the key to understanding the cultural complexity in Canada, includes the British North America Act (BNA), Indian Act, evolving immigration legislation, Multiculturalism Act, and Charter of Rights and Freedoms. The BNA of 1867 (later renamed the Constitution Act) divided provincial and federal responsibilities for areas such as education and health care in ways that persist today. Current laws and policies for First Nations originated in the 1876 Indian Act, which categorized First Nations as status or nonstatus Indians to distinguish those who receive legal recognition by the state from those who do not. Today, "registered" or "status" Indians receive some limited prescription, dental, and vision benefits not covered by provincial health insurance plans. Amendments to the Indian Act over the past 130 years have removed many overtly racist and sexist policies, but the Act continues as the overarching governing policy for "status" First Nations people.

Canada has had racist and gender-biased immigration laws, including those outlawing black immigrants (Mathieu, 1995), the infamous "Chinese Head Tax," and prohibition of female immigrants from China. Such practices created fertile ground for exploitation, disruption of families, and interpersonal violence.

Since 2002, immigration legislation emphasizes economic priorities and includes refugees and the following categories of immigrants:

- Skilled workers and professionals

- Investors, entrepreneurs, and self-employed persons

- Family class

Although the legislation is often touted as nondiscriminatory, the level of education and material resources required means that wealthy, well-educated people have the best chances of immigrating. Ironically, many find that when they arrive in Canada, they cannot find employment in their fields. Newcomers often experience "downward mobility" in their employment, job security and standard of living.

Gender bias persists in legislation, because "family class immigration" supports the notion of marriage and systematically devalues women. Women who immigrate may be multiply disadvantaged by gender discrimination in their countries of origin, Canadian immigration practices, and gender discrimination in Canada. Some have fewer resources and skills, little or no social support, and greater challenges in acquiring language skills and employment (MacKinnon & Howard, 2000). For example, in 2001, 21% of "visible minority" women 15 years or older had a university degree, compared with 14% of other women. Although visible minority women are generally better educated, they are somewhat less likely to be employed. In addition, visible minority women generally earn less at their jobs than do other women (Statistics Canada, 2006e).

Multiculturalism and respect for diversity are official policies of the federal government. Currently, a framework of policies and laws underlies Canadian support for diversity and multiculturalism. Examples include the Canadian Charter of Rights and Freedoms, Canadian Human Rights Act (1988), Employment Equity Act, Official Languages Act, Pay Equity Act, and Multiculturalism Act (1988).

The *Canadian Charter of Rights and Freedoms* is the first part of the Canadian Constitution Act of 1982, the set of laws containing the basic rules about how Canada is governed. Each of these shapes how we understand culture in Canada. Some rights and freedoms contained in the Charter include freedom of expression; right to a democratic government; right to live and to seek employment anywhere in Canada; legal rights of people accused of crimes; Aboriginal peoples' rights; right to equality, including the equality of men and women; right to use either of Canada's official languages; right of French and English linguistic minorities to an education in their language; and protection of Canada's multicultural heritage. Canada is also a signatory to multiple international declarations that commit to human rights and equity.

Importance for Health Assessment: Section 15 of the Charter makes it clear that every individual in Canada—regardless of "race," religion, national or ethnic origin, colour, sex, age, or physical or mental disability—is to be considered equal. However, as a nurse, you need to understand that although *equality means treating people the same, equity refers to fairness in treatment.* When you are completing a health assessment, treating everyone "the same" means you will not consider the unique situations and needs of various groups and individuals and thus will not be effective. To optimize your health assessments, you need to recognize that while all people may be "equal" under the law, they have varied circumstances that need to be addressed. It is important to treat people equitably, not the same.

CANADIAN DEMOGRAPHICS

Clearly, Canada is a country of diversity. This is true not only in terms of ethnicities and languages but also in terms of history, spiritual and religious affiliations, geography, and material resources, all of which shape the cultures of individuals and groups.

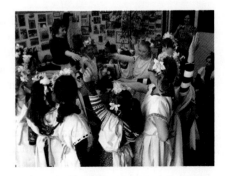

Ethnic Diversity.   Canada is one of the most *ethnically diverse* countries in the world (Statistics Canada, 2003a). Although Canadians often pride themselves on valuing diversity, the Ethnicity Diversity Survey (Statistics Canada, 2003a) found that 2.2 million people (10%) felt uncomfortable or out of place sometimes, most of the time, or all of the time because of their ethnocultural characteristics. People who self-identified as "visible minorities" were more likely to feel out of place.

Linguistic Diversity. Canada's diversity includes *languages* spoken. Colonizing practices have steadily eroded Aboriginal languages in Canada. In 2001, one in four people who identified as Aboriginal had enough knowledge of an Aboriginal language to carry on a conversation. This number will continue to decline as elders with language knowledge die, unless current efforts to reclaim languages are successful. The two "official" languages in Canada's constitution are English and French, in recognition of the two groups of early settlers who colonized Canada. A large and growing proportion of Canada's population now uses a language other than English or French as the primary means of communication (Statistics Canada, 2001). For example, 61% of immigrants who came to Canada in the 1990s used an "unofficial" language as their primary home language. Canada is becoming increasingly multilingual (Statistics Canada, 2001).

One's mother tongue is the first language a person learns and still understands (Statistics Canada, 2001). In addition to English and French, Canadians reported more than 100 mother tongues, including languages long associated with immigration to Canada such as German, Italian, Ukrainian, Dutch, and Polish. Between 1996 and 2001, language groups from Asia and the Middle East increased, and Chinese is now the third largest language group; these languages also include Punjabi, Arabic, Urdu, Tagalog, and Tamil.

Religious Diversity. Part of Canada's national character is its breadth of religions. As many as 7 out of 10 Canadians identify themselves as either Roman Catholic or Protestant (Statistics Canada, 2003b), but the trend is for fewer people to identify as Protestant and for more people to identify with Islam, Hinduism, Sikhism, and Buddhism. Much of the shift in religious affiliation during the past several decades results from changing sources of immigrants. Also, many Protestant denominations, such as Anglican and United Church, are declining, in part because fewer young people are identifying with them and their members are aging.

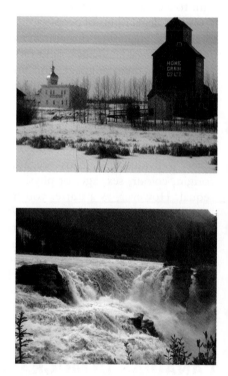

Geographical Diversity. Canada's incredibly diverse *geography* extends from the temperate climates of the Great Lakes to the far North and from the Atlantic to the Pacific Ocean. The geography of the prairies, various coasts, the North, and mountainous regions all shape cultures differently. Canada's population is concentrated primarily in southern urban centres, with just under 20% (6 million) living in rural areas (areas outside urban centres with a population of at least 10,000) (Statistics Canada, 2006b). Importantly, incomes and health indicators in rural settings are lower than in urban settings (Singh, 2004). For example, in 2001, a lower proportion of Canadians living in small towns, rural regions, and northern regions rated their health as "excellent" (compared to the national average) and had a higher prevalence of being overweight and smoking (Mitura & Bollman, 2003). People living in Northern regions had higher unmet health care needs compared to the national average, whereas people in major urban regions had lower unmet health care needs.

Income Diversity. Canada has diverse *income levels*, with the gap between rich and poor widening steadily (Statistics Canada, 2006d). Despite a strong economy, many Canadians live in poverty. In 2004, Statistics Canada estimated that 684,000 families (7.8%) were living below the low-income cutoff point (LICO). Approximately 865,000 children younger than 18 years (12.8%) were living in low-income families. Poverty has profound effects on health. Lower social and economic status and higher gaps in income equality are associated with poorer health (Raphael et al., 2006). Despite Canada's recent economic prosperity, its benefits are disproportionately distributed; the inequities between the wealthy and poor, and between the healthy and not, continue to grow (Coburn, 2006). Poverty, racialization, gendered inequities, and ageism profoundly shape patterns of ill health.

Understanding the relationship between demographic characteristics and health requires simultaneous consideration of multiple influences. For example, the differences between the health of any given group of immigrants and the general Canadian population cannot be understood by considering only the effects of migration, social class and income premigration, access to employment and income post migration, or the experiences of racism for racialized groups. Health within any given group cannot be understood without consideration of differences such as gender, class, and ability. All these intersecting influences must be considered simultaneously. Nurses need to understand the complex interaction of multiple influences when providing care to any group and to avoid making assumptions about any given person based on demographic characteristics.

Nurses also need to remember that characteristics common to a group will not necessarily apply to a specific individual. They should be careful never to confuse heredity and genetics with ethnicity when dealing with clients. Within a single ethnic designation, there can be as much or more variability in disease and in its determinants than between ethnic groups (O'Loughlin, 1999). Little, if any, scientific, biologic, or anthropologic merit exists in labels such as white, black, European, or minority.

Nurses must engage in critical self-reflection and take care to draw on *evidence* rather than stereotypes or false assumptions. For example, health care providers in British Columbia often erroneously assume that Aboriginal people drink alcohol, despite evidence that they consume less alcohol per capita than the rest of the population (Kendall, 2001).

■ *Using Knowledge of Demographics to Guide Health Assessments*

Knowledge	Example
Use knowledge of groups to inform your inquiry without drawing on stereotypes and without erroneously assuming that general trends apply to particular individuals.	Knowing about the stresses associated with immigration and relocation will lead you to inquire about individuals' experiences but to do so without assuming what the client's experience will have been.
Avoid using knowledge of demographics in ways that close your inquiry into possibilities.	Knowing that a higher percentage of women battered by partners are in common-law relationships and have lower incomes should not lead you to overlook the possibility of battering for higher-income women or those who are married, or to assume that a particular woman who is in a common-law relationship or very poor is being battered.
Ensure that you take multiple interconnecting factors into account simultaneously.	If a person has not been accessing health care, before you assume "values" are at play, consider the influences of income, transportation, racism, age, gender (perhaps the person has a partner, parent, or someone who prevents access), and the health care system itself.
Use demographic knowledge to make your approach as safe as possible. *This is the most important use of knowledge.*	If clients include political refugees, you do not need to know whether the particular individuals have experienced torture or state terrorism to act in noninvasive ways.
	If your clients include Aboriginal people, you do not need to know of their individual experiences to make your approach respectful and nontraumatizing. You might begin asking, "Would you be comfortable getting changed into this gown?"
	You might use your knowledge to challenge practices that might be routinely harmful, such as requiring people routinely to undress or asking unnecessary questions that may be invasive.

CULTURAL SAFETY: A RELATIVELY NEW CONCEPT IN CANADA

In the early 1990s, Maori leaders in nursing education in New Zealand coined the concept of *cultural safety* as an alternative to cultural sensitivity (Papps & Ramsden, 1996; Ramsden, 1993). Because it arose from the bicultural relationship between the Maoris and descendants of British colonists, cultural safety in New Zealand focuses exclusively on the relationship between indigenous peoples and early settlers. Canadians have used this concept to include all peoples.

Central Ideas of Cultural Safety

- Social, economic, and political positions of groups within society influence health and health care.
- Individual and institutional discrimination in health care creates risks for clients, particularly when people from a specific group perceive they are "demeaned, diminished or disempowered by the actions and delivery systems" including by those who typically hold the power in health care contexts (namely, health care providers) (Ramsden & Spoonley, 1994, p. 164).
- Cultural safety does *not* refer to the cataloguing of culture-specific beliefs. Rather, as Polaschek (1998) noted, in referring to the Maori people, "It is how this group is perceived and treated that is relevant rather than the different things its members think or do" (p. 452).
- The concept encourages health care providers "to reflect on their own personal and cultural history and the values and beliefs they bring in their interaction with clients, rather than an uncritical imposition of their own understandings and beliefs on clients and their families" (Anderson et al., 2003, p. 198).
- Promoting safety requires actions that *recognize*, *respect*, and *nurture* the unique cultural identity of *all* people/families and that *safely meet* their needs, expectations, and *rights*.

CULTURE AND HEALTH ASSESSMENT

A more complex and critical understanding of culture leads nurses to ask more complex questions during health assessments. From a critical perspective, one concept that helps nurses to appreciate the complexity of culture is *cultural safety*.

In Canada, cultural safety is being adapted to Canada's diverse context as an alternative to a culturalist approach (Anderson et al., 2003; Dyck & Kearns, 1995; Smye & Browne, 2002). Health care agencies are using cultural safety increasingly to orient providers to the ways that culture is embedded in historical, economic, and social contexts. This concept is relevant to the Canadian context in working with *any client population*.

> Cultural safety speaks to all of us, but not in terms of static essentialized, cultural categories . . . [I]t is a way of bringing [a critical discourse] into clinical practice, not as a set of concrete standards for practice, but as a way of questioning how we are positioned in relation to our clients and in relation to the system of health care delivery in which we practice. (Anderson et al., 2003, p. 212)

Cultural safety helps nurses pay attention to peoples' values, beliefs, and systems of meanings, within the context of their lives and the culture of health care. It helps them examine how health care practices, interactions, and policies can themselves create marginalizing conditions and inequities, particularly for those labelled as "different" (Smye & Browne, 2002). For example, when certain groups disagree with or disregard visiting hours in hospitals, health care providers sometimes see a "cultural problem" specific to clients and family members rather than a problem of difference between the group and the dominant health care culture. A cultural safety approach asks nurses to examine what it is about the culture of health care that may impede access for some groups yet facilitate access for others.

REFLEXIVITY AND SOCIAL LOCATION OF THE ASSESSOR

Critical consciousness and reflexivity are key skills for health assessment. Multiple influences shape lives and health. Nurses are likely to be privileged in relation to many clients; fluent in an official language, educated and able to afford an education, and possessing certain abilities. At the same time, they may be less privileged than their clients, perhaps in terms of gender, ethnicity, and income.

To be effective in your health assessments, you need to see how your social location shapes your view of clients and interpretation of data. To see these dynamics, you need to be reflexive. *Reflexivity* is more than self-reflection. It refers to reflecting on self in relation to others and the world around. To begin a reflexive analysis of your own social location, consider the following questions:

- What varied "cultures" are you part of? Western culture? Health care culture?

- What privileges does membership in each of these cultures extend to you?

- How does each of these cultures shape your view of the world and your clients?

For example, if you have led a primarily privileged life—with enough food, access to education and employment, and no experience of daily discrimination, it may be challenging for you to understand the circumstances of people who have not enjoyed those privileges. Otherwise, if you have had some challenges previously, you may see your current situation as a personal accomplishment and judge others negatively if they have not made similar progress. Alternatively, you can use critical analysis of your own social location to appreciate both your own and other's privileges and challenges and better understand how both affect health.

ASSESSING EXPLANATORY FRAMEWORKS AND VIEWPOINTS

"Assessment is a clinical art that combines sensitivity, judgement, and scientific knowledge" (Anderson et al., 2005, p. 338). The critical perspective on culture along with the notion of cultural safety provide a certain framework for health assessment. From this perspective, the approach to assessment of clients is different than if you see culture as determining facts (i.e., determining what a person believes and values). This perspective draws attention to the multiple cultures nurses share with clients rather than simply focusing on differences based on ethnicity or some other factor.

A proposed framework for health assessment requires that health care providers:

- be conscious about their own perspective, the ways in which their prejudices can shape *how* they see people and how they interpret what clients tell them (self-reflection—examining assumptions).
- listen to their clients' "explanatory models." Their clients become health care providers' teachers about their lives (health assessment).
- conduct their assessment informed by different domains of knowledge, including sociocultural knowledge. That is knowledge about different systems of cultural meanings, the histories from which people come, the determinants of health, and the root causes of health inequities. This knowledge informs the questions nurses ask, how they engage with clients for best practices, and most important, how they interpret what people tell them.

As early as 1980, Arthur Kleinman put forward a model for assessment, which Varcoe, Anderson, and Browne have continued to draw on in their work (e.g., see Anderson et al., 2005). They argued that, "To provide culturally responsive care, the professional needs to focus on the context of each person's life and experiences—with an immigrant even more than with a mainstream Canadian. What is different with immigrant clients is that the practitioner risks making assumptions about the client based on mainstream Canadian culture and ethnic stereotypes" (p. 326). The same can be said about working with Aboriginal people—practitioners risk making assumptions based on deep-seated prejudices toward Aboriginal people. Nurses need to start assessment with themselves.

Each nurse needs to recognize how his or her background affects interactions with clients and their families. Anderson and colleagues (2005, p. 390) proposed reflective questions that are useful to nurses:

- What are my own beliefs about newcomers to Canada [or any other group], and how might these enter into how I interact with this person?

- What assumptions am I making about this person? And about this particular cultural group?

- Why do I think this way?

- Where did I get this information?

- What might I learn if I talk to the person?

- What might we have in common?

These questions apply equally in working with *any client*. Nurses need to recognize the relations of power that exist in any health care encounter. Clients and health care providers are never on neutral terrain, but it should not be taken for granted that the nurse is always in a position of power in relation to the client. Consider the possible experiences of a female Aboriginal nurse or the immigrant nurse of colour caring for a white man or woman, an Aboriginal man, a man of colour, or a person of his or her own gender and ethnic background but from a different class background. Complex power dynamics may be manifested in several ways. For example, some white clients may demean nurses of colour by refusing to be cared for by them (Anderson et al., 2003). Racism and racialization in such cases work opposite to how it is usually conceptualized in the health care encounter. The old adage about the "power" that health providers have in the health care encounter needs to be "unpacked" and examined more closely, as nurses become more attuned to the complex social relations that operate in health care systems.

Nurses must also explore their own "explanatory models," including how they understand health and illness. Having been educated within the biomedical paradigm, nurses will have incorporated certain ideas about health, illness, and disease into their own thinking. However, they may draw on other perspectives—for example, a strong understanding of the social determinants of health—or may have incorporated other more traditional approaches to health and healing. It is useful for nurses to continuously examine their knowledge sources, critically scrutinize evidence, and be aware of the ways that knowledge shapes understanding of clients' explanatory models. Having examined their own assumptions, nurses then need to explore with the client his or her "explanatory model."

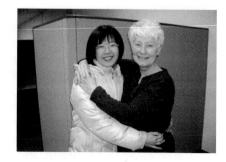

Explanatory Models of Clients. Conversing with a client to gain a deep understanding of his or her explanatory model (how a person understands his or her world and explains health and illness) assumes verbal communication between nurse and client. The starting point is to establish that client and nurse share a similar language and can speak with one another. If this is not the case, an interpreter will need to assist with assessment, a situation considered in more detail later.

The "trigger questions" that nurses can interweave sensitively in conversation with clients and their families follow. *Cautionary note:* People, including health care providers, usually do not attribute what they do to their "culture." They take for granted that people act in certain ways, and few reflect on this as their culture. Questions directed to clients about their culture may not only be confusing but may also cause clients to perceive such questions as "othering," which creates a distance or chasm between themselves and the health care provider. *The key is to establish a respectful dialogue with clients and to search for common understanding rather than to focus on differences.*

COMMUNICATING ACROSS DIFFERENCES

In every health assessment, nurses communicate across "difference." The language of health care and its disciplines is laced with terminology and jargon that are foreign to many clients. As a nurse, you must continuously adjust your language to your

■ *Trigger Questions and Rationale*	
Trigger Questions	**Rationale**
What do you think caused your illness? Why do you think it started when it did? What do you call your problem?	Such questions may reveal that the client's ideas about the body and how it works differ from biomedical perspectives. This information might help you to understand why the client makes certain decisions or, conversely, might hesitate to agree to a certain treatment. This is important for all clients because it is impossible to predict who will subscribe to biomedical ideas (or to what extent) based on ethnicity, age, nationality, or language.
Have you found any medicines or treatments that have worked for you in the past? Why do you think they helped? Are you using them now?	These questions can help you further understand the person's explanatory framework but focus on treatment.
Did you use any special medicines or treatments in your home country that worked for you?	With recent immigrants, you may want to signal your openness to hearing about therapies not available or commonly used in Canada.
Have any traditional healing methods worked for you?	You also may want to signal your interest and willingness to hear about traditional healing strategies, especially for people who identify as Aboriginal.
What do you think I need to know to give you the best care possible?	This question to ask of all clients gives the message that you are open to hearing a range of things and that you think it is important to know what they consider important. This can go a long way to building respect and understanding and will often lead clients to provide information in the health assessment that more specific questions will not. These questions are not just appropriate for clients whom you assume are different from you. They are useful for all clients and will help you challenge assumptions you might make.

(continued)

■ **Trigger Questions and Rationale** (Continued)

Trigger Questions	Rationale
What are the main problems your illness has caused you (personally, in your family, and at work)? What are the main challenges you have to deal with in managing your health? You can follow with questions such as, Are you working at the moment? Can you tell me a little about the job you now have? Can you tell me about how well life has gone for you lately? Are there any special things that you are worrying about at the moment?	These questions may lead to exploring issues around finances, the home situation, and the work situation. Assessing a client's social and economic context requires tact, and may not be explored comfortably on a first interview. Indirect ways of opening up the conversation exist. Asking direct questions about finances might be considered intrusive, but focusing on the issues caused by illness and relating the information directly to the person's ability to deal with health issues may be one way to start the discussion. Gender-related issues might surface here: trouble with adolescent children, financial support, and how the family is currently obtaining income. These questions indicate resources that may be made available to the person (Anderson et al., 2005, pp. 346–347). For both men and women try to establish whether they have experienced changes in employment or work. Health problems may exacerbate or cause such changes. Downward mobility in the market place is a key issue for many well-educated immigrants, for people with chronic illnesses or mental illnesses, and for older clients. This has enormous consequences for mental health, sometimes leading to depression, so health care providers should be alert to this.
What kinds of things do you need help with? Is there anyone you feel comfortable turning to for help? Are there other people for whom you provide help or care?	Further questions will help you learn about social support networks, whether the person has someone to turn to for help, and whether he or she is in a caregiving role. Many people, even when ill, are providing care, not only for dependent children but also for grandchildren, parents, spouses, and others. This will also draw your attention to resources available and to challenges the person might be facing. Such inquiry also will help build your understanding of the person's explanatory model.
What is your home situation like? (Related to a particular medication or other health need) How do you think you could get that? Would you need help arranging that? Is there going to be a problem for you (related to a particular need)?	As you progress toward needing to ask more directly about resources, you try to find ways to ask that will not embarrass people. Many people are very embarrassed to accept any sort of assistance from the state because they see it as charity. New immigrants are often particularly reluctant to accept any kind of state support. Nurses have heard people say, "I'd rather die than go on welfare," so great sensitivity is needed when dealing with these topics.

Source: Adapted from Anderson et al., 2005; Kleinman, 1980.

clients, seeking to be understood without being patronizing by oversimplifying. Understanding the power of language and communication in relation to your interactions *with* and *about* clients is essential for effective and respectful health assessments. It is vital to "pay attention to the subtle yet powerful ways that we communicate interpersonally, and scrutinize how our own patterns of communication are shaped by wider social forces, including the dominant culture of health care" (Hartrick-Doane & Varcoe, 2005, p. 181). It is *always* the health care provider's responsibility, not the client's, to ensure respectful communication as well as accurate and adequate sharing of information.

One way to attune yourself to the power of language and communication and their influence on health care interactions is to reflect on some assumptions that arise with a client who speaks with an accent. If that accent is British, for example, you may wonder if the person is from the United Kingdom but will not likely make judgements about his or her ability to understand what you are asking or explaining. When you encounter a person of colour with a thick accent, your assumptions may be vastly different. Through critical self-reflection you might discover that you assume that he or she is unlikely to understand English, leading you to talk in a simplified manner (much as you would to a young child). Otherwise, you may assume that this client will not understand what you want to explain, causing you to omit important information or instructions. You may find yourself speaking more loudly, assuming that will help the client understand you more clearly. You may also assume that the client holds cultural beliefs or values different from the dominant culture. Importantly, nurses are not usually conscious or aware that they are forming these kinds of assumptions based purely on a client's accent or appearance. Therefore, critical self-reflection becomes very important in the process of health assessment.

Working effectively with interpreters includes identifying *when* to use one, ensuring that adequate interpretation is available. It requires an understanding of the differences between types of interpreters and adjustment of your practice to those differences and the limitations of interpreters' practice.

When clients do not understand or speak English, it is vital to engage an interpreter for conducting an accurate health assessment and capturing clients' health concerns and priorities. Interpreter services are not used adequately even when they are clearly needed (Tang, 1999). To counter the underutilization of interpreters, you need to actively seek out their services to ensure that you are conducting a thorough, accurate, and meaningful assessment.

Reasons for neglecting to use interpreters even when they are readily available are complex. Physicians, nurses, and other health care professionals may feel pressured by time and mistakenly assume that they can collect a "good enough" history without an interpreter. They may not fully realize the serious implications of partial or inaccurate assessment information. For example, without interpreters, clients who are not proficient in English can have difficulty explaining health issues, posing questions, or understanding information that is essential to maintaining their health or managing their illness (Tang, 1999). Nurses may judge clients who do not fully

---

PROBLEMS WITH RELYING ON FAMILY MEMBERS FOR LANGUAGE INTERPRETATION

- Creates emotional and economic burdens for clients and families (Tang, 1999).
  - Adds a layer of pressure that can strain family dynamics and add to the difficulties that clients are facing.
  - Creates economic pressures when family members feel obliged to take time away from work to interpret for their relatives.
- Can result in inaccuracies during health assessments.
  - Family members are not necessarily able to interpret medical terminology and concepts.
  - Can be very embarrassing for a family member to discuss intimate aspects of their relative's health issues.

- Nurses have no way of knowing how accurately questions are being translated and answered.
- The great risk of miscommunication can be detrimental for the client and create legal consequences for the health care institution.
- Can be dangerous.
  - Intimate partner violence, child and elder abuse likely will not be identified.
  - You may contribute to such problems by giving an abusive family member more power over the client, for example, in the form of controlling access to medication, health appointments, or other needed supports.

---

understand health teaching as "noncompliant." Sometimes, providers label clients as "poor historians" when, in fact, they could have provided thorough histories with help from an interpreter. Obtaining accurate health assessments is essential. Although family members may be the only people available for interpretation in some situations, typically, this is not the case. Interpreters are now available in most institutions, but health care providers all too commonly rely on family members for language interpretation. It is imperative to use the services of paid interpreters in your health care settings, to avoid the problems outlined below, and to advocate for services if none is available.

Of course, there may be times when a family member might assist with interpretation. Examples include when the nurse has a good sense of family dynamics, the issues are more straightforward (e.g., food preferences), and major issues such as explaining surgery, assessing pain, obtaining informed consent for an operation, or assessing the home situation are not being discussed. For obvious reasons, *a child should never be used* to interpret.

Sometimes, agency staff members who speak the language in question are used to interpret. This is also inappropriate for at least three reasons (Tang, 1999).

- Although the person may have knowledge of medical language, you have no way of evaluating whether he or she even speaks the same dialect or can translate accurately.

- This pulls the person away from his or her work and adds workload.

- The person used to translate may be a part of the client's community and may not feel obliged to respect confidentiality.

Nurses must be aware that trained personnel are necessary for all health assessments that require interpretation. They use *clinical judgement* to decide when an interpreter is required and *anticipatory planning* to acquire the services when needed.

There are different types of interpreters. Some provide verbatim translation into one of the two official languages (i.e., English or French). Others interpret cultural meanings and practices and are often employed in health care settings with high numbers of people who are fluent in a language other than English or French. It is important for nurses to know what type of training an interpreter has and to discuss the extent to which he or she is familiar with medical terminology.

Nonverbal communication is in many ways more powerful than overt verbal communication, regardless of ethnocultural or social background. The chances of miscommunication increase when people are interacting across greater differences, such as when they do not speak each other's languages. Health care providers communicate according to acceptable and expected norms within the culture of biomedicine. For example, they pose quick consecutive questions as part of the health history, write notes in charts while clients are talking (instead of maintaining eye contact), or maintain an impartial (or detached) facial expression to convey a sense of "professionalism" toward clients. These ways of interacting are part of the dominant style of communication in health care, which heavily influence nurses. These communication norms can make some clients uneasy or uncomfortable.

Most (if not all) health care interactions should be considered "cross-cultural." From this perspective, nurses will realize that primary responsibility for ensuring effective communication lies with them, not clients. The onus is on nurses to convey openness and receptivity with clients whose communication styles are likely to differ from theirs.

Frequently, nonverbal communication (body posture in relation to clients, use of hand gestures, touch, facial expressions, and eye contact) conveys respect, acceptance, and openness. For example, nonverbal communication is the primary way in which nurses convey genuine interest toward clients. In contrast, clients can quickly sense dismissive attitudes, most often conveyed through nonverbal messages. As Hartrick-Doane and Varcoe (2005) described, health care providers learn to convey their availability to clients with a "busy gait" that discourages interruptions or requests for help. It is imperative that nurses develop critical self-awareness of the messages they may be conveying unwittingly.

EYE CONTACT AS NONVERBAL COMMUNICATION

Eye contact is often an issue that arises during cross-cultural encounters (Razack, 1998; Hartrick-Doane & Varcoe, 2005). Nurses frequently assume that avoidance of eye contact is a client's "cultural norm," but eye contact is more often a response to intimidation felt as a result of power inequities inherent in health care interactions. Instead of assuming that nonverbal communication patterns are "cultural," consider first the following critical question: To what extent might clients' avoidance of eye contact during a health assessment signal discomfort with people in positions of authority? Pausing to ask this question could help attune you to ways you may be inadvertently contributing to unease through tone of voice, facial expression, body posture, or lack of eye contact. Such self-reflection will be invaluable for meaningful communication with clients, family members, and significant others.

Recognizing that nurses *and* clients come to health care interactions with particular styles of communicating requires adjustment of patterns of communication in each health care interaction as nurses make an effort to remain open and responsive. This requires that nurses grapple with the difference between treating people *equally* and treating people *equitably*. When they claim that they treat everyone equally, this means that they are not treating everyone equitably (fairly). Equity requires adjusting the way they interact with others so that they can be responsive to peoples' unique cultural backgrounds, gender, age, social, or economic context. Consider how to adjust your nonverbal and verbal patterns to be as responsive as possible to clients' diverse needs and circumstances. Through this process of self-monitoring and critical self-reflection, you will develop the skills to remain open, respectful, and responsive in all your health care interactions.

Communication Among Health Care Providers   Attending to issues of language and communication is not only relevant in relation to your work with clients but also regarding your communication *about* clients to others. For example, at charting desks, in hallways, at medication counters, in supply rooms, at the receptionist's counter, and elsewhere, your style of communication is important (Browne, 2007). Nurses sometimes slip into discussions about clients in ways that objectify them because of the terms or labels they apply. To counter this tendency, remain mindful of how you are referring to particular clients when communicating with other members of the interdisciplinary team. This is not just a concern about being overheard by clients. How we speak about clients reinforces the values, attitudes, and practices of other health care providers.

For example, referring to a client as the "pregnant woman in examining room #4" tends to contribute to a fragmented view. Over time, nurses can begin to see clients only in relation to their presenting biomedical problem or situation and not in relation to their larger life context. Such a view of clients can cause you to overlook important social, cultural, or economic factors that affect health status. The language, generalizations, and labels used in relation to clients can perpetuate misperceptions and stereotypes that ultimately affect your interactions and practices. For example, when a homeless person comes into a clinic, emergency department, or hospital, you might hear comments like "homeless people should do something to improve themselves. Why doesn't he or she get a job?" Such generalizations overlook how cutbacks to social welfare programs, lack of affordable housing, or lack of mental health services lead to homelessness and impoverishment (Raphael, 2007; Raphael et al., 2006). Such generalizations form the basis of stereotypes, which in turn can lead to dismissive attitudes toward particular groups. Nurses can readily convey such dismissive attitudes to clients through their verbal and nonverbal interactions, limiting the extent to which they can conduct a complete and accurate health assessment. It is therefore important to recognize and challenge the generalizations and stereotypes you encounter at your workplace so that clients are treated with dignity and respect, and receive accurate assessments without an overlay of judgement.

HEALTH PROMOTION

Using the understanding of health promotion discussed in Chapter 1 to address cultural considerations in health assessments offers an important health-promotion approach. Health care providers can promote the following:

- *Create supportive environments for health* by working toward cultural safety for all clients by using strategies that consistently recognize, respect, and nurture the unique cultural identity of *all* people, and safely meet their needs, expectations, and rights.

- *Develop personal skills* of critically examining how our own social locations and experiences shape how we see, understand, and assess clients; listening to clients' explanations to understand the context of their lives.

- *Reorient health services* to foster cultural safety. Importantly, this includes listening to clients' explanatory frameworks and understandings, critically examining and countering assumptions and stereotypes, and ensuring that translation and interpreter services are available and used appropriately.

- *Strengthen community action* for health by advocating for diverse input into health services.

- Build *healthy public policy* by addressing patterns in social determinants of health as they affect clients. This might include facilitating health care access for those who face particular barriers (e.g., poverty, transportation, child care) or advocating broader policy initiatives that affect health (e.g., income-related policies).

Treating all clients in ways that recognize, respect, and nurture their unique identities and advocating for social conditions and health care environments that do so are key strategies for promoting health. These strategies also set the stage for equitable, effective, and efficient nurse–client relationships.

INTERDISCIPLINARY APPROACH

You are currently in an urban clinical practice setting where you are about to see a woman named Ms. Lee. She has visited twice previously, and the chart indicates that she has diabetes and depression. The dietician has seen her already and has written that she has not been testing her blood glucose level as directed. Ms. Lee has had two visits to the ER in the past month, both for hyperglycemia. You notice that the intake form on the chart has several areas of missing information, including those for next of kin and ethnicity. The client's address is the name of a hotel downtown, far from your clinic. The social worker has been asked to see her about any concerns regarding housing.

As you meet Ms. Lee, you notice that she appears to be about 40 years old, but the age on her chart says 32. She has brown, deeply lined skin and looks thin. She looks at you warily; when you say hello, she looks away and down. You begin by asking for the missing information. In response to next of kin, she says "none," and when you ask her "how would you describe your ethnicity?" she replies "I don't know."

Critical Thinking Exercise

Think about your current or most recent clinical practice setting. Consider the characteristics of the workplace: What are the "demographics?" How do staff demographics compare with those of the clients served? What is the morale like? What is the workload like? Thinking about this workplace and Ms. Lee, answer the following questions:

- What are key differences between the culturalist and critical cultural approaches? What do these differences mean for your encounter with Ms. Lee? (*Knowledge*)
- What are the implications of drawing on stereotypes in health assessment for your encounter with Ms. Lee? (*Comprehension*)

- How would you use cultural safety to assess clients who use illegal drugs? (*Application*)
- What is your evaluation of the availability and quality of interpreter services in your practice setting? How will you assess the need for an interpreter for your time with Ms. Lee? (*Analysis*)
- What are the key features of your personal "culture" and experiences that are likely to shape your approach to clients who are different from you in terms of ethnicity, class, and gender? How might these affect your interaction with Ms. Lee? (*Synthesis*)
- What is your evaluation of the characteristics of your workplace/learning environment in terms of fostering cultural safety? (*Evaluation*)

Canadian Research

Anderson, J. M., Tang, S., & Blue, C. (2007). Health care reform and the paradox of efficiency: "Writing in" culture. *International Journal of Health Services, 37*(2), 291–320.

Browne, A. J. (2007). Clinical encounters between nurses and First Nations women in a Western Canadian hospital. *Social Science & Medicine, 64*(10), 2165–2176.

Guruge, S., & Collins, E. (2008). *Working with immigrant women: Issues and strategies for mental health professionals.* Toronto, ON: Canadian Center for Addictions and Mental Health.

Reimer-Kirkham, S. (2003). The politics of belonging and intercultural health care provision. *Western Journal of Nursing Research, 25*(7), 762–780.

Srivastava, R. (2007). *The healthcare professional's guide to clinical cultural competence.* Toronto, ON: Elsevier Canada.

Test Questions

1. If a client does not speak English, a trained interpreter is required
   a. for any meaningful communication, including pain assessment or client teaching.
   b. when a family member is not available.
   c. for legal purposes such as obtaining informed consent.
   d. when there is no one on staff who speaks the person's language.

2. If a client seems reluctant to make eye contact, a health care provider should consider the possibility that this is a(n):

   a. feature of the person's culture.
   b. indicator of respect.
   c. indication of discomfort or intimidation.
   d. feature of the person's racial group.

3. From a critical cultural perspective, culture refers to
   a. values, beliefs, and practices of specific groups.
   b. genetically inherited behavioural traits.
   c. a web of connections among ethnically related persons.
   d. a dynamic process enacted between people and their families.

4. In Canada, the Indian Act
   a. outlined the relationship between the state and Aboriginal peoples.
   b. is no longer in effect.
   c. identified who qualifies as "Aboriginal."
   d. insured fair and equitable treatment of Aboriginal people.

5. A primary goal of cultural safety is to
   a. treat everyone the same in health care.
   b. develop and use knowledge about the practices of different cultures.
   c. develop sensitivity to differences among ethnic groups.
   d. examine how our own perspectives shape how we see clients.

Bibliography

CITATIONS

Anderson, J. M., Kirkham, S. R., Waxler-Morrison, N., Herbert, C., Murphy, M., & Richardson, E. (2005). Conclusion. In: N. Waxler-Morrison, J. M. Anderson, E. Richardson, & N. Chambers (Eds.), *Cross-cultural caring: A handbook for health professionals* (2nd ed., pp. 323–352). Vancouver, Toronto, ON: UBC Press.

Anderson, J. M., Perry, J., Blue, C., Browne, A. J., Henderson, A., Khan, K. B., et al. (2003). "Rewriting" cultural safety within the postcolonial and postnational feminist project: Toward new epistemologies of healing. *Advances in Nursing Science, 26*(3), 196–214.

Anderson, J. M., Tang, S., & Blue, C. (2007). Health care reform and the paradox of efficiency: "Writing in" culture. *International Journal of health Services, 37*(2), 291–320.

Arat-Koc, S. (1999). Gender and race in "non-discriminatory" immigration policies in Canada. In: E. Dua & A. Robertson (Eds.), *Scratching the surface: Canadian anti-racist thought* (pp. 207–233). Toronto, ON: Women's Press.

Assembly of First Nations. (2007). *The reality for First Nations in Canada.* Retrieved August 13, 2007, from http://www.afn.ca/article.asp?id=764.

Benoit, C., Carroll, D., & Westfall, R. (2007). Women's access to maternity services in Canada: Historical developments and contemporary challenges. In: M. Morrow, O. Hankivsky, & C. Varcoe (Eds.), *Women's health in Canada: Critical perspectives on theory and policy* (pp. 507–527). Toronto, ON: University of Toronto.

British Columbia Immigration Policy & Intergovernmental Relations Division. Multiculturalism and Immigration Branch. Ministry of Attorney General and Minister Responsible for Multiculturalism. (2007). *Immigration trends 2006.* Retrieved September 5, 2007, from www.ag.gov.bc.ca/immigration

Browne, A. J. (2007). Clinical encounters between nurses and First Nations women in a Western Canadian hospital. *Social Science & Medicine, 64*(10), 2165–2176.

Browne, A. J., & Fiske, J. (2001). First Nations women's encounters with mainstream health care services. *Western Journal of Nursing Research, 23*(2), 126–147.

Browne, A. J., & Varcoe, C. (2006). A critical cultural approach to health care for Aboriginal people. *Contemporary Nurse, 22*(2), 155–168.

Brownridge, D. (2003). Male partner violence against Aboriginal women in Canada: An empirical analysis. *Journal of Interpersonal Violence, 18*(1), 65–83.

Canadian Nurses Association. (2004). *Promoting culturally competent care, position statement.* Retrieved September 9, 2008, from http://www.cna-aiic.ca/CNA/issues/position/practice/default_e.aspx.

Carty, L. (1991). Black women in academia: A statement form the periphery. In H. Bannerji, L. Carty, K. Dehli, S. Heald, & K. McKenna (Eds.), *Unsettling relations: The university as a site of feminist struggles* (pp. 13–44). Toronto: Women's Press.

Coburn, D. (2006). Health and health care: A political economy perspective. In: D. Raphael, T. Bryant, & M. Rioux (Eds.), *Staying alive: Critical perspectives on health, illness and health care* (pp. 59–85). Toronto, ON: Canadian Scholar's Press.

Cook, E.-D., & Howe, D. (2004). Aboriginal languages of Canada. In: W. O'Grady & J. Archibald (Eds.), *Contemporary linguistic analysis* (5th ed., pp. 294–309). Toronto, ON: Addison Wesley Longman.

Dyck, I., & Kearns, R. (1995). Transforming the relations of research: Towards culturally safe geographies of health and healing. *Health & Place, 1*(3), 137–147.

Government of Canada Department of Canadian Heritage. (nd). *Canadian diversity: Respecting our differences.* Retrieved August 30, 2007, from http://www.pch.gc.ca/progs/multi/respect_e.cfm#approach

Guruge, S., & Collins, E. (2008). *Working with immigrant women: Issues and strategies for mental health professionals.* Toronto, ON: Canadian Centre for Addictions and Mental Health.

Hartrick-Doane, G., & Varcoe, C. (2005). *Family nursing as relational inquiry: Developing health-promoting practice.* Philadelphia, PA: Lippincott Williams & Wilkins.

Health Canada. (2007). *First Nations, Inuits and Aboriginal health, diseases and conditions.* Retrieved September 8, 2008, from http://www.hc-sc.gc.ca/fniah-spnia/diseases-maladies/index-eng.php.

Henry, F., Tator, C., with Mattis, W., & Rees, T. (2006). *The colour of democracy: Racism in Canadian society.* Toronto, ON: Nelson.

Indian and Northern Affairs Canada. (1996). *Report of the Royal Commission on Aboriginal Peoples.* Ottawa, ON: Minister of Supply and Services Canada.

Kaufert, P. A., & O'Neil, J. (1993). Analysis of a dialogue on risks in childbirth: Clinicians, epidemiologists and Inuit women. In S. Lindenbaum & M. Lock (Eds.), *Knowledge, power and practice: The anthropology of medicine in everyday life* (pp. 32–54). Los Angeles: University of California Press.

Kendall, P. (2001). *The health and wellbeing of Aboriginal people in British Columbia: Report on the health of British Columbians—Provincial Health Officer's Annual Report, 2001.* Victoria: Office of the Provincial Health Officer, Province of British Columbia.

Kleinman, A. (1980). *Patients and healers in the context of culture.* Berkley: University of California Press.

LaRocque, E. (1993). *Violence in Aboriginal communities—Reprinted with permission from the Royal Commission on Aboriginal Peoples—Report of the National Round Table on Aboriginal Health and Social Issues.* Retrieved December 15, 2008, from http://www.phac-aspc.gc.ca/ncfv-cnivf/familyviolence/pdfs/fv-abor-communit_e.pdf

BIBLIOGRAPHY

Leininger, M. (2002). Culture care theory: A major contribution to advance transcultural nursing and practices. *Journal of Transcultural Nursing, 13*(3), 189–192.

MacKinnon, M., & Howard, L. L. (2000). *Affirming immigrant women's health: Building inclusive policy.* Halifax, NS: Maritime Centre of Excellence for Women's Health.

Mathieu, S. (1995). *Under the lion's paw: Black migration to Canada and the development of Canadian immigration policy, 1880–1914.* Unpublished Masters Thesis, Yale University.

Mitura, V., & Bollman, R. D. (2003). The health of rural Canadians: A rural–urban comparison of health indicators. *Rural and Small Town Canada Analysis Bulletin, 4*(6), 1–23.

O'Loughlin, J. (1999). Understanding the role of ethnicity in chronic disease. *Canadian Medical Association Journal, 16*(2), 152–153.

Papps, E., & Ramsden, I. (1996). Cultural safety in nursing: The New Zealand experience. *Internal Journal for Quality in Health Care, 8*(5), 491–497.

Pederson, A., & Raphael, D. (2006). Gender, race and health inequities. In: D. Raphael, T. Bryant, & M. Rioux (Eds.), *Staying alive: Critical perspectives on health, illness and health care* (pp. 159–191). Toronto, ON: Canadian Scholar's Press.

Polaschek, N. R. (1998). Cultural safety: A new concept in nursing people of different ethnicities. *Journal of Advanced Nursing, 27,* 454–457.

Ramsden, I. (1993). Kawa Whakaruruhau: Cultural safety in nursing education in aotearoa (New Zealand). *Nursing Praxis in New Zealand, 8*(3), 4–10.

Ramsden, I., & Spoonley, P. (1994). The cultural safety debate in nursing education in Aotearoa. *New Zealand Annual Review of Education 1993,* 161–174.

Raphael, D. (2007). *Poverty and policy in Canada: Implications for health and quality of life.* Toronto, ON: Canadian Scholar's Press.

Raphael, D., Bryant, T., & Rioux, M. (2006). *Staying alive: Critical perspectives on health, illness and health care.* Toronto, ON: Canadian Scholar's Press.

Razack, S. H. (1998). *Looking white people in the eye: Gender, race, and culture in courtrooms and classrooms.* Toronto: University of Toronto Press.

Reimer-Kirkham, S. (2003). The politics of belonging and intercultural health care provision. *Western Journal of Nursing Research, 25*(7), 762–780.

Roscelli, M. (2005). Political advocacy and research both needed to address federal-provincial gaps in services. *Canadian Journal of Public Health, 96*(1), S55–S59.

Singh, V. (2004). The rural–urban income gap within provinces: An update to 2000. *Rural and Small Town Canada Analysis Bulletin, 5*(7), 1–120.

Smye, V., & Browne, A. J. (2002). Cultural safety and the analysis of health policy affecting aboriginal people. *Nurse Researcher, 9*(3), 42–56.

Srivastava, R. H. (2007). *The health care professional's guide to clinical cultural competence.* Toronto, ON: Elsevier.

Stanhope, M., Lancaster, J., Jessup-Falcioni, H., et al. (2008). Cultural influences in community health nursing. In M. Stanhope, J. Lancaster, H. Jessup-Falcioni, et al. (Eds.), *Community health nursing in Canada* (1st Canadian ed., pp. 125–152). Toronto, ON, Canada: Mosby Elsevier.

Statistics Canada. (1998, December 14). *Statistics Canada—The Daily. Canada's Aboriginal languages, 1996.* Ottawa, ON: Statistics Canada.

Statistics Canada. (2001). *Profile of languages in Canada.* Retrieved April 12, 2007, from http://www12.statcan.ca/english/census01/Products/Analytic/companion/lang/canada.cfm

Statistics Canada. (2003a). *Ethnic diversity survey: Portrait of a multicultural society.* Ottawa, ON: Statistics Canada.

Statistics Canada. (2003b). *Religions in Canada.* Ottawa, ON: Statistics Canada.

Statistics Canada. (2006a). *Definitions, data sources and methods.* Retrieved September 12, 2007, from http://www.statcan.ca/english/concepts/definitions/immigration.htm

Statistics Canada. (2006b). *Portrait of the Canadian Population in 2006: Subprovincial population dynamics. Portrait of small towns, rural areas and the territories.* Retrieved August 31, 2007, from http://www12.statcan.ca/english/census06/analysis/popdwell/Subprov7.cfm

Statistics Canada. (2006c). *Report on the demographic situation in Canada 2003–2004.* Ottawa, ON: Minister Responsible for Statistics Canada, Minister of Industry.

Statistics Canada. (2006d, March 30). *Statistics Canada—The Daily. Income of Canadians.* Retrieved July 14, 2007, from http://www.statcan.ca/Daily/English/030623/d030623c.htm

Statistics Canada. (2006e, March 7). *Statistics Canada—The Daily. Women in Canada.* Retrieved November 23, 2006, from http://www.statcan.ca/Daily/English/030623/d030623c.htm

Statistics Canada. (2007a). *Canada's ethnocultural portrait: The changing mosaic.* Retrieved August 27, 2007, from http://www12.statcan.ca/english/census01/products/analytic/companion/etoimm/canada.cfm

Statistics Canada. (2007b). *Immigration in Canada: A portrait of the foreign-born population, 2006 Census: Immigration: Driver of population growth.* Retrieved September 9, 2008, from http://www12.statcan.ca/english/census06/analysis/immcit/foreign_born.cfm

Statistics Canada. (2007c). *Immigration in Canada: A portrait of the foreign-born population, 2006 census: Immigration came from many countries.* Retrieved September 9, 2008 from http://www12.statcan.ca/english/census06/analysis/immcit/asia.cfm

Tang, S. Y. S. (1999). Interpreter services in healthcare: Policy recommendations for healthcare agencies. *Journal of Nursing Administration, 29*(6), 23–29.

ADDITIONAL RESOURCES

Statistics Canada. (1999, January 13). *Statistics Canada—The Daily: 1996 Census—Aboriginal data.* Ottawa, ON: Statistics Canada.

United Nations Educational Scientific and Cultural Organization. (1952). *The race question in modern science: The results of an inquiry—The concept of race.* Paris: Author.

World Health Organization. (1986). *Ottawa Charter for health promotion.* Geneva, Switzerland: Author.

World Health Organization. (1998). *Health promotion glossary.* Retrieved August 3, 2004, from http://www.who.int/hpr/NPH/docs/hp_glossary_en.pdf

CANADIAN ASSOCIATIONS AND WEB SITES

Culture, Race Relations, and Antiracism

Culture, Gender and Health Research Unit, School of Nursing, University of British Columbia: http://www.cghru.nursing.ubc.ca/

Canadian Race Relations Foundation: http://www.crr.ca/

Canadian Heritage: http://www.canadianheritage.gc.ca/progs/multi/index_e.cfm

Get Diversity: http://www.getdiversity.com/

National Youth Anti-racism Network: http://www.antiracism.ca/

Demographics

Statistics Canada: http://www.statcan.ca

Aboriginal Issues

Aboriginal Canada Portal: http://www.aboriginalcanada.gc.ca/acp/site.nsf/en/ao26711.html

Assembly of First Nations: http://www.afn.ca/article.asp?id=3

Indigenous Studies Portal: http://iportal.usask.ca/index.php?sid=471577458&t=about

National Aboriginal Health Organization: http://www.naho.ca/english/

Immigration Issues

Citizenship and Immigration Canada: http://www.cic.gc.ca/

Status of Women Canada: http://www.swc-cfc.gc.ca.

3

The Health History: Subjective Data

Tracey C. Stephen and Lynn S. Bickley

As you enter the realm of client assessment, you begin integrating the essential elements of clinical care: empathetic listening; the ability to interview clients of all ages, moods, and backgrounds; the techniques for examining the different body systems; and the process of clinical reasoning. Your experience with history taking and physical examination will grow and expand, and it will trigger clinical reasoning from the first moments of the client encounter. The steps of clinical reasoning include identifying key symptoms and signs with unexpected findings; linking findings to potential pathophysiology, psychopathology, or environmental concerns; and establishing a set of nursing diagnoses to begin planning effective client care. Working through these steps will reveal the multifaceted profile of the client before you. Paradoxically, the very skills that allow you to assess all clients also shape the image of the unique human being entrusted to your care.

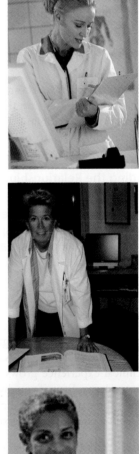

The next three chapters provide a road map to clinical proficiency in three critical areas: health history, physical examination, and the written record (documentation). In this chapter, techniques for interviewing to obtain a comprehensive, accurate account of the "client's situation," the types of health histories, and the components of the health history are discussed. The following two chapters cover the approach and overview to the physical examination and the principles and methods for documenting findings.

The health history interview is a conversation with a purpose. The health history provides the foundation for the helping relationship and guides the client care experience. It is critical to obtain comprehensive, accurate information about the client and his or her physical and mental health to develop a plan for care. As you learn to elicit the client's history, you will draw on many of the interpersonal skills that you use every day, but with unique and important differences. Unlike social conversation, in which you can freely express your own needs and interests and are responsible only for yourself, the primary goal of the nurse–client interview is to maximize the well-being of the client. At its most basic level, the purpose of conversation with a client is three-fold: to establish a trusting and supportive relationship, to gather information, and to offer information (Bird & Cohen-Cole, 1990; Cohen-Cole, 1991; Lazare et al., 1995).

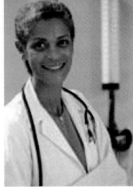

Relating effectively with clients is among the most valued skills of clinical care. As a learner, you may focus your energies on gathering information. At the same time, by using techniques that promote trust and convey respect, you will allow the client's details to unfold in its fullest and most detailed form. Establishing a supportive interaction helps the client feel more at ease when sharing information and itself becomes the foundation for helping relationships (Novack, 1995).

The following is an introduction to the essentials of interviewing. It emphasizes the approach to gathering the health history but covers all the fundamental habits that you will continually use and refine in your conversations with clients. You will learn the guiding principles for skilled interviewing and how to forge trusting client relationships. You will read about preparing for the interview, the sequence of the interviewing process, important interviewing techniques, and strategies for addressing various challenges that may arise in client encounters. To help you navigate this journey, look over the Interviewing Milestones that follow, which mark the complex tasks of a skilled interview.

INTERVIEWING MILESTONES

Getting Ready: The Approach to the Interview

Taking time for self-reflection. Reviewing the client's record. Reviewing your clinical behaviour and appearance. Adjusting the environment. Taking notes.

Learning About the Client: The Sequence of the Interview

Greeting the client and establishing rapport. Inviting the client's story. Setting the agenda for the interview. Expanding and clarifying the client's story. Creating a shared understanding of the client's concerns. Negotiating a plan. Following up and closing the interview.

Building the Relationship: The Techniques of Skilled Interviewing

Active listening. Guided questioning. Nonverbal communication. Empathetic responses. Validation. Reassurance. Partnering. Summarization. Transitions. Enabling the client.

Adapting the Interview to Specific Situations

Clients who are silent. Clients who give confusing information. Clients with altered mental capacity. Clients who are talkative. Clients who are crying. Clients who are angry or disruptive. Clients with a language barrier. Clients with low literacy. Clients with impaired hearing or vision. Clients with limited intelligence. Clients seeking personal advice.

Sensitive Topics that Call for Special Skills

The sexual history. The mental health history. Alcohol and illicit drugs. Family violence. Death and the dying client.

Societal Aspects of Interviewing

Achieving cultural safety. Maintaining professional boundaries in the nurse–client relationship. Ethical considerations.

As a nurse facilitating the client's interview, you will gather detailed information to generate a series of nursing diagnoses about the nature of the client's concerns. You will explore the client's feelings and beliefs about his or her concerns. Eventually, as your clinical experience grows, you will respond with your understanding of the client's concerns. Even if you discover that little can be done, encouraging the client to discuss the experience of illness is itself therapeutic, as shown by the following words from a client with long-standing and severe arthritis:

> The patient had never talked about what the symptoms meant to her. She had never said: "This means that I can't go to the bathroom by myself, put my clothes on, even get out of bed without calling for help." When we finished the physical examination I said something like: "Rheumatoid arthritis really has not been nice to you." She burst into tears, and her daughter did also, and I sat there, very close to losing it myself. She said: "You know, no one has ever talked about it as a personal thing before. No one's ever talked to me as if this were a thing that mattered, a personal event." That was the significant thing about the encounter. I didn't really have much else to offer.... But something really significant had happened between us, something that she valued and would carry away with her. (Hastings, 1989)

As you can see from this example, the *process* of interviewing clients requires a highly refined sensitivity to the client's feelings and behavioural cues, and is much more than just asking a series of questions. This process differs significantly from the *format* for the health history. Both are fundamental to your work with clients but serve different purposes:

- The *health history format* is a structured framework for organizing client information in *written or verbal form* for other health care providers; it focuses the clinician's attention on specific kinds of information that must be obtained from the client.

- The *interviewing process* that actually generates these pieces of information is much more fluid and demands effective communication and relational skills. It requires not only knowledge of the data that you need to obtain but also the ability to elicit accurate information and the interpersonal skills that allow you to respond to the client's feelings and concerns.

Underlying the new interviewing skills that you will learn is a mindset that allows you to collaborate with the client and build a helping relationship.

The kinds of information you seek vary according to several factors. The scope and degree of details depend on the client's needs and concerns, the clinician's goals for the encounter, and the clinical setting (e.g., inpatient or outpatient, amount of time available, primary care, subspecialty).

- For new clients, regardless of setting, you will do a *comprehensive health history* described for adults later in this chapter.

- For other clients who seek care for specific concerns (e.g., cough, painful urination), a more limited interview tailored to that specific problem may be indicated, sometimes known as a *symptom-focused assessment*.

In a primary care setting, nurses frequently choose to address issues of health promotion, such as tobacco cessation or reduction of high-risk sexual behaviours. A subspecialist may do an in-depth history to evaluate a concern that incorporates a wide range of areas of inquiry. Knowing the content and relevance of all the components of a comprehensive health history enables you to select the kinds of information most helpful for meeting both nurse and client goals. Be assured that you will fully gain the knowledge of what types of information to pursue, and when to pursue them, as you deepen your clinical experience.

GETTING READY: THE APPROACH TO THE INTERVIEW

Interviewing clients requires planning. You are undoubtedly eager to begin your relationship with the client, but first consider several steps that are crucial to success: taking time for self-reflection, reviewing the client's record, setting goals for the interview, reviewing your behaviour and appearance, adjusting the environment, and being ready to take brief notes.

TAKING TIME FOR SELF-REFLECTION

As nurses, we encounter a wide variety of individuals, each one unique. Establishing relationships with people from a broad spectrum of age, social class, genetic background, ethnicity, and states of *health or illness* is an uncommon opportunity and privilege. Being consistently respectful and open to individual differences is one of the nurse's challenges. Because we bring our own values, assumptions, and biases to every encounter, we must look inward to clarify how our own expectations and reactions may affect what we hear and how we behave. *Self-reflection is a continual part of professional development in clinical work. It brings a deepening personal awareness to our work with clients, which is one of the most rewarding aspects of client care.*

REVIEWING THE CLIENT'S RECORD

Before seeing the client, review any information that you have about the client. Doing so helps you gather information and plan what areas you need to explore with the client and also decreases the amount of information the client needs to repeat. Look closely at identifying data such as age, gender, and address, and peruse the problem list, the medication list, and details such as the documentation of allergies. The record often provides valuable information about past diagnoses and treatments, but ensure that this information does not prevent you from developing new approaches or ideas. Remember that information in the client's record comes from different observers and that standardized forms reflect different institutional norms. Moreover, it is not designed to capture the essence of the unique individual you are about to meet. Data may be incomplete or even disagree with what you learn from the client—understanding such discrepancies may prove helpful to the client's care.

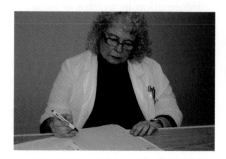

SETTING GOALS FOR THE INTERVIEW

Before you begin talking with the client, it is important to clarify your goals for the interview. As a learner, your goal may be to obtain a complete health history so that you can submit a written assignment to your teacher. As a nurse, your goals range from completing forms needed by health care institutions to following up on health care issues to testing hypotheses generated by your review of the client's record. *A clinician must balance these provider-centred goals with client-centred goals.* There can be tension between the needs of the provider, the institution, and the client and family. Part of the nurse's task is to consider these multiple agendas. By taking a few minutes to think through your goals ahead of time, you will find it easier to strike a healthy balance among the various purposes of the interview to come.

REVIEWING YOUR CLINICAL BEHAVIOUR AND APPEARANCE

Just as you carefully observe the client throughout the interview, the client will be watching you. Consciously or not, you send messages through your words and behaviour. Be sensitive to those messages and manage them as well as you can. Posture, gestures, eye contact, and tone of voice all convey the extent of your interest, attention, acceptance, and understanding. The skilled interviewer seems calm and unhurried, even when time is limited. Reactions that betray disapproval, embarrassment, impatience, or boredom block communication, as do any behaviours that condescend, stereotype, criticize, or belittle the client. Although some types of negative feelings are at times unavoidable, as a health care professional, you must take pains not to express them. Guard against these feelings not only when talking to clients but also when discussing clients with your colleagues.

Your personal appearance also affects your clinical relationships. Clients find cleanliness, neatness, conservative dress, and a name tag reassuring. Remember to keep *the client's perspective* in mind if you want to build the client's trust.

ADJUSTING THE ENVIRONMENT

Try to make the interview setting as private and comfortable as possible. Although you may have to talk with the client under difficult circumstances, such as a two-bed room or the corridor of a busy emergency department, a proper environment improves communication. If there are privacy curtains, ask permission to pull them shut. Suggest moving to an empty room instead of talking in a waiting area. *As the clinician, it is part of your job to make adjustments to the location and seating that make the client and you more comfortable.* These efforts are always worth the time.

TAKING NOTES

As a learner, you will need to write down much of what you hear during the interview. Even experienced nurses cannot remember all the details of a comprehensive history. Jot down short phrases and specific dates rather than trying to put them into a final format. Do not let note-taking or written forms distract you from the client. Maintain eye contact. Whenever the client is discussing sensitive material, put down your pen. For those who find notetaking uncomfortable, explore their concerns and explain the need for an accurate record.

LEARNING ABOUT THE CLIENT: THE SEQUENCE OF THE INTERVIEW

After you have devoted time and thought to preparing for the interview, you are fully ready to listen to the client, elicit the client's concerns, and learn about the client's health. In general, an interview moves through several stages. *Throughout this sequence, you, as the nurse, must always be attuned to the client's feelings, help the client express them, respond to their content, and validate their significance.*

As a learner, you will concentrate primarily on gathering the client's story and creating a shared understanding of the problem. As you become a practicing nurse, reaching agreement on a plan for further evaluation and treatment becomes more important. Whether the interview is comprehensive or focused, you should move through this sequence with close attention to the client's feelings and affect, always working on strengthening the relationship. A typical sequence follows.

THE SEQUENCE OF THE INTERVIEW

- Greeting the client and establishing rapport.
- Inviting the client's story.
- Establishing the agenda for the interview.
- Expanding and clarifying the client's story.
- Generating and testing diagnostic hypotheses.
- Creating a shared understanding of the problem.
- Negotiating a plan (includes further evaluation, treatment, and client education).
- Planning for follow-up and closing the interview.

GREETING THE CLIENT AND ESTABLISHING RAPPORT

The initial moments of your encounter with the client lay the foundation for your ongoing relationship. How you greet the client and other visitors in the room, provide for the client's comfort, and arrange the physical setting all shape the client's first impressions.

As you begin, *greet the client* by name and introduce yourself, giving your own name. If possible, shake hands with the client. If this is the first contact, explain your role, including your status as a student and how you will be involved in the client's care. Repeat this part of the introduction on subsequent meetings until you are confident that the client knows who you are: "Good Morning, Mr. Peters. I am Susannah Martinez, a second-year nursing student. You may remember me. I was here yesterday talking with you about your heart problems. I am a part of the health care team assisting you."

Using a formal title to address the client (e.g., Mr. O'Neil, Ms. Washington) is always best (Conant, 1998; Heller, 1987). Except with children or adolescents, avoid first names unless you have specific permission from the client or family. Addressing an unfamiliar adult as "granny" or "dear" can depersonalize and can be perceived as disrespectful. If you are unsure how to pronounce the client's name, don't be afraid to ask. You can say, "I am afraid of mispronouncing your name. Could you say it for me?" Then repeat it to make sure that you heard it correctly.

When visitors are in the room, be sure to acknowledge and greet each one in turn, inquiring about each person's name and relationship to the client. Whenever visitors are present, *you are obligated to maintain the client's confidentiality.* Let the client decide if visitors or family members should remain in the room, and ask for the client's permission before conducting the interview in their presence. For example, "I am comfortable with having your sister stay for the interview, Mrs. Jones, but I want to make sure that this is also what you want" or "Would you prefer if I spoke to you alone or with your sister present?"

Always be attuned to the client's comfort. In the office or clinic, help the client find a suitable place for coats and belongings. In the hospital, after greeting the client, ask how the client is feeling and whether you are coming at a convenient time. Arranging the bed to make the client more comfortable or allowing a few minutes for the client to say goodbye to visitors or finish using the bedpan demonstrates your awareness of the client's needs. In any setting, look for signs of discomfort such as shifting position or facial expressions showing pain or anxiety. You must attend to pain or anxiety first, both to encourage the client's trust and to allow enough ease for the interview to proceed.

Consider the best way to *arrange the room* and how far you should be from the client. Remember that cultural background and individual taste influence preferences about interpersonal space and eye contact. See Chapter 2 for more information on cultural considerations. Choose a distance that facilitates conversation and allows easy eye contact. You should probably be within several feet, close enough to be intimate but not intrusive. Pull up a chair and, if possible, sit at eye level with the client. Move any physical barriers, such as desks or bedside tables, out of the way. In an outpatient setting, sitting on a rolling stool, for example, allows you to change distances in response to client cues.

Avoid arrangements that connote disrespect or inequality of power, such as interviewing a woman already positioned for a pelvic examination. Such arrangements are unacceptable. Lighting also makes a difference. If you sit between a client and a bright light or window, although your view might be good, the client may have to squint uncomfortably to see you, making the interaction more like an interrogation than a supportive interview.

As you begin the interview, give the client your undivided attention. Spend enough time on small talk to put the client at ease, and avoid looking down to take notes or reading the chart.

INVITING THE CLIENT'S STORY

Now that you have established rapport, you are ready to pursue the client's reason for seeking health care, designated the *chief concern.* Begin with **open-ended** *questions* that allow full freedom of response: "What concerns bring you here today?" or "How can I help you?" Helpful open-ended questions are, "Was there a specific health concern that prompted you to schedule this appointment?" or "What made you decide to come in to see us today?" Note that these questions encourage the client to express any possible concerns and do not restrict the client to a minimally informative "yes" or "no" answer. Sometimes clients do not have a specific concern or problem—they may want only a blood pressure check or a routine examination. Others may say they just want a physical examination but feel uncomfortable bringing up an underlying concern. In all these situations, *it is still important to start with the client's story* (Delbanco, 1993).

Train yourself to *follow the client's leads.* Good interviewing technique includes using verbal and nonverbal cues that prompt clients to recount their stories spontaneously. If you intervene too early or ask specific questions prematurely, you risk trampling on the very information you are seeking. You should listen actively and make use of *continuers* (see p. 63), especially at the outset. These include nodding your head and phrases such as "uh huh," "go on," or "I see." Using additional guided questioning (see pp. 62–63) helps you avoid missing any of the client's concerns.

Listen to the client's answer *without interrupting.* Studies show that clinicians interrupt clients during office visits after only 18 seconds (Beckman & Frankel, 1984)! If clients are allowed to tell their concerns, most will finish within 2 minutes. After you have given the client the opportunity to respond fully, inquire again or even several times, "What else?" "Tell me more," or "Any further concerns?" You may need to lead clients back several times to elicit additional concerns or issues they may want to tell you about.

ESTABLISHING AN AGENDA

The nurse often approaches the interview with specific goals in mind. The client also has specific questions and concerns. It is important to identify all these issues at the beginning of the encounter. This allows you to use the time available most effectively and ensures that you hear all the client's issues. At times, you may have enough time to cover the breadth of both your concerns and those of the client in one visit. Often, however, time is almost always constrained. As a clinician, you may need to focus the interview by asking the client about the issue that is most pressing. For example, "You have told me about several different concerns that are important for us to discuss. I also wanted to review your blood pressure medication. We need to decide which concerns to address today. Can you tell me which one you are most concerned about?" Once you have agreed on a manageable list, let the client know that the other problems are also important and will be addressed during a future visit—this reinforces the client's confidence in your ongoing collaboration. Then proceed with questions such as, "Tell me more about that first concern that you mentioned."

EXPANDING AND CLARIFYING THE CLIENT'S STORY

You then guide the client into elaborating areas of the health history that seem most significant. Each symptom or sign has attributes that you must clarify, including context, associations, and chronology. For pain and many other symptoms, understanding these essential characteristics, summarized on the following page as the 10 key attributes of a symptom, is critical.

As you explore these attributes, be sure that you *use language that is understandable and appropriate* to the client. Although you might ask a health professional about dyspnea, the customary term for clients is "shortness of breath." It is easy to slip into

■ *The 10 Attributes of a Sign or Symptom*

Attribute	Explanation	Considerations
1. Location	The anatomical area of the body that is affected. The location may be (a) localized—in one place; (b) generalized—over a large area or the entire body; or (c) radiating—moving to or from another area.	When possible, ask the client to point to the affected area.
2. Quality or nature	What the symptom/sign is like, including consistency, colour, and type. For pain, descriptors such as crushing, aching, gnawing, and stabbing give more information about the type of pain the client is experiencing. Thick sputum, dry cough, raised rash, purple spots, and tingling weakness are other examples of words that describe quality.	If the client is having difficulty describing the quality of a symptom/sign, help him or her by suggesting several words that may be accurate descriptors.
3. Severity or quantity	How bad or how much the concern is. For pain, ask the client to rate it on a scale of 0–10 (with 0 being no pain and 10 being the worst pain) or to compare it with a previous experience (e.g., dental abscess, fracture). For bleeding, sputum, itchiness, and other symptoms/signs, ask the client to describe the quantity. For example, how much blood have you noticed?	Ask the client to describe the amount in quantifiable terms to improve understanding. For example, 100 mL of blood, two soaked hand towels, a blood clot the size of a toonie, or a lump the size of a golf ball enhance understanding of the amount.
4. Timing	Aspects about when the symptom/sign occurs: (a) onset—when the problem began and speed (slow or fast); (b) duration—the length of time; (c) constancy—whether the symptom/sign is intermittent or continuous; (d) time of day/month/year—patterns of when the problem occurs.	Assist the client to recall when the concern happens. Using familiar days such as birthdays or holidays may help the client remember when it began. Also, suggestions such as morning, night, or different seasons help the client identify aspects of timing. Inquire about relationship of the symptom/sign with work.
5. Aggravating factors	Anything that makes the symptom/sign worse. Includes exposures and activities the client has noticed that make the symptom/sign worse.	Temperature changes, altitude changes, different foods, amount of light, or chemicals are examples of exposures. Walking, sitting, reading, lifting, and bending are examples of activities.
6. Alleviating factors	Anything that makes the symptom/sign better. Includes exposures and activities the client has noticed that improve the symptom/sign.	Ask about medications, over-the-counter remedies, herbal treatments, and changes in diet or temperature that have improved the symptom/sign. Inquire about position changes, acupuncture, or massages, for example.
7. Associated symptoms and signs	Other symptoms and signs that may be related to the symptom/sign.	If the client is having difficulty recalling anything that may be related, ask about specific symptoms such as nausea, pain, weakness, or shortness of breath.
8. Environmental factors	Anything in the client's surroundings, such as home, work, or hobbies, that may be related to the symptom/sign.	Consider exposures (thermal, chemical, infectious), psychosocial aspects (stress, loss of income), recent travel, or changes in surroundings (renovations).
9. Significance to client	The effects on the client's well-being and lifestyle.	Some symptoms/signs have minimal effects on some people but major influences on

(continued)

■ The 10 Attributes of a Sign or Symptom (Continued)

Attribute	Explanation	Considerations
		others. A painful finger may cause few changes for some people but can be career-threatening for a concert pianist.
10. Client perspective	Thoughts and ideas from the client about what may be happening or causing the symptom/sign and the associated feelings.	This gives the client a chance to bring up any other information that may be related and provides insights that the nurse may not anticipate.

using medical language, but beware. Technical language may confuse the client and often blocks communication. Whenever possible, *use the client's words*, making sure you clarify their meaning.

It is important to establish *the sequence and time course* of each of the client's symptoms and signs if you are to arrive at accurate assessments. You can encourage a chronologic account by asking such questions as, "What then?" or "What happened next?" or "Please start at the beginning, or the last time you felt well, and go step by step." To fill in specific details, guide the client's story by using different types of questions and the techniques of skilled interviewing described on pp. 61–66. You will need to use some focused questions to elicit specific information that the client has not already offered (see p. 62). *In general, an interview moves back and forth from open-ended questions to increasingly focused questions and then on to another open-ended question.*

GENERATING AND TESTING DIAGNOSTIC HYPOTHESES

Eventually, as you gain experience listening to client concerns, you will develop the skills of "clinical reasoning." You will *generate and consider nursing diagnoses* about what may be happening for the client. Identifying the various attributes of the client's symptoms and pursuing specific details are fundamental to recognizing patterns of disease and to identifying nursing diagnoses. As you learn more about diagnostic patterns and epidemiology, knowing what data you are listening for and asking about specific details become more automatic. For additional data that contribute to your analysis, use items from relevant sections of the review of systems.

Appropriate questions about symptoms and signs are also suggested in each of the chapters on the system physical examinations. This is one way that you build evidence for and against various diagnostic possibilities. This kind of clinical thinking is illustrated by the tables on symptoms found in the system examination chapters and further discussed in Chapter 5. The challenge is to not let this kind of inquiry dominate the interview and displace learning about the client's perspective, conveying concern for the client's well-being, and building the relationship (Suchman & Matthews, 1988).

CREATING A SHARED UNDERSTANDING OF THE CONCERN

Recent literature makes it clear that delivering effective health care requires exploring the deeper meanings clients attach their symptoms. Although the "10 attributes of a symptom" add important details to the client's history, a good interview helps nurses fully understand the clients' experiences. Nurses bring their perspectives, which include prior knowledge and experience, to the interview that guides their interactions and helps develop nursing diagnoses, goals, and client care. Clients bring their perspectives, which include their experience of their illness, to the interview. Many factors may shape this experience, including prior personal or family health, the effect of symptoms on everyday life, individual outlook and style of coping, and expectations about health care. The melding of these perspectives forms the basis for planning goals and treatment for the client. *The clinical interview needs to take into account both of these views of reality.*

To understand the client's expectations, the nurse needs to go beyond just the attributes of a symptom or a sign. Learning about the client's perception of illness means asking client-centred questions in the six domains as listed. This information is crucial to client satisfaction, effective health care, and client follow-through (Smith et al., 1998; Smith, 2002).

The nurse should explore the client's thoughts about the cause of the problem by saying, for example, "Why do you think you have this stomachache?" To uncover the client's feelings you might ask, "What concerns you most about the pain?" A client may worry that the pain is a symptom of serious disease and want reassurance. Alternatively, the client may be less concerned about the cause of the pain and just want relief. You need to find out what the client expects from you, the nurse, or from health care in general. "I am glad that the pain is almost gone, how specifically can I help you now?" Even if the stomach pain is almost gone; the client may need a work excuse to take to an employer.

EXPLORING THE CLIENT'S PERSPECTIVE

- The client's thoughts about the nature and the cause of the problem
- The client's feelings, especially fears, about the problem
- The client's expectations of health professionals and health care
- The effect of the problem on the client's life
- Prior personal or family experiences that are similar
- Therapeutic approaches the client has already tried

It may be helpful to ask the client about prior experiences, what has been tried so far, and any related changes in daily activities.

Nurse: Has anything like this happened to you or your family before?

Client: I was worried that I might have appendicitis. My Uncle Charlie died of a ruptured appendix.

Explore what the client has done so far to take care of the concern. Most clients will have tried over-the-counter medications, traditional remedies, or advice from friends or family.

Ask how the illness has affected the client's lifestyle and level of activity. This question is especially important for clients with chronic illness. "What can't you do now that you could do before? How has your backache (shortness of breath, etc.) affected your ability to work? … Your life at home? … Your social activities? … Your role as a parent? … Your function in intimate relationships? … The way you feel about yourself as a person?"

NEGOTIATING A PLAN

Learning about the disease and conceptualizing the illness give you and the client the opportunity to create a complete and congruent picture of the concern. This multifaceted picture then forms the basis for planning further evaluation (e.g., physical examination, laboratory tests, consultations) and negotiating a treatment plan. It also plays an important role in building rapport with your client. Advanced skills, such as steps for motivating change and the therapeutic use of the helping relationship, are beyond the scope of this book.

PLANNING FOR FOLLOW-UP AND CLOSING

You may find that ending the interview is difficult. Clients often have many questions, and if you have done your job well, they are engaged and affirmed as they talk with you. Let the client know that the end of the interview is approaching to allow time for the client to ask any final questions. Make sure the client understands the mutual plans you have developed. For example, before gathering your papers or standing to leave the room, you can say, "We need to stop now. Do you have any questions about what we've covered?" As you close, reviewing future evaluation, treatments, and follow-up is helpful. "So, you will see the physician shortly, and you will likely need some tests to give us more information about what is happening. Do you have any questions about this?" Address any related concerns or questions that the client raises.

BUILDING A THERAPEUTIC RELATIONSHIP: THE TECHNIQUES OF SKILLED INTERVIEWING

You probably had many reasons to become a health professional, but one of them was undoubtedly the desire to serve others. To succeed in fulfilling this laudable goal, you must sustain this motivation throughout your rigorous educational program and transform this goal into a set of behavioural approaches to your clients. The paradigm that embeds your relationship with the client into the therapeutic process itself now has many names and models, including the biopsychosocial model and client-centred care, among others (Engel, 1977; Engel & Morgan, 1973; Smith, 2002; Suchman & Matthews, 1988). Comparing these various models reveals common elements that include interest in the client as a whole person, an enabling approach to the client role, and involvement of the clinician's self on an emotional and reflective level (Bayer-Fetzer Conference on Physician—Patient Communication in Medical Edication, 2001). There is now robust literature demonstrating that an approach to client care anchored in these principles is not only more satisfying for the client and the health professional but also more effective in achieving good health care outcomes (Stewart, 2003).

This section describes the skills that form the basic tools of interviewing. Some of these habits are purely techniques that you can readily put into practice. Some are constructs that will inform your interviewing behaviours. You will employ these interviewing skills to achieve the tasks described earlier in the Sequence of the Interview (see p. 55) more effectively. You need to practice using these tools and find ways to be observed or recorded so that you can receive feedback on your progress. A number of these fundamental skills are listed below followed by a more detailed description. Pick one or two of them to incorporate into your next client interview. Then refer back to this chapter to build your repertoire of skills.

THE TECHNIQUES OF SKILLED INTERVIEWING

Active listening	Avoiding reassurance
Guided questioning	Partnering
Nonverbal communication	Summarization
Empathetic responses	Transitions
Validation	Enabling the client

ACTIVE LISTENING

Underlying all the various techniques is the habit of *active listening*. Active listening is the process of really attending to what the client is communicating, being aware of the client's emotional state, and using verbal and nonverbal skills to encourage the speaker to continue and expand. This requires practice. It is easy to drift into thinking about your next question or lose your focus when you and the client are best served by your concentration on listening.

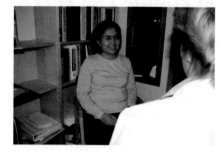

GUIDED QUESTIONING: OPTIONS FOR EXPANDING AND CLARIFYING THE CLIENT'S STORY

There are several ways you can ask for more information from the client without interfering with the flow of the client's story. Your goal is to facilitate the client's fullest communication. Learning the following specific techniques will allow you to guide clients' disclosures while minimizing the risk for distorting their ideas or missing significant details. This is how you avoid asking a series of specific questions, which takes more time and makes the client feel more passive.

GUIDED QUESTIONING: OPTIONS FOR EXPANDING AND CLARIFYING THE CLIENT'S STORY

- Moving from open-ended to focused questions
- Using questioning that elicits a graded response
- Asking a series of questions, one at a time
- Offering multiple choices for answers
- Clarifying what the client means
- Offering continuers
- Using echoing

Moving from Open-Ended to Focused Questions. Your questioning should proceed from general to specific. Start with a truly open-ended question that does not inadvertently include an answer. A possible sequence might be as follows:

"Tell me about your chest pain." (Pause)

"What else?" (Pause)

"Where did you feel it?" (Pause) "Show me."

"Anywhere else?" (Pause) "Did it travel anywhere?" (Pause) "To which arm?"

You should avoid *leading questions* that call for a "yes" or "no" answer. If a client answers "yes" to a question such as "Is your pain pressure like … ?," you run the risk of turning your words into the client's words. A better phrasing is, "Please describe your pain."

Questioning that Elicits a Graded Response. If necessary, ask questions that require *a graded response* rather than a single answer. "How many steps can you climb before you get short of breath?" is better than "Do you get short of breath climbing stairs?"

Asking a Series of Questions, One at a Time. Be sure to *ask one question at a time.* "Any tuberculosis, pleurisy, asthma, bronchitis, pneumonia?" may lead to a negative answer out of sheer confusion. Try "Do you have any of the following problems?" Be sure to pause and establish eye contact as you list each problem.

Offering Multiple Choices for Answers. Sometimes clients seem quite unable to describe their symptoms without help. To minimize bias, *offer multiple-choice answers:* "Which of the following words best describes your pain: aching, sharp, pressing, burning, shooting, or something else?" Almost any specific question can provide at least two possible answers. "Do you bring up any phlegm with your cough (pause) or is it dry?"

Clarifying What the Client Means. At times, clients use words that are ambiguous or have unclear associations. To understand their meaning, you need to *request clarification,* as in "Tell me exactly what you meant by 'the flu'" or "You said you were behaving just like your mother. What did you mean?"

Continuers. Without specifying content, you can use posture, gestures, or words to encourage the client to say more. Pausing with a nod of the head or remaining silent yet attentive and relaxed is a *cue for the client to continue.* Leaning forward, making eye contact, and using phrases, such as "Mm-hmm," or "Go on," or "I'm listening," all maintain the flow of the client's story.

Restatement. A simple repetition of the client's words, or *restating,* encourages the client to express both factual details and feelings, as in the following example:

Client: The pain got worse and began to spread. (Pause)

Response: Spread? (Pause)

Client: Yes, it went to my shoulder and down my left arm to the fingers. It was so bad that I thought I was going to die. (Pause)

Response: Going to die?

Client: Yes, it was just like the pain my father had when he had his heart attack, and I was afraid the same thing was happening to me.

This reflective technique has helped to reveal not only the location and severity of the pain but also its meaning to the client. It did not bias the story or interrupt the client's train of thought.

NONVERBAL COMMUNICATION

Communication that does not involve speech occurs continuously and provides important clues to feelings and emotions. The majority of human communication is nonverbal (Arnold & Boggs, 2007). People tend to believe nonverbal communication over verbal communication when the two are inconsistent. For example, you state that you are interested in hearing what the client is telling you yet you are yawning, looking around the room, and drumming your fingers on the table. Clients tend to believe the message in the nonverbal behaviour, which, in this case, may be disinterest. Becoming more sensitive to nonverbal messages allows you to both "read the client" more effectively and send messages of your own. Pay close attention to eye contact, facial expression, posture, head position and movement such as shaking or nodding, interpersonal distance, and placement of the arms or legs—crossed, neutral, or open. Be aware that nonverbal language is culturally bound.

Just as mirroring your position can signify the client's increasing sense of connectedness, matching your position to that of the client can signify increased rapport. You can also mirror the client's *paralanguage*, or qualities of speech, such as pacing, tone, and volume, to increase rapport. Moving closer or physical contact such as placing your hand on the client's arm can convey empathy or help the client gain control of difficult feelings. Before using touch, ensure the client feels safe and that you are respecting cultural norms. It is okay to ask the client for permission before using touch. For example, "This seems difficult for you to talk about. Is it okay if I hold your hand?" Bringing nonverbal communication to the conscious level is the first step to using this crucial form of client interaction.

EMPATHETIC RESPONSES

Conveying empathy greatly strengthens client rapport. As clients talk with you they may express—with or without words—feelings they may or may not have consciously acknowledged. These feelings are crucial to understanding their illnesses and to establishing a trusting relationship. *To empathize with your client, you must first identify the client's feelings.* This requires a willingness and even interest on your part in hearing about and eliciting emotional content. At first, this may seem unfamiliar or uncomfortable. When you sense important but unexpressed feelings from the client's face, voice, words, or behaviour, inquire about them rather than assuming that you know how he or she feels. You may simply ask, "How did you feel about that?" Unless you let clients know that you are interested in feelings as well as facts, you may miss important insights.

Once you have identified the feelings, respond with understanding and acceptance. Responses may be as simple as "I understand," "That sounds upsetting," or "You seem sad." Empathy may also be nonverbal, for example, offering a tissue to a crying client or gently placing your hand on the client's arm to show understanding. When you give an empathetic response, be sure that you are responding correctly to what the client is feeling. If your response acknowledges how upset a client must have been at the death of a parent, when in fact the death relieved the client of a long-standing financial and emotional burden, you have misunderstood the situation. Instead of making assumptions, you can ask directly about the client's emotional response. "I am sorry about the death of your father. What has that been like for you?"

VALIDATION

Another important way to make a client feel accepted is to legitimize or validate his or her emotional experience. A client who met with a car accident but has no physical injury may still be experiencing significant distress. Stating something like, "Being in that accident must have been very scary. Car accidents are always unsettling because they remind us of our vulnerability and mortality. That could explain why you feel upset," reassures the client. It helps the client feel that such emotions are legitimate and understandable.

AVOIDING REASSURANCE

When you are talking with clients who are anxious or upset, it is tempting to reassure them. You may find yourself saying, "Don't worry. Everything is going to be all right." Although this may be appropriate in nonprofessional relationships, in your role as a clinician, such comments are usually counterproductive. You have no way of really knowing if everything is going to be alright for this client. You may fall into reassuring the client about the wrong thing. Moreover, premature reassurance may block further disclosures, especially if the client feels that exposing anxiety is a weakness. Such admissions require encouragement, not a cover-up.

PARTNERING

When building your relationships with clients, one of the most useful steps is to make explicit your desire to work with them in an ongoing way. It is reassuring to state that regardless of what happens with their disease, you are committed to a helping partnership as their nurse. Even in your role as a learner, especially in a hospital setting, this support can make a big difference.

SUMMARIZATION

Giving a capsule summary of the client's concerns during the course of the interview can serve several different functions. It indicates to the client that you have been listening carefully. It can also identify what you know and what you don't know. "Now, let me make sure that I have the full story. You said you've had a cough for 3 days, that it's especially bad at night, and that you have started to bring up yellow phlegm. You have not had a fever or felt short of breath, but you do feel congested with difficulty breathing through your nose." Following with an attentive pause or stating "Anything else?" lets the client add other information and confirms that you have heard the client's concerns correctly.

You can use summarization at different points in the interview to structure the visit, especially at times of transition (see the next section). This technique also allows you, the nurse, to organize your clinical reasoning and to convey your thinking to the client, which makes the relationship more collaborative. *It is also a useful technique for learners to use when they draw a blank on what to ask the client next.*

TRANSITIONS

Clients have many reasons to feel vulnerable during a health care visit. To put them more at ease, tell them when you are changing directions during the interview. This gives clients a greater sense of control. As you move from one part of the history to another and on to the physical examination, orient the client with brief transitional phrases like, "Now I'd like to ask some questions about your past health." Make clear what the client should expect or do next. "Before we move on to reviewing all your medications, was there anything else about past health problems?"

"Now I would like to examine you. I will step out for a few minutes. Please leave your underwear and bra on, and put on this gown." Specifying that the gown should open in the back may earn the client's gratitude and save you some time.

ENABLING THE CLIENT

The nurse–client relationship is inherently unequal. Your sense of inexperience as a learner will predictably and appropriately transition over time to a sense of confidence in your knowledge and skills and confidence in your role as a nurse.

However, clients have many reasons to feel vulnerable. They may be in pain or worried about a symptom. They may be overwhelmed with the health care system or just unfamiliar with the process that you will come to take for granted.

Differences of gender, ethnicity, genetic background, or class may also create power differentials. However, ultimately, clients must be enabled to take care of themselves. They need to make lifestyle changes or follow treatment plans you recommend. They must feel confident in their ability to follow through on your advice. Listed next are principles that will help guide you. Although many of them have been discussed in other parts of this chapter, the need to enable clients is so fundamental that it is worth summarizing them here. Keep them in mind.

ENABLING THE CLIENT: PRINCIPLES OF SHARING POWER

- Inquire about the client's perspective.
- Express interest in the person, not just the problem.
- Follow the client's lead.
- Elicit emotional content.
- Share information with the client (e.g., transitions).
- Make clinical reasoning transparent to the client.
- Reveal the limits of your knowledge.

◼ ADAPTING YOUR INTERVIEW TO SPECIFIC SITUATIONS

Interviewing clients may precipitate several behaviours and situations that seem perplexing or even vexing. Your ability to handle these situations will evolve throughout your career. *Always remember the importance of listening to the client and clarifying the client's concerns.*

CLIENTS WHO ARE SILENT

Novice interviewers are often uncomfortable with periods of silence and feel obligated to keep the conversation going. Silence has many meanings and many purposes. Clients frequently fall silent for short periods to collect thoughts, remember details, or decide whether you can be trusted with certain information. The period of silence usually feels much longer to the nurse than it does to the client. The nurse should appear attentive and give brief encouragement to continue when appropriate. During periods of silence, watch the client closely for nonverbal cues such as difficulty controlling emotions.

Clients with depression or dementia may lose their usual spontaneity of expression, give short answers to questions, and then fall silent. If you have already tried guiding them through recent events or a typical day, try shifting your inquiry to the symptoms of depression or begin an exploratory mental status examination (see Chapter 9, pp. 203–237).

At times, silence may be the client's response to how you are asking questions. Are you asking too many short-answer questions in rapid succession? Have you offended the client in any way by signs of disapproval or criticism? Have you failed to recognize an overwhelming symptom such as pain, nausea, or dyspnea? If so, you may need to ask the client directly, "You seem very quiet. Have I done something to upset you?"

CLIENTS WHO GIVE CONFUSING INFORMATION

Some clients present a confusing array of *multiple symptoms*. They seem to have every symptom that you ask about, or "a positive review of systems." With these clients, focus on the meaning or function of the symptom, emphasizing the client's perspective (see p. 60), and guide the interview into a psychosocial assessment. There is little profit to exploring each symptom in detail. Although the client may have several illnesses, a somatization disorder may be in play. At other times, you may feel baffled, frustrated, and confused because you cannot make sense out of the client's story. The history is vague and difficult to understand, ideas are poorly connected, and language is hard to follow. Even though you word your questions carefully, you cannot seem to get clear answers. The client's manner of relating to you may also seem peculiar, distant, aloof, or inappropriate. Symptoms may be described in bizarre terms: "My fingernails feel too heavy" or "My stomach knots up like a snake." Perhaps there is a mental status change such as psychosis or delirium, a mental illness such as schizophrenia, or a neurologic disorder (see Chapter 9). Consider delirium in acutely ill or intoxicated clients and delirium or dementia in the elderly. Such clients give histories that are inconsistent and cannot provide a clear chronology about what has happened. Some may even confabulate to fill in the gaps in their memories.

When you suspect a psychiatric or neurologic disorder, do not spend too much time gathering a detailed history. You will only tire and frustrate the client and yourself. Shift to the mental status examination, focusing on level of consciousness, orientation, memory, and capacity to understand. You can work in the initial questions smoothly by asking, "When was your last appointment at the clinic? Let's see … that was about how long ago?" "Your address now is… ? … and your phone number?" You can check these responses against the client's record or seek permission to speak with family members or friends and then obtain their perspectives.

CLIENTS WITH ALTERED MENTAL CAPACITY

Some clients cannot provide their own histories because of delirium from illness, dementia, or other health or mental health conditions. Others are unable to relate certain parts of the history, such as events related to a febrile illness or a seizure. Under these circumstances, you need to determine whether the client has "*decision-making capacity*" or the ability to understand information related to health, to make choices based on reason and a consistent set of values, and to declare preferences about treatments. The term *capacity* is preferable to the term "*competence*," which is a legal term. You do not need to consult psychiatry to assess capacity unless mental illness impairs decision making. For many clients with psychiatric conditions or even cognitive impairments, their ability to make decisions remains intact.

For clients with impaired capacity, obtain their consent before talking about their health with others. Even if clients can communicate only with facial expressions or gestures, you must maintain confidentiality and elicit their input. Assure clients that any shared history will be kept confidential, and clarify what you can discuss with others. Your knowledge about the client can be quite comprehensive yet others may offer surprising and important information. A spouse, for example, may report significant family strains, depressive symptoms, or drinking habits that the client has not disclosed. Consider dividing the interview into two segments—one with the client and the other with both the client and a second informant. Each interview has its own value. Information from other sources often gives you helpful ideas for planning the client's care but remains confidential. Also learn the tenets of the *Freedom of Information and Protection of Privacy Legislation* enacted by the provinces in the late 1990s, which sets strict standards for disclosure for both institutions and providers when sharing client information. These can be found at http://www.efc.ca/pages/law/canada/access.html.

For clients with impaired capacity, you will often need to find a surrogate informant or decision maker to assist with the history. Check whether the client has an advance or personal directive (also known as a living will) as well as durable powers of attorney for health care, to help guide health care decisions for the client. If not, in many cases, a spouse or family member who can represent the client's wishes can fill this role. Apply the basic principles of interviewing to your conversations with clients' relatives or friends. Find a private place to talk. Introduce yourself, state your purpose, inquire how they are feeling under the circumstances, and recognize and acknowledge their concerns. As you listen to their versions of the history, assess the quality of their relationship with the client because it may colour their credibility. Establish how they know the client. For example, when a child is brought in for health care, the accompanying adult may not be the primary or even frequent caregiver—just the most available ride. Always seek the best-informed source. Occasionally, a relative or friend insists on being with the client during your evaluation. Try to find out why, and assess the client's wishes.

CLIENTS WHO ARE TALKATIVE

The client who is rambling may be just as challenging as the client who is silent or confused. Faced with limited time and the need to "get the whole story," you may grow impatient, even exasperated. Although this problem has no perfect solution, several techniques are helpful. Give the client free rein for the first 5 or 10 minutes, listening closely to the conversation. Perhaps the client simply needs a good listener and is expressing pent-up concerns. Maybe the client's style is to tell stories. Does the client seem obsessively detailed? Is the client unduly anxious or apprehensive? Is there a flight of ideas or disorganized thought process that suggests a thought disorder? What about confabulation?

Try to focus on what seems most important to the client. Show your interest by asking questions in those areas. Interrupt only if necessary but be courteous. Learn how to be directive and to set limits when needed. Remember that part of your task is structuring the interview to gain important information about the client's health. A brief summary may help you change the subject yet validate any concerns (see p. 65). "Let me make sure that I understand. You have described many concerns. In particular I heard about two kinds of pain, one on your left side that goes into your groin and is fairly new and the other in your upper abdomen after you eat that you have had for months. Let's focus just on the side pain first. Can you tell me what it feels like?"

Finally, do not show your impatience. If time runs out, explain the need for a second meeting. Setting a time limit for the next appointment may be helpful. "I know we have much more to talk about. Can you come again next week? We will have a full hour then."

CLIENTS WHO ARE CRYING

Crying signals strong emotions, ranging from sadness to anger or frustration. If the client is on the verge of tears, pausing, gentle probing, or responding with empathy gives the client permission to cry. Usually crying is therapeutic, as is your quiet acceptance of the client's distress or pain. Offer a tissue and wait for the client to recover. Make a supportive remark like, "I am glad that you got that out." Most clients will soon compose themselves and resume their story. Aside from an acute grief or loss, it is unusual for crying to escalate and become uncontrollable.

Crying makes many people uncomfortable. If this is true for you, you will need to learn how to accept displays of emotion so that as a clinician you can support clients at these significant times.

CLIENTS WHO ARE ANGRY OR DISRUPTIVE

Many clients have reasons to be angry: they are ill, they have suffered a loss, they lack their accustomed control over their own lives, and they feel relatively powerless in the health care system. They may direct this anger toward you. It is possible that this hostility toward you is justified … were you late for your appointment, inconsiderate, insensitive, or angry yourself? If so, acknowledge the fact and try to make amends. More often, however, clients displace their anger onto the nurse as a reflection of their frustration or pain.

Accept angry feelings from clients. Allow them to express such emotions without getting angry in return. Avoid joining such clients in their hostility toward another health professional, the clinic, or the hospital, even when privately you may feel sympathetic. You can validate their feelings without agreeing with their reasons. "I understand that you felt very frustrated by the long wait and answering the same questions over and over. Our complex health care system can seem very unsupportive when you are not feeling well." After the client has calmed down, help find steps that will avert such situations in the future. Rational solutions to emotional concerns are not always possible, however, and people need time to express and work through their angry feelings.

Some angry clients become overtly disruptive. Few people can disturb the clinic or emergency department more quickly than clients who are angry, belligerent, or out of control. Before approaching such clients, alert the security staff—as a nurse, maintaining a safe environment is one of your responsibilities. Stay calm, appear accepting, and avoid being confrontational in return. Keep your posture relaxed, nonthreatening, and your hands loosely open. At first do not try to make disruptive clients lower their voices or stop if they are haranguing you or the staff. Keep your voice lower and calm. Listen carefully. Try to understand what they are saying. Once you have established rapport, gently suggest moving to a different location that is more private (and will cause less disruption).

CLIENTS WITH A LANGUAGE BARRIER

Nothing will convince you more of the importance of the history than having to do without one. If your client speaks a different language, make every effort to find an interpreter. A few broken words and gestures are no substitute for the full details. The ideal interpreter is a neutral person who is familiar with both languages and cultures. Recruiting family members or friends to serve as interpreters can be hazardous—confidentiality may be violated, meanings may be distorted, and transmitted information may be incomplete. Untrained interpreters may try to speed up the interview by telescoping lengthy replies into a few words, losing much of what may be significant detail.

As you begin working with the interpreter, establish rapport and review what information would be most useful. Explain that you need the interpreter to translate everything, not to condense or summarize. *Make your questions clear, short, and simple.* You can also help the interpreter by outlining your goals for each segment of the history. After going over your plans, arrange the room so that you have easy eye contact and nonverbal communication with the client. Then speak directly to the client … "How long have you been sick?" rather than "How long has the client been sick?" Having the interpreter close by the client keeps you from moving your head back and forth as though you were watching a tennis match.

When available, bilingual written questionnaires are invaluable, especially for the review of systems. First, however, be sure that clients can read in their language; otherwise, ask for help from the interpreter. In some clinical settings, there are speakerphone translators; use them if there are no better options.

GUIDELINES FOR WORKING WITH AN INTERPRETER

- Choose a trained interpreter in preference to a hospital worker, volunteer, or family member.
- Use the interpreter as a resource for cultural information.
- Orient the interpreter to the components you plan to cover in the interview; include reminders to translate everything the client says.
- Arrange the room so that you and the client have eye contact and can read each other's nonverbal cues. Seat the interpreter next to the client.

- Allow the interpreter and the client to establish rapport.
- Address the client directly. Reinforce your questions with nonverbal behaviours.
- Keep sentences *short* and *simple.* Focus on the most important concepts to communicate.
- Verify mutual understanding by asking the client to repeat back what he or she has heard.
- Be patient. The interview will take more time and may provide less information.

CLIENTS WITH LOW LITERACY

Before giving written instructions, assess the client's ability to read. Literacy levels are highly variable, and marginal reading skills are more prevalent than commonly believed. Explore the many reasons people do not read: language barriers, learning disorders, poor vision, or lack of education. Some people may try to hide their inability to read. Asking about educational level may be helpful but can be misleading. "I understand that this may be difficult to discuss, but do you have any trouble with reading?" Ask the client to read whatever instructions you have written. (This will also address any difficulty with your handwriting.) One rapid screen is to hand the client a written text upside down—most clients who read will turn the page around immediately. Literacy skills may be the reason the client has not followed through on taking medications or adhered to recommended treatments. Respond sensitively, and remember that illiteracy and lack of intelligence are not synonymous.

CLIENTS WITH IMPAIRED HEARING

Communicating with a client who has impaired hearing presents many of the same challenges as communicating with clients who speak a different language. Find out the client's preferred method of communicating. Clients may use American Sign Language, a unique language with its own syntax or various other combinations of signs and speech and lip reading. There are several other sign languages that may be used by clients. People who are deaf have their own culture, and sign language is an element of that culture. Thus, communication is often truly cross-cultural. Ask when hearing loss occurred relative to the development of speech and other language skills. Written questionnaires are also useful. If the client prefers sign language, find an interpreter and use the principles identified earlier. At times, time-consuming handwritten questions and answers may be the only solution. Ensure that the client can read and understand the questionnaire.

Hearing deficits vary. If the client has a hearing aid, find out whether the client is using it. Make sure it is working. For clients with unilateral hearing loss, sit on the hearing side. A person who is *hard of hearing* may not be aware of the problem, a situation you will have to tactfully address. Eliminate background noise such as television or hallway conversation as much as possible. For clients who have partial hearing or can read lips, face them directly, in good light. Clients should wear their glasses to better pick up visual cues that help them understand you.

Speak at a normal volume and rate, and do not let your voice trail off at the ends of sentences. Avoid covering your mouth or looking down at papers while speaking. Remember that even the best lip readers comprehend only a percentage of what is said, so having clients repeat what you have said is important. When closing, write out any oral instructions.

CLIENTS WITH IMPAIRED VISION

When meeting with a client who is blind, shake hands to establish contact, and explain who you are and why you are there. If the room is unfamiliar, orient the client to the surroundings and report if anyone else is present. It still may be helpful to adjust the light. Encourage visually impaired clients to wear glasses whenever possible. Remember to use words because postures and gestures are unseen.

CLIENTS WITH LIMITED INTELLIGENCE

Clients of moderately limited intelligence can usually give adequate histories. If you suspect problems, however, pay special attention to the client's schooling and ability to function independently. How far have such clients gone in school? If they didn't finish, why not? What kinds of courses have they taken? How did they do? Have they had any testing done? Are they living alone? Do they need assistance with activities such as transportation or shopping? The sexual history is equally important and often overlooked. Find out if the client is sexually active and provide information that may be needed about pregnancy or sexually transmitted diseases.

If you are unsure about the client's level of intelligence, make a smooth transition to the mental status examination and assess simple calculations, vocabulary, memory, and abstract thinking (see Chapters 9 and 20).

For clients with severe mental retardation, you will have to turn to the family or caregivers to elicit the history. Identify the person who accompanies the client, but always show interest in the client first. Establish rapport, make eye contact, and engage in simple conversation. As with children, avoid "talking down" or using affectations of speech or condescending behaviour. The client, family members, caretakers, or friends will notice and appreciate your respect.

CLIENTS SEEKING PERSONAL ADVICE

Clients may ask you for advice about personal problems that fall outside the range of your clinical expertise. Should the client quit a stressful job, for example, or move out of the province/territory? Instead of responding, explore the different approaches the client has considered and related pros and cons, also with whom they have discussed the problem, and what supports are available for different choices. Letting the client talk through the problem with you is usually much more valuable and therapeutic than any answer you could give.

◼ SENSITIVE TOPICS THAT CALL FOR SPECIFIC APPROACHES

Nurses talk with clients about various subjects that are emotionally charged or sensitive. These discussions can be particularly difficult for inexperienced nurses or during evaluations of clients you do not know well. Even seasoned clinicians have some discomfort with certain topics: abuse of alcohol or drugs, sexual practices, death and dying, financial concerns, cultural and ethnic experiences, family interactions, domestic violence, psychiatric illnesses, physical deformities, bowel function, and the like. These areas are difficult to explore in part because of societal taboos. We all know, for example, that talking about bowel habits is not "polite table talk." Many of these topics evoke strong cultural, societal, and personal values. Mental illness, drug use, and same-sex practices are three obvious examples of issues that can touch on our biases and pose barriers during the interview. This section explores challenges to the interviewer in these and other important and sometimes sensitive areas, including domestic violence and the client who is dying.

Several basic principles can help guide your response to sensitive topics. Look into other strategies for becoming more comfortable with sensitive areas. Examples include general reading about these topics in medical and lay literature, talking to selected colleagues and teachers openly about your concerns, taking special courses that help you explore your own feelings and reactions, and ultimately, reflecting on your own life experience. Take advantage of all these resources. Whenever possible, listen to experienced nurses, then practice similar discussions with your own clients. The range of topics that you can explore with comfort will widen progressively.

GUIDELINES FOR BROACHING SENSITIVE TOPICS

- *The single most important rule is to be nonjudgemental.* The clinician's role is to learn about the client and help the client achieve better health. Disapproval of behaviours or elements in the health history will only interfere with this goal.
- *Explain why you need to know certain information.* This makes clients less apprehensive. For example, say to clients, "Because sexual practices put people at risk for certain diseases, I ask all of my clients the following questions."
- Find opening questions for sensitive topics and learn the specific kinds of data needed for your assessments.
- Finally, consciously acknowledge whatever discomfort you are feeling. Denying your discomfort may lead you to avoid the topic altogether.

THE SEXUAL HISTORY

Asking questions about sexual behaviour can be lifesaving. Sexual behaviours determine risks for pregnancy, sexually transmitted infections (STIs), and HIV—good interviewing helps prevent or reduce these risks. Sexual practices may be directly related to the client's symptoms and integral to both diagnosis and treatment. Many clients have questions or concerns about sexuality that they would discuss more freely if you ask about sexual health. Finally, sexual dysfunction may result from use of medication or from misinformation that, if recognized, can be readily addressed.

You can introduce questions about sexual behaviour at multiple points in an interview. If the chief concern involves genitourinary symptoms, include questions about sexual health as part of "expanding and clarifying" the client's information. For women, you can ask these questions as part of the Obstetric/Gynecologic section of the Past Medical History. You can bring them into discussions about Health Maintenance, along with diet, exercise, and screening tests, or as part of the lifestyle issues or important relationships covered in the Personal and Social History. In a comprehensive history, you can ask about sexual practices during the Review of Systems. Do not forget this area of inquiry just because the client is elderly or has a disability or chronic illness.

An orienting sentence or two is often helpful. "To assess your risk for various disorders, I need to ask you some questions about your sexual health and practices" or "I routinely ask all clients about their sexual function." For more specific concerns you might state, "To figure out why you have this discharge and what we should do about it, I need to ask some questions about your sexual activity." Try to be "matter-of-fact" in your style; the client will be likely to follow your lead. You should *use specific language*. Refer to genitalia with explicit words such as penis or vagina and avoid phrases like "private parts." Choose words that the client understands or explain what you mean. "By intercourse, I mean when a man inserts his penis into a woman's vagina."

In general, ask about both specific sexual behaviours and satisfaction with sexual function. Specific questions are included in Chapters 21, Male Genitalia and Hernias (pp. 759–783), and Chapter 22, Female Genitalia (pp. 785–828). Here are examples of questions that help guide clients to reveal their concerns in these discussions:

- "When was the last time you had intimate physical contact with someone?" "Did that contact include sexual intercourse?" Using the term "sexually active" can be ambiguous.

- "Do you have sex with men? Women? Both?" Individuals may have sex with persons of the same gender yet not consider themselves gay, lesbian, or bisexual. Some gay and lesbian clients have had sex with the opposite gender. Your questions should always be about the behaviours.

- "How many sexual partners have you had in the last 6 months? In the last 5 years? In your lifetime?" Again, these questions give the client an easy opportunity to acknowledge multiple partners. Ask also about routine use of condoms. "Do you *always* use condoms?"

- It is important to ask all clients, "Do you have any concerns about HIV infection or AIDS?" even if no explicit risk factors are evident.

Note that these questions make no assumptions about marital status, sexual preference, or attitudes toward pregnancy or contraception. Listen to each of the client's responses, and ask additional questions as indicated. To get information about sexual behaviours, you will need to ask more specific and focused questions than in other parts of the interview.

THE MENTAL HEALTH HISTORY

Cultural constructs of mental and physical illness vary widely, causing marked differences in acceptance and attitudes. Think how easy it is for clients to talk about diabetes and taking insulin compared with discussing schizophrenia and using psychotropic medications. Ask open-ended questions initially. "Have you ever had any problem with emotional or mental illnesses?" Then move to more specific questions such as, "Have you ever visited a counsellor or psychotherapist?" "Have you ever been prescribed medication for emotional issues?" "Have you or has anyone in your family ever been hospitalized for an emotional or mental health problem?"

For clients with depression or thought disorders such as schizophrenia, a careful history of their illness is in order. Depression is common worldwide but still remains underdiagnosed and undertreated. Be sensitive to reports of mood changes or symptoms such as fatigue, unusual tearfulness, appetite or weight changes, insomnia, and vague somatic complaints. Two opening screening questions are, "Over the past 2 weeks, have you felt down, depressed, or hopeless?" and "Over the past 2 weeks, have you felt little interest or pleasure in doing things?" (U.S.

Preventive Services Task Force, 2002). If the client seems depressed, also ask about thoughts of suicide, "Have you ever thought about hurting yourself or ending your life?" As with chest pain, you must evaluate severity—both depression and angina are potentially lethal. For further approaches, turn to Chapter 9.

Many clients with schizophrenia or other psychotic disorders can function in the community and tell you about their diagnoses, symptoms, hospitalizations, and current medications. You should investigate their symptoms and assess any effects on mood or daily activities.

ALCOHOL AND ILLICIT DRUGS

Many nurses hesitate to ask clients about use of alcohol and drugs, whether prescribed or illegal. Misuse of alcohol or drugs often directly contributes to symptoms and the need for care and treatment. Despite the high lifetime prevalence of substance abuse disorders—approximately 14% for alcohol and 5% for illegal drugs in Canada—they remain underdiagnosed (Canadian Addiction Survey, 2005).

Avoid letting personal feelings interfere with your role as a clinician. It is your job to gather data, assess the effects on the client's health, and plan a therapeutic response. Nurses should routinely ask about current and past use of alcohol or drugs, patterns of use, and family history. Make sure to include adolescents and older adults in your questioning.

Alcohol. Questions about alcohol and other drugs follow naturally after questions about caffeine and cigarettes. "What do you like to drink?" or "Tell me about your use of alcohol" are good opening questions that avoid the easy "yes" or "no" response. Remember to assess what the client considers alcohol—some clients do not use this term for wine or beer. To detect problem drinking, use several well-validated short screening tools that do not take much time. Two additional questions, "Have you ever had a drinking problem?" and "When was your last drink?" give information about the client's drinking habits. If the client answers yes and has had a drink within the last 24 hours, this is suspicious for problem drinking. (Cyr & Wartman, 1988). The most widely used screening questions are the **CAGE** questions about **C**utting down, **A**nnoyance if criticized, **G**uilty feelings, and **E**ye-openers.

THE CAGE QUESTIONNAIRE

Have you ever felt the need to **C**ut down on drinking?
Have you ever felt **A**nnoyed by criticism of your drinking?
Have you ever felt **G**uilty about drinking?
Have you ever taken a drink first thing in the morning (**E**ye-opener) to steady your nerves or get rid of a hangover?

Adapted from Mayfield, D., McCleod, G., & Hall, P. (1974). The CAGE questionnaire: Validation of a new alcoholism screening instrument. *American Journal of Psychiatry, 131,* 1121–1123.

Two or more affirmative answers to the CAGE questionnaire suggest alcohol misuse and have a sensitivity that ranges from 43% to 94% and specificity that ranges from 70% to 96% (Ewing, 1984; U.S. Preventive Services Task Force, 2004a). If you detect misuse, you need to ask about blackouts (loss of memory about events during drinking), seizures, accidents or injuries while drinking, job problems, conflict in personal relationships, or legal problems. Also ask specifically about drinking while driving or operating machinery.

Illicit Drugs.   As with alcohol, your questions about drugs should generally become more focused if you are to get accurate answers that help you distinguish use from misuse. A good opening question is, "Have you ever used any drugs other than those required for medical reasons?" From there, you can proceed to ask specifically about patterns of use (last use, how often, substances used, amount) or inquire about modes of consumption. "Have you ever injected a drug?" "Have you ever smoked or inhaled a drug?" "Have you ever taken a pill for nonmedical reasons?" As fashions in drugs of abuse change, it is important to stay up to date about the most current hazards and risks from overdose.

Another approach is to adapt the CAGE questions to screening for substance abuse by adding "or drugs" to each question. Once you identify substance abuse, continue with further questions like, "Are you always able to control your use of drugs?" "Have you had any bad reactions?" "What happened? . . . Any drug-related accidents, injuries, or arrests? Job or family problems?" . . . "Have you ever tried to quit? Tell me about it."

FAMILY VIOLENCE

Because of the high prevalence of physical, sexual, and emotional abuse, many authorities recommend the routine screening of all female clients for domestic violence. Other clients at increased risk are children, the elderly, and men (U.S. Preventive Services Task Force, 2004b). As with other sensitive topics, start this part of the interview with general "normalizing" questions: "Because abuse is common in many women's lives, I've begun to ask about it routinely." "Are there times in your relationships that you feel unsafe or afraid?" "Many women tell me that someone at home is hurting them in some way. Is this true for you?" "Within the last year, have you been hit, kicked, punched, or otherwise hurt by someone you know? If so, by whom?" As with other segments of the history, use a pattern that goes from general to specific, less difficult to more difficult.

Physical abuse—often not mentioned by either victim or perpetrator—should be considered in the following settings:

CLUES TO POSSIBLE PHYSICAL ABUSE

- If injuries are unexplained, seem inconsistent with the client's information, are concealed by the client, or cause embarrassment
- If the client has delayed getting treatment for trauma
- If there is a past history of repeated injuries or "accidents"
- If the client or the person close to the client has a history of alcohol or drug abuse
- If the partner tries to dominate the interview, will not leave the room, or seems unusually anxious or solicitous

---

When you suspect abuse, it is important to spend part of the encounter alone with the client. You can use the transition to the physical examination as an excuse to ask the other person to leave the room. If the client is also resistant, you should not force the situation, potentially placing the victim in jeopardy. Be attuned to diagnoses that have a higher association with abuse, such as pregnancy and somatization disorder.

Child abuse is unfortunately also common. Asking parents about their approach to discipline is a routine part of well-child care. You can also ask parents how they cope with a baby who will not stop crying or a child who misbehaves: "Most parents get very upset when their baby cries (or their child has been naughty). How do you feel when your baby cries?" "What do you do when your baby won't stop crying?" "Do you have any fears that you might hurt your child?" Find out how other caretakers or companions handle these situations as well.

DEATH AND THE DYING CLIENT

There is a growing and important emphasis in health care education on improving health professional training related to death and dying. Many nurses avoid talking about death because of their own discomforts and anxieties. Work through your own feelings with the help of reading and discussion. Basic concepts of care are appropriate even for beginning students because you will come into contact with clients of all ages near the end of their lives. (For a discussion of end-of-life decision making, grief and bereavement, and advance directives, turn to Chapter 25, The Older Adult.)

Kubler-Ross (1997) described five stages in a person's response to loss or the anticipatory grief of impending death: denial and isolation, anger, bargaining, depression or sadness, and acceptance. These stages may occur sequentially or overlap in any order or combination. At each stage, follow the same approach. Be sensitive to the client's feelings about dying; watch for cues that the client is open to talking about them. Make openings for clients to ask questions, "I wonder if you have any concerns about the procedure? . . . Your illness? . . . What it will be like when you go home?" Explore these concerns and provide whatever information the client requests. Avoid unwarranted reassurance. If you explore and accept clients' feelings, answer their questions, and demonstrate your commitment to staying with them throughout their illness, reassurance will grow where it really matters—within the clients themselves.

Clients who are dying rarely want to talk about their illnesses at each encounter; nor do they wish to confide in everyone they meet. Give them opportunities to talk, and listen receptively; however, if they stay at a social level, respect their preferences. Remember that illness—even a terminal one—is only one small part of the total person. A smile, a touch, an inquiry about a family member, a comment on the day's events, or even some gentle humour affirms and sustains the unique individual you are caring for. Communicating effectively means getting to know the whole client; it is part of the helping process.

Understanding the client's wishes about treatment at the end of life is an important responsibility. Failing to establish communication about end-of-life decisions is widely viewed as a flaw in clinical care. Even if discussions of death and dying are difficult for you, you must learn to ask specific questions. The condition of the client and the health care setting often determine what needs to be discussed. For clients who are acutely ill and in the hospital, discussions about what the client wants to have done in the event of a cardiac or respiratory arrest are usually mandatory. Asking about *Do Not Resuscitate (DNR) status* is often difficult when you have no previous relationship with the client or lack knowledge of the client's values and life experience.

In general, it is important to encourage any adult, especially the older adult or those with chronic illness, to establish a *health proxy*, who can act as the client's health decision maker (see p. 67). This part of the interview can be a "values history" that identifies what is important to the client and makes life worth living and the point when living would no longer be worthwhile. Ask how clients spend their time everyday, what brings them joy, and what they look forward to. Make sure to clarify the meaning of statements like, "You said that you don't want to be a burden to your family. What exactly do you mean by that?" Explore the client's religious or spiritual frame of reference so that you and the client can make the most appropriate decisions about health care. Assure the client that relieving pain and taking care of spiritual and physical needs will be a priority.

SOCIETAL ASPECTS OF INTERVIEWING

ACHIEVING CULTURAL SAFETY

Communicating effectively with clients from every background has always been an important professional skill. Working well with diverse clients is a career-long process built on genuine interest in learning about others, appreciation of the value of diverse cultures, and the practice of reflecting on how your own perspectives are equally shaped by culture. For more information on cultural safety, see Chapter 2.

A 28-year-old taxi driver from Ghana who had recently moved to Canada went to the clinic for fever and fatigue. He described being weighed, having his temperature taken, and having a cloth wrapped tightly, to the point of pain, around his arm. The female clinician had asked many questions and wanted to take blood, which he had refused. The client's final comment was "… and she didn't even give me chloroquine!"—his primary reason for seeking care. The man from Ghana was expecting few questions and treatment for malaria, which is what fever usually means in Ghana.

In this example, cross-cultural miscommunication is understandable and so less threatening to explore. Unconscious bias leading to miscommunication, however, occurs in many clinical interactions. Consider the following scenario.

A 16-year-old student came to the local health centre for painful menstrual cramps that were interfering with concentrating at school. She wore a tight top and short skirt and had multiple piercings. The 30-year-old male clinician asked, "What kind of job do you want after high school? What kind of birth control do you want?" The teenager felt pressured into accepting birth control pills, even though she had clearly stated that she planned to postpone sex until marriage. She was an honour student and planning to go to university, but the clinician did not elicit these goals. He glossed over her cramps by saying, "Oh, you can just take some ibuprofen. Cramps usually get better as you get older." The client will neither take the prescribed birth control pills, nor will she seek health care soon again. She experienced the encounter as an interrogation, so failed to gain trust in her clinician. In addition, the clinician made assumptions about her life and did not treat her health concern with respect.

In both these cases, the failure stems from mistaken assumptions or biases. In the first case, the clinician did not consider the many variables, including recent travel, affecting client beliefs about health and expectations for care. In the second case, the clinician allowed stereotypes to dictate the agenda instead of listening to the client and respecting her as an individual. Each of us has our own cultural background and our own biases. These do not simply fade away as we become clinicians.

As you provide care for an ever-expanding and diverse group of clients, you must recognize how culture shapes not just the client's beliefs but also your own. *Culture* is the system of shared ideas, rules, and meanings that influences how we view the world, experience it emotionally, and behave in relation to other people. It can be understood as the "lens" through which we perceive and make sense out of the world we inhabit. The meaning of culture is much broader than the term "ethnicity." Cultural influences are not limited to minority groups; they are relevant to everyone. They reflect factors such as geography, age, religion, gender, sexual orientation, ethnicity, genetic background, and socioeconomic status.

Although learning about specific cultural groups is important, avoid allowing this knowledge to turn into stereotyping rather than understanding. For example, you may have learned that clients with particular ethnic backgrounds convey their pain in a more dramatic fashion. However, it is still important for you to evaluate each person with pain as an individual, by not decreasing the amount of analgesic you would typically use, but being aware of your reactions to the client's style. Work on an appropriate and informed clinical approach to all clients by becoming aware of your own values and biases, developing communication skills that transcend cultural differences, and building therapeutic partnerships based on respect for each person's life experience. This type of framework, described in the following section, will allow you to approach each client as unique and distinct.

THE THREE DIMENSIONS OF CULTURAL ENCOUNTERS

- *Self-awareness.* Learn about your own biases ... we all have them.
- *Respectful communication.* Work to eliminate assumptions about what is "expected." Learn directly from your clients—they are the experts on their culture and illness.
- *Collaborative partnerships.* Build your client relationships on respect and mutually acceptable plans.

SELF-AWARENESS

Start by exploring your own cultural identity. How do you describe yourself in terms of ethnicity, class, region or country of origin, religion, and political affiliation? Don't forget the characteristics that we often take for granted—gender, life roles, sexual orientation, physical ability, and ethnic background—especially if we are in majority groups. What aspects of your family of origin do you identify with, and how are you different from your family of origin? How do these identities influence your beliefs and behaviours?

A more challenging task in learning about ourselves is to bring our own values and biases to a conscious level. *Values* are the standards we use to measure our own and others' beliefs and behaviours. These may appear to be absolutes. *Biases* are the attitudes or feelings that we attach to perceived differences. Being attuned to difference is expected; in fact, in the distant past, detecting differences may have preserved life. Intuitively knowing members of one's own background is a survival skill that we may have outgrown as a society but that is still actively at work.

Feeling guilty about our biases makes it hard to recognize and acknowledge them. Start with less threatening constructs, like the way an individual relates to time, a culturally determined phenomenon. Are you always on time—a positive value in the dominant Western culture? Or do you tend to run a little late? How do you feel about people whose habits are opposite to yours? Next time you attend a meeting or class, notice who is early, on time, or late. Is it predictable? Think about the role of physical appearance. Do you consider yourself thin, mid-sized, or heavy? How do you feel about your weight? What does our prevailing culture teach us to value in physique? How do you feel about people who have different weights?

RESPECTFUL COMMUNICATION

Given the complexity of culture, no one can possibly know the health beliefs and practices of every culture and subculture. Let your clients be the experts on their own unique cultural perspectives. Even if clients have trouble describing their values or beliefs in the abstract, they should be able to respond to specific questions. Find out about the client's cultural background. Use some of the same questions discussed earlier, in the section Creating a Shared Understanding of the Problem (see p. 59). Maintain an open, respectful, and inquiring attitude. "What did you hope to get from this visit?" If you have established rapport and trust, clients will be willing to teach you. Be aware of questions that contain assumptions, and always be ready to acknowledge your areas of ignorance or bias. "I know very little about Ghana. What would have happened at a clinic there if you had these concerns?" Otherwise, with the second client and with much more difficulty, "I may have made assumptions about you that are not right. I apologize. Would you be willing to tell me more about yourself and your future goals?"

Learning about cultural differences is valuable because it broadens what you, as a clinician, identify as areas you need to explore. Do some reading about the life experiences of individuals of ethnic backgrounds who live in your area. Go to movies that are filmed in different countries or explicitly present the perspective of different cultures. Learn about the concerns of different consumer groups with visible health agendas. Get to know healers of different disciplines, and learn about their practices. Most important, be open to learning from your clients. Do not assume, however, that what you have learned about a particular culture applies to the individual before you.

COLLABORATIVE PARTNERSHIPS

Through continual work on self-awareness and seeing through the "lens" of others, the nurse lays the foundation for the collaborative relationship that best supports the client's health. Communication based on trust, respect, and a willingness to reexamine assumptions allows clients to express aspects of their concerns that may run counter to the dominant culture. These concerns may be associated with strong feelings such as anger or shame. You, the nurse, must be willing to listen to and validate these feelings and not let your own feelings prevent you from exploring painful areas. You must also be willing to reexamine your beliefs about what is the "right approach" to clinical care in a given situation. Make every effort to be flexible and creative in your plans and respectful of clients' knowledge about their own best interests. By consciously distinguishing what is truly important to the client's health from what is just the standard advice; you and your clients can construct the unique approach to their health care that is in concert with their beliefs and effective clinical care. Remember that if the client stops listening, fails to follow your advice, or does not return, your health care has not been successful.

MAINTAINING PROFESSIONAL BOUNDARIES IN THE NURSE–CLIENT RELATIONSHIP

Health professionals of both genders occasionally find themselves physically attracted to their clients. Similarly, clients may make sexual overtures or exhibit flirtatious behaviour toward health professionals. The emotional and physical intimacy of the nurse–client relationship may lend itself to these sexual feelings.

If you become aware of such feelings in yourself, accept them as a human response and bring them to conscious level so they will not affect your behaviour. Denying these feelings makes it more likely for you to act inappropriately. *Any* sexual contact or romantic relationship with clients is *unethical*; keep your relationship with the client within professional bounds, and seek help if you need it.

Sometimes health professionals meet clients who are frankly seductive or make sexual advances. You may be tempted to ignore this behaviour because you are not sure that it really happened, or you are just hoping it will go away. Calmly but firmly, make it clear that your relationship is professional, not personal. If unwelcome overtures continue, leave the room and find a chaperone to continue the interview. You should also reflect on your image. Has your clothing or demeanour been unconsciously seductive? Have you been overly warm with the client? Although it is your responsibility to avoid contributing to these problems, usually you are not at fault. Often these problems reflect the client's discomfort with feeling less powerful. It may be poor judgement or failure to understand boundaries on the part of the client.

ETHICS AND PROFESSIONALISM

You may wonder why an introductory chapter on interviewing contains a section on health care ethics. The potential power of nurse–client communication calls for guidance beyond our innate sense of morality. *Ethics* are a set of principles crafted through reflection and discussion to define right and wrong. The *Code of Ethics for Registered Nurses*, which guides our professional behaviour, is neither static nor simple, but several principles have guided nurses throughout the ages. Although in most situations your gut sense of right and wrong will be all that you need, even as learners, you will face decisions that call for the application of ethical principles.

■ Nursing Values Defined

Safe, competent, and ethical care	Nurses value the ability to provide safe, competent, and ethical care that allows them to fulfill their ethical and professional obligations to the people they serve.
Health and well-being	Nurses value health promotion and well-being and assisting persons to achieve their optimum level of health in situations of normal health, illness, injury, disability, or at the end of life.
Choice	Nurses respect and promote the autonomy of persons and help them to express their health needs and values and also to obtain desired information and services so they can make informed decisions.
Dignity	Nurses recognize and respect the inherent worth of each person and advocate for respectful treatment of all persons.
Confidentiality	Nurses safeguard information learned in the context of a professional relationship, and ensure it is shared outside the health care team only with the person' informed consent, or as may be legally required, or where the failure to disclose would cause significant harm.
Justice	Nurses uphold principles of equity and fairness to assist persons in receiving a share of health services and resources proportionate to their needs and in promoting social justice.
Accountability	Nurses are answerable for their practice, and they act in a manner consistent with their professional responsibilities and standards of practice.
Quality practice environments	Nurses value and advocate for practice environments that have the organizational structures and resources necessary to ensure safety, support, and respect for all persons in the work setting.

Source: Canadian Nursing Association. 2002.

The Canadian Nurses' Association (2002) published the *Code of Ethics* to guide nursing practice in Canada. The code is organized around eight central values and guides decision making for ethical practice, provides a basis for self-evaluation and reflection of ethical nursing practice, and assists the peer-review process. Specific responsibility statements are outlined for each of the core values identified in the *Code of Ethics* to help nurses ensure ethical practice. The complete code is available at http://www.cna-aiic.ca/CNA/practice/ethics/code/default-e.aspx

As learners, you are exposed to some of the ethical challenges that you will confront later as registered nurses. However, there are dilemmas unique to learners that you will face from the time that you begin taking care of clients. The following vignettes capture some common experiences.

You are on your first clinical rotation in an acute care setting. You arrive at the unit late in the evening to complete research on your client for your shift early the next day. Part of your assignment toward your course grade includes interviewing your client and completing a health history. Your professor has asked you to give a presentation of the health history in postconference.

When you enter the client's room, you find him ready to go to sleep and exhausted. What should you do? Do you proceed with the interview and health history, which is likely to take 45–60 minutes? Do you ask permission before you start? If the client agrees to your interview, what do you include?

Here you are confronted with the tension between wanting to learn and obtain a good grade on your assignment and ensuring the health and well-being of your client. As a learner, this dilemma will arise on occasion.

Obtaining informed consent is the means to address this ethical dilemma. Making sure the client realizes that you are new at interviewing and health histories is always important. It is impressive how often people willingly let learners be involved in their care. It is an opportunity for clients to give back to their caregivers. Even when clinical activities appear to be purely for educational purposes, there may be a benefit to the client. Multiple caregivers provide multiple perspectives, and the experience of being heard can be therapeutic.

You are a fourth-year nursing student on an urgent-care unit, completing your final rotation before graduation. You are working closely with a registered nurse who will complete a portion of your final evaluation. A 16-year-old female client with a lacerated finger comes in with her mother. During the health history, the client hands you a piece of paper that says "I think I'm pregnant. Please don't tell anyone." You finish the interview and look for the registered nurse. When you approach her, she tells you that she is "really busy and you'll have to manage on your own."

Do you inform the registered nurse that you have no experience with a situation like this? Do you inform the client that you are unsure what to do? Do you try to figure out what to do? Do you pretend that you didn't get the note?

In this situation, you are being asked to take responsibility for client care that exceeds your level of comfort and possibly your competence. This can happen in several situations, such as being asked to assess a client without proper support or to draw blood or start an IV before you have done one under supervision. For the client in scenario 2, you may have many of the following thoughts: "You are pretty good at talking with young teenagers and think you might be able to address this," "There may not be much harm to the client by ignoring the information she gave you," "Maybe she'll tell someone else while she is here," and "I don't want to bother the registered nurse who is completing my evaluation." There is educational value to the learner to be challenged to solve problems and gain confidence in functioning independently. But what is the right thing to do in this situation?

Much of the tension in this scenario involves the dynamics of and your role within a health care team. You are there to help with the work of the team, but you are primarily there to learn. You need to work with your team in an honest and reliable way to do the best for the client. You can also see that such situations have no clear or easy answers.

You need to reflect on your beliefs and assess your level of comfort with a given situation. Sometimes there may be alternative solutions. For example, in Scenario 1, the client may really be willing to have an interview and health history done at that late hour, or perhaps you can renegotiate the time for the next morning. In Scenario 2, you might find another person who is more qualified to assist the client or supervise you while you help. You will need to choose which situations warrant voicing your concerns, even at the risk of a bad evaluation.

Seek coaching on how to express your reservations in a way that ensures that they will be heard. As a learner, you will need settings for discussing these immediately relevant ethical dilemmas with other learners and with more experienced teachers and nurses. Small groups structured to address these kinds of issues are particularly useful in providing validation and support. Take advantage of such opportunities whenever possible.

Sometimes the most challenging part of such dilemmas tests your will to follow through with the right course of action. Although it may appear to be a lose–lose situation, a respectful and honest discussion with your peers and more experienced faculty and nurses, respectfully articulating what is in the client's best interest, will usually be heard. Learning how to navigate difficult discussions will be a useful professional skill.

THE HEALTH HISTORY

Now that you've read about successful interviewing and ethics in nursing practice, you can apply this knowledge when conducting the health history. First, you will learn the elements of the Comprehensive Adult Health History, which includes Identifying Data and Source of the History, Chief Concern(s), Present Illness, Past History, Family History, Personal and Social History, and Review of Systems. As you talk with the client, it is critical to learn to elicit and organize all these elements. Bear in mind that during the interview this information will not spring forth in this order! However, you will quickly learn to identify where to fit in the different aspects of the client's story.

THE COMPREHENSIVE VERSUS FOCUSED HEALTH HISTORY

As you gain experience assessing clients in different settings, you will find that new clients in the clinic or in the hospital merit a *comprehensive health history;*

however, in many situations, a more flexible *focused* or *problem-oriented interview* may be appropriate. Like a tailor fitting a special garment, you will adapt the scope of the health history to several factors: the client's concerns and problems, your goals for assessment, the clinical setting (inpatient or outpatient, specialty or primary care), and the time available. Knowing the content and relevance of all components of the comprehensive health history allows you to choose those elements that will be most helpful for addressing client concerns in different contexts.

■ Components of the Adult Health History

Identifying data	■ *Identifying data*—such as age, gender, occupation, marital status ■ *Source of the history*—usually the client, but can be family member, friend, letter of referral, or the medical record ■ If appropriate, establish *source of referral* because a written report may be needed
Reliability	Varies according to the client's memory, trust, and mood
Chief concern	The one or more symptoms or signs causing the client to seek care
Present illness	■ Amplifies the *Chief Concern*; describes how each symptom or sign developed ■ Includes client's thoughts and feelings about the illness ■ Uses relevant portions of the *Review of Systems* ■ May include *medications, allergies,* habits of *smoking* and *alcohol,* which are frequently pertinent to the present illness
Past history	■ Lists childhood illnesses ■ Lists adult illnesses with dates for at least four categories: medical; surgical; obstetric/gynecologic; and psychiatric ■ Includes health maintenance practices such as immunizations, screening tests, lifestyle issues, and home safety
Family history	■ Outlines or diagrams age and health, or age and cause of death, of siblings, parents, and grandparents ■ Documents presence or absence of specific illnesses in family, such as hypertension, coronary artery disease, etc.
Personal and social history	Describes educational level, family of origin, current household, personal interests, lifestyle, and work environment
Review of systems	Documents presence or absence of common symptoms or signs related to each major body system

---

These components of the comprehensive adult health history are more fully described in the next few pages. It follows standard formats for written documentation, which you will need to learn. As you review these histories, you will encounter several technical terms for symptoms. Definitions of terms, together with ways to ask about symptoms, can be found in each of the system examination chapters.

The components of the comprehensive health history structure the client's information and the format of your written record, but the order shown should not dictate the sequence of the interview. Usually the interview will be more fluid and will follow the client's leads and cues, as described earlier in this chapter.

SUBJECTIVE VERSUS OBJECTIVE DATA

As you acquire the techniques of the history taking and physical examination, remember the important differences between **subjective information** and **objective information**, as summarized in the accompanying table. Knowing these differences helps you apply clinical reasoning and cluster client information. These distinctions are equally important for organizing written and oral presentations about the client.

Differences Between Subjective and Objective Data	
Subjective Data	**Objective Data**
What the client tells you	What you detect during the examination
The history, from Chief Concern through Review of Systems	All physical examination findings
Example: Mrs. G is a 54-year-old hairdresser who reports pressure over her left chest "like an elephant sitting there," which goes into her left neck and arm.	*Example:* Mrs. G is an older, overweight white female, who is pleasant and cooperative. BP 160/80, HR 96 and regular, respiratory rate 24, afebrile.

STRUCTURE OF THE ADULT HEALTH HISTORY

Initial Information

Date and Time of History. The date is always important. You are strongly advised to routinely document the time you interview the client, especially in urgent, emergent, or hospital settings.

Identifying Data. These include age, gender, marital status, and occupation. The *source of history* or *referral* can be the client, a family member or friend, an officer, a consultant, or the client's record. Designating the *source of referral* helps you to assess the type of information provided and any possible biases.

Reliability. This information should be documented if relevant. For example, "The client gives conflicting information when describing symptoms and cannot specify details." This statement reflects the quality of the information provided by the client and is usually made at the end of the interview.

Chief Concerns. *Make every attempt to quote the client's own words.* For example, "My stomach hurts and I feel awful." Sometimes clients have no overt concerns, in which case you should report their goals instead. For example, "I have come for my regular check-up," or "I've been admitted for a thorough evaluation of my heart."

Present Illness. This section of the history is a complete, clear, and chronologic account of the issues prompting the client to seek care. The narrative should include the onset of the concern, the setting in which it has developed, its manifestations, and any treatment. The principal symptoms should be well-characterized, with descriptions of the following:

1. Location (localized, generalized, radiating)

2. Quality or nature

3. Severity or quantity

4. Timing (onset, duration, constancy, time of day/month/year)

5. Aggravating factors

6. Alleviating factors

7. Associated symptoms/signs

8. Environmental factors

9. Significance to the client

10. Client perspective

These 10 attributes are invaluable for understanding all client symptoms (see pp. 58–59). It is also important to include the presence or absence of symptoms from sections in the Review of Systems which are relevant to the Chief Concern(s).

Other information is frequently relevant, such as risk factors for coronary artery disease in clients with chest pain or current medications in clients with syncope. The *Present Illness* should reveal the client's responses to his or her symptoms and what effect the illness has had on the client's life. Always remember, *the data flow spontaneously from the client, but the task of organization is yours.*

Clients often have more than one concern. Each merits its own paragraph and a full description.

Medications should be noted, including name, dose, route, and frequency of use. Also list home remedies, nonprescription drugs, vitamins, mineral or herbal supplements, oral contraceptives, and medicines borrowed from family members or friends. It is a good idea to ask clients to bring in all of their medications so you can see exactly what they take. ***Allergies***, including *specific reactions* to each medication, such as rash or nausea, must be recorded as well as allergies to foods, insects, or environmental factors. Note ***tobacco*** use, including the type used. Cigarettes are often reported in pack-years (a person who has smoked 1½ packs a day for 12 years has an 18-pack-year history). If someone has quit, note for how long. ***Alcohol and drug*** *use* should always be investigated (see pp. 74–75 for suggested questions). (Note that *tobacco*, *alcohol*, and *drugs* may also be included in the *Personal and Social History*; however, many clinicians find these habits pertinent to the *Present Illness*.)

Past History.   ***Childhood illnesses***, such as measles, rubella, mumps, whooping cough, chickenpox, rheumatic fever, scarlet fever, and polio, are included in the *Past History*. Also included are any chronic childhood illnesses.

You should provide information relative to ***Adult Illnesses*** in each of four areas:

- *Medical:* Illnesses such as diabetes, hypertension, hepatitis, asthma, and HIV; hospitalizations; number and gender of sexual partners; and risky sexual practices

- *Surgical:* Dates, indications, and types of operations

- *Obstetric/Gynecologic:* Obstetric history, menstrual history, methods of contraception, and sexual function

- *Psychiatric:* Illness and time frame, diagnoses, hospitalizations, and treatments

Also cover selected aspects of *Health Maintenance*, especially immunizations and screening tests. For *immunizations*, find out whether the client has received vaccines for tetanus, pertussis, diphtheria, polio, measles, rubella, mumps, influenza, varicella, hepatitis A or B, meningitis, human papillomavirus (HPV), *Haemophilus influenza* type B, and pneumococci. For *screening tests*, review tuberculin tests, Pap smears, mammograms, stool tests for occult blood, and cholesterol tests, together with results and when they were last performed. If the client does not know this information, written permission may be needed to obtain old health records.

Family History.   Under *Family History*, outline or diagram the age and health, or age and cause of death, of each immediate relative, including parents, grandparents, siblings, children, and grandchildren. Review each of the following conditions and record whether they are present or absent in the family: hypertension, coronary artery disease, elevated cholesterol levels, stroke, diabetes, thyroid or renal disease, cancer (specify type), arthritis, tuberculosis, asthma or lung disease, headache, seizure disorder, mental illness, suicide, alcohol or drug addiction, and allergies as well as symptoms or signs reported by the client.

Personal and Social History. The *Personal and Social History* captures the client's personality and interests, sources of support, coping style, strengths, and fears. It should include occupation and the last year of schooling; home situation and significant others; sources of stress, both recent and long term; important life experiences, such as military service, job history, financial situation, and retirement; leisure activities; religious affiliation and spiritual beliefs; and activities of daily living (ADLs). Baseline level of function is particularly important in clients who are older or have a disability (see p. 903 for the ADLs frequently assessed in older clients). The *Personal and Social History* also conveys lifestyle habits that promote health or create risk such as *exercise and diet*, including frequency of exercise; usual daily food intake; dietary supplements or restrictions; use of coffee, tea, and other caffeine-containing beverages; and *safety measures*, including use of seat belts, bicycle helmets, fire extinguishers, sunblock, smoke detectors, and other devices related to specific hazards. You may want to include any *alternative health care* practices.

You will come to thread personal and social questions throughout the interview to make the client feel more at ease.

Review of Systems. Understanding and using *Review of Systems* questions is often challenging for beginning learners. Think about asking series of questions going from "head to toe." It is helpful to prepare the patient for the questions to come by saying, "The next part of the history may feel like a million questions, but they are important and I want to be thorough." Most *Review of Systems* questions pertain to *symptoms*, but on occasion some clinicians also include illnesses like pneumonia or tuberculosis.

If the client remembers important illnesses as you ask questions within the *Review of Systems, record or present such illnesses as part of the Present Illness* or *Past History*.

Start with a fairly general question as you address each of the different systems. This focuses the client's attention and allows you to shift to more specific questions about systems that may be of concern. Examples of starting questions are: "How are your ears?," "How is your hearing?," "How about your lungs?," "Your breathing?," "Any trouble with your heart?," "How is your digestion?," or "How about your bowels?" Note that you will vary the need for additional questions depending on the client's age, concerns, and general state of health and your clinical judgement.

The *Review of Systems* questions may uncover problems that the client has overlooked, particularly in areas unrelated to the *present illness*. Significant health events, such as a major prior illness or a parent's death, require full exploration. Remember that *major health events should be moved to the Present Illness or Past History in your write-up*. Keep your technique flexible. Interviewing the client yields a variety of information that you organize into formal written format only after the interview and examination are completed.

Some nurses do the *Review of Systems* during the physical examination, asking about the ears, for example, as they examine them. If the client has only a few symptoms, this combination can be efficient. However, if there are multiple symptoms, the flow of both the history and the examination can be disrupted, and necessary note-taking becomes awkward. Listed is a standard series of review-of-system questions. As you gain experience, the "yes or no" questions, placed at the end of the interview, will take no more than several minutes.

■ **General:** Usual weight, recent weight change, any clothes that fit more tightly or loosely than before. Weakness, fatigue, or fever.

■ **Skin:** Rashes, lumps, sores, itching, dryness, changes in colour; changes in hair or nails; changes in size or colour of moles.

■ **Head, Eyes, Ears, Nose, Throat (HEENT):** *Head:* Headache, head injury, dizziness, lightheadedness. *Eyes:* Vision, glasses or contact lenses, last examination, pain, redness, excessive tearing, double or blurred vision, spots, specks, flashing lights, glaucoma, cataracts. *Ears:* Hearing, tinnitus, vertigo, earaches, infection, discharge. If hearing is decreased, use or nonuse of hearing aids. *Nose and sinuses:* Frequent colds; nasal stuffiness, discharge, or itching; hay fever; nosebleeds; sinus trouble. *Throat (or mouth and pharynx):* Condition of teeth and gums; bleeding gums; dentures, if any, and how they fit; last dental examination; sore tongue; dry mouth; frequent sore throats; hoarseness.

■ **Neck:** "Swollen glands"; goitre; lumps, pain, or stiffness in the neck.

■ **Breasts:** Lumps, pain, or discomfort; nipple discharge; self-examination practices.

■ **Respiratory:** Cough, sputum (colour, quantity), hemoptysis, dyspnea, wheezing, pleurisy, last chest x-ray. You may wish to include asthma, bronchitis, emphysema, pneumonia, and tuberculosis.

■ **Cardiovascular:** Heart trouble, high blood pressure, rheumatic fever, heart murmurs; chest pain or discomfort; palpitations, dyspnea, orthopnea, paroxysmal nocturnal dyspnea, edema; results of past electrocardiograms or other cardiovascular tests.

■ **Gastrointestinal:** Trouble swallowing, heartburn, appetite, nausea. Bowel movements, stool colour and size, change in bowel habits, pain with defecation, rectal bleeding or black or tarry stools, hemorrhoids, constipation, diarrhea. Abdominal pain, food intolerance, excessive belching or passing of gas. Jaundice, liver, or gallbladder trouble; hepatitis.

■ **Urinary:** Frequency of urination, polyuria, nocturia, urgency, burning or pain during urination, hematuria, urinary infections, kidney or flank pain, kidney stones, ureteral colic, suprapubic pain, incontinence; in males, reduced calibre or force of the urinary stream, hesitancy, dribbling.

■ **Genital:** *Male:* Hernias, discharge from or sores on the penis, testicular pain or masses, scrotal pain or swelling, history of STIs and their treatments. Sexual habits, interest, function, satisfaction, birth control methods, condom use, and problems. Exposure to HIV infection. *Female:* Age at menarche; regularity, frequency, and duration of periods; amount of bleeding; bleeding between periods or after intercourse; last menstrual period; dysmenorrhea; premenstrual tension. Age at menopause, menopausal symptoms, postmenopausal bleeding. If the client was born before 1971, exposure to diethylstilbestrol (DES) from maternal use during pregnancy (linked to cervical carcinoma). Vaginal discharge, itching, sores, lumps, STIs and treatments. Number of pregnancies, number and type of deliveries, number of abortions (spontaneous and induced), complications of pregnancy, birth control methods. Sexual preference, interest, function, satisfaction, any problems, including dyspareunia. Exposure to HIV infection.

- **Peripheral vascular:** Intermittent claudication; leg cramps; varicose veins; past clots in the veins; swelling in calves, legs, or feet; colour change in fingertips or toes during cold weather; swelling with redness or tenderness.

- **Musculoskeletal:** Muscle or joint pain, stiffness, arthritis, gout, and backache. If present, describe location of affected joints or muscles, any swelling, redness, pain, tenderness, stiffness, weakness, or limitation of motion or activity; include timing of symptoms (e.g., morning or evening), duration, and any history of trauma. Neck or low back pain. Joint pain with systemic features such as fever, chills, rash, anorexia, weight loss, or weakness.

- **Psychiatric:** Nervousness; tension; mood, including depression, memory change, suicide attempts, if relevant.

- **Neurologic:** Changes in mood, attention, or speech; changes in orientation, memory, insight, or judgement; headache, dizziness, vertigo; fainting, blackouts, weakness, paralysis, numbness or loss of sensation, tingling or "pins and needles," tremors or other involuntary movements; seizures.

- **Hematologic:** Anemia, easy bruising or bleeding, past transfusions, transfusion reactions.

- **Endocrine:** Thyroid trouble, heat or cold intolerance, excessive sweating, excessive thirst or hunger, polyuria, change in glove or shoe size.

DOCUMENTING FINDINGS

On completion of the health history, it is essential to document all the information you gathered in a comprehensive, accurate manner. An example of documentation of a health history and the principles of documentation are included in Chapter 5. Conducting a thorough, accurate, respectful health history interview lays the foundation for the nurse–client relationship and provides the frame-work of information that guides the planning and implementation for effective client care.

Critical Thinking Exercise

- Words such as red, raised, and burning refer to which characteristic of a symptom/sign? (*Knowledge*)
- Compare the differences between subjective and objective data. (*Comprehension*)
- How does the Freedom of Information and Protection of Privacy legislation affect how you use the information gathered in a health history? (*Application*)
- Which of the nursing values in the Code of Ethics are affected in Ethics and Professionalism Scenario #2 on page 97. (*Analysis*)
- Outline possible solutions to completing the health history for the client in Ethics and Professionalism Scenario #2. (*Synthesis*)
- How would you evaluate a successful interview and completion of the health history? (*Evaluation*)

Canadian Research

Austin, W., Bergum, V., Nuttgens, S., & Peternelj-Taylor, C. (2006). A revisioning of boundaries in professional helping relationships: Exploring other metaphors. *Ethics & Behavior, 16*(2), 77–94.

Austin, W., Rankel, M., Kagan, L., Bergum, V., & Lemermeyer, G. (2005). To stay or to go, to speak or to stay silent, to act or not to act: Moral distress as experienced by psychologists. *Ethics & Behaviour, 15*(3), 197–212.

Cossette, S., Cara, C., Ricard, N., & Pepin, J. (2005). Assessing nurse–patient interactions from a caring perspective: Report of the development and preliminary psychometric testing of the Caring Nurse–Patient Interactions Scale. *International Journal of Nursing Science, 42*(6), 673–686.

Kunyk, D., & Olson, J. (2001). Clarification of conceptualizations of empathy. *Journal of Advanced Nursing, 35*(3), 317–325.

Test Questions

1. The nurse would document driving with car seatbelt fastened, bicycling with properly fitted helmet, and installing a smoke detector in a vacation home in the client's health history under:
   a. past history.
   b. safety measures.
   c. review of systems.
   d. health-promoting activities.

2. The health history interview differs from a social conversation in that the interview:
   a. is restricted to actual or potential illnesses.
   b. permits the clinician to express his or her needs and interests.
   c. focuses on the client's needs to improve health and well-being.
   d. allows more time for the client to demonstrate self-awareness.

3. When recording the client's chief concerns during the health history, it is recommended that the interviewer:
   a. quote the client's words.
   b. summarize the client's words.
   c. paraphrase the client's words.
   d. describe the client's concerns and health goals.

4. The Review of Systems component of the health history is a:
   a. focus on diseases of the major body systems.
   b. limited number of questions about major body systems.
   c. focus on symptoms related to each of the different body systems.
   d. series of questions that start at the head and finish at the feet.

5. During the health history inquiry about alcohol intake, which of the following is a CAGE question?
   a. How often do you have a hangover?
   b. How many days per week do you drink?
   c. Describe the types of alcohol that you prefer.
   d. Have you ever felt annoyed by criticism about drinking?

Bibliography

CITATIONS

Arnold, E. C., & Boggs, K. U. (2007). *Interpersonal relationships: Professional communication skills for nurses.* St. Louis, MO: Saunders Elsevier.

Bayer–Fetzer Conference on Physician–Patient Communication in Medical Education. (2001). Essential elements of communication in medical encounters: The Kalamazoo Consensus Statement. *Academic Medicine, 76*(4), 390–393.

Beckman, H. B., & Frankel, R. M. (1984). The effect of physician behavior on the collection of data. *Annals of Internal Medicine, 101*(5), 692–696.

Bird, J., & Cohen-Cole, S. A. (1990). The three-function model of the medical interview. *Advanced Psychosometric Medicine, 20,* 65–88.

Canadian Addiction Survey. (2005). *A national survey of Canadians' use of alcohol and other drugs: Prevalence of use and related harms.* Retrieved February 27, 2008, from http://www.casa.ca/Eng/Priorities/Research/Canadian Addiction/Pages/default.aspx

Canadian Nurses Association. (2002). *Code of ethics for registered nurses.* Ottawa, ON: Author.

Cocco, K. M., & Carey, K. B. (1998). Psychometric properties of the Drug Abuse Screening Test in psychiatric outpatients. *Psychological Assessment, 10*(4), 408–414.

Cohen-Cole, S. A. (1991). *The medical interview: The three-function approach.* St. Louis, MO: Mosby–Year Book.

Conant, E. B. (1998). Addressing patients by their first names. *New England Journal of Medicine, 308*(4), 226.

Cyr, M. G., & Wartman, S. A. (1988). The effectiveness of routine screening questions in the detection of alcoholism. *Journal of the American Medical Association, 259*(1), 51–54.

Delbanco, T. L. (1993). Enriching the doctor–patient relationship by inviting the patient's perspective. *Annals of Internal Medicine, 116*(5), 414–418.

Engel, G. L. (1977). The need for a new medical model: A challenge for biomedicine. *Science, 196*(4286), 126–129.

Engel, G. L., & Morgan, W. L., Jr. (1973). *Interviewing the patient.* Philadelphia, PA: W. B. Saunders.

Ewing, J. A. (1984). Detecting alcoholism: The CAGE questionnaire. *Journal of the American Medical Association, 252*(14), 1905–1907.

Hastings, C. (1989). The lived experiences of the illness: Making contact with the patient. In: P. Benne & J. Wrubel (Eds.), *The primacy of caring: Stress and coping in health and illness.* Menlo Park, CA: Addison-Wesley pp. 9–14.

Heller, M. E. (1987). Addressing patients by their first names. *New England Journal of Medicine, 308*(18), 1107.

Kleinman, A., Eisenberg, L., & Good, B. (1978). Culture, illness, and care: Clinical lessons from anthropological and cross-cultural research. *Annals of Internal Medicine, 88*(2), 251–258.

Kubler-Ross, E. (1997). *On death and dying.* New York: Macmillan.

Lazare, A., Putnam, S. M., & Lipkin, M. Jr. (1995). Three functions of the medical interview. In: M. Lipkin Jr., S. M. Putnam, A. Lazare, et al. (Eds.), *The medical interview: Clinical care, education, and research.* New York: Springer-Verlag pp. 3–19.

Novack, D. H. (1995). Therapeutic aspects of the clinical encounter. In: M. Lipkin Jr, S. M. Putnam, A. Lazare, et al. (Eds.), *The medical interview: Clinical care, education, and research* (p. 32). New York: Springer-Verlag.

Smith, R. C. (2002). *Patient-centered interviewing: An evidence-based method.* Philadelphia: Lippincott Williams & Wilkins.

Smith, R. C., Lyles, J. S., Mettler, J., Stoffelmayr, B. E., Van Egeren, L. F., Marshall, A. A., et al. (1998). The effectiveness of an intensive teaching experience for residents in interviewing: A randomized controlled study. *Annals of Internal Medicine, 128*(2), 118–126.

Stewart, M. (2003). Questions about patient-centered care: Answers from quantitative research. In M. Stewart, J. Belle Brown, W. Weston, I. McWhinney, C. McWilliam, & T. Freeman. (Eds.) (2003). *Patient-centered medicine: Transforming the clinical method* (pp. 263–268). Abington, UK: Radcliffe Medical Press.

Suchman, A. L., & Matthews, D. A. (1988). What makes the patient–doctor relationship therapeutic? Exploring the connectional dimension of medical care. *Annals of Internal Medicine, 108*(1), 125–130.

U.S. Preventive Services Task Force. (2002). *Screening for depression: Recommendations and rationale.* Rockville, MD: Agency for Healthcare Research and Quality.

U.S. Preventive Services Task Force. (2004a). *Screening and behavioral counseling interventions in primary care to reduce alcohol misuse: Recommendation statement.* Rockville, MD: Agency for Healthcare Research and Quality.

U.S. Preventive Services Task Force. (2004b). *Screening for family and intimate partner violence: Recommendation statement.* Rockville, MD: Agency for Healthcare Research and Quality.

ADDITIONAL REFERENCES

Building a Therapeutic Relationship: The Techniques of Skilled Interviewing

Branch, W. T., & Malik, T. K. (1993). Using "windows of opportunities" in brief interviews to understand patients' concerns. *Journal of the American Medical Association, 269*(13), 1667–1668.

Fadiman, A. (1997). *The spirit catches you and you fall down.* New York: Farrar, Straus and Giroux.

Frankel, R. M., & Stein, T. S. (1996). *The four habits of highly effective clinicians: A practical guide.* Oakland, CA: Kaiser Permanente Northern California Region Physician Education and Development.

Silverman, J., Kurtz, S., & Draper, J. (1998). *Skills for communicating with patients.* Abingdon, UK: Radcliffe Medical Press Ltd.

Adapting Interviewing Techniques to Specific Situations

Barnett, S. (2002). Cross-cultural communication with patients who use American Sign Language. *Family Medicine, 34*(5), 376–382.

Committee on Disabilities of the Group for the Advancement of Psychiatry. (1997). Issues to consider in deaf and hard-of-hearing patients. *American Family Physician, 56*(8), 2057–2066.

Goldoft, M. (1992). A piece of mind: Another language. *Journal of the American Medical Association, 268*(24), 3482.

Grantmakers in Health. (2003). In the right words: Addressing language and culture in providing health care. *Issues in Brief, 18*, 1–54.

Mayeaux, E. J. Jr, Murphy, P. W., Arnold, C., Davis, T C., Jackson, R. H., & Sentell, T. (1996). Improving patient education for patients with low literacy skills. *American Family Physician, 53*(1), 205–211.

National Work Group on Literacy and Health. (1998). Communicating with patients who have limited literacy skills. Report of the National Work Group on Literacy and Health. *Journal of Family Practice, 46*(2), 168–176.

Putsch, R. W. (1985). Cross-cultural communication: The special case of interpreters in health care. *Journal of the American Medical Association, 254*(23), 3344–3348.

Sensitive Topics that Call for Specific Approaches

End of Life/Palliative Education Resource Center. Retrieved February 10, 2005, from http://www.eperc.mcw.edu/index.htm

Fiellin, D. A., Reid, M. C., & O'Connor, P. G. (2000). Screening for alcohol problems in primary care: A systematic review. *Archives in Internal Medicine, 160*(13), 1977–1989.

Societal Aspects of Interviewing

Carrillo, J. E., Green, A. R., & Betancourt, J. R. (1999). Cross-cultural primary care: A patient-based approach. *Annals of Internal Medicine, 130*, 829–834.

Doyal, L. (2001). Closing the gap between professional teaching and practice. *British Medical Journal, 322*(7288), 685–686.

Lo, B. (2000). *Resolving ethical dilemmas: A guide for clinicians.* Philadelphia: Lippincott Williams & Wilkins.

The Physical Examination: Objective Data

D. Lynn Skillen and Lynn S. Bickley

A comprehensive health history and a complete symptom/sign analysis ensure that nurses are well informed and well prepared to proceed with the physical examination of their clients. This chapter contains the foundation and essential elements for the conduct of the physical examination. It includes routine practices, additional precautions required for infection control, the underlying principles of the four basic examination modes, and specific characteristics for nurses to assess during each examination mode. It explains the anatomical position, anatomical terms, terms of comparison and movement, and characteristics of sound. The chapter also contains information about sequences for comprehensive and focused physical examinations to guide your learning. The following chapter (Chapter 5) details the principles and methods for developing the written record. Mastery of the foundation for the three critical areas of health assessment (health history, physical examination, and documentation) facilitates interdisciplinary communication and promotes best practices.

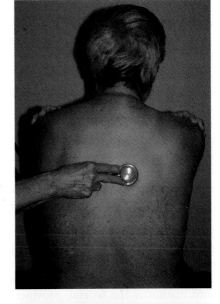

ROUTINE PRACTICES AND ADDITIONAL PRECAUTIONS

ROLE OF NURSES IN PREVENTION

Holistic health assessment by nurses integrates clients' personal, family, social, and environmental data with objective data gathered using the basic examination modes. Nurses use all acquired data to promote client health and to prevent infection and disease. Nurses must consider individual, family, environmental, and organizational factors when attempting to maximize clients' potential for health, safety, and wellness (Skillen, 1996). Throughout health assessment, nurses create opportunities for health promotion, which include client education about lifestyle practices, screening tests, immunizations, environmental hazards, and organizational practices that influence health, safety, and wellness (see Chapter 1). For example, occupational health nurses use their physical assessment skills to determine client fitness for job requirements, teach first-aid skills, identify a need for modified work, test for effects of exposure to hazards, and prevent work-related conditions, including infections (Volk & Santo, 2008).

In all environments where physical examinations occur, *routine practices* and *additional precautions* are essential to protect both clients and nurses against contact with infectious agents. Blood, body fluids, and body substances can each contribute to the transmission of infectious agents.

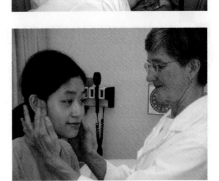

BODY COMPONENTS THAT CONTRIBUTE TO TRANSMISSION OF INFECTIOUS AGENTS

Blood

- Whole blood
- Blood components
- Blood products

Body fluids

- Saliva
- Urine
- Semen
- Vaginal secretions

- Cerebrospinal fluid
- Synovial, pleural, peritoneal, amniotic, and pericardial fluids

Body substances

- Biopsy tissue
- Vomitus
- Feces
- Sputum
- Nasal secretions

Before preparing equipment and conducting the physical examination, nurses follow routine practices such as hand hygiene using alcohol-based products or warm running water and soap. They don disposable gloves if the nurse or client has nonintact skin or if exposure to blood, body fluids, or other body substances is a possibility. They may require barriers to spray or splash exposures such as masks and safety glasses as well as gloves and gowns.

Additional precautions may include avoidance of latex gloves from a latex allergy, decision to use dedicated facilities or equipment to control airflow or maintain negative air pressure, and use of N95 respirators to prevent exposure to airborne or droplet sources of infection. As well, direct contact may be a source of infection and requires additional precautions (Health Canada, 1999). Examples of infectious agents include hepatitis A to E viruses, *Clostridium difficile*, Epstein-Barr virus, cytomegalovirus, human immunodeficiency virus (HIV), *Methacillin-resistant staphylococcus*, and *Vancomycin-resistant enterococci*.

ROLE OF INSTITUTIONS IN PREVENTION

Infection control requires compliance with legislation, guidelines, and current information at the federal, provincial, regional, or local level. Policies and procedures at the organizational level are developed within the context of relevant provincial or federal legislation. Significant leadership is provided by Health Canada (www.hc-sc.gc.ca), the Public Health Agency of Canada (www.phac-aspc.gc.ca), and the Canadian Centre for Occupational Health and Safety (www.ccohs.org). Health care providers can access these Web sites for guidelines, a biweekly journal on communicable diseases, recommendations, reports of outbreaks, and summaries related to infection control and prevention.

BASIC EXAMINATION MODES

Clinical examination is a tradition dating back 2500 years (Orient & Sapira, 2005). Throughout civilization, the art and science of applying four basic examination modes have proven useful for health assessment. *Inspection, palpation, percussion,* and *auscultation* enable health professionals to acquire first-hand objective data from their clients, develop capacity for critical analysis, and function in environments without technology.

INSPECTION IN THE PHYSICAL EXAMINATION

Inspection is either *general* or *local* and is *always* the first basic examination mode used when conducting a physical examination. General inspection *precedes* local inspection. It is likely the one basic examination mode by which most physical signs are detected. It requires that examiners consciously focus attention on numerous client characteristics. Knowledge of the specific client characteristics to assess and repetitive practice of this basic examination mode contribute to the yield of objective data about the client.

General inspection is conducted separately from percussion, palpation, and auscultation to avoid distortion or neglect of significant signs. From the first until the last moment of a client encounter, examiners have the opportunity to use their sense of sight, sense of hearing, and sense of smell to focus on client characteristics. Even when a client is unseen behind a screen or other barriers, examiners can still use hearing and olfaction. For example, nurses can hear a client wheezing or coughing from behind a bed curtain.

General inspection is used for the general survey and is presented in detail in Chapter 6. It continues throughout the client encounter. General inspection is a planned form of examination that integrates visual, auditory, and olfactory information and is maximized by the following:

■ A thorough, unhurried manner

■ Knowledge of the client characteristics to survey

■ Time to integrate inspection data into a holistic picture of the client

When an examiner uses a planned approach for general inspection, he or she minimizes the risk of failing to see or ignoring significant client signs.

Local inspection always follows general inspection, extending the data collected. Local inspection is a selective scrutiny of an anatomical region or body part with focus on specific characteristics. For example, local inspection of the thorax and lungs may reveal difficulty breathing or an increased respiratory rate.

During local inspection, *lighting* is an important consideration. Lighting used for local inspection is either *direct* or *oblique*. Diffused natural lighting is the most preferred type for local inspection, but when nurses aim an artificial light (e.g., a penlight) appropriately, it is usually adequate. Direct (perpendicular) lighting

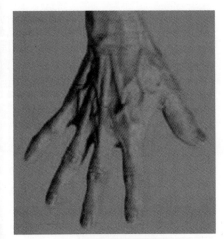

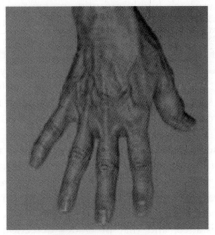

TANGENTIAL LIGHTING   **PERPENDICULAR LIGHTING**

helps detect the colouration of the integumentary system and to examine skin lesions. Direct lighting is the only lighting for detecting *colour*. Oblique (tangential) lighting casts shadows that permit detection of *movement, pulsations*, and *contour*.

CLIENT CHARACTERISTICS TO ASSESS DURING LOCAL INSPECTION

Alignment	Elevations	Movements	Secretions
Closure	Hygiene	Parasites	Shape
Colour	Integrity	Pigmentation	Size
Contraction	Integument	Pulsations	Sounds
Contour	Lesions	Range of motion	Spacing
Coordination	Lustre	Reaction to light	Symmetry
Curvature	Mass	Reflection	Vascularity
Depressions	Mobility	Reflexes	
Development	Moisture	Rhythm	

PALPATION IN THE PHYSICAL EXAMINATION

Palpation makes use of the sensory properties of examiners' hands. The second examination mode, palpation does not require equipment or depend on modern technology; when applied thoughtfully and appropriately, it yields a wealth of information. Examiners apply two types of pressure: light and deep. Light palpation is always a part of physical examination, and deep palpation is used at the discretion of the examiner. During *general* and *local inspections*, the astute examiner determines key areas to explore and decides on the amount of pressure to exert during palpation. Both light and deep palpation depends on sensory properties of the hand.

Sensory Properties of the Hand. Palpation requires the capacity for tactile, kinesthetic, vibratory, and temperature sensations and is a technique that develops with knowledge and experience. Sensory discrimination depends on the appropriate use of the examiner's hands because anatomical areas of the hand vary in their receptivity to sensations. Finger *pads* are sensitive to tactile discriminations and are used primarily to detect *texture, moisture, contour*, and *consistency*. Sensory nerve fibres are particularly abundant in the fingertips, which help in sensing finer tactile discriminations. The fingertips and pads help to determine the *fluid content of tissues, elasticity, pulsatility, thickness, turgor*, and *vascularity* of body structures. The dorsum and ulnar edge of the hands are both highly receptive to *temperature* variations as a result of their minimally keratinized skin surfaces, which means that both surfaces are thinner than other areas of the hand. The palm of the hand at the metacarpophalangeal joints (the ball of the hand) is sensitive to vibrations that originate in body organs and structures. The ulnar edge also has the sensitivity to detect vibrations, and therefore has dual sensory properties. Knowing which surface areas of the hands are to be used for specific purposes gives the examiner the knowledge and the confidence to acquire important findings.

During palpation, the examiner varies the pressure, movement, and position of the palpating hand(s) in accordance with the type of data to be collected. Bones, tendons, muscles, superficial arteries, salivary ducts, abdominal viscera, and structures accessible through body orifices are all subject to palpation. Tender areas are *always* palpated last. A client who experiences tenderness to palpation may react by voluntarily increasing muscular resistance, and that precludes detection of additional important and useful findings.

Light palpation is used to detect the characteristics of the skin surface or structures located immediately adjacent to the skin surface to a depth of about 1 cm. Begin palpation using a warm hand and light pressure to encourage the client's confidence, relaxation, and cooperation. Clients may perceive firm palpation at the beginning as roughness. By conducting light palpation first, the examiner may uncover tender areas and prevent unnecessary discomfort or muscular rigidity by clients in response. By starting with gentle palpation, the examiner facilitates continuation of the examination and collection of more data.

Deep palpation is used to elicit information about structures that are 3 cm to 4 cm deep to the surface. Examiners conduct deep palpation using firm, discontinuous pressure. Discontinuous pressure is essential because continuous pressure exerted on the examiner's finger pads reduces tactile sensitivity. Examiners conduct deep palpation by applying firm hand pressure with fingers approximated and extended and by alternating between applying and releasing the pressure. It may be necessary to employ two hands to achieve the firm pressure required for deep palpation to reach deeper structures such as the liver or colon. The hand on top exerts the pressure; the hand underneath remains relaxed in order to assess tactile sensations. Whether one or two hands are used during deep palpation, pressure is always discontinuous.

Commonly used movements in palpation include *circular* (rotary), *dipping*, *direct* (perpendicular), *gliding*, and *grasping* (pincer) motions. Examiners determine which palpation movements to use according to the information they require.

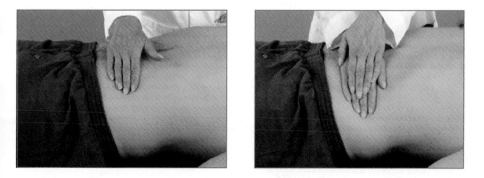

■ *Movements of Palpation*

Type of Movement	Technique	Information Obtained	Explanation
Circular (rotary) motion	With fingers approximated, roll skin surface over underlying structures to accentuate structural characteristics and masses.	■ Consistency ■ Contour ■ Discreteness ■ Mobility ■ Size ■ Shape	Move the skin, but not the fingers.
Dipping motion	Make a gentle and quick depressing movement of the approximated fingers while the hand is flat on the abdomen.	■ Consistency ■ Contour ■ Elasticity ■ Guarding ■ Mobility	Use dipping motions during abdominal palpation. Try to visualize the underlying structures of the abdomen while palpating.

(continued)

■ *Movements of Palpation (Continued)*

Type of Movement	Technique	Information Obtained	Explanation
		■ Resistance ■ Size ■ Shape ■ Status of viscera ■ Tenderness	Palpation may detect: ■ Feces in the colon ■ Cecum in right lower quadrant ■ Descending colon in left lower quadrant ■ Bladder distended with urine ■ Pregnant uterus ■ Mobile right kidney
Direct (perpendicular) pressure	Apply direct, downward, and still pressure with approximated fingers. Apply direct, downward, and still pressure with the thumb for the carotid and brachial arteries.	■ Association with respiratory movements ■ Blanching ■ Fluid content ■ Guarding ■ Pulsations ■ Resistance ■ Tenderness	Use during palpation of blood vessels, skin lesions (e.g., cherry angioma), masses, muscle, and subcutaneous tissues.
Gliding motion	Palpate the skin surface in both the horizontal and vertical planes.	■ Moisture ■ Surface contour ■ Texture	Gliding involves only the motion of the examiner's fingers that are positioned to assess both planes.
Grasping (pincer action) motion	Grasp the skin surface and structures immediately below the surface with thumb and index finger.	■ Association with respiratory movements ■ Consistency ■ Mobility ■ Pulsations ■ Size ■ Shape ■ Thickness ■ Turgor	Use anywhere on the body for assessing characteristics of masses.

SOUNDS IN THE PHYSICAL EXAMINATION

Characteristics of Sound. Audible sound created by sound pressure waves is perceived in terms of four characteristics:

■ *Pitch*—the frequency of sound pressure waves that is a measure of the number of wave cycles per second (cps), usually expressed in Hertz (Hz) in accordance with international standards

■ *Duration*—the length of time in seconds, minutes, or hours that a sound is perceived by the human ear

■ *Quality (timbre)*—the musical nature of the sound

■ *Intensity (loudness)*—the physiological perception of sound measured in decibels (dbs) on the "A" scale using an instrument calibrated to the human hearing curve

The intensity of sound can be measured objectively, independent of pitch. Intensity depends on the amplitude of vibrations produced when the source of the sound, such as a tuning fork, is stimulated. A freely vibrating source of sound is capable of producing a loud sound, and its intensity varies according to the force applied to set the vibration in motion. For example, striking a drum produces a relatively loud sound because the drum has the capacity to vibrate freely. In contrast, if the human forearm is tapped, the sound produced is always of low intensity because those tissues are relatively dense and do not vibrate freely. The force used to increase vibration may affect intensity but does not change pitch.

> **Example: Use of the Tuning Fork**
>
> - When testing *hearing*, the examiner uses a tuning fork of 1024 Hz or 512 Hz. A *1024 Hz* tuning fork has a high pitch, long duration, and a musical sound.
> - When testing *vibration*, the examiner uses a tuning fork of 256 Hz or 128 Hz. A *256 Hz* tuning fork has a low pitch, short duration, and a buzzing sound.

Sound Transmission. In the human body, audible sound is a traveling pressure wave that moves more quickly through solids and fluids than it does through gases. The sounds that are detected using the examination modes of *percussion* and *auscultation* depend not only on the nature of the tissue through which they pass (solid, fluid, or gas) but also on the elasticity of body structures. Elasticity permits vibration of body structures, which then create sound waves transmitted to the exterior of the body and perceived as sound by examiners. Examiners interpret the sounds according to their characteristics of pitch, intensity, quality, and duration.

■ Effect of Tissue Density on Sound Transmission

Density Level	Pitch	Intensity	Quality	Duration
High (solids)	Higher	Softer	Not musical	Shorter
Low (gases)	Lower	Louder	Musical	Longer

Gases are poor transmitters of sounds, fluids are better, and solids are best. Knowledge of their sound transmission capabilities permits examiners to detect deviations from expected findings in body tissues. For example, lung and other tissue changes alter breath sounds. The pitch, intensity, musical quality, and duration of sounds change as they are transmitted through solids, fluid, and air in tissues.

PERCUSSION IN THE PHYSICAL EXAMINATION

Percussion notes are sounds produced in the body as a result of the examiner percussing on body surfaces. The five percussion notes are dull, flat, resonant, hyperresonant, and tympanic. Each percussion note is characterized by pitch, intensity, quality, and duration.

■ *Characteristics of Percussion Notes*

Percussion Note	Pitch	Intensity	Quality	Duration	Example
Dull	Medium	Medium	Noise	Medium	Dullness is percussed anterior to the heart, liver, or a distended urinary bladder.
Flat	High	Soft	Noise	Short	Flatness is percussed over the thigh or scapula.
Resonant	Low	Loud	Noise	Longer	Resonance is percussed over air-filled lung tissue.
Hyperresonant	Higher than resonant	Loud	Noise	Long	Hyperresonance is percussed over hyperinflated lung tissue or a child's lung fields.
Tympanic	High	Loud	Musical Drum-like	Long	Tympany is percussed over gas-filled structures such as the bowel or stomach.

Percussion techniques are used in the following cases:

■ To determine the *density* of underlying tissues related to air, fluid, or solid

■ To locate and estimate the *size* of body organs

■ To elicit *tenderness* if present in underlying organs or structures

■ To stimulate *reflex action* when a deep tendon is partially stretched

Two methods of percussion are used in physical examination: *indirect* and *direct.*

For accuracy, clarity of the percussion note is essential, whether produced by direct or indirect percussion. Learners need to practice percussion techniques to achieve a clear percussion note before attempting to differentiate among percussion notes elicited in clients. After mastery of the technique, examiners will conclude that the percussion note they elicit is from the elasticity and density of underlying structures.

Indirect (mediated) percussion is the most commonly used method for percussion. The examiner taps with the middle (plexor) finger of the dominant hand over the middle (pleximeter) finger of the nondominant hand placed on a body surface. This elicits the percussion note. Indirect percussion may also involve striking the dorsum of one hand with the fist of the other. For example, fist percussion of the kidney in the costovertebral angle may be used to detect tenderness if first finger pressure does not.

Direct (not mediated) percussion is less commonly used. It involves percussion with the plexor finger directly on a body surface. Movement still occurs with brisk arc-like wrist action and only one or two sharp blows. The difference is that the plexor finger taps a surface such as the skin over the frontal sinuses in the head to detect tenderness, or the skin over the clavicle to detect resonance in apical lung tissue.

CRITICAL COMPONENTS OF INDIRECT PERCUSSION

- The pleximeter finger is firm and stationary on the skin surface.
- Only the distal interphalangeal (DIP) joint touches the skin, although some examiners may need to place the entire distal phalanx on the skin surface.
- The plexor fingernail is trimmed short.
- The plexor finger strikes a sharp, perpendicular blow to the pleximeter finger; the force of the blow is adjusted in accordance with the client's body build. A more forceful blow is used to percuss over a heavily muscled or obese client; a less forceful blow is required to percuss a client who is thin or emaciated.
- Brisk arc-like wrist action is used to achieve a sharp blow. A hard blow distorts the clarity of the percussion note by producing overtones; a very light blow produces a flat, muffled sound. *The ideal blow is the lightest blow that produces a clear percussion note.* By using a lighter blow, vibrations of underlying structures are limited to a small area, allowing the examiner to detect small deviations from expected findings.

- Movement occurs at the wrist and not at the elbow.
- One to two sharp blows elicit a clear percussion note. More than two blows may obscure the result and make it difficult to assess.
- Percussion is done from an area of lesser density to an area of greater density to perceive differences among percussion notes more accurately. Change from resonance to dullness is easier to detect than a change from dullness to resonance.
- A consistent technique is essential for comparing symmetrical areas.

AUSCULTATION IN THE PHYSICAL EXAMINATION

Stethoscopes detect sounds created by vibration of underlying tissues transmitted to the skin surface. To exclude environmental sounds and augment internal body sounds, René Laennec invented the first stethoscope in 1816. The binaural stethoscope is popular and has right and left ear pieces, single tubing, and a combination bell/diaphragm chestpiece. The quality of the stethoscope affects the sounds transmitted to the examiner's ears; he or she may misinterpret distorted sounds from a poor quality stethoscope. Differences among stethoscopes include ear piece configuration, tubing length, chestpiece characteristics, and tension springs (adjustable for comfort). An electronic stethoscope amplifies sound. It can be adjusted for low frequency sounds (emulating a bell) or for high frequency sounds (emulating a diaphragm).

Chestpieces of the stethoscope detect the pitch, intensity, quality, and duration of body sounds. Stethoscopes may have a single chestpiece (a bell or a diaphragm) or a paired chestpiece (a bell with a diaphragm or an adult diaphragm with a pediatric diaphragm).

The *bell* chestpiece has an outer rim, usually bordered by rubber material and a hollow centre that is not covered by a flat surface. It accentuates low frequency sounds, filtering out high pitched sounds. The bell is an open system that requires a complete seal with the skin and application of light pressure. Without a perfect seal, sound leaks occur around the bell, and environmental noise distorts the sound perceived. *When the bell is applied with firm pressure, the skin functions as a diaphragm and high pitched (rather than low pitched) sounds are accentuated.*

The *diaphragm* chestpiece detects high frequency sounds and attenuates low pitched sounds. If a chestpiece has a flat surface joining its outer rim, it is a diaphragm.

It is clinically more suitable for detecting high pitched visceral sounds. It does not require a complete seal with the skin surface, because it is a closed system, and sound leaks will not occur if an incomplete seal is made on the skin surface.

For accuracy and hygiene, examiners use their own stethoscopes. Ear pieces are large enough to fit snugly in the external opening of the ear and occlude extraneous noise yet not too small to enter further into the auditory canal and obstruct sound transmission. Ear pieces should be inserted anteriorly, nasally, and inferiorly to follow the natural curvature of the adult ear canal. They must be comfortable enough to be worn for long periods.

Tubing length is important. To maximize sound conduction, short flexible tubing is advisable. A desirable tubing length is approximately 30 cm (12 inches), although some authorities accept tubing as long as 50 cm. When tubing is too long, sound is less effectively transmitted to the examiner's ears. Single stethoscope tubing needs to be thick-walled, with approximately 3 mm diameter for transmitting sounds.

Auscultation Techniques. To maximize the sound volume of the diaphragm chestpiece, apply it directly on the client's skin with adequate pressure so that it can move in synchrony with body movements from breathing. This avoids creation of frictional noise. Coarse hair on the skin of a hirsute client may also create frictional noise. By dampening the hair so that it lies closer to the skin, examiners reduce the friction.

You also need to avoid creating extraneous noise. Do not slide or move fingers on the chestpiece, rub the tubing, breathe on the tubing, or move the chestpiece on the skin. These actions may obscure detection of significant sounds.

During auscultation, you may hear more than one sound. Concentrate on one sound at a time and allow sufficient time to listen carefully. You can enhance concentration by closing your eyes so that no environmental stimulus distracts you. Concentration helps examiners to discriminate between what *should* be heard and what *is* heard.

CRITICAL COMPONENTS OF AUSCULTATION

- Select a stethoscope with short tubing length.
- Use a stethoscope with an earpiece that fits snugly in the opening of the ear.
- Insert earpieces anteriorly, nasally, and inferiorly.
- Dampen chest hair on hirsute clients.
- Apply the chestpiece directly on the client's skin, not over a gown.
- Avoid creating frictional noise.
- Apply a chestpiece to move in synchrony with clients' respirations.
- Make a complete seal with the bell chestpiece, but use light pressure.
- Concentrate on one sound at a time.

Auscultation of Systems. During auscultation, the examiner assesses not only the characteristics of the sound (pitch, intensity, duration, and quality), but also the *location, timing, rate,* and *rhythm of sound.* The specific characteristics to assess depend on the body system being auscultated.

When auscultating the *cardiovascular system* (see Chapter 15), the examiner assesses the location of cardiac sounds according to anatomical location on the precordium and to the underlying structures of the system. The types of sounds include single first and second heart sounds, split heart sounds, fixed split sounds, murmurs, clicks, and opening snaps. It is important to establish the *timing* of heart sounds relative to systole and diastole. The *rhythm* of sounds applies to assessment in relation to the cardiac cycle. In the healthy adult, the *rhythm* of the first and second heart sounds is regular and can be observed on the electrocardiogram (ECG). The *rate* is assessed at the cardiac apex for one timed minute.

The examiner listens for a bruit when examining the *peripheral vascular system* (see Chapter 18). A bruit is an unexpected sound (e.g., rustling, crackling, creaking, rasping, ringing, or splashing) or murmur (e.g., mewing, sawing, or whooshing). It may be created by a vascular aneurysm, infection, friction, or other structural causes.

When auscultating the *respiratory system* (see Chapter 14), the examiner assesses the location of breath sounds considering the underlying lobes of the lungs or large airways. The right lower lobe of the posterior thorax is an example of a peripheral location. The expected types of sounds include vesicular breath sounds (from lung tissue), bronchovesicular breath sounds (from larger bronchi), bronchial sounds (from origins of right and left bronchi), and tracheal breath sounds (from the central trachea). It is important to establish the *timing* of breath sounds relative to inspiration and expiration. The *rate* of sounds is assessed during a defined period, usually one timed minute.

Adventitious (added) sounds are unexpected auscultated findings (e.g., crackles, wheezes, stridor, rubs, or crunches). Adventitious sounds arise from infections, partial obstructions, scarring, heart failure, narrowing of respiratory passages, secretions, inflamed surfaces, or air in the mediastinum (see Chapter 14). In addition to the four *characteristics* of sounds, the examiner identifies their *timing* in the respiratory cycle, *location*, and *ability to clear* with deep breathing.

When auscultating the *gastrointestinal system*, the examiner assesses the *location* in relation to the quadrants or regions of the abdomen and the *rate* during one timed minute. Sounds identified by auscultation may originate in the bowel, viscera, venous system, or peritoneal surface of an organ. Expected sounds include clicks, gurgles, and borborygmi (see Chapter 17). Unexpected sounds arise from diarrhea, obstruction, fluid and air under tension, increased collateral circulation, partial vascular occlusions, or inflammation. Unexpected sounds include bruits, friction rubs, venous hums, and increased or decreased bowel sounds. *A silent abdomen requires thorough assessment.*

Examiners also auscultate the *urinary system* for a renal artery bruit, the *male genitalia* for a hernia in the scrotum, and the *endocrine system* for a thyroid bruit.

ANATOMICAL TERMS IN PHYSICAL EXAMINATION

ANATOMICAL POSITION

The record of clients' subjective and objective data is a legal document that directs the activities of health care providers. To promote clear and accurate communication in both verbal and written documentations, the anatomical position has been adopted internationally to standardize descriptions of assessment findings for members of the interdisciplinary health team (Moore & Dalley, 2006). The anatomical position relates one part of the body to another so that professionals in varied jurisdictions and diverse disciplines receive understandable information in a useable mode.

The anatomical position is used to describe clients' body structures, surfaces, or functions. Whether a client is prone, supine, side-lying, or sitting for the examination—to describe expected and unexpected findings—the examiner *imagines* that the individual is standing in the anatomical position. Using the standardized anatomical position, the imagined client position is as follows:

- Posture is erect.

- Head, eyes, and toes face anteriorly.

- Great toes and heels touch one another.

- Palms face forward (anteriorly).

- Arms are at the sides.

Application of the anatomical position facilitates accurate comparisons of changes in clients over time *even when examiners do not remain constant.*

ANATOMICAL PLANES

Four major imaginary planes divide the human body so that examiners make precise written or verbal descriptions. To begin, imagine your client in the anatomical position. The four useful planes are *median, sagittal, coronal,* and *horizontal.*

The *median* plane passes through the body from back to front, dividing the body vertically (longitudinally) into imaginary right and left symmetrical and equal halves. A *sagittal* plane is *any* vertical plane that passes through the body parallel to the median plane. If a vertical plane passes right through the median plane, it is called the *midsagittal* plane. Sagittal planes are therefore all vertical and parallel to the median and midsagittal planes. The *coronal* (frontal) plane is another vertical plane that also passes through the body longitudinally and lies at *right angles* to the median plane. Beginning at the coronal suture of the skull, the coronal plane divides the body into imaginary anterior and posterior regions and passes posteriorly through the ankles and feet.

In contrast to the three vertical planes, the *horizontal* (transverse) plane lies parallel to the surface on which the client is imagined to be standing while in the anatomical position. The horizontal plane passes through the body at right angles to the median, sagittal, midsagittal, and coronal planes, dividing the body into imaginary superior and inferior regions. The reference points for the horizontal plane as it creates upper and lower body regions are the umbilicus anteriorly and the intervertebral disc between L3 (third lumbar) and L4 (fourth lumbar) vertebrae posteriorly.

ANATOMICAL SURFACES

Examiners use anatomical surfaces to describe clients' body structures in relation to other structures or to the entire body while they imagine clients to be in the anatomical position. They may use anatomical surfaces to indicate location (e.g., medial, superolateral) or direction (e.g., anteroposterior) of objective data. Anatomical surfaces are terms of relationship that incorporate the median, coronal, sagittal, and horizontal planes as points of reference. Examiners avoid using the

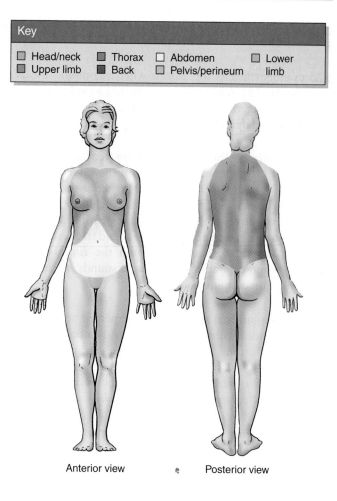

Key			
☐ Head/neck	■ Thorax	☐ Abdomen	☐ Lower
■ Upper limb	■ Back	☐ Pelvis/perineum	limb

Anterior view   Posterior view

words "on," "over," "above," and "under" to describe location. To illustrate, if an examiner records that a mass lies "under" the umbilicus, it is not clear if the mass is inferior, posterior, or deep to the umbilicus. Precise wording is fundamental for promoting client safety and well-being.

■ Anatomical Surfaces

Name of Surface	Description	Name	Explanation/Example
Anterior	The anterior region (front of the body) created by the coronal plane.	Ventral (in neuroanatomy and embryology)	The anterior thorax is a focus of the physical examination.
Dorsal	The posterior region (back of the body) created by the coronal plane or the posterior surface of a structure when in its position of function.	Posterior	To remember the back, think of the dorsal fin of a fish. It is common to refer to the posterior surface of the hand as the dorsal surface. Think of the position of function when labelling the surfaces of the tongue, hand, foot, or flaccid penis. The superior surface of the foot or tongue is referred to as the dorsal surface or dorsum, and the anterior view of the nonerect penis is referred to as the dorsum.
Inferior	On the lower region of the body. Lower than the umbilicus anteriorly and intervertebral disc between L3 and L4 posteriorly. Also indicates a structure that is closer to the foot than another structure.	Lower	Examiners avoid using "under" or "below" as indicators of location. The spleen is inferior to the diaphragm, and the suprasternal notch is inferior to the thyroid.
Lateral	Farther away from the median plane.		In the anatomical position, the thumb is lateral to the middle finger, and the little toe is lateral to the great toe. The lateral epicondyle is palpated for tenderness.
Medial	Closer to the median plane.		In the anatomical position, the little finger is medial to the thumb; the great toe is medial to the little toe. The medial epicondyle is palpated for tenderness.
Palmar	Anterior surface of the hands.	Anterior	Use is restricted to the hands.
Plantar	Inferior surface of the feet.	Inferior	Use is restricted to the feet.
Superior	On the upper region of the body. Upper to the umbilicus anteriorly and intervertebral disc between L3 and L4 posteriorly. Also indicates a structure that is closer to the head than another structure.	Upper	Examiners avoid using "on" or "above" as indicators of location. The lungs are superior to the diaphragm, and the costal margin is superior to the umbilicus.
Flexor	Anterior surface of arms. Posterior surface of legs.	Anterior	The anterior surface of the arms is involved in flexion, and the posterior surface of the legs is involved in flexion.
Extensor	Posterior surface of arms. Anterior surface of legs.	Posterior	Extensor applies to surfaces of the arms and legs that become farther away from one another during extension (straightening).

ANATOMICAL QUADRANTS AND REGIONS

Anatomical quadrants are created by imaginary intersecting vertical and horizontal lines that are in the median and horizontal planes. Usually, examiners describe the abdomen (see Chapter 17) and breasts (see Chapter 16) in terms of their quadrants. The labels for abdominal quadrants are right upper quadrant, left upper quadrant, right lower quadrant, and left lower quadrant. In contrast, labels for the breasts are upper outer quadrant, upper inner quadrant, lower outer quadrant, and lower inner quadrant.

Examiners also may use *anatomical regions* to describe findings in the abdomen. The abdomen is systematically divided into nine regions for the purposes of more specific description. Two imaginary vertical lines (sagittal planes) and two imaginary transverse lines (parallel to the horizontal plane) are used to create the following regions:

- Epigastric

- Umbilical

- Suprapubic (hypogastric)

- Right hypochondriac

- Left hypochondriac

- Right lateral (lumbar)

- Left lateral (lumbar)

- Right inguinal (iliac)

- Left inguinal (iliac)

ANATOMICAL TERMS OF COMPARISON

To use terms of comparison, examiners draw on their knowledge of the *anatomical position, planes, surfaces, quadrants,* and *regions* for relating the position of one body structure to another, one function to another, or one surface to another. When making comparisons, examiners also incorporate the two imaginary body halves created by imagining the median plane.

■ *Anatomical Terms of Comparison*

Term of Comparison	Description	Opposite Term	Explanation/Example
Proximal	Nearest to the trunk of the body. Nearest to the origin of a structure.	Distal	The upper arm is the proximal region of the arm. The elbow is proximal to the wrist. When describing a nerve, muscle, or vessel, the term proximal refers to the point nearest to the origin of the structure.
Distal	Farthest from the trunk of the body.	Proximal	The hand is the most distal part of the arm. The knee is distal to the hip.

(continued)

■ *Anatomical Terms of Comparison (Continued)*

Term of Comparison	Description	Opposite Term	Explanation/Example
	Farthest from the origin of a structure.		When describing a nerve, muscle, or vessel, *distal* refers to the point farthest from the origin of the structure.
Ipsilateral	The structure, surface, or function on the same side of the median plane as something else being described.	Contra- lateral	This term is used in neurological assessments. The right arm is ipsilateral to the right cerebral hemisphere. Ipsilateral muscle strength (upper and lower extremities) is graded 2 on a scale of 5.
Contralateral	The structure, surface, or function on the opposite side of the median plane as something else being described.	Ipsilateral	The term is used in neurological assessments. The left arm is contralateral to the right cerebral hemisphere. Contralateral sensation of upper body is intact.
Superficial	Proximity to the surface of the body.	Deep	Lactiferous ducts in the breasts are in close proximity to the surface of the breasts.
Deep	Distance from the surface of the body.	Superficial	The pectoralis major muscle is distant from the surface of the breast. The abdominal structures that are deep (>3 cm) to the surface skin are difficult to palpate.
Interior	The location of a structure within another structure OR the location with respect to the body surface.	Exterior	The cochlea is internal to the ear and interior to the postauricular surface.
Exterior	The location of a peripheral structure or the structure closer or nearer to the surface of the body.	Interior	The scrotum is exterior to the body. The epididymis is exterior to the testicle within the scrotum.
Superior	Closer to the head than another structure.	Inferior	The superior vena cava carries blood to the heart from the upper regions of the body.
Inferior	Closer to the feet than another structure.	Superior	The inferior vena cava carries blood to the heart from the lower regions of the body.

ANATOMICAL TERMS OF MOVEMENT

Body movements occur at the articulations of bones. Range of motion (movement) in the body is described in relation to the anatomical planes. The most frequently used planes of reference for terms of movement are the median and coronal planes because the medial plane creates the imaginary right and left body halves and the coronal plane creates the imaginary anterior and posterior body halves. Examiners systematically inspect body structures for the type and range of motion, guided by the standardized terms of movement, the anatomical position, and the anatomical planes. They commonly use the basic examination mode of *inspection* to compare the movements made by symmetrical areas of the body, such as the arms, shoulders, hips, and legs, or by midline structures, such as the cervical, thoracic, lumbar, and sacral spines. Range of motion is relative to a neutral position, whether midline (median plane) or in the coronal plane. The common terms of movement are described in the following table. Less common terms of movement include circumduction, depression, elevation, opposition, protraction, and retraction.

■ *Anatomical Terms of Movement*

Common Term of Movement	Description	Opposite Term	Explanation/Example
Flexion	A bending movement in the coronal plane that reduces the angle between two parts.	Extension	Flexion of the spine (as if to touch the toes) and flexion of the knee (an action used in sitting) are bending movements.
Dorsiflexion	A bending movement of the foot at the ankle in an anterior direction.	Plantarflexion	The position is used for assessing the ankle (Achilles) deep tendon reflexes.
Plantarflexion	A bending movement of the foot at the ankle in a posterior direction.	Dorsiflexion	The finding is expected when assessing the ankle (Achilles) deep tendon reflexes.
Lateral flexion	A bending movement in the coronal plane away from the midline position.		The cervical and thoracic spines are assessed for lateral flexion.
Abduction	A movement away from the median plane that increases the angle between two body parts.	Adduction	The shoulders are assessed for full abduction when the arms are moved out, away, and up.
Adduction	A movement toward the median plane that decreases the angle between two body parts.	Abduction	The hips are assessed for full adduction when the legs are moved across the midline in the coronal plane.
Medial rotation	A movement around the long axis of a body part towards the median plane.	Lateral rotation	The cervical spine rotates medially when the client turns his head from a backward looking position to look directly forward (anteriorly).
Lateral rotation	A movement around the long axis of a body part away from the median plane.	Medial rotation	When a client turns her head to look backward, she is rotating the cervical spine laterally.
Internal rotation	The combination of movements of a ball-and-socket joint in an anterior direction.	External rotation	When the client moves his hands to the small of his back, his shoulders rotate internally.
External rotation	The combination of movements of a ball-and-socket joint in a posterior direction.	Internal rotation	When the client places her hands behind her head, elbows pointing laterally, she is externally rotating her shoulders.
Eversion	A term used when the sole of the foot (plantar surface) is turned away from the median plane.	Inversion	Movement at the ankle is assessed during eversion when plantar surfaces are turned away from each other.
Inversion	A term used that involves turning the plantar surface (sole) toward the median plane.	Eversion	Movement at the ankle is assessed during inversion when plantar surfaces are turned toward each other.
Supination	The lateral rotation of the radius at the elbow around its long axis.	Pronation	Think of supination as the position of the hand to carry soup.
			The palm of the hand is turned upwards when the elbow is flexed at a right angle (90°) in the anatomical position and the radius is in a lateral rotation around its long axis.
Pronation	The medial rotation of the radius at the elbow around its long axis.	Supination	The palm of the hand is turned downwards when the radius isa medial rotation around its long axis.

SEQUENCE OF THE PHYSICAL EXAMINATION

The scope and sequence of the physical examination depend on the context. It is important to recognize that *the key to a thorough and accurate physical examination is developing a systematic sequence of examination*. Whether the examination is comprehensive or focused, organize the examination around three goals:

- Maximize client safety and comfort.

- Avoid unnecessary changes in position.

- Enhance clinical efficiency.

Your organization includes brief descriptions of what you plan to do, keeping the client informed of next steps (especially if you anticipate embarrassment or discomfort), and assessing how much the client wants to know about your methods or findings. Start by washing your hands and setting up any equipment that you may be using. Talk with the client while you are doing this, and let him or her know what you will generally be doing. When you begin your assessment, be sure your instructions are clear. For example, "I would like to examine your heart now, so please lie down." Be sensitive to your client's feelings and physical comfort, watching facial expressions or asking "Are you okay?" as you proceed through the examination. Make sure your client is comfortable when you have finished your physical examination. Wash your hands, clean your equipment, and dispose of any waste materials.

COMPREHENSIVE PHYSICAL EXAMINATION

The comprehensive examination is used not only to assess body systems but also to obtain fundamental and personalized knowledge about the client, which strengthens the nurse–client relationship. This examination provides a more complete basis for assessing client concerns and answering client questions. For evaluation of client symptoms and signs, several studies have validated the following components of the comprehensive examination: blood pressure measurement, assessment of central venous pressure from the jugular venous pulse, listening to the heart for evidence of valvular disease, detection of hepatic and splenic enlargements, and the pelvic examination with Papanicolaou smears (Culica et al., 2002; Hensrud, 2000; U.S. Preventive Services Task Force, 2000). As a screening, routine, or periodic examination, not all components of the comprehensive examination have been validated as ways to reduce future morbidity and mortality.

A new client to a facility (hospital, clinic, or continuing care facility) will have a comprehensive health history and physical examination conducted according to conventional sequences. The comprehensive physical examination always begins with the general survey and vital signs (see Chapter 6). It generally proceeds from head to toe, by region (e.g., head and neck, torso, extremities) or system. To avoid asking clients to make repeated position changes (e.g., from sitting to supine to standing), nurses often assess several systems in a region before moving on to another region. For example, when examining the upper extremities, the nurse may assess the integumentary, peripheral vascular, nervous, and musculoskeletal systems before moving on.

After completing the general survey and measurement of vital signs, one accepted sequence for conducting the comprehensive physical examination is as follows:

- Skin of the face, scalp, and hair (sitting)

- Head, eyes, ears, nose, sinuses, throat (sitting)

- Neck (sitting)

- Back (sitting)

- Posterior thorax and lungs (sitting)

- Breasts and axillae (sitting and then supine)

- Anterior thorax and lungs (supine)

- Cardiovascular system (supine)

- Abdomen (supine)

- Lower extremities (supine)

- Upper extremities (sitting)

- Lower extremities (sitting and standing)

- Rectal, genital, and pelvic (female) examinations (supine [female] standing [male])

When examining clients at bed rest, change the sequence. Examine the client's head, neck, and anterior chest with the client supine. Then roll the client onto each side to listen to the lungs, examine the back, and inspect the skin. Roll the client on to the back and finish the rest of the examination with the client again supine. With practice, you will develop your own sequence of examination, keeping in mind the need for thoroughness and client comfort.

Examine clients from the right side of the bed, examination table, or other surface. This is the standard position for the physical examination and has several advantages: It is more reliable to assess jugular veins from the right, the palpating hand rests more comfortably on the apical impulse, and the right kidney is more frequently palpable than the left. More pragmatically, examination tables are frequently positioned to permit a right-handed approach. Left-handed learners are encouraged to adopt a right-sided approach to clients but will likely use their left hand for percussing or for holding the otoscope, ophthalmoscope, and reflex hammer.

■ *Comparison of Comprehensive and Focused Physical Examinations*

The Comprehensive Examination	The Focused Examination
- Appropriate for new clients in hospitals, clinics, continuing care facilities.	- Appropriate for established clients, especially during routine or urgent examinations.
- Provides fundamental, holistic, and personalized knowledge about clients.	- Focuses on client concerns.
- Strengthens nurse–client relationship	- Builds on nurse–client relationship.
- Provides physical context of client concerns.	- Assesses symptoms/signs restricted to specific body system(s) or region(s).
- Provides baseline information for future comparisons.	- Informed by baseline information of comprehensive examination.
- Creates platform for health promotion.	- Health promotion focuses on area of client concern.
- Develops proficiency in the essential skills of physical examination.	- Makes efficient use of relevant skills of physical examination.

Individual chapters contain the detailed examination techniques. See Chapter 5 for an example of the documentation of a *comprehensive* physical examination. Examine the accompanying table for a comparison of comprehensive and focused physical examinations.

FOCUSED EXAMINATION

If the client is already known to a health care facility, the nurse's examination will focus on the client's presenting concern.

A *focused* examination starts with and builds on the nurse's analysis of the symptom or sign. After completing the symptom/sign analysis and a focused personal and family history related to the presenting concern, experienced nurses consider the most likely reasons for the symptom or sign and examine all systems related to those potential causes. Nurses generally maintain the head-to-toe approach but select only the related systems according to their analysis and interpretation of the data obtained in the symptom/sign analysis and history.

A client who is acutely ill requires an abbreviated examination focused on the presenting concern. In an emergency, the examination sequence begins with the general survey and vital signs (see Chapter 6) and proceeds according to conventions for triage and emergency care. See Chapter 5 for an example of the documentation of a *comprehensive* physical examination.

EXAMPLE OF A FOCUSED ASSESSMENT

Identifying Data: Mr. L. W. D. Robertson, 54 years, bush pilot
Presenting Concern: "My feet are sore."

Symptom Analysis:
- Describes pain on "bottom of feet"; starts in heel and moves to sole; noted especially on bottom of heel and ball of foot; does not radiate to dorsum, ankle, Achilles tendon, or lower leg.
- Reports sensation as burning and throbbing.
- On a scale of 0 = *no pain* and 10 = *worst pain,* describes pain as 9.
- States onset of pain was about 1 month ago; it occurs daily; it is better in the morning on rising but gets worse as day goes on; when standing, it is constant; it is bothersome when first going to bed.
- Reports pain aggravated by walking after resting and by daily activities and exercise.
- States pain alleviated somewhat by ice packs, elevation of feet, sticking feet out from under the bed covers on first lying down, and after lying down awhile.
- Reports no other symptoms with it, has no recall of jumping or landing hard on feet, reports no surgery.
- Considers that nothing unusual is going on in his life right now; for years as a bush pilot has taken shoes off in plane, because it helps him have better control over rudder when landing on rough terrain.

- Pain is significant to client because of its frequency and his disturbed sleep; now can only wear athletic shoes.
- Client does not know what is causing this and has no ideas about the cause.

Personal History:
- Osteoarthritis right shoulder "not bad right now."
- Appendectomy 1957.
- Current history of skipped cardiac beats and is seeing cardiologist.
- Describes low-fat diet.
- Reports no known allergies.
- Takes Mevacor 20 mg once daily, Lisinapril 5 mg once daily.
- Calcium intake 1200 mg daily (in milk).
- Denies use of over-the-counter drugs; does not use alcohol or caffeine; never smoked.

Family History:
- Mother deceased age 60; was on antimalarial drugs for rheumatoid arthritis..."heart failure."
- Father 78 years, has pacemaker because of valve problems.
- One healthy brother, no other siblings.
- Maternal aunt has diabetes.
- Maternal grandfather had a stroke.
- Denies family history of cancer.

(Continued)

EXAMPLE OF A FOCUSED ASSESSMENT *(Continued)*

Focused Physical Examination:

Client sitting

Perform general inspection (survey): Assess stated age and orientation to person, time, and place; observe for eye contact and ease of response to questions; note position assumed while answering your questions; assess reliability of responses; note signs of distress.

Vital signs:
- Measure the BP in both arms while sitting.
- Count the heart rate and assess regularity, strength; compare with radial pulse.
- Count respiratory rate and describe regularity, audible sounds.

Measure the height and weight and calculate the BMI.

Test patellar, ankle, and plantar reflexes.

Inspect integument of feet (if reddened, measure temperature).

Client standing

Spine: Inspect vertical alignment, symmetry, and range of motion. Palpate spinous processes and paravertebral muscles.

Lower extremities: Inspect integument, muscle mass, popliteal spaces, arches of feet, veins, gait, balance, posture. Palpate politeal spaces (fossae).

Client supine

Spine: [special technique— test straight leg raising]

Lower extremities: Palpate temperature of feet, lower legs, thighs. Palpate ankles, malleoli, Achilles tendon. Palpate pulses [special technique—test for chronic arterial insufficiency]. Inspect and palpate muscle tone and muscle strength of feet, legs, hips. Inspect range of motion of toes, ankles, knees, hips. Palpate joints and Achilles tendon. Test sensation.

RECORDING AND ANALYZING FINDINGS

Documentation of the comprehensive examination depends on guiding principles, organizational policies, and thoroughness of the examiner. In recent years, abbreviations and other recording practices have been subject to scrutiny in an attempt to reduce errors. Institutions develop their policies in the context of guidelines from the Public Health Agency of Canada (see Chapter 5). Similarly, documentation of the focused examination is in accordance with the principles, policies, and attention to detail of the examiner.

Critical Thinking Exercise

- Describe the anatomical position and its importance. (*Knowledge*)
- Why is general inspection important? (*Comprehension*)
- Describe how you test vibratory sensation. (*Application*)
- Compare light and deep palpation. (*Analysis*)
- What might be the challenges for conducting percussion? (*Synthesis*)
- How will you evaluate your findings from auscultation? (*Evaluation*)

Canadian Research

Gocan, S., & Fisher, A. (2005). Ontario regional stroke centres: Survey of neurological nursing assessment practices with acute stroke patients. *AXON, 26*(4), 8–13.

In 2004, researchers discovered that Ontario nurses were not using the Glasgow Coma Scale as much as in the past and were moving toward the application of standardized stroke severity scales when conducting physical assessment with clients who had suffered an acute stroke. The use of scales such as the Canadian Neurological Scale facilitated nurses' prevention of complications and identification of factors that enhance client outcomes.

Test Questions

1. When examining most body regions, nurses usually perform the four basic examination modes in which of the following sequences?
   a. Auscultation, inspection, palpation, percussion
   b. Inspection, palpation, percussion, auscultation
   c. Palpation, percussion, inspection, auscultation
   d. Inspection, percussion, palpation, auscultation

2. A general procedural rule when performing a complete physical examination is to:
   a. compare symmetrical body areas.
   b. drape primarily for examiner comfort.
   c. examine painful areas first.
   d. examine the right then left side of the body.

3. The ulnar edge of the hand is highly receptive to which of the following sensations?
   a. Moisture and contour
   b. Vibrations and moisture
   c. Contour and temperature
   d. Temperature and vibrations

4. As the density of tissue decreases, the percussion note becomes:
   a. softer.
   b. shorter.
   c. lower pitched.
   d. more melodic.

5. The median (midsagittal) plane is an imaginary line used for describing physical examination findings and passes through the body:
   a. from back to front vertically.
   b. at right angles to the midline.
   c. in any imaginary vertical line parallel to the midline.
   d. creating imaginary and equal right and left halves vertically.

Bibliography

CITATIONS

Culica, D., Rohrer, J., Ward, M., et al. (2002). Medical check-ups: Who does not get them? *American Journal of Public Health, 92*(1), 88–90.

Health Canada. (1999). Routine practices and additional precautions for preventing the transmission of infection in health care. *Canada Communicable Disease Report, 25S4*, 1–142.

Hensrud, D. D. (2000). Clinical preventive medicine in primary care: Background and practice. Rational and current preventive practices. *Mayo Clinic Proceedings, 75*, 165–172.

Moore, K. L., & Dalley, A. F. (2006). *Clinically oriented anatomy* (5th ed.). Philadelphia: Lippincott Williams & Wilkins.

Orient, J. M., & Sapira, J. D. (Eds). (2005). *Sapira's art & science of bedside diagnosis* (3rd ed.). Philadelphia: Lippincott Williams & Wilkins.

Skillen, D. L. (1996). Toward a social structural understanding of occupational hazards in public health. *International Journal of Health Services, 26*(1), 111–146.

U.S. Preventive Services Task Force. (2000). *Guide to clinical preventive services* (3rd ed.). *Recommendations and systematic evidence reviews, guide to community preventive services.* Washington, DC: Office of Public Health and Science, Office of Disease Prevention and Health Promotion.

Volk, A., & Santo, A. (2008). Occupational health nursing: Using clinical skills in the workplace. *Alberta RN, 64*(4), 11.

ADDITIONAL RESOURCES

Baid, H. (2006). The process of conducting a physical assessment: A nursing perspective. *British Journal of Nursing, 15*(13), 710–714.

Bailey, J., & Clain A. (Eds). (1986). *Hamilton Bailey's demonstrations of physical signs in clinical surgery* (17th ed.). Bristol, UK: Wright.

Coombs, M. A., & Moorse, S. E. (2002). Physical assessment skills: A developing dimension of clinical nursing practice. *Intensive and Critical Care Nursing, 18*, 200–210.

Duff, B., Gardiner, G., & Barnes, M. (2007). The impact of surgical ward nurses practicing respiratory assessment on positive patient outcomes. *Australian Journal of Advanced Nursing, 24*(4), 52–56.

Flegel, K. M. (1999). Does the physical examination have a future? *Canadian Medical Association Journal, 161*(9). Retrieved May 26, 2008, from http://www.cmaj.ca/cgi/content/full/161/9/1117

Gray, H., Standring, S., Ellis, H., & Berkovitz, B. K. B. (2005). *Gray's anatomy: The anatomical basis of clinical practice* (39th ed.). New York: Elsevier-Churchill Livingstone.

Guyton, A. C., & Hall, J. E. (2005). *Textbook of medical physiology* (11th ed.). Philadelphia: WB Saunders.

Lesa, R., & Dixon, A. (2007). Physical assessment: Implications for nurse educators and nursing practice. *International Nursing Review, 54*, 166–172.

Mandell, G. L. (2004). *Essential atlas of infectious diseases* (3rd ed.). Philadelphia: Current Medicine.

Moore, K. L., Dalley, A. F., & Agur, A. M. R. (2006). *Clinically oriented anatomy* (5th ed.). Baltimore: Lippincott Williams & Wilkins.

CANADIAN ASSOCIATIONS AND WEB SITES

Canadian Centre for Occupational Health and Safety: http://www.ccohs.org.

Health Canada: http://www.hc-sc.gc.ca.

Heart and Stroke Foundation of BC and Yukon: http://www.heartandstroke.bc.ca/

Public Health Agency of Canada: http://www.phac-aspc.gc.ca

Documenting and Analyzing Findings

Tracey C. Stephen and Lynn S. Bickley

Health assessment includes three key areas: the health history, physical examination, and written record, often referred to as the "health care record." *Documentation* is the term used to describe the process of developing the written record and is an essential aspect of nursing practice.

Florence Nightingale is considered the founder of nursing documentation. In her 19th-century publication *Notes on Nursing*, she outlined the importance of gathering and recording client information in a clear, concise, and organized manner. Over time, the progress of documentation continued. By the 1970s, nurses began to develop their own process of documentation by creating *nursing diagnoses*, which outline the standards for nursing practice based on nursing data and nursing interventions. Currently, the North American Nursing Diagnosis Association–International (NANDA-I) develops the terminology for nursing diagnoses and works in conjunction with the Nursing Intervention Classification (NIC) and Nursing Outcomes Classification (NOC) to facilitate structure for nursing practice.

FUNDAMENTALS OF DOCUMENTATION

PURPOSES OF DOCUMENTATION

The primary reason for documenting the initial health history and physical examination (*assessment*) is to provide a database for the health care team to identify health issues, *formulate diagnoses*, *plan*, *implement*, and *evaluate* client care interventions (the five steps of the nursing process). Documentation is an ongoing process that continues for the entire length of client care episodes. It "demonstrates the visible and invisible work that RNs do for each of their clients" (College and Association of Registered Nurses of Alberta, 2007, p. 12).

The health care record becomes the foundation for care of the client and facilitates communication among all members of the health care team. It is essential for nurses to ensure that they record all client data in a comprehensive and accurate manner to improve communication of plans, interventions, and evaluations of care for the client. The health care record contains the evidence that supports all aspects of care for the client; the healthcare team uses it to evaluate and enhance

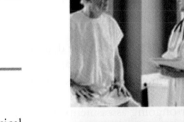

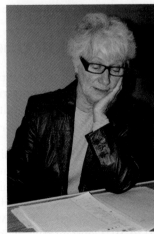

client care. The record also becomes the legal document of client care and nursing practice (Constantino, 2008; Keatings & Smith, 2000).

TYPES OF DATA

Subjective Data. Subjective data are information that clients report. They include all information that is not seen, heard, felt, or smelled by the examiner. Subjective data include the following:

- *Identifying data.* Name, age, gender, occupation, and marital status (see Chapter 3).

- *Chief concern(s).* The one or more symptoms or concerns causing the client to seek care.

- *Present illness.* Includes an analysis of the symptoms/signs that the client is reporting, medications, allergies, and the client's thoughts and feelings about the chief concern.

- *Past health history.* Includes childhood illnesses, previous hospitalizations, illnesses, surgeries, obstetrical history, and so on (see Chapter 3).

- *Family history.* Includes outlines of information about the client's biologic family (age and health; cause of death for siblings, parents, and grandparents).

- *Personal and social history.* Includes education level, family of origin, current household, safety measures, lifestyle, alcohol use, smoking, work-related information, and so on (see Chapter 3).

- *Review of systems.* The process of identifying the presence or absence of common symptoms related to each major body system.

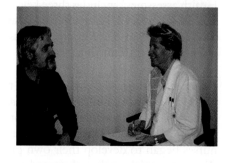

Subjective data are typically collected during the health history or interview. There may be instances of subjective data being reported during the physical examination, but data are better organized when the subjective data are recorded with the health history.

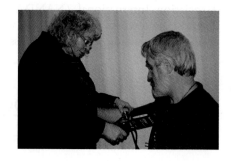

Objective Data. Objective data are information obtained during the physical examination. They include all data gathered by inspection, palpation, percussion, and auscultation. Vital signs, percussion notes, respiratory sounds, height, and weight are all examples of objective data. These data help nurses to establish a baseline for ongoing assessments, gather more information related to the client's chief concern(s), and validate the subjective data obtained in the health history.

GUIDELINES FOR DOCUMENTATION

The way that nurses document assessments, plans, interventions, and evaluations varies among different practice settings (see pp. 116–117, Comparing Health Care Recording Systems). Health care practice settings have policies to guide documentation of data; however, several guidelines apply to all practice settings:

- Record comprehensive, detailed information for all client symptoms and experiences. For example, do not record, "Client has pain in left arm." Instead, document, "Client reports pain in left wrist for 3 days. Left-hand dominant. Points to anterior aspect of left wrist, no radiation. Reports relief of pain with ibuprofen, worsened with activity, no other symptoms. Rates pain as 8 on scale of 0 to 10. Constant pain, worse in evening. States 'nothing new happening in environment.' Reports difficulty completing activities of daily living and self-care.

Thinks it is caused by tension." This description provides much more detailed information to the health care team.

- Document objectively; avoid making judgements or premature diagnoses. Use client statements when applicable to avoid jumping to conclusions and misinterpreting information. For example, avoid recording, "Client depressed about being in the hospital and missing her family." Instead, document, "Client crying in room. Avoiding eye contact. States, 'I miss my family.'"

- Record data findings, not how they were obtained. For example, do not record, "Skin pink on inspection and warm on palpation." Instead, document "Skin pink, warm." This saves time for the health care professionals writing and reading the document and makes the information easier to understand.

- Ensure documentation is legible and written in nonerasable ink. All information gathered is important and must be legible to be useful to other health care professionals. Errors in recording are usually corrected by drawing a single line through the incorrect entry, writing "error," and initialling the error. Because the heath care record is a legal document, never erase or cover the errors with opaque tape or paint.

- Use correct spelling and accepted abbreviations. Heath care practice settings include accepted abbreviations in the policies for documentation. This reduces errors resulting from incorrectly recorded or read information. For example, in some settings, examiners must record "left wrist" rather than "(L) wrist."

- Be concise. Avoid wordiness and use phrases instead of sentences. For example, do not record, "Vesicular breath sounds were auscultated in the client's upper right and left lung lobes, middle right lung lobe, and lower left and right lung lobes." Instead, document "Vesicular breath sounds present in all lung fields."

- Use detailed descriptions of findings for precision; avoid using the word "normal." What one health professional describes as "normal" could be at a different point in the range of findings expected by the person who reads the record. Consider how gender, biological variations, ethnicity, occupation, developmental stage, and age may alter the parameters of expected findings.

- Use specific measurements when applicable. For example, recording "normal bowel sounds" gives much less information than "bowel sounds present in all four quadrants." Another example is recording "large reddened area noted on right thigh," which gives less information than "reddened area on right thigh 5 cm in diameter, located in the midline, 4 cm above the patella."

- Include information about the client's response to interventions. For example, avoid recording just "Sun protection safety taught." Instead, add, "Client discusses sun protection safety and reports 'I will be using these precautions when I'm out in the sun.'"

- Follow the specific documentation policies of the health care practice setting.

TYPES OF DOCUMENTATION SYSTEMS

All health care institutions have documentation systems that include some type of recording forms. These systems may incorporate electronic recording of data or paper records, are specific to each institution, and may have varying forms for different client care areas within the institution. It is important for all health care professionals to understand the system that the health care setting uses to ensure the documentation of accurate, comprehensive, legal, and professional health care information.

■ *Comparing Health Care Recording Systems*

This table compares elements of the different health care recording systems used today. Note that the second column gives information about which systems work best in which setting.

System	Useful Setting	Parts of Health Care Record	Assessment	Plan of Care	Outcomes and Evaluations	Progress Notes Format
Narrative	■ Acute care ■ Long-term care ■ Home health care ■ Ambulatory care	■ Progress notes ■ Flow sheets to supplement care plan ■ Database	■ Initial: History and admission form ■ Ongoing: Progress notes	■ Nursing care plan based on nursing diagnoses	■ Progress notes ■ Discharge summaries	■ Narration at time of entry
Problem-oriented medical record (POMR)	■ Acute care ■ Long-term care ■ Home health care ■ Rehabilitation ■ Mental health facilities	■ Care plan ■ Problem list ■ Progress notes ■ Discharge summary	■ Initial: Database and care plan ■ Ongoing: Progress notes	■ Database ■ Nursing care plan based on problem list	■ Progress notes (under "E" in SOAPIE and SOAPIER)	SOAP, SOAPIE, SOAPIER ■ Subjective data ■ Objective data ■ Assessment data ■ Plan ■ Intervention ■ Evaluation ■ Revision
Problem-intervention-evaluation (PIE)	■ Acute care	■ Assessment flow sheets ■ Progress notes ■ Problem list	■ Initial: Assessment form ■ Ongoing: Assessment form every shift	■ None: Included in progress notes (under "P" in PIE)	■ Progress notes (under "E" in PIE)	PIE ■ Problem ■ Intervention ■ Evaluation
Focus (DAR)	■ Acute care ■ Long-term care	■ Progress notes ■ Flow sheets ■ Checklists	■ Initial: Patient history and admission assessment ■ Ongoing: Assessment form	■ Nursing care plan based on problems or nursing diagnoses	■ Progress notes (under "R" in DAR)	DAR ■ Data ■ Action ■ Response
Charting by exception (CBE)	■ Acute care ■ Long-term care	■ Care plan ■ Flow sheets, including patient-teaching health care records and patient-discharge notes ■ Graphic health care record ■ Progress notes	■ Initial: Database assessment sheet ■ Ongoing: Nursing and medical order flow sheets	■ Nursing care plan based on nursing diagnoses	■ Progress notes (under "E" in SOAPIE and SOAPIER)	■ SOAPIE or SOAPIER

(continued)

■ *Comparing Health Care Recording Systems (Continued)*

System	Useful Setting	Parts of Health Care Record	Assessment	Plan of Care	Outcomes and Evaluations	Progress Notes Format
Flow sheet, assessment, concise, timely	■ Acute care ■ Long-term care	■ Assessment sheet ■ Flow sheets ■ Progress notes	■ Initial: Baseline assessment ■ Ongoing: Flow sheets and progress notes	■ Nursing care plan based on nursing diagnoses	■ Flow sheets (under "R" in DAR)	DAR ■ Data ■ Action ■ Response
Core (with DAE)	■ Acute care ■ Long-term care	■ Kardex ■ Flow sheets ■ Progress notes	■ Initial: Baseline assessment ■ Ongoing: Progress notes	■ Nursing care plan based on nursing diagnoses	■ Progress notes (under "E" in DAE)	DAE ■ Data ■ Action ■ Evaluation
Computerized	■ Acute care ■ Long-term care ■ Home health care ■ Ambulatory care	■ Progress notes ■ Flow sheets ■ Nursing care plan ■ Database ■ Teaching plan	■ Initial: Baseline assessment ■ Ongoing: Progress notes	■ Database ■ Nursing care plan based on nursing diagnoses	■ Outcome-based care plan	■ Evaluative statements, expected outcomes, learning outcomes

Source: Health-care Recording Made Incredibly Easy! 2nd edition, Lippincott, Williams & Wilkins, 2002. Used with permission.

Narrative. This is the traditional method of recording data. Nurses record information in brief sentences using approved abbreviations. They record all information about assessment, interventions, and client responses to treatment in chronologic order. Examples of different formats of narrative charting include Subjective–Objective–Assessment–Plan–Intervention–Evaluation (SOAPIE), Assessment–Intervention–Response (AIR), and Problem–Intervention–Evaluation (PIE).

Checklist. This method of recording data is less time-consuming than the narrative approach because the health care professional selects an indicator on a checklist and checks it off as the best descriptor. The information is less comprehensive than narration, and it is challenging if there are not adequate indicators to select that accurately describe the data. A checklist can inhibit critical thinking and clinical reasoning by limiting the information collected.

Integrated Checklist and Narrative. This method incorporates both checklists and narration to achieve comprehensive recording of the data in a time-efficient manner.

DOCUMENTATION OF HEALTH HISTORY AND PHYSICAL EXAMINATION

Now you are ready to review an actual written record documenting a client's history and physical examination findings. The history and physical examination form the database for your subsequent assessment(s) of the client and your plan(s) with the client for management and next steps. Your written record organizes the information from the history and physical examination and should clearly communicate the client's clinical issues to all members of the health care team. You will find that following a standardized format is the most efficient and helpful way to transfer this information.

TIPS FOR A CLEAR AND ACCURATE WRITE-UP

You should write the record as soon as possible, before the data fade from your memory. At first, you will probably prefer to take notes when talking with the client. During the *physical examination*, make immediate note of specific measurements, such as blood pressure and heart rate. On the other hand, recording multiple items interrupts the flow of the examination, and you will soon learn to remember your findings and record them after you have finished.

Several key features distinguish a clear and well-organized written record. Pay special attention to the *order* and the *degree of detail* as you review the following record and later when you construct your own write-ups. Remember that if handwritten, a good record is always legible!

Order of the Write-Up

The order should be consistent and obvious so that future readers, including you, can easily find specific points of information. Keep subjective items of history in the history, for example, and do not let them stray into the physical examination. Offset your headings and make them clear by using indentations and spacing to accent your organization. Create emphasis by using asterisks and underlines for important points. Arrange the *present illness* in chronologic order, starting with the current episode and then filling in the relevant background information. If a client with long-standing diabetes is hospitalized in a coma, for example, begin with the events leading up to the coma and then summarize the past history of the client's diabetes.

Degree of Detail

The *degree of detail* is also a challenge. It should be pertinent to the subject or problem but not redundant. Review the record of Mrs. N. Decide if you think the order and detail included meet the standards of a complete health record.

The written record should also facilitate clinical reasoning and communicate essential information to the many health professionals involved in the client's care.

Recording the History and Physical Examination: The Case of Mrs. N, 30 August 2008

Mrs. N is a 54-year-old widowed saleswoman residing in Osoyoos, British Columbia.

Referral: None

Source and Reliability: Self; seems reliable.

Chief Concern: "My head aches."

Present Illness (Symptom Analysis): Mrs. N reports her "head is aching," with pain located in the frontal area, no radiation. "Throbbing" pain rated as 7 at present; pain increases to 9 at times. Headaches began approximately 3 months ago and occur on average once per week, lasting 4 to 6 hours each time. Reports headaches are "usually related to stress." Relieved by sleep and damp towel on forehead. No relief from aspirin. Nausea and vomiting with headaches. Denies any visual changes, motor sensory deficits, or other symptoms. Reports increased pressure at work and concern about her daughter. Has missed work on several occasions and "feels irritable with her family" because of headaches. Reports feeling concerned "because her mother died of a stroke." Feels "well other than these headaches." Thinks that the cause is "stress."

Medications: Aspirin, 1 to 2 tablets every 4 to 6 hours as needed. "Water pill" in the past for ankle swelling, none recently.

Allergies: Ampicillin causes rash.

Past History

Childhood Illnesses: Measles, chickenpox. No scarlet fever or rheumatic fever.

Adult Illnesses: Medical: Pyelonephritis, 1982, with fever and right flank pain; treated with ampicillin; develop generalized rash with itching several days later. Reports kidney x-rays were normal; no recurrence of infection. *Surgical:* Tonsillectomy, age 6; appendectomy, age 13. Sutures for laceration, 2001, after stepping on glass. *Ob/Gyn:* G3P3, with routine vaginal births. Three living children. Menarche age 12. Last menses 6 months ago. Little interest in sex, and not sexually active. No concerns about HIV infection. *Psychiatric:* None.

Health Maintenance. Immunizations: Oral polio vaccine, year uncertain; tetanus shots × 2, 1991, followed with booster 1 year later; flu vaccine, 2000, no reaction.

Screening tests: Last Pap smear, 2006, reports normal. No mammograms to date.

(continued)

Family History

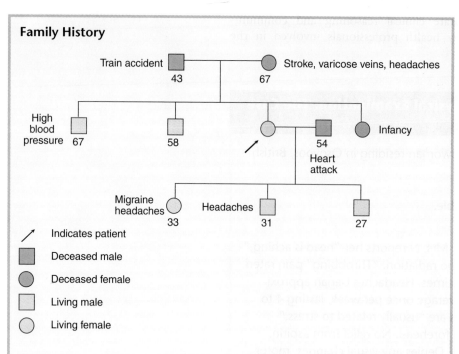

	Indicates patient
	Deceased male
	Deceased female
	Living male
	Living female

or

Father died at age 43 in train accident. Mother died at age 67 of stroke;
   had varicose veins, headaches

One brother, 61, with hypertension, otherwise well; one brother, 58, well
   except for mild arthritis; one sister, died in infancy of unknown cause

Husband died at age 54 of heart attack

Daughter, 33, with migraine headaches, otherwise well; son, 31, with
   headaches; son, 27, well

No family history of diabetes, tuberculosis, heart or kidney disease, cancer,
   anemia, epilepsy, or mental illness

Personal and Social History: Born and raised in Penticton, BC; finished
high school, married at age 19. Worked as sales clerk for 2 years, then
moved with husband to Osoyoos, had 3 children. Returned to work 15
years ago because of financial pressures. Children all married. Four years
ago Mr. N died suddenly of a heart attack, leaving "little savings." Mrs. N
has moved to a small apartment to be near daughter. Daughter's husband
"has an alcohol problem." Mrs. N's apartment now a haven for her daughter and 2 grandchildren, ages 6 and 3 years. Mrs. N feels responsible for
helping them; feels tense and nervous. She has friends but rarely discusses
family problems: "I'd rather keep them to myself. I don't like gossip."
No church or other organizational support. She is typically up at 7:00 AM,
works 9:00 to 5:30, eats dinner alone.

Tobacco use: About 1 pack of cigarettes per day since age 18 (36 pack per
   day [PPD] years).

Alcohol/drugs: Wine on rare occasions, denies use of illicit drugs.

Exercise and diet: Gets "little exercise." Diet high in carbohydrates. Eats
   three meals a day. Drinks 3 cups of coffee during the day and cola at
   night.

Safety measures: Uses seat belt regularly. Uses sunscreen. Medications
   kept in an unlocked medicine cabinet. Cleaning solutions in unlocked

(continued)

The Family History: Can record
as a diagram or a narrative. The
diagram format is more helpful
than the narrative for tracing genetic
disorders. The negatives from the
family history should follow either
format.

cabinet below sink. Mr. N's shotgun and box of shells in unlocked closet upstairs.

Review of Systems

General: Has *gained* about 5 kg in the past 4 years.

Skin: No rashes or other changes.

Head, Eyes, Ears, Nose, Throat (HEENT): See *Present Illness.* No history of head injury. *Eyes:* Reading glasses for 5 years, last checked 1 year ago. No symptoms. *Ears:* Hearing good. No tinnitus, vertigo, infections. *Nose, sinuses:* Occasional mild cold. No hay fever, sinus trouble. *Throat (or mouth and pharynx):* Some bleeding of gums recently. Last dental visit 2 years ago. Occasional canker sore.

Neck: No lumps, goitre, pain. No swollen glands bilaterally.

Breasts: No lumps, pain, discharge bilaterally. Does breast self-exam sporadically.

Respiratory: No cough, wheezing, shortness of breath. Last chest x-ray, 1996, St. Mary's Hospital; unremarkable.

Cardiovascular: No known heart disease or high blood pressure; last blood pressure taken in 2004. No dyspnea, orthopnea, chest pain, palpitations. Has never had an electrocardiogram (ECG).

Gastrointestinal: Appetite good; no nausea, vomiting, indigestion. Bowel movement about once daily, though sometimes has hard stools for 2 to 3 days when especially tense; no diarrhea or bleeding. No pain, jaundice, or gallbladder or liver problems.

Urinary: No frequency, dysuria, hematuria, or recent flank pain; nocturia× 1, large volume. Occasionally loses some urine when coughs hard.

Genital: No vaginal or pelvic infections. No dyspareunia.

Peripheral vascular: Varicose veins appeared in both legs during first pregnancy. For 10 years, has had swollen ankles after prolonged standing; wears light elastic pantyhose; tried "water pill" 5 months ago, but it did not help much; no history of phlebitis or leg pain.

Musculoskeletal: Mild, aching, low-back pain, often after a long day's work; no radiation down the legs; used to do back exercises but not now. No other joint pain.

Psychiatric: No history of depression or treatment for psychiatric disorders. See also *Present Illness* and *Personal and Social History.*

Neurologic: No fainting, seizures, motor or sensory loss. Memory good.

Hematologic: Except for bleeding gums, no easy bleeding. No anemia.

Endocrine: No known thyroid trouble, temperature intolerance. Sweating, average. No symptoms or history of diabetes.

Physical Examination: Mrs. N. is a short, overweight, middle-aged female of European genetic background, appearing stated age and in good health. She appears tense and has moist, cold hands. Her hair is fixed neatly and her clothes are clean, pressed, and appropriate for current weather. Her shoes are matching, slightly worn. Mrs. N. smiles and makes infrequent eye contact. Her posture is upright, gait is moderate. Mrs. N. mobilizes easily and sits with ease. She responds quickly and accurately to questions with recall of information and events.

Vital Signs: Ht (without shoes) 157 cm (5'2"). Wt (dressed) 65 kg (143 lb). BMI 26. BP 164/98 right arm, supine; 160/96 left arm, supine; 152/88

(continued)

right arm, supine with wide cuff. Heart rate 88 and regular. Respiratory rate 18. Temperature (oral) 36.8°C.

Skin: Palms pink, cold, and moist. Scattered cherry angiomas over upper trunk. Nails without clubbing, cyanosis.

Head, Eyes, Ears, Nose, Throat (HEENT): Head: Hair of fine texture. Scalp without lesions. *Eyes:* Vision 20/30 in each eye. Visual fields full by confrontation. Conjunctiva clear, sclera white. Pupils 4 mm constricting to 2 mm, round, regular, equally reactive to light and accommodation. Extraocular movements intact. Disc margins sharp, without hemorrhages, exudates. No arteriolar narrowing or A-V nicking. *Ears:* Yellow wax partially obscures right tympanic membrane (TM); left canal clear, TM with intact cone of light. Acuity accurate to whispered voice. Weber midline. AC > BC. *Nose:* Mucosa pink, septum midline. No sinus tenderness. *Mouth:* Oral mucosa pink. Several interdental papillae red, slightly swollen. Dentition complete. Tongue midline, with 3 × 4 mm shallow white ulcer on red base on undersurface near tip; tender but not indurated. Tonsils absent. Pharynx without exudates.

Neck: Neck supple. Trachea midline. Thyroid isthmus barely palpable, lobes not felt.

Lymph Nodes: Small (<1 cm), soft, nontender, and mobile tonsillar and posterior cervical nodes bilaterally. No axillary or epitrochlear nodes. Several small inguinal nodes bilaterally, soft and nontender.

Thorax and Lungs: Thorax symmetric with good excursion. Lungs resonant. Breath sounds vesicular with no added sounds. Diaphragms descend 4 cm bilaterally.

Cardiovascular: Jugular venous pressure 1 cm above the sternal angle, with head of examining table raised to 30°. Carotid upstrokes brisk, without bruits. Apical impulse discrete and tapping, barely palpable in the 5th left interspace, 8 cm lateral to the midsternal line. S1, S2; no S3 or S4.

Breasts: Pendulous, symmetric. No masses; nipples without discharge.

Abdomen: Protuberant. Healed 8 cm scar, right lower quadrant. Bowel sounds active in all quadrants. No tenderness or masses. Liver span 7 cm in right midclavicular line; edge smooth, palpable 1 cm below right costal margin. Spleen and kidneys not felt. No costovertebral angle tenderness.

Genitalia: External genitalia without lesions. Mild cystocele at introitus on straining. Vaginal mucosa pink. Cervix pink, parous, and without discharge. Uterus anterior, midline, smooth, not enlarged. Adnexa not palpable. No cervical or adnexal tenderness. Pap smear taken. Rectovaginal wall intact.

Rectal: Rectal vault without masses. Stool brown, negative for occult blood.

Extremities: Warm with no edema. Calves supple, nontender.

Peripheral Vascular: Trace edema at both ankles. Moderate varicosities of saphenous veins both lower extremities. No stasis pigmentation or ulcers. Pulses (2+ = brisk, or expected):

	Radial	Femoral	Popliteal	Dorsalis Pedis	Posterior Tibial
RT	2+	2+	2+	2+	2+
LT	2+	2+	2+	Absent	2+

(continued)

Musculoskeletal: No joint deformities. Full range of motion in hands, wrists, elbows, shoulders, spine, hips, knees, and ankles.

Neurologic: Mental Status: Alert and cooperative. Thought coherent. Oriented to person, place, and time. *Cranial Nerves:* II–XII intact.

Motor: Strength 5/5 throughout (see p. 116 for grading system). *Cerebellar:* Rapid alternating movements, point-to-point movements intact. Gait stable, fluid. *Sensory:* Pinprick, light touch, position sense, vibration, and stereognosis intact. Romberg negative.

Reflexes:

	Biceps	Triceps	Brachio-radialis	Patellar	Achilles	Plantar
RT	2+	2+	2+	2+	1+	↓
LT	2+	2+	2+	2+/2+	1+	↓

OR

Two methods of recording may be used, depending upon personal preference: a tabular form or a stick picture diagram, as at left. 2+ = brisk, or normal; see p. 116 for grading system.

ANALYZING DATA

VALIDATION

When they have completed and recorded the health history and physical examination, nurses begin formulating actual and potential nursing diagnoses to guide the planning, treatment, and evaluation of the client's care. One of the first steps of this process is validating the data collected from the health history and physical examination.

Validation of the data helps nurses to confirm or verify that the data collected are reliable and accurate. This process ensures the completion of planning and interventions with accurate, complete data to avoid errors during analysis. Not all data need to be validated—examples include the client's height and weight, pulse, respiratory sounds, and bowel sounds, to name a few. Occasionally, there may be a discrepancy between what the client reports and the physical examination findings. Such cases require nurses to perform another check to confirm the results. For example, a client reports never having surgery. Examination reveals that the same client has an abdominal surgical scar. It is important to check with the client to confirm that the information from the health history and the physical examination is accurate. Other instances where information needs to be validated include the following:

- *Incongruent subjective and objective data.* For example, the client may report feeling great about life but looks down and cries during the interview. Validating this information gives the nurse accurate information to ensure the development of an effective plan of care.

- *Inconsistent findings.* For example, a client is smiling and sitting with the legs crossed during the health history. The client's temperature is 40.0°C. Taking the time to confirm the data leads to more accurate analysis.

In the scenario for Mrs. N., the nurse would note that Mrs. N reported having a tonsillectomy and appendectomy in the health history. During the physical examination, the nurse would expect to find an abdominal scar in the lower right quadrant of the abdomen and absent tonsils. If these findings did not correlate with the information reported by Mrs. N., the nurse would need to validate the data.

Nurses have several options for validating data:

- Talk with the client and confirm that the recorded data were an accurate description of what he or she reported. Inform the client of the physical examination findings and ask for clarification. For example, "I notice that you have a scar on your abdomen that looks like it was from surgery. I recall you saying that you had not had any surgery. Please tell me about this scar." This encourages the client to help clarify the data. Often, clients have forgotten information or may think that the information is not necessary.

- Reassess the area of concern. For example, taking the client's temperature again with another thermometer validates the findings.

- Ask another nurse to check your findings if the data are incongruent or inconsistent.

After validating the data, the nurse checks to make sure there is no missing information or gaps. Then, he or she begins analyzing the data to formulate nursing diagnoses and plan interventions for the client.

DIAGNOSTIC REASONING AND NURSING DIAGNOSES

Diagnosis is the second step of the nursing process and is critical to identify actual and potential health concerns for the client. Once nurses have collected all the assessment data, they analyze their findings to develop nursing diagnoses.

A *nursing diagnosis* is "a clinical judgment about individuals, family or community responses to actual and potential health problems and life processes. A nursing diagnosis provides the basis for selecting nursing interventions to achieve outcomes for which the nurse is accountable" (North American Nursing Diagnosis Association International [NANDA-1], 2007, p. 332). The process of analyzing the data to formulate nursing diagnoses is called *diagnostic reasoning*.

DIAGNOSTIC REASONING AND CRITICAL THINKING

Data analysis can be challenging because nurses must interpret data accurately using diagnostic reasoning skills. This is a form of critical thinking. *Critical thinking* is the way nurses use experience, knowledge, intuition, and cognitive abilities to process the information to interpret the data and formulate conclusions that are the most appropriate decisions, options, or alternatives (Carpenito, 2005; Ignatavicius, 2001; Prideaux, 2000). Several characteristics are essential for thinking critically.

Nurses use critical thinking skills and clinical reasoning to analyze, interpret, and categorize data to identify appropriate nursing diagnoses for their clients based on the assessment data obtained from the health history and physical examination (Day, 2007).

NURSING DIAGNOSES

To select nursing diagnoses for their clients, nurses progress through several steps. Before beginning the analysis of the data to identify nursing diagnoses, nurses *determine* that the assessment data gathered are complete and validated.

Identify Deviations From Expected Findings. To *ensure* that the most appropriate nursing diagnoses are selected for the client, the nurse identifies all data that pose actual or potential health concerns from the assessment data. For example, some of the potential and actual issues for Mrs. N are as follows:

- "My head aches."

- "Increased pressure at work"

- Family history of cerebral vascular accident (CVA)

- Smoking history of 36 pack per day years

- Widow

- "Little savings"

- "Little exercise"

- Weight gain of about 5 kg in past 4 years

- "Feels tense and nervous"

- Limited outside support

This is an example of actual and potential issues for Mrs. N. After developing a complete list, the nurse identifies commonalities in the data and groups them together.

Grouping the Data. An analysis of the data gathered helps nurses to identify commonalities in them and then group the data together. Some groups of data include symptoms and signs related to a specific body system, such as smoking history, cough, shortness of breath, wheezing, and recent exposure to illness. Other groups of data include the psychosocial well-being of the client such as "avoids eye contact," crying, 10 kg weight gain in past year, and unkempt appearance. By grouping the data, the nurse can identify appropriate nursing diagnoses.

For Mrs. N., the nurse can group some of the data. For example, "my head aches," family history of CVA, and smoking history of 36 pack per day years are related to the potential development of a CVA.

Identify Possible Nursing Diagnoses. From the grouped data, the nurse can then begin to identify possible nursing diagnoses. Currently, NANDA-1 (2007) has 188 approved nursing diagnoses from which to select. Nurses infer from the grouped data and identify possible nursing diagnoses.

Each nursing diagnosis reflects seven axes:

1. The diagnostic concept

2. Subject of the diagnosis (individual, family, community)

3. Judgment (impaired, ineffective)

4. Location (e.g., bladder, auditory, cerebral)

5. Age (infant, child, adult)

6. Time (chronic, acute, intermittent)

7. Status of the diagnosis (actual, risk, wellness, health promotion)

(NANDA-1, 2007, p. 255)

One possible nursing diagnosis for Mrs. N. is ***Risk for ineffective cerebral tissue perfusion*** related to her family history, smoking history, and current symptoms ("my head aches").

From the data collected in the health history and physical examination, the nurse can identify several other possible nursing diagnoses. By grouping together "feels tense and nervous," "increased pressures at work," is a "widow," with "little savings," and "limited outside support," another possible nursing diagnosis would be:

Anxiety related to work pressures, being widowed with little savings, having limited outside support, as evidenced by Mrs. N's statement that "she feels tense and nervous."

By grouping "little exercise," "weight gain of about 5 kg in past 4 years," and "increased pressures at work," another possible nursing diagnosis would be:

Risk for imbalanced nutrition: more than body requirements related to lack of exercise, weight gain, and work pressures.

However, more data are needed in relation to Mrs. N's current weight, height, waist measurement, and body mass index before concluding that this nursing diagnosis would be appropriate.

Confirm or Exclude Nursing Diagnoses.

On completion of a list of possible nursing diagnoses, the nurse reviews the assessment data again to determine if any possible nursing diagnoses are not accurate. Then the nurse discusses each possible nursing diagnosis with the client and collaboratively confirms or excludes the diagnoses. Once the list of diagnoses is confirmed, the planning phase of the nursing process begins.

The processes of documenting findings, analyzing data, diagnostic reasoning, and formulating nursing diagnoses are challenging for beginning students. Nurses need considerable knowledge to group related symptoms and physical signs to formulate nursing diagnoses. Clinical experience, practice, knowledge, and development of critical thinking skills foster the attainment of the abilities to identify, analyze, and develop nursing diagnoses to ensure safe, effective nursing practice and client care.

ESSENTIAL ELEMENTS OF CRITICAL THINKING

- Keep an open mind.
- Use rationale to support opinions or decisions.
- Reflect on thoughts before reaching a conclusion.
- Use past clinical experiences to build knowledge.
- Acquire an adequate knowledge base that continues to build.
- Be aware of the interactions of others.
- Be aware of the environment.

Source: Weber & Kelley, 2007, p. 76.

Critical Thinking Exercise

- What type of data is collected during the health history? (*Knowledge*)
- Describe the differences between objective and subjective data. (*Comprehension*)
- Identify three possible nursing diagnoses for Mrs. N. (*Application*)

- Identify the seven axes in the following nursing diagnosis: "Potential for ineffective cerebral tissue perfusion." (*Analysis*):
- What recommendations for screening and follow-up would you suggest for Mrs. N? (*Synthesis*)
- How would you evaluate the accuracy of the nursing diagnoses identified for you client? (*Evaluation*)

Canadian Research

Howse, E., & Bailey, J. (1992). Resistance to documentation—A nursing research issue. *International Journal of Nursing Studies, 29*(4), 371-380.

Martin, A., Hinds, C., & Felix, M. (1999). Documentation practices of nurses in long-term care. *Journal of Clinical Nursing, 8* (4), 345-352.

Test Questions

1. Essential characteristics for the development of critical thinking skills include all of the following **except**:
   a. keeping an open mind.
   b. following instructions.
   c. using evidence to guide decisions.
   d. considering past experiences to plan appropriate actions.

2. Symptom analysis is recorded in which of the following sections of the health history:
   a. Personal and Social History
   b. Adult Illnesses
   c. Present Illness
   d. Family History

3. Examples of objective data include all of the following **except**:
   a. coughing.
   b. foul-smelling discharge.
   c. reddened skin.
   d. itchy skin.

4. When a client reports never having had surgery, yet physical examination reveals a 10-cm abdominal scar, the nurse needs to:
   a. confront the client.
   b. consider the client unreliable.
   c. validate the data.
   d. find a family member to give the health history.

5. All of the following associations develop the terminology for nursing diagnoses **except**:
   a. North American Nursing Diagnosis Association-International.
   b. Nursing Practice Standards International.
   c. Nursing Intervention Classification.
   d. Nursing Outcomes Classification.

Bibliography

CITATIONS

Carpenito, L. J. (2005). *Nursing diagnosis: Application to clinical practice* (11th ed.). Philadelphia: Lippincott Williams & Wilkins.

College & Association of Registered Nurses of Alberta. (2007). Documentation guidelines. *Alberta RN, 63*(1), 12–13. Edmonton, AB: Author.

Constantino, R. E. (2008). *Complete guide to documentation* (2nd ed.). Philadelphia: Lippincott Williams & Wilkins.

Day, R. A. (2007). Critical thinking, ethical decision making and the nursing process. In: R. A. Day, P. Paul, B. Williams, S. C. Smeltzer, & B. Bare (Eds.), *Brunner & Suddarth's textbook of medical-surgical nursing* (1st Canadian ed., pp. 21–42). Philadelphia: Lippincott Williams & Wilkins.

Ignatavicius, D. D. (2001). Six critical thinking skills for at-the-bedside success. *Nursing Management, 32*(1), 37–39.

Keatings, M., & Smith, O. B. (2000). *Ethical and legal issues in Canadian nursing* (2nd ed.). Toronto, ON, Canada: Elsevier.

North American Nursing Diagnosis Association International. (2007). *NANDA-I nursing diagnoses: Definitions and classifications 2007–2008* (7th ed.). Philadelphia: Author.

North American Nursing Diagnosis Association. (2005). *Nursing diagnoses: Definitions and classification, 2005–2006* (4th ed.). Philadelphia: Author.

Prideaux, D. (2000). Do you know? *Medical Teacher, 22*(6), 607.

Weber, J., & Kelley, J. H. (2007). *Health assessment in nursing* (3rd ed.). Philadelphia: Lippincott Williams & Wilkins.

ADDITIONAL RESOURCES

Agur, A. M. R., Dalley, A. F., Grant, J. C., & Boileau, J. C. (2005). *Grant's atlas anatomy* (11th ed.). Philadelphia: Lippincott Williams & Wilkins.

Barker, L. R., Burton, J. R., & Zieve, P. D. (Eds.). (2003). *Principles of ambulatory medicine* (6th ed.). Philadelphia: Lippincott Williams & Wilkins.

Berne, R. M. (2004). *Physiology* (5th ed.). St. Louis: Mosby.

Cassel, C., Leipzig, R. M., Cohen, H. J., Larson, E. B., & Meier, D. E. (2003). *Geriatric medicine: An evidence-based approach* (4th ed.). New York: Springer.

Gray, H., Standring, S., Ellis, H., & Berkovitz, B. K. B. (2005). *Gray's anatomy: The anatomical basis of clinical practice* (39th ed.). New York: Elsevier–Churchill Livingstone.

Guyton, A. C., & Hall, J. E. (2005). *Textbook of medical physiology* (11th ed.). Philadelphia: W.B. Saunders.

Hazzard, W. R. (2003). *Principles of geriatric medicine and gerontology* (5th ed.). New York: McGraw-Hill Professional.

Kasper, D. L., & Harrison, T. R. (Eds.). (2005). *Harrison's principles of internal medicine* (16th ed.). New York: McGraw-Hill.

Mandell, G. L. (2004). *Essential atlas of infectious diseases* (3rd ed.). Philadelphia: Current Medicine.

Moore, K. L., Dalley, A. F., & Agur, A. M. R. (2006). *Clinically oriented anatomy* (5th ed.). Baltimore: Lippincott Williams & Wilkins.

Orient, J. M., & Sapira, J. D. (Eds.). (2005). *Sapira's art & science of bedside diagnosis* (3rd ed.). Philadelphia: Lippincott Williams & Wilkins.

Potter, P. A., Perry, A. G., Ross-Kerr, J. C., & Wood, M. J. (Eds.). (2006). *Canadian fundamentals of nursing* (3rd ed.). Toronto, ON, Canada: Elsevier.

Youngkin, E. Q., & Davis, M. S. (2004). *Women's health: A primary care clinical guide* (3rd ed.). Upper Saddle River, NJ: Pearson/Prentice Hall, 2004.

CANADIAN ASSOCIATIONS AND WEB SITES

Canada's Health Informatics Association: http://www.coachorg.com/

Canadian Nurses Association: http://www.cna-aiic.ca/CNA/practice/standards/default_e.aspx

Canadian Nurses Protective Society (CNPS): www.cnps.ca

College of Registered Nurses of British Columbia: http://www.crnbc.ca/NursingPractice/Requirements/PracticeStandards.aspx

College of Registered Nurses of Ontario: http://www.cno.org/prac/learn/modules/documentation/slides/MeetingStandards.pdf

College of Registered Nurses of Nova Scotia: http://www.crnns.ca/documents/CRNNS%20Documentation%20Guidelines%202005.pdf

College of Registered Nurses of Alberta: http://www.nurses.ab.ca/Carna-Admin/Uploads/Documentation%20for%20Registered%20Nurses.pdf

Personal Information Protection and Electronic Documents Act: http://laws.justice.gc.ca/en/P-8.6/258031.html

6

General Survey and Vital Signs

D. Lynn Skillen and Lynn S. Bickley

Conducting the *general survey* and measuring the *vital signs* allow health providers to screen all body systems. Findings provide clues regarding the general health of a client as well as the body's response to psychological or physiological changes. The screening becomes the foundation of your assessment of the client's general state of health, growth and development, specific physical health needs, health-promotion requirements, safety needs, functional abilities, and psychosocial status. It precedes a more thorough application of all four basic examination modes (inspection, palpation, percussion, and auscultation) during the physical examination. Nurses use the general survey and vital signs to detect health deviations, monitor changes over time, and evaluate the effectiveness of interventions. They look for correlation between the observations from the general survey and vital signs, and are alert to any inconsistencies.

Inspection during the general survey begins with the very first encounter with your client, even before you initiate the health history interview (see Chapter 3). It continues throughout the health history. The general survey and vital signs are components of the first part of your documentation of the physical examination (identifying data is the first part) (see Chapter 5). The quality of the data collected from your general survey and vital signs governs the next steps that you take when you complete the physical examination using the time-honoured skills of inspection, palpation, percussion, and auscultation (see Chapter 4) for selected systems, regions, and topics (see Chapters 7–25).

Over the course of becoming an accomplished examiner, you will polish important observational skills for a lifetime. Your ability to perform a thorough general survey and accurately measure vital signs improves with practice. This chapter presents you with the essential elements and scope of the general survey and the importance and measurement of vital signs. It broadens the traditional approach to vital signs and includes client characteristics to scrutinize, techniques to apply, guidelines for interpretation, and examples of the recordings. Mastery of this component in the three critical foundational areas (health history, physical examination, and documentation) facilitates interdisciplinary communication and best practices for health assessment.

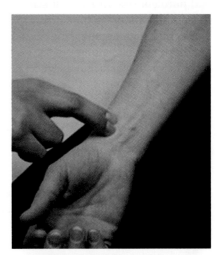

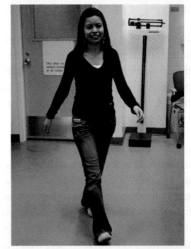

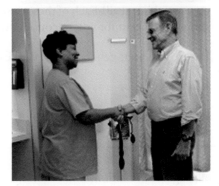

GENERAL SURVEY: INSPECTION

INTEGRATION OF SENSES (VISUAL, OLFACTORY, AND AUDITORY)

During the general survey, nurses acquire information about the client's physical, emotional, mental, social, and cultural state as well as his or her gender, ethnic background, and ability level—all information that directs the examination of systems, regions, and topics. Even before seeing your client, your senses of hearing and smell are collecting client information. You can detect many different odours with your sense of smell (olfaction)—for example, alcohol, ammonia, body odour, feces, halitosis, ketones, mustiness, urine, apocrine and eccrine perspiration, emesis, and purulent discharge. Your sense of hearing will detect accents, type of speech, speech alterations (e.g., slurring), level of vocabulary used, strength of voice, whispering, sighing, moaning, raspiness, breath sounds, Grade VI heart murmurs, and borborygmi, among others. Using your visual sense in the opening moments with the client, you begin the general survey of the client's build, height, and weight, but your observations of the client's appearance crystallize as you start the physical examination. Many factors contribute to the client's body habitus—socioeconomic status, nutrition, genetic makeup, degree of fitness, mood state, early illnesses, outstanding anatomical malformations, substance abuse, client abuse, insight and judgment, clothing, gender, geographic location, body type, and age cohort.

Nutritional status affects many of the characteristics that you scrutinize during the general survey. These include posture, mood and alertness, facial colouration, dentition and condition of the tongue and gingiva, colour of the nail beds, and muscle bulk, to name a few.

SCOPE OF GENERAL SURVEY

Nurses continually sharpen their powers of observation and description using their visual, auditory, and olfactory senses. It is important to heighten the acuity of your clinical perceptions of the client's mood, build, and behaviour. These details enrich and deepen your emerging clinical impression. When you become a skilled observer, you will describe distinguishing features of the client's general appearance so well in words that a colleague could spot the client in a crowd of strangers.

As you selectively scrutinize characteristics of the client using general inspection, recapture the observations that you made in the first moments of your interaction and sharpen them throughout your general survey. For example, does the client hear you when greeted in the examination area? Rise with ease? Walk easily or stiffly? If the client is hospitalized when you first meet, what is the client doing—sitting up and enjoying television? . . . lying in bed? . . . What occupies the bedside table—a magazine? . . . a flock of "get well" cards? . . . a Bible or a rosary? . . . an emesis basin? . . . or nothing at all? Each of these observations raises one or more tentative queries about your client for you to consider during your assessment.

Ensure that your general survey of the client includes the following categories:

- Apparent age

- Apparent state of health

- Level of consciousness

- Cognitive functions

- Insight, judgment, and thought processes

- Signs of distress

- Height, weight, and build

- Skin colour and lesions

- Dress, grooming, and personal hygiene

- Facial expression

- Odours

- Posture, gait, and motor activity

TECHNIQUES OF EXAMINATION

Apparent Age.   Although ability to evaluate age may vary widely, use your experience of others who are older, similar, or younger in age than you to assess apparent age. Consider hair colouring, skin smoothness, mobility, mode and type of dress, style of speech, types of skin lesions, and vascularity of hands.

Appearance not congruent with chronologic age.

Apparent State of Health.   Try to make a general clinical judgment based on observations throughout the encounter. Support it with the significant details.

Acutely or chronically ill, frail.

Level of Consciousness.   Is the client awake, alert, and responsive to you and others in the environment? Look for eyes opening spontaneously, an oriented verbal response, and motor response to your request. If not, assess the level of consciousness.

Irritability; eyes open only to speech, pain stimulus, or not at all; verbal response is confused, inappropriate, incomprehensible, or absent; motor response to localized pain stimulus, flexion, extension, or is flaccid.

Cognitive Functions, Insight, Judgment, and Thought Processes. Does the client seem to understand your questions and respond appropriately? Does the client recall important information and events?

Memory impairment, shortened attention span, disorientation, reduced capacity for abstract thinking, illogical problem solving.

Signs of Distress.   Does the client show evidence of health deviations, such as:

- Cardiac or respiratory distress

Clutching the chest, pallor, diaphoresis; laboured breathing, wheezing, coughing.

- Pain

Wincing, sweating, protectiveness of painful area.

- Anxiety or depression

Anxious face, fidgety movements, cold and moist palms; inexpressive or flat affect, limited eye contact, psychomotor slowing.

Height and Build.   During the general survey, you are not yet taking measurements (see Chapter 8). Does the client appear unusually short or tall? Is the build slender and lanky, muscular, or stocky? Is the client's body symmetrical? Note the general body proportions and look for any deformities.

Very short stature is seen in *Turner's syndrome,* childhood *renal failure,* and *achondroplastic and hypopituitary dwarfism.* Long limbs in proportion to the trunk are seen in *hypogonadism* and *Marfan's syndrome.* Height loss occurs with *osteoporosis* and vertebral compression fractures.

Weight. You are not yet measuring the weight (see Chapter 8). Does the client appear emaciated, slender, plump, obese, or somewhere in between? If the client is obese, is the fat distributed evenly or concentrated over the trunk, over the upper torso, or around the hips?

Causes of weight loss include malignancy, diabetes mellitus, hyperthyroidism, chronic infection, depression, diuresis, and successful dieting.

Generalized fat in simple *obesity*; truncal fat with relatively thin limbs in *Cushing's syndrome* and *metabolic (insulin-resistance) syndrome.*

Skin Colour and Obvious Lesions. Genetic background, outdoor occupations and/or sports, and illness states affect the skin colour (see Chapter 10). Illness states and age-related changes affect presence of skin lesions.

Pallor, cyanosis, jaundice, rashes, bruises.

Dress, Grooming, and Personal Hygiene. How is the client dressed? Is clothing appropriate to the temperature, weather, region, or occupation? Is it clean, properly buttoned, and zipped? How does it compare with clothing worn by people of comparable age and social group?

Excess clothing may reflect the cold intolerance of *hypothyroidism*, hide skin rash or needle marks, or signal personal lifestyle preferences.

Glance at the client's shoes. Have holes been cut in them? Are the laces tied, or is the client wearing slippers?

Cut-out holes or slippers may indicate *gout*, bunions, or other painful foot conditions. Untied laces or slippers also suggest edema.

Is the client wearing any unusual jewellery? Where? Is there any body piercing? Tattooing?

Copper bracelets are sometimes worn for *arthritis*. Piercing or tattooing may appear on any part of the body.

Note the client's hair, fingernails, and use of cosmetics. They may be clues to the client's personality, mood, or lifestyle. Nail polish and hair colouring that have "grown out" may signify decreased interest in personal appearance.

"Grown-out" hair and nail polish can help you estimate the length of an illness if the client cannot give a history. Fingernails chewed to the quick may reflect stress.

Do personal hygiene and grooming seem appropriate to the client's age, lifestyle, occupation, and socioeconomic group? These are norms that vary widely, of course.

Unkempt appearance may be seen in *depression* and *dementia*, but this appearance must be compared with the client's probable norm.

Facial Expression. Observe the facial expression at rest, during conversation about specific topics, during the physical examination, and in interaction with others. Watch for eye contact. Is it natural? Sustained and unblinking? Averted quickly? Absent?

The stare of *hyperthyroidism*; the immobile face of *parkinsonism*; the flat or sad affect of *depression*. Decreased eye contact may be cultural, or may suggest anxiety, fear, or sadness.

Odours of the Body and Breath. Odours can be important diagnostic clues, such as the fruity odour of diabetes or the scent of alcohol. The CAGE questions, p. 4 will help you determine possible misuse of alcohol.

Breath odours of alcohol, acetone (*diabetes*), pulmonary infections, uremia, or liver failure.

Never assume that alcohol on a client's breath explains changes in mental status or neurologic findings.

People with alcoholism may have other serious and potentially correctable problems such as hypoglycemia, subdural hematoma, or postictal state.

Posture, Gait, and Motor Activity. What is the client's preferred posture?

Preference for sitting up in left-sided heart failure and for leaning forward with arms braced in chronic obstructive pulmonary disease.

Is the client restless or quiet? How often does the client change position? How fast are the movements?

Is there any apparent involuntary motor activity? Are some body parts immobile? Which ones?

Does the client walk smoothly, with comfort, self-confidence, and balance; if not, is there a limp or discomfort, fear of falling, loss of balance, or any movement disorder?

Fast, frequent movements of hyperthyroidism; slowed activity of hypothyroidism.

Tremors or other involuntary movements: paralyses. See Table 20-3, Involuntary Movements (pp. 744–745).

Movements appear painful. See Table, Deviations in Gait and Posture (pp. 754–755).

DOCUMENTATION

Objective Data. See Chapter 5 for principles of documentation. When describing results of the general survey, choose vivid and graphic adjectives. Avoid clichés (e.g., "in no acute distress") because they could apply to anyone and do not convey this client's special features. Avoid evaluative comments such as "good colour," "poor hygiene," and "well-nourished."

EXAMPLE OF GENERAL SURVEY

C. M. Swarts is an elderly male of European ancestry who looks pale and chronically ill. He is alert but cautious, making frequent, fleeting eye contact. He cannot speak more than two or three words at a time due to shortness of breath. He speaks with a dry mouth and an accent. Intercostal muscle retraction occurs with inspiration, and he sits bolt upright in bed.

He is thin, with diffused muscle wasting. Wearing clean pyjamas, he smells of baby powder. His sparse yellowish hair is shaved close to the scalp. He has a number tattooed on his left wrist and a slight tremor of his left hand at rest. Fingernails of his right hand are opaque, yellowed, and thick, but nails of both hands are trimmed.

◼ VITAL SIGNS

Traditionally, measurements of the blood pressure, heart rate, respiratory rate, and temperature constituted the vital signs. Only these four were taken when nurses and other health care providers first initiated the physical examination. You assess them using inspection, palpation, and auscultation.

In the past two decades, researchers have suggested that the four vital signs be amplified. In 1995, Fiore et al. argued that smoking status should be a new vital sign. Lockwood, Conroy-Hiller, and Page (2004) found support for this in a systematic review of the literature. Pain (Jackson, 2002) (see Chapter 7) and functional ability (see Chapter 25) are commonly considered to be the fifth and sixth vital signs. Measurements of these two additional signs are both subjective and objective.

Canadian researchers propose that distress levels, measured by questionnaire, be considered the sixth vital sign for cancer patients (Alberta Heritage Foundation for Medical Research, 2008). Lockwood et al. (2004) considered pulse oximetry (oxygen saturation) and smoking status to be vital signs that were shown by the systematic review to affect client outcomes. Their review raised issues about assessing respiratory and pulse rates and emphasized the importance of correct technique for taking all measurements. Research may ultimately change the vital signs to be measured or the new digital technologies used to do so. For example, stethoscopes may be replaced with MP3 recorder/players, "smart textiles" with electrophysical properties, self-monitoring with wireless technology (e.g., see Skjodt & Hodgetts, 2008).

The vital signs provide initial information about the cardiovascular, respiratory, neurological, and endocrine systems—information that may be vital for life support, directive for interventions to improve health, and useful for health promotion education. The body's metabolic rate (rate of metabolism of nutrients and production of energy) affects the vital signs. In healthy people, sleep reduces and exercise increases the results obtained.

Always consider the physical and psychosocial environments in which you are measuring the vital signs. The *physical* environment may be noisy, hot, cold, muggy, dry, excessively illuminated, damp, mouldy, drafty, and more. As an example, in a loud or noisy environment, your client's heart rate and blood pressure may be elevated. Similarly, the *psychosocial* environment may affect the measurements. For example, too many people present, intimidating individuals, or contentious relations can all affect your results. It is always wise not to base decisions on one measurement. Do everything possible to take vital signs on a relaxed client, in a comfortable and quiet environment.

You may find that the vital signs are already taken and recorded in the client's record. If beyond expected parameters, you may wish to repeat the measurements yourself. You can also take them later as you start your examination of the cardiovascular system and the thorax and lungs, but often the vital signs provide important preliminary information that influences the direction of your evaluation.

EQUIPMENT FOR TAKING VITAL SIGNS

- Sphygmomanometer (aneroid, mercury, or digital [electronic])
- Stethoscope (acoustic [dual-frequency] or digital)
- Thermometer (mercury, tympanic, or digital)
- Pain Assessment Scale(s) (all ages)
- Functional Assessment Scale(s) (older adults)

PROMOTION OF CLIENT COMFORT, DIGNITY, AND SAFETY

Ensure that your client is in a comfortable position and can see your face clearly and hear your explanations. Assist your client to move without risk of falling or injury. You may need to ask accompanying individuals to wait in another area while you take the vital signs. Perform hand hygiene. Only expose what is absolutely necessary to ensure correct techniques are followed. You may need to cover some areas with a towel, drape, or flannel sheet. Keep the environment quiet and warm. Be patient if your client is slow to understand or move according to your instructions. Never leave a confused, weak, combative, or uncooperative client unsupervised or alone on an unprotected examination surface. Disinfect the bell or diaphragm of your stethoscope with alcohol after use.

SEQUENCE OF TAKING VITAL SIGNS

Assess the client's level of pain (see Chapter 7). Remember that pain causes alterations in all vital signs measurements. Check either the blood pressure or the pulse next.

If the blood pressure is high, measure it again later in the examination. When taking the pulse, place your fingers on the radial pulse or your stethoscope on the cardiac apex and count the rate. Continue keeping your fingers on the client's radial pulse or your stethoscope on the client's chest and then count the respiratory rate. By doing this, the client is not alerted to the nurse counting the respiratory rate. This is important because a client's breathing patterns may change if he or she becomes aware that you are watching the respirations.

Take the client's temperature using a single-use thermometer, digital electronic probe, tympanic thermometer, or mercury thermometer. The type of thermometer used depends on the availability of equipment, the age, and condition of the client. Consider the safety of the client, and do not use oral thermometers for clients with decreased capacity for understanding. As mercury is toxic, be sure to handle the glass thermometer carefully to prevent breakage. In the event that you drop a thermometer, follow approved mercury cleanup procedures immediately.

If your client is an older adult, complete a functional assessment. Consider the environment, context of your examination, age of your client, and level of pain when interpreting your findings, and make a decision about subsequent measurements. Remember that one measurement may be misleading.

BLOOD PRESSURE

Blood Pressure Cuff (Sphygmomanometer). Blood pressure results from the pressure of blood on the arteries as it is pumped through the body. The systolic blood pressure (SBP) results when the heart contracts and actively pumps blood into the arterial system. When the heart relaxes after the contraction, it results in diastolic pressure. All adult clients should be assessed by health professionals who have been specifically trained to accurately measure blood pressure (Canadian Hypertension Education Program [CHEP], 2008; http://www.hypertension.ca/chep) to determine cardiovascular risk and schedule monitoring of antihypertensive treatment.

Choice of blood pressure cuff is important for accuracy and detection of hypertension. As many as 5 million Canadians have elevated blood pressure (Blood Pressure Canada, 2008; CHEP, 2008). To measure blood pressure accurately, you must choose a cuff of appropriate size. The blood pressure gauge may be the mercury, aneroid, or digital type. The mercury sphygmomanometer is the gold standard that does not require recalibration; the aneroid instrument can become inaccurate with repeated use and should be recalibrated regularly. Because of environmental safety concerns with the use of mercury, many health care facilities use digital or aneroid sphygmomanometers.

Cuffs that are too short or too narrow may give falsely high readings. Using a regular-size cuff on an obese arm may lead to a false diagnosis of hypertension.

In addition to proper cuff size for the size of the arm, other factors that influence measurements of blood pressure include emotions, posture, activity, medications, diet, temperature, talking while the blood pressure is being taken, and alcohol consumption. When using an automated instrument for measuring blood pressure,

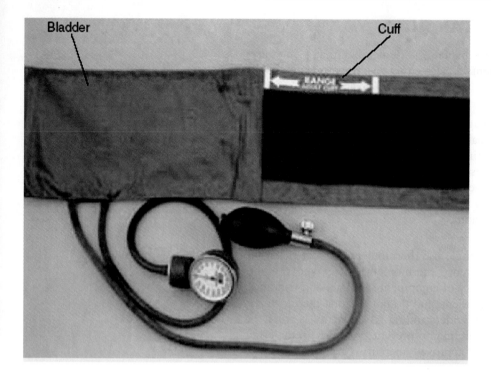

follow the recommendations for cuff size made by the manufacturer. Electronic instruments are practical for noisy environments and when frequent measurements are required.

Technique for Measuring Blood Pressure. Before assessing the blood pressure, you should take several steps to make sure your measurement will be accurate. Proper technique is important and reduces the inherent variability arising from the client, examiner, equipment, or procedure itself. The techniques that follow include the CHEP recommendations, which are evaluated annually (CHEP, 2008).

PREPARATION FOR MEASURING BLOOD PRESSURE

- Ideally, instruct the client to avoid smoking or drinking caffeinated beverages for 30 minutes before you are going to measure the blood pressure.
- Make sure the examining environment is quiet and comfortably warm.
- Ask the client to sit quietly for at least 5 minutes in a chair, rather than on the examining table, with feet on the floor. This position influences decisions about interventions. Measurements may be taken with the client supine if he or she is elderly or has diabetes. Use the standing position to examine for postural hypotension.
- Make sure the arm you select is *free of clothing*. Clothing can interfere with the cuff pressure and with your hearing of the Korotkoff sounds.
- The arm should have no arteriovenous fistulas from dialysis, scarring from prior brachial artery cutdowns, signs of lymphedema (seen after axillary node dissection), or radiation therapy. Also, do not measure blood pressure on the same side as a mastectomy or if an intravenous line is in place in the arm.

(Continued)

PREPARATION FOR MEASURING BLOOD PRESSURE (Cont'd)

- Support and position the arm so that the brachial artery, at the antecubital crease, is *at heart level*—roughly level with the fourth interspace at its junction with the sternum.
- Palpate the brachial artery to confirm that it has a viable pulse.
- If the client is seated, rest the arm on a table a little above the client's waist; if standing, try to support the client's arm at the midchest level.
- Select a sphygmomanometer known to be accurate, such as a recently calibrated aneroid or electronic instrument.
- Ensure the aneroid face head or mercury column are clearly visible at your eye level.
- Ask the client to avoid talking during the procedure.

If the brachial artery is much below heart level, systolic and diastolic blood pressures appear falsely high. The client's own effort to support the arm may raise the blood pressure.

Now you are ready to measure the blood pressure.

- Centre the inflatable bladder over the brachial artery. The lower border of the cuff should be 3 cm above the antecubital crease. Secure the cuff snugly. Position the client's arm so that it is slightly flexed at the elbow.

- To determine how high to raise the cuff pressure, first estimate the systolic pressure by palpation. As you feel the radial artery with the fingers of one hand, rapidly inflate the cuff until the radial pulse disappears. Read this pressure on the manometer and add 30 mm Hg to it. Using this sum as the target for subsequent inflations prevents discomfort from unnecessarily high cuff pressures. It also avoids the occasional error caused by a *systolic auscultatory gap*—a silent interval.

An unrecognized auscultatory gap may lead to serious underestimation of systolic pressure (e.g., 150/98 in the example that follows) or overestimation of diastolic pressure.

- Deflate the cuff promptly and completely, and wait 15 to 30 seconds.

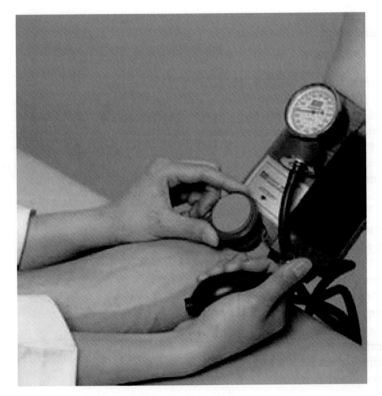

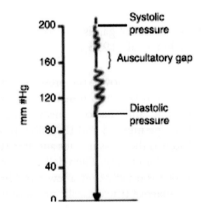

- Now place the bell or diaphragm of a stethoscope lightly over the brachial artery, taking care to make an air seal with the full bell rim. Because the *Korotkoff sounds* ("whooshing" sounds) to be heard are relatively low in pitch, they may be heard better with the bell chestpiece, but CHEP suggests using either chestpiece.

If you find an auscultatory gap, record your findings completely (e.g., 200/98 with an auscultatory gap from 170 to 150).

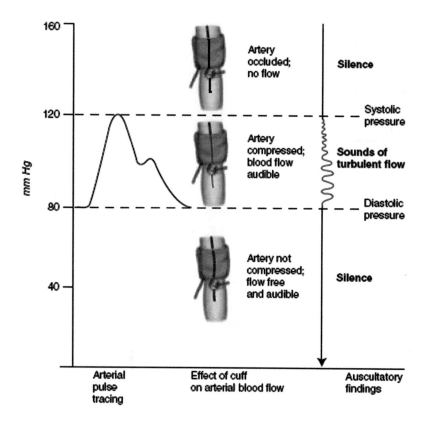

An auscultatory gap is associated with arterial stiffness and atherosclerotic disease (Cavallini et al., 1996).

- Continue to lower the pressure, opening the control valve so you achieve a cuff deflation rate of 2 mm Hg per heartbeat. This is important for estimating the systolic and diastolic measurements accurately. Continue until the sounds become muffled and then disappear. To confirm the disappearance of sounds, listen as the pressure falls another 10 to 20 mm Hg. This also excludes a *diastolic auscultatory gap.* Then deflate the cuff rapidly to zero. The disappearance point, which is usually only a few mm Hg below the muffling point, provides the best estimate of true diastolic pressure in adults.

In some people, the muffling point and the disappearance point are farther apart. Occasionally, as in aortic regurgitation, the sounds never disappear. If the difference is more than 10 mm Hg, record both figures (e.g., 154/80/68).

- Record both the systolic and the diastolic levels to the nearest 2 mm Hg. Do not round up or round down, which may make the reading inaccurate.

- To avoid venous congestion in the venous system, wait 2 or more minutes and repeat twice. Avoiding slow or repetitive inflations of the cuff reduces the risk of venous congestion, which can cause false readings.

- Discard the first reading and average your next two readings. If the first two readings differ by more than 5 mm Hg, take additional readings. Ensure that you record not only the reading but also the position of the client.

- When using a mercury sphygmomanometer, keep the manometer vertical (unless you are using a tilted floor model) and make all readings at eye level with the meniscus. When using an aneroid instrument, hold the dial so that it faces you directly.

- Blood pressure should be taken in both arms at least once. Usually, there is a difference of 5 mm Hg in pressure and sometimes up to 10 mm Hg. Make subsequent readings on the arm with the higher pressure.

- Blood pressure measurement may not include all the above steps if an automated (electronic) device is used.

Classification of Blood Pressure (Nonhypertensive to Hypertensive).
The optimal blood pressure is an SBP less than 120 mm Hg and a diastolic blood pressure (DBP) less than 80 mm Hg (Tanne, 2003). According to Blood Pressure Canada (2008), a blood pressure reading between 130/85 and 139/89 is considered to be "high normal."

The Canadian Hypertension Education Program advocates for sustained lifestyle modification to prevent and manage hypertension and cardiovascular disease. Under CHEP (see www.hypertension.ca/chep), clients are advised to

- Eat more fresh fruits and vegetables.

- Eat at restaurants less often and request that less salt be used.

- Use fewer sauces.

- Eat foods with less than 100 mg of sodium per serving.

- Have a dietary sodium intake under 2300 mg per day.

- Avoid using salt in cooking.

- Avoid heavily salted foods (e.g., pickled foods, processed meats).

In the 2008 Canadian Recommendations for the Management of Hypertension by CHEP, clients can be diagnosed as hypertensive if the SBP is 160 mm Hg or greater, the DBP is 100 mm Hg or greater *averaged across the first three office visits*, or if the SBP averages 140 mm Hg or greater or the DBP averages 90 mm Hg or greater after five visits (*Grade D level of evidence, which means that no randomized clinical trials are available to support this*). The Canadian position regarding a diagnosis of hypertension is now to average readings across several office visits and to determine target pressures according to client health states of diabetes, chronic kidney disease, diastolic and/or systolic hypertension, or isolated systolic hypertension (see www.hypertension.ca/chep).

Always interpret relatively low levels of blood pressure in the light of past readings and the client's present clinical state.

If indicated, assess *orthostatic (postural) blood pressure* (see Chapter 25, p. 889). Measure blood pressure and heart rate with the client in two positions—supine after the client is resting up to 10 minutes, then within 3 minutes after the client stands

---

By making the sounds less audible, venous congestion may produce artificially low systolic and high diastolic pressures.

Pressure difference of more than 10–15 mm Hg between arms suggests arterial compression or obstruction on the side with the lower pressure.

Assessment of hypertension also includes its effects on target organs—the eyes, heart, brain, and kidneys. Look for evidence of hypertensive retinopathy, left ventricular hypertrophy, and neurologic deficits suggesting a stroke. Renal assessment requires urinalysis and blood tests.

A pressure of 110/70 mm Hg would usually be within expected parameters, but could also indicate significant hypotension if past pressures have been high.

A fall in systolic pressure of 20 mm Hg or more, especially when accompanied by symptoms,

up. Usually, as the client rises from the horizontal to the standing position, systolic pressure drops slightly or remains unchanged, whereas diastolic pressure rises slightly.

SPECIAL SITUATIONS

Weak or Inaudible Korotkoff Sounds.   Consider technical problems such as erroneous placement of your stethoscope, failure to make full skin contact with the bell, and venous engorgement of the client's arm from repeated inflations of the cuff. Consider also the possibility of shock.

When you cannot hear Korotkoff sounds at all, you may be able to estimate the systolic pressure by palpation. Alternative methods such as Doppler techniques or direct arterial pressure tracings may be necessary.

To intensify Korotkoff sounds, one of the following methods may be helpful:

- Raise the client's arm before and while you inflate the cuff. Then lower the arm and determine the blood pressure.

- Inflate the cuff. Ask the client to make a fist several times, and then determine the blood pressure.

Arrhythmias.   Irregular rhythms produce variations in pressure and therefore unreliable measurements. Ignore the effects of an occasional premature contraction. With frequent premature contractions or atrial fibrillation, determine the average of several observations and note that your measurements are approximate.

Clients Who Are Anxious and "White Coat" Hypertension.
Anxiety is a frequent cause of DBP readings that are higher than those at home or during usual activities, occurring in 12% to 25% of clients (Bobrie et al., 2001; Kaplan & Rose, 2004). This effect may occur on several occasions. Try to relax the client and measure the blood pressure again later in the encounter.

Clients Who Are Obese or Very Thin.   For the obese arm, it is important to use a wide cuff of 15 cm. If the arm circumference exceeds 41 cm, use a thigh cuff of 18 cm. For the very thin arm, a pediatric cuff may be indicated.

Clients With Hypertension and Unequal Blood Pressures in the Arms and Legs.   To detect coarctation of the aorta, make two further blood pressure measurements at least once in every client with hypertension:

- Compare blood pressures in the arms and legs.

- Compare the volume and timing of the radial and femoral pulses. Usually, volume is equal and the pulses occur simultaneously.

To determine blood pressure in the leg, use a wide, long thigh cuff that has a bladder size of 18 × 42 cm and apply it to the midthigh. Centre the bladder over the posterior surface, wrap it securely, and listen over the popliteal artery. If possible, the client should be prone. Alternatively, ask the supine client to flex one leg slightly with the heel resting on the bed. When cuffs of the proper size are used for both the leg and the arm, blood pressures should be equal in the two areas. If an arm cuff is improperly used on the leg, it gives a falsely high reading.

indicates orthostatic (postural) hypotension. Orthostatic hypotension is a drop in SBP of ≤20 mm Hg or in DBP of ≤10 mm Hg within 3 minutes of standing (Carlson, 1999).

Causes include medications such as antihypertensive drugs, loss of blood, prolonged bed rest, chronic low blood pressure, and diseases of the autonomic nervous system.

Isolated home or ambulatory hypertension, unlike isolated hypertension in an examination environment, is associated with increased risk for cardiovascular disease (Bobrie et al., 2001; Clement et al., 2003; Kaplan & Rose, 2004).

Use of a cuff that is too small can lead to overestimation of SBP in obese clients.

Coarctation of the aorta arises from narrowing of the thoracic aorta, usually proximal but sometimes distal to the left subclavian artery. Coarctation of the aorta and occlusive aortic disease are distinguished by hypertension in the upper extremities and low blood pressure in the legs and by diminished or delayed femoral pulses (Brickner, Hillis, & Lange, 2000).

HEART RATE AND RHYTHM

Examine the arterial pulses, heart rate and rhythm, and the amplitude and contour of the pulse wave. See Table 6-1 Alterations of the Arterial Pulse and Pressure Waves (p. 145).

Heart Rate.   The radial pulse is commonly used to assess the heart rate. With the pads of your index and middle fingers, compress the radial artery until a maximal pulsation is detected. If the rhythm is regular and the rate seems within expected parameters, count the rate for 15 seconds and multiply by 4. If the rate is unusually fast or slow, count it for a full 60 seconds.

When the rhythm is irregular, evaluate the heart rate by cardiac auscultation. Beats that occur earlier than others may not be detected peripherally, and the heart rate can thus be seriously underestimated.

Irregular rhythms include atrial fibrillation and premature atrial or ventricular contractions (PACs and PVCs).

Rhythm.   To begin your assessment of rhythm, feel the radial pulse. If there are any irregularities, check the rhythm again by listening with your stethoscope at the cardiac apex. Is the rhythm regular or irregular? If irregular, try to identify a pattern: (1) Do early beats appear in a basically regular rhythm? (2) Does the irregularity vary consistently with respiration? (3) Is the rhythm totally irregular?

See Table 15-1, Selected Heart Rates and Rhythms (p. 467) and Table 15-2, Selected Irregular Rhythms (p. 468).

RESPIRATORY RATE

Observe the *rate, rhythm, depth,* and *effort of breathing.* Count the number of respirations in 1 minute either by visual inspection or by subtly listening over the client's trachea with your stethoscope during your examination of the head and neck or chest. Usually, adults take 14 to 20 breaths per minute in a quiet, regular pattern. An occasional sigh is to be expected. Check to see if expiration is prolonged.

See Table 6-2, Alterations in Rate and Rhythm of Breathing (p. 146).

Prolonged expiration suggests narrowing in the bronchioles.

TEMPERATURE

Although you may choose to omit measuring the temperature in ambulatory clients, you should check it whenever you suspect an alteration in health. The average *oral temperature,* usually quoted at 37°C, fluctuates considerably as a result of clients' metabolic rate and the time of day. In the early morning, temperature may fall as low as 35.8°C, and in the late afternoon or evening, it may rise as high as 37.3°C from muscular activity and food intake. *Rectal temperatures* are *higher* than oral temperatures by an average of 0.4 to 0.5°C and are the most accurate. In contrast, *axillary temperatures* are *lower* than oral temperatures by approximately 1°C but take 5 to 10 minutes to register and are generally considered less accurate than other measurements. Research as early as 1992 has shown that 36.8°C is the mean or average temperature of a healthy adult (see publications listed at http://hypertextbook.com/facts/LenaWong.shtml).

Fever (pyrexia) refers to an elevated body temperature. *Hyperpyrexia* refers to extreme elevation in temperature, above 41.1°C, whereas *hypothermia* refers to an abnormally low temperature, below 35°C rectally.

Most clients prefer oral to rectal temperatures. Taking oral temperatures is not recommended, however, when clients are unconscious, restless, or unable to close their mouths. Temperature readings may be inaccurate, and thermometers may be broken by unexpected movements of the client's jaw. Client safety must always be considered when selecting the type of thermometer.

Rapid respiratory rates tend to increase the discrepancy between oral and rectal temperatures. In this situation, rectal temperatures are more reliable.

For *oral temperatures*, you may choose a mercury (glass), single-use, or digital electronic thermometer. When using a glass thermometer, shake the thermometer down to 35°C or below, insert it under the tongue, instruct the client to close both lips, and wait 3 to 5 minutes. Then read the thermometer, reinsert it for a minute, and read it again. If the temperature is still rising, repeat this procedure until the reading remains stable. Note that hot or cold liquids, and even smoking, can alter the temperature reading. In these situations, it is best to delay measuring the temperature for 10 to 15 minutes.

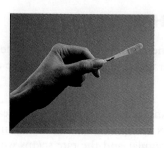

If using an electronic thermometer, carefully place the disposable cover over the probe and insert the thermometer under the tongue. Ask the client to close both lips, and then watch closely for the digital readout. An accurate temperature reading usually takes about 10 seconds.

For a *rectal temperature,* ask the client to lie on one side with the hip flexed. Select a rectal thermometer with a stubby tip, lubricate it, and insert it about 3 to 4 cm into the anal canal, in a direction pointing toward the umbilicus. Remove it after 3 minutes and read. Alternatively, use an electronic thermometer after lubricating the probe cover. Wait about 10 seconds for the digital temperature recording to appear. Single-use rectal thermometers are also available.

Taking the *tympanic membrane temperature* is an increasingly common practice, and is quick, safe, and reliable if performed properly. Use an otoscope to ensure the external auditory canal is free of cerumen. Position the probe in the canal so that the infrared beam is aimed at the tympanic membrane (otherwise the measurement will be invalid). Wait 2 to 3 seconds until the digital temperature reading appears. This method measures core body temperature, which is higher than the expected oral temperature by approximately 0.8°C.

PAIN

Pain can increase heart rate, blood pressure, respirations, restlessness, and anxiety. Pain is the most common reason clients access health care providers and is one of the most common symptoms experienced by clients in hospital. Although pain is subjective, it has objective components that nurses can observe clinically. For accuracy of vital signs and for client safety, nurses must assess pain as regularly as blood pressure, heart rate, and respirations. Chapter 7 contains a discussion of *gate control theory.* Gate control theory (Wall & Melzack, 1999) provides an explanation for the effects of pain. It addresses the differences between acute and chronic pain in their effect on the other vital signs.

FUNCTION

A primary focus for nurses is preserving the older client's functional status, the sixth vital sign. Functional status refers to the ability to perform tasks and fulfill social roles associated with daily living across a wide range of complexity (Koretz & Reuben, 2003; Reuben, 2003). During the general survey, when your client enters the room, you begin assessing functional status. You have access to several well-validated and time-efficient assessment tools (see Chapter 25) that can help you focus on these preliminary survey observations and assist you with measurement during taking of the vital signs. The 10-minute Geriatric Screener (p. 915) incorporates some functional issues. More in-depth assessment of function includes assessment of activities of daily living (ADLs) and instrumental ADLs (IADLs), and use of specific

Causes of *fever* include infection, trauma such as surgery or crush injuries, malignancy, blood disorders such as acute hemolytic anemia, drug reactions, blood transfusion reactions, and immune disorders such as collagen vascular disease.

The chief cause of *hypothermia* is exposure to cold. Other predisposing causes include reduced movement as in paralysis, interference with vasoconstriction as from sepsis or excess alcohol, starvation, *hypothyroidism*, and hypoglycemia. Elderly people are especially susceptible to hypothermia and also less likely to develop fever.

problem-focused instruments such as the Tinetti Gait and Balance Tool (Tinetti, 1986) or the Berg Balance Scale (Berg, Wood-Dauphinee, Williams, & Maki, 1992).

DOCUMENTATION OF VITAL SIGNS

It is essential to record your general survey and vital signs precisely, accurately, clearly, and at the time of your examination. As these data reflect changes in client status, the serial record is useful for early detection of physiological and psychological changes. The data also constitute a legal record of client attention. See Chapter 5 for the principles underlying documentation.

EXAMPLE OF RECORDING OF VITAL SIGNS

C. M. Swarts—BP sitting, right arm 160/95; HR 108 and irregular; RR 32 and laboured; temperature (tympanic) 38.5°C; denies pain; 10-Minute Geriatric Screener deferred.

Critical Thinking Exercise

- Describe the advantages and disadvantages of three types of sphygmomanometers. (*Knowledge*)
- Discuss the circumstances for using three different types of thermometers. (*Comprehension*)
- How would you conduct a general survey of a client who is blind or a client who is deaf? (*Application*)
- Compare the effects of using three different cuff sizes for taking blood pressure. (*Analysis*)
- What might be the challenges for completing the general survey and taking the vital signs in a client who is agitated? (*Synthesis*)
- How will you evaluate the results of client education on lifestyle modification for the purpose of reducing blood pressure? (*Evaluation*)

Canadian Research

Alberta Heritage Foundation for Medical Research. (2008). The sixth vital sign. *Research News, Summer 2008*, 18–19.
Jackson, M. (2002). *Pain: The fifth vital sign.* Toronto, ON: Random House of Canada.

Skjodt, N., & Hodgetts, B. (2008). *An MP3 recorder/player could replace the traditional stethoscope.* Paper presented September 17, 2008, at the Congress of the European Respiratory Society in Stockholm, Sweden.

Test Questions

1. The General Survey component of the physical examination is completed when the:
   a. history has been taken.
   b. client sits on the examining table.
   c. physical examination is completed.
   d. client's chief concern has been elicited.

2. The general inspection can be started:
   a. before the examiner can see the client.
   b. when the client is completely exposed.
   c. after height and weight have been taken.
   d. when the examiner has access to an examining room.

3. During general inspection, the examiner:
   a. assesses for pain and functional ability.
   b. integrates visual, auditory, and olfactory data.
   c. inquires about the occupational environment of the client.
   d. ensures the client moves from standing to lying positions.

4. When inspecting the thorax of an adult client, the expected respiratory rate in breaths per minute is:
   a. 10–16.
   b. 12–18.
   c. 14–20.
   d. none of the above.

5. During your first assessment of the client, you assess the blood pressure in both arms. Which of the following findings is an acceptable variation? The blood pressure in the right arm is:
   a. 140/90 mm Hg and 150/96 mm Hg in the left arm.
   b. 118/78 mm Hg and 130/84 mm Hg in the left arm.
   c. 118/78 mm Hg and 122/80 mm Hg in the left arm.
   d. 140/95 mm Hg and 130/85 mm Hg in the left arm.

Bibliography

CITATIONS

Alberta Heritage Foundation for Medical Research. (2008). The sixth vital sign. *Research News, Summer 2008*, 18–19.

Berg, K. O., Wood-Dauphinee, S. L., Williams, J. I., & Maki, B. (1992). Measuring balance in the elderly: Validation of an instrument. *Canadian Journal of Public Health, 83*(Suppl. 2), S7–S11.

Blood Pressure Canada. (2008). *Blood pressure information.* Retrieved August 29, 2008, from http://hypertension.ca/bpc/blood-pressure-information/meaasurements/

Bobrie, G., Genes, N., Vaur, L., Clerson, P., Vaisse, B., Mallion, J.-M., et al. (2001). Is "isolated home" hypertension as opposed to "isolated office" hypertension a sign of greater cardiovascular risk? *Archives of Internal Medicine, 161*(18), 2205–2211.

Brickner, M. E., Hillis, L. D., & Lange, R. A. (2000). Congenital heart disease in adults: First of two parts. *New England Journal of Medicine, 342*(4), 256–263.

Canadian Hypertension Education Program. (2008). *Recommendations—2008.* Retrieved August 29, 2008, from http://hypertension.ca/chep/recommendations/diagnosis-assessment/follow-up-criteria-for

Carlson, J. E. (1999). Assessment of orthostatic blood pressure: Measurement technique and clinical applications. *Southern Medical Journal, 92*(2), 167–173.

Cavallini, M. C., Roman, M. J., Blank, S. G., Pini, R., Pickering, T. G., & Devereux, R. B. (1996). Association of the auscultatory gap with vascular disease in hypertensive patients. *Annals of Internal Medicine, 124*(10), 877–883.

Clement, D. L., De Buyzere, M. L., De Bacquer, D. A., De Leeuw, P. W., Duprez, D. A., Fagard, R. H., et al. (2003). Prognostic value of ambulatory blood-pressure recordings in patients with treated hypertension. *New England Journal of Medicine, 348*(24), 2407–2415.

Fiore, M. C., Jorenby, D. E., Schensky, A. E., Smith, S. S., Bauer, R. R., & Baker, T. B. (1995). Smoking status as the new vital sign: Effect on assessment and intervention in patients who smoke. *Mayo Clinic Proceedings, 70*(3), 209–213.

Jackson, M. (2002). *Pain: The fifth vital sign.* Toronto, ON: Random House of Canada.

Kaplan, N. M., & Rose, B. C. (2004). Ambulatory blood pressure monitoring and white coat hypertension in adults. Retrieved December 11, 2004, from www.utdol.com

Koretz, B., & Reuben, D. B. (2003). Instruments to assess functional status. In C. K. Cassel, R. M. Leipzig, H. J. Cohen, E. B. Larsen, & D. E. Meier. (Eds.), *Geriatric medicine: An evidence-based approach* (4th ed., pp. 195–204). New York: Springer.

Lockwood, C., Conroy-Hiller, T., & Page, T. (2004). Vital signs. *International Journal of Evidence-Based Healthcare, 2*(6), 207–230.

Skjodt, N., & Hodgetts, B. (2008). *An MP3 recorder/player could replace the traditional stethoscope.* Paper presented September 17, 2008 at the Congress of the European Respiratory Society in Stockholm, Sweden.

Tanne, J. H. (2003). U.S. guidelines say blood pressure of 120/80 mm Hg is not "normal." *British Medical Journal, 326,* 1104.

Tinetti, M. E. (1986). Performance-oriented assessment of mobility problems in elderly patients. *Journal of the American Geriatrics Society, 34,* 119–126.

Wall, P. D., & Melzack, R. (Eds.), *Textbook of pain* (4th ed.). Edinburgh: Churchill Livingstaon.

ADDITIONAL RESOURCES

Carlson, L. E., Angen, M., Callum, J., Goodey, E., Koopmans, J., Lamont, L., et al. (2004). High levels of untreated distress and fatigue in cancer patients. *British Journal of Cancer, 90*(12), 2297–2304.

Kahn, L. H. (2008). Stethoscopes belong in museums. Retrieved August 28, 2008, from http://www.thebulletin.org/web-edition/columnists/laura-h-kahn/stethoscopes-belong-mu

McGill University Virtual Stethoscope. Retrieved February 27, 2009, from http://sprojects.mmi.mcgill.ca/mys/HowTo.htm

Reuben, D. B. (2003). Comprehensive geriatric assessment and system approaches to geriatric care. In C. K. Cassel, R. M. Leipzig, H. J. Cohen, E. B. Larsen, & D. E. Meier. (Eds.), *Geriatric Medicine: An evidence-based approach* (4th ed., pp. 195–204). New York: Springer-Verlag.

CANADIAN ASSOCIATIONS AND WEB SITES

Blood Pressure Canada: www.hypertension.ca/bpc
Canadian Hypertension Education Program: www.hypertension.ca/chep
Canadian Hypertensive Society: www.hypertension.ca/chs

TABLE 6-1   **Alterations of the Arterial Pulse and Pressure Waves**

Expected

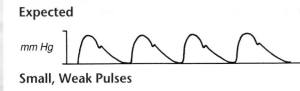

mm Hg

The pulse pressure is about 30–40 mm Hg. The pulse contour is smooth and rounded. (The notch on the descending slope of the pulse wave is not palpable.)

Small, Weak Pulses

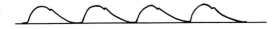

The pulse pressure is diminished, and the pulse feels weak and small. The upstroke may feel slowed, the peak prolonged. Causes include (1) decreased stroke volume, as in heart failure, hypovolemia, and severe aortic stenosis, and (2) increased peripheral resistance, as in exposure to cold and severe congestive heart failure.

Large, Bounding Pulses

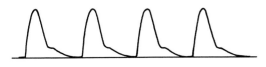

The pulse pressure is increased, and the pulse feels strong and bounding. The rise and fall may feel rapid, the peak brief. Causes include (1) an increased stroke volume, a decreased peripheral resistance, or both, as in fever, anemia, hyperthyroidism, aortic regurgitation, arteriovenous fistulas, and patent ductus arteriosus; (2) an increased stroke volume due to slow heart rates, as in bradycardia and complete heart block; and (3) decreased compliance (increased stiffness) of the aortic walls, as in aging or atherosclerosis.

Bisferiens Pulse

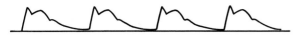

A bisferiens pulse is an increased arterial pulse with a double systolic peak. Causes include pure aortic regurgitation, combined aortic stenosis and regurgitation, and, though less commonly palpable, hypertrophic cardiomyopathy.

Pulsus Alternans

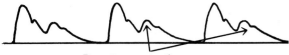

The pulse alternates in amplitude from beat to beat even though the rhythm is basically regular (and must be for you to make this judgment). When the difference between stronger and weaker beats is slight, it can be detected only by sphygmomanometry. Pulsus alternans indicates left ventricular failure and is usually accompanied by a left-sided S_3.

Bigeminal Pulse

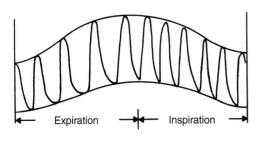

Premature contractions

This is a disorder of rhythm that may masquerade as pulsus alternans. A bigeminal pulse is caused by an expected beat alternating with a premature contraction. The stroke volume of the premature beat is diminished in relation to that of the expected beats, and the pulse varies in amplitude accordingly.

Paradoxical Pulse

A paradoxical pulse may be detected by a palpable decrease in the pulse's amplitude on quiet inspiration. If the sign is less pronounced, a blood pressure cuff is needed. Systolic pressure decreases by more than 10 mm Hg during inspiration. A paradoxical pulse is found in pericardial tamponade, constrictive pericarditis (though less commonly), and obstructive lung disease.

Expiration ◄──►│◄── Inspiration ──►

When observing respiratory patterns, think in terms of *rate, depth,* and *regularity* of the client's breathing. Describe what you see in these terms. Traditional terms, such as tachypnea, are given below so that you will understand them, but simple descriptions are recommended for use.

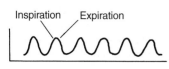

Expected

The respiratory rate is about 14–20 per min in healthy adults and up to 44 per min in infants.

Slow Breathing (*Bradypnea*)

Slow breathing may be secondary to such causes as diabetic coma, drug-induced respiratory depression, and increased intracranial pressure.

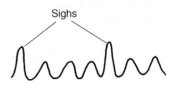

Sighing Respiration

Breathing punctuated by frequent sighs should alert you to the possibility of hyperventilation syndrome—a common cause of dyspnea and dizziness. Occasional sighs are expected.

Rapid Shallow Breathing (*Tachypnea*)

Rapid shallow breathing has a number of causes, including restrictive lung disease, pleuritic chest pain, and an elevated diaphragm.

Cheyne-Stokes Breathing

Periods of deep breathing alternate with periods of apnea (no breathing). Children and aging people typically may show this pattern in sleep. Other causes include heart failure, uremia, drug-induced respiratory depression, and brain damage (typically on both sides of the cerebral hemispheres or diencephalon).

Obstructive Breathing

In obstructive lung disease, expiration is prolonged because narrowed airways increase the resistance to air flow. Causes include asthma, chronic bronchitis, and COPD.

Rapid Deep Breathing (*Hyperpnea, Hyperventilation*)

Rapid deep breathing has several causes, including exercise, anxiety, and metabolic acidosis. In the comatose client, consider infarction, hypoxia, or hypoglycemia affecting the midbrain or pons. *Kussmaul breathing* is deep breathing due to metabolic acidosis. It may be fast, expected in rate, or slow.

Ataxic Breathing (*Biot's Breathing*)

Ataxic breathing is characterized by unpredictable irregularity. Breaths may be shallow or deep, and stop for short periods. Causes include respiratory depression and brain damage, typically at the medullary level.

Pain Assessment

Janice A. Lander

Nurses encounter people in pain in many different settings and are the professional group who spend the most time with such people. Key nursing roles related to pain include assessing the pain and the client's response to it, providing pain-relief strategies and assessing the client's response to them, monitoring for adverse effects, acting as an advocate for the client when pain-relieving strategies need alterations, and teaching the client and family about pain-relieving strategies to use at home. Nurses also consider the need for and an assessment of nonpharmaceutical measures for relieving pain, such as therapeutic touch, acupuncture, reflexology, transcutaneous electrical neural stimulation (TENS), Tai chi, and Qi gong. The overall goals are to keep the client comfortable and to prevent acute pain from becoming chronic pain.

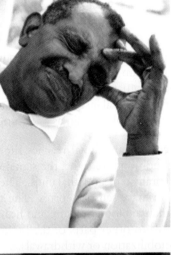

INTRODUCTION TO PAIN

Despite centuries of reflection and investigation, aspects of pain remain a mystery. Nowhere is this better reflected than in the management of chronic pain. Generally, pain (chronic pain in particular) is poorly treated and underdiagnosed. Pain is the number one reason that clients access health care (Lander, 2007) and is reported by 50% of hospitalized clients (Canadian Pain Coalition, 2005).

Pain is defined as an unpleasant sensory and emotional experience associated with actual or potential tissue damage or described in terms of such damage (Merskey & Bogduk, 1994). Pain is the outcome of biological and psychological processes that involve the peripheral nerves, spinal cord, and brain. Although pain serves as an alarm that warns of tissue damage, it also can occur long after tissue has healed.

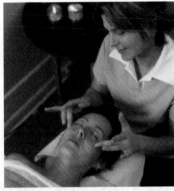

Pain has three components or dimensions. The *sensory-discriminative component*, which receives the most attention within the health care professions, refers to the severity and localization of pain. The second dimension is the *affective-motivational component*. This refers to the emotional aspects of pain, or how the pain makes us feel and what it makes us do. The third dimension is the *cognitive-evaluative component*, which is the meaning attributed to the pain.

Many organizations worked to increase the visibility of pain as a problem to be addressed. They lobbied for pain to be declared a disease by having it listed on the International Statistical Classification of Diseases and Related Health Problems (ICD) (Canadian Institute for Health Information, 2006). The rationale for this action was to draw attention to pain for improved diagnosis and management. The American Pain Society succeeded in having pain declared the fifth vital sign (2003). The aim was to draw attention to the need to assess pain with the same regularity as temperature, blood pressure, respirations, and heart rate. Accreditation Canada has

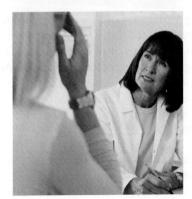

set standards for assessment and management of pain as a component of client safety that include regular pain assessments, use of standardized clinical pain measures, being knowledgeable about pain management strategies, and receiving continuing education about evidence-based pain management strategies (Canadian Pain Society, 2005).

ANATOMY AND PHYSIOLOGY

Pain receptors, which are called *nociceptors,* are located in all areas of the body except the brain itself. The density of nociceptors varies by site (more in skin and less in organs). Some body areas (e.g., the eyes, fingertips, and area around the mouth) are exquisitely sensitive to pain because they have many nerve endings. Chemical, mechanical, and thermal stimuli fire up nociceptors, as do chemical substances that are present after tissue injury. Once nociceptors have been stimulated, they send signals along peripheral sensory nerves and then to the spinal cord.

Sensory nerves for pain are of two types: high-speed A-delta fibres and slow C-fibres. A-delta fibres cause pain that is sharp, rapid in onset, and well localized and stimulate motor responses such as withdrawal or flinching. C-fibres cause dull and longer-lasting pain that is not well localized and stimulate a protective motor response (such as guarding). A- and C-fibres seem to be missing in those rare individuals with congenital insensitivity to pain. This life-threatening condition underscores the important role of pain as a warning of impending damage.

After the pain signal reaches the spinal cord, it is processed in the dorsal horn. If conditions are right, the signal will be transmitted in the spinothalamic tract to the brainstem and thalamus. The thalamus processes and relays information to the primary sensory cortex. The thalamus is also responsible for sending signals to change blood pressure and heart rate in response to acute pain, and for sending signals to other parts of the brain to bring about appropriate behaviour (such as immobilization or withdrawal).

The brain also sends signals down the spinal cord. Among these is the signal to block too much information from going upward. This is called *descending inhibition,* and it can reduce the sensation of pain. A person's state of mind can increase or decrease descending inhibition, leading to an increase or decrease in pain (by increasing or decreasing signals ascending the cord). Intense emotions such as fear or excitement increase descending inhibition and thus decrease pain. This is the explanation for tales about soldiers who were unaware of being severely injured until they reached safety. Other states such as depression and anxiety decrease inhibition and therefore increase pain.

GATE CONTROL THEORY

Ron Melzak (a Canadian psychologist) and Patrick Wall (a British physiologist) proposed the *gate control theory* in the 1960s. Before developing the theory, Melzak and Wall proved all other theories false by showing that they could not account for well-known clinical observations. Although it took a long time for the scientific community to recognize the gate control theory, it is now the only acknowledged theory of pain. Like all theories, it is a work in progress, and many changes have been made to it over time. Nonetheless, the basic elements remain the same (Melzak, 1996; Wall & Melzak, 1999).

The theory suggests that pain signals go to the spinal cord and to specialized cells that act as gatekeepers. Large, myelinated A-beta fibres interact with A-delta and C-fibres in the substantia gelatinosa of the dorsal horn. A-beta fibres carry nonnociceptive information. They inhibit pain by exciting inhibitory interneurons. This closes the gate and stops transmission of pain signals. Unmyelinated C-fibres inhibit inhibitory interneurons; this opens the gate, allowing transmission to proceed. If there is more activity in myelinated fibres, then pain is blocked; if there is more activity in C-fibres, then pain occurs. Descending information from the brain also can open or close the gate. This information can signal the release of substances that diminish pain (such as endorphins).

The gate control theory can explain many clinical observations. Among these are the effects of one's emotional state on pain sensation and the pain-reducing effect of distraction. The theory also explains how nonnociceptive information can inhibit pain. Rubbing the site of an injury seems to lessen pain because the A-beta fibres carry information about touch, which closes the gate.

SENSITIZATION OR WIND-UP

Intense or persistent pain leads to changes that sensitize the dorsal horn. Spinal cord neurons become more excitable, and areas of the brain that deal with pain may also become more sensitive to it. Messages sent from nociceptors along C-fibres become amplified and distorted. Even weak signals may be perceived as pain. This phenomenon, which is also called *wind-up*, is thought to explain chronic pain. The associated cellular changes may cause the nervous system to create a memory of the severe or prolonged pain, one that is replayed over and over. The need to prevent pain from becoming chronic is one important reason for nurses to make sure that acute pain is assessed and properly treated.

PAIN TERMS

Pain has a standard vocabulary that has been built over centuries, with contributions, from many different disciplines. These terms have agreed-upon technical meanings. Understanding the language of pain is essential to its diagnosis and management.

■ *Pain Taxonomy*

Term	Meaning
Hyperalgesia	Increased response to a painful stimulus
Hypoalgesia	Decreased response to a painful stimulus
Neuropathy	Pathological change in a nerve resulting in disturbed function
Neuropathic pain	Pain caused by damage to the nervous system
Nociceptor	Receptor that is sensitive to noxious stimuli
Nociceptive pain	Visceral and somatic pain
Noxious stimulus	A stimulus that is damaging to tissue
Pain tolerance	Greatest amount of pain that a person is willing to tolerate
Paresthesia	Abnormal sensation (spontaneous or evoked)
Hyperesthesia	Increased sensitivity to any cutaneous stimuli (e.g., increased sensitivity to heat)
Hypoesthesia	Decreased sensitivity to cutaneous stimuli
Phantom pain	Pain felt in a missing limb
Allodynia	Pain caused by a stimulus that does not normally produce pain
Radicular pain	Pain that follows the distribution of a nerve root (corresponding to dermatomes)
Referred pain	Pain in a body part or area other than where the cause of the pain is located

Interdisciplinary health professionals strive for a common language of pain terminology to aid assessment and diagnosis and to achieve a common understanding of the phenomena. The International Association for the Study of Pain (IASP) (2008) and national organizations such as the Canadian Pain Society clarify these terms and set the standards. Some common pain terms can be found in the following table. These terms describe special features associated with some types of pain.

PAIN CLASSIFICATIONS

Pain is classified in several overlapping (and perhaps confusing) ways. It can be classified based on duration (acute, chronic), frequency (intermittent, continuous), form (nociceptive, neuropathic), and association with cancer. An example of overlap in these pain classifications is chronic neuropathic pain associated with cancer (or with treatment of cancer). To add to the complexity, pain can be further defined by its special features. An example is allodynia, which is a pain response to a stimulus that does not usually cause pain.

Duration   Acute pain lasts from seconds to months. It runs a finite course and then resolves. It is typically associated with specific events (such as trauma) or disease (such as appendicitis). Acute pain drives people to seek help when it becomes uncomfortable or intense and when the cause is unknown. It is associated with tissue trauma from mechanical, thermal, chemical, or electrical stimuli. Tissue damage to nerve endings, inflammation, stretch, and ischemia cause acute pain. The body responds to severe pain with sweating, tachycardia, tachypnea, anxiety, and, perhaps, vomiting. Severe unrelieved pain is incompatible with day-to-day functioning.

Nurses observe for signs of acute pain in clients who are conscious and in those who cannot communicate verbally (Moorhead, Johnson, Maas, & Swanson, 2008; NANDA International, 2007). Behaviours that may indicate pain include the following:

- Rubbing the affected body part or area

- Pacing

- Restlessness

- Agitation

- Irritability

- Facial expressions (e.g., frowning, wincing, grimacing)

- Sighing

- Moaning

- Crying

- Positioning to avoid pain (e.g., knees bent when lying on back, legs tucked up under buttocks when side lying)

- Jerking movements

- Thrashing movements

- Writhing

Pain becomes chronic when it lasts 3 months or longer. Three months is arbitrary, however, and it may be clear that pain will become chronic early in some disease processes. Unlike acute pain, chronic pain serves no useful purpose. When pain becomes chronic, it becomes a disease in its own right. Chronic pain does not warn of tissue damage because it continues long after a signal is necessary and occurs in some cases in the absence of evidence of tissue damage. The experience of chronic pain and associated pain behaviours are very different from acute pain. Signs of distress with acute pain are absent in chronic pain; the biological signs are also missing. Whereas one can see the severe distress of a person suffering intense acute pain, one cannot see severe chronic pain in the same way. Chronic pain can be associated with withdrawal from life, depression, and sleep disturbances. It can disrupt a person's life, limiting ability to care for self, earn an income, and sustain personal relationships. Chronic pain compromises enjoyment of life, sense of control, and sense of hope. If severe, chronic pain can lead to adverse psychological responses such as helplessness, hopelessness, worthlessness, fear of unbearable pain, pessimistic thoughts, suicidal thoughts, and anger (Moorhead et al., 2008, p. 535). The treatments of acute and chronic pain also differ.

Frequency Some pain is continuous or nearly continuous, and other pain is intermittent or episodic. Pain from arthritis can be continuous (although not necessarily with the same intensity all the time), whereas the pain from migraine headaches is episodic. Episodic pain may be associated with particular events or times. For instance, some women experience migraines linked to their menstrual cycles.

Location Nociceptive pain is associated with tissue damage in viscera, bones, joints, muscles, ligaments, or skin. This tissue damage arises from inflammation, stretch, or ischemia. Nociceptive pain is classified as somatic or visceral. Somatic nociceptive pain comes from activation of nociceptors in the skin or musculoskeletal system; therefore, it may be referred to as musculoskeletal pain. When skin nociceptors are involved, pain is described as sharp. When pain comes from musculoskeletal tissues, it is often described as dull and aching. Visceral pain is associated with organs located in the thorax, abdomen, and pelvis. The pain may not be localized and may be referred or experienced at sites far from the tissue damage. This is quite typical of abdominal organ disease. Pressure, squeezing, cramping pain is often visceral. Parietal pain refers to pain located in the wall of a body cavity. It is also nociceptive.

Neuropathic pain is caused by a lesion to or dysfunction of nerve fibres in the peripheral or central nervous system. Damage to the nerve from pressure, infection, or degenerative conditions causes it to fire erratically. The brain misinterprets the erratic signals as pain and hypersensitivity. Neuropathic pain is described as burning, tingling, numbness, stabbing, shooting, or electric, and different approaches to treating this type of pain are necessary (Lander, 2007). If the problem is in the central nervous system, the pain may be labelled as central pain. An example is central poststroke pain. The stroke has damaged the thalamus or other parts of the brain, causing the sensation of pain in parts of the body contralateral to the site of damage in the brain. Any stimuli can cause damage to nerve fibres. Some examples are mechanical injury of the spinal cord and peripheral nerve damage from chemotherapy and radiation treatment. Regardless of the origin of the signals, the brain interprets them as pain. Sympathetic pain, a special case of neuropathic pain, results from overactivity of the sympathetic nervous system and central or peripheral nervous systems. This type of pain may follow typically minor muscle or soft tissue injury. Some characteristics of sympathetic pain are sweating of the affected tissues, poor temperature control in the area of pain, and extreme hypersensitivity of skin in the affected area. The terms used currently are complex regional pain syndrome I (i.e., RSD) and complex regional pain syndrome II (i.e., causalgia). Common findings with RSD include edema, changes in blood flow to the skin, abnormal sweating of the tissues, allodynia, and hyperalgesia.

A mixed pain syndrome also has been reported. This type of pain has neuropathic and nociceptive features. Myofascial pain syndrome is an example. People with this syndrome have muscle pain and tenderness, and trigger points.

Association With Cancer At one time, chronic pain was described as malignant or benign; however, these terms have fallen into disuse. Use of the term "benign" does not represent the experience of clients with chronic pain that disrupts their lives. Today, pain can be classified as chronic pain or chronic cancer pain. Pain that arises from treatment of cancer is still classified as cancer pain.

The World Health Organization (WHO) has a three-step ladder approach to managing cancer pain (Lander, 2007, p. 224):

Step 1: For mild pain, a nonopioid and an adjuvant drug are suggested.

Step 2: For moderate pain, use of a weak opioid, a nonopioid, and an adjuvant drug are indicated.

Step 3: For severe pain, a strong opioid, a nonopioid, and an adjuvant drug are required.

THE HEALTH HISTORY: SUBJECTIVE DATA

Key Symptoms and Signs Reported by Client

Acute Pain

- Sweating
- Rapid heart rate (tachycardia)
- Rapid breathing (tachypnea)
- Feeling anxious
- Vomiting
- Feeling restless
- Holding, supporting, protecting the pain site (guarding)
- Seeking help
- Muscle spasms

Chronic Pain

- Sleep disturbances
- Feeling apathetic
- Decreased concentration
- Withdrawal from life
- Decreased functional activities
- Feeling depressed
- Decreased interest in sex (decreased libido)
- Suicidal thoughts
- Feeling lethargic
- Lack or loss of appetite (anorexia)
- Wondering what is wrong and what will fix it (diagnosis/cure seeking)

VERBAL COMMUNICATION OF PAIN

An evaluation of pain must include a comprehensive history. Ask the client to provide information about the pain. Ensure that the environment for the interview is quiet and private. Listen carefully to what the client says—to the words that he or she uses to describe the pain. Pain can be difficult to describe because the language is so vivid and extensive. Is the pain like walking on a bed of hot coals? Is it like being skewered? The nurse should be aware of possible differences in vocabulary depending on age and education. Describing pain may be very difficult for some people, such as those whose first language is not English or those with little formal education. Some clients also have trouble finding the right words when the pain is overwhelming. The nurse may have to suggest some words as potential examples.

Melzak and colleagues itemized 78 words that refer to pain and grouped them into 20 categories to be used as part of the McGill Pain Questionnaire (Melzak, 1975). Although language usage changes over time (and some words become archaic and unfamiliar to younger generations), people still use most of these words to describe the pain and its meaning.

■ Pain Categories and Terms from the McGill Pain Questionnaire

Dimension	Subcategory	Pain Words
Sensory	Temporal	Flickering, quivering, pulsing, throbbing, beating, pounding
	Spatial	Jumping, flashing, shooting
	Punctuate pressure	Pricking, boring, drilling, stabbing, lancinating
	Incisive pressure	Sharp, cutting, lacerating
	Constrictive pressure	Pinching, pressing, gnawing, cramping, crushing
	Traction pressure	Tugging, pulling, wrenching
	Thermal	Hot, boring, scalding, searing
	Brightness	Tingling, itchy, smarting, stinging
	Dullness	Dull, sore, hurting, aching, heavy
	Sensory	Tender, taut, rasping, splitting
Affective	Tension	Tiring, exhausting
	Autonomic	Sickening, suffocating
	Fear	Fearful, frightful, terrifying
	Punishment	Punishing, gruelling, cruel, vicious, killing
	Affective Evaluative sensory	Wretched, blinding
Evaluative	Evaluative	Annoying, troublesome, miserable, intense, unbearable
Miscellaneous	Sensory miscellaneous	Spreading, radiating, penetrating, piercing
	Sensory miscellaneous	Tight, numb, drawing, squeezing, tearing
	Sensory	Cool, cold, freezing
	Affective Evaluative	Nagging, nauseating, agonizing, dreadful, torturing

Source: Melzak, 1975.

Begin with the sign or symptom reported by the client. Ask open-ended questions. Probe with additional questions such as those used in a symptom analysis. Pain is *the* symptom that is often used to illustrate all aspects of a symptom analysis. What follows is a comprehensive set of potential questions to use to gain an understanding of a client's pain. Health professionals choose the questions most appropriate for a particular client.

Example of Questions for Symptom Analysis—Pain

- "Where is the pain located?" "Can you point to where it is?" "Does the pain move to another place in your body?" "Can you point to that place?" [*If the client mentions more than one site*], ask: "Which site is most troubling?" "Which site is the next most troubling?" (*Location, Radiation*)
- "What is the pain like?" *First allow the client to answer without any prompts. It is very important to record exactly how the client describes the pain. If the* client is having difficulty describing the pain, then ask: "Is the pain sharp?" "Prickling?" "Burning?" "Shock-like?" "Dull?" "Aching?" "Cramping?" "Jabbing?" "Squeezing?" "Rhythmic pulsating?" "Plateau – pain that rises and then plateaus?" (*Quality*)
- "On a scale from 0 to 10, with 10 being the worst possible pain, how would you rate your pain?" [*A scale of 0 to 5 can also be used*] (*Quantity*)

(continued)

- "When did you first notice the pain?" "What were you doing when you first noticed the pain?" "Did the pain start slowly? Or suddenly?" "Is there a time of day when the pain seems worse?" "Or a time of the night the pain seems worse?" "Or a time in the day when the pain seems better?" "Or a time in the night when the pain seems better?" "Is the pain always present?" "Does it come and go?" "How often are you having the pain" "Are there times when you are free of the pain?" "Have you had previous experience with pain?" (*Timing*)
- "Where were you when you first noticed the pain?" (*Setting*)
- "What other symptoms have you noticed besides the pain?" [*Allow the client to describe other symptoms first. Then ask about other symptoms.*] "Nausea?" "Vomiting?" "Coughing?" "Shortness of breath?" "Dizziness?" "Inadequate sleeping?" "Fatigue?" "Exhaustion?" "Do you feel anxious?" "Depressed?" "Exhausted?" "Do you have increased sensitivity to pain (hyperalgesia)?" "How is your appetite?" "Do you have constipation?" "Diarrhea?" (*Associated symptoms*)
- "What makes the pain worse?" "Movement?' "Breathing?" (*Aggravating factors*)
- "What makes the pain better?" "What have you tried that relieved the pain?" "Does a warm room help?" "Using heat?" "Using cold?" "Use of prescribed medications?" [names of medications, dose, amount used daily] "Use of over-the-counter medications?" [name of medications, dose, amount used daily] "Use of herbal remedies?" [names of remedies, dose, amount used daily] "Measures other than medications— Massage? Acupuncture? Other?" "Does a certain position make the pain better?" (*Alleviating factors*)
- "Are there things in your home environment that affect the pain?" "Does anyone in your family experience pain?" "Are there things in your work environment that affect the pain?" "How much stress is in your life right now?" (*Environmental factors*)
- "How is this pain affecting your daily life?" "Work?" "Study?" "Financial implications?" "The things you enjoy doing?" "How is the pain affecting your family?" "Or other interpersonal relationships?" (*Significance to client*)
- "What do you think is the meaning of your pain?" "What is happening with your pain?" "Are you concerned it might mean the presence of disease?" "Does it mean increasing disease?" "Presence of infection?" (*Client perspective*)

PAIN MEASUREMENT SCALES AND PAIN ASSESSMENT

Pain measurement refers to the collection of specific data about pain. Pain measurement scales are often one-dimensional, typically limited to pain intensity. Nurses may be interested in measuring pain intensity only when they want to determine whether a client requires an analgesic or whether a medication has been effective in relieving pain.

Many pain measurement scales are research tools as opposed to clinical tools. The visual analogue scale is a research tool (that measures pain in millimetres with a ruler) that has also been used in practice. Simple numerical scales can be used as clinical tools (e.g., "On a scale of 0 to 10, how much pain do you have?"). A numerical scale may be simplified for use by children or by adults with developmental or cognitive disabilities (0 is *no pain* and 4 is *the worst it could be*). Verbal scales (categorical pain scales) may be easiest for some clients ("No pain," "Is your pain mild?," "Is it moderate?," "Or is it severe?"). A simple yes–no measure may be all that can be used in some situations. The Wong–Baker Faces pain rating scale consists of drawings of six faces (with scores of 1–10 attached for the rater's use) (Wong, Hockenberry-Eaton, Wilson, Winkelstein, & Schwartz, 2001). Although this tool is designed for children 3 years and older, it can be used with adults in emergency situations and when there are challenges with communication. As well, some simple pain scales have been translated into many languages and can be accessed through the Internet.

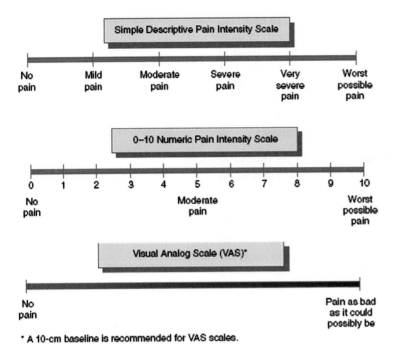

* A 10-cm baseline is recommended for VAS scales.

Pain assessment is broader than pain measurement because assessment is multidimensional and includes sensory, affective, and cognitive aspects as well as the effect of pain on activities of daily living and relationships. Other key considerations are past treatments and their effectiveness as well as treatment expectations. Thorough pain assessment is required as part of the health history.

Numerous pain assessment scales have been developed to help gather information about pain. Some have specific and narrow purposes, such as the assessment of pain disability or determination of neuropathic features to pain (Bouhassira et al., 2005; see Box 7-1). Other scales are used for a broad pain assessment. Some tools such as the Brief Pain Inventory (BPI) (Cleeland, 1991) include measurement of current pain and a drawing of the body so the client can shade in the locations of pain and mark the most painful area. No single scale gathers all required data. Scales are merely aids to, not replacements for, proper pain assessment.

The person suffering with pain ought not to be overtaxed with a lengthy, complicated assessment tool. The health professional also needs a scale that is easy to evaluate. An example of a scale that is complex to use and score, but has

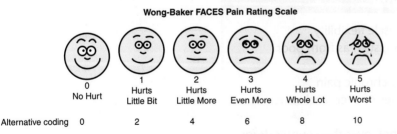

Explain to the person that each face is for a person who feels happy because he has no pain (hurt) or sad because he has some or a lot of pain. Face 0 is very happy because he doesn't hurt at all. Face 1 hurts just a little bit. Face 2 hurts a little more. Face 3 hurts even more. Face 4 hurts a whole lot. Face 5 hurts as much as you can imagine, although you don't have to be crying to feel this bad. Ask the person to choose the face that best describes how he is feeling.

Rating scale is recommended for persons age 3 years and older.

Brief word instructions : Point to each face using the words to describe the pain intensity. Ask the child to choose face that best describes own pain and record the appropriate number.

Source: Wong, 2001.

little clinical utility, is the McGill Pain Questionnaire (Melzak, 1975). In contrast, the BPI is used to assess pain location, pain severity, the effects of pain on daily functioning, use of medications for pain, and the degree of pain relief obtained in the previous 24 hours (Cleeland, 1991). The tool can be used to measure acute pain (e.g., postoperative) as well as chronic conditions (e.g., cancer, osteoarthritis, low-back pain). Nurses can use the BPI either as an interview or as a client self-report. The short form of the tool is recommended and can be completed in 5 minutes. An additional advantage of the BPI is that it has been validated in 25 languages.

Another assessment tool is the West Haven–Yale Multidimensional Pain Inventory (WHYMPI) (Kerns, Turk, & Rudy, 1985). It consists of three parts. Questions in Part 1 relate to interference of the pain, support, pain severity, control over life, and affective distress. Questions in Part 2 ask the client how his or her significant other responds when he or she knows the client is in pain. Responses are scored as *Negative* (e.g., *ignores me, expresses frustration at me*), *Solicitous* (e.g., *asks me what he or she can do to help, tries to get me to rest*), or *Distracting* (e.g., *talks to me about something else to take my mind off the pain, tries to involve me in some activity*). Questions in Part 3 ask the client how often he or she does 18 common daily activities in five categories: household chores, outdoor work, activities away from home, social activities, and general activities.

Numbers on pain scales are often treated as though they mean the same thing to all people. Health care professionals might view a 5 on a 10-point numerical scale as the point at which analgesics should be administered. Anchors must be determined for each client to individualize the assessment. Ask the question, "At what level of pain would you need to have something done to relieve it?" This point could be a 3 for some and a 7 or more for others. It is also necessary to occasionally reconfirm the pain treatment anchor. It is possible that as pain continues, one's tolerance of it lessens and the anchor will change.

Once nurses have assessed and initiated treatments for pain, they use a developmentally appropriate method (e.g., flow sheet, daily diary) to monitor changes in pain. Nurses consider the type and source of pain in deciding on the frequency of assessing the severity of a client's pain, the effectiveness of the pain control strategies, and the client's satisfaction or dissatisfaction with the pain management (Bulechek, Butcher, & Dochterman, 2008).

HEALTH PROMOTION

Important Topics for Health Promotion

- Prevention of loss of core strength and of muscle flexibility
- Prevention of development of secondary pain, such as from poor posture, change in gait
- Adequate treatment of acute pain to prevent chronic pain
- Correct self-administration of analgesics (issues of over- and under-administration)
- Reduction of risk associated with use of alcohol, over-the-counter drugs, recreational drugs

Pain affects people of all ages. The rate of adult Canadians suffering from chronic pain is 22% to 50% (Queen's News Centre, 2004), and approximately 10% of the population has disabling chronic pain (Birse & Lander, 1998). More than 15% of Canadians have chronic pain with neuropathic features (ACTION, 2008).

Pain specialists have put much effort into creating awareness of pain, changing negative stereotypes, and improving treatment. They have focused fewer efforts on pain prevention, although this is changing.

RISK FACTOR ASSESSMENT

Demographics. The prevalence of chronic pain is greater in women than in men, primarily because the prevalence of various chronic diseases that coexist with chronic pain is greater for women. For example, women have more musculoskeletal problems, possibly because they have smaller frames and less muscle mass compared with men. More women than men have migraine headaches, osteoarthritis, rheumatoid arthritis, and fibromyalgia (Unruh, 1996; Unruh, Ritchie, & Merskey, 1999). Several researchers have examined the effects of age on pain perceptions (Li et al., 2001; Miakowski, 2000). Researchers have explored gender differences on the Visual Analog Pain Scale (Kelly, 1998), sex-specific effects of pain-related anxiety and chronic pain (Edwards, Augustson, & Fillingim, 2000), and the influence of gender roles and pain (Riley et al., 2002). Men were more anxious about their pain (Edwards et al., 2000) and reported higher intensity of pain during the night (Morin, Lund, Villarroel, Clokie, & Feine, 2000). Women tended to report higher levels of pain than men and higher intensity of daytime pain (Morin et al., 2000).

There may also be a genetic explanation for women being more sensitive to pain. Recent genetic research has led to suggestions of gender differences in pain and response to analgesics (Mogil, 2004, 2005). People with red hair have a different sensitivity to pain than the rest of the population. It has not been established whether genetic background offers protection. Differences in responses to nonsteroidal anti-inflammatory drugs and opioids are related to genetic factors (Desmeules, Piquet, Ehert, & Dayer, 2004). Green and colleagues (2003) have studied ethnic disparities and pain.

As people age, they are more likely to suffer from pain because their bodies experience cumulative damage and they are prone to acquiring diseases that cause pain. At the same time, some of the intensity of pain, especially cutaneous pain, may wane as people become less sensitive to painful stimuli. Some older clients may think that pain is an expected part of aging. As well, older adults may be afraid to say they have pain because they fear that use of pain medications will lead to addiction. If an older adult becomes confused after surgery, it is likely from inadequate pain control and impaired sleep related to pain rather than from the effects of the medication. After the pain is managed, the confusion usually clears.

Cultural aspects of pain have been studied, but methodological weaknesses and flaws (Lasch, 2000) and lack of clarity about ethnicity, culture, and race have made results difficult to interpret. Some factors related to differences in a cultural group include age, gender, educational level, and income. It is also important to know whether the client identifies closely with a cultural group (e.g., continues with traditional health beliefs and practices) or has adopted new health behaviours (Lander, 2007). It is critical that a nurse react to a client's pain perception rather than his or her pain behaviour (which is culturally related). Useful questions to consider when working with a client from a background different from the nurse's are as follows (Lander, 2007, p. 230):

■ What does the illness mean to you?

■ Are there culturally or socially based stigmas related to this disease or pain?

■ What is the role of your family in your health care decisions?

■ What traditional pain-relief remedies do you use?

■ What is the role of stoicism in your family and community?

■ Are there culturally or socially determined ways of expressing and communicating pain?

■ Do you have any fears about the pain?

■ Have you seen or do you want to see a traditional healer?

The client's past experience with pain is important to discuss. People with previous experience with pain may be anxious and fearful about a new painful situation, especially if pain was not previously well controlled. Other clients with previous positive experiences with pain may feel confident that their pain will be managed in the new situation. Those clients who have experienced severe pain know how bad the pain can be, whereas those without previous experience with pain may not fear how severe the pain might be. If pain is properly assessed and relieved, the client may feel less fearful about future episodes of pain.

Workplace/Lifestyle Issues. Because pain is the outcome of damaged tissues or nerves, prevention of such damage is important. Therefore, strategies that reduce or prevent injury will also reduce acute and chronic pain. Areas for prevention include high-risk behaviours, overuse or repetitive-strain injuries, and loss of core strength and flexibility. Clients in pain may try to relieve the pain by adjusting their posture or by changing their gait. These changes inflict strain on joints and muscles and can result in the development of secondary pain. Control of obesity and overall improvement of fitness and balance are other key pain-prevention strategies.

Coexisting Diseases. Strategies to prevent diseases associated with pain are also essential. Many chronic diseases include pain as a symptom or outcome. For example, neuropathic pain can be an outcome of end-stage renal disease and diabetes.

Adequacy of Pain Treatment. Nurses need to deal more effectively with acute and chronic pain. By treating acute pain properly, they may be able to decrease the risk of pain becoming chronic. Currently, with the preventive approach to relieving pain, nurses give analgesics at set intervals. Using a time basis rather than when the client reports pain means that nurses give medication before pain becomes severe and before serum levels of the opioid fall to subtherapeutic levels. If pain is expected over a 24-hour period and nurses administer medication on a schedule around the clock, the client will have more pain relief as the peaks and valleys of the serum level are reduced. In the end, the client may require less medication. As well, comprehensive treatment of chronic pain is necessary to prevent the psychosocial and economic outcomes associated with chronic pain.

SCREENING AND MAINTENANCE

Medication Use or Abuse. There are two types of problems—overuse and underuse of medications. Fear of addiction (usually unfounded) is a factor in underuse of analgesics. People may misinterpret the development of tolerance to opioids as a sign of addiction. As people take opioids, they become used to them and require higher doses to achieve previous levels of pain relief. Concerned family members may pressure clients to limit use of analgesics because of fear that their loved one will become addicted. Even at the end of life, family may be reluctant to give enough medication because of the stigma of addiction. In palliative care settings, pain medication usually is administered at regular intervals and rules related to administering narcotics (e.g., respirations must be at least 6 per minute) may not be relevant. The priority must be comfort, which means adequate pain relief through the dying process, ending in a "comfortable death" (Moorhead et al., 2008) or a "good death" (Lander, 2007).

Overuse or improper use may well be the outcome of poorly managed pain. Desperate for pain relief, people may use over-the-counter drugs excessively or use alcohol to potentiate the effects of prescribed drugs. Clients may consume excessive amounts of alcohol to dull the pain. Infrequently, people in desperation may seek street drugs, including marijuana. Proper management and education about tolerance, addiction, and drug effects are solutions.

EMERGENCY CONCERNS

Clients in severe pain unrelieved by over-the-counter analgesics need immediate attention to investigate the cause of the pain and to provide pain relief. Sudden onset of pain may indicate life-threatening conditions, including aortic aneurysm, cardiac disease, pneumothorax, deep vein thrombosis, or pulmonary embolus. Emergency assessment and treatment are required. Clients with acute severe back pain and headache also require assessment and treatment to minimize the risk of severe disability. (See the Emergency Concerns sections in other chapters for additional information.)

TECHNIQUES OF EXAMINATION: OBJECTIVE DATA

PROMOTING CLIENT COMFORT AND SAFETY

Pain is the subjective outcome of a biological and psychological process. No clinical test or apparatus directly measures pain. With pain, the gold standard is the client's report. This is why nurses say, "Pain is what the client says it is." Despite this, some health care professionals want to judge the accuracy of the client's report by rating the pain they have. This is then referred to as objective data, but it is not. Trying to rate the client's pain often leads to clients feeling they are not believed and the suspicion that pain is all in the head (is psychogenic).

Health care professionals are poor at rating someone else's pain. Assessing the face (or expression on the face) and posture to determine whether the client is in pain is very unsatisfactory, especially for a client with chronic pain. People learn how to control facial expressions at early ages. In contrast, the newborn's response to a pain stimulus (e.g., needles) is instinctive and can therefore be observed and rated.

Pain expression is learned. People can learn from family and the community to be stoic or intolerant in the face of pain. Many gender and cultural differences in pain can be linked to learned behaviour.

PROFESSIONAL CONDUCT

The needs of clients to find the cause of and a cure for their pain can make them defensive and desperate. They may embellish pain and its effects so that others take them seriously. They may also appear demanding or overly agreeable, or apprehensive or needy. These behaviours can raise suspicions. Behaviours of clients under these circumstances can lead health professionals to question the authenticity of the pain. This makes health professionals look to the client's face and body language for clues about the pain. Too often, health professionals treat clients with disdain. Every health professional who works with this population has heard stories of unprofessional conduct. Clients with chronic pain have been ejected from emergency departments and physicians' offices, been told they are wasting health care dollars, and called drug addicts and other names. To clients who relate these stories, the events are as clear today as when they happened, sometimes decades ago. The effect of not being believed and being badly treated by health professionals is more than many can bear. They view it as a breach of trust.

Hardly anyone wants to live with pain. People want it diagnosed and fixed. Finding a cause authenticates the pain and makes it *real*. Clients need to hear that they are believed. They also need to hear that it may not be possible to find the cause and a cure but that everything that can be done will be done. They also need to know that the future may bring new diagnostic procedures and treatments. This can help the client to move forward in life.

Having chronic pain and getting it treated are challenges. In many Canadian provinces, access to a special pain clinic for assessment and treatment involves a 2- to 3-year wait or longer. Clinics are few and far between, and clients often have to travel to receive the care they need. (See Canadian Pain Society for a list of pain clinics at http://www.canadianpainsociety.ca/PainClinics_List.pdf.)

Equipment

- Tongue blade—broken
- Test tubes with stoppers (one for hot water, one for cold water)
- Cotton balls
- Tuning fork—128 Hz or 256 Hz
- Disposable gloves (for use if a rash or wound drainage is expected)

ASSESSMENT OF PAIN

When carrying out a health systems assessment, nurses use the skills of inspection, palpation, percussion, and auscultation to look for indications of pain and associated changes. It is important to note that using physiological signs to identify pain is unreliable. The body quickly adapts to the stress of the pain; therefore, blood pressure, heart rate, and respirations decrease. Observation of pain behaviours is necessary, but their absence does not mean the absence of pain.

When the client presents with a concern about pain, give close attention to the painful areas and those nearby. Inspect the skin in the area. Look for trophic changes such as absent or excessive sweating, atrophic skin, and cutaneous ulcerations. Carefully examine the area for signs such as hypo- and hyperalgesia, parasthesia, and allodynia. Administer the DN4 Questionnaire (Bouhassira et al., 2005) to determine whether the pain has neuropathic features. Also look at the nearby joints for signs of redness and edema. Check the muscles for tone, strength, and signs of wasting.

Test for pain (broken tongue blade for sharp and rounded end for dull), temperature (two test tubes [one with hot water and one with cold]), and touch sensations (light touch), always comparing symmetrical areas (right and left side of the body) and distal with proximal areas of extremities. Scatter to test most of the dermatomes and major peripheral nerves (see Chapter 20). For example, include both shoulders (C4), inner and outer aspects of forearms (C6 and T1), fronts of both thumbs and little fingers (C6 and C8), fronts of both thighs (L2), medial and lateral aspects of both calves (L4 and L5), little toes (S1), and medial aspects of each buttock (S3). Test vibratory sense bilaterally with a tuning fork (128 Hz or 256 Hz), beginning with finger joints and moving proximally to the wrists, elbows, and shoulders, stopping when sensation is noted. Then test the toe joints bilaterally, again moving proximally to ankles, knees, and hips, stopping when sensation is noted.

DN4 (DOULEUR NEUROPATHIQUE EN 4 QUESTIONS)

Does your pain have one or more of the following characteristics?

- Burning
- Painful cold
- Electric shocks

Source: Bouhassira et al., 2005.

Is your pain associated with one or more of the following symptoms in the same area?

- Tingling
- Pins and needles
- Numbness
- Itching

If an area of sensory loss or hypersensitivity is detected, map out the boundaries in detail, using a cotton wisp for light touch and a broken tongue blade for "sharp" and "dull." Start with the point of reduced sensation and move until the client detects a change. Ask the client, "Does this feel the same as this? For infection control purposes, be sure to dispose of the cotton and tongue blade."

RECORDING AND ANALYZING FINDINGS

■ *Examples of Documentation for Pain*

Area	Expected Findings	Unexpected Findings
Temperature	37°C	38°C
Blood Pressure	118/78	156/96
Heart Rate	76 per min	104 per min
Respirations	16 per min	24 per min, shallow breaths
Pain	No pain reported in hands, arms, or shoulders, bilaterally	No pain reported in left hand, arm, or shoulder. Client reports "excruciating pain" in right hand. The hand is hypersensitive to movement of air, touch, and vibration.
Skin	White tones, moist—both arms and hands. Black hair evenly distributed over both arms. Warm skin temperature over both hands and arms.	Left hand—white tone, moist. Right hand—skin is red and the hand is edematous. Black hair over left arm; black hair from mid-right forearm to shoulder. Skin temperature over left hand and arm is slightly warm; right hand and wrist are hot to touch.
Muscles	Muscle mass symmetrical in size and contour bilaterally— hands, forearms, upper arms, and shoulder girdle	Muscle mass of left hand, forearm, upper arms and shoulder girdle greater than on right side.
Nails	Short and manicured, with no lesions bilaterally.	Long finger nails with rough uneven edges, no lesions bilaterally.
Range of Motion (ROM)	Full ROM bilaterally of thumbs, fingers, wrists, elbows, and shoulders without discomfort.	Full ROM on left (thumb, fingers, wrist), with more movement at elbow and shoulder. Limited ROM on right) thumb, fingers, and wrist, with more movement at elbow and shoulder.

(continued)

■ Examples of Documentation for Pain (Continued)

Area	Expected Findings	Unexpected Findings
Joints	No pain, swelling, or bogginess noted bilaterally over distal interphalangeal (DIP) joints, proximal interphalangeal (PIP) joints, metacarpophalangeal (MCP) joints, wrists, elbows, nd shoulder girdle. Temperature over all joints bilaterally the same as surrounding skin.	Pain and swelling noted over DIP joint, PIP joint, MCP joint, and wrist on right side. No pain or swelling noted over joints of left hand, arm, and shoulder. Temperature over joints of right hand and wrist is the same as the surrounding skin—hot to touch. Temperature over all joints of left hand and arm is the same as surrounding skin—slightly warm.
Muscle Tone	Slight resistance felt bilaterally with passive movement.	Slight resistance felt on left upper extremity with passive movement. Unable to test right extremity because of intense pain.
Muscle Strength	Strong, 5+ bilaterally—fingers, wrists, elbows, and shoulders.	Muscle strength strong, 5+ on left fingers, wrist, elbow, and shoulder. Unable to test right fingers, wrist, elbow, and shoulder because of pain.
Coordination	Rapid alternating movements performed smoothly, with even rhythm, with dominant left side somewhat faster than right. Point-to-point testing accurate bilaterally with eyes open and closed.	Rapid alternating movements performed smoothly, with even rhythm, with dominant left hand and arm. Right side was slow and awkward. Point-to-point testing was accurate bilaterally with eyes open and closed, but right side movements were shaky.
Pulses	Radial and brachial pulses 2+ bilaterally with regular rhythm.	Left radial and brachial pulses 2+. Right radial and brachial pulses 1+. Regular rhythm bilaterally.
Epitrochlear Nodes	Epitrochlear nodes not palpable bilaterally.	A small, smooth, firm, and mobile node noted on left side. Nodes not palpable on right side.
Sensation	Both superficial pain and light touch intact bilaterally over dermatomes C4 to C8 and T1. Vibratory sense and position sense intact bilaterally at fingers.	Superficial pain and light touch intact over dermatomes C4 to C8 and T1 on left side. On right side, light touch intact over dermatomes C4 to C8 and T1. Client refused the test of superficial pain and vibratory sense because the tests would be too painful.
Tactile Discrimination	Stereognosis, graphesthesia, and extinction intact bilaterally.	Stereognosis, graphesthesia, and extinction intact on left upper extremity and impaired on right upper extremity due to pain.
Reflexes	All reflexes (biceps, triceps, and brachioradialis) 2+ bilaterally.	Biceps and triceps 2+ bilaterally. Brachioradialis 2+ on left arm, but unable to test on right wrist because of pain.

ANALYZING FINDINGS FROM HEALTH HISTORY AND PHYSICAL EXAMINATION

Analysis of the subjective and objective data from the health history and examination leads to the formulation of a nursing diagnosis and a plan for interdisciplinary care. Central to this care are the unique aspects of the individual client and his or her input into the proposed plan. For example:

Gary Kroeger, 27 years old, is receiving Worker's Compensation Board (WCB) benefits, reduced by the amount of Canada Pension Plan disability benefits that he receives. One year ago, a heavy piece of equipment crushed his right hand in a work accident. He had emergency surgery to repair the hand fractures and crushed median nerve. Within 1 week, he was receiving physiotherapy to improve his fine motor skills and strengthen the muscles of his hand and arm. After the initial pain from the trauma had disappeared, Gary experienced pain only when he bumped his hand. He reports that this felt like an intense electric shock. After a few months, the skin on his hand became red and swollen. He now experiences nearly constant pain that feels like his hand is caught in a red-hot clamp. He arrives with a wet cloth wrapped around his hand, explaining that without this he could not survive the pain. A gentle breeze blowing on his hand and vibrations cause excruciating pain. Gary looks lethargic and grimaces and flinches when you touch his hand. During the assessment he tells you that he wants to have his hand amputated because he cannot go on like this.

You develop the following nursing diagnosis: **Possible chronic pain syndrome** *following traumatic injury as manifested by skin changes, subjective report of pain, and radical remedy requested.*

Gary requires help from an interdisciplinary pain service. His first point of contact will be the nurse practitioner, who will assess him and begin treatment. His medical condition needs evaluation by physicians who specialize in nerve blocks, neurosurgery, and pain management. Gary also needs to be evaluated by a clinical psychologist for mood disorder and treated as necessary. He needs help to learn cognitive–behavioural pain management strategies. The pain team, including the advanced practice clinical pharmacist, needs to evaluate the client's medications to determine suitability and to change them as necessary. A physical therapist will assess Gary's fitness and develop a treatment plan to strengthen his muscles. Later, he will need assistance from the WCB to evaluate occupational opportunities and to begin a work-hardening program. The team social worker will evaluate Gary's finances and look for public resources and programs to help him and his family. A registered nurse will facilitate the care plan as well as follow up on all aspects of care and work with the family to assess the effects of Gary's pain and how all members respond to it. The nurse will connect Gary with the Chronic Pain Association of Canada (a national support group) and direct him to informative Internet sites (such as the Canadian Pain Coalition).

Critical Thinking Exercise

Answer the following questions about Mr. Kroeger:

- Describe the mechanisms of pain. (*Knowledge*)
- Differentiate between neuropathic and nociceptive pain. (*Comprehension*)
- How would you assess pain if Mr. Kroeger were a mentally challenged young adult or a cognitively impaired older adult? (*Application*)
- What factors might contribute to observations made during the pain assessment? (*Analysis*)
- What data would you use to plan client education for the prevention of pain? (*Synthesis*)
- How would you assess the effectiveness of health promotion in a client who experiences chronic pain? (*Evaluation*)

Canadian Nursing Research

Call-Schmidt, T. A., & Richardson, S. J. (2003). Prevalence of sleep disturbance and its relationship to pain in adults with chronic pain. *Pain Management Nursing, 4*(3), 124–133.

Dysvik, E., Lindstrom, T. C., Eikland, O., & Natvig, G. K. (2004). Health-related quality of life and pain beliefs among people suffering from chronic pain. *Pain Management Nursing, 5*(2), 66–74.

Horgas, A. L., & Dunn, K. (2001). Pain in nursing home residents: Comparison of residents' self-report and nursing assistants' perceptions. Incongruencies exist in resident and caregiver reports of pain; therefore, pain management education is needed to prevent suffering. *Journal of Gerontological Nursing, 27*(3), 44–53.

INTERNATIONAL NURSING RESEARCH

Hurley, A. C., Volicer, B. J., Hanrahan, P. A., Houde, S., & Volcer, L. (1992). Assessment of discomfort in advanced Alzheimer's patients. *Research in Nursing and Health, 15*(5), 369–377.

Lasch, K., Greenhill, A., Wilkes, G., Carr, D., Lee, M., & Blanchard, R. (2002). Why study pain? A qualitative analysis of medical and nursing faculty and students' knowledge of and attitudes to cancer pain management. *Journal of Palliative Medicine, 5*(1), 57–71.

McCaffery, M., Ferrell, B. R., & Pasaro, C. (2000). Nurses' personal opinions about patients' pain and their effect on recorded assessments and titration of opioid doses. *Pain Management Nursing, 1*(3), 79–87.

Morse, J. M., Beres, M. A., Spiers, J. A., Mayan, M., & Olson, K. (2003). Identifying signals of suffering by linking verbal and facial cues. *Qualitative Health Research, 13*(8), 1063–1077.

Puntillo, K., Neighbor, M., O'Neil, N., & Nixon, R. (2003). Accuracy of emergency nurses in assessment of patient's pain. *Pain Management Nursing, 4*(4), 171–175.

Puntillo, K. A., Stannard, D., Miaskowski, C., Kehrle, K., & Gleeson, S. (2002). Use of a pain assessment and intervention notation (P.A.I.N.) tool in critical care nursing practice: Nurses' evaluations. *Heart & Lung, 31*(4), 303–314.

Stotts, N. A., Puntillo, K., Morris, A. B., Stanik-Hutt, J., Thompson, C. L., White, C., et al. (2004). Wound care pain in hospitalized adult patients. *Heart & Lung, 33*(5), 321–332.

Test Questions

1. All of the following are components/dimensions of pain **except**:
   a. sensory–discriminative.
   b. reactive–protective.
   c. cognitive–evaluative.
   d. affective–motivational.

2. Areas of the body that are highly sensitive to pain include all of the following **except**:
   a. fingertips.
   b. dorsum of the hand.
   c. around the mouth.
   d. eyes.

3. Which of the following best describes neuropathic pain?
   a. Associated with organs in the thorax, abdomen, and pelvis
   b. Labelled as musculoskeletal pain
   c. Described as sharp, or dull and aching
   d. Labelled as central pain

4. All of the following are signs or symptoms reported by clients with chronic pain **except**:
   a. apathy.
   b. anxiety.
   c. depression.
   d. lethargy.

5. Pain assessment includes all of the following aspects **except**:
   a. effects of pain on activities of daily living.
   b. intensity of pain.
   c. treatment expectations.
   d. effectiveness of treatment.

Bibliography

CITATIONS

ACTION. (2008). *Chronic and neuropathic pain.* Retrieved February 27, 2008, from http://www.nepaction.ca/main.htm

American Pain Society. (2003). Progress and directions for the agenda for pain management. *American Pain Society Bulletin 14*(5). Retrieved September 27, 2008, from http://www.ampainsoc.org/pub/bulletin/sep04/pres2.htm

Birse, T. M., & Lander, J. (1998). Prevalence of chronic pain. *Canadian Journal of Public Health, 89,* 129–131.

Bouhassira, D., Attal, N., Alchaar, H., Boureau, F., Bruxelle, J., Cunin, G., et al. (2005). Comparison of pain syndromes associated with nervous or somatic lesions and development of a new neuropathic pain diagnostic questionnaire (DN4). *Pain, 114*(1-2), 29–36.

Bulechek, G. M., Butcher, H. K., & Dochterman, J. M. (Eds.). (2008). *Nursing intervention classification (NIC)* (5th ed.). St. Louis, MO: Mosby Elsevier.

Canadian Institute for Health Information. (2006). *International statistical classification of diseases and related health problems (ICD)* (10th rev.). Ottawa, ON: Author.

Canadian Pain Coalition. (2005). *About Pain Awareness Week.* Retrieved September 27, 2008, from http://www.canadianpaincoalition.ca/index.php/en/national-pain-awareness-week/about

Canadian Pain Society. (2001). *Patient pain manifesto.* Retrieved July 5, 2008, from http://www.canadianpainsociety.ca/patient_pain.html

Canadian Pain Society. (2005). *Accreditation pain standard: Making it happen!* Retrieved September 27, 2008, from http://www.canadianpainsociety.ca/accreditation_manual.pdf

Cleeland, C. S. (1991). *Brief pain inventory.* Retrieved July 31, 2008 from, http://www.mdanderson.org/departments/prg/display.cfm?id=0EE7830A-6646-11D5-812400508B603A14&pn=0EE78204-6646-11D5-812400508B603A14& method=displayfull

Desmeules, J. A., Piquet, V., Ehert, G. B., & Dayer, P. (2004). Pharmacogenetics, pharmacokinetics, and analgesia. In: J. S. Mogil (Ed.), *The genetics of pain* (pp. 211–237). Seattle, WA: IASP Press.

Edwards, R., Augustson, E. M., & Fillingim, R. (2000). Sex-specific effects of pain-related anxiety on adjustment to chronic pain. *Clinical Journal of Pain, 16*(1), 46–53.

Green, C. R., Anderson, K. O., Baker, T. A., Campbell, L. C., Decker, S., Fillingim, R. B., et al. (2003). The unequal burden of pain: Confronting racial and ethnic disparities in pain. *Pain Medicine, 4*(3), 277–294.

International Association for Studies of Pain. (2008). *What's new IASP pain terminology?* Retrieved September 25, 2008, from http://www.iasp-pain.org/AM/Template.cfm?Section=Home&template=/CM/HTMLDisplay.cfm&ContentID=6649

Kelly, A. M. (1998). Does the clinically significant difference in visual analog scale pain scores vary with gender, age, or cause of pain? *Academy of Emergency Medicine, 5*(11), 1086–1090.

Kerns, R. D., Turk, D. C., & Ruby, T. E. (1985). The West Haven–Yale Multidimensional Pain Inventory (WHYMPI). *Pain, 23*, 345–356.

Lander, J. A. (2007). Pain management. In: R. A. Day, P. Paul, B. Williams, S. C. Smeltzer, & B. Bare (Eds.), *Brunner & Suddarth's textbook of medical–surgical nursing* (1st Canadian ed., pp. 222–255). Philadelphia: Lippincott Williams & Wilkins.

Lasch, K. E. (2000). Culture, pain and culturally sensitive pain care. *Pain Management Nursing, 1*(3), S1, 16–22.

Li, S. F., Greenwald, P. W., Gennis, P., Bijur, P. E., & Gallagher, E. J. (2001). Effect of age on acute pain perception of a standardized stimulus in the emergency department. *Annals of Emergency Medicine, 38*(6), 644–647.

Melzak, R. (1975). The McGill Pain Questionnaire: Major properties and scoring methods. *Pain, 1*(3), 277–299.

Melzak, R. (1996). Gate control theory: On the evaluation of pain concept. *Pain Forum, 5*(1), 128–138.

Merskey, H., & Bogduk, N. (1994). *Classification of chronic pain.* Seattle, WA: IASP Press. Retrieved July 13, 2008, from http://www.iasp-pain.org/AM/Template.cfm?Section=Home&TEMPLATE=/CM/HTMLDisplay.cfm&CONTENTID=4781

Miaskowski, C. (2000). The impact of age on a patient's perception of pain and ways it can be managed. *Pain Management Nursing, 1*(3), S1, 2–7.

Mogil, J. (Vol. Ed.). (2004). *Progress in pain research and management: Vol. 28. The genetics of pain.* Seattle, WA: IASP Press.

Mogil, J. S. (2005). The study of the genetics of pain in humans and animals. In: H. Merskey, J. D. Loeser, & R. Dubner (Eds.), *The paths of pain 1975–2005* (pp. 69–84). Seattle, WA: IASP Press.

Moorhead, S., Johnson, M., Maas, M., & Swanson, E. (Eds.). (2008). *Nursing outcomes classifications (NIC)* (4th ed.). St. Louis, MO: Mosby Elsevier.

Morin, C., Lund, J. P., Villarroel, T., Clokie, C. M. L., & Feine, J. S. (2000). Differences between the sexes in post-surgical pain. *Pain, 85*(1–2), 79–85.

NANDA International. (2007). *Nursing diagnoses. Definitions & classification 2007–2008.* Philadelphia: Author.

Queen's News Centre. (2004). *Chronic pain incidence in S.E. Ontario higher than average.* Retrieved September 27, 2008, from http://qnc.queensu.ca/story_loader.php?id=40bf31d155807

Riley, J. L., 3rd, Wade, J. B., Myers, C. D., Sheffield, D., Papas, R. K., & Price, D. D. (2002). Racial/ethnic differences in the experience of chronic pain. *Pain, 100*(3), 291–298.

Unruh, A. (1996). Gender variations in clinical pain experience. *Pain, 65*(2,3), 123–167.

Unruh, A. M., Ritchie, J., & Merskey, H. (1999). Does gender affect appraisal of pain and pain coping strategies? *Clinical Journal of Pain, 15*(1), 31–40.

Wall, P. D., & Melzak, R. (Eds.). (1999). *Textbook of pain* (4th ed.). New York: Churchill Livingstone.

Wong, D. L., Hockenberry-Eaton, M., Wilson, D., Winkelstein, M. L., & Schwartz, P. (2001). *Wong's essentials of pediatric nursing* (6th ed.). St. Louis, MO: Mosby Elsevier.

ADDITIONAL REFERENCES

Bair, M. J., Robinson, R. L., Katon, W., & Kroenke, K. (2003). Depression and pain comorbidity: A literature review. *Archives of Internal Medicine, 163*(20), 2433–2445.

Canadian Nurses Association. (2008). *Code of ethics for registered nurses.* Retrieved February 26, 2008, from http://www.cna-aiic.ca/CNA/practice/ethics/code/default_e.aspx

Dillon, P. N. (2007). *Nursing health assessment: Clinical pocket guide* (2nd ed.). Philadelphia: F. A. Davis Company.

Fries, B. E., Simon, S. E., Morris, J. N., Flodstrom, C., & Bookstein, F. L. (2001). Pain in U.S. nursing homes: Validating a pain scale for the minimum data set. *Gerontologist, 41*(2), 173–179.

Gordon, D. B., Pellino, T. A., Enloe, M. G., & Foley, D. K. (2000). A nurse-run inpatient pain consultation service. *Pain Management Nursing, 1*(2), 29–33.

Gunnarsdottir, S., Donovan, H., & Ward, S. (2003). Interventions to overcome clinician- and patient-related barriers to pain management. *Nursing Clinics of North America, 38*(1), 419–434.

Keefe, F. J., Rumble, M. E., Scipio, C. D., Giordano, L. A., & Perri, L. M. (2004). Psychological aspects of persistent pain: Current state of the science. *Journal of Pain, 5*(4), 195–211.

Kundermann, B., Krieg, J. C., Schreiber, W., & Lautenbacher, S. (2004). The effect of sleep deprivation on pain. *Pain Research Management, 9*(1), 25–32.

Lasch, K. E., Wilkes, G., Montuori, L. M., Chew, P., Leonard, C., & Hilton, S. (2000). Using focus group methods to develop multicultural cancer patient education materials. *Pain Management Nursing, 1*(4), 129–138.

Pasero, C. (2002). The challenge of pain assessment in the PACU. *Journal of Perianesthesia Nursing, 17*(5), 348–350.

Rakel, B., & Herr, K. (2004). Assessment and treatment of postoperative pain in older adults. *Journal of Perianesthesia Nursing, 19*(3), 194–208.

Robinson, M. E., Wise, E. A., Gagnon, C., Fillingim, R., B., & Price, D. D. (2004). Influences of gender role and anxiety on sex differences in temporal summation of pain. *Journal of Pain, 5*(2), 77–82.

Teno, J. M., Kabumoto, G., Wetle, T., Roy, J., & Mor, V. (2004). Daily pain that was excruciating at some time in the previous week: Prevalence, characteristics, and outcomes in nursing home residents. *Journal of American Geriatrics Society, 52*(5), 762–767.

Tripp, D. (2006). *Biopsychosocial factors in chronic pain management.* Retrieved September 27, 2008, from http://meds.queensu.ca/courses/msk/documents/tripp_2006.pdf

Watson, A. C., & Coyne, P. (2003). Recognizing the faces of cancer pain. *Nursing, 33*(4), 32hn1–32hn8.

Watt-Watson, J., Stevens, B., Garfinkel, P., Streiner, D., & Gallop, R. (2001). Relationship between nurses' pain knowledge and pain management outcomes for their postoperative cardiac patients. *Journal of Advanced Nursing, 36*(4), 535–545.

Weber, J. R. (2008). *Nurses' handbook of health assessment* (6th ed.). Philadelphia: Lippincott Williams &Wilkins.

Weiner, D. K. (2004). Pain in nursing home residents: What does it really mean, and how can we help? *Journal of the American Geriatrics Society, 52*(6), 1020–1022.

Wise, E. A., Price, D. D., Myers, C. D., Heft, M. W., & Robinson, M. E. (2002). Gender role expectations of pain: Relationship to experimental pain perception. *Pain, 96*(3), 335–342.

RESOURCES: CANADIAN WEB SITES AND ASSOCIATIONS

ACTION (2008) Chronic and neuropathic pain: http://www.nepaction.ca/main.htm

Accreditation Canada: www.accreditation-canada.ca/Default.aspx

Canadian Institute for Relief of Pain and Disability: http://www.cirpd.org

Canadian Institutes of Health Research: www.cihr-irsc.gc.ca

Canadian Neuropathy Association: www.canadianneuropathy association.org

Canadian Pain Coalition: www.canadianpaincoalition.ca

Canadian Pain Society/Société Canadienne de la Douleur: www.canadianpainsociety.ca

North American Chronic Pain Association of Canada: http://www.chronicpaincanada.com/

Pain Explained: www.painexplained.ca/

INTERNATIONAL WEB SITES AND ASSOCIATIONS

American Society of Pain Management Nurses: http://www.aspmn.org

International Association for Studies of Pain. IASP Secretariat: http://www.iasp-pain.org

Tame the Pain: Information for chronic pain sufferers; Metronic Inc., USA: http://www.tamethepain.co.uk

Nutritional Assessment

KIM BRUNET, RENE A. DAY, AND DIANA MAGER

Registered dietitians are experts in assessing the adequacy of food and fluid intake across the life cycle and developing dietary approaches for clients with wide-ranging health concerns. These roles require extensive core knowledge about the biochemical and nutritional contents of foods and how these may influence metabolic and physiological processes. Dietitians also are highly trained to understand the feeding environment and underlying psychosocial, economic, and health determinants that influence food intake at individual, societal, and global levels. These important skills are essential to assist clinicians to meet the needs of clients in all health care settings.

Nurses also play an invaluable role in nutritional care. In many practice settings, they are the first team members to assess overall health status. Hence, they often assist the team to determine nutritional status and to set the stage for the development of nutrition care plans. Nurses take the client's health history, including an initial review of weight history, general dietary changes (fluid and food intake), urine and bowel concerns and continence, and any symptoms that may contribute to changes in nutritional status. Nurses are typically responsible for assessing vital signs and measuring height, weight, and waist circumference—all of which are required to determine overall health status. Because nurses frequently initiate referrals for client assessment by dietitians, it is necessary for nurses to develop skills in nutrition screening to ensure that clients' needs are met in a timely and efficient manner. Dietitians and nurses collaborate to assist clients to learn about and manage their dietary intake and activity levels.

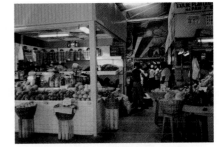

This chapter addresses major determinants that influence the nutritional well-being of clients and how this influences nutritional requirements and treatment. Knowing how aging influences body composition, organ function, and psychosocial variables is an important consideration. Content in this chapter will also present the fundamentals of nutrition screening and nutrition assessment from both the nursing and dietitian perspectives within the health care team.

ANATOMY AND PHYSIOLOGY

NUTRIENT DIGESTION AND ABSORPTION

Mouth and Stomach. The preparation of food for digestion and absorption begins when food enters the mouth and chewing commences. Food is minced into small particles and mixed with oral secretions (saliva) released from the parotid, submandibular, and sublingual salivary glands (see Chapter 13). Mucous secretions within saliva coat the food particles and protect the oral mucosa. Saliva consists predominantly of water, some electrolytes (sodium, potassium, and chloride), and α-amylase. This important enzyme breaks down internal α-1-4 bonds within starch. The mincing and mixing of food stuffs in the mouth represents the voluntary stage in nutrient digestion, while the involuntary nervous system controls the remaining steps.

Once food passes from the oral cavity and through the pharynx, the involuntary swallow occurs, encompassing two major events: (1) the esophageal sphincter relaxes, allowing the esophagus to open and (2) the larynx moves upwards and forwards, enabling the epiglottis to fall forward over the airway. Both mechanisms protect the airway and promote movement of food into the esophagus. Once food passes into the esophagus, the lower esophageal sphincter relaxes, allowing food to enter the stomach.

Within the stomach, several actions promote further digestion. Active peristalsis churns food particles into smaller particles and contributes to the release of gastric secretions from parietal cells lining the stomach antrum. The gastric secretions consist mainly of hydrochloric acid, which helps to convert several pre-enzymes (zymogens) into their active forms and promotes the denaturation (breakdown) of protein bonds in polypeptides. Such denaturation enables further digestion within the small intestine.

In addition to zymogens, gastric secretions include α-amylase and mucins. These compounds are important for subsequent digestion of complex carbohydrates (α-amylase) and for protecting the gastric mucosa from mechanical and chemical damage. Tight junctions between parietal cells also help minimize risk for damage to the gastric mucosa from ulceration (Groff & Gropper, 2000).

Small Intestine. The small intestine contains three portions: duodenum, jejunum, and ileum. Because of the large concentration of digestive enzymes released, the *duodenum* is the major site of nutrient fat (carbohydrate, and protein) digestion. Although few nutrients are absorbed in the duodenum, it is the major site for absorption of divalent ions (calcium, iron, magnesium, zinc), water-soluble vitamins (e.g., vitamin B_{12}), and, to a lesser extent, some macronutrients and trace elements. The major sites of nutrient absorption in the small intestine are the *jejunum* and *ileum*.

The surface area of the jejunum is characterized by long villi, with a large absorptive capacity and high concentration of transport protein (Bueno et al., 1999; Dibaise et al., 2004a,b). It is the primary site for absorption of macronutrients (fat, protein, and carbohydrates); water-soluble vitamins (folate, thiamine, riboflavin, niacin, pyridoxine); electrolytes; iron; calcium; and some water.

The ileum consists of shorter villi, more lymphoid tissue with less absorptive capacity, and a tighter epithelium. It is the main site for absorption of vitamin B_{12}, bile salts, fat-soluble vitamins (A, D, E, and K), cholesterol, fat, and some electrolytes. The highly adaptable ileum may take on some jejunal functions (e.g., increase absorption of fat-soluble vitamins) in situations of gut resection of the jejunum. Major gastrointestinal hormones that affect gut motility (enteroglucagen and peptide YY) are produced in the ileum, thus providing a mechanism to slow down gastric emptying when luminal fat is present (Bueno et al., 1999; Dibaise et al., 2004a, 2004b).

The Large Bowel. The large bowel, or colon, is the major site for water and electrolyte absorption and fermentation of nondigested starches (fibre) to short-chain fatty acids (Bueno et al., 1999; Dibaise et al., 2004a, 2004b).

MACRONUTRIENT DIGESTION, ABSORPTION, AND UTILIZATION

Protein. Protein digestion begins when parietal cells lining the stomach secrete hydrochloric acid to promote denaturation of the helical protein structure. The low pH in the stomach activates the release of pepsin, which denatures proteins into large polypeptide derivatives by hydrolysing peptide bonds within the main polypeptide structure, particularly those close to the carboxyl end (Groff & Gropper, 2000).

The end products of gastric digestion of proteins are primarily large polypeptides with some oligopeptides and free amino acids. Most polypeptides are digested and broken down in the small intestine by trypsin, chymotrypsin, and elastase. These enzymes rapidly attack peptide bonds to further break down protein into di- and tripeptides and amino acid residues, which are absorbed by active transport and facilitative diffusion, primarily in the jejunum. Once absorbed, amino acids are sent via the portal circulation to the liver for synthesis of protein, diversion of amino acid skeletons for converting amino acids to glucose (gluconeogenesis), or release into the systemic circulation.

Fats. Fat digestion begins in the oral cavity and stomach, stimulated by two enzymes: lingual lipase and pancreatic lipase. Lingual lipase accounts for <10% of fat digestion and acts preferentially on triacylglycerols with short- and medium-chain lengths plus some longer-chain unsaturated long-chain fatty acids. The end product of lingual lipase digestion is free fatty acids and 1,2-diacylglycerols (Groff & Gropper, 2000). The acid pH of the stomach and gastric contractions promote emulsification of these fats and partial fat breakdown.

When fat is released into the duodenum further emulsification occurs in response to bile acid release from the gallbladder. Bile acids are required to stimulate the formation of fat micelles (one of the ultramicroscopic units of protoplasm). Release of cholecystokinin stimulates bile acid release and bicarbonate release from the pancreas. The net result is increased duodenal pH, which is needed to activate pancreatic lipase, the primary enzyme responsible for fat digestion (Groff & Gropper, 2000).

Pancreatic lipase breaks down triacylglycerols (TAGs) into a mixture of diacylglycerols, monoacylglycerols, and free fatty acids. Typically co-lipase (activated by trypsin) assists in fat digestion by facilitating the action of lipase in the duodenum (Groff & Gropper, 2000). Once long-chain triglycerides are partially broken down, they combine with bile acids to form fat micelles. Formation of micellar particles is critical because it allows nonpolar long-chain fats to penetrate the polar unstirred water layer of the small intestine so that fat can be absorbed, primarily in the distal duodenum and proximal jejunum. Once this occurs, released bile acids travel to the distal ileum where they are reabsorbed via the portal circulation and returned to the liver (Groff & Gropper, 2000).

Fat is absorbed into the enterocytes lining primarily the jejunum as free fatty acids and 2-monoacylglyerols. They are resynthesized within the enterocyte into TAGs, phospholipids, or cholesterol esters (cholesterols). For TAGs with chain lengths <12 carbons, most are bound to albumin and transported directly to the liver via the portal circulation. For TAGs with carbon lengths >12 carbons, most are coupled to coenzyme A and transported via the lymphatic system as chylomicrons to the liver.

In the liver, TAGS, phospholipids, and cholesterol are repackaged into various lipoproteins that facilitate transport of fat into the systemic circulation. The types of

Protein-losing enteropathy (PLE) results in loss of serum proteins (primarily albumin) into the gastrointestinal tract. The cause may be lymphatic obstruction or is secondary to mucosal erosion or ulceration (e.g., Crohn's disease or severe viral insult). If loss of serum proteins exceeds the rate of hepatic synthesis, hypoalbuminemia, and edema develop. It is critical to take a careful dietary history to quantitate protein intake. To rule out renal, bladder, liver, and GI causes for PLE, review of the health history should include urinary frequency and colour of urine, blood pressure, bowel movements, hematochezia (stools containing red blood rather than being tarry), abdominal pain, fatigue, and jaundice (Ferrante et al., 2006).

lipoproteins include very low-density lipoproteins (VLDL), low-density lipoproteins (LDL), and high-density lipoproteins (HDL). These proteins are responsible for the transportation of fat, phospholipids, and cholesterol in the systemic circulation (Groff & Gropper, 2000).

VLDL is predominantly responsible for the transportation of triglycerides, while LDL and HDL tend to carry more polar lipids such as cholesterol and phospholipids. The major role of LDL is to bind cholesterol (>60%) for transport to peripheral cells, where it can be used to synthesize steroid hormones and other compounds needed for cell function (Groff & Gropper, 2000). The major role of HDL is to remove unesterified cholesterol from cells and other lipoproteins and return excess cholesterol to the liver for excretion into the bile (Groff & Gropper, 2000). The net effect is that LDL is responsible for depositing cholesterol in the body, and HDL is responsible for excreting or removing cholesterol from the body.

Elevated serum LDL is an early warning of excess cholesterol deposition in the arteries, which can lead to *atherosclerosis*. Thus, monitoring serum LDL and VLDL is clinically important, particularly in clients who are overweight or obese and with a family history of elevated cholesterol, triglycerides, or both. High LDL and low HDL levels are major risk factors for development of cardiovascular disease and warrant further investigation (McPherson et al., 2006). Restriction of total, saturated, and trans fats is typically recommended. Assistance from a registered dietitian to make appropriate dietary modifications is warrented.

Although high-fat diets have been associated with an increased incidence of cholelithiasis, there is *no* evidence that dietary fat restriction will prevent biliary colic from recurrence of gallstone formation (Lai et al., 2002; Misciagna et al., 1999; Wudel et al., 2002).

Carbohydrates.

Dietary starch digestion typically starts in the mouth by salivary α-amylase (Groff & Gropper, 2000). It continues into the stomach, where the acid environment inactivates this enzyme. Typically, the result is partial breakdown of dietary starches into dextrins (short-chain polysaccharides and maltose). Further digestion of dextrins occurs in the small intestine by pancreatic α-amylase. The extent of digestion depends on the form of dietary starch (amylase versus amylopectin). If the source is amylase, pancreatic α-amylase, breaks it down to maltoseand the trisaccharide maltotriose, which is further hydrolysed to maltose and glucose. However, if the source is amylopectin, then pancreatic α-amylase breaks it down into disaccharide units called isomaltose. These disaccharide units (typically sucrose, lactose, maltose) are broken down into their respective monosaccharides (glucose, fructose, galactose) by disaccharidases (e.g., sucrase, lactase, maltase, and isomaltase) found on the microvilli of the small intestine (Groff & Gropper, 2000).

Excess or abnormally high bile salt levels can contribute to gallbladder stones (*cholelithiasis*). These typically develop when bile becomes supersaturated with cholesterol. Gallstones blocking biliary ducts lead to nausea, vomiting, and abdominal pain. Predisposing factors include obesity, rapid weight loss, physical inactivity, frequent fasting, diabetes, and use of medications such as octreotide, estrogens, and fibrates. Gallstones are more common in women of northern European or Hispanic descent.

Active transport mechanisms work to absorb glucose and galactose into the mucosal cells lining the small intestine, while facilitated diffusion is the method of absorption of fructose. Active transport requires energy in the form of adenosine triphosphate (ATP) and the involvement of specific carrier proteins. The glucose–galactose carrier protein is known as SGLT-1. Less is known about the absorption of fructose. Once absorbed, all monosaccharides are transported to the liver, where fructose and galactose are converted to glucose derivatives and then either stored as liver glycogen or transported to the circulation to meet the body's energy needs. As with fructose and galactose, glucose is typically converted to liver glycogen or transported in the circulation to meet energy needs in the systemic circulation (Groff & Gropper, 2000).

Lactose intolerance (LI) is an inability to digest significant amounts of lactose, the major sugar in milk and milk products. The typical cause is shortage of the sucrose–isomaltase enzyme (lactase), which breaks down lactose into glucose and galactose. In affected clients, lactose in the small intestine causes bloating, gas, nausea, diarrhea, and cramping. Severity depends on how much lactose a person can tolerate, age, ethnicity, and digestion rate.

NUTRITION CARE PROCESS

Canadian dietitians use the four-step nutrition care process developed by the American Dietetic Association (ADA): (1) nutrition assessment, (2) nutrition diagnosis, (3) nutrition intervention, and (4) nutrition monitoring and evaluation. This standardized language allows practitioners to communicate treatment strategies with health care team members to evaluate care effectively.

■ IDENTIFICATION OF CLIENTS (NUTRITION SCREENING)

Before beginning the nutrition care process, nutrition screening is the first step in identifying clients who are currently malnourished or at risk for becoming malnourished. Nutrition screening by nurses, nurse practitioners, and physicians targets clients who require further assessment and treatment, streamlines referrals, and helps prioritize those in greatest need of service (Keller, Brockest, & Haresign, 2006). Validated nutrition screening tools exist for target populations. An example is the Mini Nutritional Assessment (MNA) used to identify clients 65 years or older who are malnourished or are at risk. It provides a scoring system and triage criteria. More information can be found at www.mna-elderly.com. Once a client has been identified, the nutrition care process would direct the dietitian to complete a nutrition assessment.

■ NUTRITION ASSESSMENT

Nutrition assessment (the first step in the nutrition care process) is a method of collecting and evaluating data to make decisions about a nutrition-related problem or diagnosis. The assessment data are compared to reliable norms and standards for evaluation when possible. Nutrition assessment initiates the data collection process, which continues throughout the nutrition care process and provides the framework for reassessment and reanalysis of data in step 4, nutrition monitoring and evaluation.

Nutrition assessment can include subjective data such as health history; symptoms; concerns; dietary intake; psychosocial, behavioural, and functional factors; knowledge; readiness; potential for change; and objective data (e.g., anthropometric and biochemical measurements).

LI is often confused with cow's milk protein intolerance, which is an allergic reaction to a specific milk protein. LI, however, represents a defect in absorption and digestion of milk sugar. A careful history to rule out any respiratory or dermatological symptoms (e.g., urticaria) will assist nurses to determine an accurate nursing diagnosis.

Typical treatment of LI includes restriction of dietary sources of lactose and requires consultation with a registered dietitian for nutritional adequacy. Dietary restrictions vary based on individual tolerance. Consumption of lactose-reduced products (e.g., lactose-reduced milk) can promote nutritional adequacy. For those who react to very small amounts of lactose or have trouble limiting intake of foods containing it, the nonprescription lactase enzyme is available. Clients take the tablets with the first bite of lactose-containing food to make the lactose more digestible. Lactase enzyme is also available as a liquid that can be added as drops to milk. A careful review of symptoms by the nurse can facilitate client education regarding use (Matthews et al., 2005; Suarez et al., 1995).

HEALTH HISTORY: SUBJECTIVE DATA

Key Symptoms and Signs Reported by the Client

- Body weight changes
- Access to healthy foods (e.g., economic constraints, cultural or religious practices)
- Food intolerances/aversions
- Appetite or taste changes (e.g., anorexia, nausea, vomiting)
- Psychological symptoms (e.g., depression, disordered eating)
- Physical impairments that limit ability to independently consume food/fluids
- Medications that affect intake

Nurses collect specific data by using an analysis-of-a-symptom approach. Weight gain is used below with sample questions related to the components of a symptom analysis.

Examples of Questions for Symptom Analysis—Weight Gain

- "How has your weight changed over the past year?" (*Timing*)
- "Tell me where you notice the weight gain." (*Location*)
- "How has the weight gain affected your activities?" "Has your weight gain created any other difficulties?" (*Quantity/severity*)
- "What other symptoms have you noticed?" (*Associated symptoms*)
- "Has anything changed in your life that has precipitated this weight gain?" "How is the stress in your life right now?" (*Environmental factors*)

- "Is this weight gain a concern for you?" "Have you ever attempted weight loss before?" "What was helpful?" "What kinds of challenges would you expect in making those changes now?" "How do you think you could deal with them?" (*Client's perception*)
- "Can you imagine how your weight may cause problems in the future?" "What does this weight gain mean to you?" (*Significance to the client*)

Assessing Dietary Intake.   Such assessment includes evaluating the amount, type, and frequency of foods the client eats. It also requires noting lifestyle factors that could influence food intake. Examples are economic status, living conditions, ethnicity, eating alone or with others, setting for eating, food preferences and restrictions, and transportation issues. Health concerns may affect mobility for shopping or preparing food.

Various methods are available to gather information about food intake. Two of the most common include *food records* (3- to 7-day client-recorded diary) and *24-hour recall* (detailed interview with a client/caregiver to determine amounts and types of foods eaten). The accuracy depends on the interviewer's skill and the client's memory and cooperation. This process can be time-consuming. The focus is to recognize nutritional problems, intervene when necessary, and refer the client to a dietitian as indicated.

Canada's Food Guide (Health Canada, 2007a) was developed to provide Canadians with guidelines to achieve a healthy eating pattern that meets the nutrient standards

---

Recommended Numbers of Food Guide Servings per Day						
Age in Years	**Teens (14–18 Years)**		**Adults (19–50 Years)**		**Older Adults (51+ Years)**	
Gender	Females	Males	Females	Males	Females	Males
Vegetables & Fruits	7	8	7–8	8–10	7	7
Grain Products	6	7	6–7	8	6	7
Milk & Alternatives	3–4	3–4	2	2	3	3
Meat & Alternatives	2	3	2	3	2	3

Source: Adapted from Health Canada, 2007a.

CANADA FOOD GUIDE SERVING SIZES AND GUIDELINES

Vegetables and Fruits: One serving is 125 mL of fresh, frozen, or canned vegetables or fruits; one fruit; or 125 mL of juice.

- Eat one orange and one dark green vegetable daily.
- Vegetables and fruits are preferable to juices.

Grain Products: One serving is a slice of bread; half a bagel, pita, or tortilla; 125 mL of cooked rice, bulgar, or quinoa; 30 g of cold cereal or 175 mL of hot cereal; 125 mL of cooked pasta or couscous.

- Select primarily whole grain products that are low in fat, sugar, and salt, and are high in fibre.

Milk and Alternatives: One serving is 250 mL of milk or fortified soy beverages daily, 175 g of yogurt or kefir, 50 g of cheese.

- Drink milk (skim, 1% or 2%) or fortified soy beverages daily.
- Choose low-fat milk alternatives.

Meat and Alternatives: One serving is 75 g of cooked fish, poultry, lean meat; 175 mL of cooked legumes; 150 g or 175 mL of tofu; 2 eggs; 30 mL of peanut or nut butter; 60 mL of shelled nuts or seeds.

- Choose lean meats and prepare with minimal fat or salt.
- Select beans, lentils, and tofu frequently.
- Consume at least two servings of "fatty" fish every week (e.g., salmon, sardines, trout, mackerel, char, or herring).

Oils and Fats: Use a maximum of 30 to 45 mL of unsaturated fats daily in cooking, margarine, salad dressings, and mayonnaise.

- Use canola, olive, and soybean oils.
- Select soft margarines that are low in saturated fats and ideally have no trans fats.
- Limit intake of butter, hard margarine, shortening, and lard.

Source: Adapted from Health Canada, 2007a.

---

called dietary reference intakes (DRIs) (Health Canada, 2006). "The DRIs summarize research findings about the amount of each nutrient and calories (energy) needed for good health and the prevention of chronic disease, while avoiding the negative effects of consuming too much of any individual nutrient" (Health Canada, 2007b, p. 4). These nutrients have been translated into a pattern that includes foods from each of four groups: vegetables and fruits, grain products, milk and alternatives, and meat and alternatives, plus a certain amount of added oils and fats. If a client avoids food groups or does not eat minimum servings, then the nurse is alerted to refer the client to a dietitian for in-depth analysis and counselling.

Canada's Food Guide is available online in multiple languages (including French) at http://www.hc-sc.gc.ca/fn-an/food-guide-aliment/index_e.html and First Nations, Inuit, and Metis at http://www.hc-sc.gc.ca/fn-an/pub/fnim-pnim/index_e.html.

OBJECTIVE DATA

Anthropometric Measurements. These important physical data provide information about nutritional status and relative body fat. A healthy body weight promotes general health and reduces the risk for some chronic diseases. Client self-reported height and weight have been found to be inaccurate (Brener et al., 2003; Engstrom et al., 2003; Kucamarski et al., 2001) and may lead to incorrect assessment of weight for height. Height and weight should be measured in all clients using standardized techniques.

Anthropometric measurements include height, weight, and waist circumference. A dietitian also may take skin-fold measurements when difficulties such as fluid overload or renal failure interfere with obtaining an accurate weight. These measures can provide additional information about fat and muscle stores. Height and weight measurements are used initially to evaluate baseline nutritional status and serially to evaluate response to the nutrition care plan.

Height and Build.   Is the client unusually short or tall? Is the build slender and lanky, muscular, or stocky? Is the body symmetric? Note general body proportions. Look for any deformities. If possible, measure height with the client in stocking or bare feet. Have the client stand backwards on the balance beam scale, with heels together, back straight, and looking forward. Lift the L-shaped measuring attachment above and lower it until it is flat on the client's head. Record the height. If a scale is not available, have the client stand with feet together, touching a wall. Measure the distance from the floor to the top of the client's head (Weber & Keliey, 2007).

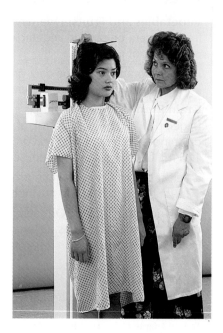

Height loss accompanies *osteoporosis* and *vertebral compression fractures*.

Nurses work with many clients who are in wheelchairs, bedridden, or elderly with kyphosis, and cannot stand upright. In such cases, use one of three measurements to estimate height: forearm length (Mitchell & Lipschitz, 1982); knee height (Chumlea, Roche, & Steinbaugh, 1985); or demispan (Bassey, 1986). All methods involve measuring long bones that do not lose length with aging.

Knee height is used particularly with older clients who are bedridden. With the client supine, use a special caliper placed under the heel and behind the knee to hold the knee and ankle areas at a 90-degree angle. Measure on the lateral side of the leg from bottom of the heel to top of the knee. Height in centimetres for women is 84.88 − (0.24 × age) + (1.83 × knee height). Height in centimetres for men is 64.19 − (0.04 × age) + (2.02 × knee height). Measurement can also be made as the client sits with feet flat on the floor.

The demi-span, a clinically useful and easy estimate of height, is recommended by the MNA tool (www.mna-elderly.com). Only a tape measure is needed. Demi-span is the distance from the middle of the sternal notch to the tip of the middle finger (palm facing forward), usually with the left arm. The arm needs to be horizontal and aligned with the shoulders. Height in centimetres is 1.35 × demi-span in cm + 60.1 for females and 1.40 × demi-span in cm + 57.8 for males. Demi-span is based on maximum height obtained at age 35 rather than current height (Bassey, 1986).

Weight.   Is the client emaciated, slender, plump, obese, or somewhere in between? If the client is obese, is fat distributed evenly or concentrated over the trunk, upper torso, or hips? Whenever possible, weigh the client with his or her shoes off and without heavy sweaters or jackets. Move the weights on a balance beam scale until the balance is level. Once the client is on the scale, move the weights until they are balanced. Record the weight (Weber & Kelley, 2007). Weight provides one index of caloric intake, and changes over time yield other valuable diagnostic data. Remember that changes in weight can accompany changes in body fluid status, as well as in fat or muscle mass.

Generalized fat in simple obesity; truncal fat with relatively thin limbs in *Cushing's syndrome* and metabolic (insulin-resistance) syndrome.

Causes of weight loss include malignancy, *diabetes mellitus*, *hyperthyroidism*, chronic infection, *depression*, diuresis, and successful dieting.

Use weight and height measurements to calculate body mass index (BMI), a ratio based on *weight (in kilograms) divided by height (in square metres)*. The BMI is widely accepted as a simple and accurate way to assess body weight in relation to health risk in clients associated with being underweight or overweight (Kirk et al., 2009).

CALCULATING BODY MASS INDEX (BMI)

$$BMI = \frac{Weight\ in\ kilograms}{(Height\ in\ metres)^2}$$

Example: Susan weighs 60 kg and is 160 cm (1.6 m) in height.

$$60/(1.6)^2 = 60/2.56 = BMI\ of\ 23.4$$

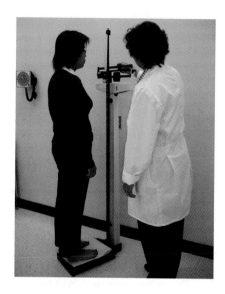

A Health Canada Website for calculating BMI is available at http://www.hc-sc.gc.ca/fn-an/nutrition/weights-poids/guide-Id-adult/bmi_chart_java-graph_imc_java-eng.php

Screening for overweight and obesity should be considered integral to routine health assessment (Canadian Medical Association, 2005). Risk for health problems increases the further BMI falls outside the "normal" category. Note that sudden or considerable weight gains or losses may also indicate health risk, even if this occurs with a "normal" BMI. In adults aged 18 to 65 years, interpretation of BMI should be based on Canadian guidelines.

People with a high BMI and who are overweight or obese are at increased risk for *type 2 diabetes mellitus*, *hypertension*, dyslipidemia, *coronary artery disease*, *stroke*, *sleep apnea*, *osteoarthritis*, *gallstones*, stress incontinence, depression, and certain cancers (Douketis et al., 2005). Low BMI is associated with *osteoporosis*, malnutrition, and eating disorders (Katzmarzyk, Craig, & Bouchard, 2001).

	Body Mass Index (kg/m²)	Risk of Developing Health Problems
Underweight	<18.5	Increased
Normal	18.5–24.9	Lowest
Overweight	25–29.9	Increased
Obesity Class I	30–34.9	High
Obesity Class II	35–39.9	Very high
Obesity Class III	≥40	Extremely high

Source: Adapted from Douketis et al., 2005.

Caution is required when interpreting BMI for those 65 years or older. They may not be at increased risk for health problems with a BMI <30, whereas those with a "low normal" BMI (18.5–20) may be at increased risk. Normal-weight or low-risk BMI range may be 22 to 29 for older adults. Weight loss in older people, especially loss of muscle, regardless of baseline BMI, is associated with increased risk of morbidity. Screening for weight loss may be a more useful means of determining health risk in older clients (American Dietetic Association, 2005; Douketis et al., 2005).

The body weight classification was intended to apply to all ethnic groups in Canada; however, there may be limitations in applying this classification to nonwhite people. A study in the Asian population (WHO Expert Consultation, 2004) suggests that BMI cut-offs for assessing health risk of overweight and obesity start at lower levels (23 and 27, respectively) (WHO Expert Consultation, 2004).

In Canadian First Nations and Inuit populations, >50% have obesity or type 2 diabetes. BMI cut-offs used for the general population may not be appropriate for Aboriginal populations.

Waist Circumference. Waist circumference measures abdominal fat content.

Excess abdominal fat relative to total body fat is an independent predictor of disease risk and morbidity.

INSTRUCTIONS FOR MEASURING WAIST CIRCUMFERENCE

- A measuring tape is placed around the trunk, at a point midway between the lower costal margin and the iliac crest, while the client is standing with feet about 25–30 cm (10–12 in.) apart.
- The measuring tape is fit snugly around the abdomen but without compressing underlying soft tissues.
- The waist circumference is recorded to the nearest 0.5 cm (1/4 in.) at the end of a usual expiration.

Source: Canadian Medical Association, 2005.

BMI and waist circumference are related; however, waist circumference provides additional information on health risk beyond that determined by the BMI. It is particularly useful to consider both measures when assessing a client's disease risk.

Increased waist circumference with a "normal" BMI may indicate abdominal body fat distribution that increases risk of health problems (Janssen, Katzmarzyk, & Ross, 2002). Increased relative disease risk occurs when waist circumference is >102 cm for males and >88 cm for females. Waist circumference is valid for a BMI of 25 to 34.9, but does not add value to predict disease risk if BMI is >35.

Waist Circumference	BMI		
	Normal	*Overweight*	*Obesity Class I*
Men ≤102 cm (≤40 in.) Women ≤88 cm (≤35 in.)	Least risk	Increased risk	High risk
Men >102 cm (>40 in.) Women >88 cm (>35 in.)	Increased risk	High risk	Very high risk

Source: Health Canada, 2003.

In addition to physical measurements, the client's other risk factors for diseases and conditions associated with obesity (e.g., high blood pressure or physical inactivity) should also be determined.

Clinical Examination. To determine general nutritional status, nurses inspect the oral cavity and assess the skin for turgor, edema, elasticity, dryness, lesions, stage of healing of wounds or ulcers, and bruising (Day, 2007).

See Tables 8-1 and 8-2 and Chapter 10.

Biochemical Assessment. Biochemical tests help provide added objective measures of nutritional status (Marshall, 2008). Some common and useful screening measures include hemoglobin and hematocrit to assess iron status, and serum proteins (albumin, prealbumin) to assess visceral protein status. Interpretation of these laboratory values must include the client's overall health.

Albumin and prealbumin have limited value in clients with chronic liver or renal disease and are influenced by hydration level. Complete blood cell count can provide useful information about

NUTRITION DIAGNOSIS

The second step in the nutrition care process is **nutrition diagnosis**—the identification and labelling that describes the actual occurrence or potential for developing a nutrition problem that requires treatment. Succinctly stated diagnoses guide clinicians to develop a care plan. For example, according to the NANDA International (2007), the nurse determines that the nursing diagnosis is *imbalanced nutrition: less than body requirements related to reported intake less than daily requirements and a BMI of 18.*

The nurse refers the client to a dietitian. The dietitian completes an in-depth nutrition assessment and determines that the nutrition diagnosis is *inadequate protein and energy intake related to recent exacerbation of Crohn's disease as evidenced by intake less than 50% of requirements, loss of 5 kilograms over the past month and a current BMI of 18.*

iron status, but caution must be used in interpreting these laboratory values in clients with chronic disease, because decreases in hematocrit and hemoglobin may be associated with anemia of chronic disease. Additional markers of iron status, such as serum ferritin or transferrin, may be warranted (Marshall, 2008).

NUTRITION INTERVENTION

Step 3 is **nutrition intervention**—a specific set of purposefully planned activities to address a problem and to meet the client's nutrition needs. Interventions are based on scientific principles, but this step is largely a client-driven process to create a realistic plan with good probability of success.

NUTRITION MONITORING AND EVALUATION

The last step is **nutrition monitoring and evaluation**. Monitoring refers to the review and measurement of the client's status at a preplanned follow-up point. Evaluation is comparison of current findings with previous status or a reference standard. The purpose is to determine the degree to which progress is being made and goals are being met. This step requires commitment to active recording of outcomes and altering intervention plans if outcomes are less than expected.

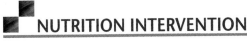
HEALTH PROMOTION: NUTRITION IN THE LIFE CYCLE

During periods of rapid growth (pregnancy, infancy, and adolescence), energy and protein needs increase to ensure sufficient growth. In early adulthood, optimal nutrient intake (particularly vitamin D, calcium, and protein) is important to ensure accretion of lean body mass and bone mineral density (BMD). This is critical to prevent problems with BMD depletion in later years. In the adult years, energy balance is essential to ensure prevention of overweight and obesity and onset of chronic disease, particularly with aging. Major body compositional changes that accompany aging are in lean body and fat masses, as well in organ function.

PREGNANCY AND LACTATION

Nutrition is directly related to outcomes in pregnancy. The following are important factors to consider and monitor. These are also discussed in Chapter 24.

Weight Gain. Maternal weight gain is an expected and important determinant of birth outcomes. Prepregnancy BMI should be evaluated and goal setting

Inadequate gestational weight gain may result in fetal growth restriction with appropriate weight ranges discussed with clients. Based on prepregnancy BMI alone, healthy-weight women are at lowest risk for giving birth to a low-birthweight or high-birthweight baby. Two or three weight recordings over the second and third trimesters are sufficient to monitor weight gain of healthy-weight women.

Guidelines for gestational weight gain based on those published by Health Canada (1999) and the Institute of Medicine (2004) are listed in Chapter 24. In general, during the first trimester, women typically gain 1.0 to 3.5 kilograms. In the second and third trimesters, weight gain is steady and incremental, from 0.3 to 0.5 kilograms per week depending on BMI category. Erratic patterns of high or low weight gain require further evaluation.

Healthy Postpartum Weights. Weight loss after pregnancy varies. Women who gain more weight than recommended and fail to lose it are at risk for long-term weight changes and higher BMI many years after pregnancy (Olson et al., 2003; Rooney & Schauberger, 2002). One study that followed women for 10 years postpartum found that those who breastfed and engaged in physical activity were more successful in controlling long-term weight gain (Rooney & Schauberger, 2002).

Nutrients of Special Concern

Folic Acid. Folic acid is a preventive nutrient against neural tube defects (NTDs). Mandatory food fortification with folic acid in Canadian provinces has been shown to reduce NTDs by 46% (Society of Obstetricians and Gynaecologists of Canada [SOGC], 2003). The SOGC (2003) recommends that all women planning to become pregnant should take a multivitamin with folic acid in amounts of 0.4 to 1.0 mg/day to reduce the risk of NTDs. Women at intermediate to high risk for having a baby with NTDs (e.g., previous NTD-affected pregnancy, maternal or paternal family history of NTD, insulin-dependent diabetes mellitus, epilepsy treatment with valproic acid or carbamazepine) should take a high dose of folic acid under medical supervision: 4.0 to 5.0 mg/day as a supplement only.

Lactating women require 0.5 mg of folic acid daily (Health Canada, 2003) and should continue taking a multivitamin with folic acid while breastfeeding.

and increased perinatal mortality. Factors that predispose women to insufficient gestational weight gain may include low socioeconomic status, teen pregnancy, limited support network, physical abuse, low educational level, severe nausea/vomiting, multiple gestation, excess dieting, and eating disorders (Health Canada, 1999).

Women with excess gestational weight gain may give birth to infants with high birth weights. Possible consequences (especially >4500 g) are prolonged labour and birth, birth trauma, birth asphyxia, caesarean birth, and perinatal mortality (Health Canada, 1999). These women may be predisposed to retaining weight after pregnancy, and may have children at higher risk for being overweight in childhood (Oken et al., 2007).

Pregnant women with low or high BMI before pregnancy should be referred to a registered dietitian for dietary assessment and counselling. Weight gain should be monitored at each prenatal visit.

Women who retain >4 to 5 kg one year postpartum should receive follow-up assistance with healthy eating and active living strategies. Risks of morbidity and mortality associated with being overweight (breast cancer, heart disease, and diabetes) make factors associated with weight gain in women an important public health concern.

Iron. Iron needs increase during pregnancy to increase maternal red blood cell mass and to supply the fetus and placenta. Adequate iron stores, if present prior to pregnancy, and a healthy eating pattern provide sufficient iron to meet these increased needs. Health Canada (2007b) recommends a multivitamin with iron for all pregnant women on the assumption that pre-pregnancy stores are inadequate. A recent Cochrane Review (Pena-Rosas & Viteri, 2006) concluded that evidence is insufficient to recommend routine prenatal iron supplementation at this time. However, in geographical regions with prevalent pre-gestational iron deficiency and anemia, routine supplementation is advisable.

Calcium/Vitamin D. Pregnant and lactating women require calcium and vitamin D to provide substrate for fetal skeletal development, for production of breast milk, and to maintain their own skeletal integrity. Calcium needs in pregnancy do not differ from age-adjusted guidelines, because pregnancy causes alterations in vitamin D synthesis that increase intestinal calcium absorption (Health Canada, 2006). However, many women, particularly teens, do not consume adequate calcium prior to pregnancy (Baker et al., 1999).

Vitamin D insufficiency exists in Canada from the low angle of the sun's rays, particularly from October to April (Hanley & Davidson, 2005). The emphasis is no longer just prevention of vitamin D deficiency, which is expressed as rickets in children and osteomalacia in adults. Deficiency can generally be prevented by following *Canada's Food Guide* servings of milk and alternatives (Health Canada, 2007a). The emphasis recently has been on prevention of associated childhood and adult diseases that are related to vitamin D insufficiency. Maternal vitamin D status during gestation and lactation may influence the health status of the child later in life. Examples include reduced bone density (Javaid et al., 2006) and susceptibility to type 1 diabetes (Hypponen et al., 2001).

Dental caries may also have their beginnings in early life. Infants of mothers who are vitamin D- or calcium-deficient during pregnancy may be at risk for enamel defects despite adequate supplementation later (Aine et al., 2000). Aboriginal communities with a high incidence of vitamin D deficiency have an associated high prevalence of dental caries (Canadian Paediatric Society, 2007). No studies demonstrating cause and effect have been published. The Canadian Paediatric Society (2007) recommends supplementing vitamin D in excess of the amounts that could be consumed from Canada's Food Guide portions (Health Canada, 2006) for pregnant and lactating women, to maintain vitamin D sufficiency. The effectiveness of this regimen and possible side effects should be checked with periodic biochemical assessments of vitamin D and calcium.

Essential Fatty Acids. Fatty acids are the major form of dietary fat. Humans cannot synthesize omega-3 and omega-6 fatty acids and thus must consume dietary sources. Recent evidence has advanced the understanding of the importance of omega-3 fatty acids in health and disease. Researchers first noticed the health benefits of omega-3 fatty acids when they observed that populations with high fish consumption (e.g., Inuit) had significantly lower rates of coronary heart disease (CHD) than the general Canadian population. Large epidemiological and longitudinal studies (National Heart, Lung, and Blood Institute Family Heart Study, 2001; Nurses Health Study, 1999) also associated significant reductions in disease risk for CHD in people with higher intakes of fish and omega-3 fatty acids.

Major types of omega-3 fatty acids are alpha-linoleic acid (ALA), eicosapentaenoic acid (EPA), and docosahexaenoic acid (DHA).The metabolic roles of each are different and, currently, incompletely understood. Good dietary sources of EPA and

Women with LI can drink only small amounts of milk without discomfort. Some women erroneously view milk products as culprits in weight gain. Women who cannot meet *Canada's Food Guide* guidelines for milk and alternatives (Health Canada, 2007) need advice from a dietitian to determine whether supplements are necessary.

DHA are fatty fish, shellfish, fish oil supplements, and omega-3-enriched eggs. ALA is found in flaxseed oil, canola oil or seeds, and nuts such as walnuts. Omega-3 fatty acids should not be confused with another family of essential polyunsaturated fatty acid—linoleic acid—which is an omega-6 fatty acid. Omega-6 fatty acids are found in corn, evening primrose, safflower, sesame, soybean, canola, and sunflower oils. These fatty acids are also essential for cellular membrane structures, but compete with omega-3 fatty acids for the same metabolic pathways in the body to form their active metabolites. To experience the full health benefits of both types of fats, it is important to eat the right balance of omega-6 and omega-3 fatty acids. The exact ratio has not been established. What is clear is that intake of omega-3 fatty acids is lower than most scientists and health professionals see as optimal for health.

These essential omega-3 fatty acids are important for neural and visual development in the first 2 years of life (ADA and Dieticians of Canada, 2007). Long-term benefits of early exposure to omega-3 fatty acids are uncertain, but food sources of DHA are known to reduce the risk of coronary death and total mortality in adults. Because of the potential benefits and lack of adverse effects in the fetus, ADA and Dietitians of Canada (2007) recommend a food-based approach to ensuring adequate intake. Pregnant and breastfeeding women should consume up to four food guide servings (75 g) per week of fish and shellfish low in methylmercury (ADA and Dieticians of Canada, 2007).

Chronic exposure to low-level methylmercury has some negative health effects. Neurodevelopmental abnormalities occur in children who had very high exposure in utero from highly contaminated food. Other neurodevelopmental deficits may also occur at chronic lower exposure levels. Therefore, an upper limit of intake is 0.1 μg/kg/day (~50 μg/for a 70-kg woman) (Mozaffarian & Rimm, 2006).

Women who do not consume fish may use fish oil supplements, which vary in the level of EPA and DHA they contain (200–800 mg/g). They should be used with caution in anyone who takes anticoagulants or hypoglycemic medications.

Fish liver oil supplements (e.g., cod liver oil) contain additional vitamins A and D but higher levels of toxins (e.g., PCBs) than fish oil supplements; thus, pregnant or breastfeeding women should not use them.

Breastfeeding. Exclusive breastfeeding should be encouraged for the first 6 months of life, because breast milk is the best food for optimal growth of the infant. This practice provides added protection against gastrointestinal infections (Kramer et al., 2003). Healthy term infants who are breastfed exclusively for 6 months grow at similar rates and show similar iron status as infants who are breastfed exclusively for 3 to 4 months and then continue partial breastfeeding to 6 months. Health Canada encourages all health professionals to promote and implement this revised recommendation at national, provincial, and community levels.

Some mothers may not exclusively breastfeed to 6 months for physiological (not enough milk production), personal, economic, and/or social reasons. They should also be supported to optimize their infant's nutritional well-being. Parents need to be supported and given appropriate information to enable informed decisions to ensure optimal infant nutrition.

Potential contraindications to breastfeeding:

- HIV/AIDS

- Active herpes lesions on or near the nipple

- Drug/alcohol abuse

- Whenever drugs are prescribed or infection detected, assess each case individually.

Mothers should maintain a well-balanced diet according to *Canada's Food Guide* (Health Canada, 2007a) and consume sufficient energy (additional 500 kcal per day) while breastfeeding. They can obtain these increased calories by including an extra 2 to 3 food guide servings each day. Implementation of this recommendation can be maximized through provision of adequate social supports to breastfeeding women by increasing community, public health, hospital, and workplace efforts.

Other Considerations

Alcohol. Use of alcohol during pregnancy is actively discouraged, and breastfeeding mothers who choose to consume alcohol should limit its use (Canadian Paediatric Society, 2006). Occasional or light use of alcoholic beverages

At-risk drinking is more than two alcoholic drinks per day or more than nine alcoholic drinks per week (Sanchez-Craig, 1996). One drink is defined as 145 mL wine, 340 mL

(two or fewer drinks per day) has not been found harmful to the nursing baby and does not warrant discontinuing breastfeeding (Canadian Paediatric Society, Dietitians of Canada and Health Canada, 2005).

While there is individual variation, alcohol concentration is highest in breast milk 30 to 60 minutes after drinking an alcoholic beverage. To allow time for alcohol concentration in breast milk to decrease, women should wait at least 2 hours per drink before breastfeeding. After 1 hour, the concentration in breast milk begins to decrease. Hungry infants during the waiting period can be fed with previously collected breast milk or infant formula. Any breast milk containing alcohol should be expressed and discarded.

Caffeine. Excess caffeine can pass through breast milk and accumulate in the infant's system. This can cause caffeine stimulation, shown as a wide-eyed, alert, and irritable infant. Women who breastfeed should consume no more than 300 mg/day of caffeine, which equals approximately two 237-mL cups of coffee (Health Canada, 2007c).

Breastfeeding women should be advised to consider all sources of caffeine, such as coffee, tea, chocolate, or cola, as well as over-the-counter medications (stimulants, pain relievers, diuretics, cold remedies, weight-loss aids). Caffeine-free items may be appropriate alternatives.

Allergy. Breastfeeding women do not need to avoid any highly allergenic foods (e.g., nuts, cow's milk). However, it is necessary for them to avoid foods to which they or their infants have a diagnosed allergy (Muraro et al., 2004).

Exclusive breastfeeding for 6 months may decrease incidence of some allergic reactions. After 6 months of age, no evidence shows that delaying any foods will prevent allergies; delayed introduction of a food may only postpone a child's allergic reaction (Zeiger & Heller, 1995).

THE ADULT YEARS

Physiological and Anatomical Changes. Major physiological changes during adulthood are declining lean body mass (2–3% per decade) and BMD. Basal metabolic rate declines with the changes in fat-free mass experienced, increasing the potential for energy imbalance. Energy intake, physical activity levels, and gender influence weight control throughout the life cycle.

The most recent Canadian surveys indicate that about 36% of Canadian adults are overweight and about 23% are obese (Katzmarzyk, 2007; Tjepkema, 2005). Prevalence of overweight has increased dramatically over the last 20 years. For example, currently, in Alberta (Edmonton), ~50% of adults are overweight or obese, and 25% of children are overweight (Després & Tchernof, 2007).

beer, or 42 mL of hard liquor (Alberta Drug and Alcohol Commission, 2007), all of which have the same amount of alcohol. Alcohol is transferred into the breast milk as long as the mother has alcohol in her blood (Mennella, 2004). Alcohol is not trapped in the breast milk but is constantly removed as it diffuses into the bloodstream.

Breastfeeding is contraindicated in women who regularly consume more than two alcoholic drinks per day. The breastfed infant may become so sleepy from alcohol in the mother's milk that he or she may sleep through feedings or suck less effectively (Canadian Paediatric Society, Dietitians of Canada, and Health Canada, 2005). The breastfed infant may have slow weight gain, failure to thrive, impaired motor development (Little et al., 1989), or disrupted sleep patterns (Mennella & Gerrish, 1998) and decreased milk intake (Mennella & Beauchamp, 1991).

If a breastfed infant has food allergy symptoms, the woman should consult a physician and eliminate the suspected food from her diet. To ensure diet adequacy, a registered dietitian should be consulted if this results in avoidance of a whole food group or multiple foods.

Energy imbalance with coinciding overweight/obesity increases risks for *CVD, hypertension, type 2 diabetes, degenerative osteoarthritis, chronic renal disease*, and certain cancers (Fernandez et at., 2004; Groeneveld, Solomons, & Doak, 2007; Rudolpf et al., 2004; Rudolpf, Walker, & Cole, 2007). Obesity is an independent risk factor for CVD, causing detrimental changes to LDL, triglyceride, HDL, blood glucose, and blood pressure levels (Klein et al., 2007).

Risk factors for increasing rates of obesity in adults include sedentary lifestyles and diets characterized by high energy, fat, sodium, simple sugars, and low fibre (Després & Tchernof, 2007; Katzmarzyk, 2007; Lau, 2007; Klein et al., 2007; Tjepkema, 2005). Lifestyle modification that focuses on dietary and physical activity in individual and small-group counselling has been shown most effective in preventing obesity (Katzmarzyk & Reeder, 2007). Controversy remains over the "best" approach to prevent obesity at community and global levels.

Anthropometric measures including height, weight, BMI, and waist circumference should be monitored regularly as outlined in Nutrition Assessment: Anthropometric Measurements.

Dietary Recommendations for Chronic Disease Prevention.
Nutrition counselling is key to prevention of overweight and obesity. Current dietary recommendations include a focus on "healthy eating patterns" (Health Canada, 2007), which fall within the Acceptable Macronutrient Distribution Ranges (AMDR) for carbohydrate (45–65%), protein (10–35%), and fat (20–35%), with consumption of moderate fat (low in saturated and trans fat) and sodium, and higher amounts of dietary fibre (20–30 g daily).

These recommendations evolved from research that demonstrated a lower risk of CVD and hypertension in those consuming more omega-3 fatty acids (fish oil) and less saturated and trans fatty acid and sodium (ADA, 2002; McPherson et al., 2006; National Heart, Lung, and Blood Institute, 1998).

Fat. Fats in foods are made up of four different types of fatty acids— polyunsaturated, monounsaturated, saturated, and trans. While the DRIs do not provide a specific limit for daily intake of saturated or trans fat (McPherson et al., 2006), the American Heart Association (AHA) recommends limiting saturated fat to <7% of total daily calories for adults.

Trans Fats. Although found naturally in some animal-based foods, major dietary contributors are from hydrogenated fats (formed when liquid oils are made into semisolid fats, like shortening and hard margarine). They are added to foods to provide a longer shelf life and give baked goods a desirable texture. Food products containing trans fat have the words "trans" or "hydrogenated" on the label and include commercially fried and breaded foods and bakery products and snacks, such as crackers, cookies, donuts, cakes, pastries, muffins, and croissants.

In early 2005, a Canadian Task Force assembled with a mandate to develop recommendations and strategies to effectively eliminate or reduce processed trans fats in Canadian foods to the lowest level possible. On December 12, 2005, Canada became the first country to regulate mandatory labelling of trans fats on pre-packaged foods.

The WHO (2003) recommends that trans fat intake be no more than 1% of total energy intake. For example, a person eating 2000 calories per day should not have more than 2.2 grams of trans fat per day.

Calorie Level per Day	Maximum Recommended Saturated Fat for Adults (grams per day)	Maximum Recommended Trans Fat for Children and Adults (grams per day)
2000 calories	15.5	2.2
1800 calories	14.0	2.0
1500 calories	11.6	1.7

Abdominal obesity in particular is associated with increased risk for CVD and diabetes and increased mortality and morbidity associated with these conditions (WHO, 1995).

Waist circumference >102 cm (40 in.) in men and >88 cm (35 in.) in women poses increased risk for type 2 diabetes, CVD, and hypertension. Note: When BMI is >35, waist circumference is beneficial to measure visceral fat changes.

Lower sodium intake is also associated with reduced risk for heart attack, heart failure, stroke, and kidney disease, and prevention of hypertension in normotensive people (Chobanian et al., 2003; Khan et al., 2006). Unfortunately, most Canadians consume a diet high in saturated and trans fats and sodium and low in omega-3 fats and fibre (Tjepkema, 2005).

Scientific evidence has shown that dietary trans fats can increase risk of CVD by adversely affecting serum lipid and lipoprotein patterns (Ascherio et al., 1999).

Dietary Fish Oil. Canadian and American heart health guidelines recommend regular consumption of fish high in omega-3 fats; the AHA (2006) suggests eating a variety of fatty fish, at least two servrings a week. Increasing fish intake increases the healthier fats in the diet and displaces foods higher in unhealthy (saturated and trans) fats (National Heart, Lung, and Blood Institute, 1998). Dietary recommendations for essential fatty acid intakes of linoleic acid (LA) and α-linolenic (ALA) acid are summarized in the following table.

■ *Dietary Reference Intake Recommendations*

	AMDR (% of Total Energy)	Adequate Intake for Men	Adequate Intake for Women
α-Linolenic acid (ALA)*	0.6–1.2%	1.6 g/day	1.1 g/day
Linoleic acid (LA)	5–10%	17 g/day	12 g/day

AMDR, Acceptable Macronutrient Distribution Ranges
*Up to 10% of the AMDR for ALA can be consumed as EPA and/or DHA (0.06–0.12%)

Sodium. Intake should be limited to 2300 mg of sodium (1 tsp) per day (National Academy of Science, 2005). Most sodium (about 75%) consumed comes from processed/packaged foods or restaurant foods.

According to the National Academy of Science (2005), an adequate intake for sodium is:

■ 9 to 50 years: 1500 mg

■ 50 to 70 years: 1300 mg

■ >70 years: 1200 mg

Dietary counselling typically focuses on reducing the consumption of sodium and sodium-containing foods, additions at the table, and in cooking. Recommendations for reading food labels include the following:

■ Check the ingredient list. If sodium, salt, or soda is listed near the beginning, the product may be high in salt.

■ Check the Nutrition Facts panel on food labels. Read the sodium content and take note of the serving size listed.

■ If the % daily value (DV) is **5** or less, the food is considered low in sodium. *Choose these foods **more** often.*

■ If the % DV is higher than **20**, the food is considered high in sodium. *Choose these foods **less** often.*

■ Compare the sodium content of similar products (e.g., different brands of canned tomatoes, canned soup) and choose items with less sodium.

Food labels show the following categories of sodium content:

Most Canadians eat more than double the recommended daily amount of sodium (4000–6000 mg/day depending on food choices).

Nutrition Facts
Valeur nutritive
Per 20 g (approx 13 crackers)/Par 20 g (enviorn 13 raquelins)

Amount Teneur		% Daily Value % valeur quotidienne
Calories / Calories 80		
Fat / Lipides 1 g		2 %
Saturated / saturés 0.2 g + Trans / trans 0 g		1 %
Cholesterol / Cholestérol 0 mg		
Sodium / Sodium 103 mg		4 %
Carbohydrate / Glucides 17 g		6 %
Fibre / Fibres 0.4 g		2 %
Sugars / Sucres 0.1 g		
Protein / Protéines 1.6 g		
Vitamin A / Vitamine A		0 %
Vitamin C / Vitamine C		0 %
Calcium / Calcium		0 %
Iron / Fer		3 %

INGREDIENTS: BROWN JAPONICA RICE, JAPONICA RICE, CORN OIL, SEA SALT, INULIN, LIQUORICE POWDER.

Sodium-free	5 mg or less of sodium per serving
Low sodium	140 mg or less of sodium per 100 g serving
Reduced or less sodium	At least 25% less sodium than regular version
Lightly salted	At least 50% less sodium than the regular version

Weight Management: Treating Obesity. The health benefits of weight loss in overweight or obese adults include reduced risks for diabetes, hypertension, CVD, and certain cancers (breast cancer in females; colon cancer in males) and improved serum levels of triglycerides and total cholesterol (ADA, 2002, 2006; Appel et al., 2006; Leaf, 1999; Lichtenstein et al., 2006). Three major components to any weight management approach are nutrition, physical activity, and behaviour modification. The combination of all three is more successful than any one intervention alone.

A greater frequency of contacts between client and practitioner may lead to more successful weight loss and maintenance (ADA, 2008). Individualized goals of weight loss therapy should be to reduce body weight at an optimal rate of 0.5 kg (1–2 lbs) per week for the first 6 months and to achieve an initial weight loss goal of 5% to 10% from baseline. These goals are realistic, achievable, and sustainable.

Weight reduction is not recommended during pregnancy and lactation or with unstable or untreated mental or physical illness (e.g., cancer).

Dietary Approach. Nutrition recommendations include a dietary reduction of 500 to 1000 kcal daily from current intake (ADA, 2008). Intake should be spread throughout the day with consumption of three balanced meals and one or two snacks. It may be beneficial to consume more calories throughout the day as opposed to in the evening (National Heart, Lung, and Blood Institute, 1998). Portion control (weighing and measuring foods) at meals and snacks results in reduced energy intake and weight loss, and counters a tendency towards underestimating portion sizes.

Energy intakes of <1200 kcal/day may not meet nutrient requirements and may require supplementation.

- Calorie reductions (deficit of 500–1000 calories per day of current or usual intake)

- 55% or more of total daily energy intake from carbohydrate

- >30% of total daily calories from fat

- 8% to 10% of total calories from saturated fat

- >300 mg cholesterol per day

- 15% of total calories from protein

- No more than ~2400 milligrams of sodium

- 20 to 30 grams of fibre daily

- 1000 to 1500 milligrams calcium per day

Physical Activity. For weight loss and maintenance, regular physical activity is necessary. The amount depends on activities performed.

- For light activities like walking (strolling in a mall), easy gardening, and stretching, 60 minutes 4 to 7 days per week is recommended.

- If performing moderate activities like brisk walking, biking, raking leaves, swimming, dancing, and water aerobics, then 30 to 40 minutes 4 to 7 days per week is recommended (Public Health Agency of Canada, 2003).

- Add up activities throughout the day in periods of at least 10 minutes at a time.

If previously inactive, start slowly and build up over time. If performing some light activities, progress to moderate ones (Health Canada, 2003b).

Other Nutritional Concerns

Iron Intake. Iron deficiency continues to be a concern throughout the life cycle; particularly in adolescent and adult women. This is because of iron losses during menses and poor dietary intake. Foods high in iron include heme sources (e.g., found in organ meats) and nonheme sources (e.g., iron-enriched whole grains, raisins).

From 29% to 84% of young Canadian women do not consume the recommended amount of iron (Chapman, 1994). Serious consequences of iron deficiency are negative effects on work and intellectual performance (Halterman et al., 2001).

Calcium and Vitamin D. Adult bone mass is a strong predictor of future osteoporotic fracture risk. It can be defined as the peak bone mass of early adulthood, minus the bone loss experienced in the adult and senior years. Adequate dietary intake during this period is critical to ensure that peak bone mass in adulthood is attained. Dietary calcium and vitamin D have the potential to be limiting factors in skeletal growth, because virtually all of the body's calcium resides in the skeleton. Other dietary factors, such as increased soft drink intake and inadequate fruits and vegetables intake, have also been shown to negatively affect bone mass accrual (Whiting et al., 2004). A healthy diet according to *Canada's Food Guide* should be encouraged. Supplemental intake of vitamin D may be necessary during critical periods of the life cycle: pregnancy, lactation, and for Canadians particularly from October to April.

Risk of osteoporosis in later life has been related to inadequate development of bone mass in the adolescent period.

Eating Disorders.
Eating disorders are psychological disorders characterized by abnormal eating patterns (Merriam-Webster Medical Dictionary, 2008). Anorexia nervosa, bulimia nervosa, binge-eating disorder, and eating disorders not otherwise specified are all considered eating disorders but differ in manifestation and symptomatology.

Potential negative health outcomes associated with eating disorders stress the need for primary prevention efforts and early diagnosis and treatment (see Table 8-3).

A 19-year-old female with an eating disorder diets, exercises 4 hours daily, and/or eats excessively and purges as a way to cope with the physical and emotional changes of adolescence.

OLDER ADULTS

Body Composition. Major body compositional changes with aging include loss of lean body mass and BMD and increased fat mass (Nair, 2005; Russell, 2000). Likely influences are declining activity, hormonal levels, and the presence of chronic disease. Regular physical activity and adequate dietary intake can attenuate increases in body fat, particularly visceral fat (Blanc et al., 2004; Kinney, 2004).

Healthy BMI for adults older than 65 years is 22 to 26.9. Weight loss in obese older adults may improve functional status and quality of life, and should be recommended as appropriate. However, need for dietary restriction or modification should be evaluated based on quality of life, risk versus benefit, and effects on overall nutrition status.

Bone Mineral Density. BMD decreases in both men and woman as they age. Reduced BMD results in bone characterized by disconnected trabeculae and thinning of outer cortical surfaces, which leads to osteoporosis (Brown et al., 2002; Kanis et al., 1994; WHO, 1994). In older adults, this leads to reduced bone strength and increased susceptibility to fracture from only mild to moderate trauma. Influences on patterns of bone loss in older adults include age, gender, ethnicity, skeletal site, and peak bone mass obtained in young adulthood. Longitudinal studies indicate that rapid bone loss follows menopause in women for the first 1 to 5 years, and then stabilizes at 1% to 2% per year. In males, bone mass starts to fall at about 50 years and continues at a rate of 1% to 2% per year.

Typically, BMD is assessed by comparing the client's BMD against the average score of a 30-year old. Ideal BMD is a T-score between +2.5 and −1 (i.e., client's BMD is between 2.5 standard deviations [SD] above and 1 SD below the mean).

Organ Function. Major organ changes include declines in cerebral and cardiovascular function. Cardiac output, stroke volume, and cardiac reserve decrease, resulting in diminished blood output to all body organs. Increased peripheral vascular resistance from decreased smooth muscle elasticity also increases the risk for hypertension. Major changes in the kidneys include impaired clearance of nitrogenous wastes from the plasma and an impaired ability to reabsorb water, resulting in increased frequency of urination. In the gastrointestinal tract, bowel motility decreases, increasing the client's risk for constipation. Basal and maximal gastric acid output decreases in the stomach, resulting in atrophic gastritis. This may influence the absorption and digestion of vitamin B_{12} (cobalamin), B_6 (pyridoxine), iron, calcium, folate, and zinc, resulting in the potential for decreased nutrient bioavailability and nutrient deficiency. Hence, it is important to assess the physiological effects of aging on nutrient requirements, use, and absorption in this population.

Oral Motor Function. Changes in chewing and mastication and acuity of taste and smell are very common in older adults and can lead to decreased appetite and food intake.

Nutritional Considerations. Major variables influencing food intake and nutritional status in older adults are physiological, psychological, and socioeconomic factors; ethnic and cultural influences; functional capacity to self-feed; and use of polypharmacy. The major nutritional issues associated with healthy aging include weight loss, obesity, dehydration, constipation, and vitamin and mineral deficiencies (Allison & Lobo, 2004; American Dietetic Association, 2005; Bates, Prentice, & Finch, 1999; Nair, 2005; Russell, 2000).

Weight loss with aging is usually associated with reduced food intake and is one of the key variables associated with increases in co-morbid conditions. Other factors include psychosocial variables such as depression and food security. Although obesity remains an important nutritional issue throughout the life cycle, it appears to decrease in incidence in clients older than 80 years, in whom weight loss is more common. Obesity is associated with an increased risk of cardiovascular and cancer risk in this population. Dehydration is also a common issue from a decline in thirst sensation and fluid intake, particularly for those exposed to environmental extremes (Allison & Lobo, 2004). Constipation from delayed gastrointestinal motility and decreased fluid intake is also very common. This typically causes early satiety resulting in decreased food intake, and may contribute to the increased risk for

Falls cause >90% of fractures in older adults (Brown et al., 2002; Dennison, Cole, & Cooper, 2005; Kanis et al., 1994; Wold et al., 2005; WHO, 1994).

Females of Caucasian/Asian ancestry, smokers, and those with low calcium and vitamin D intake during peak bone mass years are at highest risk for developing osteoporosis with age (Brown et al., 2002; Dennison et al., 2005; Wold et al., 2005).

Osteopenia (low BMD) is associated with a T-score of −1 to −2.5. *Osteoporosis* is defined as a T-score <−2.5, while severe osteoporosis is a T-score <−2.5 in a client who has also suffered a fragility fracture (Brown et al., 2002; Dennison et al., 2005; Kanis et al., 1994; Wold et al., 2005; WHO, 1994).

Problems may include chipped/ broken teeth or ill-fitting dentures, making chewing of hard foods and meats painful. Swallowing problems from stroke or neurological disability may be exacerbated by the use of over-the-counter medications causing mouth dryness (e.g., diphenhydramine).

Unexplained weight loss may indicate an unexplained pathology (Hoffman, 2002). Other contributors to unexpected weight loss include *depression* associated with loss of a loved one, *dementia*, dysphagia or swallowing problems, dysfunction from inability to perform activities of daily life (functional capacity), and use of medications that alter substrate use or interfere with

vitamin and mineral deficiency in this stage of the life cycle (Bailey et al., 1997; Chernoff, 2005; Kinney, 2004).

Psychosocial and Socioeconomic Determinants of Food Intake.

Common influences on food intake in older adults include depression, dementia, chronic use/abuse of alcohol and/or drugs, and food insecurity. All of these variables may significantly influence meal patterns and the ability to prepare and access food.

For clients with depression, a change in feeding environment (e.g., eating in family dining rooms) may help increase consumption. For clients with dementia, however, increased stimuli in a group environment may distract them from eating, while a quiet feeding environment may facilitate dietary improvements. Dietary intake may also improve with feeding assistance and dietary strategies focused on food texture and nutrient alteration. Typically, these require consultation with the registered dietitian to ensure nutritional adequacy.

Chronic drug/alcohol abuse is another concern. It may lead to reductions in appetite, displacement of financial resources for purchase of alcohol/drugs, and increased risk of malnutrition from decreased intake. Clients consuming >30% of their total calories as alcohol typically consume suboptimal levels of carbohydrate, protein, thiamine, folate, pyridoxine, calcium, iron, and vitamins A, D, E, and C (Leo & Lieber, 1999; Levy et al., 2002).

Food insecurity may exacerbate all of the previously mentioned variables (Allison & Lobo, 2004; ADA, 2005; Bates et al., 1999; Kennedy, Chokkalingham, & Srinivasan, 2004; Nair, 2005; Russell, 2000). Food insecurity can occur in any age group and typically means an inability to access a safe food supply that meets the person's nutritional needs (Russell, 2000). For older adults, this can be viewed in the context of overall mobility and the financial and physical ability to purchase and prepare safe and nutritious foods (Kinney, 2004; Russell, 2000). Between 20% and 40% of older Canadians have issues related to food insecurity (Kinney, 2004).

Ethnic and Cultural Factors.

Ethnic and cultural factors directly influence food selection and preparation and are important to acknowledge when examining food intake in older adults. Prior education is another variable that also directly influences attitudes towards nutritional intake and should be considered when counselling clients. The client's economic and geographical status can influence food security, as discussed earlier, because it may be more difficult for an older person living in geographical isolation to purchase food. A comprehensive nutritional assessment of an older client includes these variables.

Functional Capacity.

Functional capacity refers to the ability to perform the usual activities of daily living, which include the ability to access food, prepare food, and feed one's self independently or with assistance. Various factors can influence functional capacity, including fine motor and gross motor skills and/or vision, which may directly influence the ability to prepare and access food, as well as the ability to self-feed.

nutrient absorption or dietary intake (Hoffman, 2002). Consider all these factors. Many chronic conditions such as *cancers*, *CVD*, *rheumatoid arthritis*, and neurodegenerative disorders (e.g., *Parkinson's disease*) are expressed in early stages as unexplained weight loss (Blanc et al., 2004; Hoffman, 2002).

Depression in older clients may be associated with loss of a spouse or friends or change in location, but may result from side effects of prescribed and over-the-counter medications.

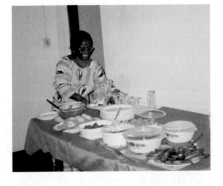

Chronic diseases such as *Parkinson's disease* or *osteoarthritis* may directly impair the client's ability to perform activities of daily living. *Dementia* or problems with swallowing may also directly influence the client's ability to self-feed.

The consequence of problems related to functional capacity may be a long-term dependence on feeding assistance. In general, the older person with a functional incapacity to self-feed requires feeding assistance either at home or in a care facility. Strategies aimed at optimizing food intake in this population are critical to ensure that nutritional needs are met. These may include alteration of food texture to facilitate ease of food preparation and swallowing, use of adaptive feeding devices to facilitate self-feeding by the individual experiencing fine motor and visual impairments, and alteration of nutrient density of food. Examples of density alterations include adding extra fat to increase energy density or adding carbohydrates, proteins, and vitamins and minerals to enhance micro- and macronutrient density of foods. Consultation with a registered dietitian is vital to ensure nutritional adequacy of dietary intake under these conditions.

Dysphagia in Older Adults.

Certainly the inability to swallow or impaired swallowing (*dysphagia*) can lead to significant feeding inefficiency and reduced dietary intake and weight loss. Dysphagia may result from various causes: a neurological insult secondary to chronic disease (as in Parkinson's disease or stroke) or structural causes related to tumours or their resections. Dysphagia needs to be carefully ruled out. Routine assessment of swallowing is appropriate for adults older than 65 years. Treatment strategies for older clients with dysphagia may include food texture modification to promote safe swallowing. This may be problematic for meeting energy requirements, because many older adults dislike alterations in food textures, particularly transitions to pureed solids or thickened liquids. It is critical that the registered dietitian be involved in the clinical care of any person diagnosed with dysphagia to ensure nutritional adequacy of dietary intake and sufficiency of hydration. If the client cannot meet nutritional needs safely with food texture modification, insertion of an enteral feeding device (e.g., nasogastric or gastrostomy feeding tube) may be necessary. Supplemental feeding via these enterostomy devices may assist the older adult in meeting nutritional and hydrational needs. The interdisciplinary health care team including, but not limited to, the registered dietitian, nurse, occupational therapist, swallowing therapist, physiotherapist, and social worker, can facilitate nutrition support in the community.

Signs and symptoms of dysphagia in older adults are:

- Wet phonation after the swallow

- Drooling or excessive saliva production

- Shortness of breath during and after the swallow

- Possible coughing during and after the swallow

- Repeated history of unexplained chest infections

Many older adults do not demonstrate an active cough during or after the swallow, even with a swallowing abnormality. Absence of this sign does NOT imply an abnormal swallow, but suggests an abnormal neuronal response to food in the airway. The older adult may still aspirate food contents into the airway in the absence of sensory stimuli, particularly if he or she has a recent history of fever and chest infection. If so, further investigation is warranted.

Polypharmacy.

Polypharmacy typically refers to the administration of numerous medicines, often for multiple indications, and may include the use of both prescribed and nonprescribed medications. The major concern about polypharmacy is its potential for harmful drug reactions and interactions. Older clients are particularly susceptible to the dangers of polypharmacy (Beilory, 2004; Brager & Sloand, 2005; Bruno & Ellis, 2005; Kishiyam et al., 2005; McCabe, 2004). They may contribute to improper medication use because of deficits in memory, vision, or functional ability. In addition, information overload may compromise the client's ability to comprehend instructions. Ailments such as arthritis, insomnia, and constipation are among the main reasons why the older consumer has increased consumption of supplements. Reduced dietary intake from nausea and vomiting, constipation, or changes in taste acuity is a common drug side effect. The use of pain medications containing codeine may cause constipation, resulting in decreased food

A client with a history of constipation develops a cough, self-medicates, and suddenly develops diarrhea. Many over-the-counter cough and cold remedies contain sorbitol, a sugar alcohol that causes diarrhea. A careful health history and review of prescribed and nonprescribed medications is important to determine the cause of a sudden change in bowel movements.

intake. Treatment with anti-hypertensives using diuretics is typically associated with reduced fluid intake and increased frequency of urination. Other examples of adverse nutritional sequelae include the use of non-steroidal anti-inflammatory drugs (NSAIDs) on iron bioavailability, anticoagulants on vitamin K metabolism, and antibiotic use with calcium bioavailability (Brager & Sloand, 2005). Hence, it is critical for the nurse to ask about the use of both prescribed and over-the-counter medications and supplements in a health history.

Health History. Review functional and mental status with the client and family members and other caregivers. Focus the history on each of the following:

■ Previous gastrointestinal condition or surgeries (for evidence of malabsorption)

■ Renal, hepatic, cardiac, and respiratory disease (for evidence of organ failure)

■ Rheumatologic diseases (chronic inflammation)

■ Recurrent infections

■ Previous psychiatric illness.

Thoroughly review prescribed and nonprescribed medications and nutritional supplements to identify the potential effects of these agents on appetite, taste, and gastrointestinal and cognitive functions. Also include the potential for drug–nutrient interactions and prescribed drug therapeutic action.

Use of sedatives and narcotic analgesics may interfere with cognition and ability to eat, along with causing significant gastrointestinal dysfunction (e.g., constipation).

Clinical and Physical Assessment. Physical examination includes a review of dentition and oral motor function, looking for evidence of altered food intake from difficulty with chewing and swallowing. Often clues to the etiology of changes in food intake can be obtained by watching a client eat part of a meal. For example, the client may be distracted by stimuli in the room or by being presented with food textures that he or she cannot eat (Hoffman, 2002; Roubenoff et al., 1996). Examine physical findings that suggest vitamin, mineral, and protein–energy deficiencies/excess in the context of clinical and medical history, anthropometric, and laboratory findings. Assess mental health status, social and economic factors, as well as cultural and religious beliefs because of their effects on dietary intake.

The finding of *follicular hyperkeratosis* isolated to the back of the arm is a widespread finding that may not be attributed to a specific vitamin deficiency. If it is diffuse in the body of a person with an extremely low intake of fruits and vegetables, it warrants comprehensive assessment by a registered dietitian to determine if laboratory testing is required to confirm a vitamin C deficiency.

Compare current weight and height measurements to minimum and maximum adult weights. Low body weights are often defined as <80% of the recommended body weight.

BMI <22 in older women and <23.5 in older men is associated with increased mortality.

Although stable weight parameters are the goal for the healthy older adult, they do not indicate appropriate muscle and fat mass. Many older adults with expected or increased body weight have marked reduction in fat-free mass and/or excess in fat mass.

Sarcopenia or skeletal muscle atrophy is common in older adults and is strongly associated with disability (Kinney, 2004).

Anthropometric assessment should include a review of any alterations in weight to rule out unexplained changes.

Difficulties in accurate height measures may be from gross motor dysfunction or vertebral compressions associated with osteoporosis. Nurses recognize that these problems may affect estimates of BMI. Waist and hip circumference

Involuntary weight loss can lead to muscle wasting, decreased immunocompetence, depression, and increased rate of disease complications. A weight loss of ~5% to 10% of body weight over

can provide important information regarding any central obesity. Alternative measurements, such as skin-fold and upper-arm measures, to assess body fat or fat-free mass may be warranted to identify risk for functional decline. However, changes in skin elasticity and compressibility of skin folds that occur with aging influence the accuracy of these measures, and they should be performed only by registered dietitians.

Nutrients of Concern

Calcium and Vitamin D. Currently, there is controversy in the literature regarding calcium and vitamin D requirements. Evidence supports the need for calcium intake at 1200 to 1500 milligrams/day in the presence of osteoporosis. Age-related changes in calcium absorption and decreases in calcium intake place the older female, in particular, at high risk for suboptimal calcium intake, especially if suboptimal vitamin D status exists.

Current recommendations for adults older than 70 years are 1200 milligrams/day of calcium and 600 International Units (IU)/day of vitamin D. Older adults are encouraged to follow *Canada's Food Guide* and to increase their intake of calcium-rich foods. However, most older adults require calcium and vitamin D supplementation to achieve the daily recommended intake (DRI) (Health Canada, 2007).

Canadian clinical practice guidelines (2002) recommend nutrition and physical activity, in conjunction with pharmaceutical therapy, for prevention and treatment of osteoporosis (Brown et al., 2002). Other authors concur (de Groot & van Staveren, 1996; Dennison et al., 2005; Institute of Medicine, 1997, 1998, 2004a, 2004b; Kanis et al., 1994; Trumbo et al., 2002; WHO, 1994; Wold et al., 2005).

Vitamin B_{12}. Causes of deficiency are decreased gastric acid production (hypochlorhydria in up to 15% of persons older than 65 years) and *Helicobacter pylori* infection of the stomach. Alternatively, it can be from low consumption of B_{12}-containing foods. The DRI for vitamin B_{12} is 2.4 micrograms daily. Vitamin B_{12} is found naturally only in animal products such as meat, milk products, and eggs. Because it is not known which cases will progress to anemia or neurological injury if untreated, screening and treatment are recommended. Oral and nasal replacement forms of vitamin B_{12} are available, but generally older persons with symptoms or signs of deficiency are given monthly intramuscular (IM) injections of vitamin B_{12}. A systematic review found that 2000-microgram doses of oral vitamin B_{12} daily, and 1000-microgram doses initially daily and thereafter weekly and then monthly, may be as effective as IM administration in obtaining short-term hematological and neurological responses in vitamin B_{12}-deficient clients (WHO, 1994).

Zinc. Zinc is needed for adequate wound healing, immunity, and a healthy appetite (DRI = 12 to 15 mg). It may also slow progression of age-related macular degeneration.

the previous 12 months can indicate a problem and should not be considered part of the aging process.

Vitamin B_{12} deficiency causes hematological and neurological signs and symptoms. Hematological signs include anemia with macrocytosis and megaloblastic changes noted as hypersegmented polymorphonuclear leukocytes. Neurological damage is independent of the hematological changes and results in nonspecific paresthesia (e.g., numbness) of the extremities, abnormal position and vibration sense, difficulty walking (i.e., gait ataxia from degeneration of the posterior–lateral columns of the spinal cord), and mental confusion, each of which can occur in many other age-related diseases.

Zinc deficiency is common among malnourished elderly persons, particularly among those who also have cirrhosis or diabetes mellitus or who are taking diuretics (Allison & Lobo, 2004).

NUTRITION POLICY

Research clearly indicates that nutrition plays an important role in the prevention of chronic diseases and obesity. For example, the imbalance between physical inactivity and high energy intake is a main determinant of the obesity epidemic (WHO, 2003). Strategies to increase physical activity and improve diet quality can prevent unhealthy weight gain. However, the lack of adherence to these patterns continues, despite the best efforts of healthcare practitioners and public health campaigns to promote appropriate nutrition education. Some evidence shows that Canadians understand several aspects of Health Canada's dietary guidelines (Paquette, 2005), but why does this not translate to action? Existing food and eating environments are likely contributors to this difficulty, over and above individual factors like motivation, knowledge, and skill. Environmental interventions may be the most effective strategies for creating improvements in diet patterns (Story et al., 2008).

Humphries, Traci, and Seekins (2004) found that the menus of group homes and pantries in Montana had less than 45% of the recommended daily amount of vegetables available for consumption. In other words, teaching people to eat more vegetables only works if vegetables are available; the environment in this case did not allow people to follow accepted nutrition recommendations.

Schools exert a large influence over the dietary habits of teens who eat at least one meal and two snacks in that environment daily. School food policy can affect students' eating patterns and reinforce nutrition education if written policies about foods in cafeterias and vending machines permit only "healthy" foods. All regions of Canada recognize that policy can make a difference. While some provinces are further along in developing these guidelines, all are in the process of developing and/or implementing school nutrition policies. The *Alberta Nutrition Guidelines* is a good example of a school nutrition policy and can be accessed at: http://www.healthyalberta.com/Documents/AB_Nutri_Guidelines_2008(1).pdf.

Reduction in chronic disease incidence will require a sustained public health effort, where the ultimate end point should be to structure environments so that healthy behaviours are the optimal choice.

RECORDING AND ANALYZING FINDINGS

The collection, recording, and analysis of data must be accurate, comprehensive, and organized, and use terminology that all the members of the interprofessional team understand. Documentation of expected and unexpected findings regarding nutritional status of a female client follows.

ANALYZING FINDINGS FROM HISTORY AND PHYSICAL EXAMINATION

Nurses and dietitians analyze findings from a client's history (subjective data) and physical examination (objective data) to arrive at nursing and nutritional diagnoses. The following case study provides an example of the plan of care for Mrs. Chrissie McCulloch.

Mrs. McCulloch, 81 years old, has recently lost weight. She reports that her dentures keep falling out, making chewing difficult. She lives with her currently unemployed son Chad. Her husband died 2 months ago. She makes all the meals for Chad and buys all the groceries. She recently slipped on ice on the way to the

■ *Examples of Documentation and Analysis of Findings: Nutritional Status*

Areas of Assessment	Expected Findings	Unexpected Findings
Height	170 cm (1.7 m) at age 35 years	162 cm (1.62 m) at age 60 years
Weight	59 kg at age 35 years	89 kg at age 60 years
Body Mass Index	20.4 at age 35 years	34.0 at age 60 years
Waist Circumference	71 cm at age 35 years	90 cm at age 60 years
Blood Pressure	118/76	150/100
Inspection of Oral Cavity	Own teeth, in good repair Gums: pink, no bleeding Lips: moist, no lesions in corners of mouth	Dentures: poorly fitting Gums: bleed easily Lips: dry, cracks in corners of mouth
24-Hour Food Recall (using *Canada's Food Guide* for no. of servings per day)	Vegetables and fruits: 7–8 Grain Products: 6–7 (particularly whole grain) Milk and alternates: 2 Meat and alternates: 2 Fats: 30–45 mL of unsaturated fat Snacks; apple, peapods	Vegetables & fruits: 3 Grain Products: 9 (mainly white bread, pasta) Milk and alternates: 0 Meat and alternates: 4 Fats: 45 mL of butter Snacks: Two pieces of chocolate cake, potato chips
Comfort Foods	Fruits, milk, raw vegetables	Bread and butter, chocolate bars, donuts
Dietary Restrictions	None	Allergic to eggs, all nuts, and sesame seeds; Lactose intolerant
Caffeine Intake	1 cup of coffee daily	1400 mL of diet cola daily
Alcohol Intake	1 glass of red wine daily	12 beers every weekend
Exercise	Treadmill × 30 minutes, 5 days per week	Walking very restricted due to osteoarthritis in both knees. Uses walker outside of house. No other exercise.
Ability to Shop for Food	Has transportation to grocery store	A family member shops for groceries
Resources for Food	Has resources to purchase all types of food: fruits, vegetables, grain products, and milk and meat alternatives	Has food insecurity because of limited resources. Purchases little fruits, some vegetables such as carrots, potatoes; day-old white bread, macaroni and other pasta, occasional meat and cheese
Physical Ability to Prepare Food	Can prepare all types of foods	Limited ability to stand and prepare food—uses mostly canned and packaged foods

store and has asked Chad to buy the groceries until she recovers from her sprained ankle. Mrs. McCulloch and Chad enjoy drinking coffee and tea and snacking on cookies as they watch their favourite television shows. She is currently well (other than her ankle) and eats regularly, but thinks her son should get a job so they can eat better.

Nursing Diagnosis: *Imbalanced nutrition related to decreased mobility due to a fall, change in family unit, and limited financial resources.*

Nutritional Diagnosis: *Imbalanced nutrition related to decreased mobility due to a fall, change in family unit, and limited financial resources.*

Critical Thinking Exercise

Answer the following questions related to Mrs. McCulloch's present situation:

- What substance is of concern in the coffee Mrs. McCulloch is drinking? (*Knowledge*)
- What nutrients are likely to be at risk in Mrs. McCulloch's diet? (*Comprehension*)
- What would you teach Mrs. McCulloch about how to improve her intake? (*Application*)
- What factors are contributing to Mrs. McCulloch's weight loss? (*Analysis*)
- What recommendations for screening and follow-up would you suggest for Mrs. McCulloch? (*Synthesis*)
- How would you evaluate the success of your client teaching for Mrs. McCulloch? (*Evaluation*)

Test Questions

1. The major sites for nutrient absorption in the small intestine are:
   a. the jejunum and ileum.
   b. the duodenum and ileum.
   c. the jejunum and duodenum.
   d. the jejunum and epithelium.

2. Which BMI indicates the lowest risk of developing health problems in a 40 year old?
   a. 18
   b. 23
   c. 28
   d. 33

3. Foods rich in iron include all of the following **except**:
   a. almonds.
   b. meats.

Canadian Research

*Chang, C.-C., & Roberts, B. L. (2008). Cultural perspectives in feeding difficulty in Taiwanese elderly with dementia. *Journal of Nursing Scholarship, 40*(3), 235–240.

*Johnson, R. L., Williams, S. M., & Spruill, I. J. (2006). Genomics, nutrition, obesity, and diabetes. *Journal of Nursing Scholarship, 38*(1), 11–18.

*Kara, B., Caglar, K., & Kilic, S. (2007). Nonadherence with diet and fluid restrictions and perceived social support in patients receiving hemodialysis. *Journal of Nursing Scholarship, 39*(3), 243–248.

Lamarche, B. (2008). Nutrition bites. Natural trans fat and cardiovascular disease: Important new findings. *Canadian Nurse, 104*(7), 36.

*Indicates nursing research.

   c. fortified cereals/grains.
   d. legumes.

4. Vitamins requiring a fat source to be absorbed and stored by the body include all of the following **except:**
   a. vitamin A.
   b. vitamin B.
   c. vitamin D.
   d. vitamin E.

5. Higher sodium intake is associated with all of the following **except:**
   a. hypertension.
   b. stroke and kidney disease.
   c. heart failure.
   d. osteomalacia.

Bibliography

CITATIONS

Aine, L., Backström, M. C., Mäki, R., Kuusela, A. L., Koivisto, A. M., Ikonen, R.S., et al. (2000). Enamel defects in primary and permanent teeth of children born prematurely. *Journal of Oral Pathology & Medicine, 29*, 403–409.

Alberta Alcohol and Drug Abuse Commission. (2007). *The ABCs–alcohol.* Retrieved November 13, 2008, from http://www.aadac.com/87_149.asp[0]

Allison, S. P., & Lobo, D. N. (2004). Fluid and electrolytes in the elderly. *Current Opinions in Clinical Nutrition Metabolic Care, 7*, 27–33.

American Dietetic Association. (2002). Position on Weight Management. *Journal of the American Dietetic Association, 102*, 1145–1155.

American Dietetic Association. (2005). Nutrition across the spectrum of aging. *Journal of the American Dietetic Association, 105*, 613–623.

American Dietetic Association. (2008). *Adult weight management evidence–based nutrition practice guideline.* Retrieved November 14, 2008, from http://www.adaevidencelibrary.com/topic.cfm?format_tables=0&cat=3014

American Dietetic Association and Dietitians of Canada. (2007). Position statement: Dietary fatty acids. *Journal of the American Dietetic Association, 107*(9), 1599–1611.

American Psychiatric Association. (2000). *Diagnostic and statistical manual of mental disorders: DSM–IV–TR* (4th ed., Text Rev.). Washington, DC: Author.

Appel, L. J., Brand, M. W., Daniels, S. R., Daranja, N., Elmer, P. J., & Sacks, F. M. (2006). Dietary approaches to prevent and treat hypertension. A scientific statement from the American Heart Association. *Hypertension, 47*, 296–308.

Ascherio, A., Katan, M. B., Stampfer, M. J., & Willett, W. C. (1999).Trans fatty acids and coronary heart disease. *New England Journal of Medicine, 340*, 1994–1997.

Bailey, A., Maisey, S., Southon, S., Wright, A. J. A., Finglas, P. M., & Fulcher, R. A. (1997). Relationships between micronutrient intake and biochemical indicators of nutrient adequacy in a "free–living" elderly UK population. *British Journal of Nutrition, 77*, 225–242.

Baker, S. S., Cochran, W. J., Flores, C. A., Georgieff, M. K., Jacobson, M. S., Jaksic, T., et al. American Academy of Pediatrics, Committee on Nutrition. (1999). Calcium requirements of infants, children, and adolescents. *Pediatrics 104* (5, Pt. 1), 1152–1157.

Balkau, B., Deanfield, J. E., Després, J.-P., Bassand, J.-P., Fox, K. A. A., Smith, S. C., et al. (2007). International day for the evaluation of abdominal obesity (IDEA): A study of waist circumference, cardiovascular disease and diabetes mellitus in 168,000 primary care patients in 63 countries. *Circulation, 116*(17), 1942–1951.

Barrett, B., Brown, R., Miundt, M., Dye, L., Alt, J., Safdar, N., et al. (2005).Using benefit harm tradeoffs to estimate sufficiently important difference: The case of the common cold. *Medical Decision Making, 25*, 47–55.

Bassey, E. J. (1986). Demi-span as a measure of skeletal size. *Annals of Human Biology, 13*(5), 499–502.

Bates, C. J., Prentice, A., & Finch, S. (1999). Gender differences in food and nutrient intakes and status indices from the National Diet and Nutrition Survey of people aged 65 years and over. *European Journal of Clinical Nutrition, 53*, 694–699.

Beilory, L. (2004). Complementary and alternative interventions in asthma, allergy and immunology. *Annals of Allergy Asthma Immunology, 93*(Suppl. 1), S45–S54.

Berkel, L. A. (2005). Behavioural interventions for obesity. *Journal of the American Medical Association, 105* (5 Suppl. 1), S35–S43.

Blanc, S., Schoeller, D. A., Bauer, D., Danielson, M. E., Tylavsky, F., Simonsick, E. M., et al. (2004). Energy requirements in the eighth decade of life. *American Journal of Clinical Nutrition, 79*, 303–310.

Brager, R., & Sloand, E. (2005). The spectrum of polypharmacy. *Nurse Practitioner, 30*, 44–50.

Brener, N. D., McManus, T., Galuska, D. A., Lowry, R., & Wechsler, H. (2003) Reliability and validity of self-reported height and weight among high school students. *Journal of Adolescent Health, 32*(4), 281–287.

Brown, J. P., Josse, R. G., for the Scientific Advisory Council of the Osteoporosis Society of Canada. (2002). *Canadian Medical Association Journal, 167* (Suppl. 10), S1–S34.

Bruno, J. J., & Ellis, J. J. (2005). Herbal use among U.S. elderly: 2002 national health interview survey. *Annals of Pharmacotherapeutics, 39*, 643–648.

Bueno, J., Ohwada, S., Kocoshis, S., Mazariegos, G. V., Dvorchik, I., Sigurdsson, L., et al. (1999). Factors impacting the survival of children with intestinal failure referred for intestinal transplantation. *Journal of Pediatric Surgery, 34*(1), 27–33.

Canadian Medical Association. (2005). Canadian guidelines for body weight classification in adults: Application in clinical practice to screen for overweight and obesity and to assess disease risk. *Canadian Medical Association Journal, 172*(8), 995–998.

Canadian Paediatric Society, Dietitians of Canada and Health Canada. (2005). *Nutrition for healthy term infants.* Ottawa, ON: Minister of Public Works and Government Services. Retrieved November 13, 2008, from http://www.hc-sc.gc.ca/fn-an/pubs/infant-nourrisson/nut_infant_nourrisson_term-eng.php

Canadian Paediatric Society. (2007). Vitamin D supplementation: Recommendations for Canadian mothers and infants. *Paediatrics and Child Health, 12*(7), 583–589.

Canadian Paediatric Society. (2008). *Breastfeeding.* Retrieved November 13, 2008, from http://www.caringforkids.cps.ca/pregnancy&babies/breastfeeding.htm

Capital Health. (2007). *Nutrition for Healthy Term Infants.* Edmonton, AB: Author.

Chapman, G. (1994). *Food practices and concerns of teenage girls.* Ottawa, ON, Canada: National Institute of Nutrition.

Chernoff, R. (2005). Micronutrient requirements in older women. *American Journal of Clinical Nutrition, 81*(Suppl. 1), 1240S–1245S.

Chobanian, A. V., Bakris, G. L., Black, H. R., Cushman, W. C., Green, L. A., Izzo, J. L., Jr., et al. (2003). Seventh Report of the Joint National Committee on Prevention, Detection, Evaluation, and Treatment of High Blood Pressure. *Hypertension, 42*, 1206–1252.

Chumlea, W. C., Roche, A. F., & Steinbaugh, M. L. (1985). Estimating stature from knee height for persons 60-90 years of age. *Journal of the American Geriatric Society, 33*, 116–120.

Day, R. A. (2007). Health assessment. In R. A. Day, P. Paul, B. Williams, S. C. Smeltzer, & B. Bare (Eds.), *Brunner & Suddarth's textbook of medical–surgical nursing* (1st Canadian edn., pp. 68–74). Philadelphia: Lippincott Williams & Wilkins.

de Groot, L., & van Staveren, W. A. (1996). Low protein intakes and protein turnover in elderly women. *Nutrition Review, 1*, 58–65.

Dennison, E., Cole, Z., & Cooper, C. (2005). Diagnosis and epidemiology of osteoporosis. *Current Opinions in Rheumatology, 17*(4), 456–461.

Després, J.-P., & Tchernof, A. (2007). Classification of overweight and obesity in adults. *Canadian Medical Association Journal, 176*(1), 21–26.

De Wals, P., Tairou, F., Van Allen, M. I., Uh, S. H., Lowry, R. B., Sibbald, B., et al. (2007). Reduction in neural-tube defects after folic acid fortification in Canada. *New England Journal of Medicine, 357*(2), 135–142. Retrieved December 18, 2008, from http://content.nejm.org/cgi/content/short/357/2/135?query=TOC

DiBaise, J. K., Young, R. J., Vanderhoof, J. A. (2004a). Intestinal rehabilitation and the short bowel syndrome: part 1. *American Journal of Gastroenterology 99*(7), 1386–1395.

DiBaise, J. K., Young, R. J., Vanderhoof, J. A. (2004b). Intestinal rehabilitation and the short bowel syndrome: part 2. *American Journal of Gastroenterology 99*(9):1823–1832.

Douketis, J. D., Paradis, G., Keller, H., & Martineau, C. (2005). Canadian guidelines for body weight classification in adults: Application in clinical practice to screen for overweight and obesity and to assess disease risk. *Canadian Medical Association Journal, 172*(8), 995–998.

Engstrom, J. L., Paterson, S. A., Doherty, A., Trabulsi, M., & Speer, K. L. (2003). Accuracy of self-reported height and weight in women: an integrative review of the literature. *Journal of Midwifery & Women's Health, 48*(5), 338–345.

Expert Panel on Detection, Evaluation, and Treatment of High Blood Cholesterol in Adults. (2001). Executive summary of the third report of the National Cholesterol Education Program (NCEP) expert panel on detection, evaluation, and treatment of high blood cholesterol in adults (Adult Treatment

Panel III). *Journal of the American Medical Association, 285*(19), 2486–2497.

Fernandez, J. R., Redden, D. T., Pietrobelli, A., & Allison, D. B. (2004). Waist circumference percentiles in nationally representative samples of African–American, European–American, and Mexican–American children and adolescents. *Journal of Pediatrics, 45,* 439–444.

Groeneveld, I., Solomons, N. W., & Doak, C. M. (2007). Determination of central body fat by measuring natural waist and umbilical abdominal circumference in Guatemalan schoolchildren. *International Journal of Pediatric Obesity, 2,* 114–121.

Groff, J. L., & Gropper, S. S. (2000). *Advanced nutrition and human metabolism* (3rd ed.). Scarborough, ON: Wadsworth Thomson Learning.

Halterman, J. S., Kaczorowski, J. M., Aligne, A., Auinger, P., & Szilagyi, P. G. (2001). Iron deficiency and cognitive achievement among school–aged children and adolescents in the United States. *Pediatrics, 107*(60), 1381–1386.

Hanley, D. A., & Davidson, K. S. (2005). Vitamin D insufficiency in North America. *The Journal of Nutrition, 135,* 332–337.

Health and Welfare Canada. (1988). *Canadian guidelines for healthy weight: Report of an expert group.* Ottawa, ON: Minister of Supply and Services Canada.

Health Canada. (1999). *Nutrition for a healthy pregnancy–National Guidelines for the childbearing years.* Retrieved November 8, 2007, from http://www.hc–sc.gc.ca/fn–an/nutrition/prenatal/national_guidelines_tc–lignes_directrices_nationales_tm_e.html

Health Canada. (2003). *Canadian guidelines for body weight classification in adults.* Ottawa, ON: Minister of Public Works and Government Services. Retrieved November 23, 2008, from http://www.hc–sc.gc.ca/fn–an/nutrition/weights–poids/guide–ld–adult/index–eng.php

Health Canada. (2004). *Exclusive breastfeeding duration: 2004 Health Canada recommendation.* Ottawa. Retrieved November 13, 2008, from http://www.hc–sc.gc.ca/fn–an/nutrition/child–enfant/infant–nourisson/excl_bf_dur–dur_am_excl_eng.html

Health Canada. (2006). *Dietary reference intakes.* Retrieved November 8, 2008, from http://www.hc-sc.gc.ca/fn–an/alt_formats/hpfb-dgpsa/pdf/nutrition/dri_tables-eng.pdf

Health Canada. (2007a). *Eating well with Canada's food guide.* Ottawa, ON: Minister of Health Canada. Retrieved November 13, 2008, from http://www.hc-sc.gc.ca/fn–an/alt_formats/hpfb-dgpsa/pdf/food-guide-aliment/print_eatwell_bienmang-eng.pdf

Health Canada. (2007b). *Eating well with Canada's food guide—First Nations, Inuit and Metis.* Retrieved December 1, 2008, from http://hc-sc.gc.ca/fn–an/pubs/fnim-pnim/index-eng.php

Health Canada. (2007c). *It's your health: Caffeine.* Retrieved November 13, 2008, from http://www.hc-sc.gc.ca/hl-vs/iyh-vsv/food-aliment/caffeine-eng.php

Health Canada. (2007d). *Eating well with Canada's food guide: A resource for educators and communicators.* Ottawa, ON: Minister of Health Canada.

Health Canada. (2007e). *Eating well with Canada's food guide. Milk and alternatives.* Ottawa, ON: Author. Retrieved November 13, 2007, from http://www.hc-sc.gc.ca/fn–an/food-guide-aliment/choose-choix/milk-lait/index-eng.php

Hickson, M., & Frost, G. (2003). A comparison of three methods for estimating height in the acutely ill elderly population. *Journal of Human Nutrition and Dietetics, 16,* 13–20.

Hoffman, G. B. (2002). Evaluating and treating unintentional weight loss in the elderly. *American Family Physician, 65,* 640–650.

Humphries, K., Traci, M. A., & Seekins, T. (2004). A preliminary assessment of the nutrition and food–system environment of adults with intellectual disabilities living in supported arrangements in the community. *Ecology of Food and Nutrition, 43,* 517–532.

Hypponen, E., Laara, E., Reuanen, A., Jarvelin, M. R., & Virtanen, S. M. (2001). Intake of vitamin D and risk of type 1 diabetes: A birth cohort study. *The Lancet, 358,* 1500–1503.

Institute of Medicine. (1997). *Dietary reference intakes for calcium, phosphorus, magnesium, vitamin D and fluoride.* Food and Nutrition Board, Washington, DC: National Academy Press.

Institute of Medicine. (1998). *Dietary reference intakes for thiamin, riboflavin, niacin, vitamin B6, folate, vitamin B12, pantothenic acid, biotin and choline.* Food and Nutrition Board, Washington, DC: National Academy Press.

Institute of Medicine. (2004a). *Dietary reference intakes for water, potassium, sodium, chloride and sulfate.* Food and Nutrition Board, Washington, DC: National Academy Press.

Institute of Medicine. (2004b). *Nutrition during pregnancy.* Washington, DC: National Academy Press.

Janssen, I., Katzmarzyk, P. T., & Ross, R. (2002). Body mass index, waist circumference, and health risk: Evidence in support of current National Institutes of Health guidelines. *Archives of Internal Medicine, 162,* 2074–2079.

Javaid, M. K., Crozier, S. R., Harvey, N. C., Gale, C. R., Dennison, E. M., Boucher, B. J., et al. (2006). Maternal vitamin D status during pregnancy and childhood bone mass at age 9 years: A longitudinal study. *The Lancet, 367*(9504), 36–43.

Jones, J. M., Bennett, S., Olmsted, M. P., Lawson, M. L, & Rodin, G. (2001). Disordered eating attitudes and behaviours in teenaged girls: A school–based study. *Canadian Medical Association Journal, 165*(5), 547–552.

Kanis, J. A., Melton, L. G., Christiansen, C., Johnson, C. C., & Khaltaev, N. (1994). The diagnosis of osteoporosis. *Journal of Bone Mineral Research, 9,* 1137–1141.

Katzmarzyk, P. T. (2007). The metabolic syndrome: An introduction. *Applied Physiology, Nutrition & Metabolism, 32*(1), 1–3.

Katzmarzyk, P. T., Craig, C. L., & Bouchard, C. (2001). Underweight, overweight and obesity: Relationships with mortality in the 13-year follow-up of the Canada Fitness Survey. *Journal of Clinical Epidemiology, 54,* 916–920.

Katzmarzyk, P. T., & Ardern, C. I. (2004). Overweight and obesity mortality trends in Canada, 1985–2000. *Canadian Medical Association Journal, 95*(1), 16–20.

Katzmarzyk, P. T., Tremblay, A., Pérusse, L., Després, J. P., & Bouchard, C. (2003). The utility of the international child and adolescent overweight guidelines for predicting coronary heart disease risk factors. *Journal of Clinical Epidemiology, 56*(5), 456–462.

Kavey, R. W., Daniels, S. R., Lauer, R. M., Atkins, D. L., Hayman, L. L., & Taubert, K. (2003). American Heart Association guidelines for primary prevention of atherosclerotic cardiovascular disease beginning in childhood. *Journal of Pediatrics, 142*(4), 368–372.

Keller, H., Brockest, B., & Haresign, H. (2006). Building capacity for nutrition screening. *Nutrition Today, 41*(4), 164–170.

Kennedy, R. L., Chokkalingham, K., & Srinivasan, R. (2004). Obesity in the elderly: Who should we be treating and why, and how? *Current Opinions in Clinical Nutrition Metabolic Care, 7,* 3–9.

Khan, N. A., McAlister, F. A., Rabkin, S. W., Padwal, R., Feldman, R. D., Campbell, N. R., et al. (2006). The 2006 Canadian Hypertension Education Program recommendations for the management of hypertension: Part II – Therapy. *The Canadian Journal of Cardiology, 22*(7), 583–593.

Kinney, J. M. (2004). Nutritional frailty, sarcopenia and falls in the elderly. *Current Opinions in Clinical Nutrition Metabolic Care, 7,* 15–20.

Kirk, S. F. L., Cramm, C. L., Price, S. L., Penney, T. L., Jarvie, L., & Power, H. (2009). BMI: A vital sign for patients and health professionals. *Canadian Nurse, 105*(1), 25–28.

Kishiyam, S. S., Leahy, M. J., Zitzelberger, T. A., Guariglia, R., Zajdel, D. P., Calvert, J. E., et al. (2005). Patterns of dietary supplement usage in demographically diverse older people. *Alternative Therapy in Health and Medicine, 11,* 48–53.

Klein, S., Allison, D. B., Heymsfield, S. B., Kelley, D. E., Leibel, R. L., Nonas, C., et al. (2007). Waist circumference and cardiometabolic risk: A consensus statement for shaping America's health: Association for Weight Management and Obesity Prevention, NAASO, The Obesity Society; the American Society for Nutrition, and the American Diabetes Association. *Diabetes Care, 30,* 1647–1652.

Kramer, M. S., Guo, T., Platt, R. W., Sevkovskava, Z., Dzikovich, I., Collet, J. P., et al. (2003). Infant growth and health outcomes associated with 3 compared with 6 months exclusive breast-feeding. *American Journal of Clinical Nutrition, 78,* 291–295.

Kuczmarski, M. F., Kuczmarski, R. J., & Najjar, M. (2001). Effects of age on validity of self-reported height, weight, and body mass index: findings from the Third National Health and Nutrition Examination Survey, 1988-1994. *Journal of the American Dietetic Association, 101*(1), 28–36.

Lai, K. H., Peng, N. J., Lo, G. H., Lin, C. K., Chan, H. H., Hsu, P. I., et al. (2002). Does a fatty meal improve hepatic clearance in patients after endoscopic sphincterotomy? *Journal of Gastroenterology and Hepatology, 17*(3), 337–341.

Lau, D. C. W. (2007). Synopsis of the 2006 Canadian clinical practice guidelines on the management and prevention of obesity in adults and children. *Canadian Medical Association Journal, 176*(8), 1103–1106.

Leaf, A. (1999). Dietary prevention of coronary heart disease: The Lyon Diet Heart Study. *Circulation, 99,* 733–735.

Leo, M. A., & Lieber, C. S. (1999). Alcohol, vitamin A, and beta–carotene: Adverse interactions, including hepatotoxicity and carcinogenicity. *American Journal of Clinical Nutrition, 69,* 1071–1085.

Levy, S., Herve, C., Delacoux, E., & Erlinger, S. (2002). Thiamine deficiency in hepatitis C virus and alcohol–related liver diseases. *Digestive Diseases and Sciences, 47,* 543–548.

Lichtenstein, A. H., Appel, L. J., Brands, M., Carnethon, M., Daniels, S., Franch, H. A., et al. (2006). American Heart Association Nutrition Committee. Diet and lifestyle recommendations revision 2006: A scientific statement from the American Heart Association. *Circulation, 114,* 82–96.

Lin, B. H., Guthrie, J., & Frazao, E. (2001). American children's diet not making the grade. *Food Review, 24*(2), 8–17.

Little, R. E., Anderson, K. W., Ervin, C. H., Worthington–Roberts, B., & Clarren, S. K. (1989). Maternal alcohol use during breastfeeding and infant mental and motor development at one year. *New England Journal of Medicine, 321*(7), 425–430.

Malina, R. M., & Katzmarzyk, P. T. (2006). Physical activity and fitness in an international growth standard for preadolescent and adolescent children. *Food and Nutrition Bulletin, 27*(4 Suppl. Growth Standard), S295–S313.

Marshall, W. J. (2008). Nutrition assessment: Its role in the provision of nutrition support. *Journal of Clinical Pathology, 61*(10), 1083–1088.

Mattes, R. D., & Donnelly, D. (1991). Relative contributions of dietary sodium sources. *Journal of the American College of Nutrition, 10,* 383–393.

McCabe, B. J. (2004). Prevention of food–drug interactions with special emphasis on older adults. *Current Opinion in Clinical Nutrition Metabolic Care, 7,* 21–26.

McPherson, R., Frohlich, J., Fodor, G., & Genest, J. (2006). Canadian Cardiovascular Society position statement—Recom-mendations for the diagnosis and treatment of dyslipidemia and prevention of cardiovascular disease. *The Canadian Journal of Cardiology, 22*(11), 913–927.

Mennella, J. (2001). Alcohol's effect on lactation. *Alcohol Research & Health, 25*(3), 230–234.

Mennella, J. A., & Beauchamp, G. K. (1991). The transfer of alcohol to human milk. Effects on flavor and the infant's behaviour. *New England Journal of Medicine, 325*(14), 981–985.

Mennella, J. A., & Gerrish, C. J. (1998). Effects of exposure to alcohol in mother's milk on infant sleep. *Pediatrics, 101*(5), E2.

Merriam-Webster medical dictionary. Retrieved November 10, 2008, from http://medical.merriamwebster.com/medical/eating%20disorder

Misciagna, G., Centonze, S., Leoci, C., Guerra, V., Cisternino, A. M., Ceo, R., et al. (1999). Diet, physical activity, and gallstones–a population-based, case-control study in southern Italy. *The American Journal of Clinical Nutrition, 69,* 120–126.

Mitchell, C. O., & Lipschitz, D. A. (1982). Arm length measurement as an alternative to height in nutritional assessment of the elderly. *Journal of Parenteral and Enteral Nutrition, 6*(3), 226–229.

Mozaffarian, D., & Rimm, E. B. (2006). Fish intake, contaminants and human health: Evaluating the risks and benefits. *Journal of the American Medical Association, 296,* 1885–1899.

Muraro, A., Dreborg, S., Halken, S., Host, A., Niggemann, B., Aalberse, R., et al. (2004). Dietary prevention of allergic diseases in infants and small children. Part III: Critical review of published peer reviewed observational and interventional studies and final recommendations. *Pediatric Allergy and Immunology, 15,* 291–307.

Nair, K. S. (2005). Aging muscle. *American Journal of Clinical Nutrition, 81,* 953–963.

NANDA International. (2007). *NANDA–1 nursing diagnoses: Definitions & classifications 2007–2008* (7th ed.). Philadelphia: Author.

National Academy of Science. (2005a). *Dietary reference intakes for energy, carbohydrates, fiber, fat, fatty acids, protein and amino acids (macronutrients).* Retrieved November 14, 2008, from http://books.nap.edu/catalog.php?record_id=10490

National Academy of Science. (2004). *Dietary reference intakes for water, potassium, sodium, chloride and sulfate.* Retrieved November 15, 2008, from http://books.nap.edu/catalog.php?record_id=10925

National Heart, Lung, and Blood Institute, National Institutes of Health, Department of Health and Human Services. Produced in cooperation with the National Institute of Diabetes and Digestive and Kidney Diseases. (1998). *Clinical guidelines on the identification, evaluation, and treatment of overweight and obesity in adults: The evidence report.* NIH Publication No. 98–4083. Retrieved November 14, 2008, from http://www.nhlbi.nih.gov/guidelines/obesity/ob_gdlns.htm

Nonas, C. A., & Foster, G. D. (2005). Setting achievable goals for weight loss. *Journal of the American Dietetic Association, 105*(5 Suppl 1), S118–S123.

Nutrition Recommendations Update: Dietary Fat and Children. (1991). Report of the Joint Working Group of the Canadian Paediatric Society (CPS) and Health Canada. Reference No. N94–01.

Oken, E., Taveras, E. M., Kleinman, K. P., Rich–Edwards, J. W., & Gillman, M. W. (2007). Gestational weight gain and child adiposity at age 3 years. *American Journal of Obstetrics & Gynecolology, 196*(4), 322.e1–322.e8.

Olson, C. M., Strawderman, M. S., Hinton, P. S., & Pearson, T. A. (2003). Gestational weight gain and postpartum behaviours associated with weight change from early pregnancy to 1 year postpartum. *International Journal of Obesity, 27*, 117–127.

Paquette, M.-C. (2005). Perceptions of healthy eating: State of knowledge and research gaps. *Canadian Journal of Public Health, 96* (Suppl. 3), S15–S19.

Pena–Rosas, J. P., & Viteri, F. E. (2006). Effects of routine iron supplementation with or without folic acid for women during pregnancy. *Cochrane Database of Systematic Reviews (Online), 3*, CD004736.

Public Health Agency of Canada (2003). *Canada's Physical Activity Guide to Healthy Active Living.* Retrieved November 15, 2008, from http://www.phac–aspc.gc.ca/pau–uap/paguide/index.html

Rooney, B. L., & Schauberger, C. W. (2002). Excess pregnancy weight gain and long–term obesity: One decade later. *Obstetrics & Gynecology, 100*, 245–252.

Ross, R., Berentzen, T., Bradshaw, A. J., Janssen, I., Kahn, H. S., Katzmarzyk, P. T., et al. (2008). Does the relationship between waist circumference, morbidity and mortality depend on measurement protocol for waist circumference? *Obesity Review, 9*(4), 312–325.

Roubenoff, R., Giacoppe, J., Richardson, S., & Hoffman, P. J. (1996). Nutrition assessment in long–term care facilities. *Nutrition Review, 54*, S40–S42.

Rudolf, M. C., Greenwood, D. C., Cole, T. J., Levine, R., Sahota, P., Walker, J., et al. (2004). Rising obesity and expanding waistlines in schoolchildren: A cohort study. *Archives of Disease in Childhood, 89*, 235–237.

Rudolf, M., Walker, J, W., & Cole, T. J. (2007). What is the best way to measure waist circumference? *International Journal of Pediatric Obesity, 2*, 58–71.

Russell, R. M. (2000). The aging process as a modifier of metabolism. *American Journal of Clinical Nutrition, 72*(2 Suppl.), 529S–532S.

Sanchez–Craig, M. (1996). *A therapist's manual: Secondary prevention of alcohol problems.* Toronto, ON: Addiction Research Foundation.

Skelly, A. H., Leeman, J., Carlson, J., Soward, A. C. M., & Burns, D. (2008). Conceptual model of symptom–focused diabetes care for African Americans. *Journal of Nursing Scholarship, 40*(3), 261–267.

Society of Obstetricians and Gynaecologists of Canada. (2003). Clinical practice guideline: The use of folic acid for prevention of neural tube defects and other congenital abnormalities. *Journal of Obstetrics and Gynaecology Canada, 25*(11), 959–965.

Story, M., Kaphingst, K., Robinson–O'Brien, R., & Glanz, K. (2008). Creating healthy food and eating environments: Policy and environmental approaches. *Annual Review of Public Health, 29*, 253–272.

Strychar, I. (2006). Diet in the management of weight loss. *Canadian Medical Association Journal, 174*(1), 56–63.

Suarez, F. L., Savaiano, D. A., & Levitt, M. D. (1995). A comparison of symptoms after the consumption of milk or lactose-hydrolyzed milk by people with self-reported severe lactose intolerance. *New England Journal of Medicine, 333*(1), 1–4.

Sutcliffe, T., Khambalia, A., Westergard, S., Jacobson Peer, M., & Parkin, P. (2006). Iron depletion is associated with daytime bottle-feeding in the second and third years of life. *Archives of Pediatric Adolescent Medicine, 160*, 1114–1120.

Taylor, R. W., Jones, I. E., Williams, S. M., & Goulding, A. (2000). Evaluation of waist circumference, waist–to–hip ratio, and the conicity index as screening tools for high trunk fat mass, as measured by dual–energy X–ray absorptiometry, in children aged 3–19 y. *American Journal of Clinical Nutrition, 72*(2), 490–495.

Tjepkema, M. (2005). Adult obesity in Canada: Measured height and weight. In: *Nutrition: Findings from the Canadian Community Health Survey.* Issue 1. Ottawa, ON: Statistics Canada. Cat No 82–620–MWE2005001.

Trumbo, P., Schlicker, S., Yates, A. A., & Poos, M. (2002). Dietary reference intakes for energy, carbohydrate, fiber, fat, fatty acids, cholesterol, protein, and amino acids. *Journal of the American Dietetic Association, 102*, 1621–1630.

Walsh, B. T., & Devlin, M. J. (1998). Eating disorders: Progress and problems. *Science, 280*, 1387–1390.

Weber, J., & Kelley, J. (2007). *Health assessment in nursing* (3rd ed.). Philadelphia: Lippincott Williams & Wilkins.

Whiting, S. J., Vatanparast, H., Baxter–Jones, A., Faulkner, R. A., Mirwald, R., & Bailey, D. A. (2004). Factors that affect bone mineral accrual in the adolescent growth spurt. *The Journal of Nutrition, 134*, 696S–700S.

Wold, R. S., Lopez, S. T., Yau, L. C., Butler, L. M., Pareo-Tubbeh, S. L., Waters, D. L., et al. (2005). Increasing trends in elderly persons' use of nonvitamin, nonmineral dietary supplements and concurrent use of medications. *Journal of the American Dietetic Association, 105*, 54–63.

World Health Organization. (1994). Assessment of fracture risk and its application to screening for postmenopausal osteoporosis: Report of a WHO study group. *World Health Organization Technical Report Series*, 843. Geneva, Switzerland: Author.

World Health Organization. (1995). The use and interpretation of anthropometry. Report of a WHO expert committee. *World Health Organization Technical Report Series*, 854. Geneva, Switzerland: Author.

World Health Organization. (2003). Diet, nutrition and the prevention of chronic diseases. Report of a Joint WHO/FAO Expert Consultation. *World Health Organization Technical Report Series*, 916. Geneva, Switzerland: Author.

World Health Organization. (2008). *The WHO Child Growth Standards.* Retrieved November 23, 2008, from http://www.who.int/childgrowth/standards/en/

World Health Organization Expert Consultation. (2004). Appropriate body-mass index for Asian populations and its implications for policy and intervention strategies. *Lancet 363*(9414), 1077.

Wudel, L. J. Jr., Wright, J. K., Debelak, J. P., Allos, T. M., Shyr, Y., & Chapman, W. C. (2002). Prevention of gallstone formation in morbidly obese patients undergoing rapid weight loss: Results of a randomized controlled pilot study. *The Journal of Surgical Research, 102*, 50–56.

Yokoyama, M., Origasa, H., Matsuzaki, M., Matsuzawa, Y., Saito, Y., Ishikawa, Y., et al. for the Japan EPA Lipid Intervention Study (JELIS). (2007). Effects of eicosapentaenoic acid on major coronary events in hypercholesterolaemic patients (JELIS): A randomised open–label, blinded endpoint analysis. *The Lancet, 369*(9567), 1090–1098.

Zeiger, R. S., & Heller, S. (1995). The development and prediction of atopy in high–risk children: Follow–up at age seven years in a prospective randomized study of combined maternal and infant food allergen avoidance. *The Journal of Allergy and Clinical Immunology, 95*(6), 1179–1190.

ADDITIONAL REFERENCES

Mager, D., Smits, M., Turbico, F., & Roberts, E. A. (2006). What is the most informative simple anthropometric measure of abdominal adiposity in children with nonalcoholic fatty liver disease? *Hepatology, 44*, 661A.

Standing Committee on the Scientific Evaluation of Dietary Reference Intakes, Food and Nutrition Board, Institute of Medicine, National Academy of Sciences. (2001). *Dietary reference intakes for vitamin A, vitamin K, arsenic, boron, chromium, copper, iodine, iron, manganese, molybdenum, nickel, silicon, vanadium, and zinc: A report of the Panel on Micronutrients. National Academy of Sciences.* Retrieved March 22, 2008, from http://books.nap.edu/catalogue.php?record_id=10026#toc

	Signs of Good Nutrition	Signs of Poor Nutrition
TABLE 8-1	**Physical Signs Indicative of Nutritional Status**	
General appearance	Alert, responsive, energetic	Listless, apathetic, appears acutely or chronically ill
Hair	Shiny, lustrous, minimal loss	Dull and dry, brittle, depigmented, easily plucked, thin and sparse
Face	Skin colour uniform; smooth, moist	Skin dark over cheeks and under eyes, skin flaky, face swollen or hollow/sunken cheeks
Eyes	Bright, clear, moist	Eye membranes pale, dry; increased vascularity
Lips	Pink colour, smooth, moist	Edematous, cracks, angular lesions at corners of mouth (cheilosis)
Tongue	Deep red in appearance; surface papillae present	Smooth, edematous, beefy red, atrophic papillae
Teeth	Straight, no crowding, no dental caries, uniform colour	Dental caries, missing teeth, mottled appearance (fluorosis), malpositioned, dentures no longer fit
Gums	Firm, pink colour; margins tight around teeth	Spongy; bleed easily; marginal redness, recession
Thyroid	No enlargement of the thyroid	Thyroid enlargement (simple goitre)
Skin	Smooth, uniform colour; moist, warm	Rough, dry, flaky; edema present; pale, pigmented; lack of fat under skin or excess fat under skin
Nails	Firm, pink	Spoon-shaped, ridged, brittle
Skeleton	Good posture, no malformation	Poor posture, stooped, bending of ribs, bowed legs, or knock knees
Muscles	Well developed, firm	Flaccid, poor tone, wasted, underdeveloped
Extremities	No tenderness	Weak and tender, edematous
Abdomen	Flat	Concave or hollowed (scaphoid), protruding
Nervous system	Reflexes present	Decreased or absent ankle and knee reflexes
Weight	Appropriate for height, age, and body build	Overweight or underweight

Source: Day, R. A., 2007.

TABLE 8-2   Factors Associated With Potential Nutritional Deficits

Factors	Possible Consequences
Dental and oral problems (missing teeth, ill-fitting dentures, impaired swallowing or chewing)	Inadequate caloric and protein intake
NPO for diagnostic testing	Inadequate caloric and protein intake; dehydration
Prolonged use of glucose and saline IV fluids	Inadequate caloric and protein intake
Nausea and vomiting	Inadequate caloric and protein intake; loss of fluid, electrolytes, and minerals
Stress of illness, surgery, and/or hospitalization	Increased protein and caloric requirement; increased catabolism
Wound drainage	Loss of protein, fluid, electrolytes, and minerals
Pain	Loss of appetite; inability to shop, cook, eat
Fever	Increased caloric, protein, and fluid requirement; increased catabolism
Gastrointestinal disease	Inadequate intake and malabsorption of nutrients
Alcoholism	Inadequate intake of nutrients; increased consumption of calories without other nutrients; vitamin deficiencies
Depression	Loss of appetite; inability to shop, cook, eat
Eating disorders (anorexia, bulimia)	Inadequate caloric and protein intake; loss of fluid, electrolytes, and minerals
Medications	Inadequate intake due to medication side effects, such as dry mouth, loss of appetite, decreased taste perception, difficulty swallowing, nausea and vomiting
Restricted ambulation or disability	Physical problems that limit shopping, cooking, eating; inability to help self to food, liquids, or other nutrients; malabsorption of nutrients

Source: Adapted from Day, R. A., 2007.

TABLE 8-3   Eating Disorders and Excessively Low BMI

Estimates are that 3% of all women in industrialized countries will suffer from an eating disorder during their lifetime (Walsh & Devlin, 1998). Disordered eating has been reported in >27% of Canadian girls 12 to 18 years old and has been seen to increase gradually throughout adolescence (Jones et al., 2001). Although the rates of eating disorders among men are lower, these illnesses can affect both men and women. These severe disturbances of eating behaviour are often difficult to detect, especially in teens wearing baggy clothes or in individuals who binge then induce vomiting or evacuation.

Be familiar with the two principal eating disorders, *anorexia nervosa* and *bulimia nervosa*. Both conditions are characterized by distorted perceptions of body image and weight. Early detection is important, because prognosis improves when treatment occurs in the early stages of these disorders.

Clinical Features

Anorexia Nervosa

- Refusal to maintain minimally normal body weight (or **BMI** above **17.5kg/m²**)
- Afraid of appearing fat
- Frequently starving but in denial; lacking insight
- Often brought in by family members
- May present as failure to make expected weight gains in childhood or adolescence, amenorrhea in women, loss of libido or potency in men
- Associated with depressive symptoms such as depressed mood, irritability, social withdrawal, insomnia, decreased libido
- Additional features supporting diagnosis: self-induced vomiting or purging, excessive exercise, use of appetite suppressants and/or diuretics
- Biologic complications
  - *Neuroendocrine changes:* amenorrhea, increased corticotropin-releasing factor, cortisol, growth hormone, serotonin; decreased diurnal cortisol fluctuation, luteinizing hormone, follicle-stimulating hormone, thyroid-stimulating hormone
  - *Cardiovascular disorders:* bradycardia, hypotension, arrhythmias, cardiomyopathy
  - *Metabolic disorders:* hypokalemia, hypochloremic metabolic alkalosis, increased **BUN**, edema
  - *Other:* dry skin, dental caries, delayed gastric emptying, constipation, anemia, osteoporosis

Bulimia Nervosa

- Repeated binge eating followed by self-induced vomiting, misuse of laxatives, diuretics or other medications, fasting; or excesssive exercise
- Often with normal weight
- Overeating at least twice a week during 3-month period; large amounts of food consumed in short period (– 2 hrs)
- Preoccupation with eating; craving and compulsion to eat; lack of control over eating; alternating with periods of starvation
- Dread of fatness but may be obese
- Subtypes of
  - *Purging:* bulimic episodes accompanied by self-induced vomiting or use of laxatives, diuretics, or enemas
  - *Non-purging:* bulimic episodes accompanied by compensatory behaviour, such as fasting, exercise, but without purging
  - Biologic complications

See changes listed for anorexia nervosa, especially weakness, fatigue, mild cognitive disorder, also erosion of dental enamel, parotitis, pancreatic inflammation with elevated amylase, mild neuropathies, seizures, hypokalemia, hypochloremic metabolic acidosis, hypomagnesemia

Sources: Walsh, B. T., & Devlin, M. J., 1998; Jones, J. M., Bennett, S., Olmsted, M. P., Lawson, M. L., & Rodin, G., 2001.

Psychosocial and Mental Status Assessment

GERRI C. LASIUK AND LYNN S. BICKLEY

Along with the physical examination, a psychosocial nursing and mental status assessment contributes to a comprehensive understanding of the client's health status, which is the basis of his or her care plan. Ongoing assessment, diagnosis, and monitoring are fundamental to the nurse's role and require a broad base of theoretical knowledge, as well as skills grounded in the biological, social, and nursing sciences. Psychosocial/mental status assessment is not a discrete one-time activity; rather, it encompasses systematic, purposeful, and dynamic processes that are part of all encounters nurses have with clients in their care.

THEORETICAL BASIS FOR PSYCHOSOCIAL ASSESSMENT

By its nature, psychosocial assessment is holistic and addresses genetic, physiological, psychological, developmental, emotional, and spiritual dimensions of clients within the context of their physical and social environments. In performing psychosocial assessments, nurses continually collect, validate, analyze, synthesize, and document objective and subjective data about the changing health status of clients. Nurses endeavour to understand the meaning of the client's experience; identify needs and problems, strengths, and resources; and ascertain how these things interact to affect well-being and function. At each encounter, nurses consider new information along with existing information to use in the ongoing reevaluation of the client's responses to treatments and interventions, nursing diagnoses, and the plan of care.

Although the discipline of nursing endorses a view of the individual as a unique and whole being living in continuous and reciprocal relationship with the environment, too often nurses tend to focus on a particular body system or part, as if it existed in isolation. This might be because of the influence of the "biomedical model" on traditional Western health care (see Chapter 1). The physical body is central in this paradigm, which emphasizes biological data, physical assessment, and disease care over holism, psychosocial assessment, and health care. Assessment and diagnostic activities are divided by speciality (e.g., orthopedics and physical therapy for musculoskeletal care; urology, obstetrics, and gynecology for urogenital and reproductive care) in many hospitals and clinics. The result tends to be a fragmented or incomplete understanding of the client's health–illness experience. Inherent risks to this approach include overlooking information, misdiagnosis, and lack of continuity of care.

The next section contains two constructs that underpin this chapter's approach to psychosocial assessment: Erik Erikson's (1997) theory of psychosocial development

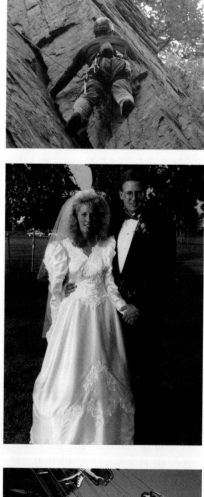

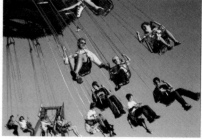

and Hardy, Titchen, Maley, and McCormack's (2006) description of nursing expertise. Erikson's work underscores the person's dynamic and reciprocal relationships with the environment and offers a lens through which to view the contextual nature of the health–illness experience. Hardy and colleagues offer an empirically based description of the unique qualities that nurses enact in their care of the individual-in-context.

ERIKSON'S THEORY OF PSYCHOSOCIAL DEVELOPMENT

Although Erikson, a psychoanalyst, accepted Freud's ideas about the ego, Oedipal complex, and development of the self through various stages, he rejected the notion that universal drives could account for cognitive development and personality. Instead, he looked for anthropological explanations of how society and culture shape human development. During his research, Erikson observed that children in various cultural groups receive different kinds of nurturing and guidance and learn different values and goals, which he believed shaped the development of their psyche and influenced how they navigated life's challenges.

Erikson (1980, 1997) articulated a theory of development with eight distinct phases. Unlike Freud, who believed that personality is fixed by 5 years of age, Erikson thought that personality continued to evolve from birth until death. He identified a series of natural and inevitable crises at various points in the life cycle and hypothesized that their resolution drives ego development and influences happiness, psychological adjustment, and mental health. At the centre of each crisis is a conflict

■ Summary of Erikson's Psychosocial Theory of Development

Stage (Age)	Psychosocial Crisis	Significant Relationships	Psychosocial Modalities	Ego Strength	Maladaptations
I Infant (0–1)	Trust vs. mistrust	Mother	To get, to give in return	Hope, faith	Sensory distortion withdrawal
II Toddler (1–3)	Autonomy vs. shame and doubt	Parents	To hold on, to let go	Will, determination	Impulsivity compulsion
III Preschooler (3–6)	Initiative vs. guilt	Family	To go after, to play	Purpose, courage	Ruthlessness inhibition
IV School-aged child (7–12)	Industry vs. inferiority	Neighbourhood and school	To complete, to make things together	Competence	Narrow virtuosity inertia
V Adolescence (12–18)	Ego identity vs. role confusion	Peer groups, role models	To be oneself, to share oneself	Fidelity, loyalty	Fanaticism repudiation
VI Young adult (20s)	Intimacy vs. isolation	Partners, friends	To lose and find oneself in another	Love	Promiscuity exclusivity
VII Middle adult (30–50)	Generativity vs. self-absorption	Household, workmates	To make be, to take care of	Care	Overextension rejectivity
VIII Older adult (50+)	Integrity vs. despair	Mankind or "my kind"	To be, through having been, to face not being	Wisdom	Presumption despair

Source: Adapted from Erikson, 1980.

that requires development of a specific ego strength to resolve it. For example, in stage one, an infant must find a balance between trust and mistrust, so that she or he has the capacity to trust, while concurrently maintaining enough distrust to avoid being disadvantaged. The strengths and skills required to resolve successive crises builds on those developed in earlier stages; similarly, the inability to resolve early developmental crises interferes with the successful resolution of later ones.

Among the many contributions of Erikson's theory is its ecological view of humans. One that informs the approach of this chapter is the emphasis on the inter-relationship between the person and his or her physical/social environment. This theory offers a framework for understanding the implications of experience for emotional and cognitive development and provides nurses with a way to identify issues and skills that clients may need to address.

ATTRIBUTES OF NURSING EXPERTISE

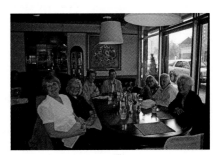

A second work that contributes to the theoretical basis of this chapter is from the Expertise in Practice Project (EPP; Hardy et al., 2006), which began 10 years ago during upheaval in the United Kingdom's health care system. A directive from the National Health Service defining quality health care as *patient-centred* precipitated a cascade of other changes in health professional education, continuing professional development, clinical and research governance, and workplace effectiveness (Manley, Hardy, Titchen, Garbett, & McCormack, 2005). These changes sparked the recognition that because the social sciences, humanities, and medicine heavily influence nursing, nurses often lack the language to articulate the complexity of their expertise. The EPP employed action research to identify a language that nurses can use to capture and articulate the dimensions and impact of their practice. The study revealed five attributes of expert nursing practice: *holistic practice knowledge*, *saliency*, *knowing the patient/client*, *moral agency*, and *skilled know-how*. The accompanying table describes each attribute more fully and offers supporting quotes from the EPP. As nurses develop in their own practice and acquire these attributes, they can enact them and perform psychosocial assessments knowledgeably, with sensitivity and tact.

■ *Attributes of Practice Expertise*

Attribute	Description	Examples Cited by EPP Participants
Holistic practice knowledge	Ongoing learning and evaluation from new situations Using all forms of knowledge in practice Drawing from a range of knowledge bases to assess situations and inform appropriate action with consideration of consequences Embedding new knowledge and accessing it in future similar situations	"I had to draw on all dimensions of thinking, feeling, and sensing to help him feel more in control again. I was very aware I was tailoring information to allow him to assume his coping strategy for his own normality of life. Sharing my knowledge appeared to give him comfort. I was very aware that the time taken to listen and utilize my feelings, to explore this problem, well, the outcome could have been very different."
Saliency	Observing nonverbal cues to understand the person's situation Listening and responding to verbal cues; regarding the client as a whole to inform treatment process Recognizing the needs of client, colleagues, and others in actions taken Picking up cues that others can miss or dismiss, to inform the situation	"His wife asked how I knew something was wrong and I explained it was his body language, the way he looked uninterested in the discussion, and the way he avoided eye contact when I looked directly at him when we were talking."

(continued)

■ Attributes of Practice Expertise (Continued)

Attribute	Description	Examples Cited by EPP Participants
Knowing the client	Respecting people and their views, understandings, and ways of being Respecting clients' unique perspective on their illnesses or situation Promoting and maintaining dignity at all times Using self to promote a helping relationship Promoting the client's own decisions and relinquishing efforts to "control" him or her; recognizing the person's own expertise	"Days when I was not on the ward she [client] may ask to see me—sometimes this can make the others on the ward feel undermined. However, through teaching and supporting them [colleagues] I have helped them realize that the client's own knowledge is valuable to listen to as well. At times she can become angry and cross with anyone who may not know what she can be like in times of particular ill health."
Moral agency	Providing information to enhance people's ability to problem solve and make decisions Working at a level of consciousness that promotes another person's dignity, respect, and individuality Being conscientiously aware of integrity in one's own work Actualizing values and beliefs, while not forcing them on others	"I gave her some information, which I know I'd given her before and she said, 'It's really useful to know that.' I am adopting an empowering approach that I know will help her with her confidence in dealing with her diabetes and encourages her to take more responsibility to the level she wishes."
Skilled know-how	Enabling others through willingness to share knowledge and skills Adapting and responding with consideration to each individual situation Mobilizing and using all available resources Envisioning a path through a problem or situation and inviting others on that journey	"He [a colleague] was looking after a child with a deep head injury. The child was only four. Each time anyone tried to get near, the child became very upset and would not cooperate. He managed to find the child an anaesthetic and explain to the parents what would happen, and to the child that he would feel a little dizzy, in such a way that the child allowed him to stitch him and he waited until the child was OK. I think that was acting as an expert because next time, if the child ever has to come back, he won't be as frightened."

Source: Adapted from Hardy et al., 2006, p. 262.

COMPONENTS OF PSYCHOSOCIAL ASSESSMENT

Psychosocial assessment typically takes the form of a semistructured or conversational interview. Effective interviewing is far more than bombarding clients with a series of predetermined questions; it is both an art and a science. As well as being an opportunity to collect information, psychosocial assessment interviews are a time to establish rapport; clarify and validate observations, perceptions, and meanings; and validate understandings.

Novice interviewers are often so anxious about "getting it right" that they focus more on asking questions than on listening to responses. In contrast, adept interviewers are respectful, warm, and genuinely interested in clients. They approach clients as collaborators with the same goals and engage in what Carl Rogers (1980) called *empathic listening*, which is entering the private perceptual world of the other and becoming thoroughly at home in it. [Empathic listening] involves being sensitive, moment by moment, to the changing felt meanings which flow in the other person, to the fear or rage or tenderness or confusion or whatever he or she is experiencing. It means temporarily living in the other's life, moving about in it delicately without making judgments. (p. 142)

Arrange to perform the psychosocial assessment in a private space where you will not be interrupted and cannot be overheard; turn off your mobile phone or pager and ask the client to do so, too. Sit at eye level, facing the client at a comfortable distance apart (~1 metre)—any closer may seem invasive, but any farther away may make conversation awkward. Explain your intention, rationale for the assessment, and how long it will take—*I'd like to spend the next hour or so talking about you and things that affect your life and health. Is that okay?* If the client agrees, explain that he or she can choose not to answer any question. Doing so acknowledges autonomy and the right to privacy and your willingness to negotiate all aspects of the encounter.

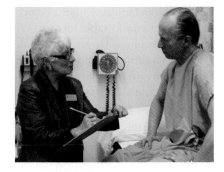

Because many people have a poor understanding of what nurses actually do in their day-to-day work, consider inviting clients to ask questions they may have about you (e.g., *Before we begin, would you like to ask me anything about my role or the work I do?*). If you intend to take notes during the interview, make this clear (e.g., *I will take notes as we talk to summarize what you tell me. That summary will become part of your confidential record here*). Proceed with questions only after the client has given consent.

Clients may decline to answer a question, not because they are being "difficult" or hiding something, but because sufficient rapport has not been established for them to reveal certain things. They may be more willing to discuss sensitive issues as their trust in you builds. Holding back information from strangers (even health professionals) may be a sign of judicious ego boundary integrity. Conversely, being too willing to share private information before determining the trustworthiness of others may indicate poor boundary maintenance, lack of attention to personal safety, or both. At the same time, nurses must remain cognizant of the power difference that exists between them and clients, many of whom regard all health professionals as authority figures. This may leave clients feeling conflicted—wanting to please an authority figure, while at the same time protecting their self.

Although verbal communication is vital to assessment, nonverbal cues also communicate important information about clients, their responses to life events, and their health status. Train yourself to focus full attention on the client to observe posture, behaviour, facial expression, voice tone, and verbal fluency. Consider the congruity between *what* clients say (content) and *how* they say it (behaviour, mannerisms, body position, skin tone, voice quality). For example, when people talk about a positive experience, their face, body, and voice are expected to be animated. Similarly, if they are relating something sad, expected facial expression would be downcast, with slumped posture, slow movements, and low or constricted voices. Crying or lengthy pauses in speech would be expected as well.

Incongruities between content and behaviour and/or abrupt changes in a client's presentation present opportunities for deeper exploration of a topic. If you notice such things as alterations in skin tone (e.g., pallor, flushing); sudden turning away, fidgeting, or stillness; or long pauses in conversation, reflect your observation back to the client. For instance, if a man tells you in a matter-of-fact or upbeat voice that he has just lost his job, saying something like *Losing a job is often a big concern, yet you don't seem too upset about it* invites him to explain what the experience means to him. He may report that he has been waiting for this opportunity to change careers or return to school. If he is suddenly very quiet and his eyes fill with tears, you might infer that the experience is much more difficult than he initially indicated. In this case, ask if he is willing to discuss it (e.g., *It seems like this is difficult for you. Do you want to talk about it?*). If he agrees, listen as he says as much as he chooses to; if he says no, give him time to compose himself and then say, *Shall we move on?* He may decide to reveal more about this issue as the interview progresses.

The following is intended as a guide for organizing a psychosocial assessment. As you become more familiar with the topics addressed, you will be able to phrase questions in a manner comfortable for you. When broaching a particular topic, it is generally better to begin with an open-ended question and proceed with closed-ended questions for more details. If a response is unclear, invite the client to restate it (e.g., *I am not sure what you mean. Can you say it another way?*) or ask for a specific example (e.g., *Tell me about a time when that happened*). Brief pauses between questions give the client time to add details or to raise topics you have not yet addressed. Keep in mind that if you forget to ask something, you can always return to it later.

Examples of Questions for Symptom Analysis: "Stressed Out, Nervous, or Anxious"

- "Think about a time when you felt particularly 'stressed out,' nervous, or anxious—where do you feel it in your body?" "Do these sensations or feelings move or are they always in the same place(s)?" (*Location/radiation*)
- "Describe what being 'stressed-out,' nervous, or anxious is like for you." "Complete this phrase—being 'stressed-out,' nervous, or anxious is like . . ." [The intent is to invite the client to offer a metaphor or compare these sensations to something else (e.g., "having a big knot in my gut" or "like I am vibrating all of the time").] "On a scale of 0–10 with 0 being no stress, nervousness, or anxiety and 10 being the most you have ever experienced, where would you rate yourself right now?" "Using this same scale, where are you on an average day?" (*Quality*)
- "When did this stress, nervousness, or anxiety begin?" (*Onset*) "Did it start suddenly?" "Or did it start gradually?" "Are there times when you feel 'stressed-out,' nervous, or anxious?" "How long do those feelings last?" (*Duration*). "How often do they come?" (*Frequency*). "Is there a time of day that it seems worse?" "Or better?" "Has this stress, nervousness, or anxiety ever gone completely away?" (*Timing*)

- "Where were you when you first noticed being 'stressed-out,' nervous, or anxious?" (*Setting*)
- "What other symptoms have you noticed?" (*Associated symptoms*)
- "What makes it (stress, nervousness, or anxiety) worse?" (*Aggravating factors*)
- "What makes it (stress, nervousness, or anxiety) better?" (*Alleviating factors*)
- "What was going on in your life when this stress, nervousness, or anxiety began? [Probe for details about developmental, relationship, health, or career changes; use of prescribed medications or other substances; and traumatic or extremely distressing events.]" Do things in your home environment make you feel stressed, nervous, or anxious? "Do things in your work environment make you feel stressed, nervous, or anxious?" (*Environmental/situational factors*)
- "Tell me how this stress, nervousness, or anxiety is affecting your daily life." "Your work?" "Are there financial implications?" "How is it affecting your family?" "Or other interpersonal relationships?" (*Significance to client*)
- "What do you think is happening?" (*Client perspective*)

IDENTIFICATION/DEMOGRAPHIC INFORMATION

Demographic information identifies clients, their place of residence, and other personal information. This relatively nonthreatening information is a good place to begin a psychosocial assessment. If the client has provided some data elsewhere (e.g., on a registration or intake form), review it and ask for missing information or clarification as necessary. It can be annoying to be asked the same questions when it seems that no one is actually tracking your responses.

- *What is your full legal name?*

- *Nickname or preferred name?*

- *Date of birth?*

- *Address and telephone numbers (home, work, mobile)?*

- *Provincial/territorial health insurance number?*

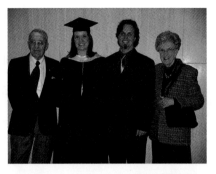

Education/Employment. Responses to these questions inform an understanding of the client's interests, skills, intellectual abilities, motivation, volition, economic status, and quality of life.

- *How many years of schooling have you completed?* (Probe for details about early withdrawal or expulsion from school.)

- *What are your plans after you complete your programme?*

- *Are you currently employed?* (If yes, ask where, how long, number of hours worked in 1 week, and job satisfaction.)

- If not employed, ask *Would you like to be employed?*

- *Have you ever been in the military?* (If yes, ask about active combat.)

- *What are your sources of income? Is it sufficient for your needs?*

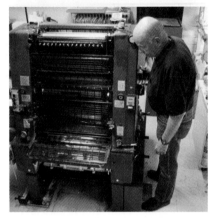

Family of Origin. Discussion of clients' family of origin provides details about early development, learned social roles, availability of social support, and family resources or stressors. Early parental death or separation may be associated with difficulties with attachment and later relationship difficulties.

- *Tell me about the family into which you were born* (i.e., family of origin). *Who are the members of that family?*

- *Did anyone else live in your home when you were growing up?*

- *Are your family members still living?* (If a family member is deceased, note the date and cause of death; ask about experience of grief/loss. For example, *What was it like for you after he (she) died? And now?*)

- *Where do they live?*

- *How often do you see each other?*

- *What is your place in your family?* (Consider both birth order and social roles.)

- *How would you describe your relationships with your parents and siblings?*

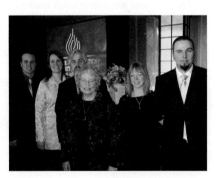

Developmental History. A developmental history can alert the nurse to clients' personal resources and strengths as well as to longstanding behavioural, social, or educational difficulties and failure to achieve expected milestones. Of particular interest is a chaotic family environment and childhood infections, illness, or injury.

- *What do you know about your birth?* (Probe for details about complicated birth such as prolonged labour, difficult delivery, caesarean section, anoxia, etc.)

- *How was your mother's health when she was pregnant with you?* (Probe for details about infections, accidents, illnesses, alcohol or drug use, and unexpected/ untoward experiences.)

- *Were you born before the expected due date?* If yes, probe for details about prematurity.

- *Were you a healthy child?* If no, probe for details.

- *What are your memories of your childhood?*

- *What are the favourite family stories about you?*

- *What was school like for you?*

- *Who were the three most important people in your life when you were a child?*

Significant Relationships.   Questions offer clues about the client's affiliation needs, ability to form and maintain satisfying relationships, and social roles. Frame questions in a gender-neutral manner to invite information about same-sex relationships.

- *Are you currently in a relationship?* (If the client is in a same-sex relationship, ask if he or she is open with others about it.)

- *What is your partner/spouse's name?*

- *How long have you been together?*

- *Have you had other long-term relationships? With whom? How long did they last? What caused them to end?*

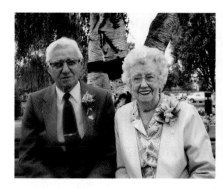

- *Do you have any children? If yes, what are their names and ages?*

- *Do they live with you all of the time? If no, where do they live? What is your relationship with them like? How often do you see them?*

- *How do you get along with your co-workers?*

- *Do you belong to any clubs or social groups?* (Consider community or faith-based groups or organizations, service clubs, sports teams, etc.)

- *Do you have social and emotional support? From whom? Is it adequate?*

ETHNICITY, IDENTITY, AND MEANING

Statistics Canada (2006) defines *ethnicity* as a multidimensional construct that includes race, origin or ancestry, identity, language, and religion. It also includes more subtle dimensions, such as culture, the arts, customs, and beliefs, and even practices such as dress and food preparation. It is also dynamic and in a constant state of flux. It will change because of new immigration flows, blending, and intermarriage—new identities may be formed.

Ethnicity.   Ethnicity offers insight into the client's history, meaning systems, social roles, and lifestyle choices and practices.

- *Where were you born?*

- *What is your citizenship or immigration status?*

- *What is your first or preferred language?*

- *What language(s) do you speak at home?*

- *With which ethnic group(s) do you identify?*

- *What does it mean to you to be "healthy?" To be "ill?"*

- *Do you engage in special health practices (e.g., traditional medicines/practices, healers)?*

- *Does your background prohibit certain things* (e.g., premarital sex, surgery, relationships with those of different ethnicity)? If yes, explore whether this has caused conflicts or problems in the client's life.

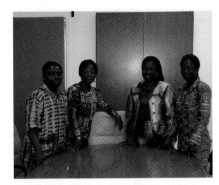

If the client identifies himself or herself as First Nations or Métis, ask:

- *To which nation or band do you belong?*

- *What place does your Aboriginal background have in your life?*

- *Do you live on a reserve? Or in an urban setting?*

- *Did your parents attend residential schools?* (If yes, ask how it has affected the family.)

Identity.   To get a sense of a client's personal identity, self-concept, and meaning structures, ask:

- *How do you describe yourself to others?* (Probe for specificity, detail, and examples.)

- *What do you like best about yourself? Like least?* (People with a negative self-concept or low self-esteem often have difficulty identifying what they like about themselves. Note whether the list of things they dislike is more forthcoming or longer than the list of things they like.)

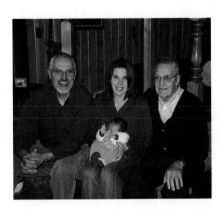

- *Do you identify with a particular spiritual group or religious denomination?*

- *What gives meaning to your life?*

- *How do you deal with everyday challenges?*

- *How do you respond to change?*

SEXUALITY

Sexuality is central to self-perception and interactions with others and the world. Although it influences all the ways people experience and express themselves, it is a topic that some people have difficulty discussing, and is fraught with uncertainty and misconception. Because humans take social cues from others, if you approach questions about sexuality in a matter-of-fact manner, clients will likely relax and follow your lead. If a client seems very reluctant to answer such questions, defer them to later in the interview when he or she may feel more comfortable (e.g., *You seem a bit uncomfortable with this topic. Shall we save these questions until later?*). See the accompanying box of definitions of common sexuality-related terms.

SEXUALITY-RELATED DEFINITIONS

Sex: Biological characteristics that define an individual as female or male.

Sexuality: Shaped by biological, psychological, socio-economic, cultural, ethical, and religious/spiritual factors. It is manifest through sex, gender, gender and sexual identity, sex roles, sexual orientation, eroticism, pleasure, intimacy, and reproduction, which are experienced and expressed in thoughts, fantasies, desires, beliefs, attitudes, values, behaviours, practices, roles, and relationships.

Gender: The holistic expression of cultural values, attitudes, roles, practices, and characteristics based on sex. Historically, cross-culturally, and in contemporary societies, gender reflects and perpetuates power relations between men and women.

Gender Identity: The degree to which individuals identify themselves as male, female, or some combination. It is an internal framework, constructed over time and influences self-concept, gender roles, and relationships with others.

Sexual Orientation: The enduring emotional, romantic, sexual, or affectional attraction an individual feels towards others. It exists along a continuum that ranges from exclusively same-sex to exclusively opposite-sex, with various forms of bisexuality in between. It includes thoughts, fantasies, desire, and/or behaviour.

Sexual Identity: Encompasses all aspects of sexual self identity, including how an individual identifies as male/female, masculine/feminine/some combination, and sexual orientation.

Sexual Health: A state of physical, emotional, mental, and social well-being in relation to sexuality; it is not merely the absence of disease, dysfunction, or infirmity. Sexual health requires a positive and respectful approach to sexuality and sexual relationships, as well as the possibility of having pleasurable and safe sexual experiences, free of coercion, discrimination, and violence. For sexual health to be attained and maintained, the sexual rights of all persons must be respected, protected, and fulfilled.

Sexual Rights: Embraces human rights that are already recognized in national laws, international human rights documents, and other consensus statements. They include the right of all persons, free of coercion, discrimination and violence, to (1) the highest attainable standard of sexual health, including access to sexual and reproductive health care services; (2) seek, receive, and impart information related to sexuality; (3) sexuality education; (4) respect for bodily integrity; (5) choose their partner; (6) decide to be sexually active or not; (7) consensual sexual relations; (8) consensual marriage; (9) decide whether or not, and when, to have children; and (10) pursue a satisfying, safe, and pleasurable sexual life.

Source: Adapted from Pan American Health Organization and World Health Organization, 2000.

Questions to Ask Women.   (In addition to questions in Chapter 22):

- *Are you sexually active?* (If yes, ask age at first sexual experience, number, and gender of partners.)

- *Do you consider yourself heterosexual, homosexual, or bisexual?*

- *Do you use contraception?* (If yes, ask about the type.)

- *Do you or a partner use protection from sexually transmitted infections?*

- *Have you ever been pregnant?* (Note number of pregnancies, live births, miscarriages, abortions.) If the client responds that she has never been pregnant, consider whether infertility or personal choice may be the reason.

- *Are you satisfied with your sex life?* (If no, probe for details about level of sexual desire, frequency of sexual activity, satisfaction with sexual relationships, etc.)

Questions to Ask Men.   (In addition to questions in Chapter 21):

- *Are you sexually active?* (If yes, ask about age at first sexual experience, number, and gender of partners.)

- *Have you ever had any problems having or sustaining an erection? Ejaculating?*

■ *Do you consider yourself heterosexual, homosexual, or bisexual?*

■ *Do you use contraception?*

■ *Do you or a partner use protection from sexually transmitted infections?*

■ *Do you have any biological children?* (If no, consider infertility or personal choice.)

■ *Are you satisfied with your sex life?* (If no, probe for details about level of sexual desire, frequency of sexual activity, satisfaction with sexual relationships, etc.)

ENVIRONMENTAL SAFETY

Safety and security are fundamental human needs affected by the various environments in which people live, work, and conduct daily affairs.

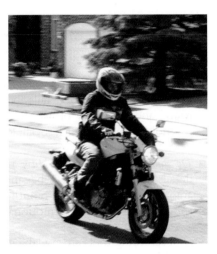

■ *How adequate is your home for your needs? How safe is it?* (If responses are negative, probe for details about overcrowding, noise, structural integrity, heating, ventilation, infestations, and/or chemical hazards.)

■ *Which of the following do you have in your home, vehicle, or both? First aid kit? Fire extinguisher? Working smoke detectors? Working carbon monoxide detectors?*

■ *Tell me about your neighbourhood. How safe is it?* (If negative, probe for details.)

■ *Is safety a concern in your work environment?* (Follow with probes.)

■ *How much time do you spend daily travelling in a car? How often do you use a seat belt?*

■ *How often do you use a mobile phone while driving?*

EXERCISE AND LEISURE ACTIVITIES

Regular exercise and leisure activities enhance health, improve quality of life, and reduce stress. Changes in energy or withdrawal from these things may be early signs of illness.

■ *Do you exercise regularly?* (Ask about type of activities, frequency, duration, and intensity.)

■ *Are there any restrictions on the types of exercise you can do?*

■ *How much leisure time do you usually have in a week?*

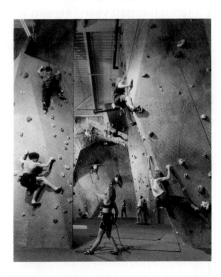

■ *What are your favourite leisure activities?* (Probe for details about frequency, duration, and level of enjoyment.)

■ *How satisfied are you with the balance of work and play in your life?*

■ *Have there been any recent changes in your patterns of exercise or leisure activities?*

■ *Are there any barriers to your engaging in exercise or leisure activities?* (Consider level of energy, cost, transportation, child care, etc.)

■ *Do you enjoy your life?*

TOBACCO, ALCOHOL, AND ILLICIT DRUG USE AND PROBLEM GAMBLING

Many people use exogenous substances or activities to feel good, manage stress, cope with unpleasant emotions, or help with sleep disturbances. Tobacco, alcohol, and illicit drug use and activities like problem gambling have important health implications to explore. It is also important to find out whether the client or others believe that these behaviours are a problem.

- *Do you currently smoke? Have you ever smoked? Or chewed tobacco?* [If yes, probe for details about type of tobacco use (e.g., cigarettes, cigars, or pipe smoking) or use of chewing tobacco; age at first use; frequency; and health effects.]

- *Do you currently use alcohol? Have you ever used alcohol?* [If yes, ask about age at first use; preferred type of alcohol (beer, wine, or spirits); usual pattern of drinking; and any recent changes to that pattern.]

- *Do you currently use nonprescription drugs? Have you ever used nonprescription drugs?* [If yes, probe for details about the age of first use, drug(s) of choice, dose, route, and frequency of use. Inquire about the effects of drug use (physical, psychological, emotional, social, legal, and economic).]

- *Do you currently gamble? Have you ever gambled regularly?* [If yes, probe for details about age when it began, game(s) of choice, frequency, and average amount of money lost per month. Ask for information about the consequences (physical, psychological, emotional, social, legal, and economic)].

Several screening tools are available to aid the assessment of excessive alcohol use. Two of the most widely used are the CAGE (Ewing, 1984) (see Chapter 3) and the Alcohol Use Disorders Identification Test or AUDIT (Babor, Higgins-Biddle, Saunders, & Monteiro, 2001). Research comparing the two concludes that the

---

THE AUDIT: INTERVIEW VERSION

Read questions as written. Record answers carefully. Begin the audit by saying "Now I am going to ask you some questions about your use of alcoholic beverages during this past year." Explain what is meant by "standard drinks" and how to calculate them. Code answers in terms of "standard drinks."

1. How often do you have a drink containing alcohol?
   (0) Never (Skip to Qs 9–10)
   (1) Monthly or less
   (2) 2–4 times a month
   (3) 2–3 times a week
   (4) 4 or more times a week
2. How many drinks containing alcohol do you have on a typical day when you are drinking?
   (0) 1 or 2
   (1) 3 or 4
   (2) 5 or 6
   (3) 7, 8, or 9
   (4) 10 or more

3. How often do you have six or more drinks on one occasion?
   (0) Never
   (1) Less than monthly
   (2) Monthly
   (3) Weekly
   (4) Daily or almost daily
   Skip to Question 9 and 10 if total score for Questions 2 and 3 = 0
4. How often during the last year have you found that you were not able to stop drinking once you had started?
   (0) Never
   (1) Less than monthly
   (2) Monthly
   (3) Weekly
   (4) Daily or almost daily

(Continued)

THE AUDIT: INTERVIEW VERSION (Continued)

5. How often during the last year have you failed to do what was normally expected from you because of drinking?
   - (0) Never
   - (1) Less than monthly
   - (2) Monthly
   - (3) Weekly
   - (4) Daily or almost daily

6. How often during the last year have you needed a first drink in the morning to get yourself going after a heavy drinking session?
   - (0) Never
   - (1) Less than monthly
   - (2) Monthly
   - (3) Weekly
   - (4) Daily or almost daily

7. How often during the last year have you had a feeling of guilt or remorse after drinking?
   - (0) Never
   - (1) Less than monthly
   - (2) Monthly
   - (3) Weekly
   - (4) Daily or almost daily

8. How often during the last year have you been unable to remember what happened the night before because you had been drinking?
   - (0) Never
   - (1) Less than monthly
   - (2) Monthly
   - (3) Weekly
   - (4) Daily or almost daily

9. Have you or someone else been injured as a result of your drinking?
   - (0) No
   - (2) Yes, but not in the last year
   - (4) Yes, during the last year

10. Has a relative or friend or a doctor or another health worker been concerned about your drinking or suggested you cut down?
    - (0) No
    - (2) Yes, but not in the last year
    - (4) Yes, during the last year

    Record total of items 1 to 10.

11. Do you think you presently have a problem with drinking?
    - (a) No
    - (b) Probably not
    - (c) Unsure
    - (d) Possibly
    - (e) Definitely

12. In the next 3 months, how difficult would you find it to cut down or stop drinking?
    - (a) Very easy
    - (b) Fairly easy
    - (c) Neither difficult nor easy
    - (d) Fairly difficult
    - (e) Very Difficult

    Do not score questions 11 and 12. These questions provide an indication of the client's "readiness to change" or motivation to change their alcohol use. This will assist you in deciding what level of intervention is appropriate.

Scoring:

A total score of 8 or more indicates harmful alcohol use and possible alcohol dependence for men and women under the age of 65 years.

A total score of 7 or more indicates harmful alcohol use and possible alcohol dependence for men and women over the age of 65 years.

Source: Babor et al., 2001.

AUDIT is more sensitive and reliable, particularly among adolescents and people older than 65 years (McCusker, Basquille, Khwaja, Murray-Lyon, & Catalan, 2002; Sheilds, 2003). The WHO developed the AUDIT as a brief screening tool for excessive drinking and to guide assessment. According to its authors (Babor et al., 2001), its purpose is to identify excessive drinking and to provide a framework for intervention to help risky drinkers reduce or cease alcohol consumption. It is designed for use by health care practitioners in a range of settings, but with instruction it can be administered by non-health professionals or be self-administered.

SLEEP/REST

The sleep–wake cycle is a function of the body's circadian (Latin for *around a day*) rhythm, which is regulated by the suprachiasmatic nuclei (SCN)—two clusters of

~20,000 neurons in the hypothalamus (Buijs, van Eden, Goncharuk & Kalsbeek, 2003). The SCN sends signals to several brain regions, including the pineal gland, which is responsible for production of the hormone melatonin. Levels of melatonin normally decrease in response to morning light and increase in the evening as darkness falls, making people feel drowsy. The SCN also governs functions associated with the sleep–wake cycle, such as body temperature, hormone secretion, urine production, and changes in blood pressure.

Sleep–wake alterations are common responses to stress and are associated with illnesses; psychiatric disorders such as depression, mania, and schizophrenia (Abad & Guilleminault, 2005), and pain syndromes (Roehrs & Roth, 2005). When inquiring about sleep–wake patterns, it is important to ask about sleep onset (latency between going to bed and falling asleep); sleep maintenance (ability to stay asleep, frequency of night wakenings, and ease of falling back to sleep); early morning wakening; and whether the client generally feels rested/refreshed.

- *What time do you usually go to bed?*

- *How long does it usually take you to fall asleep?*

- *Do you wake up during the night? Why?* (Consider physical discomfort, emotional factors, child care activities, etc.)

- *If you wake during the night, how long does it take you to fall back to sleep?*

- *What time do you usually wake up in the morning?*

- *Do you wake up on your own? Or to an alarm clock?*

- *How rested do you feel in the morning?*

- *Do you use sleep aids?*

- *Do you walk, talk, or grind your teeth in your sleep?*

- *Do you have vivid dreams or nightmares?*

- *Do you snore?*

- *Do you nap or rest during the day?*

NUTRITION

Physical, psychological, emotional, social, cultural, and economic factors interact to influence nutrition and eating habits. A complete nutrition assessment includes both objective and subjective data related to dietary intake, lifestyle, medical conditions, and health–illness status. Data come from the health history and physical examination and include allergies/intolerances, height, weight, body mass index (BMI), waist circumference, and results of labouratory and other diagnostic tests (see Chapter 8). Information about dietary intake typically comes from a 24-hour food recall (i.e., asking what the client ate during the previous 24 hours) or a food log (i.e., for 1 week the client records what he or she eats and drinks). Psychosocial aspects of nutrition focus on clients' perceptions, beliefs, and feelings about body size and shape and psychological, emotional, and social factors that influence food choices and eating behaviours.

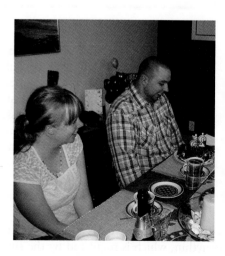

■ *How would you describe your appetite?*

■ *What place do food and eating have in your life?*

■ *Are there foods that you do not eat?* (If yes, probe for details; consider economic, cultural, food sensitivities/allergies, and personal preferences.)

■ *What is your caffeine intake on an average day?* (Consider coffee, tea, cola, chocolate, and energy drinks.)

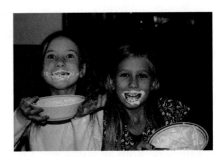

■ *Do you ever have cravings for certain foods? Or nonfood substances?* (If yes, ask about frequency, types of foods or non-food substances (e.g., clay, dirt, starch), precipitating factors, and feelings about this behaviour.)

■ *Has your weight fluctuated more than 10 lbs up or down in your adult life?* (If yes, probe for details about cause [e.g., pregnancy, dieting, illness, stress, etc.].)

■ *Would you describe your body as average, underweight, or overweight for your height and bone structure?*

■ *Have family, close friends, or a health care provider ever expressed concern about your being over- or underweight?*

■ *How do you feel about your body?*

■ *Do you ever eat when you are not hungry?* (Consider boredom, stress, depression, social circumstances.)

■ *Do you ever sneak food? Or eat in secret?*

■ *Do you ever engage in binge eating* (i.e., *uncontrollable* ingestion of large amounts of food)? (If yes, consider the possibility of a clinical eating disorder; probe for details about frequency, precipitating factors, feelings about this behaviour, treatment.)

■ *Do you ever engage in purging behaviours such as self-induced vomiting, laxative use, or strenuous exercise to lose weight?* (If yes, consider the possibility of a clinical eating disorder; probe for details about frequency, precipitating factors, feelings about this behaviour, treatment.)

MENTAL STATUS ASSESSMENT

Assessment of the client's mental status begins with the first words of the interview. As you gather the health history, you will quickly discern the client's level of *alertness* and *orientation, mood, attention,* and *memory.* As the history unfolds, you will learn about the client's *insight* and *judgment* and any *recurring or unusual thoughts or perceptions.* For some, you will need to supplement the interview with specific questions and a more formal evaluation of mental status. Just as symptoms, blood pressure, and valvular murmurs help you to distinguish, for example, health from disease in the cardiovascular system, specific components of mental function illuminate the workings of the mind. Although these components do not encompass all aspects of human thought and feeling, they serve as useful and continually important clinical tools. Many terms used to describe the mental status examination are familiar from social conversation. Take time to learn their precise meanings within the formal evaluation of mental status.

TERMINOLOGY: THE MENTAL STATUS EXAMINATION

Level of consciousness: Alertness or state of awareness of the environment.

Attention: Ability to focus or concentrate over time on one task or activity—an inattentive or distractible person has difficulty giving a history or responding to questions.

Memory: Both an entity and a process; the latter involves registering or encoding information into memory, storing information over time, and retrieval. Assessments evaluate registration and immediate recall; recent or short-term memory (retention and recall over days–weeks), long-term memory (retention and recall over weeks–years), and working memory.

Orientation: Awareness of personal identity, place, and time; requires memory and attention.

Perception: Processes involved in interpreting and organizing sensory stimuli (sensations) into a meaningful experience of the world.

Thought process: Logic, coherence, and goal-directedness of ideas, symbolic representations, and associations in relation to a problem or task.

Thought content: What the client thinks about—beliefs, obsessions, delusions, phobias.

Insight: Clients' understandings of their circumstances; includes awareness of thoughts, feelings, and behaviours and ability in relation to the thoughts, feelings, and behaviours of others (i.e., typical/expected vs. atypical/unexpected). Assessment of insight also considers clients' awareness and understanding of their illness.

Judgment: Ability to generate and evaluate alternatives in light of outcomes. Does the client understand the implications of behaviour? Is he or she influenced by this understanding?

Affect: Client's emotional responsiveness during the interview, inferred from facial expression, verbal responses, and behaviour.

Mood: A more pervasive and sustained feeling state that shapes the client's perceptions and world view (mood is to affect as climate is to weather).

Language: Speech is a general term for patterned verbal behaviour. Language is a set of rules for generating speech. More specifically, language is a learned system of communication based on shared symbols and their associated meanings. Assessment considers both receptive language (e.g., understanding the meaning of spoken and/or written anguage) and expressive language (e.g., correctness and fluency and correctness of content and grammar). See Table 9-1.

Cognition: Includes all the complex mental operations involved in acquiring information, comprehension, thinking, knowing, memory, judging, and problem solving, all of which relate to sensation, perception, language, imagination, memory, and planning.

Distinguishing the interplay of body and mind in relation to these attributes is very important but not always easy. For example, anxiety or depression may manifest as somatic complaints. Likewise, physical illness can cause mental and emotional responses; in older clients, illness can impair mental function without causing typical symptoms or signs (e.g., fever, pain). Always look carefully for physical or pharmacologic causes as you try to understand the context and meaning of changes in mental status. Some mental status evaluations are complicated by personality factors, psychodynamics, or the client's personal experiences, areas that can be explored during the interview. By integrating and correlating all relevant data from all these sources, the clinician tries to understand the person as a whole.

Students may feel reluctant to perform mental status examinations, wondering if they will upset clients, invade their privacy, or result in labelling their thoughts or behaviour as pathologic. Such concerns are understandable and appropriate. Insensitive mental status examinations may alarm clients—even skilful examinations may bring to awareness embarrassing or upsetting deficits that clients are trying to ignore. Discuss any concerns with your instructor or other experienced clinicians. As with other realms of interviewing and assessment, your skills and confidence will improve with practice. Clients appreciate understanding listeners, and some will owe their health, their safety, or even their lives to your attention.

THE HEALTH HISTORY: SUBJECTIVE DATA

Key Symptoms and Signs Reported by Client

- Changes in thought content or process
- Changes in mood and affect
- Behavioural changes
- Recent changes, losses, and/or extremely stressful life events
- Past physical, psychological, and/or sexual abuse/assault

Much information about *mental status* becomes evident during the interview. When you first meet the client, note your general impression of his or her *appearance, mood and affect, behaviour,* and *attitude toward you.* Throughout the conversation, attend to his or her *level of consciousness, ability to attend and participate, comprehension, memory, speech,* and *language.* By placing the client's vocabulary and general fund of information in the context of his or her cultural and educational background, you can often roughly estimate intelligence. Likewise, the client's responses to illness and life circumstances often tell you about his or her degree of *insight and judgment.* If you suspect a problem in orientation and memory, ask, "Let's see, your last clinic appointment was when . . . ?" "And the date today?" The more you integrate your exploration of mental status into a sensitive health history, the less it will seem like an interrogation.

See Table 9-1, Disorders of Speech, p. 238, and Table 9-2, Disorders of Mood, p. 239.

Explore unusual thoughts, preoccupations, beliefs, or perceptions as they arise. For example, reports of intense and persistent fear or worry that seem disproportionate to the actual threat or danger suggest an *anxiety disorder.* In Canada, the 1-year incidence of all anxiety disorders is 12%; of these, 9% occur in men and 16% in women (Ansseau et al., 2004; Health Canada, 2002). Anxiety disorders are thus among the most common mental health problems, imposing a significant burden on clients, families, and society. In time, you will begin to recognize the specific anxiety disorders summarized in Table 9-3. For such clients, you will need to supplement your interview with questions in specific areas; you may need to perform a formal mental status examination.

See Table 9-3, Anxiety Disorders, p. 240 and Table 9-4, Psychotic Disorders, p. 241.

All clients with documented or suspected brain lesions, psychiatric symptoms, or reports from family members of vague, unusual, or distressing behaviours need further systematic assessment. Clients may have subtle behavioural changes, difficulty taking medications properly, problems attending to chores or paying bills, or loss of interest in usual activities. Some may behave strangely after surgery or during acute illness. Each problem should be identified as expeditiously as possible. Mental function influences all aspects of day-to-day functions, social interactions, and quality of life.

Possible signs of *depression* or *dementia.*

HEALTH PROMOTION

Regardless of presenting concern, many people seeking primary care have mental health issues. *Generalized anxiety disorder (GAD)* is higher among clients in primary care settings than in the general population, suggesting that these clients are high users of primary care resources (Toft et al., 2005). In a study of 965 primary care

---

Important Topics for Health Promotion

- Alterations in interest in life, motivation, energy, sleep patterns, appetite, and sexual desire/behaviour
- Current stressors and coping abilities
- Past or current physical, sexual, or psychological abuse/assault
- Pervasive or prolonged worry or anxiety
- Alterations in affect or mood
- Thoughts or behaviours of self-harm or suicide
- Alcohol or drug use
- Memory, concentration, and problem-solving abilities

---

clients (Kroenke, Spitzer, Williams, Monahan, & Löwe, 2007), 19.5% had at least one anxiety disorder; 8.6% met the diagnostic criteria for post-traumatic stress disorder (PTSD), 7.6% for GAD, 6.8% for panic disorder, and 6.2% for social anxiety disorder. Each disorder was associated with substantial impairment that increased with the number of anxiety disorders. Furthermore, almost half (41%) of these clients reported no current treatment (medications, counselling, or psychotherapy) for anxiety.

Anxiety disorders impose a considerable burden on affected clients, their families, and general society. The U.S. National Comorbidity Study (NCS) (Kessler, Du Pont, Berglund, & Wittchen, 1999), a large population-based study, estimated the direct and indirect cost of anxiety disorders as $42 billion dollars per year. *Direct costs* are those associated with use of health-care resources (e.g., medications; visits to physicians, emergency departments, specialists), while *indirect costs* relate to absenteeism, reduced productivity, reliance on social assistance, and caregiver burden (Koerner et al., 2004). Secondary analysis of NCS data (Greenberg et al., 1999) found that in the year preceding the study, people with anxiety disorders consulted all sectors of the health care system, leading the authors to conclude that the largest proportion of the total economic cost of anxiety disorders is attributable to primary care and not to mental health services. Although data on the cost of anxiety disorders in Canada are limited, existing information reflects similar findings.

The burden of suffering imposed by these disorders is great, yet they are often underdiagnosed and not adequately treated. For the general population, focus health promotion on anxiety, depression, suicidality, and dementia, four important conditions often overlooked. Also screen routinely for addiction to alcohol or drugs (see pp. 214–215).

Depressive disorders are also common and frequently coexist with physical and mental illnesses/disorders (See Table 9-2 for a summary of common disorders of mood). Epidemiologic studies (Bland, Newman, & Orn, 1988; Murphy, Laird, Monson, Sobol, & Leighton, 2000; Parikh, Wasylenki, Goering, & Wong, 1996) conducted over the past five decades report that approximately 8% to 9% of Canadians will have at least one episode of *major depressive disorder (MDD)* in their lifetime.

More recently, preliminary data from the 2003 Joint Canada/U.S. Survey of Health (Vasiliadis, Lesage, Adair, Wang, & Kessler, 2007) found that rates of depression were similar in both countries at approximately 8.5%. The same study found a positive correlation between mental health needs and service use in Canada, but not for those without medical insurance in the United States. Around the globe, MDD is twice as common in women as it is in men (Lopez, Mathers, Ezzati, Jamison, & Murray, 2006).

Research tells us that primary care providers fail to diagnose MDD at alarming rates (Baik, Bowers, Oakley, & Susman, 2005), which can negatively affect the development and persistence of unexplained medical symptoms (e.g., pain), social and occupational functioning, self-care, and medical outcomes, not to mention economic costs and quality of life (Seelig & Katon, 2008). Clinicians often miss early clues such as changes in vegetative function (i.e., sleep, appetite, energy, and sexual desire), low self-esteem, anhedonia or the failure to experience pleasure, and difficulty concentrating or making decisions. Although the exact cause of depression is unknown, it clearly involves an interaction of genetic, biological, social, and psychological factors. Depression affects people of all ages, but at higher risk are clients who have (Parikh & Lam, 2001):

■ A history of depression

■ Female gender

■ A family history of depression and/or suicide

■ Major life stress (e.g., relationship conflict, interpersonal violence, death of a loved one, economic strain)

■ Serious or chronic disease/illness (e.g., hypertension, type 2 diabetes, arthritis, chronic pain)

■ Particular personality traits (e.g., poor self-esteem, dependent, self-critical, or pessimistic)

■ Recently given birth

Screening helps to identify clients with depression in primary care settings, and treatment reduces clinical morbidity (Greenberg et al., 1999; Murphy et al., 2000). The U.S. Preventative Services Task Force (2002) recommends routine screening of adults for depression in clinical practices that have systems in place to ensure accurate diagnosis, effective treatment, and follow-up. Two questions that may be as effective as more formal screening tools are: "Over the past 2 weeks, have you felt down, depressed, or hopeless?" and "Over the past 2 weeks, have you felt little interest or pleasure in doing things?" Screening tools suitable for the office are also readily available. Positive screening warrants more formal diagnostic evaluation. Failure to diagnose depression can have fatal consequences—suicide rates in clients with major depression are eight times higher than in the general population (Health Canada, 2002).

According to Health Canada's (2002) *Report on Mental Illnesses in Canada*:

■ Suicide accounts for 24% of all deaths among 15- to 24-year-olds and 16% among 25- to 44-year-olds.

■ In 1998, almost 3700 Canadians died from self-inflicted causes.

■ Although more women than men attempt suicide, the mortality rate is four times higher among men (women most commonly choose an overdose of pills, with the possibility of being rescued, while men choose firearms or hanging).

■ People age 15 to 44 account for 73% of hospital admissions for attempted suicide.

■ Women are hospitalized in general hospitals for attempted suicide at 1.5 times the rate of men. Women 15- to 19-year-olds have the highest hospitalization rate for attempted suicide.

- Men 80 years of age and older have the highest risk for suicide.

- Aboriginal-Canadians have 3 to 6 times the rate for suicide than the rest of the population. Treatment received in residential schools continues to be a contributing factor of sexual abuse, family violence, substance abuse, poverty, and access to firearms.

Risk factors include suicidal or homicidal ideation, intent, or plan; access to the means for suicide; current symptoms of psychosis or severe anxiety; any history of psychiatric illness, especially if linked to hospital admission; substance abuse or personality disorder; and prior history or family history of suicide. Clients with these risk factors should be immediately referred for psychiatric assessment.

If you suspect depression, assess its duration and intensity as well as associated risk of self-harm or suicide. The following questions can guide your inquiry; continue to probe as the person's positive answers warrant.

- *Do you get discouraged? ("Down?" "Depressed?" "Or blue?")*

- *On a scale of 0–10 (with 0 being low and 10 being high), how discouraged (down, depressed, or blue) are you right now?*

- *Do you ever feel that life is not worth living?*

- *If you died in your sleep, would that be all right with you?* (Many depressed people do not actively think about suicide, but passively wish for death. Without intervention, this may progress to active suicidal ideation.)

- *Have you ever thought of harming yourself? Or killing yourself?*

- *Do you have a plan for committing suicide?* (Probe to determine if the person has a specific and concrete plan and the means to carry out that plan.)

- *What stops you from harming yourself? Or killing yourself?* (Most clients have some degree of ambivalence about self-harm/suicide; identifying why they have not acted on their thoughts offers clues about their reasons for living.)

Many clinicians avoid the topic of self-harm (Sutton & Martinson, 2007; Wysong, 2007) or suicide because they worry that broaching it will implant the idea in the client's mind. There is little risk that talking about suicide with someone who is not already thinking about it will prompt him or her to do it (Canadian Mental Health Association, n.d.). Openly discussing this can be a relief and may reduce the likelihood that a client will act on suicidal thoughts/feelings.

Dementia is an acquired decline in cognitive function, especially memory, but also language, visual-spatial, or executive function, sufficient to interfere with social or occupational activities (American Psychiatric Association, 2000). It affects 3% to 11% of Americans older than 65 years and is highly correlated with age, rising to 25% to 45% of those older than 85 years (U.S. Preventive Services Task Force, 2003). Early results from the *Canadian Study of Health and Aging* (CSHA; 2000) estimate that approximately 500,000 Canadians have some form of dementia, a figure that will double over the next three decades. Apolipoprotein E, hypertension, and mild cognitive impairment may also increase risk (Kawas, 2003). Most dementias (roughly 60–70%) are associated with Alzheimer's disease or vascular or multi-infarct dementia (20–30% of cases; U.S. Preventive Services Task Force, 2003). Although clients with a positive family history have a three times higher risk for dementia than the general population, the U.S. Preventative Services Task Force has deferred recommendations for screening because of inconclusive evidence related to accuracy of diagnosis, feasibility of routine screening and treatment, and potential harms of screening (e.g., labelling effects; Boustani, Peterson, Hanson, Harris, & Lohr, 2003). The Alzheimer Society of Canada (2005) encourages people to self-refer (or have family members refer them) to a health professional for early assessment to rule out other conditions with similar symptoms (e.g., depression, infections, thyroid disease, heart disease, drug interactions, alcohol abuse). Assessment may include a health history, mental status examination, physical examination, laboratory and diagnostic tests, and psychiatric and psychological evaluations. A diagnosis of "probable" Alzheimer's disease may be made. Having a "probable" diagnosis allows clients and families to understand the source of the symptoms; receive appropriate care, treatment (possibly beginning medications), and support; and plan for the future.

TECHNIQUES OF EXAMINATION: OBJECTIVE DATA

Important Areas of Examination

- Appearance and behaviour
- Speech and language
- Mood
- Thoughts and perceptions
- Cognition, including memory, attention, information and vocabulary, calculations, abstract thinking, and constructional ability

Your approach to examination centres on three important questions. Keep all these in mind throughout each segment, even though you begin by focusing on mental status and behaviour:

- Is mental status intact?

- Are right-sided and left-sided findings symmetric?

- If findings are asymmetric or otherwise abnormal, does the causative lesion lie in the central or peripheral nervous system?

The mental status examination consists of (1) appearance and behaviour; (2) speech and language; (3) mood; (4) thoughts and perceptions; and (5) cognitive function, including memory, attention, information/vocabulary, calculations, and abstract thinking/constructional ability. The following format should help you organize observations, but it is not intended as a step-by-step guide. When a full examination is indicated, be flexible in your approach but thorough in what you cover. In some situations, sequence is important. If during the initial interview, the client's consciousness, attention, word comprehension, or speech seems impaired, assess this attribute promptly. Such a client cannot give a reliable history, and you will not be able to test most other mental functions.

APPEARANCE AND BEHAVIOUR

When asserting appearance and behaviour, use all relevant observations made throughout the history and examination. Include these areas:

Level of Consciousness. Is the client awake and alert? Does the client seem to understand your questions and respond appropriately and reasonably quickly, or does he or she tend to lose track of the topic and fall silent (even asleep)?

See Table 20-1, Syncope and Similar Disorders.

If the client does not respond to questions, escalate the stimulus in steps:

■ Speak to the client by name and in a loud voice.

Lethargic clients are drowsy but open their eyes and look at you, respond to questions, and then fall asleep.

■ Shake the client gently, as if awakening a sleeper.

Obtunded clients open their eyes and look at you, but respond slowly and are somewhat confused.

If there is no response to these stimuli, promptly assess the client for stupor or coma—severe reductions in the level of consciousness (see Chapter 20).

Posture and Motor Behaviour.

Does the client lie in bed or prefer to walk around? Note body posture and ability to relax. Observe the pace, range, and character of movements. Do they seem under voluntary control? Are certain parts immobile? Do posture and motor activity change with topics discussed or with activities or people around the client?

Tense posture, restlessness, and fidgeting of *anxiety*; crying, pacing, and handwringing of agitated *depression*; hopeless, slumped posture, and slowed movements of *depression*; singing, dancing, and expansive movements of *mania*.

Dress, Grooming, and Personal Hygiene.

How is the client dressed? Is clothing clean, pressed, and properly fastened? How does it compare with clothing worn by people of comparable age and social group? Note the client's hair, nails, teeth, skin, and, if present, beard. Are they groomed?

How do grooming and hygiene compare with others of comparable age, lifestyle, and socioeconomic group? Compare one side of the body with the other.

Grooming and hygiene may deteriorate in *depression*, *schizophrenia*, and *dementia*. Fastidiousness may accompany *obsessive–compulsive disorder*. One-sided neglect may result from a lesion in the opposite parietal cortex (usually the nondominant side).

Facial Expression.

Observe the face, both at rest and during interaction with others. Watch for variations in expression with topics under discussion. Are they appropriate? Or is the face relatively immobile throughout?

Expressions of anxiety, depression, apathy, anger, elation. Facial immobility of parkinsonism.

Manner, Affect, and Relationship to Persons and Things.

Using your observations of facial expressions, voice, and body movements, assess the client's affect. Does it vary appropriately with topics discussed, or is it labile, blunted, or flat? Does it seem inappropriate or extreme at certain points? If so, how? Note the client's openness, approachability, and reactions to others and surroundings. Does the client seem to hear or see things that you do not or seem to be conversing with someone who is not there?

Anger, hostility, suspiciousness, or evasiveness of clients with *paranoia*. Elation and euphoria of *mania*. Flat affect and remoteness of *schizophrenia*. Apathy (dulled affect with detachment and indifference) of *dementia*. Anxiety, depression.

SPEECH AND LANGUAGE

Throughout the interview, note the characteristics of the client's speech, including the following:

Quantity.

Is the client talkative or relatively silent? Are comments spontaneous or only responsive to direct questions?

Rate.

Is speech fast or slow?

Slow speech of *depression*; rapid, loud speech in *mania*.

Loudness.

Is speech loud or soft?

Dysarthria refers to defective articulation. *Aphasia* refers to a disorder of language. See Table 9-1, Disorders of Speech, p. 238.

Articulation of Words.

Are words spoken clearly and distinctly? Is there a nasal quality to the speech?

Fluency. This involves the rate, flow, and melody of speech and content and use of words. Be alert for abnormalities of spontaneous speech such as:

- Hesitancies and gaps in the flow and rhythm of words

- Disturbed inflections, such as a monotone

- Circumlocutions, in which phrases or sentences are substituted for a word the person cannot think of, such as "what you write with" for "pen"

- Paraphasias, in which words are malformed ("I write with a den"), wrong ("I write with a bar"), or invented ("I write with a dar")

If the client's speech lacks meaning or fluency, proceed with further testing as outlined in the following table.

These abnormalities suggest *aphasia.* The client may have so much difficulty talking or understanding others that you may not be able to obtain a history. You may also falsely suspect a psychotic disorder.

■ Testing for Aphasia

Word Comprehension	Ask the client to follow a one-stage command, such as "Point to your nose." Try a two-stage command: "Point to your mouth, then your knee."
Repetition	Ask the client to repeat a phrase of one-syllable words (the most difficult repetition task): "No ifs, ands, or buts."
Naming	Ask the client to name the parts of a watch.
Reading Comprehension	Ask the client to read a paragraph aloud.
Writing	Ask the client to write a sentence.

These tests help you to decide what kind of aphasia the client may have. Remember that deficiencies in vision, hearing, intelligence, and education may also affect performance. Two common kinds of aphasia—Wernicke's and Broca's—are compared in Table 9-1, p. 238.

A person who can write a correct sentence does not have aphasia.

MOOD

Assess mood during the interview by exploring the client's perceptions of it. Ask about the client's usual mood level and how it has varied with life events. "How did you feel about that?" or, more generally, "How are your spirits?" The reports of relatives and friends may be of great value.

What has the client's mood been like? How intense has it been? Has it been labile or fairly unchanging? How long has it lasted? Is it appropriate to circumstances? In case of depression, have there also been episodes of an elevated mood, suggesting a bipolar disorder?

For depressive and bipolar disorders, see Table 9-2, Disorders of Mood, p. 239.

THOUGHT AND PERCEPTIONS

Thought Processes. Assess the logic, relevance, organization, and coherence of thought processes as clients reveal them in words and speech throughout the interview. Does speech progress logically toward a goal? Here you use speech as a window into the client's mind. Listen for speech patterns that suggest disorders of thought processes, as outlined in the following table.

Thought Content. You should assess information relevant to thought content during the interview. Follow appropriate leads as they occur rather than using stereotyped lists of specific questions. For example, "You mentioned a few minutes ago that a neighbour was responsible for your entire illness. Can you tell me more about that?" Or, "What do you think about at times like these?"

■ *Variations and Abnormalities in Thought Processes*

Circumstantiality	Speech characterized by indirection and delay in reaching the point because of unnecessary detail, although components of the description have a meaningful connection. Many people without mental disorders speak circumstantially.	Observed in people with obsessions and mania.
Derailment (Loosening of Associations)	Speech in which a person shifts from one subject to others that are unrelated or related only obliquely without realizing that the subjects are not meaningfully connected. Ideas slip off the track between clauses, not within them.	Observed in *schizophrenia, manic episodes,* and other *psychotic disorders.*
Flight of Ideas	An almost continuous flow of accelerated speech in which a person changes abruptly from topic to topic. Changes are usually based on understandable associations, plays on words, or distracting stimuli, but the ideas do not progress to sensible conversation.	Most frequently noted in *manic episodes.*
Neolograms	Invented or distorted words, or words with new and highly idiosyncratic meanings	Observed in *schizophrenia,* other *psychotic disorders,* and *aphasia.*
Incoherence	Speech that is largely incomprehensible because of illogic, lack of meaningful connections, abrupt changes in topic, or disordered grammar or word use. Shifts in meaning occur within clauses. Flight of ideas, when severe, may produce incoherence.	Observed in severe psychotic disturbances (usually *schizophrenia*).
Blocking	Sudden pauses or interruption of speech in midsentence or before completion of an idea. The person attributes this to losing the thought. Blocking can occur in mentally healthy people.	Blocking may be striking in *schizophrenia.*
Confabulation	Fabrication of facts or events in response to questions, to fill in the gaps in an impaired memory	Common with *amnesia* and damage to the basal forebrain or frontal lobes.
Perseveration	Persistent repetition of words or ideas	Occurs in *schizophrenia* and other *psychotic disorders.*
Echolalia	Repetition of the words and phrases of others	Occurs in manic episodes and *schizophrenia.*
Clanging	Speech in which a person chooses a word on the basis of sound rather than meaning, as in rhyming and punning speech. For example, "Look at my eyes and nose, wise eyes and rosy nose. Two to one, the ayes have it!"	Occurs in *schizophrenia* and *manic episodes.*

When you may need to make more specific inquiries, couch them in tactful and accepting terms. "When people are upset, they sometimes can't keep certain thoughts out of their minds," or ". . . things seem unreal. Have you experienced anything like this?"

In these ways, find out about any of the patterns shown in the following table.

■ *Unexpected Thought Content*

Compulsions	Repetitive behaviours or mental acts that a person feels driven to perform in order to produce or prevent some future state of affairs, although expectation of such an effect is unrealistic
Obsessions	Recurrent, uncontrollable thoughts, images, or impulses that a person considers unacceptable and alien
Phobias	Persistent, irrational fears, accompanied by a compelling desire to avoid the stimulus
Anxieties	Apprehensions, fears, tensions, or uneasiness that may be focused (phobia) or free floating (a general sense of ill-defined dread or impending doom)
Feelings of Unreality	A sense that things in the environment are strange, unreal, or remote
Feelings of Depersonalization	A sense that one's self is different, changed, or unreal, or has lost identity or become detached from one's mind or body
Delusions	False, fixed, personal beliefs that are not shared by other members of the person's culture or subculture. Examples include: ■ *Delusions of persecution* ■ *Delusions of grandeur* ■ *Delusional jealousy* ■ *Delusions of reference*, in which a person believes that external events, objects, or people have a particular and unusual personal significance (e.g., that the radio or television might be commenting on or giving instructions to the person) ■ *Delusions of being controlled* by an outside force ■ *Somatic delusions* of having a disease, disorder, or physical defect ■ *Systematized delusions*, a single delusion with many elaborations or a cluster of related delusions around a single theme, all systematized into a complex network

Compulsions, obsessions, phobias, and *anxiety* are key features of anxiety disorder. See Table 9-3, Anxiety Disorders (p. 240).

Delusions and feelings of unreality or depersonalization are more often associated with *psychotic disorders.* See Table 9-4, Psychotic Disorders (p. 241). Delusions may also occur in delirium, severe mood disorders, and dementia.

Perceptions. Inquire about unusual perceptions in a manner similar to that used for thought content. For example, "When you heard the voice speaking, what did it say? How did it make you feel?" Or, "After you've been drinking a lot, do you ever see things that aren't really there?" Or, "Sometimes after surgery, people hear peculiar or frightening things. Have you experienced anything like that?" In these ways, find out about the following unexpected perceptions.

Command hallucinations are orders or commands an individual feels obligated to obey or unable to resist (e.g., to harm or kill him - or herself or someone else).

■ Alterations of Perception

Illusions	Misinterpretations of real external stimuli	Illusions may occur in grief reactions, *delirium,* acute and *posttraumatic stress disorders,* and *schizophrenia.*
Hallucinations	Subjective sensory perceptions in the absence of relevant external stimuli. The person may or may not recognize the experiences as false. Hallucinations may be auditory, visual, olfactory, gustatory, tactile, or somatic. (False perceptions associated with dreaming, falling asleep, and awakening are not classified as hallucinations.)	Hallucinations may occur in *delirium, dementia* (less commonly), *posttraumatic stress disorder, schizophrenia,* and alcoholism.

Insight and Judgment. These attributes are usually best assessed during the interview.

Insight. Some of your very first questions to the client often yield important information about insight: "What brings you to the hospital?" "What seems to be the trouble?" "What do you think is wrong?" More specifically, note whether the client is aware that a particular mood, thought, or perception is unusual or part of an illness.

Clients with psychotic disorders often lack insight. Denial of impairment may accompany some neurologic disorders.

Judgment. You can usually assess judgment by noting the client's responses to family situations, jobs, use of money, and interpersonal conflicts. "How do you plan to get the help you'll need after leaving the hospital?" "How are you going to manage if you lose your job?" "If your husband starts to abuse you again, what will you do?" "Who will attend to your finances while you are in the nursing home?" "How will you manage to shop for food?" "Prepare meals?"

Judgment may be poor in *delirium, dementia, mental retardation,* frontal lobe lesions, and psychotic states. Anxiety, *mood disorders,* intelligence, education, income, and cultural values also influence judgment.

Note whether decisions and actions are based on reality, for example, on impulse, wish fulfilment, or disordered thought content. What values seem to underlie the client's decisions and behaviour? Allowing for cultural variations, how do these compare with mature adult standards? Because judgment reflects maturity, it may be variable and unpredictable during adolescence.

Disorientation occurs especially when memory or attention is impaired, as in *delirium.*

COGNITIVE FUNCTIONS

Orientation. By skillful questioning, you can often determine the client's orientation in the context of the interview. For example, you can ask quite naturally for specific dates and times, home address and telephone number, names of family members, or route taken to the hospital. At times—when rechecking the status of a client with delirium, for example—simple, direct questions may be indicated.

"Can you tell me what time it is now . . . and what day is it?" In either of these ways, determine the client's orientation for:

■ *Time*—the time of day, day of week, month, season, date and year, duration of hospitalization

■ *Place*—client's residence, names of the hospital, city, and province

■ *Person*—client's own name; names of relatives and professional personnel

Attention. These tests of attention are commonly used.

Digit Span. Explain that you would like to test the client's ability to concentrate, perhaps adding that this can be difficult when people are in pain, ill, or feverish. Recite a series of digits, starting with two at a time and speaking each number clearly at approximately one per second. Ask the client to repeat the numbers back to you. If this repetition is accurate, try a series of three numbers, then four, and so on as long as the client responds correctly. Jot down the numbers as you say them to ensure accuracy. If the client makes a mistake, try once more with another series of the same length. Stop after a second failure in a single series.

In choosing digits you may use street numbers, telephone numbers, and other numerical sequences that are familiar to you, but avoid consecutive numbers, easily recognized dates, and sequences that possibly are familiar to the client.

Now, starting again with a series of two, ask the client to repeat the numbers to you backward. Usually, a person can repeat correctly at least five digits forward and four backward.

Serial 7s. Instruct the client, "Starting from a hundred, subtract 7, and keep subtracting 7...." Note the effort required and the speed and accuracy of responses. Writing down the answers helps you keep up with the arithmetic. Usually, a person can complete serial 7s in 1½ minutes, with fewer than four errors. If the client cannot do serial 7s, try 3s or counting backward.

Spelling Backward. This can substitute for serial 7s. Say a five-letter word, spell it, for example, W-O-R-L-D, and ask the client to spell it backward.

Remote Memory. Inquire about birthdays, anniversaries, insurance number, names of schools attended, jobs held, or past historical events such as wars relevant to the client's past.

Recent Memory. This involves events of the day. Ask questions with answers you can check against other sources so you can see if the client is confabulating (making up facts to compensate for a defective memory). These might include the weather, today's appointment time, and medications or laboratory tests taken during the day. (Asking what the client had for breakfast may be a waste of time unless you can check the accuracy of the answer.)

New Learning Ability. Give the client three or four words, such as "83 Water Street and blue," or "table, flower, green, and hamburger." Ask the client to repeat them so that you know that the information has been heard and registered. Like digit span, this step tests registration and immediate recall. Proceed to other parts of the examination. After about 3 to 5 minutes, ask the client to repeat the words. Note the accuracy of the response, awareness of whether it is correct, and any tendency to confabulate. Usually, a person should be able to remember the words.

Set Test. This test was developed for use with clients 65 years or older to screen for dementia (Isaacs & Kennie, 1973). Do not use it if the client has hearing loss or aphasia. Ask the client to name 10 items in each of four categories, one category at a time: fruits, animals, colours, and towns/cities. There is no time limit. Give no prompts. Each correct answer is 1 point. Total possible score is 40. If the score is 25 or more, dementia is unlikely. Examples of responses that indicate that the test is challenging for the client include "apples . . . oranges." and then the client's voice trails off; others might say "apples, oranges . . . Oh I could tell you lots more if I wanted to!" The Set Test is holistic in terms of what is being assessed—" the client is asked to categorize, name, remember, and count items in the test—this means the

Causes of impaired performance include *delirium, dementia, mental retardation,* and performance anxiety.

Impaired performance may be from *delirium,* the late stage of *dementia,* mental retardation, loss of calculating ability, anxiety, or depression. Also consider the possibility of limited education.

Remote memory may be impaired in the late stage of *dementia.*

Recent memory is impaired in *dementia* and *delirium. Amnestic disorders* impair memory or new learning ability significantly and reduce social or occupational functioning, but do not have the global features of delirium or dementia. Anxiety, depression, and mental retardation may also impair recent memory.

examiner is really assessing the client's alertness, motivation, concentration, short-term memory, and problem-solving ability" (Jarvis 2004, p. 114).

HIGHER COGNITIVE FUNCTIONS

Information and Vocabulary. Information and vocabulary, when observed clinically, provide a rough estimate of intelligence. Assess them during the interview. Ask a student, for example, about favourite courses, or inquire about work, hobbies, reading, favourite television programs, or current events. Explore such topics first with simple questions, then with more difficult ones. Note the person's grasp of information, complexity of the ideas expressed, and vocabulary used. More directly, you can ask about specific facts such as:

- The name of the Prime Minister of Canada, Premier of Province, or Lieutenant Governor

- The names of the last four or five prime ministers

- The names of five large cities in Canada

If considered in the context of cultural and educational background, information and vocabulary are fairly good indicators of intelligence. They are relatively unaffected by any but the most severe psychiatric disorders, and may be helpful for distinguishing mentally retarded adults (with limited information and vocabulary) from those with mild or moderate *dementia* (with fairly well-preserved information and vocabulary).

Calculating Ability. Test the client's ability to do arithmetical calculations, starting at the rote level with simple addition ("What is 4 + 1? . . . 8 + 7?") and multiplication ("What is 5 × 6? . . . 9 × 7?"). The task can be made more difficult by using two-digit numbers ("15 + 12" or "25 × 6") or longer, written examples.

Alternatively, pose practical and functionally important questions, such as "If something costs 78 cents and you give the clerk 1 dollar, how much should you get back?"

Impaired performance may be a useful sign of dementia or may accompany *aphasia*, but it must be assessed in terms of the client's intelligence and education.

Abstract Thinking. Test the capacity to think abstractly in two ways.

   Proverbs. Ask the client what people mean when they use some of the following proverbs:

- A stitch in time saves nine.

- Don't count your chickens before they're hatched.

- The proof of the pudding is in the eating.

- A rolling stone gathers no moss.

- The squeaking wheel gets the grease.

Note the relevance of the answers and their degree of concreteness or abstractness. For example, "You should sew a rip before it gets bigger" is concrete, whereas "Prompt attention to a problem prevents trouble" is abstract. Average clients should give abstract or semi-abstract responses.

   Similarities. Ask the client to tell you how the following are alike:

An orange and an apple

A church and a theatre

A cat and a mouse

A piano and a violin

A child and a dwarf

Wood and coal

Concrete responses are often given by people with mental retardation, *delirium,* or *dementia,* but may also be a function of limited education. Clients with *schizophrenia* may respond concretely or with personal, bizarre interpretations.

Note the accuracy and relevance of the answers and their degree of concreteness or abstractness. For example, "A cat and a mouse are both animals" is abstract, "They both have tails" is concrete, and "A cat chases a mouse" is not relevant.

Constructional Ability. The task here is to copy figures of increasing complexity onto a piece of blank unlined paper. Show each figure one at a time and ask the client to copy it as well as possible.

The three diamonds below are rated poor, fair, and good (but not excellent).

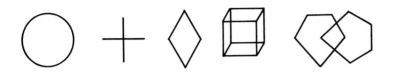

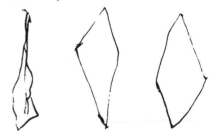

In another approach, ask the client to draw a clock face complete with numbers and hands. The example below is rated excellent.

These three clocks are poor, fair, and good.

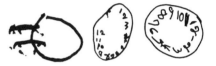

If vision and motor ability are intact, poor constructional ability suggests dementia or parietal lobe damage. Mental retardation may also impair performance.

SPECIAL TECHNIQUES

Mini-Mental State Examination (MMSE). This brief test is useful in screening for cognitive dysfunction or dementia and following their course over time. For more detailed information regarding the MMSE, contact the publisher, Psychological Assessment Resources, Inc., 16204 North Florida Avenue, Lutz, Florida 33549. Some sample questions are presented in the following box.

MMSE SAMPLE ITEMS

Orientation to Time
"What is the date?"

Registration
"Listen carefully, I am going to say three words. You say them back after I stop. Ready? Here they are . . .
HOUSE (pause), CAR (pause), LAKE (pause). Now repeat those words back to me." [Repeat up to five times, but score only the first trial.]

Naming
"What is this?" [Point to a pencil or pen.]

Reading
"Please read this and do what it says." [Show examinee the words on the stimulus form.]
CLOSE YOUR EYES

RECORDING AND ANALYZING FINDINGS

Documentation of a psychosocial and mental health assessment needs to be descriptive and supported with specific examples or client quotes to contribute meaningfully to accurate diagnosis and care planning. Depending on the policies of the clinical setting, this documentation may be done on a standardized form or in narrative form.

Psychosocial and mental health assessments are highly subjective; what nurses notice and how they understand and articulate observations and conclusions about the world is filtered through their own experience, culture, education, social roles, values, beliefs, and worldview. Because humans can never be completely objective, the best nurses can offer is a thoughtful and informed impression of a client's psychosocial function and mental status. Maintain an attitude of genuine and respectful curiosity about the individuals with whom you work and the ways that they understand and relate to the world. By sharing and validating observations and perceptions with the client and other members of the health-care team, nurses create a dynamic and contextual understanding of patients' health–illness status.

■ *Documentation of a Mental Status Examination*

Area of Assessment	Expected Findings	Unexpected Findings
Appearance and behaviour: *Level of consciousness; dress, grooming, and hygiene; facial expression; manner, affect, and relationship to persons and things in the environment*	Alert and oriented. Attire is clean, neat, and appropriate to setting, time of day, and season. Attitude toward the interview/interview process is positive and cooperative. Movements are coordinated and purposeful.	Face is pale and expression is downcast. Cried frequently, especially when talking about recent marital separation. Posture is rigid; seemed restless (e.g., client shifted frequently in her chair and hands were always moving—ran her fingers through her hair, tapped her fingers, adjusted clothing).
Speech and language	Nothing unusual about the quantity, rate, tone, and fluency of speech when client talks about matters unrelated to her recent separation.	Voice tone dropped and speech production slowed when discussing her relationship. Long pauses in speech as she attempted to compose herself. Sighed frequently and loudly.
Mood	Reports feeling "content" with life, smiling frequently.	"As far as I can remember, I have always been an extremely nervous person." "Worried about everything" as a child.
Thoughts and perceptions	Thought process is reality focused, logical, and rational. No evidence of perceptual disturbances, delusions, or hallucinations.	Thought content very focused on her marital relationship; moves back and forth between how to repair the relationship ("What should I do?") and how difficult it will be to live alone for the rest of her life ("I can't do this").
Insight and judgment	Insight and judgment intact. Came to emergency department because she believed she was having a heart attack. Accepts the explanation that her chest pain is likely related to anxiety. Stated "I guess it's time to do something about this [her anxiety]"; requested a referral for mental health counselling.	Arrived at emergency department because she needed help accepting her marital situation. Believes that her chest pain is all her husband's fault. Wants a social worker to call him in for counselling.

(continued)

■ *Documentation of a Mental Status Examination (Continued)*

Area of Assessment	Expected Findings	Unexpected Findings
Cognitive function: *orientation, attention (serial 7's), memory (recent, remote), new learning ability, Set test*	Oriented to person, place, and time. Accurately completed serial 7s from 100 to 72. Recent and remote memory intact. Able to recall the words *flower, telephone,* and *hot dog* immediately, and at 7 and 45 minutes. Set test—able to name 10 items in each category: (*fruits, animals, colours, towns/cities:* Total score of 40/40).	Oriented to person and place, not time. Serial 7s incorrect after 93. Recalled 3 out of 4 words immediately and at 10 minutes. Unable to recall words at 30 minutes. On the Set Test, able to list 5 *fruits*, 4 *animals*, 6 *colours*, and 3 *towns/cities* for a total score of 18/40.
Higher cognitive functions: *information and vocabulary, calculations, proverbs*	Vocabulary consistent with a university education. Accurately named last three prime ministers and five provincial capitals. Abstract thinking intact. Interpreted "A stitch in time saves nine" to mean "If you look after things before they need attention, it will be less work in the long run."	Identified one of five prime ministers and named three provinces. Responded "you should fix things" for interpretation of "the squeaking wheel gets the grease."

NARRATIVE DOCUMENTATION OF A PSYCHOSOCIAL ASSESSMENT

Barbara M., a 45-year-old Caucasian woman, arrives at the emergency department by ambulance at 2130 hours, reporting chest pain and shortness of breath. She states that she's been feeling tired and unwell for several weeks. A physical examination and diagnostic testing yield expected findings.

Three weeks ago, her husband of 15 years told her that he found her worry and constant need for reassurance exhausting and moved out for a "trial separation." Since then, Barbara has been on leave from her job as an art teacher at a private high school. Her chest pain began when she was composing an email to her husband asking him to consider marriage counselling.

The client states, "For as long as I can remember, I've always been very nervous." She is an only child, born to parents of English descent when they were in their 40s. A shy child, she had so much difficulty separating from her parents that her mother home-schooled her until grade 9. She describes her parents as "gentle and loving" and family life as "happy." Barbara had one or two close friends in high school, but spent most of her time alone reading, doing art, or playing with her cat. Up through her teen years, she "worried about everything" including her parents' health, grades, the dark, insects, and thunderstorms, most of which she "outgrew" except for an ongoing

fear of snakes. She denies any abuse and states that apart from her worrying, she was healthy.

Barbara's anxiety became more problematic when she began university at age 19; that same year her mother died suddenly. She was so distressed that she left school for 1 year. Upon her return the next fall, she was still crying often and could not focus on her studies. Her roommate insisted that Barbara go to the student health centre where she attended a cognitive behavioural therapy (CBT) group and was prescribed as-needed Ativan to "take the edge off" her anxiety.

After university, Barbara moved home to live with her father. She took her current job teaching art and married "the boy next door" at age 30. She states that she was attracted to her husband's calm manner, stable job, and dependability. The couple have no children by choice. Over the years, he has "lectured" her regularly "for worrying too much" and has gradually become distant. Although they have few conflicts, they do not spend much time together. Barbara states that while they both enjoyed sex early in their marriage, "it has been nonexistent" for at least 5 years. The home is safe; they are "financially secure" and both enjoy their work.

With the CBT strategies that she learned, her art, and increasing doses of Ativan, Barbara says that she

(Continued)

ANALYZING FINDINGS FROM PSYCHOSOCIAL ASSESSMENT AND MENTAL STATUS EXAMINATION

Once nurses have documented and analyzed findings from the psychosocial assessment and mental status examination, they use information to make a nursing diagnosis and develop an interdisciplinary care plan. Potential nursing diagnoses include the following:

Severe anxiety related to situational crisis

Chronic anxiety related to heredity/constitutional factors

Grieving related to threatened loss of marital relationship

In developing a comprehensive and interprofessional care plan, Barbara M. requires further assessment by other mental health practitioners (i.e., psychologist, social worker, clinical nurse specialist, psychiatrist) and her primary care physician. Because her primary concern is her marital situation, the clinician should begin there with the aim of helping her to manage her distress and do short-term problem solving. Once her distress abates, it will be important to rule out any physical problems that might contribute to her anxiety, to assess the depth and accuracy of her knowledge about anxiety, and to determine the effectiveness of her coping strategies. This information will highlight her need for further intervention (e.g., relationship counselling, stress management program, CBT refresher, anxiolytics).

Critical Thinking Exercise

Answer the following questions about Barbara M.

- List three types of anxiety disorders. (*Knowledge*)
- What is the underlying reason for Barbara M.'s repeated visits to her primary care physician? (*Comprehension*)
- What elements of Erikson's theory of development could guide the nurse in her further interactions with Barbara M.? (*Application*)
- What developmental and behavioural factors and life choices might contribute to Barbara M.'s symptom(s)? (*Analysis*)
- What recommendations for follow-up would you suggest for Barbara M.? Explain. (*Synthesis*)
- How would you evaluate the effectiveness of your teaching for Barbara M.? (*Evaluation*)

BIBLIOGRAPHY

Canadian Research

Bender, A., & Kennedy, S. (2004). Mental health and mental illness in the workplace: Diagnostic and treatment issues. *Healthcare Papers, 5*(2), 54–67.

Cairney, J., Corna, L. M., Veldhuizen, S., Herrmann, N., & Streiner, D. L. (2008). Comorbid depression and anxiety in later life: Patterns of association, subjective well-being, and impairment. *American Journal of Geriatric Psychiatry, 16*(3), 201–208.

Currie, S. R., Hodgins, D. C., Wang, J., el-Guebaly, N., Wynne, H., & Chen, S. (2006). Risk of harm among gamblers in the general population as a function of level of participation in gambling activities. *Addiction, 101*(4), 570–580.

Dunn, J. R., Hayes, M. V., Hulchanski, J. D., Hwang, S. W., & Potvin, L. (2006). Housing as a socio-economic determinant of health: Findings of a national needs, gaps and opportunities assessment. *Canadian Journal of Public Health, 97*(Suppl. 3), S11–S15, S12–S17.

Gadalla, T., & Piran, N. (2007). Eating disorders and substance abuse in Canadian men and women: A national study. *Eating Disorders, 15*(3), 189–203.

Jarvis, G. E., Kirmayer, L. J., Weinfeld, M., & Lasry, J. (2005). Religious practice and psychological distress: The importance of gender, ethnicity and immigrant status. *Transcultural Psychiatry, 42*(4), 657–675.

Kates, N., & Mach, M. (2007). Chronic disease management for depression in primary care: A summary of the current literature and implications for practice. *Canadian Journal of Psychiatry, 52*(2), 77–85.

O'Reilly, R., Bishop, J., Maddox, K., Hutchinson, L., Fisman, M., & Takhar, J. (2007). Is telepsychiatry equivalent to face-to-face psychiatry? Results from a randomized controlled equivalence trial. *Psychiatric Services, 58*(6), 836–843.

Ryan-Nicholls, K. D., & Haggarty, J. M. (2007). A pilot study of a Canadian shared mental health care programme: Changes in client symptoms and disability. *Journal of Psychosocial Nursing & Mental Health Services, 45*(12), 37–45.

Schachter, C. L., Stalker, C. A., & Teram, E. (2001). *Handbook on sensitive practice for health professionals: Lessons from women survivors of sexual abuse.* Retrieved July 21, 2008, from http://www.phac-aspc.gc.ca/ncfv-cnivf/familyviolence/html/nfntsxsensi_e.html

Test Questions

1. During the health history interview, the nurse can quickly assess which of the following components of cognitive function:
   a. Memory and attention
   b. Judgment and behaviour
   c. Calculation and language
   d. Abstract thinking and perceptions

2. One of the most important types of skills a nurse needs when conducting a mental status assessment is:
   a. rapid interpretive skills.
   b. effective listening skills.
   c. thorough assessment skills.
   d. well-developed writing skills

3. If a nurse suspects that a client is depressed, asking the client about the presence of suicidal thoughts:
   a. will stimulate thoughts of suicide.
   b. is important, but is not the first priority.
   c. will stimulate clients to act on suicidal ideation.
   d. is important and will not stimulate the thought of suicide.

4. When assessing the client's ability to make sound judgments, ask:
   a. "Do you eat breakfast?"
   b. "How many dimes are in one dollar?"
   c. "How do you plan to pay rent if you lose your job?"
   d. "Can you keep track of your finances on an ongoing basis?"

5. The nurse asks the client to draw the face of a clock with numbers and hands and to make it read 3:00. Completion of this task tests:
   a. visual spatial ability.
   b. new learning ability.
   c. constructional ability.
   d. information about clocks.

Bibliography

CITATIONS

Abad, V. C., & Guilleminault, C. (2005). Sleep and psychiatry. *Dialogues in Clinical Neuroscience, 7*(4), 291–303.

Alzheimer Society (2005). *Alzheimer's disease—Getting a diagnosis: Finding out if it is Alzheimer's disease.* Retrieved July 3, 2008, from http://alzheimer.ca/english/disease/diagnosis.htm

American Psychiatric Association. (2000). *Diagnostic and Statistical Manual of Mental Disorders* (4th ed., text Rev.). Washington, DC: Author.

Ansseau, M., Dierick, M., Buntinkx, F., Cnockaert, P., De Smedt, J., Van Den Haute, M., et al. (2004). High prevalence of mental disorders in primary care. *Journal of Affective Disorders, 78*(1), 49–55.

Babor, T. F., Higgins-Biddle, J. C., Saunders, J. B., & Monteiro, M. G. (2001). *AUDIT. The alcohol use disorders identification test: Guidelines for use in primary care* (2nd ed.). Geneva, Switzerland: World Health Organization, Department of Mental Health and Substance Dependence.

Baik, S., Bowers, B. J., Oakley, L. D., & Susman, J. L. (2005). The recognition of depression: The primary care clinician's perspective. *Annals of Family Medicine, 3*(1), 31–37.

Bland, R. C., Newman, S. C., & Orn, H. (1988). Period prevalence of psychiatric disorders in Edmonton. *Acta Psychiatrica Scandinavica, Supplementum, 338*, 33–42.

Boustani, M., Peterson, B., Hanson, L., Harris, R., & Lohr, K. N. (2003). Screening for dementia in primary care: A summary of the evidence for the U.S. Preventive Services Task Force. *Annals of Internal Medicine, 138*(11), 927–937.

Buijs, R. M., van Eden, C. G., Goncharuk, V. D., & Kalsbeek, A. (2003). The biological clock tunes the organs of the body: Timing by hormones and the autonomic nervous system. *Journal of Endocrinology, 177*(1), 17–26.

Canadian Mental Health Association. (n.d.). *Preventing suicide.* Retrieved July 15, 2008, from http://www.cmha.ca/bins/content_page.asp?cid=3-101-102

Canadian Study of Health and Aging Working Group. (2000). The incidence of dementia in Canada. *Neurology, 55*(1), 66–73.

Erikson, E. H. (1997). *The life cycle completed.* New York: W.W. Norton.

Erikson, E. H. (1980). *Identity and the life cycle.* New York: W. W. Norton.

Ewing, J. A. (1984). Detecting alcoholism. The CAGE questionnaire. *Journal of the American Medical Association, 252*(14), 1905–1907.

Greenberg, P. E., Sisitsky, T., Kessler, R. C., Finkelstein, S. N., Berndt, E. R., Davidson J. R. T., et al. (1999). The economic burden of anxiety disorders in the 1990s. *Journal of Clinical Psychiatry, 60*(7), 427–435.

Hardy, S., Titchen, A., Maley, K., & McCormack, B. (2006). Re-defining nursing expertise in the United Kingdom. *Nursing Science Quarterly, 19*(3), 260–264.

Health Canada. (2002). *A report on mental illnesses in Canada.* Ottawa, ON: Author. Retrieved July 15, 2008, from http://www.phac-aspc.gc.ca/publicat/miic-mmac/pdf/men_ill_e.pdf

Isaacs, B., & Kennie, A. (1973). The Set Test as an aid to the detection of dementia in old people. *British Journal of Psychiatry, 123*, 467–470.

Jarvis, C. (2004). *Physical examination and health assessment* (4th ed., p. 114). St. Louis: Elsevier Science.

Kawas, C. H. (2003). Early Alzheimer's disease. *New England Journal of Medicine, 349*(11), 1056–1063.

Kessler, R., Du Pont, R., Berglund, P., & Wittchen, H. (1999). Impairment in pure and comorbid generalized anxiety disorder and major depression at 12 months in two national surveys. *American Journal of Psychiatry, 156*, 1915–1923.

Koerner, N., Dugas, M. J., Savard, P., Gaudet, A., Turcotte, J., & Marchand, A. (2004). The economic burden of anxiety disorders in Canada. *Canadian Psychology, 45*(3), 191–201.

Kroenke, K., Spitzer, R. L., Williams, J. B., Monahan, P. O., & Löwe, B. (2007). Anxiety disorders in primary care: Prevalence, impairment, comorbidity, and detection. *Annals of Internal Medicine, 146*(5), 317–325.

Lopez, A. D., Mathers, C. D., Ezzati, M., Jamison, D. T., & Murray, C. J. (2006). Global and regional burden of disease and risk factors, 2001: Systematic analysis of population health data. *Lancet, 367*(9524), 1747–1757.

Manley, K., Hardy, S., Titchen, A., Garbett, R., & McCormack, B. (2005). *Changing patients' worlds through nursing practice expertise: Exploring nursing practice expertise through emancipator action research and fourth generation evaluation.* A Royal College of Nursing Research Report, 1998 – 2004. London: Royal College of Nursing.

McCusker, M. T., Basquille, J., Khwaja, M., Murray-Lyon, I. M., & Catalan, J. (2002). Hazardous and harmful drinking: A comparison of the AUDIT and CAGE screening questionnaires. *Quality Journal of Medicine: An International Journal of Medicine, 95*(9), 591–595.

Murphy, J. M., Laird, N. M., Monson, R. R., Sobol, A. M., & Leighton, A. H. (2000). A 40-year perspective on the prevalence of depression: The Stirling County study. *Archives of General Psychiatry, 57*(3), 209–215.

Pan American Health Organization and World Health Organization. (2000). *Promotion of sexual health: Recommendations for action.* Proceedings of a regional consultation convened by the Pan American Health Organization and the World Health Organization in collaboration with the World Association for Sexology. Antigua Guatemala, Guatemala: Author.

Parikh, S. V., & Lam, R. L. (2001). The CANMAT Depression Work Group. Clinical guidelines for the treatment of depressive disorders. I. Definitions, prevalence, and health burden. *Canadian Journal of Psychiatry, 46*(Suppl. 1), 13S–20S.

Parikh, S. V., Wasylenki, D., Goering, P., & Wong, J. (1996). Mood disorders: Rural/urban differences in prevalence, health care utilization, and disability in Ontario. *Journal of Affective Disorders, 38*(1), 57–65.

Roehrs, T., & Roth, T. (2005). Sleep and pain: Interaction of two vital functions. *Seminars in Neurology, 25*(1), 106–116.

Rogers, C. R. (1980). *A way of being.* Boston: Houghton Mifflin.

Seelig, M. D., & Katon, W. (2008). Gaps in depression care: Why primary care physicians should hone their depression screening, diagnosis, and management skills. *Journal of Occupational and Environmental Medicine, 50*(4), 451–458.

Shields, A. L. (2003). *Reliability generalizations of three alcohol screening measures: The Alcohol use Disorders Identification Test, the CAGE Questionnaire, and the Michigan Alcoholism Screening Test.* Unpublished doctoral dissertation. University of Montana, Missoula.

Statistics Canada. (2006). *Concept: Ethnicity.* Ottawa, ON. Retrieved July 15, 2008, from http://www.statcan.ca/english/concepts/definitions/ethnicity.htm

Sutton, J., & Martinson, D. (2008). *Self-Injury: You are not the only one.* Retrieved August 2, 2008, from www.palace.net/~llama/psych/injury.html

Toft, T., Fink, P., Oernboel, E., Christensen, K., Frostholm, L., & Olesen, F. (2005). Mental disorders in primary care: Prevalence and co-morbidity among disorders. Results from the functional illness in primary care (FIP) study. *Psychological Medicine, 35*(8), 1175–1184.

U.S. Preventative Services Task Force. (2002). Screening for depression: Recommendations and rationale. *Annals of Internal Medicine, 36*(10), 760–764.

U.S. Preventive Services Task Force. (2003). Screening for dementia: Recommendations and rationale. *Annals of Internal Medicine, 138*(11), 925–926.

BIBLIOGRAPHY

Vasiliadis, H.-M., Lesage, A., Adair, C., Wang, P. S., & Kessler, R. C. (2007). Do Canada and the United States differ in prevalence of depression and utilization of services? *Psychiatric Services, 58*(1), 63–71.

Wysong, P. (2007). Bodily harm—understanding self-injury. *Canadian Living, 32*(9), 105–106, 108, 110.

ADDITIONAL REFERENCES

Austin, W. J., & Boyd, M. A. (Eds.). (2008). *Psychiatric nursing for Canadian practice.* Philadelphia: Lippincott Williams & Wilkins.

Belmaker, R. H. (2004). Bipolar disorder. *New England Journal of Medicine, 351*(5), 476–486, 518.

Berry, P. D. (Ed.). (1996). *Psychosocial nursing: Care of physically ill patients and their families* (3rd ed.). Philadelphia: Lippincott.

Long, L.G., Higgins, P. G., & Brady, D. (1988). *Psychosocial assessment: A pocket guide for data collection.* Norwalk, CT: Appleton & Lange.

RESOURCES: CANADIAN ASSOCIATIONS AND WEB SITES

Alzheimer Society: http://www.alzheimer.ca/

Canadian Alliance on Mental Illness and Mental Health: http://www.camimh.ca/

Canadian Coalition for Seniors' Mental Health: http://www.ccsmh.ca/en/default.cfm

Canadian Collaborative Mental Health Initiative. The College of Family Physicians of Canada (Project Sponsor): http://www.ccmhi.ca/

Canadian Federation of Mental Health Nurses: http://www.cfmhn.ca/

Canadian Mental Health Association: http://www.cmha.ca/bins/index.asp

Canadian Psychiatric Association: http://www.cpa-apc.org/

Centre for Addiction and Mental Health: http://www.camh.net/

Cool Nurse: www.coolnurse.com/self-injury.htm

Interdisciplinary National Self-Injury in Youth Network Canada (INSYNC): www.insync-group.ca/

Mood Disorders Society of Canada: http://www.mooddisorderscanada.ca/

National Eating Disorder Information Centre: http://www.nedic.ca/index.shtml

Registered Psychiatric Nurses of Canada: http://www.rpnc.ca/pages/home.php

Schizophrenia Society of Canada: http://www.schizophrenia.ca/

The Health of Canadians—The Federal Role: Final Report (The Kirby Report): http://www.parl.gc.ca/37/2/parlbus/commbus/senate/Com-e/soci-e/rep-e/repoct02vol6-e.htm

World Federation for Mental Health: http://www.wfmh.com/index.html

TABLE 9-1   Disorders of Speech

Disorders of speech fall into three groups: those affecting (1) the voice, (2) the articulation of words, and (3) the production and comprehension of language.

Aphonia refers to a loss of voice that accompanies disease affecting the larynx or its nerve supply. *Dysphonia* refers to less severe impairment in the volume, quality, or pitch of the voice. For example, a person may be hoarse or only able to speak in a whisper. Causes include laryngitis, laryngeal tumors, and a unilateral vocal cord paralysis (Cranial Nerve X).

Dysarthria refers to a defect in the muscular control of the speech apparatus (lips, tongue, palate, or pharynx). Words may be nasal, slurred, or indistinct, but the central symbolic aspect of language remains intact. Causes include motor lesions of the central or peripheral nervous system, parkinsonism, and cerebellar disease.

Aphasia refers to a disorder in producing or understanding language. It is often caused by lesions in the dominant cerebral hemisphere, usually the left.

Compared below are two common types of aphasia: (1) Wernicke's, a fluent (receptive) aphasia, and (2) Broca's, a nonfluent (or expressive) aphasia. There are other less common kinds of aphasia, which are distinguished by differing responses on the specific tests listed. Neurologic consultation is usually indicated.

	Wernicke's Aphasia	Broca's Aphasia
Qualities of Spontaneous Speech	Fluent; often rapid, voluble, and effortless. Inflection and articulation are good, but sentences lack meaning and words are malformed (paraphasias) or invented (neologisms). Speech may be totally incomprehensible.	Nonfluent; slow, with few words and laborious effort. Inflection and articulation are impaired, but words are meaningful, with nouns, transitive verbs, and important adjectives. Small grammatical words are often dropped.
Word Comprehension	Impaired	Fair to good
Repetition	Impaired	Impaired
Naming	Impaired	Impaired, though the client recognizes objects
Reading Comprehension	Impaired	Fair to good
Writing	Impaired	Impaired
Location of Lesion	Posterior superior temporal lobe	Posterior inferior frontal lobe

Although it is important to recognize aphasia early in your encounter with a client, its full diagnostic meaning does not become clear until you integrate this information with your neurologic examination.

TABLE 9-2　Disorders of Mood

Mood disorders may be either depressive or bipolar. A bipolar disorder can include manic, hypomanic, or depressive features. Four types of episodes, described below, are combined in different ways in diagnosis of mood disorders. A major depressive disorder includes only one or more major depressive episodes. A bipolar I disorder includes one or more manic or mixed episodes, usually accompanied by major depressive episodes. A bipolar II disorder includes one or more major depressive episodes accompanied by at least one hypomanic episode.

Dysthymic and cyclothymic disorders are chronic and less severe conditions that do not meet the criteria of the other disorders. Mood disorders due to general medical conditions or substance abuse are classified separately.

Major Depressive Episode

At least five of the symptoms listed here (including one of the first two) must be present during the same 2-week period. They must also represent a change from the person's previous state.

- Depressed mood (may be an irritable mood in children and adolescents) most of the day, nearly every day
- Markedly diminished interest or pleasure in almost all activities most of the day, nearly every day
- Significant weight gain or loss (not dieting) or increased or decreased appetite nearly every day
- Insomnia or hypersomnia nearly every day
- Psychomotor agitation or retardation nearly every day
- Fatigue or loss of energy nearly every day
- Feelings of worthlessness or inappropriate guilt nearly every day
- Inability to think or concentrate or indecisiveness nearly every day
- Recurrent thoughts of death or suicide, or a specific plan for or attempt at suicide

The symptoms cause significant distress or impair social, occupational, or other important functions. In severe cases, hallucinations and delusions may occur.

Mixed Episode

A mixed episode, which must last at least 1 week, meets the criteria for both major and manic depressive episodes.

Dysthymic Disorder

A depressed mood and symptoms for most of the day, for more days than not, over at least 2 years (1 year in children and adolescents). Freedom from symptoms lasts no more than 2 months at a time.

Manic Episode

A distinct period of abnormally and persistently elevated, expansive, or irritable mood must be present for at least a week (any duration if hospitalization is necessary). During this time, at least three of the symptoms listed here have been persistent and significant. (Four of these symptoms are required if the mood is only irritable).

- Inflated self-esteem or grandiosity
- Decreased need for sleep (feels rested after sleeping 3 hours)
- More talkative than usual or pressure to keep talking
- Flight of ideas or racing thoughts
- Distractibility
- Increased goal-directed activity (either socially at work or school, or sexually) or psychomotor agitation
- Excessive involvement in pleasurable high-risk activities (buying sprees, foolish business ventures, sexual indiscretions)

The disturbance is severe enough to impair social or occupational functions or relationships. It may necessitate hospitalization for the protection of self or others. In severe cases, hallucinations and delusions may occur.

Hypomanic Episode

The mood and symptoms resemble those in a manic episode but are less impairing, do not require hospitalization, do not include hallucinations or delusions, and have a shorter minimum duration—4 days.

Cyclothymic Episode

Numerous periods of hypomanic and depressive symptoms that last for at least 2 years (1 year in children and adolescents). Freedom from symptoms lasts no more than 2 months at a time.

Source: Tables 9-2, 9-3, and 9-4 are based, with permission, on the Diagnostic and Statistical Manual of Mental Disorders, 4th ed., text revision (DSM IV-TR). Washington, D.C. American Psychiatric Association, 2000. For further details and criteria, the reader should consult this manual, its successor, or comprehensive textbooks of psychiatry.

TABLE 9-3	Anxiety Disorders

Panic Disorder

A *panic disorder* is defined by recurrent, unexpected panic attacks, at least one of which has been followed by a month or more of persistent concern about further attacks, worry over their implications or consequences, or a significant change in behaviour in relation to the attacks. A *panic attack* is a discrete period of intense fear or discomfort that develops abruptly and peaks within 10 minutes. It involves at least four of the following symptoms: (1) palpitations, pounding heart, or accelerated heart rate; (2) sweating; (3) trembling or shaking; (4) shortness of breath or a sense of smothering; (5) a feeling of choking; (6) chest pain or discomfort; (7) nausea or abdominal distress; (8) feeling dizzy, unsteady, lightheaded, or faint; (9) feelings of unreality or depersonalization; (10) fear of losing control or going crazy; (11) fear of dying; (12) paresthesias (numbness or tingling); (13) chills or hot flushes. Panic disorder may occur with or without *agoraphobia*.

Agoraphobia

Agoraphobia is an anxiety about being in places or situations where escape may be difficult or embarrassing or help unavailable. Such situations are avoided, require a companion, or cause marked anxiety.

Specific Phobia

A specific phobia is a marked, persistent, and excessive or unreasonable fear that is cued by the presence or anticipation of a specific object or situation, such as dogs, injections, or flying. The person recognizes the fear as excessive or unreasonable, but exposure to the cue provokes immediate anxiety. Avoidance or fear impairs the person's usual routine, occupational or academic functioning, or social activities or relationships.

Social Phobia

A social phobia is a marked, persistent fear of one or more social or performance situations that involve exposure to unfamiliar people or to scrutiny by others. Those afflicted fear that they will act in embarrassing or humiliating ways, as by showing their anxiety. Exposure creates anxiety and possibly a panic attack, and the person avoids precipitating situations. He or she recognizes the fear as excessive or unreasonable. Usual routines, occupational or academic functioning, or social activities or relationships are impaired.

Obsessive–Compulsive Disorder

This disorder involves obsessions or compulsions that cause marked anxiety or distress. Although they are recognized at some point as excessive or unreasonable, they are very time-consuming and interfere with the person's usual routine, occupational functioning, or social activities or relationships.

Acute Stress Disorder

The person has been exposed to a traumatic event that involved actual or threatened death or serious injury to self or others and responded with intense fear, helplessness, or horror. During or immediately after this event, the person has at least three of these dissociative symptoms: (1) a subjective sense of numbing, detachment, or absence of emotional responsiveness; (2) a reduced awareness of surroundings, as in a daze; (3) feelings of unreality; (4) feelings of depersonalization; and (5) amnesia for an important part of the event. The event is persistently reexperienced, as in thoughts, images, dreams, illusions, and flashbacks, or distress from reminders of the event. The person is very anxious or shows increased arousal and tries to avoid stimuli that evoke memories of the event. The disturbance causes marked distress or impairs social, occupational, or other important functions. The symptoms occur within 4 weeks of the event and last from 2 days to 4 weeks.

Posttraumatic Stress Disorder

The event, the fearful response, and the persistent reexperiencing of the traumatic event resemble those in acute stress disorder. Hallucinations may occur. The person has increased arousal, tries to avoid stimuli related to the trauma, and has numbing of general responsiveness. The disturbance causes marked distress; impairs social, occupational, or other important functions; and lasts for more than a month.

Generalized Anxiety Disorder

This disorder lacks a specific traumatic event or focus for concern. Excessive anxiety and worry, which the person finds hard to control, are about a number of events or activities. At least three of the following symptoms are associated: (1) feeling restless, keyed up, or on edge; (2) being easily fatigued; (3) difficulty in concentrating or mind going blank; (4) irritability; (5) muscle tension; (6) difficulty in falling or staying asleep, or restless, unsatisfying sleep. The disturbance causes significant distress or impairs social, occupational, or other important functions.

TABLE 9-4   **Psychotic Disorders**

Psychotic disorders involve grossly impaired reality testing. Specific diagnoses depend on the nature and duration of the symptoms and on a cause when it can be identified. Seven disorders are outlined here.

Schizophrenia	Schizophrenia impairs major functioning, as at work or school or in interpersonal relations or self-care. For this diagnosis, performance of one or more of these functions must have decreased for a significant time to a level markedly below prior achievement. In addition, the person must manifest at least two of the following for a significant part of 1 month: (1) delusions, (2) hallucinations, (3) disorganized speech, (4) grossly disorganized or catatonic behavior,* and (5) negative symptoms such as a flat affect, alogia (lack of content in speech), or avolition (lack of interest, drive, and ability to set and pursue goals). Continuous signs of the disturbance must persist for at least 6 months.
	Subtypes of this disorder include paranoid, disorganized, and catatonic schizophrenia.
Schizophreniform Disorder	A schizophreniform disorder has symptoms similar to those of schizophrenia, but they last less than 6 months and the functional impairment seen in schizophrenia need not be present.
Schizoaffective Disorder	A schizoaffective disorder has features of both a major mood disturbance and schizophrenia. The mood disturbance (depressive, manic, or mixed) is present during most of the illness and must, for a time, be concurrent with symptoms of schizophrenia (listed above). During the same period of time, there must also be delusions or hallucinations for at least 2 weeks without prominent mood symptoms.
Delusional Disorder	A delusional disorder is characterized by nonbizarre delusions that involve situations in real life, such as having a disease or being deceived by a lover. The delusion has persisted for at least a month, but the person's functioning is not markedly impaired, and behaviour is not obviously odd or bizarre. The symptoms of schizophrenia, except for tactile and olfactory hallucinations related to the delusion, have not been present.
Brief Psychotic Disorder	In this disorder, at least one of the following psychotic symptoms must be present: delusions, hallucinations, disordered speech such as frequent derailment or incoherence, or grossly disorganized or catatonic behavior. The disturbance lasts at least 1 day but less than 1 month, and the person returns to his or her prior functional level.
Psychotic Disorder Due to a General Medical Condition	Prominent hallucinations or delusions may be experienced during a medical illness. For this diagnosis, they should not occur exclusively during the course of delirium. The medical condition should be documented and judged to be causally related to the symptoms.
Substance-Induced Psychotic Disorder	Prominent hallucinations or delusions may be induced by intoxication or withdrawal from a substance such as alcohol, cocaine, or opioids. For this diagnosis, these symptoms should not occur exclusively during the course of delirium. The substance should be judged to be causally related to the symptoms.

*Catatonic behaviors are psychomotor abnormalities that include stupor, mutism, negativistic resistance to instructions or attempts to move the person, rigid or bizarre postures, and excited, apparently purposeless activity.

10

The Skin, Hair, and Nails

TRACEY C. STEPHEN AND LYNN S. BICKLEY

The skin, hair, and nails are the three major components of the integumentary system. The sebaceous glands and sweat glands (apocrine and eccrine) are the other essential components of this system. Much of the integumentary system is publicly visible and plays an essential role in self-image. Assessment of the integumentary system provides clues about a client's general state of health, age, and specific disease processes.

ANATOMY AND PHYSIOLOGY

The major function of the skin is to keep the body in homeostasis despite daily assaults from the environment. The skin provides boundaries for body fluids while protecting underlying tissues from microorganisms, harmful substances, and radiation. It modulates body temperature and is the largest sensory organ that synthesizes vitamin D. *Hair*, *nails*, and *sebaceous* and *sweat glands* are considered appendages of the skin. The skin and its appendages undergo many changes during aging. Turn to Chapter 26, The Older Adult, to review normal and abnormal changes of the skin with aging.

SKIN

The skin is the heaviest single organ of the body, accounting for approximately 16% of body weight and covering an area of roughly 1.2 to 2.3 metres squared comprising three layers: the epidermis, the dermis, and the subcutaneous tissues.

The most superficial layer, the *epidermis*, is thin, devoid of blood vessels, and is divided into two layers: an outer horny layer of dead keratinized cells and an inner cellular layer, where melanin and keratin are formed. Migration from the inner layer to the outer layer of the epidermis takes approximately 1 month.

The epidermis depends on the underlying *dermis* for its nutrition. The dermis is well supplied with blood. It contains connective tissue, sebaceous

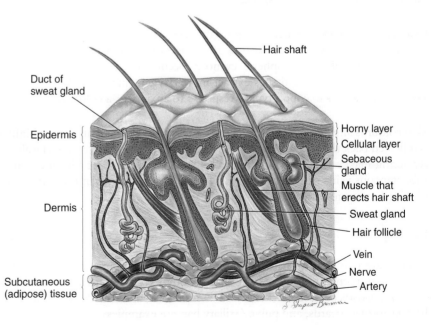

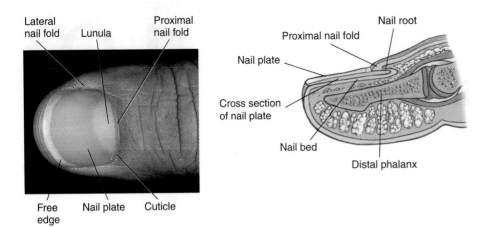

glands, sweat glands, and hair follicles. It merges below with *subcutaneous tissue*, or *adipose*, also known as fat.

The colour of skin depends primarily on four pigments: melanin, carotene, oxyhemoglobin, and deoxyhemoglobin. The amount of *melanin*, the brownish pigment of the skin, is genetically determined and is increased by sunlight. *Carotene* is a golden yellow pigment that exists in subcutaneous fat and in heavily keratinized areas such as the palms and soles.

Hemoglobin, which circulates in the red cells and carries most of the oxygen of the blood, exists in two forms. *Oxyhemoglobin*, a bright red pigment, predominates in the arteries and capillaries. An increase in blood flow through the arteries to the capillaries of the skin causes a reddening of the skin, whereas the opposite change usually produces pallor. The skin of light-coloured people is usually redder on the palms, soles, face, neck, and upper chest.

As blood passes through the capillary bed, oxyhemoglobin loses its oxygen to the tissues and changes to *deoxyhemoglobin*—a darker and somewhat bluer pigment. An increased concentration of deoxyhemoglobin in cutaneous blood vessels gives the skin a bluish cast known as *cyanosis*.

Cyanosis is of two kinds, depending on the level of oxygen in the arterial blood. If this level is low, cyanosis is *central*. If the level is within expected parameters, cyanosis is *peripheral*. Peripheral cyanosis occurs when cutaneous blood flow decreases and slows, and tissues extract more oxygen than usual from the blood. Peripheral cyanosis may be a typical response to anxiety or a cold environment.

Skin colour is affected not only by pigments, but also by the scattering of light as it is reflected back through the turbid superficial layers of the skin or vessel walls. This scattering makes the colour look more blue and less red. The bluish colour of a subcutaneous vein is a result of this effect; it is much bluer than the venous blood obtained on venipuncture.

HAIR

Adults have two types of hair: *vellus hair,* which is short, fine, inconspicuous, and relatively unpigmented, covers the entire body except for the soles and palms. *Terminal hair* is coarser, thicker, more conspicuous, and usually pigmented. Scalp hair, eyebrows, beards, and pubic/axillary hair are examples.

Cultural Considerations

Clients of Asian and First Nation descent have less terminal hair on the body.

NAILS

Nails protect the distal ends of the fingers and toes. The firm, rectangular, and usually curving *nail plate* gets its pink colour from the vascular *nail bed* to which the plate is firmly attached. Note the whitish moon, or *lunula*, and the free edge of the nail plate. Roughly one-fourth of the nail plate (the *nail root*) is covered by the *proximal nail fold*. The *cuticle* extends from this fold and, functioning as a seal, protects the space between the fold and the plate from external moisture. *Lateral nail folds* cover the sides of the nail plate. Note that the angle between the proximal nail fold and the nail plate is normally less than 180°.

Fingernails grow approximately 0.1 millimetres daily; toenails grow more slowly.

SEBACEOUS GLANDS AND SWEAT GLANDS

Sebaceous glands produce a fatty substance that is secreted onto the skin surface through the hair follicles. These glands are present on all skin surfaces except the palms and soles.

Sweat glands are of two types: eccrine and apocrine. The *eccrine glands* are widely distributed, open directly onto the skin surface, and by their sweat production help to control body temperature. In contrast, the *apocrine glands* are found chiefly in the axillary and genital regions, usually open into hair follicles, and are stimulated by emotional stress. Bacterial decomposition of apocrine sweat is responsible for adult body odour.

THE HEALTH HISTORY: SUBJECTIVE DATA

Key Signs and Symptoms Reported by Client

- Hair loss
- Moles
- Rashes
- Lesions
- Dryness of skin
- Excessive sweating

Begin the health history with a few open-ended questions: "How are you feeling today?," "Have you been having any concerns about how you are feeling?" Use the information from the client's responses to guide the rest of the health history. "What concerns have brought you here today?" It is essential to start with the client's concerns and work from this point.

Start your inquiry about the skin with a few open-ended questions: "Have you noticed any changes in your skin? . . . your hair? . . . your nails? . . . Have you had any rashes? . . . sores? . . . lumps? . . . itching?"

Causes of generalized itching without obvious reason include dry skin, aging, pregnancy, uremia, jaundice, lymphomas and leukemia, drug reaction, and lice.

Ask, "Have you noticed any moles you are concerned about? Do you have any moles that have changed in size, shape, colour, or sensation? What about any new moles?" If clients have such moles, pursue any personal or family history of melanoma and results of any prior biopsies of the skin.

Approximately half of melanomas are initially detected by the client (Whited & Grichnek, 1998).

You may wish to defer further questions about the skin until the physical examination, when you inspect the skin and identify the lesions that the client is concerned about.

Examples of Questions for Sign/Symptom Analysis—Rash

- "Where is the rash?" "Where did the rash start?" "Has the rash spread?" "Is it all over your legs?" (*Location, Radiation*)
- "Describe what the rash is like." "Is it raised?" "Scaly?" "Itchy?" "Painful?" (*Quality*)
- "Describe how itchy (or painful) the rash is." (*Severity*)
- "When did the rash start?" "Did it start suddenly?" "Did you notice it starting over time?" (*Onset*)
- "Has the rash stayed since you first noticed it?" (*Duration*)
- "Have there been times when it got better?" "Or worse?" (*Constancy*)
- "Is there a time of day that it (rash) seems worse? Or better?" (*Time of day/month/year*)

- "What makes the rash worse?" (*Aggravating factors*)
- "What makes the rash better?" (*Alleviating factors*)
- "What other symptoms have you noticed?" (*Associated symptoms*)
- "Have you been exposed to any chemicals?" "Or other substances?" "Have you recently changed anything in your house or office such as laundry detergent or soap?" "Have you been experiencing more stress than usual?" (*Environmental factors*)
- "Describe how this is affecting your life." (*Significance to client*)
- "What do you think may be happening?" (*Client perspective*)

HEALTH PROMOTION

Important Topics for Health Promotion

- Risk factors for skin cancer
- Sun safety
- Self-assessment of skin
- Vitamin D deficiency
- Work-related skin disorders
- Body art (tattooing and piercing)
- Psoriasis

Clinicians play an important role in educating clients about self-examination of the skin and reduction of risk factors for skin cancer and other disorders of the integument. They also help clients to understand measures for the early detection of suspicious moles, protective skin care, and the hazards of excessive sun exposure.

SPECIFIC PREVENTION FOR SPECIFIC DISEASES

Skin Cancer. Incidence of skin cancer in Canadians has risen steadily over the past 30 years, with cases increasing by more than 60% in the past 10 years (Canadian

Cancer Society, 2008a). Skin cancer usually arises on sun-exposed areas, particularly the head, neck, and hands, and is now the leading type of cancer in Canadian men and women (Canadian Cancer Society, 2008a). In 2005, there were 78,000 new cases of basal cell and squamous cell carcinoma and 4400 new cases of malignant melanoma (Canadian Dermatology Association [CDA], 2008a). Almost all skin cancers are of three types:

- *Basal cell carcinoma*, arising in the lowest—or basal—level of the epidermis, accounts for approximately 80% of skin cancers. These shiny and translucent cancers tend to grow slowly and rarely metastasize.

- *Squamous cell carcinoma*, in the upper layer of the epidermis, accounts for approximately 15% of skin cancers. These are often crusted and scaly, with a red, inflamed, or ulcerated appearance, and can metastasize.

- *Malignant melanoma*, arising from the pigment-producing melanocytes in the epidermis, accounts for approximately 5% of skin cancers and is the most lethal type. Although rare, melanomas are the most rapidly increasing malignancy. They can spread rapidly to the lymph system and internal organs. Mortality rates from melanoma are highest in Caucasian men, possibly because of less "skin awareness" and lower rates of self-examination.

Actinic keratoses are not actual cancerous lesions, but they have the potential to turn into squamous cell carcinomas. These lesions appear as red, rough, scaling spots usually on sun-exposed areas such as the hands, forearms, legs, face, scalp, and ears.

Risk Factor Assessment. Risk arises from exposure to the sun's ultraviolet (UV) radiation, which is categorized by wave length as UVA, UVB, and UVC. UVC radiation does not penetrate the earth's ozone layer, UVB affects the outer layer of the skin, and UVA (which penetrates glass) affects even deeper skin layers to cause damage.

Educating clients about risk factors for skin cancer helps decrease associated mortality rates. Fair-skinned people with blonde or red hair are at highest risk. Clients with 50 or more common moles and 1 to 4 or more atypical or unusual moles, especially if atypical, are also at increased risk. Other risk factors include presence of actinic lentigenes or brown or tan spots usually on sun-exposed areas, heavy sun exposure, history of sunburns, light eye colour, skin that freckles or burns easily, previous skin cancer history, and positive family history of skin cancer. Also, clients who are immunosuppressed from HIV, other disorders, or organ transplantation are at increased risk.

Incidence of skin cancer increases with age, especially past 50 years. Increasingly, however, skin cancers are appearing in teenagers and adults in their 20s (CDA, 2008b).

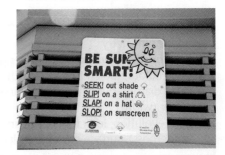

Clients who spend extended hours outdoors for work, sports, or hobbies are at increased risk for skin cancer. The CDA (2008c) developed a program of sun safety for outdoor workers. Information is available at http://www.dermatology.ca/outdoorworkers/index.html.

Almost all skin cancers are preventable (Canadian Cancer Society, 2008a). Most prevention techniques focus on limiting exposure to harmful UV radiation. Examples include:

- Limit time spent in the sun, especially from 1000 to 1600 hours when the sun's radiation is strongest.

- Wear UV-protective clothes or clothes that cover as much of the body as possible.

- Apply a broad-spectrum (protective against UVA and UVB rays) sunscreen with a minimum SPF 15; reapply every $1\frac{1}{2}$ to 2 hours. Use 30 to 60 mL of sunscreen for each application. Apply more often if perspiring heavily or playing in the water. Recognized sunscreens have the CDA label on the product.

- Apply sunscreen 30 minutes before exposure to sun.

- Wear a broad-brimmed hat with cover for the back of the neck and ears.

- Apply a broad-spectrum SPF 30 lip balm.

- Seek shade from trees, buildings, and the like.

- Wear protective sunglasses.

Skin cancer may develop over 10 to 30 years, so it is essential to promote early prevention. Parents need to protect children from the sun and encourage them to wear sunscreen, hats, and appropriate clothing at all times when outdoors. Ultraviolet protective clothing is available for babies and children.

The CDA (2008b) has developed the Sun Safety program to help protect children and teenagers from UV radiation. The principles are designed to be easy to remember and follow: SEEK out shade, SLIP on a shirt, SLAP on a hat, and SLOP on sunscreen. Details are available at http://www.dermatology.ca/sap/safety_resources/sun_exposure/kids_teens.html.

Screening and Maintenance. Although incidence of skin cancer has increased over the past three decades, mortality rates from it have declined. Early detection is essential to ensure prompt treatment with the best possible outcomes. The most commonly recommended screening measure for skin cancer is total-body skin examination by a clinician, although data on the utility of this method by nondermatologists are limited. Only a few studies have shown that self-examination of the skin enhances detection, but this low-cost method of client education can promote health awareness in at-risk clients. The CDA recommends monthly skin self-examinations and yearly examinations by a family physician or a dermatologist.

The CDA (2008a) recommends the ABCDE method for screening moles for possible melanoma by clients and health care professionals.

ABCDE: SCREENING MOLES FOR POSSIBLE MELANOMA

- A for asymmetry
- B for borders; look for irregular edges, ragged or notched, and imprecise
- C for colour; look for change with brown, black, red, grey, or white areas
- D for diameter; look for growth in size of the lesion larger than a pencil eraser (width)
- E for evolution; look for change in size, shape, symptoms (itchiness, tenderness), surface elevation, bleeding, or colour

---

Vitamin D Deficiency. One of the functions of the skin is to synthesize vitamin D, which requires exposure to sunlight. If exposure is limited, clients need to increase intake of vitamin D through foods fortified with it or vitamin supplements. Canadians may not get enough vitamin D because of the country's northern latitude and its relationship to the weakness of the sun's rays, especially during fall and winter (Canadian Cancer Society, 2008b). Vitamin D is required for healthy bones and muscles and has been shown to prevent some cancers (colorectal, breast, and prostate). It is recommended that adults take a daily supplement with 1000 international units (IU) of vitamin D during the fall and winter.

Work-Related Skin Disorders. Skin disorders related to the workplace are frequently reported, second only to workplace trauma. Exposure to hot and humid conditions and substances such as solvents, heavy oils, cleaners, ionizing radiation, acids, detergents, infectious agents, and latex cause several skin disorders. Sweat, friction, and nonhygienic work environments contribute to acne, contact dermatitis, heat rashes, and sports-related skin disorders. Clients with existing skin conditions are at increased risk to hazardous exposures in the workplace.

Latex allergies are becoming increasingly common. Skin allergies begin with a process of sensitization and may continue throughout the client's life.

During the health history, ensure the collection of comprehensive information related to exposures to substances of concern, including frequency, duration, and type. Discuss preventive measures with the client:

- Perform careful personal hygiene, including handwashing with mild soap or appropriate cleansing agents (waterless hand cleaners).

- Use showers at the end of work shifts.

- Wear protective clothing (gloves, aprons, coveralls, masks).

- Apply protective creams or moisturizers.

- Ensure cleanliness of worksite.

- Reduce all hazardous exposures (toxic substances, infectious agents, thermal exposures).

- Wear nonlatex gloves.

- Provide education programs such as Workplace Hazardous Materials Information System WHMIS training.

- Review Material Safety Data Sheets (MSDS) on designated hazardous substances.

Body Art (Tattooing and Piercing). Body piercing and tattooing are increasingly popular among Canadians, especially those 18 to 22 years old (Health Canada, 2008). Although no recent statistics are available that outline the numbers of Canadians who have undergone these procedures, a 2002 survey completed by Leger Marketing found that nearly 20% of all Canadians have some form of tattoo or body piercing, excluding traditional earlobe piercing. Ear piercing accounts for 85% of all body piercing.

Tattooing and body piercing are procedures that pierce the skin. Tattooing uses a machine with a cluster of needles 1 to 2 mm to permanently deposit pigment beneath the skin to create a design. Body piercing inserts metal jewellery into skin tissue through a piercing gun or long needles. Because both procedures penetrate the skin, they carry several risks (Canadian Broadcasting Corporation, 2004; Eastern Ontario Health Unit, 2005). These include transmitted diseases such as hepatitis B, hepatitis C, herpes, toxic shock syndrome, HIV/AIDS, skin tuberculosis, inoculation leprosy, warts, and bacterial skin infections; allergic reactions to the tattoo pigments; reactions to the metals in body piercing; and scar tissue. Malignant melanoma has also been linked to tattooing (Canadian Broadcasting Corporation, 2004). The Public Health Agency of Canada (1999) has published safety guidelines to prevent infection during these procedures, available at http://www.phac-aspc.gc.ca.

Psoriasis. Psoriasis, a recurrent and chronic skin disorder, affects approximately 1 million Canadians and 80 million people worldwide. It occurs more often in people of European descent. It can manifest at any age and begins with small red bumps that gradually grow and form scales. These scales can form tender lesions prone to bleeding. Approximately one-third of people with psoriasis experience symptoms of arthritis and may have some disability in the joints covered by psoriasis such as knees and elbows. The cause of psoriasis is unknown, but treatments such as lotions, creams, oral medications, and light therapy are available to control it.

SPECIAL CONSIDERATIONS FOR DISORDERS OF THE SKIN AND INTEGUMENT

Several other disorders of the skin and integument commonly affect millions of Canadians. Acne, alopecia, rosacea, pruritis, excessive sweating, and winter skin are examples. Many of these problems contribute to altered self-image, low self-esteem, depression, anxiety, and feelings of helplessness. Canadians spend millions of dollars on skin treatments, hairstyling, hair colouring, manicures, and pedicures to enhance their appearance. Disorders of the skin and integument are usually very visible and may result in diminished self-concept and feelings of embarrassment.

EMERGENCY CONCERNS

Many signs and symptoms of disorders of the integument require attention from a physician or dermatologist; however, most do not require emergency treatment. Examples of problems that necessitate emergency attention are as follows:

- Deep lacerations requiring stitches

- Burn injuries

- Extensive crush injuries to the nails

Most rashes can be attended to on a nonurgent basis except those that occur with other symptoms that may indicate serious illness. For example, red inflamed areas of the skin with symptoms of anaphylactic shock may indicate anaphylaxis, or a purple spotted rash along with neck pain may signify meningitis. Skin rashes or lesions that suddenly appear and are accompanied by fever and general malaise require emergency assessment.

TECHNIQUES OF EXAMINATION: OBJECTIVE DATA

PROMOTING CLIENT COMFORT AND SAFETY

Examination of the skin, hair, and nails begins with the general survey and continues throughout the physical examination. Ensure the client wears a gown and is draped to provide privacy and warmth. Also, expose only one area at a time during full skin assessments to ensure warmth and privacy for the client. Remain attentive to any signs of physical or emotional discomfort from the client. Appropriate draping facilitates close inspection of the hair, anterior and posterior surfaces of the body, palms, soles, and web spaces between the fingers and toes.

Equipment	
■ Penlight	■ Disposable gloves
■ Ruler	■ Magnifying glass

Inspect the entire skin surface in good light, preferably natural light or artificial light that resembles it. Correlate your findings with observations of the mucous membranes, especially when assessing skin colour, because diseases may appear in both areas. Techniques for examining these membranes are described in later chapters.

Artificial light often distorts colours and masks jaundice.

To sharpen your observations, you may wish to turn to the tables at the end of the chapter to better identify skin colours and patterns and types of lesions that you may encounter during the examination.

SKIN

Inspect and palpate the skin, and note the following characteristics.

Colour.   Clients may notice a change in their skin colour before the clinician does. Ask about it. Look for increased pigmentation (brownness), loss of pigmentation, redness, pallor, cyanosis, and yellowing of the skin.

See Table 10-1, Skin Colours (p. 259).

The red colour of oxyhemoglobin and the pallor in its absence are best assessed where the horny layer of the epidermis is thinnest and causes the least scatter: the fingernails, the lips, and the mucous membranes, particularly those of the mouth and the palpebral conjunctiva. In dark-skinned people, inspecting the palms and soles may also be useful.

Pallor from decreased redness in *anemia* and in decreased blood flow, as occurs in fainting or arterial insufficiency.

Central cyanosis is best identified in the lips, oral mucosa, and tongue. The lips, however, may turn blue in the cold, and melanin in the lips may simulate cyanosis in darker-skinned people.

Causes of *central cyanosis* include advanced lung disease, congenital heart disease, and abnormal hemoglobins.

Look for the yellow colour of jaundice in the sclera. Jaundice may also appear in the palpebral conjunctiva, lips, hard palate, undersurface of the tongue, tympanic membrane, and skin.

Jaundice suggests liver disease or excessive hemolysis of red blood cells.

Cyanosis of the nails, hands, and feet may be central or peripheral in origin. Anxiety or a cold examining room may cause peripheral cyanosis.

Cyanosis in congestive heart failure is usually peripheral, reflecting decreased blood flow, but in pulmonary edema, it may also be central. Venous obstruction may cause peripheral cyanosis.

For the yellow colour that accompanies high levels of carotene, look at the palms, soles, and face.

Carotenemia

Moisture.   Examples are dryness, sweating, and oiliness.

Dryness in hypothyroidism; oiliness in acne.

Temperature.   Use the backs of your fingers to make this assessment. In addition to identifying generalized warmth or coolness of the skin, note the temperature of any red areas.

Generalized warmth in fever, *hyperthyroidism*; coolness in *hypothyroidism*. Local warmth of inflammation or cellulitis.

Texture.   Examples are roughness and smoothness.

Roughness in hypothyroidism; velvety texture in hyperthyroidism.

Mobility and Turgor.   Lift a fold of skin and note the ease with which it lifts up (mobility) and the speed with which it returns into place (turgor).

Decreased mobility in edema, *scleroderma*; decreased turgor in dehydration.

Lesions. Observe any lesions of the skin, noting their characteristics:

- Their *anatomic location and distribution* over the body. Are they generalized or localized? Do they, for example, involve the exposed surfaces, the intertriginous or skin fold areas, extensor or flexor areas, or acral (peripheral) areas? Do they involve areas exposed to specific allergens or irritants, such as wrist bands, rings, or industrial chemicals?

- Their *patterns and shapes.* For example, are they linear, clustered, annular (in a ring), arciform (in an arc), geographic, or serpiginous (serpent or worm-like)? Are they dermatomal, covering a skin band that corresponds to a sensory nerve root (see p. 262)?

- The *types of skin lesions* (e.g., macules, papules, vesicles, nevi). If possible, find representative and recent lesions that have not been traumatized by scratching or otherwise altered. Inspect them carefully and feel them.

- Their *colour.*

SKIN LESIONS IN CONTEXT

After familiarizing yourself with the basic types of lesions, review their appearances, as described in Tables 10-9 and 10-10 and in a well-illustrated textbook of dermatology. Primary skin lesions originate from previously healthy skin. Secondary skin lesions may arise from primary skin lesions and are the progression of the primary disease. Whenever you see a skin lesion, look it up in such a text. The type of lesions, their location, and their distribution, together with other information from the history and the examination, should equip you well for this search and, in time, for arriving at specific dermatologic diagnoses.

Assessing the Immobilized Client. People who are confined to bed, especially when they are emaciated, elderly, or neurologically impaired, are particularly susceptible to skin damage and ulceration. *Pressure sores* result when sustained compression obliterates arteriolar and capillary blood flow to the skin. Sores may also result from the shearing forces created by bodily movements. When a person slides down in bed from a partially sitting position, for example, or is dragged rather than lifted up from a supine position, the movements may distort the soft tissues of the buttocks and close off the arteries and arterioles within. Friction and moisture further increase the risk.

Assess every susceptible client by carefully inspecting the skin that overlies the sacrum, buttocks, greater trochanters, knees, and heels. Roll the client onto one side to see the sacrum and buttocks.

HAIR

Inspect and palpate the hair. Note its quantity, distribution, and texture.

Many skin disorders have typical distributions. Acne affects the face, upper chest, and back; psoriasis, the knees and elbows (among other areas); and *Candida* infections, the intertriginous areas. See patterns in Table 10-2, Skin Lesions—Anatomic Location and Distribution (p. 261).

Vesicles in a unilateral dermatomal pattern are typical of herpes zoster (Gnann & Whitley, 2002). See patterns in Table 10-3, Skin Lesions—Patterns and Shapes (p. 262).

See Table 10-4, Elevated Skin Lesions (pp. 263–264); Table 10-5, Depressed Skin Lesions (p. 267); Table 10-6, Vascular and Purpuric Lesions of the Skin (p. 268); Table 10-7, Skin Tumours (p. 269); and Table 10-8, Benign and Malignant Nevi (p. 270).

See Table 10-9, Skin Lesions in Context (pp. 271–272), and Table 10-10, Diseases and Related Skin Conditions (pp. 273-274).

See Table 10-11, Pressure Ulcers (p. 275).

Local redness of the skin warns of impending necrosis, although some deep pressure sores develop without antecedent redness. Ulcers may be seen.

Alopecia refers to hair loss—diffuse, patchy, or total. Sparse hair in hypothyroidism; fine silky hair in hyperthyroidism.

NAILS

Inspect and palpate the fingernails and toenails. Note their colour and shape and any lesions. Longitudinal bands of pigment may be seen in the nails of people who have darker skin.

See Table 10-12, Hair Loss (p. 276).

See Table 10-13, Findings in or Near the Nails (pp. 277–278).

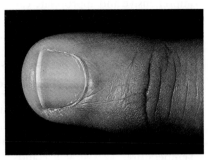

SPECIAL TECHNIQUES

Instructions for the Skin Self-Examination.
The CDA recommends regular self-examination of the skin using the following techniques. The client will need a full-length mirror, a hand-held mirror, and a well-lit room that provides privacy. Teach the client the **ABCDE** method for assessing moles (see p. XX), and show the client the photos of benign and malignant nevi presented in Table 10-8 on p. 270.

A Guide to Skin Cancer Self-Examination

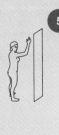

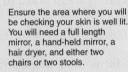
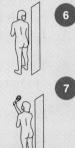

1. Ensure the area where you will be checking your skin is well lit. You will need a full length mirror, a hand-held mirror, a hair dryer, and either two chairs or two stools.

2. Remove all your clothing. To begin, raise your arms to waist height with your palms facing upwards. Examine your palms, fingers and forearms. Open your fingers and check the skin in between them. Turn your hands over and look at the backs of your hands, fingers, fingernails and forearms. Again, open your fingers and look at the skin in between them.

3. Now stand in front of the full length mirror. Raise your arms toward your chest. Your palms should be toward you. Look in the mirror to check the backs of your forearms and elbows.

4. Now lower your arms to your sides, with palms facing away from the mirror. You should be able to see the whole front of your body. Check your face, neck and arms. Turn your palms toward the mirror and check your upper arms and shoulders. Examine your chest, stomach, pubic area, thighs and lower legs.

5. Now turn your body sideways to the left. Raise your arms over your head. Your palms should be facing each other. Check the whole side of your body, starting at the top with your hands, moving to your arms, underarms, torso area, thighs, and calves. Finally, turn to the right and check the other side of your body in the same way.

6. Next, stand with your back toward the full length mirror. Check your buttocks and the backs of your thighs and calves.

7. For this step, you will need the hand-held mirror. Holding up the mirror in front of you and standing again with your back to the full length mirror, look at the back of your neck, your back and buttocks. Check the backs of your arms also.

8. Staying in the same position, examine your scalp. It is recommended that you use a hair dryer (on a cold air setting) to part your hair to reveal the skin. You may find this step difficult and are encouraged to have your partner or a friend conduct your scalp examination with the aid of the hair dryer.

9. Sitting down on the chair and with your right leg resting on the other chair or stool, look at the inside of your leg from the top of your thigh right down to your ankle, using the hand-held mirror if necessary. Now do the same with your left leg.

10. Remaining seated, bring your right leg over the left leg, resting your foot on your left knee. Using the hand-held mirror, if necessary, look at the top of your foot, your toes, toenails and the skin in between your toes. Check the bottom of your foot also. Now do the same so you can examine your left foot.

For more information or to view photos of what to look for, go to www.dermatology.ca.

Source: Used with permission from Canadian Dermatology Association.

RECORDING AND ANALYZING FINDINGS

Accurate documentation of the information obtained during the health history and physical examination of the skin needs to be thorough and clear for all members of the interdisciplinary team to ensure the planning and implementation of comprehensive and appropriate care for the client.

■ Examples of Documentation for Skin, Hair, and Nails

Area of Assessment	Expected Findings	Unexpected Findings
Skin colour	Pink, uniform colour bilaterally	Pale, bluish tinge around lips
Moisture	Moist, dry areas noted to elbows bilaterally	Excessive sweating noted to forehead and bilateral axillary areas
Temperature	Hands, forearms, shoulders warm bilaterally	Right hand, forearm, and shoulder warm. Left forearm and hand cool
Texture	Uniformly smooth, rough areas to elbows bilaterally	3-cm diameter rough area noted to dorsal surface of left hand
Mobility and turgor	Fold of skin returns of original position <1 second	Fold of skin remains tented for >5 seconds
Lesions	Smooth, uniform, no lesions noted bilaterally. Freckles to nose and cheeks bilaterally	1 cm × 2 cm bicoloured, irregularly shaped lesion to right upper cheek
Hair	Uniformly distributed over scalp (coarse, black, curly)	Patches of alopecia to left side of scalp
Nails	Intact, white with pinkish undertones, angle <180° bilaterally	Thickened, yellow with ragged edges, angle >180° bilaterally

ANALYZING FINDINGS FROM HEALTH HISTORY AND PHYSICAL EXAMINATION

After documenting the findings from the health history and physical examination, the nurse completes an analysis of the findings to identify a nursing diagnosis and plan an interdisciplinary approach. For example:

Ms. Jones, 23 years old, comes to the clinic with reports of dry, itchy, irritated skin over both hands and episodic blisters. She reports no previous health conditions, allergies, or medications. Ms. Jones recently completed a certificate program and began working as a lab technician in a major hospital. She reports no changes in the detergents, soaps, or cleaning solutions she uses in her household. From this information, you develop the following nursing diagnosis:

Impaired skin integrity *evidenced by open areas of skin on hands related to environmental exposures with potential for infection.*

To ensure comprehensive care for Ms. Jones, a physician or a dermatologist needs to perform a complete skin assessment and the nurse specializing in occupational health and environmental care needs to complete an assessment of exposure to hazardous substances.

Critical Thinking Exercise

Answer the following questions about Ms. Jones.

- What are the major functions of the skin? (*Knowledge*)
- What additional questions could you ask Ms. Jones to clarify her symptoms? (*Comprehension*)
- What information would you teach Ms. Jones about promoting healthy skin? (*Application*)

- What factors at the client's workplace might be aggravating the skin problems? (*Analysis*)
- What precautions at work, home, and leisure would benefit Ms. Jones? (*Synthesis*)
- How would you evaluate Ms. Jones' understanding of the teaching you have done? (*Evaluation*)

Canadian Research

Dutz, J. P. (2006). The skin as a site of initiation of systemic autoimmune disease: New opportunities for treatment. *The Journal of Investigative Dermatology, 126*(6), 1209–1212.

Freiman, A., Kalia, S., & O'Brien, E. A. (2006). Dermatologic signs. *Journal of Cutaneous Medicine and Surgery, 10*(4), 175–182.

Humphrey, S., Bergman J. N., & Au, S. (2006). Practical management strategies for diaper dermatitis. *Skin Therapy Letter, 11*(7), 1–6.

Lee, T. K., Rivers, J. K., & Gallagher, R. P. (2005). Site-specific protective effect of broad-spectrum sunscreen on nevus development among white schoolchildren in a randomized trial. *Journal of the American Academy of Dermatology, 52*(5), 786–792.

Lupin, M. H. (2006). Common bacterial skin infections. *Skin Therapy Letter. Family Practice Edition, 2*(2), 1–3.

Provost, N., Landells, I., & Maddin, S. (2006). Sunscreens—past, present, and future. *Journal of Cutaneous Medicine and Surgery*, (Suppl. 1), S14–S21.

Rivers, J. K., Wang, B., & Marcoux, D. (2006). Ultraviolet radiation exposure, public health concerns. *Journal of Cutaneous Medicine and Surgery*, (Suppl. 1), S8–S13.

Tan, A. W., & Dutz, J. P. (2006). Sclerotic skin disease: When smooth skin is unwelcome. *Expert Review of Dermatology, 1*(4), 487–492.

Yu, M., Finner, A., Shaprio, J., Lo, B., Barekatain, A., & McElwee, K. J. (2006). Hair follicles and their role in skin health. *Expert Review of Dermatology, 1*(6), 855–871.

Test Questions

1. Recommended protective measures to avoid skin cancer include which of the following?
   a. Avoiding sun exposure
   b. Knowing signs of skin cancer
   c. Performing monthly skin self-examinations
   d. Seeking biannual examination by clinician after age 40

2. One of the important functions of the skin is:
   a. synthesis of vitamin D.
   b. production of carotene.
   c. destruction of microorganisms.
   d. protection against melanin deposits.

3. When assessing a client's terminal hair distribution, the nurse inspects all of the following areas **except**:
   a. limbs.
   b. vertex.
   c. temples.
   d. palmar surfaces.

4. Which of the following terms refers to the arrangement of skin lesions?
   a. Annular
   b. Exposed
   c. Localized
   d. Generalized

5. The terms *generalized*, *exposed surfaces*, *upper arms*, and *skin folds* are used to describe which major characteristic of skin lesions?
   a. Type
   b. Colour
   c. Distribution
   d. Arrangement

Bibliography

CITATIONS

Canadian Broadcasting Corporation. (2004). *Body art: The story behind tattooing and piercing in Canada.* Retrieved March 7, 2008, from www.cbc.ca/news/background/tattoo/

Canadian Cancer Society. (2008a). *What is non-melanoma skin cancer?* Retrieved March 2, 2009, from www.cancer.ca/ccs/internet/standard/0,2939,3278_10175_87619_langID-en,00.html

Canadian Cancer Society. (2008b). *Vitamin D.* Retrieved June 15, 2007, from www.cancer.ca/ccs/internet/standard/0,3182,3225_1176359459_langID-en,00.html

Canadian Dermatology Association. (2008a). *Malignant melanoma.* Retrieved March 2, 2009, from www.dermatology.ca/patients_public/info_patients/skin_cancer/malignant_melanoma.html

Canadian Dermatology Association. (2008b). *Sun protection for children and teenagers.* Retrieved March 7, 2008, from www.dermatology.ca/sap/safety_resources/cancer/melanoma.html

Canadian Dermatology Association. (2008c). *Sun safety for outdoor workers.* Retrieved June 15, 2007, from www.dermatology.ca/outdoorworkers/index.html

Eastern Ontario Health Unit. (2005). *Adults: Tattooing and body piercing.* Retrieved March 7, 2008, from www.eohu.ca/segments/topics_e.php?segmentID=2&topicID=128

Gnann, J. G., & Whitley, R. J. (2002). Herpes zoster. *New England Journal of Medicine, 3247*(5), 340–346.

Health Canada. (2008). *It's your health: Tattooing and piercing.* Retrieved March 7, 2008, from www.hc-sc.gc.ca/iyh-vsv/life-vie/tat_e.html

Leger Marketing. (2002). *How Canadians feel about tattoos and body piercing.* Retrieved March 7, 2008, from www.legermarketing.com/documents/SPCLM/021230ENG.pdf

Public Health Agency of Canada. (1999). *Infection prevention and control practices for personal services: Tattooing, ear/body piercing, and electrolysis.* Retrieved March 7, 2008, from http://www.phac-aspc.gc.ca/publicat/ccdr-rmtc/99vol25/25s3/

Whited, J. D., & Grichnik, J. M. (1998). Does this client have a mole or a melanoma? The rational clinical examination. *Journal of the American Medical Association, 279*(9), 696–701.

ADDITIONAL READINGS

Bigby, M. C., Arndt, K. A., & Coopman, S. A. (2000). Skin disorders. In B. S. Levy & D. H. Wegman (Eds.), *Occupational health: Recognizing and preventing work-related disease and injury* (4th ed., pp. 537–552). Philadelphia: Lippincott Williams & Wilkins.

Canadian Dermatology Association. (2007). *Psoriasis.* Retrieved June 15, 2007, from www.dermatology.ca/patients_public/info_patients/psoriasis/index.html

Canadian Dermatology Association. (2007). *A guide to skin cancer self-examination.* Retrieved June 15, 2007, from www.dermatology.ca/patients_public/info_patients/skin_cancer/index.html

Canadian Dermatology Association. (2007). *Recognized sunscreens.* Retrieved June 15, 2007, from www.dermatology.ca/patients_public/info_patients/sun_safety/recognizedsunscreens/index.html

Canadian Dermatology Association. (2007). *Sunscreen FAQs.* Retrieved June 15, 2007, from www.dermatology.ca/patients_public/info_patients/sun_safety/sunscreen_faq.html

Canadian Dermatology Association. (2007). *Actinic (solar) keratoses.* Retrieved June 15, 2007, from www.dermatology.ca/patients_public/info_patients/skin_cancer/actinic_keratosis.html

Canadian Dermatology Association. (2007). *Basal cell skin cancer.* Retrieved June 15, 2007, from www.dermatology.ca/patients_public/info_patients/skin_cancer/basal_cell_skin_cancer.html

Canadian Dermatology Association. (2007). *Squamous cell skin cancer.* Retrieved June 15, 2007, from www.dermatology.ca/patients_public/info_patients/skin_cancer/squamous_cell_skin_cancer.html

Health Unit. (2007). *Sun safety.* Retrieved June 15, 2007, from www.healthunit.org/sunsafety/skincancerfacts.htm

Psoriasis Society of Canada. (2007). *Living with psoriasis.* Retrieved July 12, 2007, from www.psoriasissociety.org/living.htm

Stephen, T. C. (1997). Symptom analysis. In *Adult health assessment series* [CD-ROM]. Edmonton, AB: DataStar Education Systems & Services.

Stephen, T. C. (2004). Documentation. In *Health assessment self-test modules* (WebCT Vista). Edmonton, AB: Faculty of Nursing, University of Alberta.

Stephen, T.C. (2007). Assessment of integumentary function. In R. A. Day, P. Paul, B. Williams, S. C. Smeltzer, & B. G. Bare (Eds.), *Brunner and Suddarth's textbook of medical-surgical nursing* (1st Canadian ed., pp. 1646–1661). Philadelphia: Lippincott Williams & Wilkins.

Stephen, T. C. (2007). Management of clients with dermatologic problems. In R. A. Day, P. Paul, B. Williams, S. C. Smeltzer, & B. G. Bare (Eds.), *Brunner and Suddarth's textbook of medical surgical nursing* (1st Canadian ed., pp. 1662–1711). Philadelphia: Lippincott Williams & Wilkins.

Thompson, W. & Shapiro, J. (2002). Alopecia areata: Understanding and coping with hair loss. The John Hopkins University Press: Baltimore: MA.

Weber, J., & Kelley, J. (2007). *Health assessment in nursing* (3rd ed). Philadelphia: Lippincott Williams & Wilkins.

WEB SITES AND ASSOCIATIONS

Canadian Alopecia Areata Association: www.kumc.edu/gec/support/alopecia.html

The Canadian Association of Wound Care: www.cawc.net

Canadian Dermatology Association: www.dermatology.ca

Eczema Society of Canada: www.eczemacanada.ca

Health Canada: www.hc-sc.gc.ca/fn-an/index-eng.php

Lupus Canada: www.lupuscanada.org

Psoriasis Society of Canada: www.psoriasissociety.org

Rosacea Awareness Program: www.about-rosacea.com, www.rosacea.org

Sun Safety: www.healthunit.org

TABLE 10-1	Skin Colours

Changes in Pigmentation

Addison's disease (hypofunction of the adrenal cortex) or some pituitary tumours may cause a widespread increase in *melanin*. More common are local areas of increased or decreased pigment:

Café-Au-Lait Spot

A slightly but uniformly pigmented macule or patch with a somewhat irregular border, usually 0.5–1.5 cm in diameter and of no consequence. Six or more such spots, each with a diameter of >1.5 cm, however, suggest neurofibromatosis (p. 272). (The small, darker macules are unrelated.)

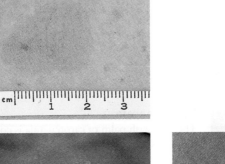

Tinea Versicolour

Common superficial fungal infection of the skin, causing hypopigmented, slightly scaly macules on the trunk, neck, and upper arms (short-sleeved shirt distribution). They are easier to see in darker skin and in some are more obvious after tanning. In lighter skin, macules may look reddish or tan instead of pale.

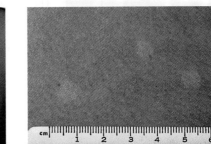

Vitiligo

In vitiligo, depigmented macules appear on the face, hands, feet, extensor surfaces, and other regions and may coalesce into extensive areas that lack melanin. The brown pigment is normal skin colour; the pale areas are vitiligo. The condition may be hereditary. These changes may be distressing to the client.

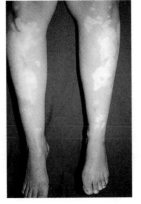

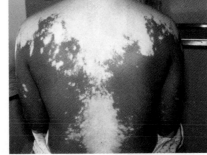

Cyanosis

Cyanosis is the somewhat bluish colour that is visible in the toenails and toes. Compare this colour with the pink fingernails and fingers of the same client. Impaired venous return in the leg caused this example of peripheral cyanosis. Cyanosis, especially when slight, may be hard to distinguish from typical skin colour.

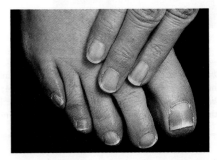

(table continues on next page)

TABLE 10-1 **Skin Colours** *(Continued)*

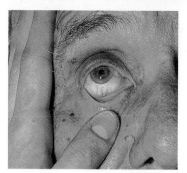

Jaundice

Jaundice makes the skin diffusely yellow. Note this client's skin colour, contrasted with the examiner's hand. The colour of jaundice is seen most easily and reliably in the sclera, as shown here. It may also be visible in mucous membranes. Causes include liver disease and hemolysis of red blood cells.

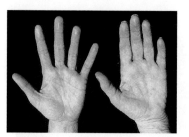

Carotenemia

The yellowish palm of carotenemia is compared with a pink palm, sometimes a subtle finding. Unlike jaundice, carotenemia does not affect the sclera, which remains white. The cause is a diet high in carrots and other yellow vegetables or fruits. Carotenemia is not harmful, but indicates the need for assessing dietary intake.

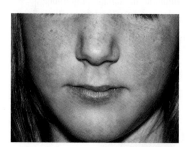

Erythema

Red hue, increased blood flow, seen here as the "slapped cheeks" of erythema infectiosum ("fifth disease").

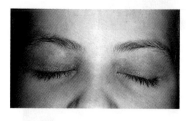

Heliotrope

Violaceous eruption over the eyelids in the collagen vascular disease dermatomyositis.

Photo sources: Tinea versicolour, Ostler, H. B., Mailbach, H. I., Hoke, A. W., & Schwab, I. R. *Diseases of the Eye and Skin: A Colour Atlas.* Philadelphia: Lippincott Williams & Wilkins, 2004; Vitiligo, erythema, Goodheart, H. P. *Goodheart's Photoguide of Common Skin Disorders: Diagnosis and Management,* 2nd ed. Philadelphia: Lippincott Williams & Wilkins, 2003; Heliotrope, Hall, J. C. *Sauer's Manual of Skin Diseases,* 9th ed. Philadelphia: Lippincott Williams & Wilkins, 2006.

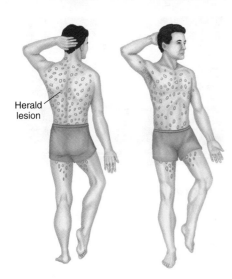

Pityriasis Rosea

Reddish oval ringworm-like lesions

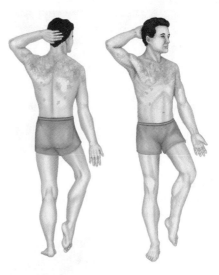

Tinea Versicolour

Tan, flat, scaly lesions

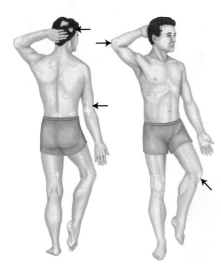

Psoriasis

Silvery scaly lesions, mainly on the
extensor surfaces

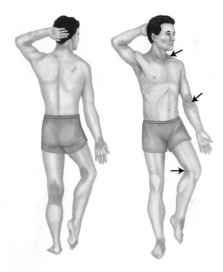

Atopic Eczema (adult form)

Appears mainly on flexor surfaces

Source: Hall, J. C., 2006.

| TABLE 10-3 | Skin Lesions—Patterns and Shapes |

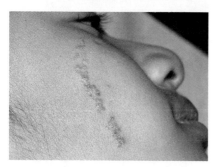

Linear

Example: Linear epidermal nevus

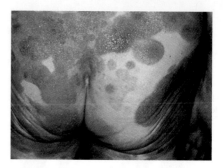

Geographic

Example: Mycosis fungoides

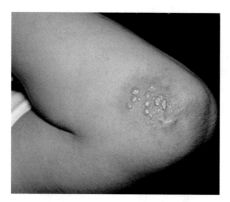

Clustered

Example: Grouped lesions of herpes simplex

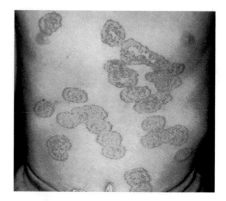

Serpiginous

Example: Tinea corporis

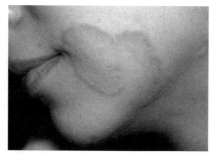

Annular, arciform

Example: Annular lesion of tinea faciale (ringworm)

Photo sources: Linear epidermal nevus, herpes simplex, tinea faciale, Goodheart, H. P. *Goodheart's Photoguide of Common Skin Disorders: Diagnosis and Management*, 2nd ed. Philadelphia: Lippincott Williams & Wilkins, 2003; Mycosis fungoides, tinea corporis, Hall, J. C. *Sauer's Manual of Skin Diseases*, 9th ed. Philadelphia: Lippincott Williams & Wilkins, 2006.

TABLE 10-4   Skin Lesions

Primary Lesions
Flat, Nonpalpable Lesions With Changes in Skin Colour
Macule—Small flat spot, up to 1.0 cm

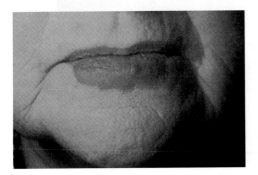

Hemangioma

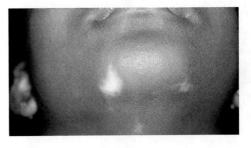

Vitiligo

Patch—Flat spot, 1.0 cm or larger

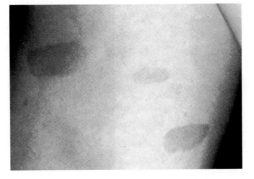

Café-au-lait spot

Palpable Elevations: Solid Masses
Plaque—Elevated superficial lesion 1.0 cm or larger, often formed by coalescence of papules

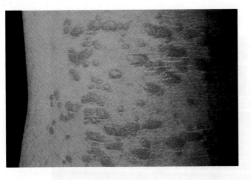

Psoriasis

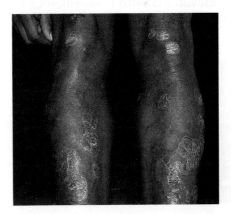

Psoriasis

(table continues on next page)

TABLE 10-4   **Skin Lesions** *(Continued)*

Papule—Up to 1.0 cm

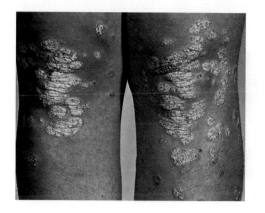

Psoriasis

Cyst—Nodule filled with expressible material, either liquid or semisolid

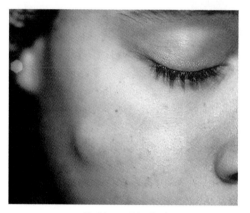

Epidermal inclusion cyst

Palpable Elevations With Fluid-Filled Cavities
Vesicle—Up to 1.0 cm; filled with serous fluid

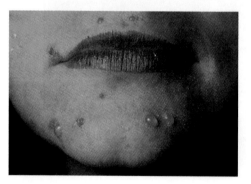

Herpes simplex

Nodule—Marble-like lesion larger than 0.5 cm, often deeper and firmer than a papule

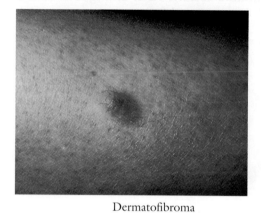

Dermatofibroma

Wheal—A somewhat irregular, relatively transient, superficial area of localized skin edema

Urticaria

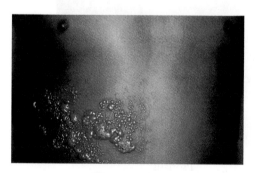

Herpes zoster

(table continues on next page)

TABLE 10-4   **Skin Lesions** *(Continued)*

Bulla—1.0 cm or larger; filled with serous fluid

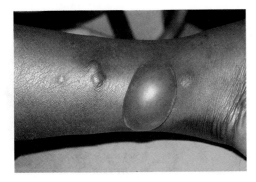

Insect bite

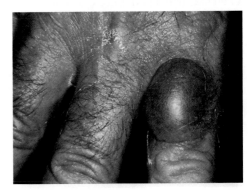

Insect bite

Pustule—Filled with pus

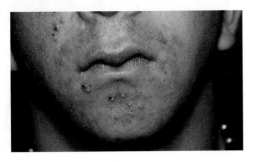

Acne

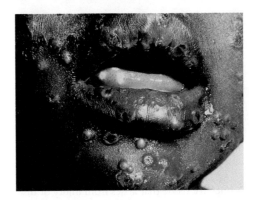

Smallpox

Burrow (scabies)—A minute, slightly raised tunnel in the epidermis, commonly found on the finger webs and on the sides of the fingers. It looks like a short (5–15 mm), linear, or curved grey line and may end in a tiny vesicle. Skin lesions include small papules, pustules, lichenified areas, and excoriations. With a magnifying lens, look for the *burrow* of the mite that causes scabies.

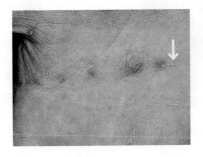

Scabies

(table continues on next page)

TABLE 10-4 | **Skin Lesions** *(Continued)*

Secondary Lesions (may arise from primary lesions)

Scale—A thin flake of dead exfoliated epidermis.

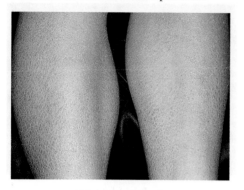

Ichthyosis vulgaris

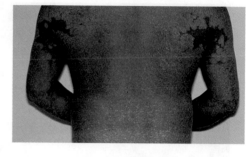

Dry skin

Crust—The dried residue of skin exudates such as serum, pus, or blood

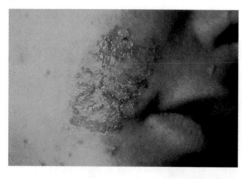

Impetigo

Lichenification—Visible and palpable thickening of the epidermis and roughening of the skin with increased visibility of the skin furrows (often from chronic rubbing)

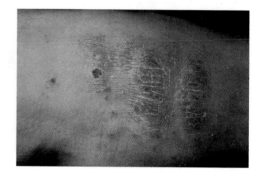

Neurodermatitis

Scars—Connective tissue that arises from injury or disease

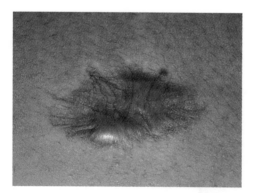

Hypertrophic scar from steroid injections

Keloids—Hypertrophic scarring that extends beyond the borders of the initiating injury

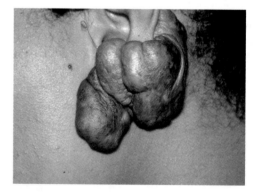

Keloid—ear lobe

Photo sources: Hemangioma, café-au-lait spot, elevated nevus, psoriasis (bottom), dermatofibroma, herpes simplex, insect bite (bottom), impetigo, lichenification, Hall, J. C. *Sauer's Manual of Skin Diseases,* 9th ed. Philadelphia: Lippincott Williams & Wilkins, 2000; Vitiligo, psoriasis (top), epidermal inclusion cyst, urticaria, insect bite (top), acne, ichthyosis, psoriasis, hypertrophic scar, keloids, Goodheart, H. P. *Goodheart's Photoguide of Common Skin Disorders: Diagnosis and Management,* 2nd ed. Philadelphia: Lippincott Williams & Wilkins, 2003; Small pox, Ostler, H. B., Mailbach, H. I., Hoke, A. W., & Schwab, I. R. *Diseases of the Eye and Skin: A Colour Atlas.* Philadelphia: Lippincott Williams & Wilkins, 2004.

TABLE 10-5   **Depressed Skin Lesions***

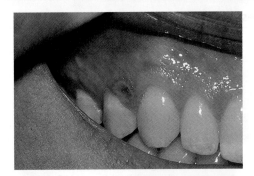

Erosion—Nonscarring loss of the superficial epidermis; surface is moist but does not bleed

Example: Aphthous stomatitis, moist area after the rupture of a vesicle, as in chickenpox

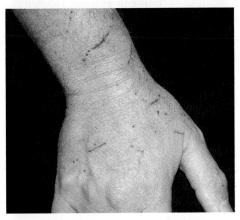

Excoriation—Linear or punctate erosions caused by scratching

Example: Cat scratches

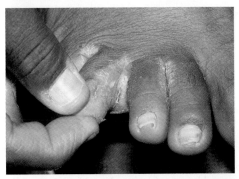

Fissure—A linear crack in the skin, often resulting from excessive dryness

Example: Athlete's foot

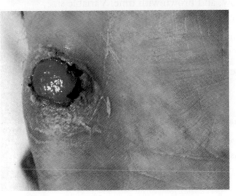

Ulcer—A deeper loss of epidermis and dermis; may bleed and scar

Examples: Stasis ulcer of venous insufficiency, syphilitic chancre

---

*These are secondary lesions (resulting from primary lesions).

Photo sources: Erosion, excoriation, fissure, Goodheart, H. P. *Goodheart's Photoguide of Common Skin Disorders: Diagnosis and Management,* 2nd ed. Philadelphia: Lippincott Williams & Wilkins, 2003; Ulcer, Hall, J. C. *Sauer's Manual of Skin Diseases,* 9th ed. Philadelphia: Lippincott Williams & Wilkins, 2006.

TABLE 10-6 Vascular and Purpuric Lesions of the Skin

Vascular Lesions

	Spider Angioma*	Spider Vein*	Cherry Angioma
	(image)	(image)	(image)
Colour and Size	Fiery red. From very small to 2 cm.	Bluish. Size variable, from very small to several inches.	Bright or ruby red; may become brownish with age. 1–3 mm.
Shape	Central body, sometimes raised, surrounded by erythema and radiating legs.	Variable. May resemble a spider or be linear, irregular, cascading.	Round, flat, or sometimes raised, may be surrounded by a pale halo.
Pulsatility and Effect of Pressure	Often seen in centre of the spider, when pressure with a glass slide is applied. Pressure on the body causes blanching of the spider.	Absent. Pressure over the centre does not cause blanching, but diffuse pressure blanches the veins.	Absent. May show partial blanching, especially if pressure applied with edge of a pinpoint.
Distribution	Face, neck, arms, and upper trunk; almost never below the waist.	Most often on the legs, near veins; also on the anterior chest.	Trunk; also extremities.
Significance	Liver disease, pregnancy, vitamin B deficiency; also occurs without associated illness in some people.	Often accompanies increased pressure in the superficial veins, as in varicose veins.	None; increase in size and numbers with aging.

Purpuric Lesions

	Petechia/Purpura	Ecchymosis
	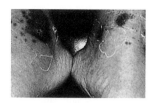	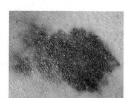
Colour and Size	Deep red or reddish purple, fading away over time. Petechia, 1–3 mm; purpura, larger.	Purple or purplish blue, fading to green, yellow, and brown with time. Variable size, larger than petechiae, >3 mm.
Shape	Rounded, sometimes irregular; flat.	Rounded, oval, or irregular; may have a central subcutaneous flat nodule (a hematoma).
Pulsatility and Effect of Pressure	Absent. No effect from pressure.	Absent. No effect from pressure.
Distribution	Variable.	Variable.
Significance	Blood outside the vessels; may suggest a bleeding disorder or, if petechiae, emboli to skin; palpable purpura in *vasculitis*.	Blood outside the vessels; often secondary to bruising or trauma; also seen in bleeding disorders.

*These are telangiectasias or dilated small vessels that look red or bluish.

Photo sources: Spider angioma, Marks, R. *Skin Disease in Old Age.* Philadelphia: JB Lippincott, 1987; Petechia/purpura, Kelley, W. N. *Textbook of Internal Medicine.* Philadelphia: JB Lippincott, 1989.

TABLE 10-7	Skin Tumours

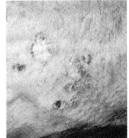
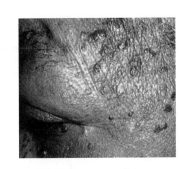

Actinic Keratosis

Superficial, flattened papules covered by a dry scale. Often multiple; can be round or irregular; pink, tan, or greyish. Appear on sun-exposed skin of older, fair-skinned people. Though benign, 1 of every 1000 per year develop into squamous cell carcinoma (suggested by rapid growth, induration, redness at the base, and ulceration). Keratoses on face and hand, typical locations, are shown.

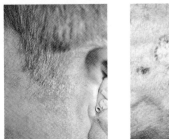

Seborrheic Keratosis

Common, benign, yellowish to brown raised lesions that feel slightly greasy and velvety or warty and have a "stuck on" appearance. Typically multiple and symmetrically distributed on the trunk of older people but may also appear on the face and elsewhere. In black people, often younger women, may appear as small, deeply pigmented papules on the cheeks and temples (dermatosis papulosa nigra).

Basal Cell Carcinoma

A basal cell carcinoma, although malignant, grows slowly and seldom metastasizes. It is most common in fair-skinned adults older than 40 years and usually appears on the face. An initial translucent nodule spreads, leaving a depressed centre and a firm, elevated border. Telangiectatic vessels are often visible.

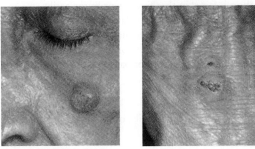
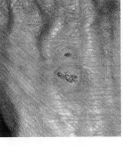

Squamous Cell Carcinoma

Usually appears on sun-exposed skin of fair-skinned adults older than 60 years. May develop in an actinic keratosis. Usually grows more quickly than a basal cell carcinoma, is firmer, and looks redder. The face and the back of the hand are often affected, as shown here.

TABLE 10-8   Benign and Malignant Nevi

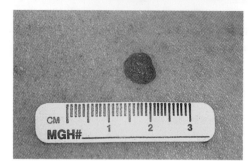

Benign Nevus

The *benign nevus*, or common mole, usually appears in the first few decades. Several nevi may arise at the same time, but their appearance usually remains unchanged. Note the following typical features and contrast them with those of atypical nevi and melanoma:

- Round or oval shape
- Sharply defined borders
- Uniform colour, especially tan or brown
- Diameter <6 mm
- Flat or raised surface

Changes in these features raise the spectre of *atypical (dysplastic) nevi* or melanoma. Atypical nevi are varied in colour but often dark and larger than 6 mm, with irregular borders that fade into the surrounding skin. Look for atypical nevi primarily on the trunk. They may number more than 50–100.

Malignant Melanoma

ABCDE: Screening Moles for Possible Melanoma

A for asymmetry (Fig. A)

B for borders; look for irregular edges, ragged or notched, and imprecise (Fig. B)

C for colour; look for variation or change in colour with brown, black, red, grey, or white areas (Fig. C)

D for diameter; look for growth in size of the lesion larger than a pencil eraser (width)

E for evolution; look for change in size, shape, symptoms (itchiness, tenderness), surface elevation, bleeding, or colour

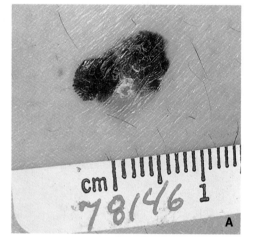

Review melanoma risk factors such as intense year-round sun exposure, blistering sunburns in childhood, fair skin that freckles or burns easily (especially if blond or red hair), family history of melanoma, and nevi that are changing or atypical, especially if the client is older than 50 years. Changing nevi may have new swelling or redness beyond the border, scaling, oozing, or bleeding, or sensations such as itching, burning, or pain.

On darker skin, look for melanomas under the nails, on the hands, or on the soles of the feet.

Source: Courtesy of American Cancer Society; American Academy of Dermatology.

TABLE 10-9   **Skin Lesions in Context**

This table shows a variety of primary and secondary skin lesions. Try to identify them, including those indicated by letters, before reading the accompanying text.

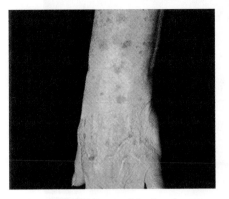

Macules on the dorsum of the hand, wrist, and forearm (*actinic lentigines*)

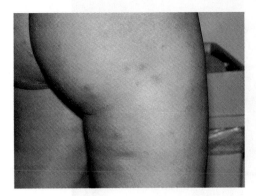

Papules and pustules (in hot tub folliculitis from *Pseudomonas*)

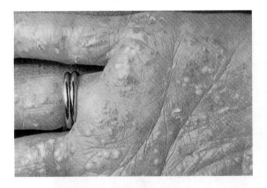

Pustules on the palm (in *pustular psoriasis*)

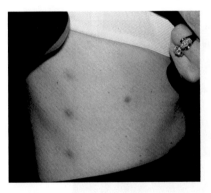

Vesicles (*chicken pox*)

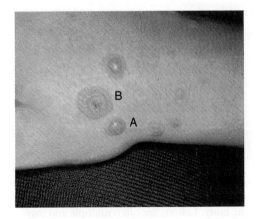

(A) Bulla, (B) target (or iris) lesion (in *erythema multiforme*)

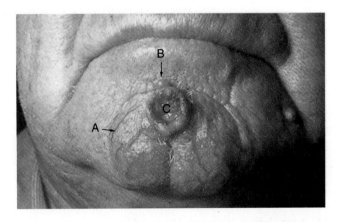

(A) Telangiectasia, (B) nodule, (C) ulcer (in *squamous cell carcinoma*)

(table continues on next page)

TABLE 10-9   **Skin Lesions in Context** *(Continued)*

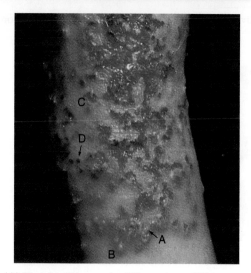

(A) Vesicle, (B) pustule, (C) erosions, (D) crust, on the back of a knee (in *infected atopic dermatitis*)

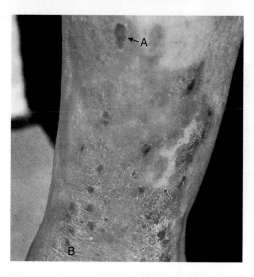

(A) Excoriation, (B) lichenification on the leg (in *atopic dermatitis*)

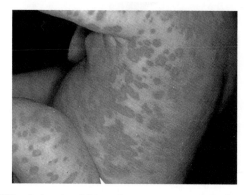

Wheals (*urticaria*) in a drug eruption in an infant

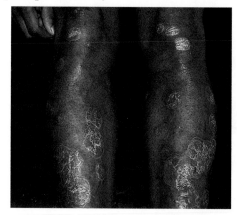

Plaques with scales on knee (*psoriasis*) and legs

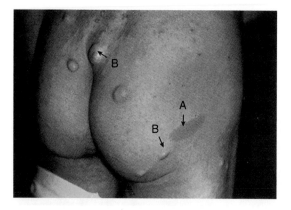

(A) Patch (café-au-lait spots), (B) nodules—a combination typical of neurofibromatosis.

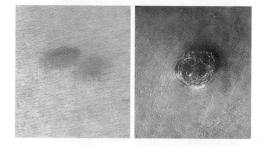

Kaposi's sarcoma in AIDS: This malignant tumour may appear in many forms: macules, papules, plaques, or nodules almost anywhere on the body. Lesions are often multiple and may involve internal structures. On left: ovoid, pinkish red plaques that typically lengthen along the skin line may become pigmented. On right: a purplish red nodule on the foot.

Photo sources: Hall, J. C. *Sauer's: Manual of Skin Diseases*, 9th ed. Philadelphia: Williams & Wilkins, Lippincott, 2006; Kaposi's sarcoma in AIDS, DeVita, V. T. Jr., Hellman, S., & Rosenberg, S. A. [eds]: *AIDS: Etiology, Diagnosis, Treatment, and Prevention*. Philadelphia: JB Lippincott, 1985; Psoriasis, papules, vesicles (chicken pox), Goodheart, H. P. *Goodheart's Photoguide of Common Skin Disorders: Diagnosis and Management*, 2nd ed. Philadelphia: Lippincott Williams & Wilkins, 2003.

TABLE 10-10   **Diseases and Related Skin Conditions**

Addison's disease	Hyperpigmentation of skin and mucous membranes
AIDS	Hairy leukoplakia, Kaposi's sarcoma, herpes simplex virus (HSV), human papillomavirus (HPV), cytomegalovirus (CMV), molluscum contagiosum, mycobacterial skin infections, candidiasis and other cutaneous fungal infections, oral and anal squamous cell carcinoma, acquired ichthyosis, bacterial abscesses, psoriasis (often severe), erythroderma, seborrheic dermatitis (often severe)
Chronic renal disease	Pallor, xerosis, pruritus, hyperpigmentation, uremic frost, metastatic calcification in the skin, calciphylaxis, "half-and-half" nails, hemodialysis-related skin disease
CREST syndrome	Calcinosis, Raynaud's phenomenon, sclerodactyly, telangiectasias
Crohn's disease	Erythema nodosum, pyoderma gangrenosum, enterocutaneous fistulas, aphthous ulcers
Cushing's disease	Striae, skin atrophy, purpura, ecchymoses, telangiectasias, acne, moon facies, buffalo hump, hypertrichosis
Dermatomyositis	Heliotrope rash, Gottron's papules, periungual telangiectasias, alopecia, poikiloderma in sun-exposed areas, Raynaud's phenomenon
Diabetes	Necrobiosis lipoidica diabeticorum, diabetic bullae, diabetic dermopathy, granuloma annulare, acanthosis nigricans, candidiasis, neuropathic ulcers, eruptive xanthomas, peripheral vascular disease
Disseminated intravascular coagulation	Skin necrosis, petechiae, ecchymoses, hemorrhagic bullae, purpura fulminans
Dyslipidemias	Xanthomas (tendon, eruptive, and tuberous), xanthelasma (may occur in healthy people)
Gonococcemia	Erythematous macules to hemorrhagic pustules; lesions in acral distribution that can involve palms and soles
Hemochromatosis	Skin bronzing and hyperpigmentation
Hypothyroidism	Dry, rough, and pale skin; coarse and brittle hair; myxedema; alopecia (lateral third of the eyebrows to diffuse); skin cool to touch; thin and brittle nails
Hyperthyroidism	Warm, moist, soft, and velvety skin; thin and fine hair; alopecia; vitiligo; pretibial myxedema (in Graves' disease); hyperpigmentation (local or generalized)
Infective endocarditis	Janeway lesions, Osler nodes, splinter hemorrhages, petechiae
Kawasaki disease	Mucosal erythema (lips, tongue, and pharynx), strawberry tongue, cherry red lips, polymorphous rash (primarily on trunk), erythema of palms and soles with later desquamation of fingertips
Liver disease	Jaundice, spider angiomas and other telangiectasias, palmar erythema, Terry's nails, pruritus, purpura, caput medusae
Leukemia/lymphoma	Pallor, exfoliative erythroderma, nodules, petechiae, ecchymoses, pruritus, vasculitis, pyoderma gangrenosum, bullous diseases
Meningococcemia	Pink macules and papules, petechiae, hemorrhagic petechiae, hemorrhagic bullae, purpura fulminans
Neurofibromatoses 1 (von Recklinghausen's syndrome)	Neurofibromas, café au lait, freckling in the axillary and inguinal areas, plexiform neurofibroma
Pancreatitis (hemorrhagic)	Grey Turner sign, Cullen's sign, panniculitis
Pancreatic carcinoma	Panniculitis, migratory thrombophlebitis
Peripheral vascular disease	Dry, scaly, shiny atrophic skin; dystrophic, brittle toenails; cool skin; hairless shins; ulcers; pallor; cyanosis; gangrene

(table continues on next page)

TABLE 10-10   Diseases and Related Skin Conditions *(Continued)*

Pregnancy (physiologic changes)	Melasma, increased pigmentation of areolae, linea nigra, palmar erythema, varicose veins, striae, spider angiomas, hirsutism, pyogenic granuloma
Reiter's syndrome	Psoriasis-like skin and mucous membrane lesions, keratoderma blennorrhagicum, balanitis circinata
Rheumatoid arthritis	Vasculitis, Raynaud's phenomenon, rheumatoid nodules, pyoderma gangrenosum, rheumatoid papules, erythematous to salmon-coloured rashes
Rocky Mountain spotted fever	Erythematous rash that begins on wrists and ankles, then spreads to palms and soles; becomes more purpuric as it generalizes
Scleroderma	Thickened, taut, and shiny skin; ulcerations and pitted scars on fingertips; sclerodactyly; telangiectasias; Raynaud's phenomenon
Sickle cell	Jaundice, leg ulcers (malleolar regions), pallor
Syphilis	*1°:* Chancre (painless)
	2°: Rash ("the great imitator")—ham- to bronze-coloured, generalized, maculopapular rash that involves the palms and soles; pustules; condylomata lata; alopecia ("moth-eaten"); white plaques on oral and genital mucosa
	3°: Gummas, granulomas
Systemic lupus erythematosus	Photosensitivity, malar (butterfly) rash, discoid rash, alopecia, vasculitis, oral ulcers, Raynaud's phenomenon
Thrombocytopenic purpura	Petechiae, ecchymoses
Tuberous sclerosis	Adenoma sebaceum (angiofibromas), ash-leaf spots, shagreen patch, perungual fibromas
Ulcerative colitis	Erythema nodosum, pyoderma gangrenosum
Viral exanthems	*Coxsackie A (hand, foot, and mouth):* Oral ulcers; macules, papules, and vesicles on hands, feet, and buttocks
	Erythema infectiosum (fifth disease): Erythema of cheeks ("slapped cheeks") followed by erythematous, pruritic, reticulated (net-like) rash that starts on trunk and proximal extremities (rash worsens with sun, fever, and temperature changes)
	Roseola infantum (HSV 6): Erythematous, maculopapular, discrete rash (often fever present) that begins on head and spreads to involve trunk and extremities; petechiae on soft palate
	Rubella (German measles): Erythematous, maculopapular, discrete rash (often fever present) that begins on head and spreads to involve trunk and extremities, petechiae on soft palate
	Rubeola (measles): Erythematous, maculopapular rash that begins on head and spreads to involve trunk and extremities (lesions become confluent on face and trunk, but are discrete on extremities); Koplik spots on buccal mucosa
	Varicella (chicken pox): Generalized, pruritic, vesicular (vesicles on an erythematous base, "dewdrop on a rose petal") rash begins on trunk and spreads peripherally, lesions appear in crops and are in different stages of healing
	Herpes zoster (shingles): Pruritic, vesicular rash (vesicles on an erythematous base) in a dermatomal distribution

TABLE 10-11   **Pressure Ulcers**

Pressure ulcers, also termed *decubitus* ulcers, usually develop over body prominences subject to unrelieved pressure, resulting in ischemic damage to underlying tissue. Prevention is important: inspect the skin thoroughly for *early warning signs* of erythema that blanches with pressure, especially in clients with risk factors.

Pressure ulcers form most commonly over the sacrum, ischial tuberosities, greater trochanters, and heels. A commonly applied staging system, based on depth of destroyed tissue, is illustrated here. Note that necrosis or eschar must be debrided before ulcers can be staged; ulcers may not progress sequentially through the four stages.

Inspect ulcers for signs of infection (drainage, odour, cellulitis, or necrosis). Fever, chills, and pain suggest underlying osteomyelitis. Address the client's overall health, including *comorbid conditions* such as vascular disease, diabetes, immune deficiencies, collagen vascular disease, malignancy, psychosis, or depression; nutritional status; pain and level of analgesia; risk for recurrence; psychosocial factors such as learning ability, social supports, and lifestyle; and evidence of polypharmacy, overmedication, or abuse of alcohol, tobacco, or illicit drugs.

Risk Factors for Pressure Ulcers

- Decreased mobility, especially if accompanied by increased pressure or movement causing friction or shear stress
- Decreased sensation, from brain or spinal cord lesions or peripheral nerve disease

- Decreased blood flow from hypotension or microvascular disease such as diabetes or atherosclerosis
- Fecal or urinary incontinence
- Presence of fracture
- Poor nutritional status or low albumin

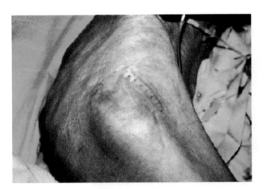

Stage I
Pressure-related alteration of intact skin, with changes in temperature (warmth or coolness), consistency (firm or boggy), sensation (pain or itching), or colour (red, blue, or purple on darker skin; red on lighter skin)

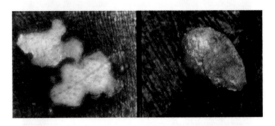

Stage II
Partial-thickness skin loss or ulceration involving the epidermis, dermis, or both

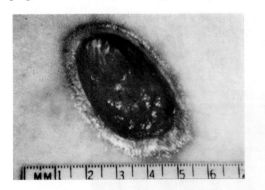

Stage III
Full-thickness skin loss, with damage to or necrosis of subcutaneous tissue that may extend to, but not through, underlying muscle

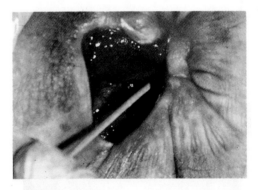

Stage IV
Full-thickness skin loss, with destruction, tissue necrosis, or damage to underlying muscle, bone, or supporting structures

Source: National Pressure Ulcer Advisory Panel, Reston, VA.

TABLE 10-12   Hair Loss

Alopecia Areata

Clearly demarcated round or oval patches of hair loss, usually affecting young adults and children. There is no visible scaling or inflammation.

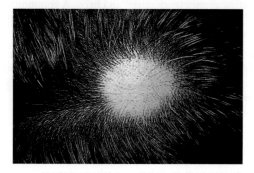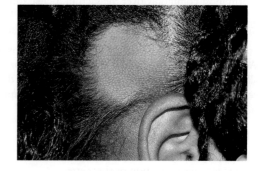

Trichotillomania

Hair loss from pulling, plucking, or twisting hair. Hair shafts are broken and of varying lengths. More common in children, often in settings of family or psychosocial stress.

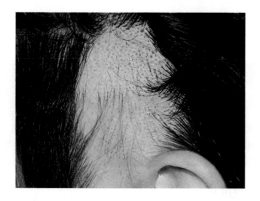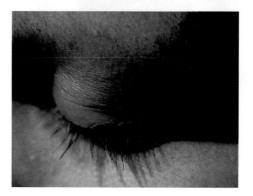

Tinea Capitis ("Ringworm")

Round scaling patches of alopecia. Hairs are broken off close to the surface of the scalp. Usually caused by fungal infection from *tinea tonsurans*. Mimics seborrheic dermatitis.

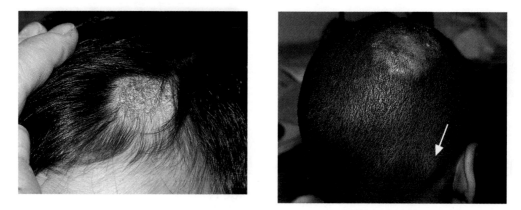

TABLE 10-13   **Findings In or Near the Nails**

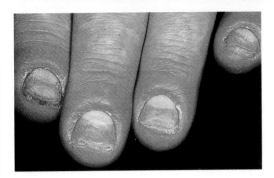

Paronychia

An inflammation of the proximal and lateral nail folds that may be acute or, as illustrated, chronic. The folds are red, swollen, and often tender. The cuticle may not be visible. People who frequently immerse their nails in water are especially susceptible. Multiple nails are often affected.

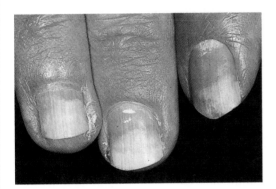

Onycholysis

A painless separation of the nail plate from the nail bed. It starts distally, enlarging the free edge of the nail to a varying degree. Several or all nails are usually affected. There are many causes.

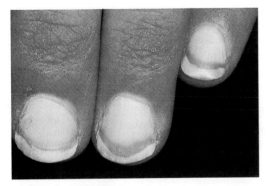

Terry's Nails

Nails are mostly whitish with a distal band of reddish brown. The lunulae of the nails may not be visible. Seen with aging and in people with chronic diseases such as cirrhosis of the liver, congestive heart failure, and type 2 diabetes.

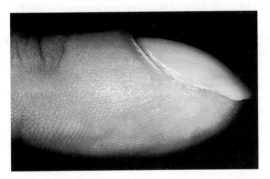

Clubbing of the Fingers

The distal phalanx of each finger is rounded and bulbous. The nail plate is more convex, and the angle between the plate and the proximal nail fold increases to 180° or more. The proximal nail fold, when palpated, feels spongy or floating. Causes are many, including chronic hypoxia from heart disease or lung cancer and hepatic cirrhosis.

(table continues on next page)

TABLE 10-13   **Findings In or Near the Nails** *(Continued)*

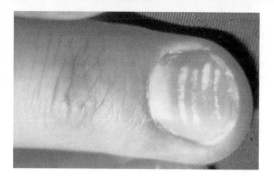

White Spots (Leukonychia)

Trauma to the nails is commonly followed by white spots that grow slowly out with the nail. Spots in the pattern illustrated are typical of overly vigorous and repeated manicuring. The curves in this example resemble the curve of the cuticle and proximal nail fold.

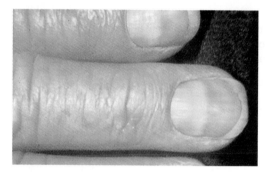

Transverse White Lines (Mees' Lines)

These are transverse lines, not spots, and their curves are similar to those of the lunula, not the cuticle. These uncommon lines may follow an acute or severe illness. They emerge from under the proximal nail folds and grow out with the nails.

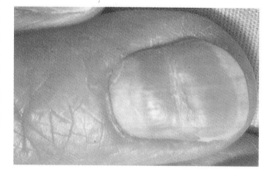

Beau's Lines

Beau's lines are transverse depressions in the nails associated with acute severe illness. The lines emerge from under the proximal nail folds weeks later and grow gradually out with the nails. As with Mees' lines, clinicians may be able to estimate the timing of a causal illness.

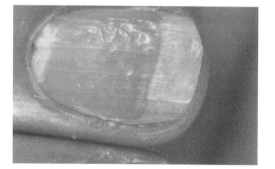

Psoriasis

Small pits in the nails may be early signs of psoriasis, but are not specific for it. Additional findings, not shown here, include onycholysis and a circumscribed yellowish tan discoloration known as an "oil spot" lesion. Marked thickening of the nails may develop.

Photo sources: Clubbing of the fingers, paronychia, onycholysis, Terry's nails, Habif, T. P. *Clinical Dermatology: A Colour Guide to Diagnosis and Therapy,* 2nd ed. St. Louis, MO: CV Mosby, 1990; White spots, transverse white lines, psoriasis, Beau's lines, Sams, W. M. Jr., & Lynch, P. J. *Principles and Practice of Dermatology.* New York, Churchill Livingstone, 1990.

The Head and Neck

11

Sheri Roach, Pat Roddick, and Lynn S. Bickley

Assessment of the head and neck focuses on the cranium, face, regional lymph nodes, and thyroid gland. Although it is neither desirable nor practical to ignore the eyes, ears, nose, and mouth during examination of this region, the focus of this chapter is the head and neck. It is essential not to overlook the remainder of the head and neck. Assessment of the eyes is covered in Chapter 12 and assessment of the ears, nose, mouth, and throat is described in Chapter 13.

There are several functions of the head and neck. The bone structure of the head protects the brain as well as the organs of vision, hearing, smell, and taste. The face is an important instrument of communication and the most immediate representation of the self to the world. Lymph nodes play a vital role in immune processes. The neck houses the trachea and upper esophagus, routes by which the body accesses oxygen and nourishment. The neck also contains the thyroid, the largest endocrine gland.

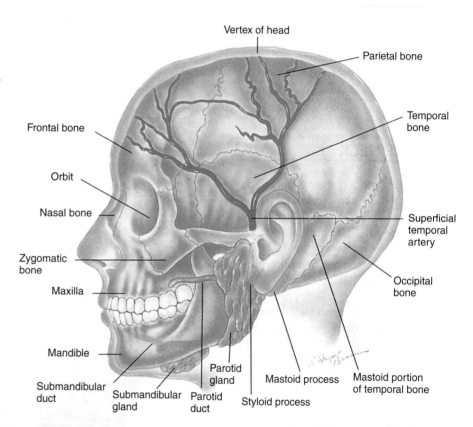

Vertex of head
Parietal bone
Temporal bone
Frontal bone
Orbit
Nasal bone
Superficial temporal artery
Zygomatic bone
Occipital bone
Maxilla
Mandible
Parotid gland
Mastoid process
Mastoid portion of temporal bone
Submandibular duct
Submandibular gland
Parotid duct
Styloid process

ANATOMY AND PHYSIOLOGY

THE HEAD

Regions of the head take their names from the underlying bones of the skull, for example, the frontal area. Knowing this anatomy helps to locate and describe physical findings.

The skull is covered by muscle and skin commonly called the *scalp*, which is nurtured by blood vessels. The facial bones provide protective cavities for sensory organs and structure for the face, whereas the many facial muscles enable movement and expression.

The temporomandibular joint, where the mandible attaches to the rest of the face, facilitates the movements required for chewing and talking. Two sets of paired salivary glands lie near the mandible: the *parotid glands*, on either side of the face, superficial to and behind the mandible (both visible and palpable when enlarged); and the *submandibular glands*, located inferior to the mandible underneath the base of the tongue. The openings for the parotid and submandibular ducts are visible within the oral cavity (see p. XX).

The *superficial temporal artery* passes upward just in front of the ear, where it is readily palpable. In many people, especially those who are thin and elderly, the tortuous course of one of its branches can be traced across the forehead.

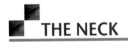

THE NECK

The neck supports the cranium. It consists of the seven cervical vertebrae as well as muscles and ligaments, covered by skin. The neck has several major blood vessels, the hyoid bone, the larynx, the trachea, lymph nodes, and the thyroid gland.

Muscles. The primary neck muscles are the *sternomastoid* (*sternocleidomastoid*), which rotates and flexes the head, and the *trapezius*, which extends the head and moves the shoulders.

For descriptive purposes, divide each side of the neck into two triangles bounded by the sternomastoid. Visualize the borders of the two triangles as follows:

- For the *anterior triangle:* the mandible above, the sternomastoid laterally, and the midline of the neck medially.

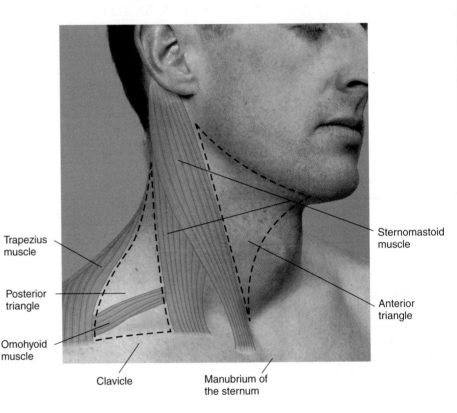

Trapezius muscle

Posterior triangle

Omohyoid muscle

Clavicle

Sternomastoid muscle

Anterior triangle

Manubrium of the sternum

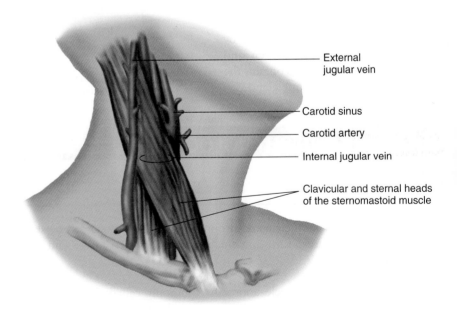

External jugular vein

Carotid sinus

Carotid artery

Internal jugular vein

Clavicular and sternal heads of the sternomastoid muscle

■ For the *posterior triangle:* the sterno-mastoid muscle, the trapezius, and the clavicle. Note that a portion of the omohyoid muscle crosses the lower portion of this triangle and can be mistaken for a lymph node or mass.

Great Vessels. Deep to the sterno-mastoids run the great vessels of the neck: the *carotid artery* and the *internal jugular vein.* The *external jugular vein* passes diagonally over the surface of the sternomastoid and may be helpful when trying to identify the jugular venous pressure (see p. 433).

Midline Structures and Thyroid Gland. Now identify the following midline structures: (1) the mobile *hyoid bone* just below the mandible, (2) the *thyroid cartilage*, readily identified by the notch on the superior edge (larger in males than in females), (3) the *cricoid cartilage*, (4) the *tracheal rings*, and (5) the *thyroid gland*.

The isthmus, which connects the right and left lobes of the thyroid gland, lies across the trachea below the cricoid. The lateral lobes of the thyroid gland curve posteriorly around the sides of the trachea and esophagus. Except in the midline, thin strap-like muscles cover the thyroid gland, among which only the sternomastoids are visible. Women have larger and more easily palpable thyroids than men.

Lymph Nodes. The *lymph nodes* of the head and neck have been classified in various ways. One classification is shown here, together with the directions of lymphatic drainage. The deep cervical chain is largely obscured by the overlying sternomastoid muscle, but at its two extremes, the tonsillar node and supraclavicular nodes may be palpable. The submandibular nodes lie superficial to the submandibular gland, from which they should be differentiated. Nodes are normally round or ovoid, smooth, and smaller than this gland. The gland is larger and has a lobulated, slightly irregular surface (see p. 279).

Note that the tonsillar, submandibular, and submental nodes drain portions of the mouth and throat as well as the face.

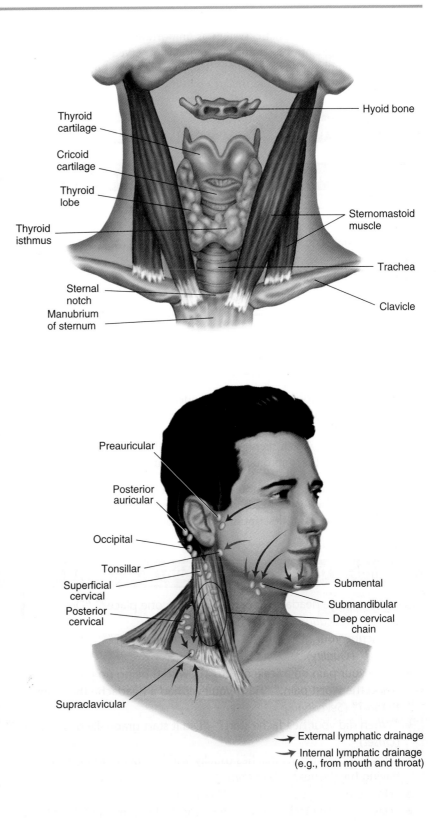

Thyroid cartilage
Cricoid cartilage
Thyroid lobe
Thyroid isthmus
Sternal notch
Manubrium of sternum
Hyoid bone
Sternomastoid muscle
Trachea
Clavicle

Preauricular
Posterior auricular
Occipital
Tonsillar
Superficial cervical
Posterior cervical
Supraclavicular
Submental
Submandibular
Deep cervical chain

→ External lymphatic drainage
→ Internal lymphatic drainage (e.g., from mouth and throat)

Knowledge of the lymphatic system is important to a sound clinical habit: Whenever a malignant or inflammatory lesion is observed, look for involvement of the regional lymph nodes that drain it; whenever a node is enlarged or tender, look for a source such as infection in the area that it drains.

THE HEALTH HISTORY: SUBJECTIVE DATA

Key Symptoms and Signs Reported by Client

- Headache
- Neck pain
- Scalp itchiness
- Swollen glands (salivary, lymphatic, or thyroid)
- Increased sweating
- Weight gain or loss

THE HEAD

Begin the health history by asking open-ended questions, such as "What concerns bring you to the clinic today?" or "Describe any concerns about how you are feeling." Responses to these questions allow the examiner to identify what concerns the client the most, which then guides the health history. If the client identifies a symptom, analyze the symptom to gain as much information as possible.

Headache is an extremely common symptom that always requires careful evaluation because a small fraction of headaches arise from life-threatening conditions. It is important to elicit a full description of the headache and all 10 attributes of the client's pain.

Example of Questions for Symptom/Sign Analysis—Headache

- "Where is the headache located?" "Is it in one place?" "Does it change places?" (*Location, Radiating*)
- "Describe your headache." "Is the pain throbbing?" "Steady?" "Sharp?" "Dull?" (*Quality*)
- "Rate your pain on a scale of 0 to 10, with 0 being no pain and 10 being the worst pain." "Have you ever had a headache this painful before?" (*Severity*)
- "When did your headache start?" "Did it start gradually or suddenly?" (*Onset*)
- "How long do the headaches usually last?" "How long have you been having headaches?" (*Duration*)
- "How often do you have them?" (*Frequency*)
- "Have your headaches stayed the same?" "Do they get better then worse?" (*Constancy*)
- "Do your headaches occur at a particular time of day?" (*Time of day/month/year*)
- "What makes your headache worse?" "Does anything trigger your headaches?" (*Aggravating factors*)

(continued)

See Tables 11-1, Primary Headaches (p. 294) and 11-3 Secondary Headaches (p. 296). *Tension* and *migraine headaches* are the most common kinds of recurring headaches.

Tension headaches often arise in the temporal areas; cluster headaches may be retro-orbital.

Changing or progressively severe headaches increase the likelihood of *tumour, abscess,* or other *mass lesion.* Extremely severe headaches suggest *subarachnoid hemorrhage* or *meningitis.*

Visual aura or scintillating scotomas with *migraine* (Goadsby, Lipton, & Ferrari, 2002). Nausea and vomiting are common with migraine but also occur with brain tumours and subarachnoid hemorrhage.

Coughing, sneezing, or changing head position may increase pain from brain tumour and acute sinusitis.

Family history may be positive in clients with migraine.

- "What makes it (headache) better?" (*Alleviating factors*)
- "Do you have any other symptoms, such as nausea? Vomiting? Dizziness? Vision changes with your headache?" (*Associated symptoms*)
- "Have you recently changed anything in your home or office?" "Have you had any recent head injuries?" "How much stress is in your life right now?" (*Environmental factors*)
- "How do your headaches affect your life?" (*Significance to client*)

THE NECK

Assess neck pain, stiffness, or restricted motion and investigate underlying causes.

Neck pain may indicate problems with musculature or the cervical spinal cord. Stress and tension may exacerbate neck pain. Sudden onset of head and neck pain or stiffness with elevated temperature could indicate *meningitis*.

Inquire about neck range of motion.

Older clients with *osteoporosis* or *arthritis* may have decreased range of motion.

Ask "Have you noticed any swollen glands or lumps in your neck?" because clients are more familiar with the lay terms than with "lymph nodes."

Enlarged tender lymph nodes commonly accompany pharyngitis.

Assess thyroid function and ask about any evidence of an enlarged thyroid gland or *goitre*. To evaluate thyroid function, ask about *temperature intolerance* and *sweating*. Opening questions include, "Do you prefer hot or cold weather?" "Do you dress more warmly or less warmly than other people?" "What about blankets . . . do you use more or fewer than others at home?" "Do you perspire more or less than others?" "Any new palpitations or change in weight?" Note that as people grow older, they sweat less, have less tolerance for cold, and tend to prefer warmer environments.

With goitre thyroid function may be increased, decreased, or normal.

Intolerance to cold, preference for warm clothing and many blankets, and decreased sweating suggest *hypothyroidism*; the opposite symptoms, palpitations and involuntary weight loss, suggest *hyperthyroidism* (p. 285).

HEALTH PROMOTION

Important Topics for Health Promotion

- Injury prevention
- Thyroid health

SPECIFIC PREVENTION FOR SPECIFIC DISEASES

Head and Neck Injuries. The skull, approximately 2 centimetres thick, is the only protection for the human brain. Each year, more than 11,000 Canadians die from traumatic brain injuries (TBIs) (Brain Injury Awareness Month, 2004). Brain injuries following a blow to the head or spinning forces on the brain are the leading cause of death in Canadian children (Brain Injury Awareness Month, 2004). The positive effects of health-promotion activities are evident in the decreased

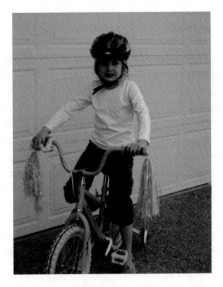

number of hospital admissions related to head trauma following the introduction of bike-helmet legislation in several provinces between 1994 and 2004. That decade saw 50% fewer people younger than 19 years admitted to hospitals for TBIs (Canadian Institute for Health Information, 2006a). Falls and motor vehicle collisions cause the vast majority of TBIs in Canadian adults (Canadian Institute for Health Information, 2006b). Health-promotion activities related to both of these preventable events are essential. Health care providers should note that the risk of a second TBI is three times greater following an initial TBI.

TBIs accounted for 45% of 488 work-related fatalities in Ontario from 1996 to 2000. Work-related deaths from TBIs were most often a consequence of falls (Tricco, Colantonio, Chipman, Liss, & McLellan, 2006).

Spinal cord injuries affect approximately 900 Canadians each year (Canadian Paraplegic Association [CPA], 2007). Causes include motor vehicle collisions (35%), falls (16.5%), medical conditions (10.8%), sports (6.7%), diving (5.3%), work-related injuries (5.3%), and other (14.2%). People engaging in high-risk sports and activities (e.g., skydiving, contact sports, climbing, auto racing) are at higher risk for injuries to the head and neck. Workers in construction and other environments with exposure to heavy equipment and falls, as well as clients who do not follow appropriate use of protective equipment during leisure and activities, have an increased risk for head and neck injuries.

Health promotion related to head and neck injuries includes teaching clients about several elements of harm prevention:

■ Wear seatbelts in vehicles.

■ Avoid driving under the influence of alcohol or drugs.

■ Maintain awareness of the distracting influences of cell phones, loud music, food and beverages, and passengers when driving.

■ Wear appropriate helmets for cycling and other sports; replace helmets at recommended intervals or when damaged.

■ Use harnesses and hard hats as required at worksites.

■ Take advantage of safety training in occupational and recreational settings.

■ Assess environmental hazards and ensure the availability of adequate safety equipment to help prevent falls in the older adult population.

■ Do not dive into water of unknown depth.

Thyroid Health.   Studies indicate that 30% of Canadians have some problem involving the thyroid gland (Thyroid Foundation of Canada, 2007a). Clients at higher risk for thyroid dysfunction include postpartum women, the elderly, those with high levels of exposure to radiation, and clients with Down syndrome (Thyroid Foundation of Canada, 2007a). Thyroid dysfunction is associated with numerous health issues, including cardiac disease, lupus, reproductive difficulties, diabetes, and arthritis. Research has shown that early thyroid assessment may reduce the incidence or severity of these problems. Thyroid disease is more common in women than in men and develops more frequently in both sexes after 60 years. Important aspects of health promotion include supporting client awareness of thyroid health, improving client awareness of symptoms associated with a poorly functioning thyroid gland, and screening for thyroid dysfunction. A blood test for thyroid-stimulating hormone (TSH) usually can accurately determine thyroid activity.

To date, no recommendations in North America exist for routine screening for thyroid disorders. Studies have shown no conclusive evidence of benefits or risks of thyroid function screening (U.S. Preventive Services Task Force, 2004). Current practice recommends that clinicians be aware of clients at increased risk of problems and identify early signs of dysfunction.

Hyperthyroidism. *Hyperthyroidism* results from an overactive thyroid gland. Most cases (90%) are related to Graves' disease, an autoimmune disorder in which an overstimulated thyroid releases too much thyroid hormone. Signs and symptoms of hyperthyroidism include rapid, forceful heartbeat; tremor; muscular weakness; weight loss despite increased appetite; anxiety; nervousness; irritability; insomnia; profuse sweating; diarrhea; eye changes; and goitre. Hyperthyroidism has no standard treatment; however, some options include antithyroid drugs, thyroidectomy, and administration of radioactive iodine.

Hypothyroidism. *Hypothyroidism* occurs when the thyroid gland does not produce enough hormones to maintain adequate metabolism and body functioning. Because the pituitary and hypothalamus glands stimulate the thyroid gland, disorders of these glands may lead to hypothyroidism. Other causes include thyroid disease, treatment for hyperthyroidism, and iodine deficiency because iodine is the main component of thyroid hormones.

Signs and symptoms of hypothyroidism include slow, weak heartbeat; muscular weakness; fatigue; increased sensitivity to cold; thick and puffy skin; mental sluggishness; depression; poor memory; constipation; and goitre (Thyroid Foundation of Canada, 2007b). Hypothyroidism is treated with a thyroid hormone replacement, which clients must take for the rest of their lives.

Cultural Considerations

Water and food intake provide the body with iodine. Some geographical areas have iodine deficiencies: for example, the Great Lakes areas of Canada and the United States. Although iodized salt is commonly used throughout North America, lack of dietary iodine may lead to increased incidence of thyroid disease in immigrant populations. Also, hypothyroidism is more prevalent in Caucasians than in African Canadians.

Goitre. *Goitre* is an enlargement of the thyroid gland. Clients may describe it as a swelling or lump in the neck; it may be one-sided or midline. Although it merits assessment, goitre does not always indicate disease. Physiological changes, such as during puberty or pregnancy, can cause goitre.

Thyroid Nodules. Thyroid nodules are common, treatable, and usually benign. Nevertheless, they should always be investigated because some cases are cancerous.

EMERGENCY CONCERNS

Careful assessment of the head and neck is necessary to ensure the prompt identification and treatment of potentially life-threatening or debilitating conditions. Several of the signs and symptoms of cerebral vascular accidents (strokes), aneurysms, brain injuries, infections, and spinal cord injuries are identified in the assessment of the head and neck. Severe headache (localized or not), facial paralysis or unilateral drooping, painful neck movement, sudden numbness or tingling, loss of consciousness, and sudden decrease in orientation may indicate serious problems requiring emergency assessment and intervention. Clients reporting that they are experiencing the "worst headache they have ever had" require immediate assessment. Head and neck injuries from motor vehicle collisions, sports injuries, falls, or other incidents also require emergency assessment. Lacerations to the head and face tend to bleed profusely because these areas are highly vascular. They may require emergency treatment to ensure cessation of blood loss and also for cosmetic considerations.

TECHNIQUES OF EXAMINATION: OBJECTIVE DATA

PROMOTING CLIENT COMFORT AND SAFETY

During examination of the head and neck, ask the client to sit comfortably on the edge of a bed or examination table, with the client's head at the nurse's eye level. Then, stand in front of the client, and move to either side as necessary. If the positioning of the bed or examination table in the room does not allow the examiner to stand behind the client to palpate the thyroid, ask the client to reposition himself or herself at this time. If repositioning is not possible, use the anterior approach.

Cultural Considerations

Muslim women from parts of the Persian Gulf, North Africa, Southeast Asia, and India may wear veils or head scarves that cover a part or most of their faces. These clients regard this apparel as a symbol of modesty and piety. Wearing such clothing is often a personal choice of Canadian immigrants from these regions. The veil and head coverings may be removed for the purposes of examination, when required. Consideration must be given to the relationship of any male who is present when the client's head is not covered.

Clients from some cultures, such as those of Southeast Asian descent, may prohibit others from touching their heads. Remember to consider the cultural norms for touch when assessing the head and neck.

Equipment

■ Disposable gloves
■ Glass of water

THE HEAD

Prior to examination ask the client to remove any hair coverings: hairpieces, wigs, jewelery, and hair accessories. Because abnormalities covered by the hair are easily missed, ask whether the client has noticed anything wrong with the scalp or hair.

Examine:

The Hair. Note its quantity, distribution, texture, and pattern of loss, if any. You may see loose flakes of dandruff.

Fine hair in *hyperthyroidism*; coarse hair in *hypothyroidism*. Tiny white ovoid granules that adhere to hairs may be nits, or lice eggs.

TECHNIQUES OF EXAMINATION: OBJECTIVE DATA	UNEXPECTED FINDINGS

The Scalp. Part the hair in several places and look for scaliness, lumps, nevi, or other lesions.

Redness and scaling in *seborrheic dermatitis*, *psoriasis*; *soft lumps of pilar cysts* (wens).

The Skull. Observe the general size and contour of the skull. Note any deformities, depressions, lumps, or tenderness. Learn to recognize the irregularities in a normal skull, such as those near the suture lines between the parietal and occipital bones.

Enlarged skull in *hydrocephalus*, *Paget's disease* of bone. Tenderness after trauma.

The Face. Note the client's facial expression and contours. Observe for asymmetry, involuntary movements, edema, and masses.

See Table 11-2, Selected Facies, p. 295.

 Cultural Considerations

Facial structures and features vary widely among people from different cultures.

The Skin. Observe the skin, noting its colour, pigmentation, texture, thickness, hair distribution, and any lesions.

Acne in many adolescents. *Hirsutism* (excessive facial hair) in some women with *polycystic ovary syndrome*.

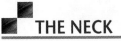 **THE NECK**

Inspect the neck, noting its symmetry and any masses or scars. Look for enlargement of the parotid or submandibular glands, and note any visible lymph nodes.

A scar of past thyroid surgery is often a clue to unsuspected thyroid disease.

The Lymph Nodes. *Palpate the lymph nodes.* Using the pads of your index and middle fingers, move the skin over the underlying tissues in each area. The client should be relaxed, with the neck flexed slightly forward and, if needed, slightly toward the side being examined. You can usually examine both sides at once. For the submental node, however, it is helpful to feel with one hand while bracing the top of the head with the other.

Feel in sequence for the following nodes:

1. *Preauricular*—in front of the ear.

2. *Posterior auricular*—superficial to the mastoid process.

3. *Occipital*—at the base of the skull posteriorly.

4. *Tonsillar*—at the angle of the mandible.

5. *Submandibular*—midway between the angle and the tip of the mandible. These nodes are usually smaller and smoother than the lobulated submandibular gland against which they lie.

A "tonsillar node" that pulsates is really the carotid artery. A small, hard, tender "tonsillar node" high and deep between the mandible and the sternomastoid is probably a styloid process.

6. *Submental*—in the midline a few centimetres behind the tip of the mandible.

7. *Superficial cervical*—superficial to the sternomastoid.

8. *Posterior cervical*—along the anterior edge of the trapezius.

9. *Deep cervical chain*—deep to the sternomastoid and often inaccessible to examination. Hook your thumb and fingers around either side of the sternomastoid muscle to find them.

10. *Supraclavicular*—deep in the angle formed by the clavicle and the sternomastoid.

Note their size, shape, delimitation (discrete or matted together), mobility, consistency, and any tenderness. Small, mobile, discrete, nontender nodes, sometimes termed "shotty," are frequently found.

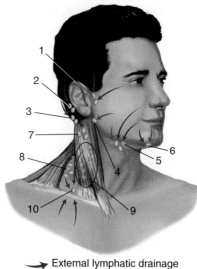

→ External lymphatic drainage
→ Internal lymphatic drainage
(e.g., from mouth and throat)

Enlargement of a supraclavicular node, especially on the left, suggests possible metastasis from a thoracic or an abdominal malignancy.

■ Using the pads of the second and third fingers, palpate the preauricular nodes with a gentle rotary motion. Then examine the posterior auricular and occipital lymph nodes.

■ Palpate the anterior cervical chain, located anterior and superficial to the sternomastoid. Then palpate the posterior cervical chain along the trapezius (anterior edge) and along the sternomastoid (posterior edge). Flex the client's neck slightly forward toward the side being examined. Examine the supraclavicular nodes in the angle between the clavicle and the sternomastoid.

Enlarged or tender nodes, if unexplained, call for (1) reexamination of the regions they drain and (2) careful assessment of lymph nodes elsewhere so that you can distinguish between regional and generalized lymphadenopathy.

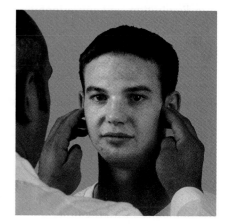

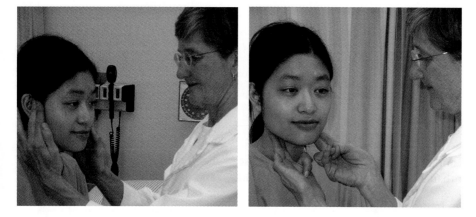

Occasionally, you may mistake a band of muscle or an artery for a lymph node. You should be able to roll a node in two directions: up and down, and side to side. Neither a muscle nor an artery will pass this test.

The Trachea and the Thyroid Gland.
To orient yourself to the neck, identify the thyroid and cricoid cartilages and the trachea below them.

Diffuse lymphadenopathy raises the suspicion of *HIV* or *AIDS*.

- *Inspect the trachea* for any deviation from its usual midline position. Then *feel for any deviation*. Place your finger along one side of the trachea and note the space between it and the sternomastoid. Compare it with the other side. The spaces should be symmetric.

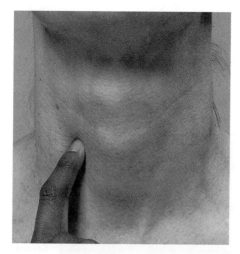

- *Inspect the neck for the thyroid gland.* Tip the client's head back a bit. Using tangential lighting directed downward from the tip of the client's chin, *inspect the region below the cricoid cartilage* for the gland. The lower, shadowed border of each thyroid gland shown here is outlined by arrows.

Tender nodes suggest inflammation; hard or fixed nodes suggest malignancy.

Masses in the neck may push the trachea to one side. Tracheal deviation may also signify important problems in the thorax, such as a mediastinal mass, atelectasis, or a large pneumothorax (see pp. 399).

The lower border of this large thyroid gland is outlined by tangential lighting. *Goitre* is a general term for an enlarged thyroid gland (McGuirt, 1989; Siminoski, 1995).

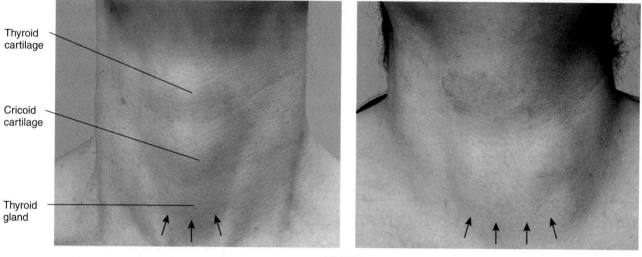

Thyroid cartilage

Cricoid cartilage

Thyroid gland

AT REST

Ask the client to sip some water and to extend the neck again and swallow. Watch for upward movement of the thyroid gland, noting its contour and symmetry. The thyroid cartilage, the cricoid cartilage, and the thyroid gland all rise with swallowing and then fall to their resting positions.

With swallowing, the lower border of this large gland rises and looks less symmetric.

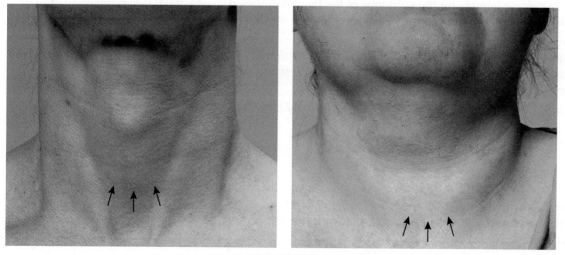

SWALLOWING

Until you become familiar with this examination, check your visual observations with your fingers from in front of the client. This will orient you to the next step.

You are now ready to *palpate the thyroid gland*. This may seem difficult at first. Use the cues from visual inspection. Find your landmarks—the notched thyroid cartilage and the cricoid cartilage below it. Locate the *thyroid isthmus*, usually overlying the second, third, and fourth tracheal rings.

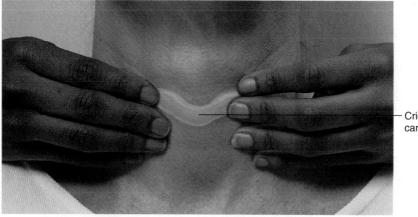

Cricoid cartilage

Adopt good technique, and follow the steps described, which outline the posterior approach (technique for the anterior approach is similar). With experience you will become more adept. The thyroid gland is usually easier to feel in a long slender neck than in a short stocky one. In shorter necks, added extension of the neck may help. In some people, however, the thyroid gland is partially or wholly substernal and not amenable to physical examination.

STEPS FOR PALPATING THE THYROID GLAND

- Ask the client to flex the neck slightly forward to relax the sternomastoid muscles.
- Place the fingers of both hands on the client's neck so that your index fingers are just below the cricoid cartilage.
- Ask the client to sip and swallow water as before. Feel for the thyroid isthmus rising up under your finger pads. It is often but not always palpable.
- Displace the trachea to the right with the fingers of the left hand; with the right-hand fingers, palpate laterally for the right lobe of the thyroid in the space between the displaced trachea and the relaxed sternomastoid. Find the lateral margin. In similar fashion, examine the left lobe.

  The lobes are somewhat harder to feel than the isthmus, so practice is needed. The anterior surface of a lateral lobe is approximately the size of the distal phalanx of the thumb and feels somewhat rubbery.

- Note the *size, shape,* and *consistency* of the gland and identify any *nodules* or *tenderness*.

If the thyroid gland is enlarged, listen over the lateral lobes with a stethoscope to detect a *bruit*, a sound similar to a cardiac murmur but of noncardiac origin.

Although physical characteristics of the thyroid gland, such as size, shape, and consistency, are diagnostically important, assessment of thyroid function depends on symptoms, signs elsewhere in the body, and labouratory tests (Surks et al., 2004; U.S. Preventive Services Task Force, 2004). See Table 11-4, Thyroid Enlargement and Function (p. 298).

Soft in Graves' disease; firm in Hashimoto's thyroiditis, malignancy. Benign and malignant nodules, (Hegedus, 2004) tenderness in thyroiditis.

A localized systolic or continuous bruit may be heard in hyperthyroidism.

The Carotid Arteries and Jugular Veins.   Defer a detailed examination of these vessels until the client lies down for the cardiovascular examination. Jugular venous distention, however, may be visible in the sitting position and should not be overlooked. You should also be alert to unusually prominent arterial pulsations. See Chapter 15 for further discussion.

Note: Many clinicians would complete examination of the cranial nerves (see pp. 362) at this point.

RECORDING AND ANALYZING FINDINGS

Documentation of findings related to client history and assessment of the head and neck are often combined with information gathered about the eyes, ears, nose, and throat. Accuracy and clear organization will ensure that information is easily accessible to all members of the health care team.

■ *Examples of Documentation for Head and Neck*

Area of Assessment	Expected Findings	Unexpected Findings
Hair	Evenly distributed, clean, brown	Thinning and patchy, lice visualized
Scalp	Even colouration, skin intact	Soft lump superior to right mastoid process that is painful to touch
Skull	Size proportional to body, symmetrical	Depressed, tender area on left temporal bone
Face	Symmetrical movement of facial muscles	Involuntary muscle spasms inferior to left eye
Skin	Smooth, consistent colour, intact	Excessive facial hair (hirsutism), acne on face and anterior neck
Neck	Full range of motion, symmetrical	Limited forward flexion of neck, enlargement on left side of trachea
Lymph nodes and salivary glands	Nonpalpable, nontender	Tonsillar lymph nodes palpable and tender to touch
Trachea and thyroid	Trachea midline, thyroid isthmus midline with palpable, nontender lobes	Trachea deviates to right; enlarged, visible thyroid gland with nodular tissue palpated on left side

■ ANALYZING FINDINGS FROM HEALTH HISTORY AND PHYSICAL EXAMINATION

Following collection of and documentation of assessment data, the nurse analyzes the information to determine a nursing diagnosis and form a holistic plan for client care. For example,

Mrs. White, 65 years old, comes to the clinic reporting that she has been feeling "generally unwell" for the past several months. She says her energy level is much lower than usual, she tires easily, and she often feels sad. Mrs. White also confides that although she has not changed her diet, she has recently had ongoing constipation. She had planned on working until she turned 70, but is considering earlier retirement because of how she has been feeling. Mrs. White has already cut back on volunteering at her community league and has stopped golfing weekly with her friends. Upon examination, you note swelling on the anterior neck. From this information, you develop the following nursing diagnosis:

Altered lifestyle related to potential thyroid dysfunction

To develop a holistic plan of care for Mrs. White, the nurse should refer the client to a physician for a thorough examination and blood tests for thyroid hormone levels. Mrs. White may also benefit from a psychological consultation to assess for depression. A dietary consultation could help Mrs. White address the constipation as well as potential deficiencies, such as iodine, that could be contributing to her health issues. If she is prescribed a thyroid hormone supplement such as levothyroxine, important follow-up would include assessing the client's understanding of the medication and the necessity for taking it for the rest of her life. In addition, the nurse must assess the effectiveness of the medication. Indicators of effectiveness would include reduced symptoms and the client's verbalization of improved quality of life.

Critical Thinking Exercise

Answer the following questions about Mrs. White.

- What might be causing Mrs. White's symptoms? What medical diagnosis would you anticipate for Mrs. White? (*Knowledge*)
- How do hyperthyroidism and hypothyroidism differ? How are these differences manifested in client symptoms? (*Comprehension*)
- Mrs. White is alarmed about her symptoms and says that she can't stand to go on like this. How would you address her health concerns? (*Analysis*)
- Mrs. White starts taking levothyroxine as prescribed by her physician. What questions would you ask Mrs. White when she comes to the clinic for a follow-up visit? (*Synthesis*)
- Once a diagnosis has been established for Mrs. White, how would you evaluate her understanding of it and determine any additional needed teaching? (*Evaluation*)

Canadian Research

Dooley, J. M., Gordon K. E., & Wood E. P. (2005). Self-reported headache frequency in Canadian adolescents: Validation and follow-up headache. *The Journal of Head and Face Pain, 45*(2), 127–131.

Meneilly, G. S. (2005). Should subclinical hypothyroidism in elderly clients be treated? *Canadian Medical Association Journal, 172*(5), 633.

Molgat, C. V., & Patten, S. V. (2005). Comorbidity of major depression and migraine—A Canadian population-based study. *Canadian Journal of Psychiatry, 50*(13), 832–837.

Pryse-Phillips, W., Dodick, D., Edmeads, J., Gawel, M., Nelson, R., Purdy, R. A., et al. (1997). Guidelines for the diagnosis and management of migraine in clinical practice. *Canadian Medical Association Journal, 156,* 1273–1287.

Stiell, I. G., Grimshaw, J., Wells, G. A., Coyle, D., Lesiuk, H. J., Rowe, B. H., et al. (2007). A matched-pair cluster design study protocol to evaluate implementation of the Canadian C-spine rule in hospital emergency departments: Phase III. *Implementation Science, 2*(4).

Tricco, A. C., Colantonio, A., Chipman, M., Liss, G., & McLellan, B. (2006). Work-related deaths and traumatic brain injury. *Brain Injury, 20*(7), 719–724.

Test Questions

1. When examining the head, the nurse remembers that the anatomic regions of the cranium take their names from:
   a. noted anatomists.
   b. the underlying bones.
   c. their anatomical positions.
   d. the underlying vascular network.

2. When identifying the midline structures of the neck from the mandible to the sternal notch, the nurse notes the structures in the following order:
   a. Cricoid cartilage, hyoid bone, tracheal rings, thyroid isthmus
   b. Thyroid cartilage, thyroid isthmus, cricoid cartilage, hyoid bone
   c. Hyoid bone, thyroid cartilage, cricoid cartilage, isthmus of the thyroid
   d. Hyoid bone, tracheal rings, cricoid cartilage, lobes of the thyroid gland

3. When palpating the lymph nodes of the neck, which of the following characteristics does the nurse assesses for?
   a. Congruency, induration, size, turgor
   b. Delineation, integrity, shape, colour
   c. Consistency, delineation, mobility tenderness
   d. Configuration, discreteness, temperature, colour

4. When palpating the neck, which of the following techniques will help differentiate lymph nodes from a band of muscles?
   a. Applying pressure and assessing for induration
   b. Attempting to roll the structure up and down and side to side
   c. Palpating for lateral movement when the client swallows a sip of water

d. Observing for hypertrophy when the client turns the head against resistance

5. Lymph from the scalp and face drains into which of the following nodes?
   a. Occipital, preauricular, submandibular
   b. Submandibular, deep cervical, tonsillar
   c. Deep cervical, supraclavicular, tonsillar
   d. Submental, posterior cervical, superficial cervical

Bibliography

CITATIONS

Brain Injury Awareness Month. (2004). *About brain injury.* Retrieved May 15, 2007, from http://www.biam.ca/about.htm

Canadian Institute for Health Information. (2006a). *Hospitalizations due to traumatic head injuries down 35% over a decade.* Retrieved May 15, 2007, from http://secure.cihi.ca/cihiweb/dispPage.jsp?cw_page=media_30aug2006_e

Canadian Institute for Health Information. (2006b). *Causes of head injury hospitalizations, overall (2003–2004).* Retrieved May 15, 2007, from http://secure.cihi.ca/cihiweb/en/media_30aug2006_fig1_e.html

Canadian Paraplegic Association. (2007). *Overview on SCI and its consequences.* Retrieved June 25, 2007, from http://www.canparaplegic.org/en/SCI_Facts_67/items/t.html

Goadsby, P. J., Lipton, R. B., & Ferrari, M. D. (2002). Migraine: Current understanding and treatment. *New England Journal of Medicine, 346*(4), 257–270.

Haas, D. C. (1996). Chronic post-traumatic headaches classified and compared with natural headaches. *Cephalalgia, 16*(7), 486–493.

Headache Classification Subcommittee of the International Headache Society. (2004). The international headache classification. *Cephalalgia, 24*(Suppl. 1), 1–160.

Hegedus, L. (2004). The thyroid nodule. *New England Journal of Medicine, 351*(17), 1764–1771.

McGuirt, W. F. (1989). The neck mass. *Medical Clinics of North America, 83,* 219–234.

Rollnik, J. D., Karst, M., Fink, M., & Dengler, R. (2001). Botulinum toxin type A and EMG: A key to the understanding of chronic tension-type headaches? *Headache, 41*(10), 985–989.

Siminoski, K. (1995). Does this client have a goitre? *Journal of the American Medical Association, 273*(10), 813–817.

Smetana, G. W., & Shmerling, R. H. (2002). Does this client have temporal arteritis? *Journal of the American Medical Association, 287*(1), 92–101.

Surks, M. I., Ortiz, E., Daniels, G. H., Sawin, C. T., Col, N. F., Cobin, R. H., et al. (2004). Subclinical thyroid disease: Scientific review and guidelines for diagnosis and management. *Journal of the American Medical Association, 291*(2), 228–238.

Thyroid Foundation of Canada. (2007a). *Thyroid health—It's not black and white.* Retrieved May 18, 2007, from http://www.thyroid.ca/Thyroid_Health.html

Thyroid Foundation of Canada. (2007b). *Thyroid disease … Know the facts.* Retrieved May 18, 2007, from http://www.thyroid.ca/Guides/HG00.html#3

Tricco, A. C., Colantonio, A., Chipman, M., Liss, G., & McLellan, B. (2006). Work-related deaths and traumatic brain injury. *Brain Injury, 20*(7), 719–724.

US Preventive Services Task Force. (2004). Screening for thyroid disease: Recommendation statement. *Annals of Internal Medicine, 140*(2), 125–127.

ADDITIONAL RESOURCES

Bahra, A., & May, A. (2002). Cluster headache: A prospective clinical study with diagnostic implications. *Neurology, 58*(3), 354–361.

Bliss, S. J., Flanders, S. A., & Saint, S. (2004). A pain in the neck. *New England Journal of Medicine, 350*(10), 1037–1042.

Dussault, J. (1999). The anecdotal history for screening of congenital hypothyroidism. *The Journal of Clinical Endocrinology and Metabolism, 84*(12), 4332–4334.

Henry, P. H., & Long, D. L. (2005). Enlargement of the lymph nodes and spleen. In D. L. Kasper, A. S. Fauci, D. L Longo, et al. (Eds.), *Harrison's principles of internal medicine* (16th ed.). New York: McGraw Hill. 343–366.

Prisco, M. K. (2000). Evaluating neck masses. *Nurse Practitioner, 25*(4), 30–32, 35–36, 38.

Schwetschenau, E., & Kelley, D. J. (2003). The adult neck mass. *American Family Physician, 67*(6), 1190, 1192, 1195.

Weber, J., & Kelley, J. (2007). *Health assessment in nursing* (3rd ed.). Philadelphia: Lippincott Williams & Wilkins.

WEB SITES AND ASSOCIATIONS

The Brain Injury Association of Canada: http://www.biac-aclc.ca/

The Canadian Headache Society and Headache Network Canada: http://www.headachenetwork.ca/

Canadian Paraplegic Association: http://www.canparaplegic.org

Canadian Thyroid Cancer Support Group: http://www.thryvors.org/

Help for Headaches: http://www.headache-help.org

Lymphoma Foundation of Canada: http://www.lymphoma.ca

Meningitis Research Foundation of Canada: http://www.meningitis.ca

Think First Foundation of Canada: http://www.thinkfirst.ca/

Thyroid Foundation of Canada: http://www.thyroid.ca

Victoria Headache Clinic: http://www.victoriaheadacheclinic.com

TABLE 11-1   Primary Headaches

	Migraines (with aura, without aura, variants)	Tension	Cluster
Process	Primary neuronal dysfunction, possibly of brainstem origin, causing imbalance of excitatory and inhibitory neurotransmitters and affecting craniovascular modulation (Goadsby et al., 2002)	Unclear—muscle contraction or vasoconstriction unlikely (Rollnik, Karst, Fink, & Dengler, 2001)	Unclear—possibly extracranial vasodilation from neural dysfunction with trigeminovascular pain
Location	Unilateral in ~70%; bifrontal or global in ~30%	Usually bilateral; may be generalized or localized to the back of the head and upper neck or to the frontotemporal area	Unilateral, usually behind or around the eye
Quality and Severity	Throbbing or aching, variable in severity	Pressing or tightening pain; mild to moderate intensity	Deep, continuous, severe
Timing *Onset*	Fairly rapid, reaching a peak in 1–2 h	Gradual	Abrupt, peaks within minutes
Duration	4–72 h	Minutes to days	Up to 3 h
Course	Peak incidence early to mid-adolescence; prevalence is ~6% in men and ~15% in women. Recurrent—usually monthly, but weekly in ~10%	Often recurrent or persistent over long periods; annual prevalence ~40%	Episodic, clustered in time with several each day for 4–8 weeks and then relief for 6–12 months; prevalence <1%, more common in men
Associated Factors	Nausea, vomiting, photophobia, phonophobia, visual auras (flickering zig-zagging lines), motor auras affecting hand or arm, sensory auras (numbness, tingling usually precede attack)	Sometimes photophobia, phonophobia; nausea absent	Lacrimation, rhinorrhea, miosis, ptosis, eyelid edema, conjunctival infection
Factors That Aggravate or Provoke	Alcohol, certain foods, or tension may provoke; more common premenstrually; aggravated by noise and bright light	Sustained muscle tension, as in driving or typing	During attack, sensitivity to alcohol may increase
Factors That Relieve	Quiet, dark room; sleep; sometimes transient relief from pressure on the involved artery, if early in the course	Possible massage, relaxation	

Source: Headache Classification Subcommittee of the International Headache Society, 2004.

TABLE 11-2   Selected Facies

Facial Swelling

Cushing's Syndrome	Nephrotic Syndrome	Myxedema

The increased adrenal hormone production of Cushing's syndrome produces a round or "moon" face with red cheeks. Excessive hair growth may be present in the mustache and sideburn areas and on the chin.

The face is edematous and often pale. Swelling usually appears first around the eyes and in the morning. The eyes may become slit like when edema is severe.

The client with severe hypothyroidism (*myxedema*) has a dull, puffy facies. The edema, often particularly pronounced around the eyes, does not pit with pressure. The hair and eyebrows are dry, coarse, and thinned. The skin is dry.

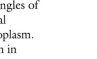

Red cheeks
Hirsutism
Moon face

Periorbital edema
Puffy pale face
Lips may be swollen

Hair dry, coarse, sparse
Lateral eyebrows thin
Periorbital edema
Puffy, dull face with dry skin

Other Facies

Parotid Gland Enlargement	Acromegaly	Parkinson's Disease

Chronic bilateral asymptomatic parotid gland enlargement may be associated with obesity, diabetes, cirrhosis, and other conditions. Note the swellings anterior to the ear lobes and above the angles of the jaw. Gradual unilateral enlargement suggests neoplasm. Acute enlargement is seen in mumps.

The increased growth hormone of acromegaly produces enlargement of both bone and soft tissues. The head is elongated, with bony prominence of the forehead, nose, and lower jaw. Soft tissues of the nose, lips, and ears also enlarge. The facial features appear generally coarsened.

Decreased facial mobility blunts expression. A mask-like face may result, with decreased blinking and a characteristic stare. Since the neck and upper trunk tend to flex forward, the client seems to peer upward toward the observer. Facial skin becomes oily, and drooling may occur.

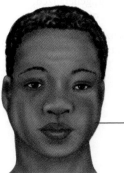
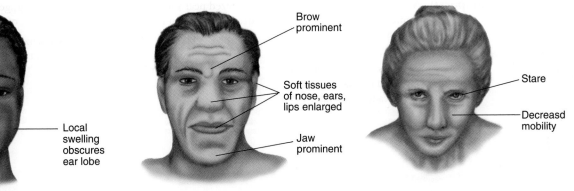

Local swelling obscures ear lobe

Brow prominent
Soft tissues of nose, ears, lips enlarged
Jaw prominent

Stare
Decreasd mobility

TABLE 11-3   Secondary Headaches

Type	Process	Location	Quality and Severity
Analgesic Rebound	Withdrawal of medication	Previous headache pattern	Variable
Headaches From Eye Disorders			
Errors of Refraction (farsightedness and astigmatism, but not nearsightedness)	Probably the sustained contraction of the extraocular muscles, and possibly of the frontal, temporal, and occipital muscles	Around and over the eyes, may radiate to the occipital area	Steady, aching, dull
Acute Glaucoma	Sudden increase in intraocular pressure (see p. 308)	In and around one eye	Steady, aching, often severe
Headache from Sinusitis	Mucosal inflammation of the paranasal sinuses	Usually above the eye (frontal sinus) or over the maxillary sinus	Aching or throbbing, variable in severity; consider possible migraine
Meningitis	Infection of the meninges surrounding the brain	Generalized	Steady or throbbing, very severe
Subarachnoid Hemorrhage	Bleeding, most often from a ruptured intracranial aneurysm	Generalized	Very severe, "the worst of my life"
Brain Tumour	Displacement of or traction on pain-sensitive arteries and veins or pressure on nerves	Varies with the location of the tumour	Aching, steady, variable in intensity
Cranial Neuralgias			
Trigeminal Neuralgia (CNV)	Compression of CNV, often by aberrant loop or artery of vein	Cheek, jaws, lips, or gums; trigeminal nerve divisions 2 and 3 >1	Shocklike, stabbing, burning; severe
Giant Cell (Temporal) Arteritis*	Vasculitis from cell-mediated immune response to elastic lamina of artery	Localized near the involved artery, most often the temporal, also the occipital; age-related	Throbbing, generalized, persistent; often severe
Posttraumatic Headache	Mechanism unclear; episodes similar to tension-type and migraine without aura headaches (Haas, 1996)	May be localized to the injured area, but not necessarily	Generalized, dull, aching, constant

Note: Blanks appear in this table when the categories are not applicable or not usually helpful in assessing the problem.

Sources: Smetana & Shmerling, 2002; Headache Classification Subcommittee of the International Headache Society (2004).

Timing			Associated Factors	Factors That Aggravate or Provoke	Factors That Relieve
Onset	Duration	Course			
Variable	Depends on prior headache pattern	Depends on frequency of "mini-withdrawals"	Depends on prior headache pattern	Fever, carbon monoxide, hypoxia, withdrawal of caffeine, other headache triggers	Depends on cause
Gradual	Variable	Variable	Eye fatigue, "sandy" sensations in the eyes, redness of the conjunctiva	Prolonged use of the eyes, particularly for close work	Resting the eyes
Often rapid	Variable, may depend on treatment	Variable, may depend on treatment	Diminished vision, sometimes nausea and vomiting	Sometimes provoked by drops that dilate the pupils	
Variable	Often several hours at a time, recurring over days or longer	Often recurrent in a repetitive daily pattern	Local tenderness, nasal congestion, discharge, and fever	May be aggravated by coughing, sneezing, or jarring the head	Nasal decongestants, antibiotics
Fairly rapid	Variable, usually days	A persistent headache in an acute illness	Fever, stiff neck		
Usually abrupt, severe; prodromal symptoms may occur	Variable, usually days	A persistent headache in an acute illness	Nausea, vomiting, possibly loss of consciousness, neck pain		
Variable	Often brief	Often inter-mittent but progressive	May be aggravated by cough-ing, sneezing, or sudden movements of the head		
Abrupt, paroxysmal	Each jab lasts seconds but recurs at intervals of seconds or minutes	May last for months, then disappear for months, but often recurs; it is uncommon at night	Exhaustion from recurrent pain	Touching certain areas of the lower face or mouth; chewing, talking, brushing teeth	
Gradual or rapid	Variable	Recurrent or persistent over weeks to months	Tenderness of the adjacent scalp; fever (in ~50%), fatigue, weight loss; new headache (~60%), jaw claudication (~50%), visual loss or blindness (~15%–20%), polymyalgia rheumatica (~50%)	Movement of neck and shoulders	
Within hours to 1–2 days of the injury	Weeks, months, or even years	Tends to diminish over time	Poor concentration, problems with memory, vertigo, irritability, restlessness, fatigue	Mental and physical exertion, straining, stooping, emotional excitement, alcohol	Rest

TABLE 11-4   **Thyroid Enlargement and Function**

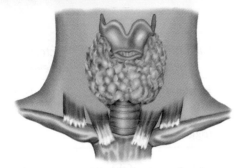

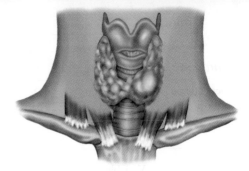

Diffuse Enlargement. Includes the isthmus and lateral lobes; there are no discretely palpable nodules. Causes include Graves' disease, Hashimoto's thyroiditis, and endemic goitre.

Single Nodule. May be a cyst, a benign tumour, or one nodule within a multinodular gland. It raises the question of malignancy. Risk factors are prior irradiation, hardness, rapid growth, fixation to surrounding tissues, enlarged cervical nodes, and occurrence in males (Hegedus, 2004).

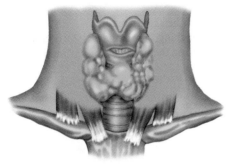

Multinodular Goitre. An enlarged thyroid gland with two or more nodules suggests a metabolic rather than a neoplastic process. Positive family history and continuing nodular enlargement are additional risk factors for malignancy.

	Hyperthyroidism	Hypothyroidism
Symptoms	Nervousness	Fatigue, lethargy
	Weight loss despite increased appetite	Modest weight gain with anorexia
	Excessive sweating and heat intolerance	Dry, coarse skin and cold intolerance
	Palpitations	Swelling of face, hands, and legs
	Frequent bowel movements	Constipation
	Muscular weakness of the proximal type and tremor	Weakness, muscle cramps, arthralgias, paresthesias, impaired memory and hearing
Signs	Warm, smooth, moist skin	Dry, coarse, cool skin, sometimes yellowish from carotene, with nonpitting edema and loss of hair
	With Graves' disease, eye signs such as stare, lid lag, and exophthalmos	Periorbital puffiness
	Increased systolic and decreased diastolic blood pressures	Decreased systolic and increased diastolic blood pressures
	Tachycardia or atrial fibrillation	Bradycardia and, in late stages, hypothermia
	Hyperdynamic cardiac pulsations with an accentuated S_1	Intensity of heart sounds sometimes decreased
	Tremor and proximal muscle weakness	Impaired memory, mixed hearing loss, somnolence, peripheral neuropathy, carpal tunnel syndrome

Sources: Surks, 2004; U.S. Preventive Services Task Force, 2004.

The Eyes

Tracey C. Stephen and Lynn S. Bickley

The eye is the highly specialized organ of vision and is complex in its function and assessment. We use our eyes to see the world around us and to experience aspects of our environment that would not otherwise be accessible to us.

ANATOMY AND PHYSIOLOGY

The eyes sit in a protective bony structure called the *orbit*. Each eyeball, or *globe*, is protected superiorly by the *frontal bone*, laterally by the *temporal* and *nasal* bones, and inferiorly by the *zygomatic* bones. The orbits contain muscle, connective, and adipose tissues and are approximately 4 centimetres in height, width, and depth.

The illustration at right shows the structures of the external eye. The upper and lower eyelids comprise striated and smooth muscle covered with skin. Within the eyelids lie firm strips of connective tissue called *tarsal plates*. Each plate contains a parallel row of *meibomian glands*, which open on the lid margin. The eyelids open and close to help protect the eyeball and control the amount of light entering the eye. The opening and closing of the eyelids also help distribute tears to lubricate the eye. Note that the upper eyelid covers a portion of the iris but does not normally overlie the pupil. The opening between the eyelids is called the *palpebral fissure*. On each eyelid are stiff hairs (the eyelashes) that curve outward from the eyes and help prevent dirt and foreign objects from entering.

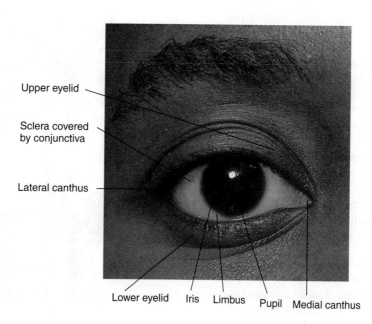

Upper eyelid

Sclera covered by conjunctiva

Lateral canthus

Lower eyelid   Iris   Limbus   Pupil   Medial canthus

The internal structures of the eyes include the three layers of the eyeball. The outermost layer comprises the *cornea* and the *sclera*. The clear cornea covers the *anterior chamber* and *iris* in the anterior portion of the outer layer.

The *cornea* permits light to enter the eye through the *lens* and focus on the *retina* for vision. The *sclera* is the white portion of the eyeball and consists of a dense fibrous tissue that helps maintain the shape of the eyeball and protect the intraocular components. The colour of the *sclera* may differ from slightly bluish in young children to dull white in adults to pale yellow in the elderly.

The middle layer comprises the *choroid* posteriorly and the *iris* and *ciliary body* anteriorly. The *choroid* layer contains blood vessels that supply nourishment to the eye. The iris is the coloured portion of the eye surrounding the pupil. The muscle fibres in the *iris* control the size of the *pupil*, which in turn controls the amount of light entering the eye. Immediately behind the *iris* is the *lens*. The lens is attached by *suspensory ligaments* to the *ciliary body*. The function of the lens is to refract (bend) light on to the *retina* for visualizing an object. The amount of refraction required is determined by the size or the distance of the object. The lens changes shape to adjust the amount of refraction needed. For close objects, the lens bulges; for far objects, the lens flattens. Muscles of the ciliary body control the changing of the lens shape.

The inner layer of the eye is the *retina*: This posterior inner portion of the eyeball extends to the *ciliary body*. The retina comprises specialized nerve cells called *photoreceptors*, which receive visual stimuli and transmit them to the brain. The first type of photoreceptors is the *rods*, which are highly sensitive to light and aid vision in dimly lit environments. The second type of photoreceptors is the *cones*, which are sensitive to colour and function in bright light.

The *conjunctiva* is a clear mucous membrane with two easily visible components. The *bulbar conjunctiva* covers most of the anterior eyeball, adhering loosely to the underlying tissue. It meets the cornea at the *limbus*. The *palpebral conjunctiva* lines the eyelids. The two parts of the conjunctiva merge in a folded recess that permits movement of the eyeball.

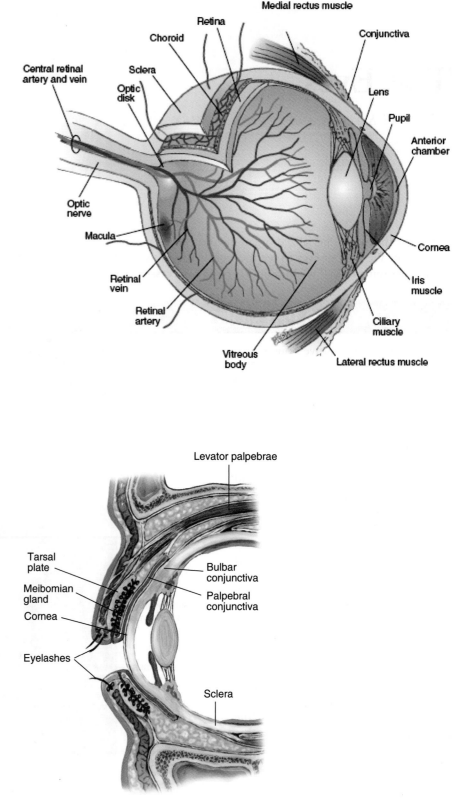

SAGITTAL SECTION OF ANTERIOR EYE WITH LIDS CLOSED

A film of tear fluid protects the conjunctiva and cornea from drying, inhibits microbial growth, and gives a smooth optical surface to the cornea. This fluid comes from the meibomian glands, conjunctival glands, and the lacrimal gland. The *lacrimal gland* lies mostly within the bony orbit, above and lateral to the eyeball. The tear fluid spreads across the eye and drains medially through two tiny holes called *lacrimal puncta*. The tears then pass into the *lacrimal sac* and on into the nose through the *nasolacrimal duct*. You can easily find a *punctum* atop the small elevation of the lower lid medially. The lacrimal sac rests in a small depression inside the bony orbit and is not visible.

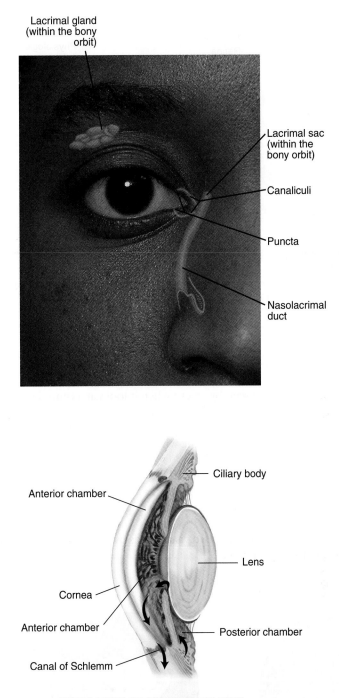

A clear liquid called **aqueous humour** fills the anterior and posterior chambers of the eye. Aqueous humour is produced by the *ciliary body*, circulates from the posterior chamber through the pupil into the anterior chamber, and drains out through the *canal of Schlemm*. This circulatory system helps to control the pressure inside the eye. When the production of aqueous fluid equals the amount of drainage of aqueous fluid, the intraocular pressure is stable. If drainage is impeded, the intraocular pressure increases.

The posterior part of the eye that is seen through an ophthalmoscope is often called the *fundus* of the eye. Structures here include the retina, choroid, fovea, macula, optic disc, and retinal vessels. The optic nerve with its retinal vessels enters the eyeball posteriorly. You can find it with an ophthalmoscope at the *optic disc*. Lateral and slightly inferior to the disc, there is a small depression in the retinal surface that marks the point of central vision. Around it is a darkened circular area called the *fovea*. The roughly circular *macula* (named for a microscopic yellow spot) surrounds the fovea but has no discernible margins. It does not quite reach the optic disc. You do not usually see the *vitreous body*, a transparent mass of gelatinous material that fills the eyeball behind the lens. It helps to maintain the shape of the eye.

CIRCULATION OF AQUEOUS HUMOUR

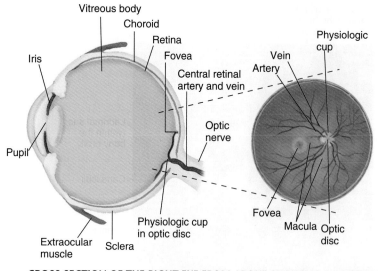

CROSS SECTION OF THE RIGHT EYE FROM ABOVE SHOWING A PORTION OF THE FUNDUS COMMONLY SEEN WITH THE OPHTHALMOSCOPE

VISUAL FIELDS

A *visual field* is the entire area seen by an eye when it looks at a central point. Fields are conventionally diagrammed on circles from the client's point of view. The centre of the circle represents the focus of gaze. The circumference is 90 degrees from the line of gaze. Each visual field, shown by the white areas in the illustration, is divided into quadrants. Note that the fields extend farthest on the temporal sides. Visual fields are limited by the brows above, the cheeks below, and the nose medially. A lack of retinal receptors at the optic disc produces an oval blind spot in the normal field of each eye, 15 degrees temporal to the line of gaze.

When a person is using both eyes, the two visual fields overlap in an area of binocular vision. Laterally, vision is monocular.

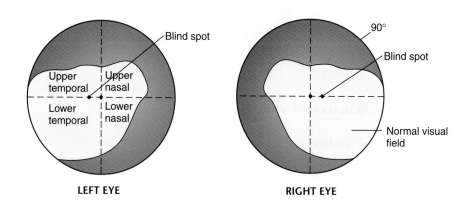

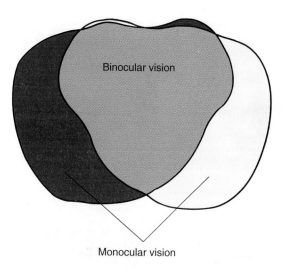

Binocular vision

Monocular vision

VISUAL PATHWAYS

To see an image, light reflected from the image must pass through the pupil and be focused on sensory neurons in the retina. The image projected there is upside down and reversed right to left. An image from the upper nasal visual field thus strikes the lower temporal quadrant of the retina.

Nerve impulses, stimulated by light, are conducted through the retina, optic nerve, and optic tract on each side, then on through a curving tract called the *optic radiation*. This ends in the visual cortex, a part of the occipital lobe of the brain.

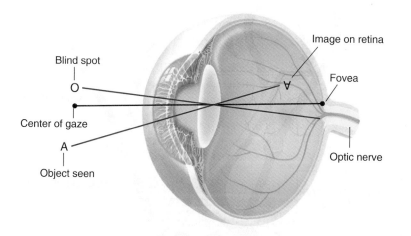

Blind spot

O

Center of gaze

A

Object seen

Image on retina

Fovea

Optic nerve

PUPILLARY REACTIONS

Pupillary size changes in response to light and to the effort of focusing on a near object.

The Near Reaction. When a person shifts gaze from a far object to a near one, the pupils constrict. This response, like the light reaction (discussed next), is mediated by the oculomotor nerve. Coincident with this pupillary reaction, but not part of it, are (1) *convergence* of the eyes, an extraocular movement; and (2) *accommodation*, convexity of the lenses caused by contraction of the ciliary muscles. This change in shape of the lenses brings near objects into focus but is not visible to the examiner.

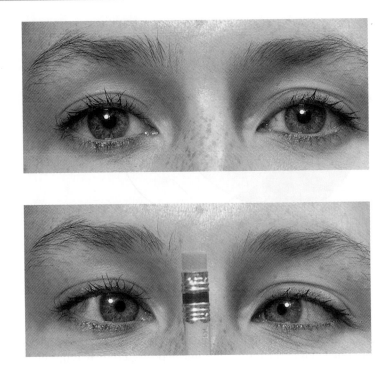

The Light Reaction. A light beam shining onto one retina causes pupillary constriction both in the eye the light is shone, termed the *direct reaction* to light, and in the opposite eye, the *consensual reaction.* The initial sensory pathways are similar to those described for vision: retina, optic nerve, and optic tract. The pathways diverge in the midbrain, however, and impulses are transmitted through the oculomotor nerve to the constrictor muscles of the iris of each eye.

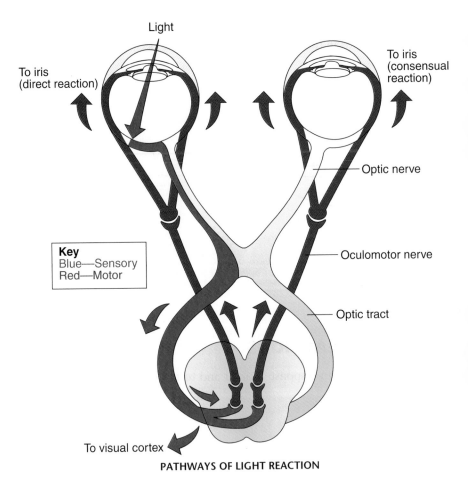

PATHWAYS OF LIGHT REACTION

AUTONOMIC NERVE SUPPLY TO THE EYES

Fibres travelling in the oculomotor nerve and producing pupillary constriction are part of the parasympathetic nervous system. The iris is also supplied by sympathetic fibres. When these are stimulated, the pupil dilates and the upper eyelid rises a little, as if from fear. The sympathetic pathway starts in the hypothalamus and passes down through the brainstem and cervical cord into the neck. From there, it follows the carotid artery or its branches into the orbit. A lesion anywhere along this pathway may impair sympathetic effects on the pupil.

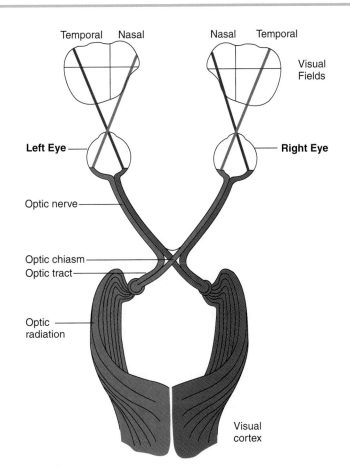

VISUAL PATHWAYS FROM THE RETINA TO THE VISUAL CORTEX

EXTRAOCULAR MOVEMENTS

The movement of each eye is controlled by the coordinated action of six muscles, the four rectus and two oblique muscles. You can test the function of each muscle and the nerve that supplies it by asking the client to move the eye in the direction controlled by that muscle. There are six such *cardinal directions*, indicated by the lines in the following figure. When a person looks down and to the right, for example, the right inferior rectus (Cranial Nerve [CN] III) is principally responsible for moving the right eye, whereas the left superior oblique (Cranial Nerve IV) is principally responsible for moving the left. If one of these muscles is paralyzed, the eye will deviate from its position in that direction of gaze, and the eyes will no longer appear conjugate or parallel.

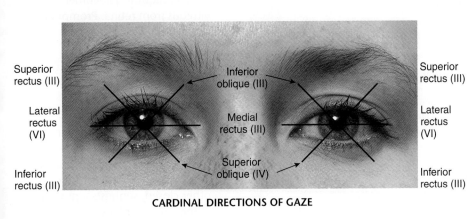

CARDINAL DIRECTIONS OF GAZE

THE HEALTH HISTORY: SUBJECTIVE DATA

Key Symptoms and Signs Reported by Client

- Changes in vision (blurred vision, spots in visual field, loss of vision, flashing lights, floaters)
- Double vision
- Headache
- Eye pain
- Sensitivity to light
- Redness
- Inflammation

Begin the health history by asking open-ended questions, such as "What concerns have brought you to the clinic today?" or "Tell me how you are feeling." These questions allow the client to give responses that help guide the rest of the examination. When a client reports a sign or a symptom, it is analyzed further to gain more information.

Start your inquiry about eye and vision problems with open-ended questions such as "How is your vision?" and "Have you had any trouble with your eyes?" If the client reports a change in vision, pursue the related details:

- Is the problem worse during close work or at distances?

- Are there specks in the vision or areas where the client cannot see (scotomas)? If so, do they move around in visual field with shifts in gaze or are they fixed?

- Has the client seen lights flashing in the field of vision? Vitreous floaters may accompany this symptom.
- When was the client's last eye examination?
- Does the client wear glasses?
- Does the client wear contact lenses?

Ask about *pain* in or around the eyes, *redness*, and *excessive tearing or watering* (see p. 329).

Check for presence of *diplopia*, or double vision. If present, find out whether the images are side by side (horizontal diplopia) or on top of each other (vertical diplopia). Does diplopia persist with one eye closed? Which eye is affected?

Refractive errors most commonly explain gradual blurring. High blood glucose levels may cause blurring (Shingleton & O'Donoghue, 2000).

Sudden visual loss suggests *retinal detachment, vitreous hemorrhage,* or *occlusion of the central retinal artery.*

Slow central loss occurs in *nuclear cataract* (p. 330) *macular degeneration* (Fine et al., 2000) (p. 308); peripheral loss occurs in advanced *open-angle glaucoma* (p. 314); one-sided loss occurs in *hemianopsia* and *quadrantic defects* (p. 326).

Difficulty with close work suggests *hyperopia* (farsightedness) or *presbyopia* (aging vision); with distances, *myopia* (near-sightedness).

Moving specks or strands suggest vitreous floaters; fixed defects (scotomas) suggest lesions in the retina or visual pathways.

Flashing lights or new vitreous floaters suggest detachment of vitreous from retina. Prompt eye consultation is indicated.

Diplopia in adults may arise from a lesion in the brainstem or cerebellum, or from weakness or paralysis of extraocular muscles. Diplopia in one eye, with the other closed, suggests a problem in the cornea or lens.

Example of Questions for Symptom/Sign Analysis—Blurred Vision

- "When you look at something, what areas are blurry?" "Is the blurred vision in both eyes?" "Is the blurred vision in your entire field of vision?" "Is one part of your vision blurry?" "Is the same part of your vision blurry or does it change?" (*Location/radiating*)
- "Describe what the blurred vision is like." (*Quality*)
- "Describe how much blurriness you have." "Can you see large objects?" "Can you see large printed letters?" (*Severity*)
- "When did your blurred vision start?" "Did it start suddenly or gradually?" (*Onset*)
- "Has your vision been consistently blurry ever since the problem started?" (*Duration*)
- "Have there been times when your vision seemed more blurry or less blurry?" (*Constancy*)
- "Is there a time of day that it (blurred vision) seems worse? Or better?" (*Time of day/month/year*)

- "What makes it (blurred vision) worse?" (*Aggravating factors*)
- "What makes it (blurred vision) better?" (*Alleviating factors*)
- "What other symptoms have you noticed?" (*Associated symptoms*)
- "Have you recently changed anything in your home or office?" "Have you had any recent injuries to your eyes or head?" "Have your eyes been exposed to any chemicals or other substances?" "How much stress is in your life right now?" (*Environmental factors*)
- "Tell me how this is affecting your life." (*Significance to client*)
- "What do you think is happening?" (*Client perspective*)

HEALTH PROMOTION

Important Topics for Health Promotion

- Changes in vision: cataracts, macular degeneration, glaucoma, diabetic retinopathy
- Prevention of eye injury
- Reduction of risk factors

Vision is a critical sense for experiencing the world around us and is an area of special importance for health promotion and education. A recent study showed that only 25% of working-age Canadians with vision loss are employed (Canadian National Institute for the Blind [CNIB], 2007a).

Our vision changes as we age. The types of disorders of vision that are most common vary according to age group and as people age. Healthy young adults generally have some refractive errors requiring correction. Many visual disorders are related to aging. One in nine Canadians older than 65 years and one in four Canadians older than 80 years have significant vision loss that requires special attention (CNIB, 2007b). These disorders reduce awareness of the social and physical environments and contribute to falls, injuries, and even social isolation. In Canada, the four most prevalent medical conditions that contribute to vision loss are *age-related macular degeneration (AMD)*, *glaucoma*, *diabetic retinopathy*, and *cataracts*. The leading cause of vision loss in North Americans older than 50 years is AMD, with 78,000 Canadians diagnosed with this problem each year (Canadian Ophthalmological Society [COS], 2007). This number is expected to triple within the next 25 years.

Blindness in developing countries has increased recently as a result of noncommunicable chronic diseases and increased longevity. The World Health Organization (WHO, 2007) has developed a plan called *Vision 2020* aimed at decreasing preventable blindness for all member states.

RISK FACTOR ASSESSMENT

The leading overall risk factors for vision loss include smoking, age, exposure to ultraviolet (UV) radiation (sun exposure), heredity, diet, African descent, and diabetes (CNIB, 2007a; COS, 2007). Inquiring about these risk factors during the health history provides essential information. Family history, demographics, and workplace/lifestyle issues should be assessed for increased risk factors. For example, clients who work in construction may be exposed to more eye injuries or UV rays, which put them at greater risk for some eye disorders.

Promoting healthy vision and preventing eye disease include attention to the following recommendations:

- Ensuring healthy nutrition (including fruits and vegetables)

- Quitting smoking

- Maintaining a healthy weight

- Ensuring blood pressure is within expected parameters

- Avoiding eye injuries (*chemical, thermal, traumatic, infectious*) by use of protective eyewear

- Decreasing exposure to UV rays by wearing protective sunglasses or goggles (select sunglasses that block 99–100% of UVA and UVB rays)

- Stabilizing blood glucose levels for clients with diabetes through diet, exercise, blood glucose monitoring, and adherence to medication regimens

SPECIFIC PREVENTION FOR SPECIFIC DISEASES

Macular Degeneration. *Macular degeneration* is the leading cause of vision loss (one out of every three cases) in Canadians. *Age-related macular degeneration* is the most common form of the disease and occurs after the age of 55 years. The result of macular degeneration is the loss of central vision accompanied by blurry details of vision. The causes of macular degeneration are unknown, but it may be linked to conditions such as infections, high blood pressure, diabetes, and nearsightedness. Exposure to toxic light, such as a solar eclipse, and eye injuries that affect the attachment of the retina can also damage the macula. A positive family history is also a risk factor. Ingestion of vitamins C and E, beta carotene, and zinc may help delay the progression of macular degeneration, but more research is needed in this area. Screening tests include a complete eye examination and ophthalmoscopy (fundoscopy), with particular attention to mottling of the macula, variations in the retinal pigmentation, and subretinal hemorrhage or exudates.

Glaucoma. *Glaucoma* is one of the leading causes of blindness in Canada, affecting 1 in 100 Canadians older than 40 years (CNIB, 2007c). It is caused by increased pressure within the eye that results in damage to the optic nerve. Specific risk factors for glaucoma include age, family history of glaucoma, general poor health, and *myopia*, although the exact cause is unknown. Screening tests include tonometry to measure intraocular pressure, ophthalmoscopy to identify a change in size and colour of the optic cup, slit-lamp examination of the optic nerve head, and perimetry to map the visual fields.

Diabetic Retinopathy. For clients with diabetes, the complication of *diabetic retinopathy* may result in vision loss. This type of vision loss is the cause of blindness for 400 Canadians each year (CNIB, 2007a). In diabetic retinopathy, the vessels that feed the retina change and become weakened. Eventually, they may become blocked and cause bleeding into the eye, which blocks vision. Screening tests include regular fundoscopic examination of the retina, with particular attention to the vessels. The best prevention for diabetic retinopathy is the maintenance of stable blood glucose levels through appropriate diet, exercise, and adherence to medication regimens.

Cataracts. *Cataracts* are one of the main causes of vision loss in Canadians, but they do not lead to permanent blindness. Cataracts cause the lens to become cloudy or opaque, resulting in decreased vision. In North America, more than 1.5 million cataract surgeries are completed each year (COS, 2007). Aging, eye injuries, certain diseases such as diabetes, certain medications, and exposure to UV rays are the most common causes of cataracts. Screening tests include a complete eye examination with fundoscopy to identify and locate cataracts.

SCREENING AND MAINTENANCE

The Canadian Ophthalmology Society (2007) outlines the following recommendations for screening examinations:

- Low-risk clients

  - 19 to 40 years, at least every 10 years

  - 41 to 55 years, at least every 5 years

  - 56 to 65 years, at least every 3 years

  - >65 years, at least every 2 years

- High-risk clients

  - >40 years, at least every 3 years

  - >50 years, at least every 2 years

  - >60 years, at least annually

It is recommended that an eye specialist, such as an ophthalmologist or optometrist, complete these screening tests.

EMERGENCY CONCERNS

For any client noticing any changes in vision, assessment of the eye should be done as soon as possible. Sudden onset of blurred or double vision, eye pain, loss of vision, flashing lights, redness around the limbus, change in visual field, or change in peripheral vision requires immediate attention by a physician. Eye injuries such as lacerations to the eye or eyelid; blunt force trauma; foreign objects in the eye; scratches on the eyeball; or exposure to infectious, thermal, or chemical agents need emergency assessment and treatment.

TECHNIQUES OF EXAMINATION: OBJECTIVE DATA

Throughout the eye examination, ensure that the client is comfortable. Position the client seated, preferably at eye level of the examiner. If the client is unable to sit unassisted on an examination table, provide a chair with armrests to ensure safety for the client. Inquire about sensitivity to light and areas of pain or discomfort before beginning any of the techniques of examination. Remain attentive to any areas of pain or discomfort, and adjust examination techniques as needed to ensure client comfort.

IMPORTANT AREAS OF EXAMINATION

- Visual acuity
- Visual fields
- Conjunctiva and sclera
- Cornea, lens, and pupils
- Extraocular movements
- Fundi, including optic disc and cup, retina, retina vessels

---

Visual Acuity.   To test the acuity of central vision, use a Snellen eye chart, if possible, and light it well. Position the client 6.1 metres from the chart.

Equipment

- Snellen or E chart
- Disposable gloves (use when needed to prevent contact with exudate or fluid)
- Penlight
- Opaque cards
- Ophthalmoscope
- Pen

Clients who use glasses other than for reading should put them on all the time. Ask the client to cover one eye with a card (to prevent peeking through the fingers) and to read the smallest line of print possible. Coaxing to attempt the next line may improve performance. A client who cannot read the largest letter should be positioned closer to the chart; note the intervening distance. Determine the smallest line of print from which the client can identify more than half the letters. Record the visual acuity designated at the side of this line, along with use of glasses, if any. Visual acuity is expressed as two numbers (e.g., 20/30): The first indicates the distance of client from chart and the second, the distance at which a healthy eye can read the line of letters.

Testing near vision with a special hand-held card helps identify the need for reading glasses or bifocals in clients older than age 45. You can also use this card to test visual acuity at the bedside. Held 35 cm from the client's eyes, the card simulates a Snellen chart. You may, however, let clients choose their own distance.

If you have no charts, screen visual acuity with any available print. If clients cannot read even the largest letters, test their ability to count your upraised fingers and distinguish light (such as your flashlight) from dark.

Cultural Considerations

Visual acuity varies with race. Asians have the poorest corrected vision, followed by people of African and Hispanic descent. First Nations and Caucasians have the best-corrected visual acuity.

Vision of 20/200 means that at 6.1 metres (20 feet) the client can read print that a person with normal vision could read at 200 feet. The larger the second number, the worse the vision. "20/40 corrected" means the client could read the 40 line with glasses (a correction).

Myopia is impaired far vision.

Presbyopia is the impaired near vision, found in middle-aged and older people. A presbyopic person often sees better when the card is farther away.

In Canada, a person is usually considered legally blind when vision in the better eye, corrected by glasses, is 20/200 or less. Legal blindness also results from a constricted field of vision: 20° or less in the better eye.

Visual Fields by Confrontation

Screening. Screening starts in the temporal fields because most defects involve these areas. Imagine the client's visual fields projected onto a glass bowl that encircles the front of the client's head. Ask the client to look with both eyes into your eyes. While you return the client's gaze, place your hands about 60 centimetres apart, lateral to the client's ears. Instruct the client to point to your fingers as soon as they are seen. Then slowly move the wiggling fingers of both your hands along the imaginary bowl and toward the line of gaze until the client identifies them. Repeat this pattern in the upper and lower temporal quadrants.

Usually a person sees both sets of fingers at the same time.

Field defects that are all temporal or partly temporal include those shown in the following illustration:

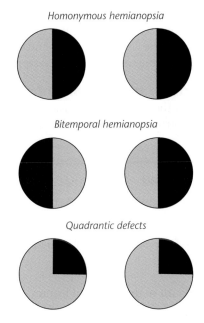

Homonymous hemianopsia

Bitemporal hemianopsia

Quadrantic defects

Review these patterns in Table 12-1, Visual Field Defects, p. 326.

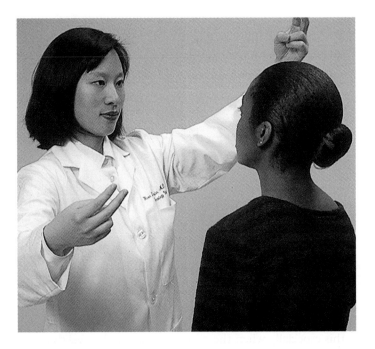

Further Testing. If you find a defect, try to establish its boundaries. Test one eye at a time. If you suspect a temporal defect in the left visual field, for example, ask the client to cover the right eye and, with the left one, to look into your eye directly opposite. Then slowly move your wiggling fingers from the defective area toward the better vision, noting where the client first responds. Repeat this at several levels to define the border.

When the client's left eye repeatedly does not see your fingers until they have crossed the line of gaze, a left temporal hemianopsia is present. It is diagrammed from the client's viewpoint.

A left homonymous hemianopsia may thus be established.

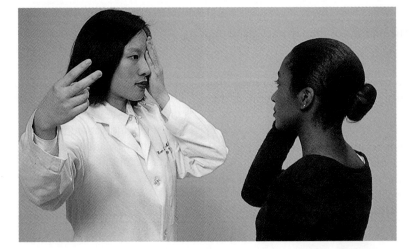

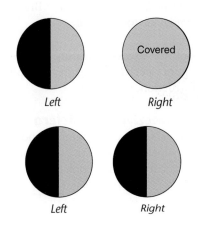

Left · Right

Left · Right

A temporal defect in the visual field of one eye suggests a nasal defect in the other eye. To test this hypothesis, examine the other eye in a similar way, again moving from the anticipated defect toward the better vision.

Small visual field defects and enlarged blind spots require a finer stimulus. Using a small red object such as a red-headed matchstick or the red eraser on a pencil, test one eye at a time. As the client looks into your eye directly opposite, move the object about in the visual field. The blind spot can usually be found 15° temporal to the line of gaze—the small red object disappears. (Find your own blind spots for practice.)

An enlarged blind spot occurs in conditions affecting the optic nerve, for example, glaucoma, optic neuritis, and papilledema.

Position and Alignment of the Eyes.
Stand in front of the client and survey the eyes for position and alignment with each other. If one or both eyes seem to protrude, assess them from above (see p. 320).

Unexpected findings are inward or outward deviation of the eyes; excessive protrusion may be found in Graves' disease or ocular tumours.

Eyebrows.
Inspect the eyebrows, noting their quantity and distribution and any scaliness of the underlying skin.

Scaliness accompanies *seborrheic dermatitis;* lateral sparseness is seen in hypothyroidism.

Eyelids.
Note the position of the lids in relation to the eyeballs. Inspect for the following:

See Table 12-2, Variations of the Eyelids (p. 327).

■ Width of the palpebral fissures

Red inflamed lid margins occur with blepharitis, often with crusting.

■ Edema of the lids

■ Colour of the lids

■ Lesions

■ Condition and direction of the eyelashes

■ Adequacy with which the eyelids close. Look for this especially when the eyes are unusually prominent, when there is facial paralysis, or when the client is unconscious.

Failure of the eyelids to close exposes the corneas to serious damage.

See Table 12-3, Lumps and Swellings in and Around the Eyes (p. 328).

Cultural Considerations

The eyes of clients of African descent protrude more than the eyes of Caucasians.

Lacrimal Apparatus.
Briefly inspect the regions of the lacrimal gland and lacrimal sac for swelling.

Look for excessive tearing or dryness of the eyes. Assessment of dryness may require special testing by an ophthalmologist. To test for nasolacrimal duct obstruction, see p. 321.

Excessive tearing may result from increased production or impaired drainage of tears. In the first group, causes include conjunctival inflammation and corneal irritation; in the second, ectropion (p. 327) and nasolacrimal duct obstruction.

Conjunctiva and Sclera.
Ask the client to look up as you depress both lower lids with your thumbs, exposing the sclera and conjunctiva. Inspect the sclera and palpebral conjunctiva for colour, and note the vascular pattern against the white scleral background. Look for any nodules or swelling.

A yellow sclera indicates jaundice.

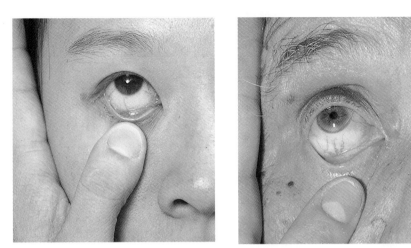

 ### Cultural Considerations

The sclera in darker-skinned clients may have yellow or pigmented freckles.

If you need a fuller view of the eye, rest your thumb and finger on the bones of the cheek and brow, respectively, and spread the lids.

Ask the client to look to each side and down. This technique gives you a good view of the sclera and bulbar conjunctiva, but not of the palpebral conjunctiva of the upper lid.

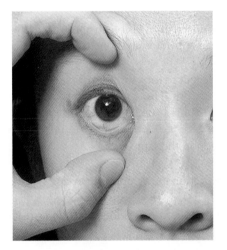

The local redness below is from *nodular episcleritis:*

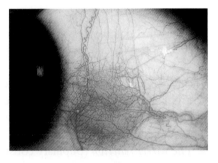

For comparisons, see Table 12-4, Red Eyes (p. 329).

Cornea and Lens. With oblique lighting, inspect the cornea of each eye for opacities and note any opacity in the lens that may be visible through the pupil.

See Table 12-5, Opacities of the Cornea and Lens (p. 330).

Iris. At the same time, inspect each iris. The markings should be clearly defined. With your light shining directly from the temporal side, look for a crescentic shadow on the medial side of the iris. Because the iris is usually fairly flat and forms a relatively open angle with the cornea, this lighting casts no shadow.

Occasionally the iris bows far forward, forming a very narrow angle with the cornea. The light then casts a crescentic shadow.

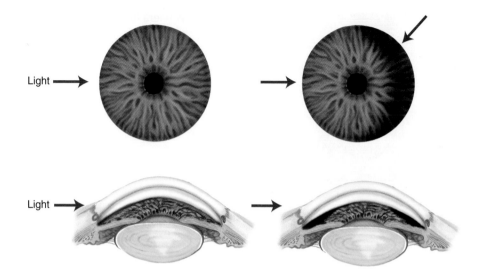

This narrow angle increases the risk for acute *narrow-angle glaucoma*—a sudden increase in intraocular pressure when drainage of the aqueous humour is blocked.

In *open-angle glaucoma*—the common form of glaucoma—the spatial relation between iris and cornea is preserved and the iris is fully lit.

Pupils. Inspect the *size, shape,* and *symmetry* of the pupils. If the pupils are large (>5 mm), small (<3 mm), or unequal, measure them. A card with black circles of varying sizes facilitates measurement.

Miosis refers to constriction of the pupils, *mydriasis* to dilation.

| 1 | 2 | 3 | 4 | 5 | 6 | 7 mm |

Pupillary inequality of less than 0.5 mm (*anisocoria*) is visible in approximately 20% of people. If pupillary reactions are brisk, anisocoria is considered benign.

Compare benign anisocoria with *Horner's syndrome, oculomotor nerve paralysis,* and *tonic pupil.* See Table 12-6, Pupillary Variations (p. 331).

Test the *pupillary reaction to light.* Ask the client to look into the distance, and shine a bright light obliquely into each pupil in turn. (Both the distant gaze and the oblique lighting help to prevent a near reaction.) Look for the following:

■ The *direct reaction* (pupillary constriction in the same eye)

■ The *consensual reaction* (pupillary constriction in the opposite eye)

Always darken the room and use a bright light before deciding that a light reaction is absent.

If the reaction to light is impaired or questionable, test the *near reaction* in room light. Testing one eye at a time makes it easier to concentrate on pupillary responses, without the distraction of extraocular movement. Hold your finger or pencil approximately 10 cm from the client's eye. Ask the client to look alternately at it and into the distance directly behind it. Watch for pupillary constriction with near effort.

Testing the near reaction is helpful in diagnosing *Argyll Robertson* and *tonic (Adie's) pupils* (see p. 331).

Extraocular Muscles. From approximately 60 centimetres directly in front of the client, shine a light onto the client's eyes and ask the client to look at it. *Inspect the reflections in the corneas.* They should be visible slightly nasal to the centre of the pupils.

Asymmetry of the corneal reflections indicates a deviation from ocular alignment. A temporal light reflection on one cornea, for example, indicates a nasal deviation of that eye. See Table 12-7, Dysconjugate Gaze (p. 332).

A *cover–uncover test* may reveal a slight or latent muscle imbalance not otherwise seen (see p. 332).

Now *assess the extraocular movements* by looking for the following:

- The normal *conjugate movements* of the eyes in each direction or any *deviation*.

- *Nystagmus*, a fine rhythmic oscillation of the eyes. A few beats of nystagmus on extreme lateral gaze are expected. If you see it, bring your finger in to within the field of binocular vision and look again.

- *Lid lag* as the eyes move from up to down.

To make these observations, *ask the client to follow your finger or pencil* as you sweep through the six cardinal directions of gaze. Making a wide H in the air, lead the client's gaze (1) to the client's extreme right, (2) to the right and upward, and (3) down on the right; then (4) without pausing in the middle, to the extreme left, (5) to the left and upward, and (6) down on the left. Pause during upward

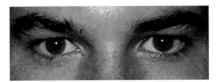

See Table 12-7, Dysconjugate Gaze (p. 332).

Sustained nystagmus within the binocular field of gaze is seen with various neurologic conditions.

Lid lag accompanies *hyperthyroidism.*

In paralysis of the CN VI, illustrated below, the eyes are conjugate in right lateral gaze but not in left lateral gaze, *left infranuclear ophthalmoplegia.*

LOOKING RIGHT

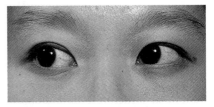

LOOKING LEFT

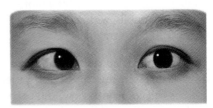

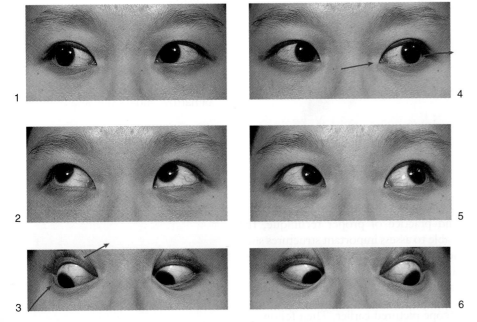

and lateral gaze to detect nystagmus. Move your finger or pencil at a comfortable distance from the client. Because middle-aged or older people may have difficulty focusing on near objects, make this distance greater for them than for young people. Some clients move their heads to follow your finger. If necessary, hold the head in the proper midline position. Ensure that you do not hold the client's eyes in any extreme position.

If you suspect a lid lag or hyperthyroidism, ask the client to follow your finger again as you move it slowly from up to down in the midline. The lid should overlap the iris slightly throughout this movement.

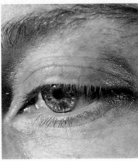

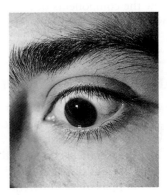

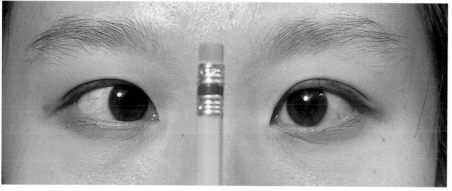

CONVERGENCE

Finally, test for *convergence*. Ask the client to follow your finger or pencil as you move it in toward the bridge of the nose. The converging eyes usually follow the object to within 5 cm to 8 cm of the nose.

Ophthalmoscopic Examination. In general health care, you usually examine your client's eyes *without dilating the pupils*. Your view is therefore limited to the posterior structures of the retina. To see more peripheral structures, to evaluate the macula well, or to investigate unexplained visual loss, ophthalmologists dilate the pupils with mydriatic drops unless this is contraindicated.

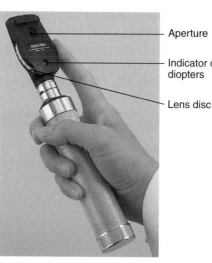

Aperture

Indicator of diopters

Lens disc

In the lid lag of hyperthyroidism, a rim of sclera is seen between the upper lid and iris; the lid seems to lag behind the eyeball.

Convergence is poor in *hyperthyroidism.*

Contraindications for mydriatic drops include (1) head injury and coma, in which continuing observations of pupillary reactions are essential and (2) any suspicion of narrow-angle glaucoma.

At first, using the ophthalmoscope may seem awkward, and it may be difficult to visualize the fundus. With patience and practice of proper technique, the fundus will come into view, and you will be able to assess important structures such as the optic disc and the retinal vessels. Remove your glasses unless you have marked nearsightedness or severe astigmatism. (However, if the client's refractive errors make it difficult to focus on the fundi, it may be easier to keep your glasses on.)

Review the components of the ophthalmoscope pictured earlier. Then follow the steps for using the ophthalmoscope, and your examination skills will improve over time.

STEPS FOR USING THE OPHTHALMOSCOPE

- Darken the room. Switch on the ophthalmoscope light and turn the lens disc until you see the large round beam of white light.* Shine the light on the back of your hand to check the type of light, its desired brightness, and the electrical charge of the ophthalmoscope.
- Turn the lens disc to the 0 diopter (a diopter is a unit that measures the power of a lens to converge or diverge light). At this diopter, the lens neither converges nor diverges light. Keep your finger on the edge of the lens disc so you can turn the disc to focus the lens when you examine the fundus.

(Continued)

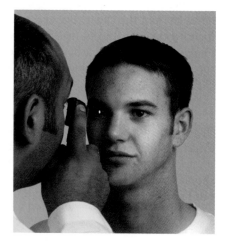

STEPS FOR USING THE OPHTHALMOSCOPE (Continued)

- Remember, hold the ophthalmoscope *in your right hand* to examine *the client's right eye*; hold it *in your left hand* to examine *the client's left eye*. This keeps you from bumping the client's nose and gives you more mobility and closer range for visualizing the fundus. At first, you may have difficulty using the nondominant eye, but this will abate with practice.
- Hold the ophthalmoscope firmly braced against the medial aspect of your bony orbit, with the handle tilted laterally at about a 20° slant from the vertical. Check to make sure you can see clearly through the aperture. Instruct the client to look slightly up and over your shoulder at a point directly ahead on the wall.
- Place yourself 35 cm away from the client and at an angle 15° lateral to the client's line of vision. Shine the light beam on the pupil and look for the orange glow in the pupil—the *red reflex*. Note any opacity interrupting the red reflex.
- Now, place the thumb of your other hand across the client's eyebrow (this technique helps keep you steady but is not essential). Keeping the light beam focused on the red reflex, move in with the ophthalmoscope on the 15° angle toward the pupil until you are very close it, almost touching the client's eyelashes.

Try to keep both eyes open and relaxed, as if gazing into the distance, to help minimize any fluctuating blurriness as your eyes attempt to accommodate.

You may need to lower the brightness of the light beam to make the examination more comfortable for the client, avoid *hippus* (spasm of the pupil), and improve your observations.

*Some clinicians like to use the large round beam for large pupils, the small round beam for small pupils. The other beams are rarely helpful. The slit-like beam is sometimes used to assess elevations or concavities in the retina, the green (or red-free) beam to detect small red lesions, and the grid to make measurements. Ignore the last three lights and practice with the large round white beam.

Absence of *a red reflex* suggests opacity of the lens (cataract) or possibly of the vitreous. Less commonly, *a detached retina* or, in children, a *retinoblastoma* may obscure this reflex. Do not be fooled by an artificial eye, which has no red reflex.

Now you are ready to inspect the *optic disc* and the *retina*. You should be seeing the optic disc—a yellowish orange to creamy pink oval or round structure that may fill your field of gaze or even exceed it. Of interest, the ophthalmoscope magnifies the retina about 15 times and the iris about 4 times. The optic disc actually measures about 1.5 mm. The following table outlines this important segment of the physical examination.

When the lens has been removed surgically, its magnifying effect is lost. Retinal structures then look much smaller than usual, and you can see a much larger expanse of fundus.

STEPS FOR EXAMINING THE OPTIC DISC AND THE RETINA

The Optic Disc

- First, *locate the optic disc.* Look for the round yellowish orange structure described previously. If you do not see it at first, follow a blood vessel centrally until you do. You can tell which direction is central by noting the angles at which vessels branch—the vessel size becomes progressively larger at each junction as you approach the disc.

(Continued)

STEPS FOR EXAMINING THE OPTIC DISC AND THE RETINA (Continued)

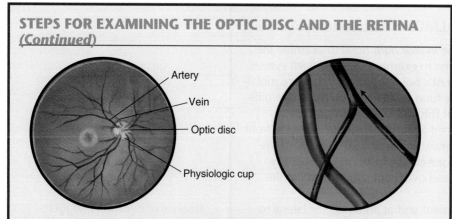

Artery
Vein
Optic disc
Physiologic cup

- Now, *bring the optic disc into sharp focus* by adjusting the lens of your ophthalmoscope. If both you and the client have no refractive errors, the retina should be in focus at 0 diopter. If structures are blurred, rotate the lens disc until you find the sharpest focus.

    For example, if the client is myopic (nearsighted), rotate the lens disc counterclockwise to the minus diopters; in a hyperopic (farsighted) client, move the disc clockwise to the plus diopters. You can correct your own refractive error in the same way.

- *Inspect the optic disc.* Note the following features:
  - *The sharpness or clarity of the disc outline.* The nasal portion of the disc margin may be somewhat blurred, are expected finding.
  - *The colour of the disc,* normally yellowish orange to creamy pink. White or pigmented crescents may ring the disc, an expected finding.

  - *The size of the central physiologic cup,* if present. It is usually yellowish white. The horizontal diameter is usually less than half the horizontal diameter of the disc.
  - *The comparative symmetry* of the eyes and findings in the fundi.

Detecting Papilledema

Papilledema describes swelling of the optic disc and anterior bulging of the physiologic cup. Increased intracranial pressure is transmitted to the optic nerve, causing stasis of axoplasmic flow, intra-axonal edema, and swelling of the optic nerve head. Papilledema often signals serious disorders of the brain, such as meningitis, subarachnoid hemorrhage, trauma, and mass lesions, so searching for this important disorder is a priority during all your fundoscopic examinations.

    If you detect papilledema, measure elevation of the optic disc by subtracting the difference in the diopters of the two lenses needed to focus clearly on the elevated disc and on the uninvolved retina. *Note that at the retina, 3 diopters = 1 mm.*

    Venous pulsations, seen in many but not all normal eyegrounds, may also be obliterated.

The Retina—Arteries, Veins, Fovea, and Macula

Inspect the retina, including arteries and veins as they extend to the periphery, arteriovenous crossings, the fovea, and the macula. Distinguish arteries from veins based on the features listed here.

(Continued)

In a refractive error, light rays from a distance do not focus on the retina. In myopia, they focus anterior to it; in hyperopia, posterior to it. Retinal structures in a myopic eye look larger than usual.

See Table 12-8, Expected Variations of the Optic Disc (p. 333), and Table 12-9, Variations of the Optic Disc (p. 334).

An enlarged cup suggests chronic open-angle glaucoma.

Loss of venous pulsations in pathologic conditions such as head trauma, meningitis, or mass lesions may be an early sign of elevated intracranial pressure.

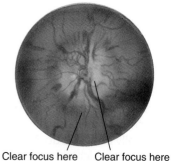

Clear focus here at −1 diopter   Clear focus here at + 3 diopters

+ 3 − (−1) = 4, therefore, a disc elevation of 4 diopters

STEPS FOR EXAMINING THE OPTIC DISC AND THE RETINA *(Continued)*

	Arteries	*Veins*
Colour	Light red	Dark red
Size	Smaller ($^2/_3$ to $^4/_5$ the diameter of veins)	Larger
Light reflex (reflection)	Bright	Inconspicuous or absent

- *Follow the vessels peripherally in each of four directions*, noting their relative sizes and the character of the arteriovenous crossings.

  Identify any lesions of the surrounding *retina* and note their size, shape, colour, and distribution. As you search the retina, *move your head and instrument as a unit*, using the client's pupil as an imaginary fulcrum. At first, you may repeatedly lose your view of the retina because your light falls out of the pupil. You will improve with practice.

  Lesions of the retina can be measured in terms of "disc diameters" from the optic disc. For example, among the cotton-wool patches illustrated on the right, note the irregular patches between 11 and 12 o'clock, 1 to 2 disc diameters from the disc. Each measures about one-half by one-half disc diameters.

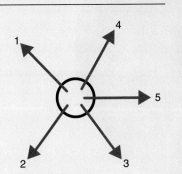

Sequence of inspection from disc to macula

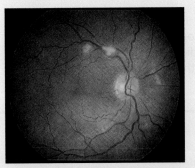

COTTON-WOOL PATCHES

See Table 12-10, Retinal Arteries and Arteriovenous Crossings: Healthy and Hypertensive (p. 335); Table 12-11, Red Spots and Streaks in the Fundi (p. 336); Table 12-12, Ocular Fundi (pp. 337); Table 12-13, Light-Coloured Spots in the Fundi.

- Inspect the *fovea and surrounding macula.* Direct your light beam laterally or by asking the client to look directly into the light. Except in older people, the tiny bright reflection at the centre of the fovea helps to orient you. Shimmering light reflections in the macular area are common in young people

Macular degeneration is an important cause of poor central vision in the elderly. Types include *dry atrophic* (more common but less severe) and *wet exudative,* or neovascular. Undigested cellular debris, called *drusen,* may be hard and sharply defined, as seen below, or soft and confluent with altered pigmentation (see p. 339).

(Continued)

STEPS FOR EXAMINING THE OPTIC DISC AND THE RETINA
(Continued)

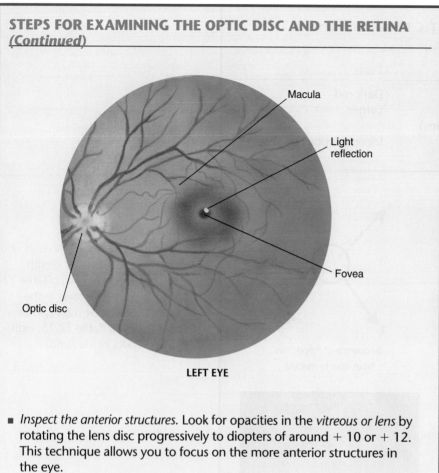

Macula

Light reflection

Fovea

Optic disc

LEFT EYE

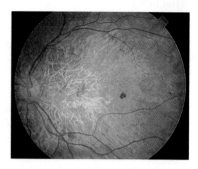

Photo from Tasman W, Jaeger E (eds). The Wills Eye Hospital Atlas of Clinical Ophthalmology, 2nd ed. Philadelphia, Lippincott Williams & Wilkins, 2001.

- *Inspect the anterior structures.* Look for opacities in the *vitreous or lens* by rotating the lens disc progressively to diopters of around + 10 or + 12. This technique allows you to focus on the more anterior structures in the eye.

Vitreous floaters may be seen as dark specks or strands between the fundus and the lens. Cataracts are densities in the lens (see p. 309).

Cultural Considerations

First Nations clients, Asian Canadians, and African Canadians have larger optic nerve discs than Caucasians.

SPECIAL TECHNIQUES

For Assessing Protruding Eyes (Proptosis or Exophthalmos). For eyes that seem unusually prominent, stand behind the seated client and inspect from above. Draw the upper lids gently upward, then compare the protrusion of the eyes and the relationship of the corneas to the lower lids. For objective measurement, use an exophthalmometer. This instrument measures the distance between the lateral angle of the orbit and an imaginary line across the most anterior point of the cornea. The upper limits are 20 millimetres in whites and 22 millimetres in blacks (Bartley et al., 1996; Gladstone, 1998).

When protrusion exceeds the expected measurement, further evaluation by ultrasound or computerized tomography scan often follows (Hallin & Feldon, 1988).

Exophthalmos is excessive protrusion of the eye.

For Nasolacrimal Duct Obstruction. This test helps identify the cause of excessive tearing. Ask the client to look up. Press on the lower lid close to the medial canthus, just inside the rim of the bony orbit—this compresses the lacrimal sac. Look for fluid regurgitated out of the puncta into the eye. Avoid this test if the area is inflamed and tender.

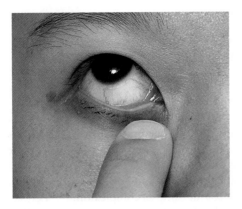

Discharge of mucopurulent fluid from the puncta suggests an obstructed nasolacrimal duct.

When the optic nerve is damaged, as in the left eye below, the sensory or afferent stimulus sent to the brainstem is reduced. The pupil dilates instead of constricting when the light moves from the good right eye into the left eye. This response is an *afferent pupillary defect,* sometimes termed a *Marcus Gunn pupil.* The opposite eye responds consensually.

Swinging Flashlight Test. The swinging flashlight test is a clinical test for functional impairment in the optic nerves. In dim light, note the size of the pupils. After asking the client to gaze into the distance, swing the beam of a penlight first into one pupil, then into the other. Each illuminated eye looks or promptly becomes constricted. The opposite eye also constricts consensually.

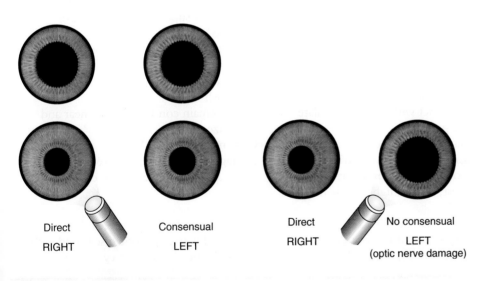

Direct RIGHT — Consensual LEFT

Direct RIGHT — No consensual LEFT (optic nerve damage)

RECORDING AND ANALYZING FINDINGS

Documentation of the information obtained through the client history and the physical examination of the eyes needs to be thorough, accurate, and clear for all members of the interdisciplinary team to ensure that comprehensive and appropriate care can be planned and implemented for the client.

■ *Examples of Documentation for Eyes*

Area of Assessment	Expected Findings	Unexpected Findings
Visual acuity	20/20 bilaterally, 20/200 in left eye, 20/20 in right eye	
Fields of confrontation	Visual fields full bilaterally	Vision absent in right superotemporal field
Position and alignment of the eyes	Symmetrical, equally spaced from nose. Outer canthus of eye aligned with superior aspect of helix.	Left eye slightly lower than right eye. Left eye deviates medially.
Eyebrows	Symmetrical hair distribution	Patchy, asymmetrical hair distribution
Eyelids	Full closure, colour same as complexion, symmetrical blinking, overlie pupils slightly and symmetrically	Left lateral upper eyelid swollen with yellowish exudate along border, asymmetrical blinking
Eyelashes	Full, curl outward from upper and lower eyelids bilaterally	Right lateral eyelashes on upper eyelid curl inward, lashes missing from medial aspect of left lower eyelid
Lacrimal glands/sacs	No redness or inflammation bilaterally	Tender upon palpation bilaterally, excessive tearing in right eye
Conjunctiva	Clear, transparent bilaterally	Reddened area on lower medial margin of left eye
Sclera	White, clear bilaterally	Greyish, dull bilaterally
Cornea/lens	Shiny, clear bilaterally	Cloudy yellow opacity on right medial, superior left eye
Iris	Green/brown/blue; circular with regular border; symmetrical in size, colour, and shape	Right iris blue, left iris green; irregular border on superior lateral aspect of left iris
Pupils	Round and equal at 2 mm, direct and consensual reactions brisk bilaterally	Right pupil at 2 mm, left pupil at 4 mm
Pupillary reaction to light	PERRLA (pupils equal, round, reactive to light and accommodation)	Pupils unequal, left pupil fixed, right pupil sluggish
Accommodation (near reaction)	Pupils constrict with near gaze, dilate with far gaze	Pupils remain constricted with near and far gaze
Convergence	Gaze maintained to 4 cm	Gaze maintained to 10 cm
Extraocular muscles	Conjugate tracking in six cardinal directions, no eye movement noted in cover test, corneal light symmetrically reflected	Nystagmus present in left eye in all directions, left eye movement in cover test
Ophthalmoscopic (lens, vessels, optic discs)	Lens clear, bilateral red reflex, arterioles 2/3 size of veins with smooth crossings, optic discs round, yellowish pink	Absent red reflex in left eye, A/V nicking present bilaterally, optic disc round with irregular border in right eye

◢ ANALYZING FINDINGS FROM HEALTH HISTORY AND PHYSICAL EXAMINATION

Once findings from the physical examination are documented, their analysis combined with a review of information from the health history is completed to identify one or more nursing diagnoses and plan an interdisciplinary approach for treatment. For example:

Mr. Smith, 55 years old, presents to the clinic with concerns about his "vision getting worse." He has a 20-year history of insulin-dependent diabetes mellitus and reports having high blood pressure. During the ophthalmoscopic examination you note tiny red dots on the retina. From this information, you develop the following nursing diagnosis:

Potential for vision loss related to complications from diabetes mellitus and hypertension

To ensure comprehensive care for Mr. Smith, an eye specialist (ophthalmologist or optometrist) needs to perform a complete eye examination. A physician specializing in diabetes needs to conduct an assessment of Mr. Smith's medical conditions. A dietician should develop a dietary plan that considers nutrition, exercise, and blood glucose monitoring and stabilization. A registered nurse in home care should carry out continued follow-up to facilitate all aspects of the client's care, including assessing Mr. Smith's home environment to ensure safety, assessing Mr. Smith's understanding of the treatment plan, and identifying any psychosocial considerations. Continued follow-up by a registered nurse is essential to promoting vision health for Mr. Smith.

Critical Thinking Exercise

Answer the following questions about Mr. Smith.

- What is the physiology behind the observation of tiny red dots on the retina in a client with insulin-dependent diabetes mellitus? (*Knowledge*)
- How can you distinguish between the findings for macular degeneration from the findings for diabetic retinopathy? (*Comprehension*)
- How would you teach Mr. Smith about promoting the health of his eyes and vision? What information would you include? (*Application*)
- What lifestyle factors might be contributing to Mr. Smith's vision symptom(s)? (*Analysis*)
- What recommendations for screening and follow-up would you suggest for Mr. Smith? (*Synthesis*)
- How would you evaluate the success of client teaching for Mr. Smith? (*Evaluation*)

Canadian Research

Canadian National Institute for the Blind National Service Development and Research. (2004). *Vision care and rehabilitation problems and solutions emerging through a culturally appropriate participatory action research process with First Nations Peoples—Recommendations for health service providers and policy makers.* Toronto, ON: Author.

Dhillon, S., Shapiro, C. M., & Flanagan, J. (2007). Sleep-disordered breathing and effects on ocular health. *Canadian Journal of Ophthalmology, 42*(2), 238–243.

Perruccio, A. V., Badley, E. M., & Trope, G. E. (2007). Self-reported glaucoma in Canada: Findings from population-based surveys 1994–2003. *Canadian Journal of Ophthalmology, 42*(2), 219–226.

Russell-Minda, E., Jutai, J., & Strong, G. (2006). *An evidence-based review of the research on typeface legibility for readers with low vision.* Toronto, ON: Vision Rehabilitation Evidence-Based Review and Canadian National Institute for the Blind Research Unit.

Simson, H., Gold, D., & Zuvela, B. (2005). *An unequal playing field: Report on the needs of people who are blind or visually impaired living in Canada.* Toronto, ON: Canadian National Institute for the Blind National Research Unit.

Wolffe, K. (2004). *The status of Canadian youth who are blind or visually impaired: A study of lifestyles, quality of life, and employment (2004).* Toronto, ON: Canadian National Institute for the Blind National Research Unit.

Test Questions

1. Signs of macular degeneration seen during the ophthalmoscopic examination include which of the following?
   a. Clouded lens
   b. Subretinal exudate
   c. Hemorrhage around optic disc
   d. Altered size and colour of optic disc

2. When testing the near reaction, an expected finding includes papillary:
   a. dilation on near gaze; dilation on distant gaze.
   b. dilation on near gaze; constriction on distant gaze.
   c. constriction on near gaze; dilation on distant gaze.
   d. constriction on near gaze; constriction on distant gaze.

3. When visual acuity is tested using the Snellen eye chart, which client has the better distance vision?
   a. Numerator at 20
   b. Numerator at 30
   c. Denominator at 20
   d. Denominator at 10

4. The nurse observes a middle-aged colleague fully extending her arm to read the label on a vial of medication. Which of the following age-related changes is the nurse likely to have observed?
   a. Presbyopia
   b. Cataract formation
   c. Loss of convergence
   d. Macular degeneration

5. The muscles of the ciliary body control the thickness of the lens, allowing the eye to:
   a. focus on near or distant objects.
   b. coordinate extraocular movement.
   c. adjust the pressure inside the eye.
   d. control the amount of light entering the eye.

Bibliography

CITATIONS

Bartley, G. B., et al. (1996). Clinical features of Graves' ophthalmology in an incidence cohort. *American Journal of Ophthalmology, 121*, 284–290.

Canadian National Institute for the Blind. (2007a). *Vision loss: Fast facts about vision loss*. Retrieved March 28, 2007, from www.cnib.ca/vision-health/vision-loss/fast-facts.htm

Canadian National Institute for the Blind. (2007b). *Vision loss: Cataracts*. Retrieved March 28, 2007, from www.cnib.ca/vision-health/vision-loss/cataracts.htm

Canadian National Institute for the Blind. (2007c). *Vision loss: Glaucoma the facts*. Retrieved March 28, 2007, from www.cnib.ca/vision-health/vision-loss/glaucoma.htm

Canadian Ophthalmological Society. (2007). *Age-related macular degeneration*. Retrieved March 28, 2007, from www.eyesite.ca/english/public-information/eye-conditions/pdfs/MacDegeneration_e.pdf

Fine, S. L., Berger, J. W., Macguire, M. G., & Ho, A. C. (2000). Age-related macular degeneration. *New England Journal of Medicine, 342*(7), 483–492.

Gladstone, G. J. (1998). Ophthalmological aspects of thyroid-related orbitopathy. *Endocrinological and Metabolic Clinics of North America, 27*, 91–100.

Hallin, E. S., & Feldon, S. E. (1988). Graves' ophthalmology. II. Correlation of clinical signs with measures derived from computed tomography. *British Journal of Ophthalmology, 72*, 678–682.

Shingleton, B. J., & O'Donoghue, M. W. (2000). Blurred vision. *New England Journal of Medicine, 343*(8), 556–562.

Wong, T. Y., & Mitchell, P. (2004). Hypertensive retinopathy. *New England Journal of Medicine, 351*(22), 2310–2317.

World Health Organization. (2007). *Stop the global epidemic of chronic disease*. Retrieved April 16, 2007, from www.who.int/blindness/en

ADDITIONAL RESOURCES

Albert, D. M., & Jabobieck, F. A. (2000). *Principles and practice of ophthalmology* (2nd ed.). Philadelphia: W.B. Saunders.

Congdon, N., O'Colmain, B., Klaver, C. C., Klein, R., Muñoz, B., Friedman, D. S., et al. (2004). Causes and prevalence of visual impairment among adults in the United States. *Archives of Ophthalmology, 122*(4), 477–485.

Delpero, W., Beiko, G., Casey, R., Ells, A., Kertes, P., Molgat, Y., et al. (2007). Canadian Ophthalmological Society evidence-based clinical practice guidelines for the periodic eye examination in adults in Canada. *Canadian Journal of Ophthalmology, 42*, 39–45.

Fong, D. S., Aiello, L. P., Ferris, F. L., & Klein, R. (2004). Diabetic retinopathy. *Diabetes Care, 27*(10), 2540–2553.

Gold, D. H., & Weingeist, T. A. (2001). *Colour atlas of the eye in systemic disease*. Philadelphia: Lippincott Williams & Wilkins.

McCluskey, P. J., Towler, H. M., & Lightman, S. (2000). Management of chronic uveitis. *British Medical Journal, 320*(7234), 555–558.

Ostler, H. B., Maibach, H. I., Hoke, A. W., & Schwab, I. R. (2004). *Diseases of the eye and skin: A colour atlas*. Philadelphia: Lippincott Williams & Wilkins.

Shields, S. R. (2000). Managing eye disease in primary care. Part 1. How to screen for occult disease. *Postgraduate Medicine, 108*(5), 69–72, 75–78.

Spoor, T. C. (Ed.). (2004). *Atlas of neuro-opththalmology*. New York: Taylor & Francis.

Stephen, T. C. (1997). Symptom analysis. In *Adult health assessment series* [CD-ROM]. Edmonton, AB: DataStar Education Systems & Services.

Stephen, T. C. (2004). Documentation. In *Health assessment self-test modules (WebCT Vista)*. Edmonton, AB: Faculty of Nursing, University of Alberta.

Stephen, T. C. (2007). Assessment and management of clients with eye and vision disorders. In R. A. Day, P. Paul, & B. Williams (Eds.), *Brunner and Suddarth's textbook of medical-surgical nursing* (pp. 1754–1797). Philadelphia: Lippincott Williams & Wilkins.

Tasman, W., & Jaeger, E. A. (2001). *The Wills Eye Hospital Atlas of Clinical Ophthalmology* (2nd ed.). Philadelphia: Lippincott Williams & Wilkins.

Weber, J., & Kelley, J. (2007). *Health assessment in nursing* (3rd ed.). Philadelphia: Lippincott Williams & Wilkins.

Yanoff, M., & Duker, J. S. (2004). *Ophthalmology* (2nd ed.). St. Louis: Mosby.

WEB SITES AND ASSOCIATIONS

Adaptive Technology Resource Centre: http://atrc.utoronto.ca

Alliance for Equality of Blind Canadians: http://www.blindcanadians.ca

AMD Canada: http://amdcanada.com/

Canadian Association Disability Service Providers in Post Secondary Education: http://www.cacuss.ca

Canadian Association of Independent Living Centres: http://www.cailc.ca

The Canadian Association of Optometrists: http://www.opto.ca

Canadian Braille Authority: http://www.canadianbrailleauthority.ca

Canadian Council of the Blind: http://www.ccbnational.net

Canadian Council on Social Development: http://www.ccsd.ca

Canadian Library Association: http://www.cla.ca

BIBLIOGRAPHY

Canadian Diabetes Association: http://www.diabetes.ca/

Canadian National Institute for the Blind: http://www.cnib.ca

Canadian National Society for the Deaf Blind: http://www.cnsdb.ca

Canadian Ophthalmological Society: http://www.eyesite.ca

Cancer Prevention (Sun safety)—Toronto Public Health: http://www.toronto.ca/health/sun/sunsafety_eyes.htm

Cataracts. University of Ottawa Eye Institute: http://www.eyeinstitute.net/cataracts.html

Council on Access to Information for Print-Disabled Canadians: http://www.collectionscanada.ca/accessinfo

Council of Canadians with Disabilities: http://www.ccdonline.ca

Five Steps to Eye Health:

The Foundation Fighting Blindness: Canada – http://www.ffb.ca/

Glaucoma Canada: http://www.glaucomacanada.com

Glaucoma Research Society of Canada: http://www.glaucomaresearch.ca/

Graves' disease. Thyroid Foundation of Canada: http://www.thyroid.ca/Guides/HG07.html

Health Canada – It's Your Health: http://www.hc-sc.gc.ca/iyh-vsv/index_e.html

Help the Aged Canada: http://www.helptheaged.ca

The Learning Disabilities Association of Canada (National Office): http://www.ldac-taac.ca

The National Coalition for Vision Health: http://www.visionhealth.ca/

National Educational Association of Disabled Students: http://www.neads.ca

The Pediatric Glaucoma and Cataract Family Association: http://pgcfa.org/index.htm

Public Health Agency of Canada: http://www.phac-aspc.gc.ca

Strabismus. Alberta Association of Optometrists: http://www.optometrists.ab.ca/

Veteran Affairs Canada: http://www.vac-acc.gc.ca

TABLE 12-1   Visual Field Defects

Visual Field Defects

1 Horizontal Defect Occlusion of a branch of the central retinal artery may cause a horizontal (altitudinal) defect. Shown is the lower field defect associated with occlusion of the superior branch of this artery.

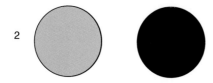

2 Blind Right Eye (right optic nerve) A lesion of the optic nerve, and of course of the eye itself, produces unilateral blindness.

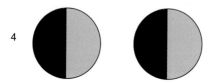

3 Bitemporal Hemianopsia (optic chiasm) A lesion at the optic chiasm may involve only fibres crossing over to the opposite side. As these fibres originate in the nasal half of each retina, visual loss involves the temporal half of each field.

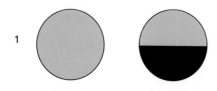

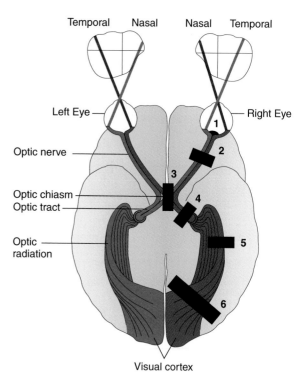

4 Left Homonymous Hemianopsia (right optic tract) A lesion of the optic tract interrupts fibres originating on the same side of both eyes. Visual loss in the eyes is therefore similar (homonymous) and involves half of each field (hemianopsia).

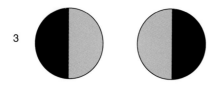

5 Homonymous Left Superior Quadrantic Defect (right optic radiation, partial) A partial lesion of the optic radiation in the temporal lobe may involve only a portion of the nerve fibres, producing, for example, a homonymous quadrantic defect.

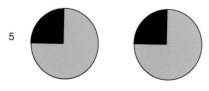

6 Left Homonymous Hemianopsia (right optic radiation) A complete interruption of fibres in the optic radiation produces a visual defect similar to that produced by a lesion of the optic tract.

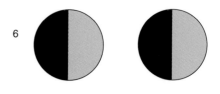

TABLE 12-2   Variations of the Eyelids

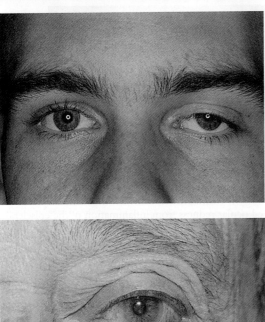

Ptosis

Ptosis is a drooping of the upper lid. Causes include myasthenia gravis, damage to the oculomotor nerve, and damage to the sympathetic nerve supply (*Horner's syndrome*). A weakened muscle, relaxed tissues, and the weight of herniated fat may cause senile ptosis. Ptosis may also be congenital.

Entropion

Entropion, more common in the elderly, is an inward turning of the lid margin. The lower lashes, which are often invisible when turned inward, irritate the conjunctiva and lower cornea. Asking the client to squeeze the lids together and then open them may reveal an entropion that is not obvious.

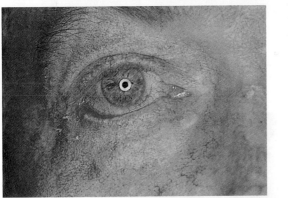

Ectropion

In ectropion the margin of the lower lid is turned outward, exposing the palpebral conjunctiva. When the punctum of the lower lid turns outward, the eye no longer drains satisfactorily and tearing occurs. Ectropion is more common in the elderly.

Lid Retraction and Exophthalmos

A wide-eyed stare suggests retracted eyelids. Note the rim of sclera between the upper lid and the iris. Retracted lids and a lid lag (p. 315) are often indicative of hyperthyroidism.

In exophthalmos, the eyeball protrudes forward. When bilateral, it suggests the infiltrative ophthalmopathy of Graves' hyperthyroidism. Edema of the eyelids and conjunctival injection may be associated. Unilateral exophthalmos seen in Graves' disease or a tumour or inflammation in the orbit.

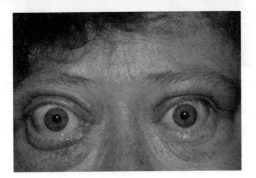

Photo source: Ptosis, ectropion, entropion: Tasman, W., & Jaeger, E. (Eds). *The Wills Eye Hospital Atlas of Clinical Ophthalmology*, 2nd ed. Philadelphia: Lippincott Williams & Wilkins, 2001.

TABLE 12-3   Lumps and Swellings in and Around the Eyes

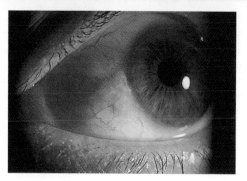

Pinguecula

A harmless yellowish triangular nodule in the bulbar conjunctiva on either side of the iris. Appears frequently with aging, first on the nasal and then on the temporal side.

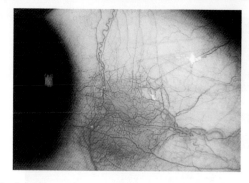

Episcleritis

A localized ocular redness from inflammation of the episcleral vessels. Vessels appear salmon pink and are movable over the scleral surface. May be nodular, as shown, or may show only redness and dilated vessels.

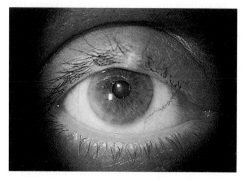

Sty

A painful, tender, red infection in a gland at the margin of the eyelid.

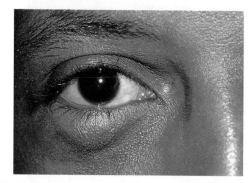

Chalazion

A subacute nontender and usually painless nodule involving a meibomian gland. May become acutely inflamed, but, unlike a sty, usually points inside the lid rather than on the lid margin.

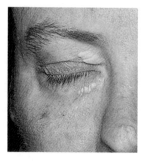

Xanthelasma

Slightly raised, yellowish, well-circumscribed plaques that appear along the nasal portions of one or both eyelids. May accompany lipid disorders.

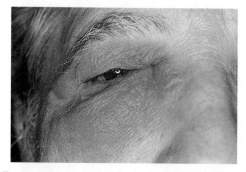

Inflammation of the Lacrimal Sac (Dacryocystitis)

A swelling between the lower eyelid and nose. An *acute* inflammation (illustrated) is painful, red, and tender. *Chronic* inflammation is associated with obstruction of the nasolacrimal duct. Tearing is prominent, and pressure on the sac produces regurgitation of material through the puncta of the eyelids.

Photo source: Tasman, W., & Jaeger, E. (Eds). *The Wills Eye Hospital Atlas of Clinical Ophthalmology*, 2nd ed. Philadelphia: Lippincott Williams & Wilkins, 2001.

TABLE 12-4   **Red Eyes**

	Conjunctivitis	Subconjunctival Hemorrhage
	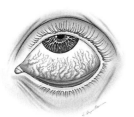	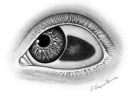
Pattern of Redness	Conjunctival injection: diffuse dilatation of conjunctival vessels with redness that tends to be maximal peripherally	Leakage of blood outside of the vessels, producing a homogeneous, sharply demarcated, red area that fades over days to yellow and then disappears
Pain	Mild discomfort rather than pain	Absent
Vision	Not affected, except for temporary mild blurring from discharge	Not affected
Ocular Discharge	Watery, mucoid, or mucopurulent	Absent
Pupil	Not affected	Not affected
Cornea	Clear	Clear
Significance	Bacterial, viral, and other infections; allergy; irritation	Often none. May result from trauma, bleeding disorders, or a sudden increase in venous pressure, as from cough.

	Corneal Injury or Infection	Acute Iritis	Glaucoma
	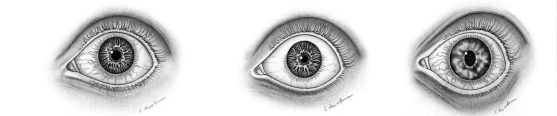		
Pattern of Redness	Ciliary injection: dilation of deeper vessels that are visible as radiating vessels or a reddish violet flush around the limbus. Ciliary injection is an important sign of these three conditions, but may not be apparent. The eye may be diffusely red instead. Other clues of these more serious disorders are pain, decreased vision, unequal pupils, and a less than perfectly clear cornea.		
Pain	Moderate to severe, superficial	Moderate, aching, deep	Severe, aching, deep
Vision	Usually decreased	Decreased	Decreased
Ocular Discharge	Watery or purulent	Absent	Absent
Pupil	Not affected unless iritis develops	May be small and, with time, irregular	Dilated, fixed
Cornea	Changes depending on cause	Clear or slightly clouded	Steamy, cloudy
Significance	Abrasions and other injuries; viral and bacterial infections	Associated with many ocular and systemic disorders	Acute increase in intraocular pressure—an emergency

TABLE 12-5   Opacities of the Cornea and Lens

Corneal Arcus

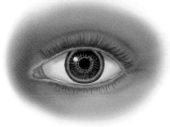

A thin greyish white arc or circle not quite at the edge of the cornea. Accompanies aging, but also seen in younger people, especially people of African descent. In young people, suggests possible hyperlipoproteinemia. Usually benign.

Corneal Scar

A superficial greyish white opacity in the cornea, secondary to an old injury or to inflammation. Size and shape are variable. Do not confuse with the opaque lens of a cataract, visible on a deeper plane and only through the pupil.

Pterygium

A triangular thickening of the bulbar conjunctiva that grows slowly across the outer surface of the cornea, usually from the nasal side. Reddening may occur. May interfere with vision as it encroaches on the pupil.

Cataracts

Opacities of the lenses visible through the pupil; most common in old age.

Nuclear cataract. A nuclear cataract looks grey when seen by a flashlight. If the pupil is widely dilated, the grey opacity is surrounded by a black rim. Through an ophthalmoscope, the cataract looks black against the red reflex.

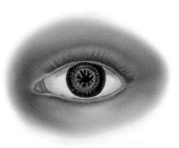

Peripheral cataract. Produces spoke-like shadows that point inward—grey against black as seen with a flashlight, or black against red with an ophthalmoscope. A dilated pupil, as shown here, facilitates this observation.

TABLE 12-6   **Variations**

Unequal Pupils (*Anisocoria*)—When anisocoria is greater in bright light than in dim light, the larger pupil cannot constrict properly. Causes include blunt trauma to the eye, open-angle glaucoma (p. 314), and impaired parasympathetic nerve supply to the iris, as in tonic pupil and oculomotor nerve paralysis. When anisocoria is greater in dim light, the smaller pupil cannot dilate properly, as in Horner's syndrome, caused by an interruption of the sympathetic nerve supply.

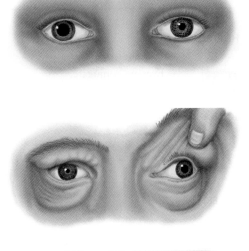

Tonic Pupil *(Adie's Pupil).* Pupil is large, regular, and usually unilateral. Reaction to light is severely reduced and slowed, or even absent. Near reaction, although very slow, is present. Slow accommodation causes blurred vision. Deep tendon reflexes are often decreased.

Oculomotor Nerve (CN III) Paralysis. The dilated pupil (6–7 mm) is fixed to light and near effort. Ptosis of the upper eyelid and lateral deviation of the eye are often, but not always, present. An even more dilated (8–9 mm) and fixed pupil may result from atropine-like eye drops.

Horner's Syndrome. The affected pupil, although small, reacts briskly to light and near effort. Ptosis of the eyelid is present, perhaps with loss of sweating on the forehead. In congenital Horner's syndrome, the involved iris is lighter in colour than its fellow (*heterochromia*).

Small, Irregular Pupils. Small, irregular pupils that accommodate but do not react to light indicate *Argyll Robertson pupils.* Seen in central nervous system syphilis.

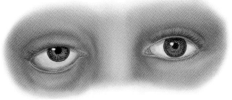

Blind eye

Light

Equal Pupils and One Blind Eye. Unilateral blindness does not cause anisocoria as long as the sympathetic and parasympathetic innervation to both irises is intact. A light directed into the seeing eye produces a direct reaction in that eye and a consensual reaction in the blind eye. A light directed into the blind eye, however, causes no response in either eye.

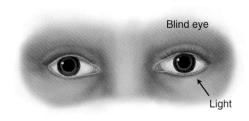

Blind eye

Light

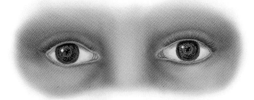

TABLE 12-7   Dysconjugate Gaze

Various gaze patterns give clinicians clues about brainstem developmental disorders and cranial nerve deviations.

Developmental Disorders

Developmental dysconjugate gaze is caused by an imbalance in ocular muscle tone. This imbalance has many causes, may be hereditary, and usually appears in early childhood. These gaze deviations are classified according to direction.

Disorders of Cranial Nerves

New onset of dysconjugate gaze in adult life is usually the result of cranial nerve injuries, lesions, or disorders from such causes as trauma, multiple sclerosis, syphilis, and others.

Esotropia   *Exotropia*

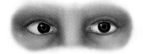

Cover–Uncover Test

A cover–uncover test may be helpful. Here is what you would see in the right monocular esotropia illustrated above.

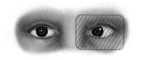

Corneal reflections are asymmetric.

COVER

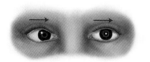

The right eye moves outward to fix on the light. (The left eye is not seen but moves inward to the same degree.)

UNCOVER

The left eye moves outward to fix on the light. The right eye deviates inward again.

A Left Cranial Nerve VI Paralysis

LOOKING TO THE RIGHT

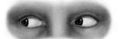

Eyes are conjugate.

LOOKING STRAIGHT AHEAD

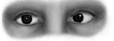

Esotropia appears.

LOOKING TO THE LEFT

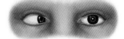

Esotropia is maximum.

A Left Cranial Nerve IV Paralysis

LOOKING DOWN AND TO THE RIGHT

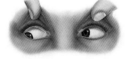

The left eye cannot look down when turned inward. Deviation is maximum in this direction.

A Left Cranial Nerve III Paralysis

LOOKING STRAIGHT AHEAD

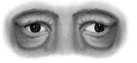

The eye is pulled outward by action of the sixth nerve. Upward, downward, and inward movements are impaired or lost. Ptosis and pupillary dilation may be associated.

TABLE 12-8	Expected Variations of the Optic Disc

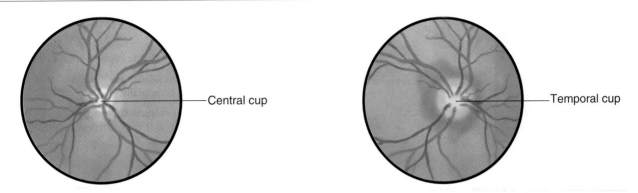

Physiologic Cupping

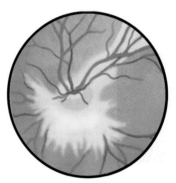

The physiologic cup is a small whitish depression in the optic disc from which the retinal vessels appear to emerge. Although sometimes absent, the cup is usually visible either centrally or toward the temporal side of the disc. Greyish spots are often seen at its base.

Rings and Crescents

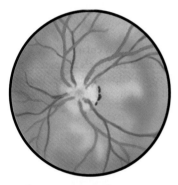

Medullated Nerve Fibres

Rings and crescents are often seen around the optic disc. These are developmental variations in which you can glimpse white sclera, black retinal pigment, or both, especially along the temporal border of the disc. Rings and crescents are not part of the disc itself and should not be included in your estimates of disc diameters.

Medullated nerve fibres are a much less common but dramatic finding. Appearing as irregular white patches with feathered margins, they obscure the disc edge and retinal vessels. They have no pathologic significance.

TABLE 12-9   Variations of the Optic Disc

	Process	Appearance
Expected	Tiny disc vessels give normal colour to the disc.	Colour yellowish orange to creamy pink. Disc vessels tiny. Disc margins sharp (except perhaps nasally). The physiologic cup is located centrally or somewhat temporally. It may be conspicuous or absent. Its diameter from side to side is usually less than half that of the disc.
Papilledema	Venous stasis leads to engorgement and swelling.	Colour pink, hyperemic. Disc vessels more visible, more numerous, curve over the borders of the disc. Disc swollen with margins blurred. The physiologic cup is not visible.
Glaucomatous Cupping	Increased pressure within the eye leads to increased cupping (backward depression of the disc) and atrophy. The base of the enlarged cup is pale.	The physiologic cup is enlarged, occupying more than half of the disc's diameter, at times extending to the edge of the disc. Retinal vessels sink in and under it, and may be displaced nasally.
Optic Atrophy	Death of optic nerve fibres. Leads to loss of the tiny disc vessels.	Colour white. Disc vessels absent.

Photo source: Tasman, W., & Jaeger, E. (Eds). *The Wills Eye Hospital Atlas of Clinical Ophthalmology*, 2nd ed. Philadelphia: Lippincott Williams & Wilkins, 2001.

Healthy Retinal Artery and Arteriovenous (A-V) Crossing

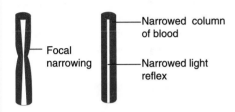

— Arterial wall (invisible)
— Column of blood
— Light reflex

The arterial wall is transparent. Only the column of blood within it can usually be seen. The light reflex is *narrow—about one-fourth the diameter of the blood column.*

Because the arterial wall is transparent, a vein crossing beneath the artery can be seen right up to the column of blood on either side.

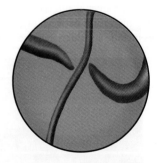

— Vein
— Arterial Wall
— Artery

Retinal Arteries in Hypertension

— Focal narrowing
— Narrowed column of blood
— Narrowed light reflex

In hypertension, the arteries may show areas of focal or generalized narrowing. The light reflex is also narrowed. The arterial wall thickens and becomes less transparent.

Copper Wiring

Sometimes the arteries, especially those close to the disc, become full and somewhat tortuous and develop an increased light reflex with a bright coppery lustre.

Silver Wiring

Occasionally a portion of a narrowed artery develops such an opaque wall that no blood is visible within it. It is then called a silver wire artery.

Arteriovenous Crossing

When the arterial walls lose their transparency, changes appear in the arteriovenous crossings. Decreased transparency of the retina probably also contributes to the first two changes shown below.

Concealment or A-V Nicking

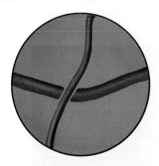

The vein appears to stop abruptly on either side of the artery.

Tapering and Banking

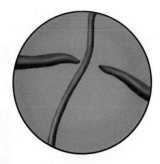

Tapering. The vein appears to taper down on either side of the artery.

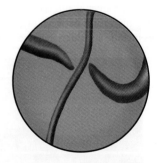

Banking. The vein is twisted on the distal side of the artery and forms a dark, wide knuckle.

TABLE 12-11   Red Spots and Streaks in the Fundi

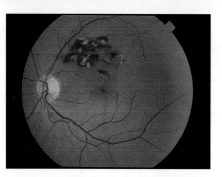

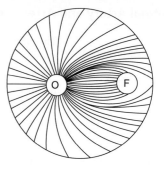

Superficial Retinal Hemorrhages—Small, linear, flame-shaped, red streaks in the fundi, shaped by the superficial bundles of nerve fibres that radiate from the optic disc in the pattern illustrated (O = optic disc; F = fovea). Sometimes the hemorrhages occur in clusters and look like a larger hemorrhage, but can be identified by the linear streaking at the edges. Superficial hemorrhages are seen in severe hypertension, papilledema, and occlusion of the retinal vein, among other conditions. An occasional superficial hemorrhage has a white center consisting of fibrin. White-centered retinal hemorrhages have many causes.

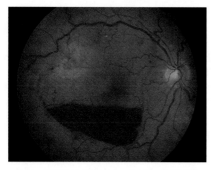

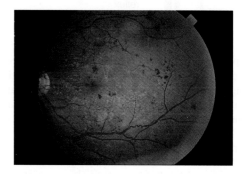

Preretinal Hemorrhage—Develops when blood escapes into the potential space between retina and vitreous. This hemorrhage is typically larger than retinal hemorrhages. Because it is anterior to the retina, it obscures any underlying retinal vessels. In an erect client, red cells settle, creating a horizontal line of demarcation between plasma above and cells below. Causes include a sudden increase in intracranial pressure.

Microaneurysms—Tiny, round, red spots seen commonly, but not exclusively, in and around the macular area. They are minute dilatations of very small retinal vessels, but the vascular connections are too small to be seen ophthalmoscopically. They arise from diabetic retinopathy, but have other causes.

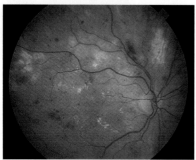

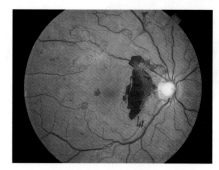

Deep Retinal Hemorrhages—Small, rounded, slightly irregular red spots that are sometimes called dot or blot hemorrhages. They occur in a deeper layer of the retina than flame-shaped hemorrhages. Diabetes is a common cause.

Neovascularization—Refers to the formation of new blood vessels. They are more numerous, more tortuous, and narrower than other blood vessels in the area and form disorderly looking red arcades. A common cause is the late, proliferative stage of diabetic retinopathy. The vessels may grow into the vitreous, where retinal detachment or hemorrhage may cause loss of vision.

Photo source: Tasman, W., & Jaeger, E. (Eds). *The Wills Eye Hospital Atlas of Clinical Ophthalmology*, 2nd ed. Philadelphia: Lippincott Williams & Wilkins, 2001.

TABLE 12-12   Ocular Fundi

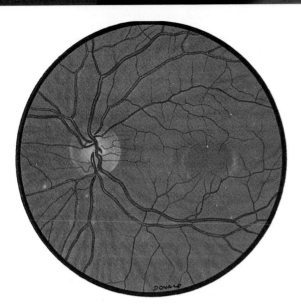

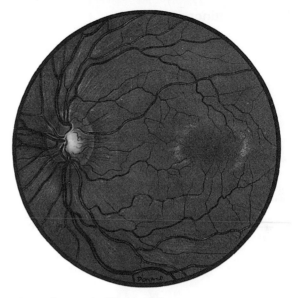

Fundus of a Fair-Skinned Person

Inspect the optic disc. Follow the major vessels in four directions, noting their relative sizes and any arteriovenous crossings. Inspect the macular area. The slightly darker fovea is just discernible; no light reflex is visible in this subject. Look for any lesions in the retina. Note the striped, or tessellated, character of the fundus, especially in the lower field that comes from underlying choroidal vessels.

Fundus of a Dark-Skinned Person

Again, inspect the disc, vessels, macula, and retina. The ring around the fovea is a light reflection. The colour of the fundus has a greyish brown, almost purplish cast, which comes from pigment in the retina and the choroid that characteristically obscures the choroidal vessels; no tessellation is visible. The fundus of a light-skinned person with brunette colouring is redder.

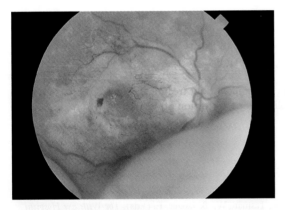

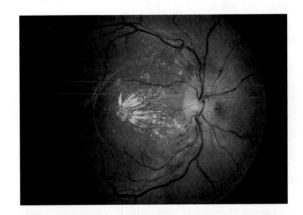

Hypertensive Retinopathy

Inspect the fundus. The nasal border of the optic disc is blurred. The light reflexes from the arteries just above and below the disc are increased. Note venous tapering—at the A-V crossing, about 1 disc diameter above the disc (Wong & Mitchell, 2004).

Hypertensive Retinopathy With Macular Star

Punctate exudates are readily visible: Some are scattered; others radiate from the fovea to form a macular star. Note the two small, soft exudates about 1 disc diameter from the disc. Find the flame-shaped hemorrhages sweeping toward 7 o'clock and 8 o'clock; a few more may be seen toward 10 o'clock. These fundi show changes typical of accelerated (malignant) hypertension and are often accompanied by a papilledema (p. 318).

(table continues on next page)

TABLE 12-12   **Ocular Fundi** *(Continued)*

Diabetic Retinopathy

Study carefully the fundi in the series of photographs below. They represent a standard used by ophthalmologists to assess diabetic retinopathy.

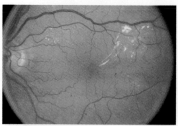

Nonproliferative Retinopathy, Moderately Severe

Note tiny red dots or microaneurysms. Note also the ring of hard exudates (white spots) located superotemporally. Retinal thickening or edema in the area of the hard exudates can impair visual acuity if it extends into the centre of the macula (detection requires specialized stereoscopic examination).

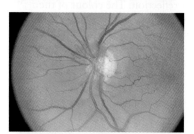

Nonproliferative Retinopathy, Severe

In the superior temporal quadrant, note the large retinal hemorrhage between two cotton-wool patches, beading of the retinal vein just above them, and tiny tortuous retinal vessels above the superior temporal artery.

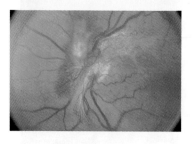

Proliferative Retinopathy, With Neovascularization

Note new preretinal vessels arising on the disc and extending across the disc margins. Visual acuity is still healthy but the risk for visual loss is high (photocoagulation reduces this risk by more than 50%).

Proliferative Retinopathy, Advanced

This is the same eye, but 2 years later and without treatment. Neovascularization has increased, now with fibrous proliferations, distortion of the macula, and reduced visual acuity.

Photo sources: Hypertensive retinopathy, hypertensive retinopathy with macular star, Tasman, W., & Jaeger, E. (Eds). *The Wills Eye Hospital Atlas of Clinical Ophthalmology,* 2nd ed. Philadelphia: Lippincott Williams & Wilkins, 2001; Nonproliferative retinopathy (moderately severe), proliferative retinopathy with neovascularization, nonproliferative retinopathy (severe), proliferative retinopathy (advanced) courtesy of Early Treatment Diabetic Retinopathy Study Research Group, MF Davis, MD, University of Wisconsin, Madison,

TABLE 12-13   Light-Coloured Spots in the Fundi

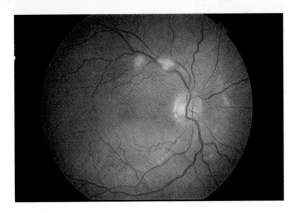

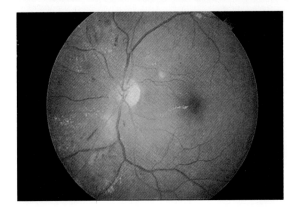

Cotton-Wool Patches (Soft Exudates)

Cotton-wool patches are white or greyish, ovoid lesions with irregular "soft" borders. They are moderate in size but usually smaller than the disc. They result from infarcted nerve fibres and are seen in hypertension and many other conditions.

Hard Exudates

Hard exudates are creamy or yellowish, often bright lesions with well-defined "hard" borders. They are small and round (as shown in the lower group of exudates), but may coalesce into larger irregular spots (as shown in the upper group). They often occur in clusters or in circular, linear, or star-shaped patterns. Causes include diabetes and hypertension.

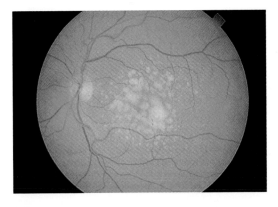

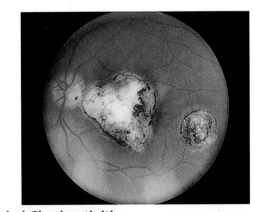

Drusen

Drusen are yellowish round spots that vary from tiny to small. The edges may be soft, as here, or hard. They are haphazardly distributed, but may concentrate at the posterior pole. Drusen appear with aging, but may also accompany various conditions, including age-related macular degeneration.

Healed Chorioretinitis

Here inflammation has destroyed the superficial tissues to reveal a well-defined, irregular patch of white sclera marked with dark pigment. Size varies from small to very large. *Toxoplasmosis* is illustrated. Multiple, small, somewhat similar-looking areas may result from laser treatments. Here there is also a temporal scar near the macula.

Photo source: Tasman, W., & Jaeger, E. (eds). *The Wills Eye Hospital Atlas of Clinical Ophthalmology*, 2nd ed. Philadelphia: Lippincott Williams & Wilkins, 2001.

The Ear, Nose, Mouth, and Throat

Sheri Roach, Pat Roddick, and Lynn S. Bickley

The ears, nose, mouth, and throat, while functionally distinct from one another, are grouped together because of their anatomical connectedness and tendency to affect one another. The ear, the organ of hearing and equilibrium, maintains its inner pressure balance through the eustachian tube, which connects to the nasopharynx, or upper portion of the throat. The nose functions as a filter and humidifier for air that enters the lungs, and shares the pharynx with the mouth. In addition, the senses of smell and taste are intimately connected. The mouth may also serve as a portal for respiration, and is the starting point of digestion, where the body takes in food and liquids for sustenance and growth. The throat is a muscular passage for both food and air and houses the large lymphatic structures called the tonsils.

ANATOMY AND PHYSIOLOGY

THE EAR

Anatomy. The ear has three compartments: the external ear, the middle ear, and the inner ear.

The *external ear* comprises the auricle and ear canal. The *auricle* consists chiefly of cartilage covered by skin and has a firm elastic consistency. Its prominent curved outer ridge is the *helix*. Parallel and anterior to the helix is another curved prominence, the *antihelix*. Inferiorly lies the fleshy projection of the earlobe, or *lobule*. The ear canal opens behind the *tragus*, a nodular eminence that points backward over the entrance to the canal.

The *ear canal* curves inward approximately 24 mm. Cartilage surrounds its outer portion. The skin in this outer portion is hairy and contains glands that produce cerumen (wax). The inner portion of the canal is surrounded by bone and lined by thin, hairless skin. Pressure on this latter area causes pain—a point to remember when you examine the ear. Pressure may also cause the client to cough and to move the head during examination.

Behind and below the ear canal is the mastoid part of the temporal bone. The lowest portion of this bone, the *mastoid process*, is palpable behind the lobule.

At the end of the ear canal lies the *tympanic membrane*, or eardrum, marking the lateral limits of the middle ear. The *middle ear* is an air-filled cavity that transmits sound from the outer ear to the inner ear by way of three tiny bones, or *ossicles*: the malleus, incus, and stapes. It is connected by the *eustachian tube* to the nasopharynx.

The eardrum is an oblique membrane held inward at its centre by the *malleus*, one of its three ossicles. Find the *handle* and the *short process* of the malleus—the two chief landmarks. From the *umbo*, where the eardrum meets the tip of the malleus, a light reflection called the *cone of light* fans downward and anteriorly.

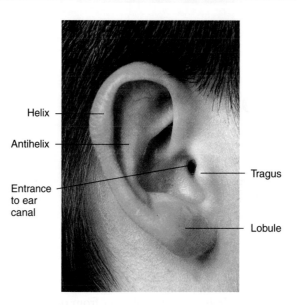

Above the short process lies a small portion of the eardrum called the *pars flaccida*. The remainder of the drum is the *pars tensa*. The incus can sometimes be seen through the drum.

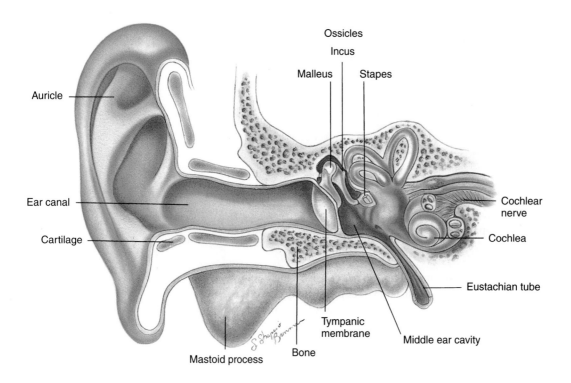

The inner ear contains the bony labyrinth, consisting of a central cavity called the *vestibule*, the three *semicircular canals*, and the *cochlea*. Receptors in the vestibule and semicircular canals sense position and head movement to help maintain static and dynamic equilibrium. The spiral-shaped cochlea houses the *organ of Corti*, the sensory organ for hearing. Hair cells in the cochlea are an essential component of hearing.

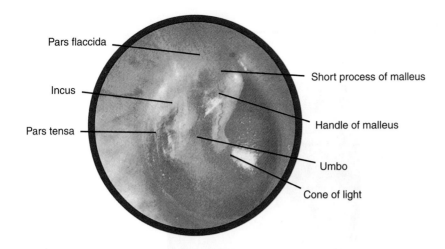

Pars flaccida

Incus

Pars tensa

Short process of malleus

Handle of malleus

Umbo

Cone of light

Much of the middle ear and all of the inner ear are inaccessible to direct examination. Some inferences concerning their condition can be made, however, by testing auditory function.

Pathways of Hearing. Vibrations of sound pass through the air of the external ear and are transmitted through the eardrum and ossicles of the middle ear to the *cochlea*. The cochlea senses and codes the vibrations, and nerve impulses are sent to the brain through the cochlear nerve. The first part of this pathway—from the external ear through the middle ear—is known as the *conductive* phase, and a disorder here causes conductive hearing loss. The second part of the pathway, involving the cochlea and the cochlear nerve, is called the *sensorineural* phase; a disorder here causes sensorineural hearing loss.

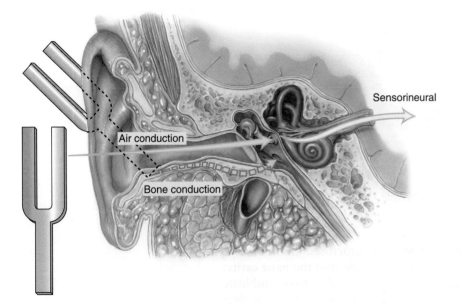

Sensorineural

Air conduction

Bone conduction

Air conduction describes the usual first phase in the hearing pathway. An alternate pathway, known as *bone conduction*, bypasses the external and the middle ear and is used to test for conduction hearing loss. A vibrating tuning fork, placed on the head, sets the bone of the skull into vibration and stimulates the cochlea directly. In a client with no hearing disorders or deviations, air conduction is more sensitive.

■ THE NOSE AND PARANASAL SINUSES

Review the terms used to describe the external anatomy of the nose.

Approximately the upper one-third of the nose is supported by bone and the lower two-thirds by cartilage. Air enters the nasal cavity by way of the *anterior naris* on either side, then passes into a widened area known as the *vestibule* and on through the narrow nasal passage to the nasopharynx. The medial wall of each nasal cavity is formed by the *nasal septum*, which, similar to the external nose, is supported by both bone and cartilage. A mucous membrane well supplied with blood covers it. The vestibule, unlike the rest of the nasal cavity, is lined with hair-bearing skin, not mucosa.

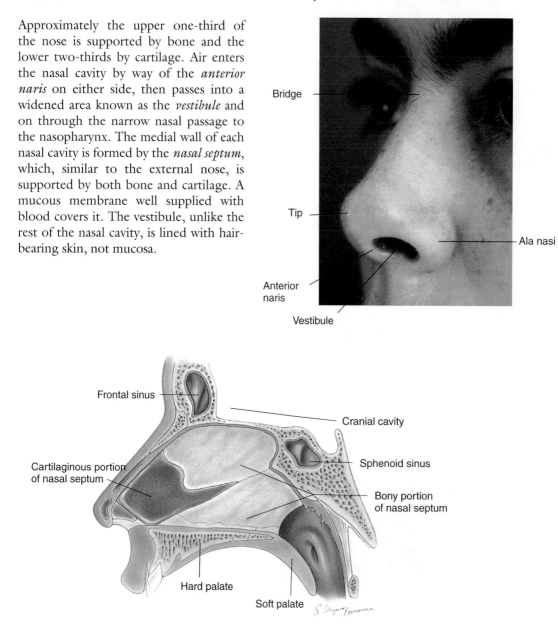

Laterally, the anatomy is more complex. Curving bony structures, the *turbinates*, covered by a highly vascular mucous membrane, protrude into the nasal cavity. Below each turbinate is a groove, or meatus, each named according to the turbinate above it. Into the inferior meatus drains the nasolacrimal duct; into the middle meatus drain most of the paranasal sinuses. Their openings are not usually visible.

The additional surface area provided by the turbinates and the mucosa covering them aids the nasal cavities in their principal functions: cleansing, humidification, and temperature control of inspired air.

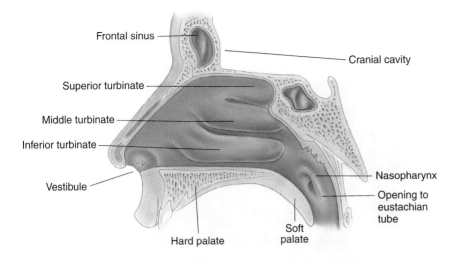

The *paranasal sinuses* are air-filled cavities within the bones of the skull. Similar to the nasal cavities into which they drain, they are lined with mucous membrane. Their locations are diagrammed. Only the frontal and maxillary sinuses are readily accessible to clinical examination. Beyond functioning as an airway, the nose and sinuses also provide resonance for the voice and house the olfactory receptors.

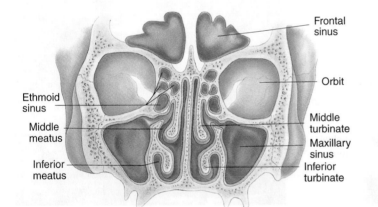

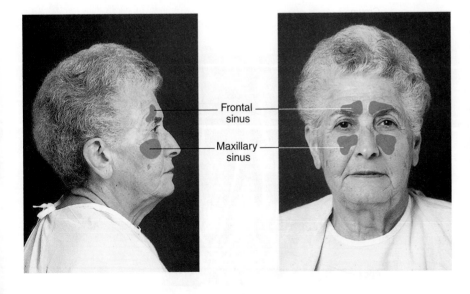

THE MOUTH AND PHARYNX

The *lips* are muscular folds that surround the entrance to the mouth. When opened, the gums (gingival) and teeth are visible. Note the scalloped shape of the *gingival margins* and the pointed *interdental papillae*.

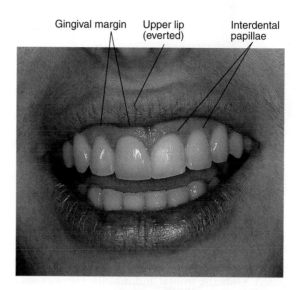

The gingiva is firmly attached to the teeth and to the maxilla or mandible in which they are seated. In lighter-skinned people, the gingival is pale or coral pink and lightly stippled. In darker-skinned people, it may be diffusely or partly brown, as shown below. A midline mucosal fold, called a *labial frenulum*, connects each lip with the gingiva. A shallow *gingiva sulcus* between the

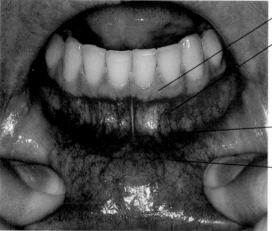

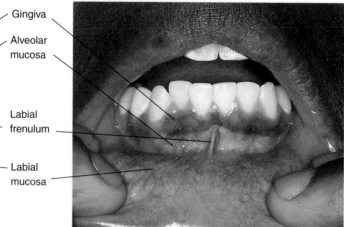

gum's thin margin and each tooth is not readily visible (but is probed and measured by dentists). Adjacent to the gingiva is the *alveolar mucosa*, which merges with the *labial mucosa* of the lip.

Each tooth, composed chiefly of dentin, lies rooted in a bony socket with only its enamel-covered crown exposed. Small blood vessels and nerves enter the tooth through its apex and pass into the pulp canal and pulp chamber.

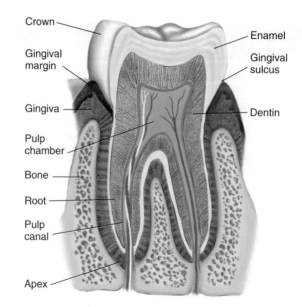

Note the terms designating the 32 adult teeth, 16 in each jaw.

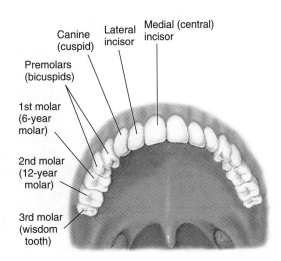

The dorsum of the *tongue* is covered with papillae, giving it a rough surface. Some of these papillae look like red dots, which contrast with the thin white coat that often covers the tongue. The undersurface of the tongue has no papillae. Note the midline *lingual frenulum* that connects the tongue to the floor of the mouth. At the base of the tongue, the *ducts of the submandibular gland* (Wharton's ducts) pass forward and medially. They open on papillae that lie on each side of the lingual frenulum.

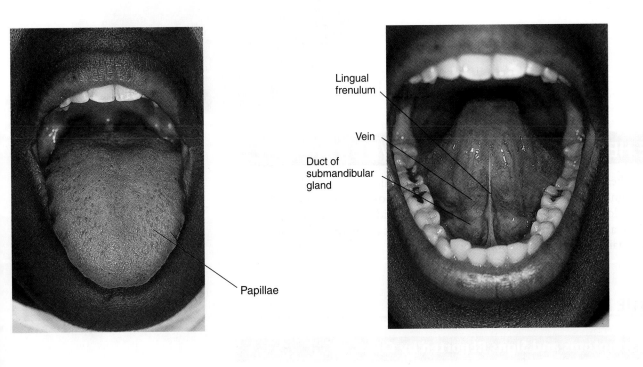

Above and behind the tongue rises an arch formed by the *anterior* and *posterior pillars*, the *soft palate*, and the *uvula*. A meshwork of small blood vessels may web the soft palate. The *pharynx* is visible in the recess behind the soft palate and tongue.

In the adjacent photograph, note the right tonsil protruding from the hollowed *tonsillar fossa*, or cavity, between the anterior and posterior pillars. In adults, tonsils are often small or absent, as in the empty left tonsillar fossa here.

The *buccal mucosa* lines the cheeks. Each *parotid duct*, sometimes termed *Stenson's duct*, opens on to the buccal mucosa near the upper second molar. Its location is frequently marked by its own small papilla.

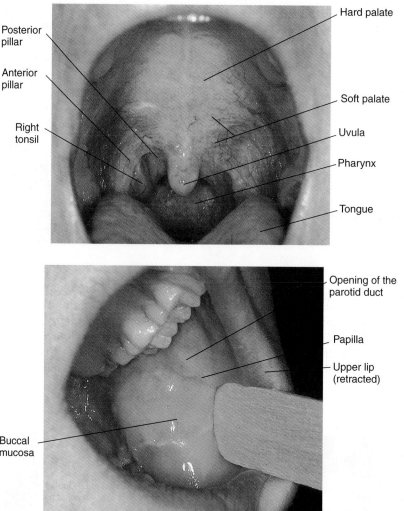

THE HEALTH HISTORY: SUBJECTIVE DATA

Begin the health history by asking open-ended questions, such as "What concerns have brought you to the clinic today?" or "Tell me how you are feeling." These questions allow the client to give responses that help guide the rest of the health history. When a client reports a sign or symptom, conduct an analysis of the symptom or sign to gain as much information as possible.

THE EARS

Key Symptoms and Signs Reported by Client

- Earache
- Discharge from the ears
- Ringing in the ears, rushing sounds
- Changes in hearing or hearing loss
- Feeling lightheaded or dizzy
- Changes in balance

Opening questions are "How is your hearing?," "Have you had any trouble with your ears?," "Do you work in a noisy environment?"

Try to distinguish between two basic types of hearing impairment: *conductive loss*, which results from problems in the external or middle ear, and *sensorineural loss*, resulting from problems in the inner ear, the cochlear nerve, or its central connections in the brain. Two questions may be helpful: "Do you have special difficulty understanding people as they talk?" and "What difference does a noisy environment make?"

People with sensorineural loss have particular trouble understanding speech, often complaining that others mumble; noisy environments make hearing worse. In conductive loss, noisy environments may help. Noise-induced hearing loss may derive from workplace or recreational exposures.

Symptoms associated with hearing loss, such as earache or vertigo, help you to assess most probable causes. In addition, inquire specifically about medications that might affect hearing and ask about sustained exposure to loud noise.

Medications that affect hearing include aminoglycosides, aspirin, NSAIDs, quinine, furosemide, and others.

Complaints of *earache*, or *pain in the ear*, are especially common. Ask about associated fever, sore throat, cough, and concurrent upper respiratory infection.

Pain suggests a problem in the external ear, such as *otitis externa*, or, if associated with symptoms of respiratory infection, in the inner ear, as in *otitis media*. It may also be referred from other structures in the mouth, throat, or neck.

Ask about *discharge from the ear*, especially if associated with earache or trauma.

Unusually soft wax, debris from inflammation or rash in the ear canal, or discharge through a perforated eardrum secondary to *acute* or *chronic otitis media*.

Tinnitus is a perceived sound with no external stimulus—commonly a musical ringing or a rushing or roaring noise. It can involve one or both ears. Tinnitus may accompany hearing loss and often remains unexplained. Occasionally, popping sounds originating in the temporomandibular joint or vascular noises from the neck may be audible.

Tinnitus is a common symptom, increasing in frequency with age. When associated with hearing loss and vertigo, it suggests *Ménière's disease*. Excessive use of aspirin may contribute to tinnitus.

Vertigo refers to the perception that the client or the environment is rotating or spinning. These sensations point primarily to a problem in the labyrinths of the inner ear, peripheral lesions of CN VIII, or lesions in its central pathways or nuclei in the brain.

See Table 13-1, Dizziness and Vertigo, p. 367.

Vertigo is a challenging symptom for you as clinician, because clients differ widely in what they mean by the word "dizzy." "Are there times when you feel dizzy?" is an appropriate first question, but clients often find it difficult to be more specific. Ask "Do you feel unsteady, as if you are going to fall or black out? ... Or do you feel the room is spinning (true vertigo)?" Get the information without biasing it. You may need to offer the client several choices of wording. Ask if the client feels pulled to the ground or off to one side. Ask if the dizziness is related to a change in body position. Pursue any associated feelings of clamminess or flushing, nausea, or vomiting. Check if any medications may be contributing.

Feeling unsteady, lightheaded, or "dizzy in the legs" sometimes suggests a cardiovascular etiology. A feeling of being pulled suggests true vertigo from an inner ear problem or a central or peripheral lesion of CN VIII.

■ *Example of Questions for Symptom/Sign Analysis—Hearing Loss*

- "Does your hearing loss involve both ears?" (*Location*)
- "Describe your hearing." "What types of sounds do you hear?" (*Quality*)
- "Do you have difficulty hearing people when they talk?" "What difference does a noisy environment make?" (*Severity*)
- "When did you start to notice the hearing loss?" "Did it happen suddenly or gradually?" (*Onset*)
- "Has your hearing loss continued since it started?" (*Duration*)
- "Do you feel like it is getting better or worse over time?" (*Constancy*)
- "Is your hearing better at different times of the day? "Or worse?" (*Time of day/month/year*)
- "Does anything make it more difficult for you to hear?" (*Aggravating factors*)
- "What makes it easier for you to hear?" (*Alleviating factors*)
- "Do you have any pain in your ears?" "Do you feel dizzy?" "Nauseated?" (*Associated symptoms*)
- "Have you had any exposure to loud noises?" "At work?" "Do you have any hobbies that have resulted in loud noise?" "Have you had any head injuries?" (*Environmental factors*)
- "How does your hearing loss affect your life?" (*Significance to client*)
- "Tell me what you think is happening." (*Client perspective*)

◢ THE NOSE AND SINUSES

Key Symptoms and Signs Reported by Client

- Nasal congestion or stuffiness
- Runny nose
- Sneezing
- Facial pain or tenderness on cheeks, around eyes, or forehead
- Nosebleed

Rhinorrhea refers to drainage from the nose and is often associated with *nasal congestion*, a sense of stuffiness or obstruction. These symptoms are frequently accompanied by *sneezing*, watery eyes, and throat discomfort, and also by *itching* in the eyes, nose, and throat.

Causes include viral infections, *allergic rhinitis* ("hay fever"), and *vasomotor rhinitis*. Itching favours an allergic cause.

Assess the chronology of the illness. Does it last for a week or so, especially when common colds and related syndromes are prevalent, or does it occur seasonally when pollens are in the air? Is it associated with specific contacts or environments? What remedies has the client used? For how long? And how well do they work?

Relation to seasons or environmental contacts suggests allergy.

Excessive use of decongestants can worsen the symptoms, causing rhinitis medicamentosa.

Inquire about drugs that might cause stuffiness.

Oral contraceptives, reserpine, guanethidine, and alcohol; excessive use of nasal sprays may produce rebound stuffiness.

Are there symptoms in addition to rhinorrhea or congestion, such as pain and tenderness in the face or over the sinuses, local headache, or fever?

Is the client's nasal congestion limited to one side? If so, you may be dealing with a different problem that requires careful physical examination.

Consider a deviated nasal septum, foreign body, or tumour.

Epistaxis means bleeding from the nose. The blood usually originates from the nose itself, but may come from a paranasal sinus or the nasopharynx. In clients who are lying down, or whose bleeding originates in posterior structures, blood may pass into the throat instead of out through the nostrils. You must identify the source of the bleeding carefully—is it from the nose, or has it been coughed up or vomited? Assess the site of bleeding, its severity, and associated symptoms. Is it a recurrent problem? Has there been easy bruising or bleeding elsewhere in the body?

Local causes of epistaxis include trauma (especially nose picking), inflammation, drying and crusting of the nasal mucosa, tumours, and foreign bodies.

Bleeding disorders and anticoagulants used to prevent clot formation may contribute to epistaxis.

◢ THE MOUTH AND THROAT

Key Symptoms and Signs Reported by Client

- Bleeding from gums
- Sore throat
- Hoarseness
- Swelling in throat
- Changes in voice
- Scratchy throat
- Sore tongue

Sore throat is a frequent concern, usually associated with acute upper respiratory symptoms.

Fever, pharyngeal exudates, and anterior lymphadenopathy, especially in the absence of cough, suggest streptococcal pharyngitis, or strep throat (p. 374)

A *sore tongue* may be caused by local lesions as well as by systemic illness.

Aphthous ulcers (p. 380); sore smooth tongue caused by nutritional deficiency (p. 379)

Bleeding from the gums is a common symptom, especially when brushing teeth. Ask about local lesions and any tendency to bleed or bruise elsewhere.

Bleeding gums are most often caused by *gingivitis* (p. 377).

Hoarseness refers to an altered quality of the voice, often described as husky, rough, or harsh. The pitch may be lower than before. Hoarseness usually arises from disease of the larynx, but may also develop as extralaryngeal lesions press on the laryngeal nerves. Check for overuse of the voice, allergy, smoking or other inhaled irritants, and any associated symptoms. Is the problem acute or chronic? Frequently trying to clear the throat may aggravate the problem. Encourage clients to "hum" instead. If hoarseness lasts more than 2 weeks, visual examination of the larynx by indirect or direct laryngoscopy is advisable.

Overuse of the voice (as in cheering) and acute infections are the most probable causes.

Causes of chronic hoarseness include smoking, allergy, voice abuse, hypothyroidism, chronic infections such as tuberculosis, and tumours.

HEALTH PROMOTION

Important Topics for Health Promotion

- Hearing loss, screening, and preventive measures
- Tinnitus
- Vestibular dysfunction
- Oral health

HEARING LOSS

Hearing, a critical sense, requires special attention from nurses relative to health promotion. Hearing loss is Canada's most rapidly increasing chronic disability. Loss of hearing can damage mental processing, emotional and mental health, and educational and occupational abilities. Especially in older adults, hearing loss may lead to social isolation, depression, withdrawal from daily activities, and frustration with and among family and friends (Manohar, 2007).

A pervasive societal belief exists that hearing loss is directly related to advancing age. Although more than 33% of Canadians older than 65 years have detectable hearing deficits, approximately 80% of Canadians with hearing loss are younger than 65 years, and significant hearing loss is now being detected in people as young as 30 years. The increasing exposure of younger people to occupational- and leisure-related noise at levels associated with hearing loss creates a need for health-promotion teaching about hearing for clients of all age groups. Noise-induced hearing loss is irreversible when it damages the tiny hair cells in the cochlea. Canadian provinces legislate 85 to 90 decibels on the A scale as the maximum exposure for an 8-hour period.

Risk Factor Assessment. *Conductive hearing loss* involves a problem with the outer or middle ear. Usual causes are wax build-up or infection, and appropriate treatment of the cause commonly resolves the problem with hearing. *Sensorineural hearing loss*, which results from degeneration of the inner ear or auditory nerve, represents 90% of cases of hearing impairment in adults. Other causes include aging; hereditary factors; infection with syphilis, rubella, or meningitis; head trauma; and noise exposure. A key health-promotion consideration is that 99% of cases of hearing loss from noise exposure are preventable (Canadian Association of Speech-Language Pathologists and Audiologists, 2000).

The main categories that contribute to hearing loss are work-related and leisure-associated noise. Work-related noise is significant in several occupational settings where power tools and heavy machinery are in constant use, such as construction sites and manufacturing plants. Recent Canadian legislation has required these types of industries to improve their health-promotion approach. For example, the Canadian Centre for Occupational Health and Safety (2006) requires these workplaces to provide education and enforcement in addition to appropriate personal protective equipment (PPE) for hearing protection, such as fitted earplugs or earmuffs. Although industrial areas are recognized as having noise levels that require hearing protection, workers in the service and entertainment industries, many of whom are younger adults, are also exposed to noise levels above those considered safe for extended periods. Workplaces such as race tracks, sporting arenas, concert halls, and dance clubs all have increased levels of noise.

One simple way to assess whether noise at work is affecting a client's hearing is to ask if he or she turns the radio up in the vehicle on the way home from work and then down again on the way to work the next day. The need to increase the radio volume can indicate hearing damage from work-related noise. Other simple ways to assess any effect of work-related noise on hearing is to ask the client about ringing in the ears after work or if he or she needs to shout at someone to be heard when 1 metre away while in a noisy environment.

Leisure-associated noise can affect all clients; however, Health Canada (2006) has identified this potential hearing risk as especially relevant for teenagers and young adults. Personal stereo systems with headphones are particularly concerning, because they pose a risk to hearing when played above the halfway point on the volume dial (Health Canada, 2006). Other contributors to hearing problems may include home and car sound systems, music in fitness classes or dance clubs, music and crowd noise at concerts or sporting events, and noise in bars. Many younger clients view hearing protection as unnecessary or embarrassing; some never consider the issue. Thus, it is essential for nurses to communicate the risks to hearing that everyday work and leisure activities impose to all clients, and the importance of protecting against hearing loss.

Screening and Maintenance. Currently, Canada has no universal newborn hearing screening test; the average age of identification for hearing difficulties is $2\frac{1}{2}$ to 3 years (Hearing Foundation of Canada, 2009a). Earlier recognition and intervention regarding hearing problems can vastly increase a child's language, speech, and social development (Hearing Foundation of Canada, 2007a). Nurses can advocate for infants and children by making parents aware that noninvasive testing is available for children of all ages, including newborns. In the broader scope of population health, nurses can lobby for mandatory newborn hearing screening legislation, which was available only to residents of Ontario, New Brunswick, Prince Edward Island, and the Yukon as of 2007 (Hearing Foundation of Canada, 2009b).

Hearing screening remains important throughout childhood and adulthood. Up to 30% of young adults entering the workforce have some degree of hearing loss (Political Hear-it, 2007). Hearing tests at least every 2 years help health care providers note incremental changes before they evolve into more obvious and life-altering problems. In addition, many workplaces with hearing loss prevention programmes now offer yearly hearing screening to their employees, as outlined under mandatory provincial legislation.

Despite the social stigmas that associate loss of hearing with advanced age, hearing loss often goes undetected in older adults. Unlike vision prerequisites for driving, there is no mandate for widespread testing, and many seniors avoid hearing aids. Statistics show that only 1 in 6 Canadians who would benefit from a hearing aid actually wears one (Hearing Foundation of Canada, 2009c). Audiologists use hand-held audioscopes to diagnose hearing deficits. Occupational health nurses use computerized hearing assessment booths in the workplace. Less sensitive tests, such as the whisper test and the use of tuning forks, as well as hearing questionnaires, are readily available for periodic screening and are sufficient to identify clients who would benefit from further medical attention.

TINNITUS

People who suffer from tinnitus have reported 50 different sounds, including ringing, thumping, chirping, and sizzling (Tinnitus Association of Canada, n.d.). Tinnitus can happen at any age. It may be continuous or intermittent, and physiological or biochemical. Some causes include hearing loss, head trauma, aspirin intake, and physical or emotional stress. Nurses should refer clients with tinnitus to a physician to assess for reversible causes; however, most cases of tinnitus have no "cure." Health promotion should focus on clients' experiences and on helping them access support and develop coping skills as needed (Davis, et al., 2002).

VESTIBULAR DYSFUNCTION

The vestibular system in the inner ear controls balance. Diseases such as Meniere's disease may alter the vestibular sense, resulting in acute onset of violent vertigo, nausea, and tinnitus. Vestibular senses also can diminish slowly over time from aging. In this latter case, clients may not be aware of a problem until they fall unexpectedly. Decreasing vestibular function, more common in older adults, can be compounded by the ototoxic effects of many medications, such as aspirin; aminoglycoside antibiotics, such as gentamicin; loop diuretics, such as furosemide; and anti-cancer drugs, such as carboplatin (Vestibular Disorders Association, 2005). Symptoms of ototoxicity include fullness in the ears, dizziness, and difficulty with movement. Medications that cause ototoxicity have a compounded effect when used simultaneously, which has significant implications for many older adults, who often take several medications at one time (*polypharmacy*) (see Chapter 25). Health-promotion education about the possible side effects of these drugs and awareness of symptoms of ototoxicity may allow clients to get assistance before experiencing a fall that causes major injury. Research shows that effective interventions for balance problems from vestibular dysfunction include physiotherapy, occupational therapy, and physical aids to daily living such as canes or walkers (Vestibular Disorders Association, 2005).

ORAL HEALTH

Oral health, often overlooked by nurses, merits attention. Approximately 60% of Canadians 5 to 17 years have dental decay, 9% of Canadians older than 15 years have lost all their natural teeth, and gum disease affects 80% of Canadians at some point in their lives (Canadian Dental Association, 2005). Poor oral health can affect psychological and social well-being by reducing enjoyment of eating; it can also compromise communication, social relationships, and other daily activities. Poor oral hygiene also has systemic physical implications. For example, bacteria in dental plaque can move into the bloodstream and contribute to arteriosclerosis, or travel via the blood to the lungs and cause infection or aggravate existing lung conditions (Health Canada, 2007a).

Risk Factor Assessment. Alcohol and tobacco use, changes in salivary flow from medications, and denture use are some risk factors affecting oral health. Tobacco products and excess alcohol are the principal risk factors for oral cancer; clients should avoid their use. Saliva cleanses and lubricates the mouth. Many medications reduce salivary flow, increasing the risk for tooth decay, mucositis, and gum disease, especially in the elderly. As with children, adults should avoid excessive intake of foods high in refined sugars, such as sucrose, which enhance attachment and colonization of cariogenic bacteria. For those wearing dentures, encourage removal and cleaning each night to reduce bacterial plaque and potential malodor. Regular massage of the gums relieves soreness and pressure from dentures on underlying soft tissue. Also, regular inspection for lesions developing under dentures is important for early identification and treatment.

Screening and Maintenance. Effective screening begins with careful examination of the mouth, including inspection of the oral cavity for decayed or loose teeth, inflammation of the gingiva, lesions and leukoplakia on the tongue, and signs of periodontal disease (bleeding, pus, recession of the gums, and bad breath). To improve oral health, encourage clients to adopt daily hygiene measures, including the following recommendations (Health Canada, 2007b):

- Brush teeth daily with fluoride-containing toothpaste.

- Floss daily.

- Visit a dental professional every 6 to 12 months.

- Eat a healthy diet consistent with Canada's Food Guide.

- Avoid tobacco products.

- Brush teeth for children until they have the dexterity to write (not print) their own names.

- Drink minimal to no alcohol.

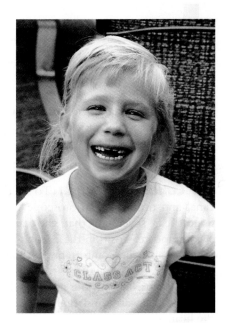

Oral health also provides clues to further health problems. For example, bleeding gums may indicate nutritional deficiencies, alcohol use, or stress; breath with a fruity odour may indicate diabetic ketoacidosis; and lesions on the lips, buccal mucosa, or tongue may signify oral cancer or infection with human immunodeficiency virus (HIV).

EMERGENCY CONCERNS

Several signs and symptoms related to hearing and balance require prompt assessment and treatment. Examples of manifestations that warrant emergency attention include bleeding from the ear, severe ear pain, sudden loss of hearing, and sudden loss of balance. Trauma to the ear or ear canal also requires emergency assessment and treatment. Purulent, bloody, or straw-coloured discharge from the ear requires emergency medical consultation—this finding may be a sign of a ruptured eardrum or internal traumatic injury.

Trauma to the teeth, mouth, nose, tongue, and throat require immediate assessment and intervention. Nosebleeds that do not stop after 20 minutes merit immediate attention, because they could indicate a bleeding disorder, dangerously high blood pressure, or a skull fracture from head trauma. Clients with difficulty speaking, slurred speech, difficulty swallowing, jaw pain, or notable swelling in their throats need referral for emergency treatment because of the potential for stroke, cardiac conditions, or anaphylaxis. Other symptoms that may not be emergencies but that require prompt attention include tooth pain unrelieved by use of non-prescription medications accompanied by facial or neck swelling, redness, or both, and bleeding associated with pain or trauma. These symptoms may indicate a dental abscess, which can have systemic implications if left untreated.

TECHNIQUES OF EXAMINATION: OBJECTIVE DATA

Equipment

- Otoscope
- Disposable speculum tips
- Tuning fork (512 or 1024 Hz)

THE EARS

The Auricle. Inspect each auricle and surrounding tissues for deformities, lumps, or skin lesions.

If ear pain, discharge, or inflammation is present, move the auricle up and down, press the tragus, and press firmly just behind the ear.

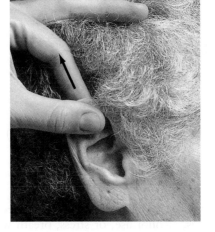

See Table 13-2, Lumps On or Near the Ear (p. 368).

Ear Canal and Drum. To see the ear canal and drum, use an otoscope with the largest ear speculum that the canal will accommodate. Position the client's head so that you can see comfortably through the instrument. To straighten the ear canal, grasp the auricle firmly but gently and pull it upward, backward, and slightly away from the head.

Movement of the auricle and tragus (the "tug test") is painful in acute *otitis externa* (inflammation of the ear canal), but not in *otitis media* (inflammation of the middle ear). Tenderness behind the ear may be present in otitis media.

Holding the otoscope handle between your thumb and fingers, brace your hand against the client's face. Your hand and instrument thus follow unexpected movements by the client. (If you are uncomfortable switching hands for the left ear, as shown below, you may reach over that ear to pull it up and back with your left hand and rest your otoscope-holding right hand on the head behind the ear.) Another option is to hold the otoscope with the handle pointing up and fingers anchored against the client's head.

Insert the speculum gently into the ear canal, directing it somewhat down and forward and through the hairs, if any.

Nontender nodular swellings covered by usual skin deep in the ear canals suggest *exostoses*. These are nonmalignant overgrowths, which may obscure the drum.

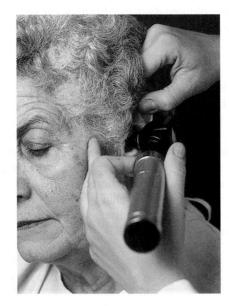

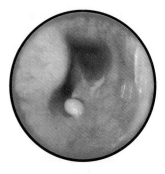

🌐 Cultural Considerations

The incidence and severity of otitis media is higher in ethnic groups with shorter, wider, and more horizontal eustachian tubes, such as aboriginal North Americans, Hispanics, and Canadian and Alaskan Inuits.

Inspect the ear canal, noting any discharge, foreign bodies, redness of the skin, or swelling. Cerumen, which varies in colour and consistency from yellow and flaky to brown and sticky or even to dark and hard, may wholly or partly obscure your view.

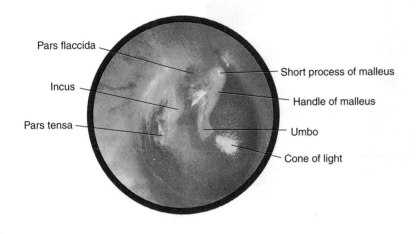

Pars flaccida — Short process of malleus
Incus — Handle of malleus
Pars tensa — Umbo
Cone of light

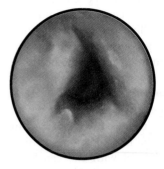

In *chronic otitis externa*, the skin of the canal is often thickened, red, and itchy.

Inspect the eardrum, noting its colour and contour. The cone of light—usually easy to see—helps to orient you.

Red bulging drum of acute purulent otitis media, amber drum of a serous effusion.

Identify the *handle of the malleus*, noting its position, and inspect the *short process of the malleus.*

An unusually prominent short process and a prominent handle that looks more horizontal suggest a retracted drum.

Gently move the speculum so that you can see as much of the drum as possible, including the *pars flaccida* superiorly and the margins of the *pars tensa*. Look for any perforations. The anterior and inferior margins of the drum may be obscured by the curving wall of the ear canal.

See Table 13-3, Unexpected Findings of the Eardrum (p. 369).

Auditory Acuity.
To estimate hearing, test one ear at a time. Occlude one of the client's ears with your finger to ensure reliable results. When auditory acuity on the two sides is different, move your finger rapidly, but gently, in the occluded canal. The noise so produced helps prevent the occluded ear from doing the work of the ear you wish to test. Then, standing 30 to 60 cm away, exhale fully (so as to minimize the intensity of your voice) and whisper softly toward the unoccluded ear. Choose numbers or other words with two equally accented syllables, such as "nine-four," or "baseball." If necessary, increase the intensity of your voice to a medium whisper; a loud whisper; and then a soft, medium, and loud voice. To make sure the client does not read your lips, hide your mouth with your hand or obstruct the client's vision.

Air and Bone Conduction.
If hearing is diminished, *try to distinguish between conductive and sensorineural hearing loss.* You need a quiet room and a tuning fork, preferably of 512 Hz or possibly 1024 Hz. These frequencies fall within the range of human speech (300 Hz to 3000 Hz)—functionally the most important range. Forks with lower pitches may lead to overestimating bone conduction and can also be felt as vibration.

Set the fork into light vibration by briskly stroking it between the thumb and index finger or by tapping it on your knuckles.

In unilateral *conductive hearing loss*, sound is heard in (lateralized to) the impaired ear. Visible explanations

■ *Test for lateralization* (Weber test). Place the base of the lightly vibrating tuning fork firmly on top of the client's head or on the midforehead.

Ask where the client hears it: on one or both sides. Usually the sound is heard in the midline or equally in both ears. If nothing is heard, try again, pressing the fork more firmly on the head.

■ *Compare air conduction (AC) and bone conduction (BC)* (Rinne test). Place the base of a lightly vibrating tuning fork on the mastoid bone, behind the ear and level with the canal. When the client can no longer hear the sound, quickly place the fork close to the ear canal and ascertain whether the sound can be heard again. Here the "U" of the fork should face forward, thus max-imizing its sound for the client. Usually the sound is heard longer through air than through bone (AC > BC).

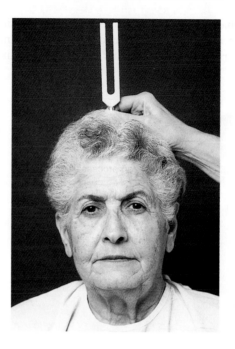

include acute otitis media, perforation of the eardrum, and obstruction of the ear canal, as by cerumen.

In unilateral *sensorineural hearing loss*, sound is heard in the good ear.

In conductive hearing loss, sound is heard through bone as long as or longer than it is through air (BC = AC or BC > AC). In sensorineural hearing loss, sound is heard longer through air (AC > BC). See Table 13-4, Patterns of Hearing Loss (p. 370).

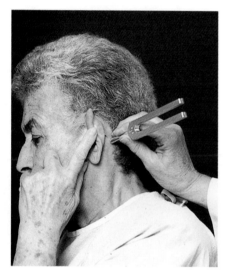

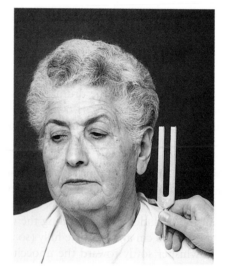

THE NOSE AND PARANASAL SINUSES

Equipment

■ Nasal speculum and penlight or
■ Otoscope with short, wide-tipped speculum

Inspect the anterior and inferior surfaces of the nose. Gentle pressure on the tip of the nose with your thumb usually widens the nostrils and, with the aid of a penlight or otoscope light, you can get a partial view of each nasal *vestibule*. If the tip is tender, be particularly gentle and manipulate the nose as little as possible.

Tenderness of the nasal tip or alae suggests local infection such as a furuncle.

Note any asymmetry or deformity of the nose.

Test for nasal obstruction, if indicated, by pressing on each ala nasi in turn and asking the client to breathe in with the mouth closed.

Inspect the inside of the nose with an otoscope and the largest ear speculum available.‡ Tilt the client's head back a bit and insert the speculum gently into the vestibule of each nostril, avoiding contact with the sensitive nasal septum. Hold the otoscope handle to one side to avoid the client's chin and improve your mobility. By directing the speculum posteriorly, then upward in small steps, try to see the inferior and middle turbinates, the nasal septum, and the narrow nasal passage between them. Some asymmetry of the two sides is expected.

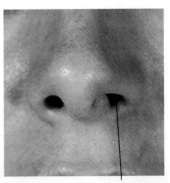

Vestibule

Deviation of the lower septum is common and may be easily visible, as illustrated above. Deviation seldom obstructs air flow, but can affect nasal ventilation.

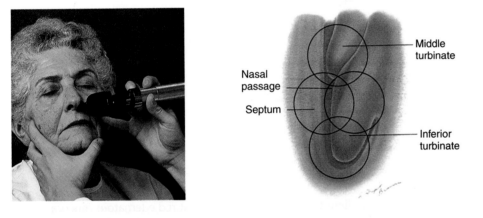

Middle turbinate

Nasal passage

Septum

Inferior turbinate

Observe the nasal mucosa and the nasal septum; look for any unexpected findings.

- The *nasal mucosa* that covers the septum and turbinates. Note its colour and any swelling, bleeding, or exudate. If exudate is present, note its character: clear, mucopurulent, or purulent. The nasal mucosa is usually somewhat redder than the oral mucosa.

- The *nasal septum*. Note any deviation, inflammation, or perforation of the septum. The lower anterior portion of the septum (where the client's finger can reach) is a common source of *epistaxis* (nosebleed).

- Any *unexpected findings* such as ulcers or polyps.

Make it a habit to place all nasal and ear specula outside your instrument case after use. Then discard them or clean and disinfect them appropriately. (Check the policies of your institution.)

In *viral rhinitis* the mucosa is reddened and swollen; in *allergic rhinitis* it may be pale, bluish, red, or pink and swollen.

Fresh blood or crusting may be seen. Causes of septal perforation include trauma, surgery, and the intranasal use of cocaine or amphetamines.

Polyps are pale, semitranslucent masses that usually come from the middle meatus and move with respiration. Ulcers may result from nasal use of cocaine.

---

‡A nasal illuminator, equipped with a short wide nasal speculum but lacking an otoscope's magnification, may also be used, but structures look much smaller. Otolaryngologists use special equipment not widely available to others.

CHAPTER 13 ■ THE EAR, NOSE, MOUTH, AND THROAT

Palpate for sinus tenderness. Press up on the *frontal sinuses* from under the bony brows, avoiding pressure on the eyes. Then press up on the *maxillary sinuses.*

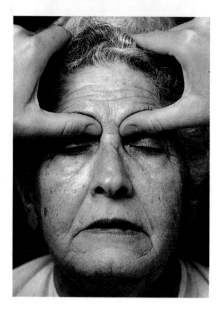

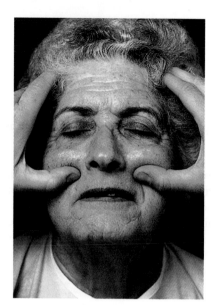

Local tenderness, together with symptoms such as pain, fever, and nasal discharge, suggests *acute sinusitis* involving the frontal or maxillary sinuses (Piccirillo, 2004; Spector et al., 1998; Williams et al., 1992). Transillumination may be diagnostically useful. For this technique, see p. 362.

THE MOUTH AND THROAT

Equipment

- Disposable gloves
- Penlight
- Tongue depressor

If the client wears dentures, offer a paper towel and ask the client to remove them so that you can see the mucosa underneath. If you detect any suspicious ulcers or nodules, put on a glove and palpate any lesions, noting especially any thickening or infiltration of the tissues that might suggest malignancy.

Bright red edematous mucosa underneath a denture suggests denture sore mouth. There may be ulcers or papillary granulation tissue.

Inspect the following:

The Lips. Observe their colour and moisture, and note any lumps, ulcers, cracking, or scaliness.

Cyanosis, pallor. See Table 13-5, Unexpected Findings of the Lips (p. 372).

The Oral Mucosa. Look into the client's mouth and, with a good light and the help of a tongue blade, inspect the oral mucosa for colour, ulcers, white patches, and nodules. The wavy white line on this buccal mucosa developed where the upper and lower teeth meet. Irritation from sucking or chewing may cause or intensify it.

An *aphthous ulcer* on the labial mucosa is shown by the client.

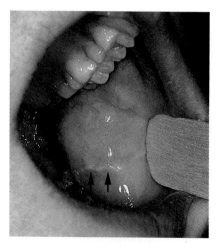

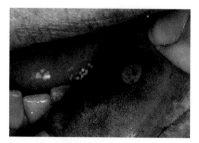

See Table 13-6, Findings in the Pharynx, Palate, and Oral Mucosa (p. 374).

The Gums and Teeth.   Note the colour of the gums, usually pink. Patchy brownness may be present, especially but not exclusively in people of African descent. Inspect the gum margins and the interdental papillae for swelling or ulceration.

Inspect the teeth. Are any of them missing, discoloured, misshapen, or abnormally positioned? You can check for looseness with your gloved thumb and index finger.

The Roof of the Mouth.   Inspect the colour and architecture of the hard palate.

The Tongue and the Floor of the Mouth.   Ask the client to put out his or her tongue. Inspect it for symmetry—a test of the hypoglossal nerve (Cranial Nerve XII).

Note the colour and texture of the dorsum of the tongue.

Redness of *gingivitis*, black line of *lead poisoning*.

Swollen interdental papillae in *gingivitis*. See Table 13-7, Findings in the Gums and Teeth (p. 377).

Torus palatinus, a midline lump (see p. 375)

Asymmetric protrusion suggests a lesion of Cranial Nerve XII, as shown below.

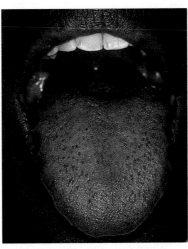

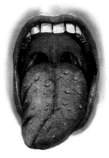

Inspect the sides and undersurface of the tongue and the floor of the mouth. These are areas where cancer most often develops. Note any white or reddened areas, nodules or ulcerations. Because cancer of the tongue is more common in men older than 50 years, especially in smokers and drinkers of alcohol, palpation is indicated. Explain what you plan to do and put on gloves. Ask the client to protrude his tongue. With your right hand, grasp the tip of the tongue with a square of gauze and gently pull it to the client's left. Inspect the side of the tongue, and then palpate it with your gloved left hand, feeling for any induration (hardness). Reverse the procedure for the other side.

Cancer of the tongue is the second most common cancer of the mouth, second only to cancer of the lip. Any persistent nodule or ulcer, red or white, must be suspect. Induration of the lesion further increases the possibility of malignancy. Cancer occurs most often on the side of the tongue, next most often at its base.

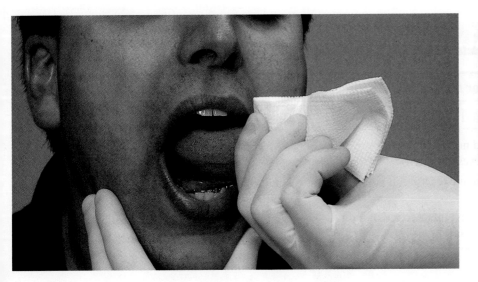

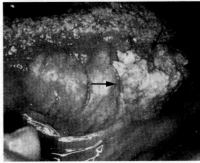

See Table 13-8, Findings In or Under the Tongue (p. 379).

The Pharynx. Now, with the client's mouth open but the tongue not protruded, ask the client to say "ah" or yawn. This action may let you see the pharynx well. If not, press a tongue blade firmly down upon the midpoint of the arched tongue—far enough back to get good visualization of the pharynx but not so far that you cause gagging. Simultaneously, ask for an "ah" or a yawn. Note the rise of the soft palate—a test of Cranial Nerve X (the vagal nerve).

In CN X paralysis, the soft palate fails to rise and the uvula deviates to the opposite side.

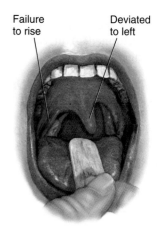

Failure to rise   Deviated to left

Inspect the soft palate, anterior and posterior pillars, uvula, tonsils, and pharynx. Note their colour and symmetry and look for exudate, swelling, ulceration, or tonsillar enlargement. If possible, palpate any suspicious area for induration or tenderness. Tonsils have crypts, or deep infoldings of squamous epithelium. Whitish spots of usual exfoliating epithelium may sometimes be seen in these crypts.

Discard your tongue blade after use.

See Table 13-6, Findings in the Pharynx, Palate, and Oral Mucosa (p. 374).

SPECIAL TECHNIQUES

Transillumination of the Sinuses. When sinus tenderness or other symptoms suggest sinusitis, this test can at times be helpful but is not highly sensitive or specific for diagnosis. The room should be thoroughly darkened. Using a strong, narrow light source, place the light snugly deep under each brow, close to the nose. Shield the light with your hand. Look for a dim red glow as light is transmitted through the air-filled frontal sinus to the forehead.

Absence of glow on one or both sides suggests a thickened mucosa or secretions in the frontal sinus, but it may also result from developmental absence of one or both sinuses.

Ask the client to tilt his or her head back with mouth opened wide. (An upper denture should first be removed.) Shine the light downward from just below the inner aspect of each eye. Look through the open mouth at the hard palate. A reddish glow indicates a usual air-filled maxillary sinus.

Absence of glow suggests thickened mucosa or secretions in the maxillary sinus.

RECORDING AND ANALYZING FINDINGS

▪ *Examples of Documentation for Ears, Nose, Mouth, and Throat*

Area of Assessment	Expected Findings	Unexpected Findings
External ear	Aligned horizontally and vertically with eyes, symmetrical bilaterally	Lower than eyes, 0.5 cm × 0.25 cm fixed mass present on upper right helix
Ear canal	Pink, minimal cerumen visible bilaterally	Left canal reddened and inflamed; soft brown cerumen obstructs entire left canal
Eardrum (tympanic membrane)	Pearly-grey, intact, cone of light visualized bilaterally	Central perforation visualized with yellow exudates on right eardrum

(continued)

■ *Examples of Documentation for Ears, Nose, Mouth, and Throat (Continued)*

Area of Assessment	Expected Findings	Unexpected Findings
Hearing acuity	Accurately identifies low whispered two-syllable words bilaterally	Identified three high-whispered words accurately bilaterally
Conduction	AC > BC bilaterally	BC > AC Left ear; AC = BC Right ear
Nose	Mucosa dark pink, septum midline, nontender, intact	Septum appears eroded, purulent discharge noted from left nare
Turbinates	Mucosa pink, moist, no lesions bilaterally	Mucosa swollen and reddened bilaterally
Smell	Correctly identifies coffee (left nare) and soap odours (right nare)	Unable to distinguish odours bilaterally
Paranasal sinuses (frontal and maxillary)	Nontender on palpation bilaterally	Tenderness over right maxillary sinus
Lips	Pink, moist, and intact	Circumoral pallor, cracking at corners
Mouth (oral mucosa)	Buccal mucosa pink and moist, no lesions	Mucosa grey; red, open, 0.5 cm × 0.5 cm lesion on right buccal mucosa
Gums and hard palate	Gingiva pink and firm, upper and lower	Bleeding from lower gums, palate rough, painful to touch
Teeth	White, 32, intact, no debris	Mottled yellow, broken left lower molar, plaque evident
Tongue	Midline, no tremors, no lesions	Thick white coating, nodules noted on upper surface
Uvula	Midline, gag reflex intact bilaterally	Deviates right, no gag reflex noted on left
Pharynx	Pink, no exudates bilaterally	White patches on pharynx, tonsils red and swollen to 2 cm × 2 cm bilaterally

ANALYZING FINDINGS FROM PHYSICAL EXAMINATION AND HEALTH HISTORY

Because of increased need for interdisciplinary collaboration relative to conditions of the ear, nose, mouth, and throat, clear and concise documentation is necessary. Following the gathering and documentation of nursing assessment information, a nursing diagnosis and care plan may be formulated, as in the following example:

Tony Binder, 23 years old, arrives at the clinic with concerns about hearing loss. Mr. Binder is a third-year university student and says he notices that he has to sit closer to the front of large lecture theatres to hear his professors. Mr. Binder works part time on the weekends in a window factory. He jogs three times a week for fitness and stress relief. Upon examination, the nurse notes that Mr. Binder has a small amount of cerumen in his ears with no excessive buildup. From this information, you develop the following nursing diagnosis:

Sensory alteration *related to potential changes in auditory function*

During Mr. Binder's visit to the clinic, the nurse collects a detailed history and performs a focused assessment of his ears and hearing function. The history includes questions directed at elements of his lifestyle that could affect hearing. He may benefit from examination by a physician or audiologist and referral to special student services at the university.

Critical Thinking Exercise

Answer the following questions about Tony Binder:

- What are some of the possible causes of his hearing loss? How would you determine whether he has sensory or conductive hearing loss? (*Knowledge*)
- What additional questions could you ask Mr. Binder to clarify his symptoms? (*Comprehension*)
- How would you teach Mr. Binder about preventing further hearing loss? (*Application*)
- What lifestyle factors might be contributing to this client's hearing loss? What adjustments might you suggest? (*Analysis*)
- What recommendations for future screening and follow-up would you recommend to Mr. Binder? (*Synthesis*)
- How would you evaluate Mr. Binder's understanding of the teaching you have done? How would you evaluate the exposures over a 1- or 2-year period? (*Evaluation*)

Canadian Research

Armstrong, R. (2005). Access and care: Towards a national oral health strategy. *Journal of the Canadian Dental Association, 71*(1), 19–22.

Ayukawa, H., Lejeune, P., & Proulx, J. F. (2002). Hearing screening outcomes in Inuit children in Nunavik, Quebec, Canada. *International Journal of Circumpolar Health, 63*(Suppl. 2), 309–311.

Canadian Hearing Society Awareness Survey. (2002). Retrieved March 14, 2009, from http://www.chs.ca/en/documents-and-publications/survey-research-studies-reports/index.php

Hawkins, R. J., Wang, E. E., & Leake, J. C. (1999). Preventative health care update: Prevention of oral cancer mortality. *Journal of the Canadian Dental Association, 65*(11), 617–628.

Statistics Canada. (2005). *Health indicators Volume 2004.* No. 1: Contact with dental professionals Report No. 82-221-XIE. Retrieved August 1, 2007, from http://www.statcan.ca/english/freepub/82-221-XIE/00604/tables/html/4295.htm

Villa, P. D. (1999). Midfacial complications of prolonged cocaine snorting. *Journal of the Canadian Dental Association, 65,* 218–223.

Test Questions

1. When inspecting the tympanic membrane, the structures that the nurse expects to identify are:
   a. cone of light, incus, umbo, cochlea.
   b. pars tensa, umbo, handle of malleus, ossicles.
   c. pars tensa, pars flaccida, vestibule, cone of light.
   d. handle of malleus, short process of malleus, cone of light.

2. When moving a client's left auricle up and back and the client reports pain, the nurse should:
   a. postpone the otoscopic examination.
   b. confine the otoscopic inspection to the right ear.
   c. press on the left tragus to confirm the presence of discharge.
   d. perform an otoscopic examination of the right ear before the left.

3. When inspecting the nose with an otoscope, the nurse:
   a. holds the handle vertically.
   b. uses the smallest speculum available.
   c. avoids contact with the nasal septum.
   d. directs the nasal speculum superiorly and medially.

4. When inspecting the mouth, the nurse focuses on lateral and vertical surfaces of the tongue and its base, because these are regions where:
   a. cancers often occur.
   b. sloughing of papillae begins.
   c. early jaundice can be detected.
   d. lesions from loose dentures are found.

5. When inspecting the mouth and pharynx, the nurse asks the client to say "ah." Which of the following findings is unexpected?
   a. Clear vocalization
   b. Stationary soft palate
   c. Scattered reddened regions
   d. Midline uvula movement

Bibliography

CITATIONS

Branch, W. (2005). *Approach to the client with dizziness.* Retrieved February 26, 2005, from http://www.utdol.com

Canadian Association of Speech-Language Pathologists and Audiologists. (2000). *Adult hearing disorders: Fact sheet.* Retrieved June 15, 2007, from http://www.caslpa.ca/PDF/fact%20sheets/adult%20hearing%20disorders.pdf

Canadian Centre for Occupational Health and Safety. (2006). *Hearing protectors.* Retrieved June 3, 2007, from http://www.ccohs.ca/oshanswers/prevention/ppe/ear_prot.html

Canadian Dental Association. (ND). *What you can't see can hurt you.* Retrieved May 15, 2007, from http://www.cda-adc.ca/_files/cda/news_events/health_month/PDFs/nohm_oralhealth_quiz.PDF

Canadian Dental Association. (2005). *Dental statistics.* Retrieved May 15, 2007, from http://www.cda-adc.ca/en/cda/news_events/statistics/default.asp

Davis, C. G., Morgan, M., & Sirois, F. (2002). *Coping with tinnitus: Severity, interpretations and adjustment.* Department of Psychology, Carleton University. Retrieved June 18, 2007, from http://www.kadis.com/ta/tinnitus.htm

Health Canada. (2007a). *It's your health: The effects of oral health on overall health.* Retrieved May 15, 2007, from http://www.hc-sc.gc.ca/iyh-vsv/life-vie/dent_e.html

Health Canada. (2007b). *Healthy living: Oral health.* Retrieved May 15, 2007, from http://www.hc-sc.gc.ca/hl-vs/oral-bucco/index_e.html

Health Canada. (2006). *It's your health: Personal stereo systems and the risk of hearing loss.* Retrieved May 10, 2007, from http://ww.hc-sc.gc.ca/iyh-vsv/life-vie/stereo-baladeur_e.html

Hearing Foundation of Canada. (2009a). *Children overview.* Retrieved March 13, 2009, from http://www.hearingfoundation.ca/cms/en/ChildrenYouth/NewbornHearingScreening.aspx?menuid=106

Hearing Foundation of Canada. (2009b). *Public education advocacy: Universal newborn hearing screening program.* Retrieved March 13, 2009, from http://www.hearingfoundation.ca/cms/en/ChildrenYouth/NewbornHearingScreening.aspx?menuid=106

Hearing Foundation of Canada. (2009c). *Hearing aids & devices.* Retrieved March 13, 2009, from http://www.hearingfoundation.ca/cms/en/ChildrenYouth/NewbornHearingScreening.aspx?menuid=106

Kroenke, K., Lucas, C. A., Rosengerg, M. L., et al. (1992). Causes of persistent dizziness: A prospective study of 100 clients in ambulatory care. *Annals of Internal Medicine, 117*(11), 898–904.

Kroenke, K., Hoffman, R. M., & Einstadter, D. (2000). How common are various causes of dizziness? A critical review. *Southern Medical Journal, 93*(2), 160–167, quiz 168.

Lockwood, A. H., Salvie, R. J., & Burkard, R. F. (2002). Tinnitus. *New England Journal of Medicine, 347*(12), 904–910.

Matthies, C., & Samii, M. (1997). Management of 1000 vestibular schwanomas (acoustic neuromas): Clinical presentation. *Neurosurgery, 1,* 1–10.

Manohar, B. (2007). Hearing and aging. *Canadian Medical Association Journal, 176*(7), 925.

Piccirillo, J. F. (2004). Acute bacterial sinusitis. *New England Journal of Medicine, 351*(9), 902–910.

Political Hear-It. (2007). Many *people suffer form hearing loss before they start workin*g. Retrieved June 2, 2007, from http://political.hear-it.org/page.dsp?page=1095

Public Health Agency of Canada. (2006). *Hearing loss info-sheet for seniors.* Retrieved May 20, 2007, from http://www.phac-aspc.gc.ca/seniors-aines/pubs/info_sheets/hearing_loss/index.htm

Spector, S. L., Bernstein, I. L., Li, J. T., et al. (1998). Parameters for the diagnosis and management of sinusitis. *Journal of Allergy and Clinical Immunology, 102*(6, part 2), S107–S114.

Tinnitus Association of Canada. (ND). *Questions and answers.* Retrieved June 3, 2007, from http://www.kadis.com/ta/tinnitus.htm

Tusa, R. J. (2001). Vertigo. *Neurological Clinics, 19*(1), 23–55.

U.S. Preventive Services Task Force. (1996a). Screening for hearing impairment. In *Guide to clinical preventive services* (2nd ed., pp. 393–405). Baltimore: Williams & Wilkins.

U.S. Preventive Services Task Force. (1996b). Counselling to prevent dental and periodontal disease. In *Guide to clinical preventive services* (2nd ed., pp. 711–721). Baltimore: Williams & Wilkins.

Vestibular Disorders Association. (2005). *Ototoxicity.* Retrieved May 15, 2007, from http://www.vestibular.org/vestibular-disorders/specific-disorders/ototoxicity.php

Williams, J. W., Simel, D. L., Roberts, L., et al. (1992). Clinical evaluation for sinusitis: Making the diagnosis by history and physical examination. *Annals of Internal Medicine, 117,* 705–710.

ADDITIONAL RESOURCES

Bevan, Y., Shapiro, N., MacLean, C. H., et al. (2003). Screening and management of adult hearing loss in primary care: scientific review. *Journal of the American Medical Association, 289*(15), 1976–1985.

Bull, T. R. (2003). *Colour atlas of ENT diagnosis* (4th ed.). New York: Thieme.

Doty, R. L. (Ed.). (2003). *Handbook of olfaction and gestation* (2nd ed., Neurological Disease and Therapy, Vol 57). New York: Marcel Dekker.

Ebell, M. H., Smith, M. A., Barry, H. C., et al. (2000). Does this client have strep throat? *Journal of the American Medical Association, 284*(22), 2912–2918.

Eisen, D., & Lynch, D. P. (1998). *The mouth: Diagnosis and treatment.* St Louis: Mosby.

Field, E. A., Longman, L., Tyldesley, W. R., et al. (2003). *Tyldesley's oral medicine* (5th ed.). New York: Oxford University Press.

Greene, J. C., & Greene, A. R. (1996). Oral health. In S. H. Woolf, S. Jonas, & R. S. Lawrence (Eds.), *Health promotion and disease prevention in clinical practice* (pp. 315–334). Baltimore: Williams & Wilkins.

Hendley, J. O. (2002). Otitis media. *New England Journal of Medicine, 347*(15), 1169–1174.

Kennedy, D. W. (2000). A 48-year-old man with recurrent sinusitis. *Journal of the American Medical Association, 283*(16), 2143–2150.

Langlais, R. P., & Miller, C. S. (2003). *Colour atlas of common oral diseases* (3rd ed.). Philadelphia: Lippincott Williams & Wilkins.

Neville, B. W., Damm, D. D., & White, D. K. (1999). *Colour atlas of clinical oral pathology* (2nd ed.). Baltimore: Williams & Wilkins.

Newman, M. F., Carranza, F. A., & Takei, H. (2002). *Carranza's clinical periodontology* (9th ed.). Philadelphia: W. B. Saunders.

O'Donoghue, G. M., Narula, A. A., & Bates, G. J. (2000). *Clinical ENT: An illustrated textbook* (2nd ed.). San Diego: Singular Pub Group.

Regezi, J. A., Sciubba, J. J., & Jordan, R. C. K. (2003). *Oral pathology: Clinical pathologic correlations* (4th ed.). St. Louis: Saunders.

Young, T., Skatrud, J., & Peppard, P. E. (2004). Risk factors for obstructive sleep apnea in adults. *Journal of the American Medical Association, 291*(16), 2013–2016.

CANADIAN WEB SITES AND ASSOCIATIONS

Canadian Academy of Audiology: http://www.canadianaudiology.ca

Canadian Association of the Deaf: http://www.cad.ca

Canadian Cancer Society: http://www.cancer.ca

Canadian Centre for Occupational Health and Safety: http://www.ccohs.ca

Canadian Dental Association: http://www.cda-adc.ca

Canadian Dental Hygienists Association: http://www.cdha.ca

Canadian Hard of Hearing Association: http://www.chha.ca

Canadian Hearing Society: http://www.chs.ca

Health Canada: http://www.hc-sc.gc.ca/iyh-vsv/med/earoreille_e.html

The Hearing Foundation of Canada: http://www.thfc.ca

Nosebleeds – What to do when your nose bleeds: http://www.cfpc.ca/English/cfpc/programs/client%20education/nosebleeds/default.asp?s=1

Silent Voice Canada: http://www.silentvoice.ca

The Tinnitus Association of Canada: http://www.kadis.com/ta/tinnitus.htm

TABLE 13-1   Dizziness and Vertigo

"Dizziness" is a nonspecific term used by clients encompassing several disorders that clinicians must carefully sort out. A detailed history usually identifies the primary etiology (Branch, 2005; Kroenke et al., 1992, 2000; Lock wood et al., 2002; Tusa, 2001). It is important to learn the specific meanings of the following terms or conditions:

- *Vertigo*—a spinning sensation accompanied by nystagmus and ataxia; usually from *peripheral vestibular dysfunction* (~40% of "dizzy" clients) but may be from a *central brainstem lesion* (~10%; causes include atherosclerosis, multiple sclerosis, vertebrobasilar migraine, or TIA)

- *Presyncope*—a near faint from "feeling faint or lightheaded"; causes include orthostatic hypotension, especially from medication, arrhythmias, and vasovagal attacks (~5%)

- *Dysequilibrium*—unsteadiness or imbalance when walking, especially in older clients (see Chapter 25); causes include fear of walking, visual loss, weakness from musculoskeletal problems, and peripheral neuropathy (up to 15%)

- *Psychiatric*—causes include anxiety, panic disorder, hyperventilation, depression, somatization disorder, alcohol, and substance abuse (~10%)

- *Multifactorial or unknown*—(up to 20%)

Peripheral and Central Vertigo

	Onset	Duration and Course	Hearing	Tinnitus	Additional Features
Peripheral Vertigo					
Benign Positional Vertigo	Sudden, on rolling on to affected side or tilting head up	Onset a few seconds to <1 minute Lasts a few weeks, may recur	Not affected	Absent	Sometimes nausea, vomiting, nystagmus
Vestibular Neuronitis (acute labyrinthitis)	Sudden	Onset hours to up to 2 weeks May recur over 12–18 months	Not affected	Absent	Nausea, vomiting, nystagmus
Ménière's Disease	Sudden	Onset several hours to ≥1 day Recurrent	Sensorineural hearing loss—recurs, eventually progresses	Present, fluctuating	Pressure or fullness in affected ear; nausea, vomiting, nystagmus
Drug Toxicity	Insidious or acute—linked to loop diuretics, aminoglycosides, salicylates, alcohol	May or may not be reversible Partial adaptation occurs	May be impaired	May be present	Nausea, vomiting
Acoustic Neuroma	Insidious from CN VIII compression, vestibular branch	Variable	Impaired, one side	Present	May involve CN V and VII
Central Vertigo	Often sudden (see causes above)	Variable but rarely continuous	Not affected	Absent	Usually with other brainstem deficits—dysarthria, ataxia, crossed motor and sensory deficits

TABLE 13-2   **Lumps On or Near the Ear**

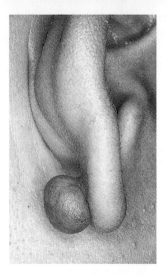

Keloid. A firm, nodular, hypertrophic mass of scar tissue extending beyond the area of injury. It may develop in any scarred area but is most common on the shoulders and upper chest. A keloid on a pierced earlobe may have troublesome cosmetic effects. Keloids are more common in darker-skinned people. Recurrence may follow treatment.

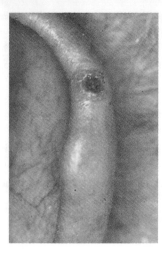

Chondrodermatitis Helicis. This chronic inflammatory lesion starts as a painful, tender papule on the helix or antihelix. Here the upper lesion is at a later stage of ulceration and crusting. Reddening may occur. Biopsy is needed to rule out carcinoma.

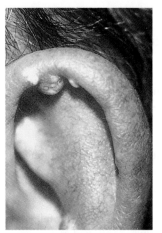

Tophi. A deposit of uric acid crystals characteristic of chronic tophaceous gout. It appears as hard nodules in the helix or antihelix and may discharge chalky white crystals through the skin. It also may appear near the joints: hands (p. 672), feet, and other areas. It usually develops after chronic sustained high blood levels of uric acid.

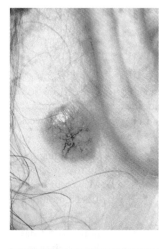

Basal Cell Carcinoma. This raised nodule shows the lustrous surface and telangiectatic vessels of basal cell carcinoma, a common slow-growing malignancy that rarely metastasizes. Growth and ulceration may occur. These are more frequent in fair-skinned people overexposed to sunlight.

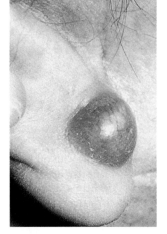

Cutaneous Cyst. Formerly called a *sebaceous cyst*, a dome-shaped lump in the dermis forms a benign, closed, firm sac attached to the epidermis. A dark dot (blackhead) may be visible on its surface. Histologically, it is usually either (1) an *epidermoid* cyst, common on the face and neck, or (2) a *pilar (trichilemmal)* cyst, common in the scalp. Both may become inflamed.

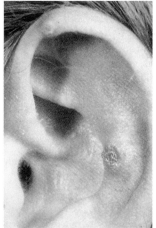

Rheumatoid Nodules. In chronic rheumatoid arthritis, look for small lumps on the helix or antihelix and additional nodules elsewhere on the hands, along the surface of the ulna distal to the elbow (p. 676), and on the knees and heels. Ulceration may result from repeated injuries. Such nodules may antedate the arthritis.

Photo sources: Keloid—Sams, W. M. Jr., & Lynch, P. J. (Eds). *Principles and Practice of Dermatology.* Edinburgh, Churchill Livingstone, 1990; *Tophi*—du Vivier, A. *Atlas of Clinical Dermatology*, 2nd ed. London: Gower Medical Publishing, 1993; *Cutaneous Cyst, Chondrodermatitis Helicis*—Young, E. M., Newcomer, V. D., & Kligman, A. M. *Geriatric Dermatology: Colour Atlas and Practitioner's Guide.* Philadelphia, Lea & Febiger, 1993; *Basal Cell Carcinoma*—*The New England Journal of Medicine*, 326:169–170, 1992; *Rheumatoid Nodules*—Champion, R. H., Burton, J. L., & Ebling, F. J. G. (Eds). *Rook/Wilkinson/Ebling Textbook of Dermatology*, 5th ed. Oxford, UK: Blackwell Scientific, 1992.

TABLE 13-3 **Unexpected Findings of the Eardrum**

Healthy Eardrum

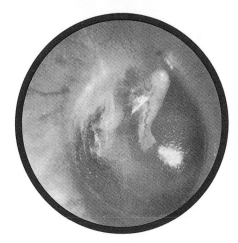

This right eardrum (tympanic membrane) is pinkish grey. Note the malleus lying behind the upper part of the drum. Above the short process lies the *pars flaccida*. The remainder of the drum is the *pars tensa*. From the umbo, the bright cone of light fans anteriorly and downward. Posterior to the malleus, part of the incus is visible behind the drum. The small blood vessels along the handle of the malleus are expected findings.

Perforation of the Drum

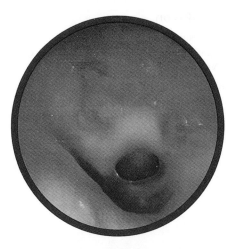

Perforations are holes in the eardrum that usually result from purulent infections of the middle ear. They are classified as *central* perforations, which do not extend to the margin of the drum, and *marginal* perforations, which do involve the margin.

The more common central perforation is illustrated here. A reddened ring of granulation tissue surrounds the perforation, indicating chronic infection. The eardrum itself is scarred, and no landmarks are visible. Discharge from the infected middle ear may drain out through such a perforation. A perforation often closes in the healing process, as in the next photo. The membrane covering the hole may be exceedingly thin and transparent.

Tympanosclerosis

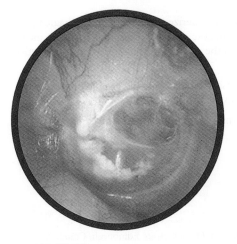

In the inferior portion of this left eardrum, there is a large, chalky white patch with irregular margins. It is typical of tympanosclerosis: a deposition of hyaline material within the layers of the tympanic membrane that sometimes follows a severe episode of otitis media. It does not usually impair hearing and is seldom clinically significant.

Other unexpected findings in this eardrum include a *healed perforation* (the large oval area in the upper posterior drum) and signs of a *retracted drum*. A retracted drum is pulled medially, away from the examiner's eye, and the malleolar folds are tightened into sharp outlines. The short process often protrudes sharply, and the handle of the malleus, pulled inward at the umbo, looks foreshortened and more horizontal.

Photo sources: Normal Eardrum—Hawke, M., Keene, M., & Alberti, P. W. *Clinical Otoscopy: A Text and Colour Atlas*. Edinburgh, Churchill Livingstone, 1984; *Perforation of the Drum, Tympanosclerosis*—Courtesy of Michael Hawke, MD, Toronto, Canada.

(table continues on next page)

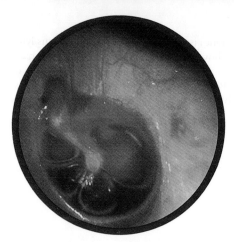

Serous Effusion

Serous effusions usually result from viral upper respiratory infections (*otitis media with serous effusion*) or sudden changes in atmospheric pressure as with flying or diving (*otitic barotrauma*). The eustachian tube cannot equalize the air pressure in the middle ear with that of the outside air. Air is partly or completely absorbed from the middle ear into the bloodstream, and serous fluid accumulates there instead. Symptoms include fullness and popping sensations in the ear, mild conduction hearing loss, and perhaps some pain.

Amber fluid behind the eardrum is characteristic, as in this client with otitic barotrauma. A fluid level, a line between air above and amber fluid below, can be seen on either side of the short process. Air bubbles (not always present) can be seen here within the amber fluid.

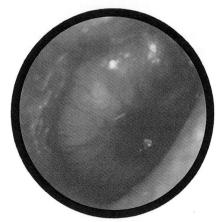

Acute Otitis Media With Purulent Effusion

Acute otitis media with purulent effusion results from bacterial infection. Symptoms include earache, fever, and hearing loss. The eardrum reddens, loses its landmarks, and bulges laterally, toward the examiner's eye.

Here the eardrum is bulging, and most landmarks are obscured. Redness is most obvious near the umbo, but dilated vessels can be seen in all segments of the drum. A diffuse redness of the entire drum often develops. Spontaneous rupture (perforation) of the drum may follow, with discharge of purulent material into the ear canal.

Hearing loss is of the conductive type. Acute purulent otitis media is much more common in children than in adults.

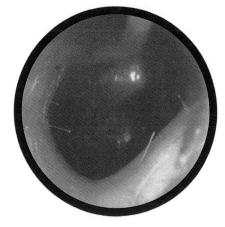

Bullous Myringitis

Bullous myringitis is a viral infection characterized by painful hemorrhagic vesicles that appear on the tympanic membrane, the ear canal, or both. Symptoms include earache, blood-tinged discharge from the ear, and hearing loss of the conductive type.

In this right ear, at least two large vesicles (bullae) are discernible on the drum. The drum is reddened, and its landmarks are obscured.

Several different viruses may cause this condition, including mycoplasma.

Photo sources: Serous Effusion—Hawke, M., Keene, M., & Alberti, P. W. *Clinical Otoscopy: A Text and Colour Atlas.* Edinburgh, Churchill Livingstone, 1984; *Acute Otitis Media, Bullous Myringitis*—The Wellcome Trust, National Medical Slide Bank, London, UK.

TABLE 13-4	Patterns of Hearing Loss

	Conductive Loss	Sensorineural Loss
	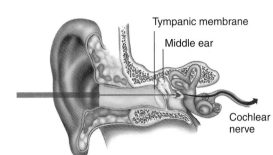	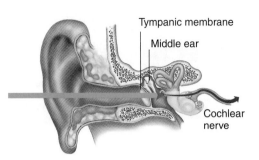
Pathophysiology	External or middle ear disorder impairs sound conduction to inner ear. Causes include foreign body, *otitis media*, perforated eardrum, and otosclerosis of ossicles.	Inner ear disorder involves cochlear nerve and neuronal impulse transmission to the brain. Causes include loud noise exposure, inner ear infections, trauma, tremors, congenital and familial disorders, and aging.
Usual Age of Onset	Childhood and young adulthood, up to age 40 years	Middle or later years
Ear Canal and Drum	Abnormality usually visible, except in otosclerosis	Problem not visible
Effects	▪ Little effect on sound. ▪ Hearing seems to improve in noisy environment. ▪ Voice becomes soft because inner ear and cochlear nerve are intact.	▪ Higher registers are lost, so sound may be distorted. ▪ Hearing worsens in noisy environment. ▪ Voice may be loud because hearing is difficult.
Weber Test (*in unilateral hearing loss*)	▪ Tuning fork at vertex. ▪ Sound lateralizes to *impaired ear*—room noise not well heard, so detection of vibrations *improves*.	▪ Tuning fork at vertex. ▪ Sound lateralizes to *good ear*—inner ear or cochlear nerve damage impairs transmission to affected ear.
Rinne Test	▪ Tuning fork at external auditory meatus, then on mastoid bone. ▪ Bone conduction longer than or equal to air conduction (BC ≥ AC). While air conduction through the external or middle ear is impaired, vibrations through bone bypass the problem to reach the cochlea.	▪ Tuning fork at external auditory meatus, then on mastoid bone. ▪ Air conduction longer than bone conduction (AC > BC). The inner ear or cochlear nerve is less able to transmit impulses, regardless of how the vibrations reach the cochlea. The expected pattern prevails.

TABLE 13-5   **Unexpected Findings of the Lips**

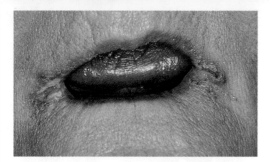

Angular Cheilitis

Angular cheilitis starts with softening of the skin at the angles of the mouth, followed by fissuring. It may be the result of nutritional deficiency or, more commonly, overclosure of the mouth, as in people with no teeth or with ill-fitting dentures. Saliva wets and macerates the infolded skin, often leading to secondary infection with *Candida*, as in this example.

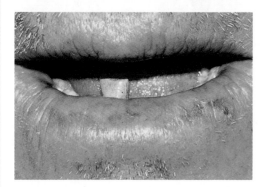

Actinic Cheilitis

Actinic cheilitis results from excessive exposure to sunlight and affects primarily the lower lip. Fair-skinned men who work outdoors are most often affected. The lip loses its usual redness and may become scaly, somewhat thickened, and slightly everted. Because solar damage also predisposes to carcinoma of the lip, be alert to this possibility.

Herpes Simplex *(Cold Sore, Fever Blister)*

The herpes simplex virus (HSV) produces recurrent and painful vesicular eruptions of the lips and surrounding skin. A small cluster of vesicles first develops. As these break, yellow-brown crusts form, and healing ensues within 10 to 14 days. Both of these stages are visible here.

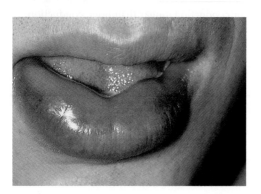

Angioedema

Angioedema is a diffuse, nonpitting, tense swelling of the dermis and subcutaneous tissue. It develops rapidly, and typically disappears over subsequent hours or days. Although usually allergic in nature and sometimes associated with hives, angioedema does not itch.

Photo sources: Angular Cheilitis, Herpes Simplex, Angioedema—Neville, B., et al. *Colour Atlas of Clinical Oral Pathology.* Philadelphia: Lea & Febiger, 1991; Used with permission; *Actinic Cheilitis*—Langlais, R. P., & Miller, C. S. *Colour Atlas of Common Oral Diseases.* Philadelphia: Lea & Febiger, 1992. Used with permission.

(table continues on next page)

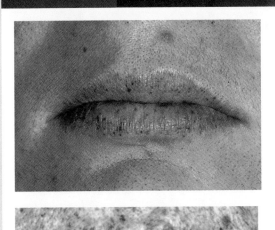

Hereditary Hemorrhagic Telangiectasia

Multiple small red spots on the lips strongly suggest hereditary hemorrhagic telangiectasia. Spots may also be visible on the face and hands and in the mouth. The spots are dilated capillaries and may bleed when traumatized. Affected people often have nosebleeds and gastrointestinal bleeding.

Peutz-Jeghers Syndrome

When pigmented spots on the lips are more prominent than freckling of the surrounding skin, suspect this syndrome. Pigment in the buccal mucosa helps to confirm the diagnosis. Pigmented spots may also be found on the face and hands. Multiple intestinal polyps are often associated.

Chancre of Syphilis

This lesion of primary syphilis may appear on the lip rather than on the genitalia. It is a firm, buttonlike lesion that ulcerates and may become crusted. A chancre may resemble a carcinoma or a crusted cold sore. Because it is infectious, use gloves to feel any suspicious lesion.

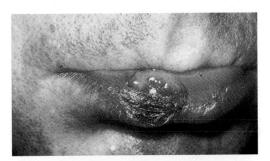

Carcinoma of the Lip
Like actinic cheilitis, carcinoma usually affects the lower lip. It may appear as a scaly plaque, as an ulcer with or without a crust, or as a nodular lesion, illustrated here. Fair skin and prolonged exposure to the sun are common risk factors.

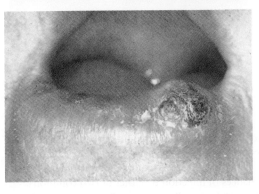

Photo sources: Hereditary Hemorrhagic Telangiectasia—Langlais, R. P., & Miller, C. S. *Colour Atlas of Common Oral Diseases.* Philadelphia: Lea & Febiger, 1992; Used with permission; *Peutz-Jeghers Syndrome*—Robinson, H. B. G., & Miller, A. S. *Colby, Kerr, and Robinson's Colour Atlas of Oral Pathology.* Philadelphia: JB Lippincott, 1990; *Chancre of Syphilis*—Wisdom, A. *A Colour Atlas of Sexually Transmitted Diseases,* 2nd ed. London: Wolfe Medical Publications, 1989; *Carcinoma of the Lip*—Tyldesley, W. R. *A Colour Atlas of Orofacial Diseases,* 2nd ed. London: Wolfe Medical Publications, 1991.

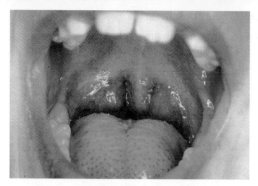

Large Healthy Tonsils

Large-size tonsils may be a healthy deviation rather than a sign of infection, especially in children. They may protrude medially beyond the pillars and even to the midline. Here they touch the sides of the uvula and obscure the pharynx. Their colour is within usual limits. The white marks are light reflections, not exudate.

Exudative Tonsillitis

This red throat has a white exudate on the tonsils. This, together with fever and enlarged cervical nodes, increases the probability of *group A streptococcal infection*, or infectious mononucleosis. Some anterior cervical lymph nodes are usually enlarged in the former, posterior nodes in the latter.

Pharyngitis

These two photos show reddened throats without exudate.

In **A**, redness and vascularity of the pillars and uvula are mild to moderate.

A

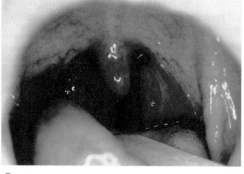

In **B**, redness is diffuse and intense. Each client would probably report a sore throat, or at least a scratchy one. Possible causes include several kinds of viruses and bacteria. If the client has no fever, exudate, or enlargement of cervical lymph node, the chances of infection by either of two common causes—*group A streptococci* and *Epstein-Barr virus* (infectious mononucleosis)—are very small.

B

Photo sources: Large Normal Tonsils, Exudative Tonsillitis, Pharyngitis [**A** and **B**]—The Wellcome Trust, National Medical Slide Bank, London, UK.)

(table continues on next page)

TABLE 13-6   **Findings in the Pharynx, Palate, and Oral Mucosa** *(Continued)*

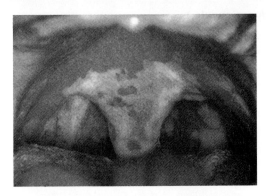

Diphtheria

Diphtheria (an acute infection caused by *Corynebacterium diphtheriae*) is now rare but still important. Prompt diagnosis may lead to life-saving treatment. The throat is dull red, and a grey exudate (pseudomembrane) is present on the uvula, pharynx, and tongue. The airway may become obstructed.

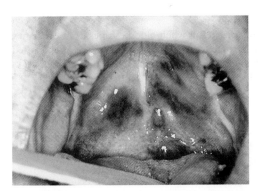

Thrush on the Palate (Candidiasis)

Thrush is a yeast infection due to *Candida*. Shown here on the palate, it may appear elsewhere in the mouth (see p. 379). Thick, white plaques are somewhat adherent to the underlying mucosa. Predisposing factors include (1) prolonged treatment with antibiotics or corticosteroids, and (2) AIDS.

Kaposi's Sarcoma in AIDS

The deep purple colour of these lesions, although not necessarily present, strongly suggests Kaposi's sarcoma. The lesions may be raised or flat. Among people with HIV and AIDS, the palate, as illustrated here, is a common site for this tumour.

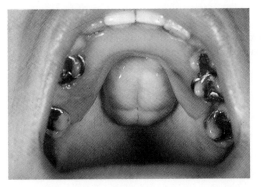

Torus Palatinus

A torus palatinus is a midline bony growth in the hard palate that is fairly common in adults. Its size and lobulation vary. Although alarming at first glance, it is harmless. In this example, an upper denture has been fitted around the torus.

Photo sources: Diphtheria—Harnisch, J. P., et al. Diphtheria among alcoholic urban adults. *Annals of Internal Medicine* 1989;111:77; *Thrush on the Palate*—The Wellcome Trust, National Medical Slide Bank, London, UK; *Kaposi's Sarcoma in AIDS*—Ioachim, H. L. *Textbook and Atlas of Disease Associated With Acquired Immune Deficiency Syndrome.* London, UK: Gower Medical Publishing, 1989.)

(table continues on next page)

TABLE 13-6   **Findings in the Pharynx, Palate, and Oral Mucosa** *(Continued)*

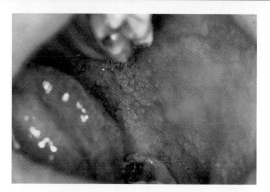

Fordyce Spots *(Fordyce Granules)*

Fordyce spots are healthy sebaceous glands that appear as small yellowish spots in the buccal mucosa or on the lips. A worried person who has suddenly noticed them may be reassured. Here they are seen best anterior to the tongue and lower jaw. These spots are usually not so numerous.

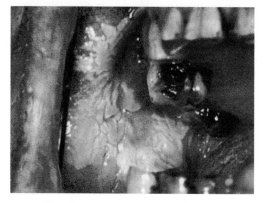

Koplik's Spots

Koplik's spots are an early sign of measles (rubeola). Search for small white specks that resemble grains of salt on a red background. They usually appear on the buccal mucosa near the first and second molars. In this photo, look also in the upper third of the mucosa. The rash of measles appears within a day.

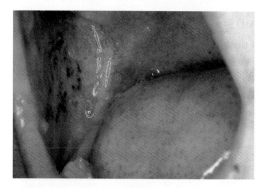

Petechiae

Petechiae are small red spots that result when blood escapes from capillaries into the tissues. Petechiae in the buccal mucosa, as shown, are often caused by accidentally biting the cheek. Oral petechiae may be from infection or decreased platelets, as well as trauma.

Leukoplakia

A thickened white patch (*leukoplakia*) may occur anywhere in the oral mucosa. The extensive example shown on this buccal mucosa resulted from frequent chewing of tobacco, a local irritant. This kind of irritation may lead to cancer.

Photo sources: Fordyce Spots—Neville, B., et al. *Colour Atlas of Clinical Oral Pathology.* Philadelphia: Lea & Febiger, 1991; Used with permission; *Koplik's Spots, Petechiae*—The Wellcome Trust, National Medical Slide Bank, London: UK; *Leukoplakia*—Robinson, H. B. G., & Miller, A. S. *Colby, Kerr, and Robinson's Colour Atlas of Oral Pathology.* Philadelphia: JB Lippincott, 1990.)

TABLE 13-7   Findings in the Gums and Teeth

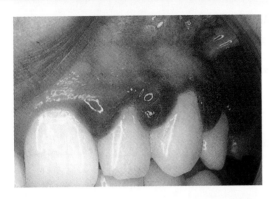

Marginal Gingivitis

Marginal gingivitis is common among teenagers and young adults. The gingival margins are reddened and swollen, and the interdental papillae are blunted, swollen, and red. Brushing the teeth often makes the gums bleed. *Plaque*—the soft white film of salivary salts, protein, and bacteria that covers the teeth and leads to gingivitis—is not readily visible.

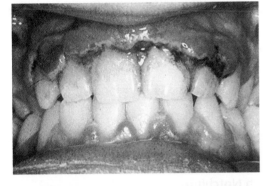

Acute Necrotizing Ulcerative Gingivitis

This uncommon form of gingivitis occurs suddenly in adolescents and young adults and is accompanied by fever, malaise, and enlarged lymph nodes. Ulcers develop in the interdental papillae. Then the destructive (necrotizing) process spreads along the gum margins, where a greyish pseudomembrane develops. The red, painful gums bleed easily; the breath is foul.

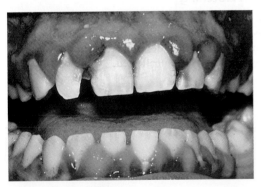

Gingival Hyperplasia

Gums enlarged by hyperplasia are swollen into heaped-up masses that may even cover the teeth. The redness of inflammation may coexist, as in this example. Causes include dilantin therapy (as in this case), puberty, pregnancy, and leukemia.

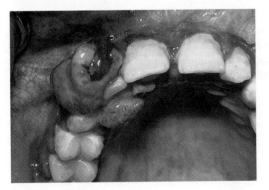

Pregnancy Tumour (Epulis, Pyogenic Granuloma)

Gingival enlargement may be localized, forming a tumourlike mass that usually originates in an interdental papilla. It is red and soft and usually bleeds easily. The estimated incidence of this lesion in pregnancy is about 1%. Note the accompanying gingivitis in this example.

Photo sources: Marginal Gingivitis, Acute Necrotizing Ulcerative Gingivitis—Tyldesley, W. R. *A Colour Atlas of Orofacial Diseases*, 2nd ed. London: Wolfe Medical Publications, 1991; *Gingival Hyperplasia*—Courtesy of Dr. James Cottone; *Pregnancy Tumour*—Langlais, R. P., & Miller, C. S. *Colour Atlas of Common Oral Diseases.* Philadelphia: Lea & Febiger, 1992. Used with permission.

(table continues on next page)

TABLE 13-7 Findings in the Gums and Teeth (Continued)

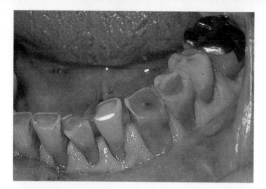

Attrition of Teeth; Recession of Gums

In many elderly people, the chewing surfaces of the teeth have been worn down by repetitive use so that the yellow-brown dentin becomes exposed—a process called *attrition*. Note also the *recession of the gums*, which has exposed the roots of the teeth, giving a "long in the tooth" appearance.

Erosion of Teeth

Teeth may be eroded by chemical action. Note here the erosion of the enamel from the lingual surfaces of the upper incisors, exposing the yellow-brown dentin. This results from recurrent regurgitation of stomach contents, as in bulimia.

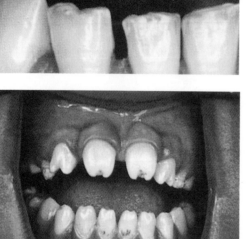

Abrasion of Teeth with Notching

The biting surface of the teeth may become abraded or notched by recurrent trauma, such as holding nails or opening bobby pins between the teeth. Unlike Hutchinson's teeth, the sides of these teeth show usual contours; size and spacing of the teeth are unaffected.

Hutchinson's Teeth

Hutchinson's teeth are smaller and more widely spaced than usual and are notched on their biting surfaces. The sides of the teeth taper toward the biting edges. The upper central incisors of the permanent (not the deciduous) teeth are most often affected. These teeth are a sign of congenital syphilis.

Photo sources: Attrition of Teeth, Erosion of Teeth—Langlais, R. P., & Miller, C. S. *Colour Atlas of Common Oral Diseases.* Philadelphia: Lea & Febiger, 1992. Used with permission; *Abrasion of Teeth, Hutchinson's Teeth*—Robinson, H. B. G., & Miller, A. S. *Colby, Kerr, and Robinson's Colour Atlas of Oral Pathology.* Philadelphia: JB Lippincott, 1990.

TABLE 13-8   Findings in or Under the Tongue

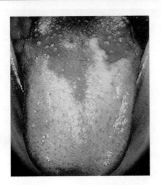

Geographic Tongue. In this benign condition, the dorsum shows scattered smooth red areas denuded of papillae. Together with the usual rough and coated areas, they give a maplike pattern that changes over time.

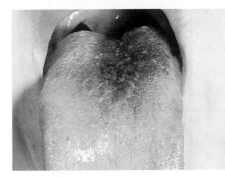

Hairy Tongue. Note the "hairy" yellowish to brown or black elongated papillae on the tongue's dorsum. This benign condition may follow antibiotic therapy; it also may occur spontaneously.

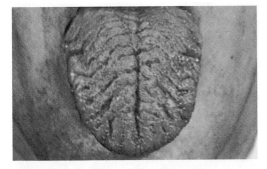

Fissured Tongue. Fissures appear with increasing age, sometimes termed *scrotal tongue*. Food debris may accumulate in the crevices and become irritating, but a fissured tongue is benign.

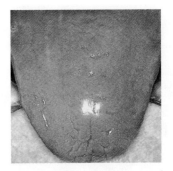

Smooth Tongue (Atrophic Glossitis). A smooth and often sore tongue that has lost its papillae suggests a deficiency in riboflavin, niacin, folic acid, vitamin B_{12}, pyridoxine, or iron, or treatment with chemotherapy.

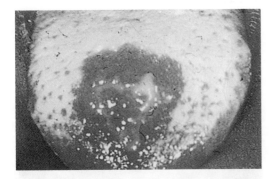

Candidiasis. Note the thick white coating from *Candida*. The raw red surface is where the coat was scraped off. Infection may also occur without the white coating. It is seen in immunosuppressed conditions.

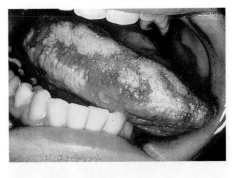

Hairy Leukoplakia. These whitish raised areas with a feathery or corrugated pattern most often affect the sides of the tongue. Unlike candidiasis, these areas cannot be scraped off. They are seen in clients with HIV and AIDS.

(table continues on next page)

TABLE 13-8 **Findings in or Under the Tongue** *(Continued)*

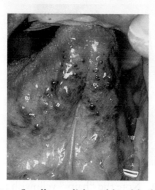

Varicose Veins. Small purplish or blue-black round swellings appear under the tongue with age. These dilatations of the lingual veins have no clinical significance.

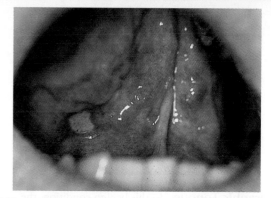

Aphthous Ulcer (Canker Sore). A painful, round or oval ulcer that is white or yellowish grey and surrounded by a halo of reddened mucosa. It may be single or multiple. It heals in 7–10 days, but may recur.

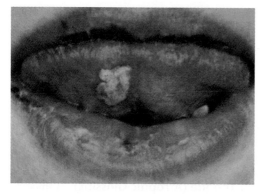

Mucous Patch of Syphilis. This painless lesion in the secondary stage of syphilis is highly infectious. It is slightly raised, oval, and covered by a greyish membrane. It may be multiple and occur elsewhere in the mouth.

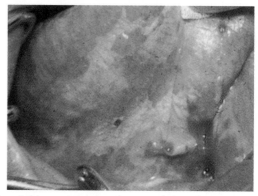

Leukoplakia. With this persisting painless white patch in the oral mucosa, the undersurface of the tongue appears painted white. Patches of any size raise the possibility of malignancy and require a biopsy.

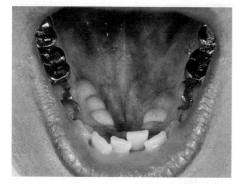

Tori Mandibulares. Rounded bony growths on the inner surfaces of the mandible are typically bilateral, asymptomatic, and harmless.

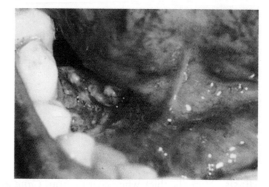

Carcinoma, Floor of the Mouth. This ulcerated lesion is in a common location for carcinoma. Medially, note the reddened area of mucosa, called *erythroplakia*, suggesting possible malignancy.

Photo sources: Fissured Tongue, Candidiasis, Mucous Patch, Leukoplakia, Carcinoma—Robinson, H. B. G., & Miller, A. S. *Colby, Kerr, and Robinson's Colour Atlas of Oral Pathology*. Philadelphia: JB Lippincott, 1990; *Smooth Tongue*—Courtesy of Dr. R. A. Cawson, from Cawson, R. A. *Oral Pathology*, 1st ed. London: Gower Medical Publishing, 1987; *Geographic Tongue*—The Wellcome Trust, National Medical Slide Bank, London, UK; *Hairy Leukoplakia*—Ioachim, H. L. *Textbook and Atlas of Disease Associated With Acquired Immune Deficiency Syndrome*. London: Gower Medical Publishing, 1989; *Varicose Veins*—Neville, B., et al. *Colour Atlas of Clinical Oral Pathology*. Philadelphia: Lea & Febiger, 1991. Used with permission.

14

The Thorax and Lungs

Dana S. Edge and Lynn S. Bickley

Ventilation, the inhaling and exhaling of ambient gases, requires intact and functioning thoracic muscles and diaphragm, as well as intricate neurological control orchestrated by the brainstem. The exchange of oxygen and carbon dioxide at the level of the alveoli constitutes *respiration*. Oxygenation of the cells is critical to sustaining life. Healthy lung function supports human activities, including recreation, sports, and exercise.

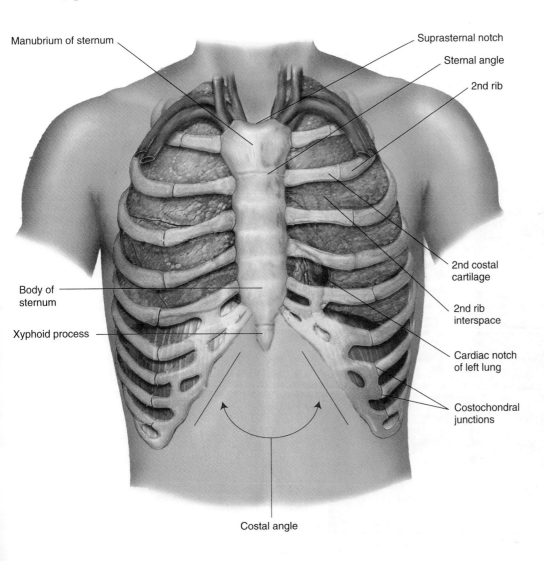

Manubrium of sternum

Suprasternal notch

Sternal angle

2nd rib

2nd costal cartilage

2nd rib interspace

Body of sternum

Xyphoid process

Cardiac notch of left lung

Costochondral junctions

Costal angle

Infection, trauma, environmental pollutants, chronic disease processes, or surgical interventions can disrupt lung functioning. Assessment of the lungs and thorax is critical in every clinical setting because severe disorders in breathing and ventilation are incompatible with life.

Nurses play a key role with clients in assessing respiratory function; providing clinical management; promoting respiratory health; assisting clients with treatments; teaching about medications, including the use of inhalers; and assessing the effectiveness of treatments, including deep breathing and coughing, as well as treatments provided by respiratory therapists and chest physiotherapists. Also, nurses understand how respiratory diseases affect the quality of life of their clients.

ANATOMY AND PHYSIOLOGY

Study the *anatomy of the chest wall*, identifying the structures illustrated. Note that an interspace between two ribs is numbered by the rib above it.

LOCATING FINDINGS ON THE CHEST

Describe unexpected findings of the chest in two dimensions: *along the vertical axis* and *around the circumference of the chest*.

To make *vertical* locations, you must be able to count the ribs and intercostal spaces. The *sternal angle*, also termed the *angle of Louis*, is the best guide. Place your finger in the hollow curve of the suprasternal notch, then move your finger down about 5 cm to the horizontal bony ridge joining the manubrium to the body of the

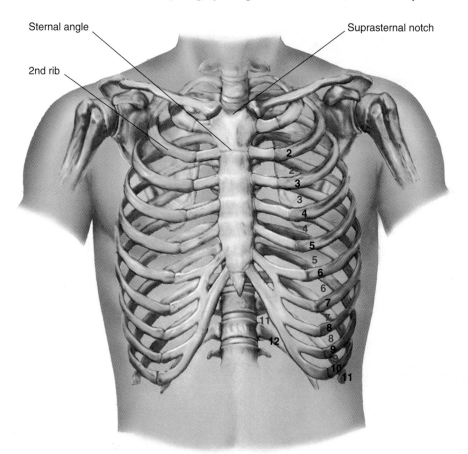

Sternal angle

Suprasternal notch

2nd rib

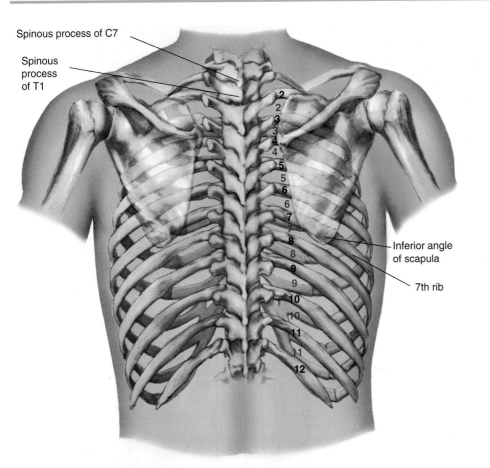

Spinous process of C7

Spinous process of T1

Inferior angle of scapula

7th rib

sternum. Then move your finger laterally and find the adjacent 2nd rib and costal cartilage. From here, using two fingers, "walk down the intercostal spaces," one space at a time, on an oblique line illustrated by the red numbers below. Do not try to count intercostal spaces along the lower edge of the sternum; the ribs there are too close together. In a woman, to find the intercostal spaces, either displace the breast laterally or palpate a little more medially than illustrated. Avoid pressing too hard on tender breast tissue.

Note that the costal cartilages of the first seven ribs articulate with the sternum; the cartilages of the 8th, 9th, and 10th ribs articulate with the costal cartilages just above them. The 11th and 12th ribs, the "floating ribs," have no anterior attachments. The cartilaginous tip of the 11th rib can usually be felt laterally, and the 12th rib may be felt posteriorly. On palpation, costal cartilages and ribs feel identical.

Posteriorly, the 12th rib is another possible starting point for counting ribs and intercostal spaces. It helps locate findings on the lower posterior chest and provides an option when the anterior approach is unsatisfactory. With the fingers of one hand, press in and up against the lower border of the 12th rib, then "walk up" the intercostal spaces numbered in red below, or follow a more oblique line up and around to the front of the chest.

The inferior tip of the scapula is another useful bony marker—it usually lies at the level of the 7th rib or intercostal space.

The spinous processes of the vertebrae are also useful anatomical landmarks. When the neck is flexed forward, the most protruding process is usually the vertebra of C7. If two processes are equally prominent, they are C7 and T1. You can often palpate and count the processes below them, especially when the spine is flexed.

To locate findings around the *circumference of the chest*, use a series of vertical lines, shown in the adjacent illustrations. The *midsternal* and *vertebral lines* are precise; the others are estimated. The *midclavicular line* (MCL) drops vertically from the midpoint of the clavicle. To find it, you must identify both ends of the clavicle accurately (see p. 382).

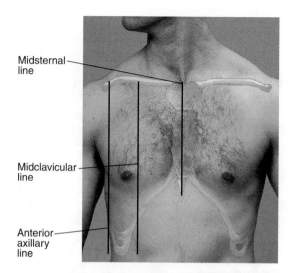

The *anterior* and *posterior axillary lines* drop vertically from the anterior and posterior axillary folds, the muscle masses that border the axilla. The *midaxillary line* drops from the apex of the axilla.

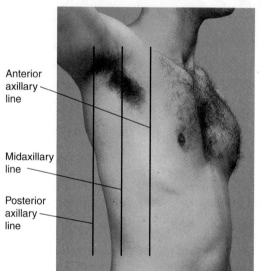

Posteriorly, the *vertebral line* overlies the spinous process of the vertebrae. The scapular line drops from the inferior angle of the scapula.

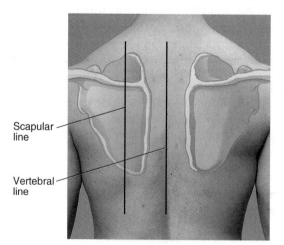

Lungs, Fissures, and Lobes. Picture the lungs and their fissures and lobes on the chest wall. Anteriorly, the apex of each lung rises about 2 cm to 4 cm above the inner third of the clavicle. The lower border of the lung crosses the 6th rib at the MCL and the 8th rib at the midaxillary line. Posteriorly, the lower border of the lung lies at about the level of the T10 spinous process. On inspiration, it descends farther.

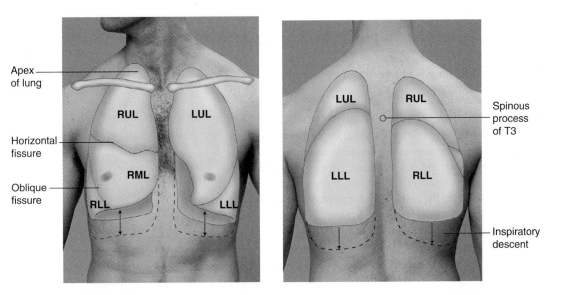

Each lung is divided roughly in half by an *oblique (major) fissure*. This fissure may be approximated by a string that runs from the T3 spinous process obliquely down and around the chest to the 6th rib at the MCL. The right lung is further divided by the *horizontal (minor) fissure*. Anteriorly, this fissure runs close to the 4th rib and meets the oblique fissure in the midaxillary line near the 5th rib. The right lung is thus divided into *upper, middle,* and *lower lobes*. The left lung has only two lobes, upper and lower.

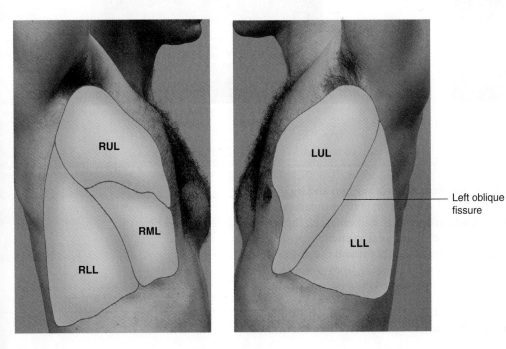

Locations on the Chest. Learn the general anatomic terms used to locate chest findings, such as:

Supraclavicular—above the clavicles
Infraclavicular—below the clavicles
Interscapular—between the scapulae
Infrascapular—below the scapulae
Bases of the lungs—the lowermost portions
Upper, middle, and lower lung fields

You may then infer what parts of the lungs are affected by an unhealthy process. Signs in the right upper lung field, for example, almost certainly originate in the right upper lobe. Signs in the right middle lung field laterally, however, could come from any of three different lobes.

The Trachea and Major Bronchi. The larger airway passages of the trachea and bronchi create a different quality of breath sounds compared to the lung parenchyma or tissue. The trachea bifurcates into its mainstem bronchi at the levels of the sternal angle anteriorly and the T4 spinous process posteriorly; clinically, these landmarks are essential to know. In addition, the right mainstem bronchus is typically more vertical than the left, resulting in a greater likelihood of aspiration of foreign bodies into the right lung (Husain & Kumar, 2005).

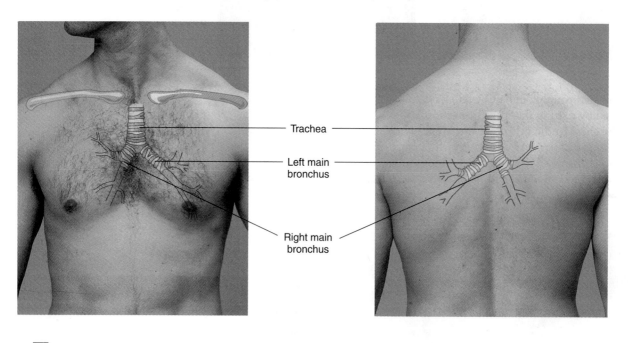

Trachea
Left main bronchus
Right main bronchus

BREATHING

Breathing is largely an automatic act, controlled in the brainstem and mediated by the muscles of respiration. The dome-shaped *diaphragm* is the primary muscle of inspiration. When it contracts, it descends in the chest and enlarges the thoracic cavity. At the same time, it compresses the abdominal contents, pushing the abdominal wall outward. Muscles in the rib cage and neck expand the thorax during inspiration, especially the *parasternals*, which run obliquely from sternum to ribs, and the *scalenes*, which run from the cervical vertebrae to the first two ribs.

During inspiration, as these muscles contract, the thorax expands. Intrathoracic pressure decreases, drawing air through the tracheobronchial tree into the *alveoli*, or distal air sacs, and expanding the lungs. Oxygen diffuses into the blood of adjacent pulmonary capillaries, and carbon dioxide diffuses from the blood into the alveoli.

After inspiratory effort stops, the expiratory phase begins. The chest wall and lungs recoil, the diaphragm relaxes and rises passively, air flows outward, and the chest and abdomen return to their resting positions.

Breathing is generally quiet and effortless—barely audible near the open mouth as a faint whish. When a healthy person lies supine, the breathing movements of the thorax are relatively slight. In contrast, the abdominal movements are usually easy to see. In the sitting position, movements of the thorax become more prominent.

During exercise and in certain diseases, extra work is required to breathe, and accessory muscles join the inspiratory effort. The sternomastoids are the most important of these, and the scalenes may become visible. Abdominal muscles assist in expiration.

 ## Cultural Considerations

Studies have shown that pulmonary function, even after adjusting for different size body frames, varies by genetic group. For instance, Caucasians have the largest thorax and the greatest lung capacity, followed by African Canadians, Asian Canadians, and Aboriginal Canadians (Overfield, 1995); these differences are significant enough that the standard norms for forced vital capacity (FVC) and forced expiratory volume (FEV) differ by genetics.

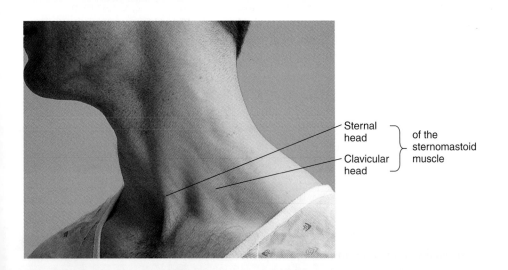

Sternal head ⎫
Clavicular head ⎬ of the sternomastoid muscle

THE HEALTH HISTORY: SUBJECTIVE DATA

Key Symptoms and Signs Reported by Client

- Difficulty breathing (dyspnea)
- Chest pain
- Cough
- Sputum production
- Blood-streaked sputum (hemoptysis)
- Wheezing

Begin the health history with the symptoms or signs reported by the client, using broad questions. Difficulty breathing, or *dyspnea*, is an uncomfortable sensation that is inappropriate for the level of exertion. Clients may refer to the sensation as shortness of breath. It warrants a full exploration and assessment because dyspnea often results from either cardiac or pulmonary disease.

See Table 14-1, Dyspnea, pp. 412–413.

Initially ask, "Have you had any trouble breathing?" Find out whether the difficulty in breathing occurred suddenly or developed gradually. Inquire when the symptom occurs (at rest or with exercise) and how much effort produces its onset. Because dyspnea is a subjective sensation and people vary in age, body weight, and physical fitness, make every effort *to quantify the severity of the dyspnea based on the person's daily activities.* Ask about the client's typical day and then how the difficulty breathing has altered his or her lifestyle and activities. Specific questions such as "How many stairs can you climb before pausing for a breath?" or "What about carrying bags of groceries? Sweeping the floor?" and "What happens to your breathing when you are outside in cold weather?" or "In windy weather?" can provide important clues to the severity of the symptom. Carefully gather information about the timing, setting, associated symptoms, and any relieving or aggravating factors related to the dyspnea.

Most clients with dyspnea relate shortness of breath to their level of activity. Anxious clients present a different picture. They may describe difficulty taking a deep enough breath or a smothering sensation with inability to get enough air, along with *paresthesias*, or sensations of tingling or "pins and needles" around the lips or in the extremities.

Anxious clients may have episodic dyspnea during both rest and exercise, and *hyperventilation*, or rapid, shallow breathing. At other times, they may have frequent sighs.

Chest discomfort or chest pain can arise from structures within the thorax, including the heart and the lungs. To assess this symptom, the nurse must pursue a dual investigation of both thoracic and cardiac causes (Cayley, 2005). Sources of chest pain are listed below (Goroll & Mulley, 2006a). For this important symptom, keep all of these in mind.

See Table 14-2, Chest Pain, pp. 414–415.

- The myocardium

  Angina pectoris, myocardial infection

- The pericardium

  Pericarditis

- The aorta

  Dissecting aortic aneurysm

- The trachea and large bronchi

  Bronchitis

- The parietal pleura

  Pericarditis, pneumonia

- The chest wall, including the musculoskeletal system and skin

  Costochondritis, herpes zoster

- The esophagus

  Reflux esophagitis, esophageal spasm

- Extrathoracic structures, such as the neck, gallbladder, and stomach

  Cervical arthritis, biliary colic, gastritis

Ask the client, "Do you have any discomfort in your chest? Or unpleasant feelings in your chest?" If the client reports any chest discomfort, explore the nature of the symptom thoroughly to distinguish among the various causes of chest pain. Ask the client to point to where the pain is in the chest; note any gestures the client uses when locating the pain.

A clenched fist over the sternum suggests *angina pectoris*; a finger pointing to a tender area on the chest wall suggests musculoskeletal pain; a hand moving from neck to epigastrum suggests heartburn.

The lung tissue itself has no pain fibres, and the pericardium typically has minimal pain receptors (Spencer & Leof, 1964). Pain associated with lung conditions, such as pneumonia or pulmonary infarction, usually arises from inflammation of the adjacent parietal pleura. Prolonged recurrent coughing can result in thoracic muscle strain, costochondritis (inflammation of the cartilage between a rib and the sternum), or both. Both situations present as chest pain. While the mechanism is not understood, chest pain is also associated with anxiety.

Idiopathic pain, or pain without a recognizable cause, is the most frequent source of chest pain in children; anxiety and costochondritis are also common (Yildirim et al., 2004).

For queries about exertional chest pain, palpitations, orthopnea, paroxysmal noctural dyspnea, and edema, see Chapter 15, The Cardiovascular System.

See Table 14-3, Cough and Hemoptysis, p. 416.

Cough is a leading symptom for visits to health care providers. The protective cough reflex is modulated in the medulla and responds to stimuli that irritate cough receptors in the respiratory tree, particularly those in the larynx, trachea, and bronchi. It is noteworthy that cough receptors are also found in the ear canals, nose, sinuses, pharynx, stomach, and diaphragm (Goroll & Mulley, 2006b). Although most coughing is reflexive, voluntary control is possible. Examples include attempts to suppress a cough or to deliberately cough (e.g., deep breathing and coughing postoperatively).

Cough can be a symptom of left-sided heart failure.

Environmental irritants, such as dust; tobacco smoke; foreign bodies; pets; pollutants; cold, hot, or dry air; high humidity; and high altitude, are external agents that can stimulate cough. Internal irritants typically arise from inflammatory processes within the respiratory tract and include mucus, pus, and blood, but may also evolve from tumours or enlarged peribronchial lymph nodes. Although cough is most often associated with a problem in the respiratory tract, the symptom may also signal a cardiovascular origin.

For reports of cough, a thorough assessment is in order. Ask whether the cough is dry or produces *sputum*, or phlegm. Ask the client to describe the volume of any sputum and its colour, odour, and consistency.

Dry hacking cough in mycoplasma pneumonia; productive cough in bronchitis, viral or bacterial pneumonia.

Mucoid sputum is translucent, white, or grey; *purulent* sputum is yellowish or greenish.

Foul-smelling sputum in anaerobic lung abscess; tenacious sputum in cystic fibrosis.

To help clients quantify volume, a multiple-choice question may be helpful: "How much do you cough up in 24 hours; a teaspoon? Tablespoon? A quarter cup? Half cup? Cupful?" If possible, ask the client to cough into a tissue; inspect the phlegm and note its characteristics. The symptoms associated with a cough often lead to its cause.

Large volumes of purulent sputum in bronchiectasis or lung abscess.

Diagnostically helpful symptoms include fever, chest pain, dyspnea, orthopnea, and wheezing.

Hemoptysis is the coughing up of blood from the lungs; it may vary from blood-streaked phlegm to frank blood. For clients reporting hemoptysis, assess the volume of blood produced as well as the other sputum attributes; ask about the related setting and activity and any associated symptoms.

See Table 14-3, Cough and Hemoptysis, p. 416. Hemoptysis is rare in infants, children, and adolescents; it is seen most often in cystic fibrosis.

Before using the term *hemoptysis*, try to confirm the source of the bleeding by both history and physical examination. Blood or blood-streaked material may originate in the mouth, pharynx, or gastrointestinal tract and is easily mislabelled. When

Blood originating in the stomach is usually darker than blood from the

vomited, it probably originates in the gastrointestinal tract. Occasionally, however, blood from the nasopharynx or the gastrointestinal tract is aspirated and then coughed out.

respiratory tract and may be mixed with food particles.

Wheezing is the production of whistling or musical respiratory sounds that result from narrowing of the lumen of a respiratory passageway. The wheeze may be audible to both the client and to others.

Wheezing suggests partial airway obstruction from secretions, tissue inflammation, or a foreign body.

If the client voices no concerns, be sure to ask in the review of systems about any chest discomfort? Any difficulty breathing? Persistent cough? Ever been told you have asthma? Ever been exposed to tuberculosis? Any workplace exposures?

Example of Questions for Symptom Analysis—Cough

- "In what part of your chest do you feel the cough?" (*Location*)
- "How you would you describe the cough?" "What does the cough sound like?" "Would you describe the cough as dry? Or moist?" (*Quality*)
- "Describe how much coughing you have." "Is the coughing disrupting your sleep?" (*Severity*)
- "Describe when you first noticed the cough." "How did the cough start?" "Suddenly (continued) or gradually?" (*Onset*)
- "How long have you had the cough?" (*Duration*)
- "Is the cough becoming more frequent?" "Or is it getting worse?" (*Constancy*)
- "When is the cough at its worst?" "Daytime or night time?" "Are there certain times of the year when your cough is worse?" (*Time of day/month/year*)
- "What have you tried to relieve the cough?" "What makes it better?" (*Alleviating factors*)
- "What makes the cough worse?" "Do you smoke?" "Does eating affect your cough?" "Do you take ACE-inhibitor pills (a type of antihypertensive medication) to manage your blood pressure?" (*Aggravating factors*)

- "What other symptoms have you noticed?" "Do you cough up sputum?" [*If the client does cough up sputum, inquire about:*] "Colour?" "Amount?" "Odour?" "Have you had a fever in the past week?" "Do you have a fever now?" "Have you had any difficulty breathing? If yes, please describe." "Any headache?" "Sore throat?" "Any sinus pain (above the eyebrows, below the eyes)?" "Do you have the sensation that fluid/discharge is running down the back of your throat?" "Are you coughing to clear your throat?" (*Associated symptoms*)
- "What type of work do you do?" "Have you ever been exposed to any chemicals?" "Dust?" "Other substances?" "At work?" "Are you exposed to cigarette smoke on a regular basis?" "How does exercise affect your cough?" "What type of heating does your residence have?" "How does cold air outside affect your cough?" "What other weather conditions affect your cough?" (*Environmental factors*)
- "How is the coughing affecting your daily activities?" (*Significance to the client*)
- "What do you think is causing the cough?" (*Client perspective*)

HEALTH PROMOTION

Important Topics for Health Promotion

- Tobacco cessation
- Influenza vaccine
- Respiratory protection in the workplace

In 2005, five serious respiratory diseases—asthma, chronic obstructive pulmonary disease (COPD), lung cancer, tuberculosis (TB), and cystic fibrosis (CF)—affected more than 3,000,000 Canadians (Public Health Agency of Canada [PHAC], 2007).

This statistic does not include people with influenza or pneumonia, which are the leading respiratory causes of hospitalization. Respiratory diseases accounted for nearly 9% of all deaths among Canadians in 2004, and the total health care cost for respiratory diseases was $8.63 billion in 2000 (PHAC, 2007).

RISK FACTOR ASSESSMENT

Smoking has been identified as the single most preventable risk factor for respiratory diseases, in particular lung cancer and COPD. Although the number of people who smoke has declined over the past 30 years, 14% of all Canadians still smoke daily (PHAC, 2007). Upon closer examination, however, the prevalence of smoking among Canadians 20 to 24 years was 27% in 2006; strikingly, among the 18- to 29-year-olds on First Nations reserves, the prevalence was much higher at 70% (PHAC, 2007).

The indirect effects of secondhand smoke associated with lung cancer among nonsmokers and sudden infant death syndrome (SIDS) have been well documented (PHAC, 2007). Environmental exposure to tobacco smoke is consistently associated with respiratory infections, asthma incidence, and exacerbation of asthma symptoms (Banerji et al., 2001; Eder, Ege, & von Mutius, 2006; Kovesi et al., 2007). Given the significance of this risk factor, it is imperative to inquire about personal smoking behaviour and potential environmental exposures at home and in the workplace during every health history.

More than 70% of smokers express interest in quitting, although less than 10% are successful (Centres for Disease Control and Prevention, 2007). Nurses should use a nonjudgemental approach when questioning smokers about quitting, focus especially on teenagers and pregnant women, and adopt the five "*A's*" (Agency for Healthcare Research and Quality, 2005; U.S. Public Health Service, n.d.):

- *Ask* about smoking at each visit.

- *Advise* clients regularly to stop smoking, using a clear personalized message.

- *Assess* client readiness to quit.

- *Assist* clients to set stop dates and provide educational materials for self-help.

- *Arrange* for follow-up visits to monitor and support client progress.

Be aware of the addictive features of nicotine (tolerance over time, physical dependence) and those of withdrawal (irritability, anger, insomnia, anxiety, and depressed mood). Learn to make effective interventions to promote sustained quit rates, such as targeted messages, group counselling, and use of nicotine-replacement strategies (Rigotti, 2003). The Canadian Lung Association (2008) and the Heather Crowe Resource Centre (n.d.) are two sources of information on smoking cessation. Combining clinician and group counselling is especially effective for clients who are highly addicted.

Relapses are common and should be expected. Help clients to learn from these experiences and work with them to identify the precipitating circumstances. From there, nurses can develop strategies for alternative responses and health-promoting behaviours. The good news for clients is that the disease risks of smoking drop significantly within 1 year of smoking cessation.

SPECIFIC PREVENTION

Asthma. Characteristics of asthma include inflammation, increased airway responsiveness, and reversible obstruction of the lung airways. The disease process results in cough, dyspnea, chest tightness, and wheezing. Worldwide incidence of asthma has increased over the past 20 years. In Canada, 1.78 million people in 1996 were diagnosed with asthma; by 2005, this number had risen to 2.25 million (Statistics Canada, 2005a). Proposed reasons for this increase centre on environmental factors, namely, tobacco exposure; air pollution (Finkelstein et al., 2003); increased exposure to allergens; obesity; lack of exposure to infectious agents as children, given the increased use of hand sanitizers and antibacterial cleansers (the "hygiene hypothesis") (Nicolle, 2007); and overuse of antibiotics (Eder et al., 2006). In addition to exposure to environmental risk factors, people with a family history of allergy, including eczema and hay fever, are at higher risk for developing asthma (PHAC, 2007). No clear causal mechanisms have emerged to date, belying the complexity of the disease.

Occupational asthma that results from workplace exposures accounts for approximately 10% of all cases of adult asthma. Most occupational exposures are classified as sensitizer-induced, and workplace sensitizers include animal proteins, flour, natural rubber latex, and low-molecular–weight compounds, such as epoxy (Tarlo, 2003). Occupational asthma should be suspected if an adult acquires new-onset asthma with decreased symptoms away from the workplace. Despite the ambiguity of the etiological mechanisms of asthma, it is clear that avoidance of direct or passive exposure to tobacco smoke reduces the risk of asthma and that modification of workplaces can lessen exacerbations.

COPD. COPD encompasses both chronic bronchitis and emphysema and has many overlapping features with asthma. Unlike asthma, however, the obstructive changes of COPD are not readily reversible. A slowly progressive disease resulting from cigarette smoking in 80% to 90% of affected people, COPD typically appears after age 55 years (PHAC, 2007). The most frequent symptoms and signs are difficulty breathing, cough, and sputum production. COPD is now more prevalent among Canadian women younger than 74 years than men of the same age group (PHAC, 2007).

Loss of productivity and decreased quality of life are hallmarks of COPD. The structural changes in the airways with subsequent obstruction predispose clients with COPD to respiratory infections. The degree of severity of COPD has been associated with several client characteristics, including obesity. The recent development of the BODE index (Body Mass Index, airflow obstruction, dyspnea, and exercise capacity) promises to have clinical application in early identification of those at risk for death from COPD (Celli et al., 2004).

Lung Cancer. Lung cancer is the second most frequently diagnosed cancer for both women and men in Canada, and is the leading cancer-related cause of death in both genders. In 2008, the estimated number of new cases of lung cancer in Canada was 23,900, with an estimated 20,200 deaths from lung cancer (Canadian Cancer Society/National Cancer Institute of Canada, 2008). The major cause of lung cancer is cigarette smoking; in 2005, 18% of males 12 years and older smoked, compared with nearly 15% of Canadian females of the same age (Statistics Canada, 2005b). Among women, lung cancer incidence and mortality rates continue to rise, while they are decreasing among men. It should be noted that occupational exposures, such as asbestos, arsenic, nickel refining, uranium mining, radon, and silica, are associated with lung cancer; risk becomes synergistic if a worker also smokes (PHAC, 2007). Public health messages and smoking cessation strategies are key to reducing the harm caused by tobacco.

Tuberculosis. While decreasing in Canada since 1940, tuberculosis (TB) remains highly prevalent worldwide. Estimates are that one third of the world's population is infected with TB, which has implications for travel and immigration policies (Long & Ellis, 2007). The TB bacterium (*Mycobacterium tuberculosis*) is highly resistant to most chemical agents and to penicillin, but is destroyed by heat, direct sunlight, and ultraviolet light (Hornick, 2007). Transmission is primarily airborne, and infected people are frequently asymptomatic. Characteristic symptoms include low-grade fever, weight loss, night sweats, fatigue, and productive cough with small amounts of sputum. Risk factors for TB infection include close contact with someone with known or suspected active TB (e.g., on airplanes) and travel in countries where TB is widespread. The homeless are at risk for TB, as are First Nations people residing in a community with active TB. About one third of the 40 million people in the world living with HIV/AIDS are coinfected with TB (Long & Ellis, 2007). Health care professionals are at risk for TB, because they may be in contact with infected people in any setting.

Cystic Fibrosis. Cystic fibrosis (CF), a chronic fatal autosomal-recessive disease, is characterized by unusual production of mucus in the lungs, with 60% of children with CF identified by 1 year of age (PHAC, 2007). Respiratory infections are the most frequent complication, and most clients with CF do not survive past 30 years. The incidence rate of CF in Canada has decreased in the past 20 years, mainly as a result of genetic testing. By 2005, the incidence rate decreased to 2.8 per 10,000 births from 3.7 per 10,000 births in 1987 (PHAC, 2007).

Influenza. The ability of influenza viruses to easily mutate causes sporadic epidemics and, occasionally, a global pandemic. Clinical diagnosis is challenging, because the classical influenza signs of fever, cough, and headache are common with other infections as well. Studies have found that the combination of cough and fever during influenza season in people older than 60 years conveys increased likelihood of truly being influenza (Call, Vollenwider, Hornung, Simel, & McKinney, 2005). Yearly influenza vaccination is recommended for the following groups:

- Those 65 years and older

- Healthy children 6 to 23 months

- Pregnant women

- Adults and children with chronic diseases such as asthma and COPD

- Family members of anyone at risk

- Caregivers and health care providers (FluWatch, n.d.)

To protect clients and their families, nurses and all other health care professionals (including nursing students) need yearly influenza immunization (National Advisory Committee on Immunization, 2006). Most long-term care facilities require their staff to be immunized.

Invasive Pneumococcal Disease (IPD). IPD (caused by *Streptococcus pneumoniae*) is a nationally reportable disease. Between 2000 and 2004, adults 60 years and older made up 37% (711 per year) of IPD cases in Canada (National Advisory Committee on Immunization, 2006). One dose of polysaccharide pneumococcal vaccine is strongly advised for all Canadians 65 years and older, as well as younger people with chronic pulmonary disease, other chronic illnesses, or impaired immune responsiveness. The vaccine is usually given once in a lifetime, but a booster may be considered for those with chronic illness who received the vaccine before 65 years of age.

SCREENING AND MAINTENANCE

Limited screening tests or procedures exist for respiratory diseases that could be applied at a population level. Instead, targeted screening is carried out for people at risk (e.g., those with TB, CF). Chest x-rays may be used for screening in some situations.

EMERGENCY CONCERNS

In most health care settings, nurses are responsible for monitoring the respiratory status of clients. Pulmonary complications are a risk postoperatively if the client:

■ Is a current smoker or has been smoking within 8 weeks of surgery

■ Is in poor general health

■ Has COPD

■ Is having upper abdominal or thoracic surgeries

■ Is having a surgical procedure lasting more than 3 hours (Smetana, 1999)

A U.S. study that evaluated the effect of nurse staffing and client outcomes among 124,204 clients found that pneumonia was the most frequent adverse event in acute care hospitals; the complication was associated with a 3.39-fold increase in the odds of death (Cho, Ketefian, Barkauskas, & Smith, 2003). By reviewing the client's health history, nurses can anticipate those at highest risk for pulmonary complications following surgical procedures or from preexisting medical conditions and institute preventive measures such as coughing and deep breathing.

Changes in respiratory rate or sudden onset of dyspnea, retrosternal pain, or both in a client warrant rapid nursing assessment and intervention. It is noteworthy that potential reversible changes in respiratory signs precede approximately 76% of cardiopulmonary arrests (Buist et al., 2002). It is incumbent upon nurses to closely monitor the pulmonary status of clients for early identification of respiratory changes and deteriorating status (Duff, Gardiner, & Barnes, 2007). Included are those clients at risk for pulmonary embolus from prolonged immobility, fractures, trauma, recent travel, pregnancy, or postpartum status, or with a history of deep vein thrombosis. See Table 14-1.

TECHNIQUES OF EXAMINATION: OBJECTIVE DATA

◼ PROMOTING CLIENT COMFORT, DIGNITY, AND SAFETY

Accurate assessment of the thorax and lungs requires a warm room and warm examiner hands. Prepare the client by describing the examination. If the client is not already in a gown, provide one, along with a drape to cover the client's lower extremities. It is helpful to examine the posterior thorax and lungs while the client is sitting and the anterior thorax and lungs with the client supine. Wash your hands thoroughly, and then proceed with inspection of the chest wall. Throughout the examination, provide ongoing explanation and attend to the comfort level of the client.

Equipment Box

- Half-sheet or bath blanket
- Stethoscope
- Felt marker
- Small ruler

Proceed in an orderly fashion: inspect, palpate, percuss, and auscultate. Try to visualize the underlying lobes and use side-to-side comparison, so that the client serves as his or her own control. For men, arrange the gown so that you can see the chest fully. For women, cover the anterior chest when you examine the back. For the anterior examination, drape the gown over each half of the chest as you examine the other; alternatively, assist the woman to switch the orientation of the gown so that the back opening and ties are now at the front.

With the client sitting, examine the posterior thorax and lungs. The client's arms should be folded across the chest with hands resting, if possible, on the opposite shoulders. This position moves the scapulae partly out of the way and increases your access to the lung fields. Then ask the client to lie down.

With the client supine, examine the anterior thorax and lungs. The supine position makes it easier to examine women because the breasts can be gently displaced. Furthermore, wheezes, if present, are more likely to be heard. (Some experts, however, prefer to examine both the back and the front of the chest with the client sitting. This technique is also satisfactory.)

For clients unable to sit up without aid, try to get help so that you can examine the posterior chest in the sitting position. If this is impossible, roll the client to one side and then to the other. Percuss the upper lung, and auscultate both lungs in each position. Because ventilation is relatively greater in the dependent lung, your chances of hearing unexpected wheezes or crackles are greater on the dependent side (see pp. 401–402).

◼ INITIAL SURVEY OF RESPIRATION AND THE THORAX

Begin with inspection of the client's overall appearance. Is the client having difficulty breathing? Any retractions or accessory muscle use? Are there signs of discomfort or pain present (e.g., grimacing, diaphoresis)? *Always inspect the client for any signs of respiratory difficulty.*

Even though you may have already recorded the respiratory rate when you took the vital signs, it is wise to again observe the *rate, rhythm, depth, and effort of breathing*.

- *Assess the client's colour* for cyanosis. Examine the shape and condition of the fingernails.

Hypoxia can present as cyanosis. Clubbing of the nails (see p. 277) in *thoracic neoplasms*, lung abscesses, *CF*, and *asbestosis* (Meyer & Farquhar, 2001). Clubbing also is visible in people who live long periods in high-altitude locations (e.g., Bolivia's altiplano).

- *Listen to the client's breathing*. Is there any audible wheezing? If so, where does it fall in the respiratory cycle?

Audible *stridor*, a high-pitched wheeze, is an ominous sign of airway obstruction in the larynx or trachea.

- *Inspect the neck*. Is the trachea midline? During inspiration, is there contraction of the sternomastoid muscles or supraclavicular retractions? During expiration, is the client using abdominal muscles to push the breath out?

Lateral displacement of the trachea in *pneumothorax, pleural effusion,* or *atelectasis*. Inspiratory contraction of the sternomastoids at rest signals severe difficulty breathing.

- *Observe the shape of the chest*. In the adult, the anterioposterior (AP) diameter is less than the transverse chest diameter. The AP diameter may increase with aging.

The AP diameter also may increase in *chronic obstructive pulmonary disease* (COPD).

EXAMINATION OF THE POSTERIOR CHEST

Inspection. From a midline position behind the client note the *shape of the chest* and *the way in which it moves*, including:

- Deformities or asymmetry

See Table 14-4, Deviations of the Thorax (p. 417).

- Retraction of the intercostal spaces during inspiration. Retraction is most apparent in the lower intercostal spaces. Supraclavicular retraction is often present.

Retraction in severe asthma, COPD, or upper airway obstruction.

- Impaired respiratory movement on one or both sides or a unilateral lag (or delay) in movement.

Unilateral impairment or lagging of respiratory movement suggests disease of the underlying lung or pleura.

Palpation. As you palpate the chest, focus on areas of tenderness and abnormalities in the overlying skin, respiratory expansion, and fremitus.

Intercostal tenderness over inflamed pleura.

Identify tender areas. Carefully palpate any area where pain has been reported or where lesions or bruises are evident.

Bruises over a fractured rib.

Assess any observed abnormalities such as masses or sinus tracts (blind, inflammatory, tube-like structures opening onto the skin).

Although rare, sinus tracts usually indicate infection of the underlying pleura and lung (as in tuberculosis, actinomycosis).

Test chest expansion. Place your thumbs at about the level of the 10th ribs, with your fingers loosely grasping and parallel to the lateral rib cage. As you position your hands, slide them medially just enough to raise a loose fold of skin on each side between your thumb and the spine.

Ask the client to inhale deeply. Watch the distance between your thumbs as they move apart during inspiration, and feel for the range and symmetry of the rib cage as it expands and contracts.

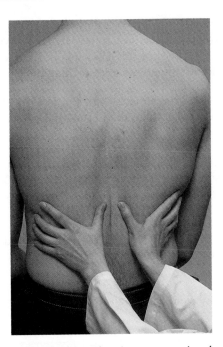

Causes of unilateral decrease or delay in chest expansion include chronic fibrotic disease of the underlying lung or pleura, pleural effusion, lobar pneumonia, pleural pain with associated splinting, and unilateral bronchial obstruction.

Feel for tactile fremitus. Fremitus refers to the palpable vibrations transmitted through the bronchopulmonary tree to the chest wall when the client speaks. To detect fremitus, use either the ball (the bony part of the palm at the base of the fingers) or the ulnar surface of your hand to optimize the vibratory sensitivity of the bones in your hand. Ask the client to repeat the words "ninety-nine" or "one-one-one." If fremitus is faint, ask the client to speak more loudly or in a deeper voice.

Use one hand until you have learned the feel of fremitus. Some clinicians find using one hand more accurate. The simultaneous use of both hands to compare sides, however, increases your speed and may facilitate detection of differences.

Palpate and compare symmetric areas of the lungs in the pattern shown in the photograph. Identify and locate any areas of increased, decreased, or absent fremitus. Fremitus is typically more prominent in the interscapular area than in the lower lung fields and is often more prominent on the right side than on the left. It disappears below the diaphragm.

Tactile fremitus is a relatively rough assessment tool, but as a scouting technique, it directs your attention to possible abnormalities. Later in the examination you will check any suggested findings by listening for breath sounds, voice sounds, and whispered voice sounds. All of these attributes tend to increase or decrease together.

Fremitus is decreased or absent when the voice is soft or when the transmission of vibrations from the larynx to the surface of the chest is impeded. Causes include an obstructed bronchus; COPD; separation of the pleural surfaces by fluid (pleural effusion), fibrosis (pleural thickening), air (pneumothorax), or an infiltrating tumour; and a very thick chest wall.

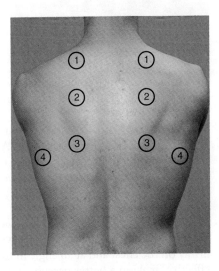

Percussion. Percussion of the chest sets the chest wall and underlying tissues into motion, producing audible sound and palpable vibrations. Percussion helps you establish whether the underlying tissues are air-filled, fluid-filled, or solid. It penetrates only about 5 cm to 7 cm into the chest, however, and will not help you to detect deep-seated lesions.

The technique of percussion can be practiced on any surface. For percussion of the lungs, it is helpful to practice on a wall, as this can simulate the client's thorax while he or she is sitting. As you practice, listen for changes in percussion notes over different types of materials or different parts of the body. The key points for good technique, described for a right-handed person, are as follows:

■ Hyperextend the middle finger of your left hand, known as the pleximeter finger. Press its distal interphalangeal joint firmly on the surface to be percussed. Avoid surface contact by any other part of the hand because this dampens out vibrations. Note that the thumb and 2nd, 4th, and 5th fingers are not touching the chest.

■ Position your right forearm quite close to the surface, with the hand cocked upward. The middle finger should be partially flexed, relaxed, and poised to strike.

■ With a *quick, sharp but relaxed wrist motion*, strike the pleximeter finger with the right middle finger, or plexor finger. Aim at your distal interphalangeal joint. You are trying to transmit vibrations through the bones of this joint to the underlying chest wall.

Strike using the *tip of the plexor finger*, not the finger pad. Your finger should be almost at right angles to the pleximeter. A short fingernail is recommended to avoid self-injury.

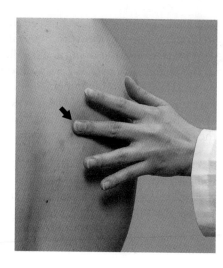

■ Withdraw your striking finger quickly to avoid damping the vibrations you have created.

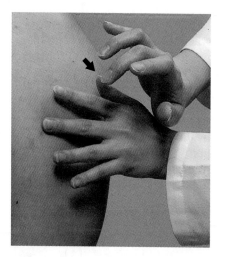

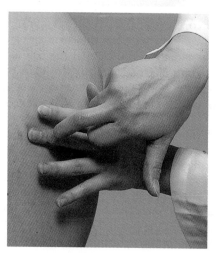

In summary, the movement is at the wrist. It is directed, brisk yet relaxed, and a bit bouncy, similar to striking a staccato note on a piano.

Percussion Notes. With your plexor or tapping finger, use the lightest percussion that produces a clear note. A thick chest wall requires stronger percussion than a thin one. However, if a *louder* note is needed, apply more pressure with the *pleximeter* finger (this is more effective for increasing percussion note volume than tapping harder with the plexor finger).

When percussing the lower posterior chest, stand somewhat to the side rather than directly behind the client. This allows you to place your pleximeter finger more firmly on the chest and at an angle in the intercostal spaces. Your plexor is also more effective, making a better percussion note.

When comparing two areas, use the same percussion technique in both areas. Percuss or strike twice in each location. It is easier to detect differences in percussion notes by comparing one area with another than by striking repetitively in one place.

Learn to identify five percussion notes. You can practice four of them on yourself. These notes differ in their basic qualities of sound: intensity, pitch, and duration.

Train your ear to distinguish these differences by concentrating on one quality at a time as you percuss first in one location, then in another. Review the following table. Lungs are usually *resonant*.

▪ Percussion Notes and Their Characteristics

	Relative Intensity	Relative Pitch	Relative Duration	Example of Location
Flatness	Soft	High	Short	Thigh
Dullness	Medium	Medium	Medium	Liver
Resonance	Loud	Low	Long	Lung
Hyperresonance	Very loud	Lower	Longer	None usually
Tympany	Loud	High*	*	Gastric air bubble or puffed-out cheek

*Distinguished mainly by its musical timbre.

While the client keeps both arms crossed in front of the chest, percuss the thorax in symmetric locations from the apices to the lung bases.

Percuss one side of the chest and then the other at each level in a ladder-like pattern, as shown by the numbers in the illustration. Omit the areas over the scapulae—the thickness of muscle and bone alters the percussion notes over the lungs. Identify and locate the area and quality of any unusual percussion note.

Dullness replaces resonance when fluid or solid tissue replaces air-containing lung or occupies the pleural space beneath your percussing fingers. Examples include lobar pneumonia, in which the alveoli are filled with fluid and blood cells, and pleural accumulations of serous fluid (pleural effusion), blood (hemothorax), pus (empyema), fibrous tissue, or tumour.

Generalized hyperresonance may be heard over the hyperinflated lungs of emphysema or asthma, but it is not a reliable sign. Unilateral hyperresonance suggests a large pneumothorax or possibly a large air-filled bulla in the lung.

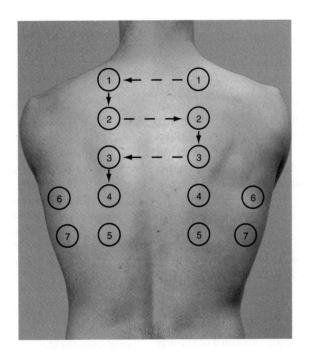

Identify the descent of the diaphragms, or diaphragmatic excursion. First, *determine the level of diaphragmatic dullness* during quiet respiration. Holding the pleximeter finger *above and parallel* to the expected level of dullness, percuss downward in progressive steps until dullness clearly replaces resonance. Confirm this level of change by percussion near the middle of the hemothorax and also more laterally.

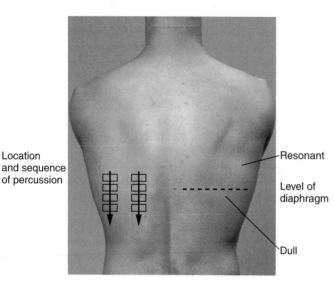

Location and sequence of percussion

Resonant

Level of diaphragm

Dull

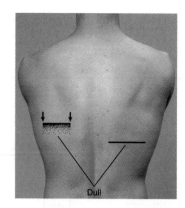

Dull

An abnormally high level suggests pleural effusion, or a high diaphragm, as in atelectasis or diaphragmatic paralysis.

Note that with this technique, you are identifying the boundary between the resonant lung tissue and the duller structures below the diaphragm. You are not percussing the diaphragm itself. You can infer the probable location of the diaphragm from the level of dullness.

Now, *estimate the extent of diaphragmatic excursion* by determining the distance between the level of dullness on full expiration and the level of dullness on full inspiration. Instruct the client to fully exhale and hold the exhalation. Percuss and then use a felt marker to mark the level of dullness. Allow the client to breathe through a few respiratory cycles. Then ask the client to fully inhale and hold the inhalation. Always hold your own breath when you ask a client to hold his or her breath. This helps you to monitor the client's need to take a breath. Repeat the percussion and mark the level of dullness. Instruct the client to then breathe as usual. Measure the distance between the two marks with a small ruler; usually the difference is 5 to 6 cm. This estimate does not correlate well, however, with radiologic assessment of diaphragmatic movement.

Auscultation. Auscultation of the lungs is the most important examining technique for assessing air flow through the tracheobronchial tree. Together with percussion, it also helps the nurse to assess the condition of the surrounding lungs and pleural space. Auscultation involves (1) listening to the sounds generated by breathing; (2) listening for any adventitious (added) sounds; and (3) if abnormalities are suspected, listening to the sounds of the client's spoken or whispered voice as they are transmitted through the chest wall.

Sounds from bedclothes, paper gowns, and the chest itself can generate confusion in auscultation. Hair on the chest may cause crackling sounds. Either press harder or wet the hair. If the client is cold or tense, you may hear muscle contraction sounds—muffled, low-pitched rumbling or roaring noises.

A change in the client's position may eliminate this noise. You can reproduce this sound on yourself by doing a Valsalva manoeuvre (straining down) as you listen to your own chest.

   Breath Sounds (Lung Sounds). You will learn to identify patterns of breath sounds by their intensity, their pitch, and the relative duration of their inspiratory and expiratory phases. Usual breath sounds are as follows:

■ *Vesicular*, or soft and low pitched. They are heard through inspiration, continue without pause through expiration, and then fade away about one third of the way through expiration.

■ *Bronchovesicular*, with inspiratory and expiratory sounds about equal in length, at times separated by a silent interval. Detecting differences in pitch and intensity is often easier during expiration.

■ *Bronchial*, or louder and higher in pitch, with a short silence between inspiratory and expiratory sounds. Expiratory sounds last longer than inspiratory sounds.

The characteristics of these three kinds of breath sounds are summarized in the following table. Also shown are the *tracheal* breath sounds—very loud, harsh sounds that are heard by listening over the trachea in the neck.

Listen to the breath sounds with the diaphragm of a stethoscope after instructing the client to breathe deeply through an open mouth. Use the pattern suggested for percussion, moving from one side to the other and comparing symmetric areas of the lungs. If you hear or suspect unusual sounds, auscultate adjacent areas so that you can fully describe the extent of any unexpected findings. Listen to at least one full breath in each location. Be alert for client discomfort due to hyperventilation (e.g., lightheadedness, faintness), and allow the client to rest as needed.

If bronchovesicular or bronchial breath sounds are heard in locations distant from those listed, suspect that air-filled lung has been replaced by fluid-filled or solid lung tissue. See Table 14-5, Expected and Altered Breath and Voice Sounds (p. 401).

■ *Characteristics of Breath Sounds*

	Duration of Sounds	Intensity of Expiratory Sound	Pitch of Expiratory Sound	Locations Where Heard Usually
Vesicular*	Inspiratory sounds last longer than expiratory ones.	Soft	Relatively low	Over most of both lungs
Bronchovesicular	Inspiratory and expiratory sounds are about equal.	Intermediate	Intermediate	Often in the 1st and 2nd intercostal spaces anteriorly and between the scapulae
Bronchial	Expiratory sounds last longer than inspiratory ones.	Loud	Relatively high	Over the manubrium, if heard at all
Tracheal	Inspiratory and expiratory sounds are about equal.	Very loud	Relatively high	Over the trachea in the neck

*The thickness of the bars indicates intensity; the steeper their incline, the higher the pitch.

Note the *intensity* of the breath sounds. Breath sounds are usually louder in the lower posterior lung fields and may also vary from area to area. If the breath sounds seem faint, ask the client to breathe more deeply. You may then hear them easily. When clients do not breathe deeply enough or have a thick chest wall, as in obesity, breath sounds may remain diminished.

Breath sounds may be decreased when air flow is decreased (as by obstructive lung disease or muscular weakness) or when the transmission of sound is poor (as in pleural effusion, pneumothorax, or emphysema).

Is there a *silent gap* between the inspiratory and expiratory sounds?

A gap suggests bronchial breath sounds.

Listen for the *pitch, intensity, and duration of the expiratory and inspiratory sounds*. Are vesicular breath sounds distributed as expected over the chest wall? Or are there bronchovesicular or bronchial breath sounds in unexpected places? If so, where are they?

For further discussion and other added sounds, see Table 14-6, Adventitious (Added) Lung Sounds: Causes and Qualities (p. 419).

Adventitious (Added) Sounds. Listen for any added, or adventitious, sounds that are superimposed on the usual breath sounds. Detection of adventitious sounds—*crackles* (sometimes called *rales*), *wheezes*, and *rhonchi*—is an important part of your examination, often leading to diagnosis of cardiac and pulmonary conditions. The most common kinds of these sounds are described in the following table:

■ *Adventitious or Added Breath Sounds*	
Crackles (or Rales)	**Wheezes and Rhonchi**
Discontinuous	*Continuous*
■ Intermittent, nonmusical, and brief	■ ≥250 msec, musical, prolonged (but not necessarily persisting throughout the respiratory cycle)
■ Like dots in time	■ Like dashes in time
■ *Fine crackles:* soft, high-pitched, very brief (5–10 msec)	■ *Wheezes:* relatively high pitched (≥400 Hz) with hissing or shrill quality
• • • • •	• • • • •
Coarse crackles: somewhat louder, lower in pitch, brief (20–30 msec)	■ *Rhonchi:* relatively low pitched (≤200 Hz) with snoring quality
⋀⋁⋀	⋀⋀⋀⋀

Crackles may be due to disorders of the lungs (pneumonia, fibrosis, early congestive heart failure) or of the airways (bronchitis, bronchiectasis).

Wheezes suggest narrowed airways, as in asthma, COPD, or bronchitis.

Rhonchi suggest secretions in large airways.

If you hear *crackles*, especially those that do not clear after cough, listen carefully for the following characteristics. These are clues to the underlying condition:

■ Loudness, pitch, and duration (summarized as fine or coarse crackles)

■ Number (few to many)

■ Timing in the respiratory cycle

■ Location on the chest wall

■ Persistence of their pattern from breath to breath

■ Any change after a cough or a change in the client's position

In some people, crackles may be heard at the lung bases anteriorly after maximal expiration. Crackles in dependent portions of the lungs may also occur after prolonged bed rest.

If you hear *wheezes* or *rhonchi*, note their timing and location. Do they change with deep breathing or coughing?

Transmitted Voice Sounds. If you hear bronchovesicular or bronchial breath sounds in the wrong locations, assess transmitted voice sounds. With a stethoscope, listen in symmetric areas over the chest wall as you:

■ Ask the client to say "ninety-nine." Usually the sounds transmitted through the chest wall are muffled and indistinct.

Fine late inspiratory crackles that persist from breath to breath suggest unhealthy lung tissue.

Clearing of crackles, wheezes, or rhonchi after cough or position change suggests inspissated (thickened) secretions, as in bronchitis or atelectasis.

Increased transmission of voice sounds suggests that air-filled lung has become airless. See Table 14-5, Expected and Altered Breath and Voice Sounds (p. 418).

Louder, clearer voice sounds are called *bronchophony*.

■ Ask the client to say, "ee." You will usually hear a muffled long E sound.

When "ee" is heard as "ay," an *E-to-A change (egophony)* is present, as in lobar consolidation from pneumonia. The quality sounds nasal.

■ Ask the client to whisper, "ninety-nine" or "one-two-three." The whispered voice is usually heard faintly and indistinctly, if at all.

Louder, clearer whispered sounds are called *whispered pectoriloquy.*

EXAMINATION OF THE ANTERIOR CHEST

When examined in the supine position, the client should lie comfortably with arms somewhat abducted. An individual who is having difficulty breathing should be examined in the sitting position or with the head of the bed elevated to a comfortable level.

Persons with severe COPD may prefer to sit leaning forward, with lips pursed during exhalation and arms supported on their knees or a table.

Inspection. Observe *the shape of the client's chest* and *the movement of the chest wall.* Note the following:

■ Deviations or asymmetry

See Table 14-4, Deviations of the Thorax (p. 417).

■ Unexpected retraction of the lower intercostal spaces during inspiration

Severe asthma, COPD, or upper airway obstruction.

■ Local lag or impairment in respiratory movement

Underlying disease of lung or pleura.

Palpation. Palpation has four potential uses:

■ *Identification of tender areas*

■ *Assessment of observed deviations*

■ *Further assessment of chest expansion.* Place your thumbs along each costal margin, your hands along the lateral rib cage. As you position your hands, slide them medially a bit to raise loose skin folds between your thumbs. Ask the client to inhale deeply. Observe how far your thumbs diverge as the thorax expands, and feel for the extent and symmetry of respiratory movement.

Tender pectoral muscles or costal cartilages tend to corroborate, but do not prove, that chest pain has a musculoskeletal origin.

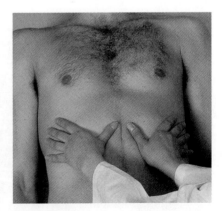

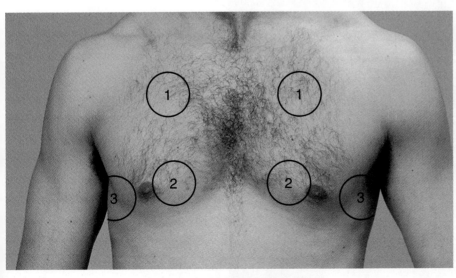

LOCATIONS FOR FEELING FREMITUS

■ *Assessment of tactile fremitus.* Compare both sides of the chest, using the ball or ulnar surface of your hand. Fremitus is usually decreased or absent over the precordium. When examining a woman, gently displace the breasts as necessary.

Percussion.   Percuss the anterior and lateral chest, again comparing both sides. It is important to percuss lung tissue in the apices above the clavicles, as shown in the circled position 1 in the photo that follows. The heart usually produces an area of dullness to the left of the sternum from the 3rd to 5th intercostal spaces. Percuss the left lung lateral to it.

Dullness replaces resonance when fluid or solid tissue replaces air-containing lung or occupies the pleural space. Because pleural fluid usually sinks to the lowest part of the pleural space (posteriorly in a supine client), only a very large effusion can be detected anteriorly.

The hyperresonance of COPD may totally replace cardiac dullness.

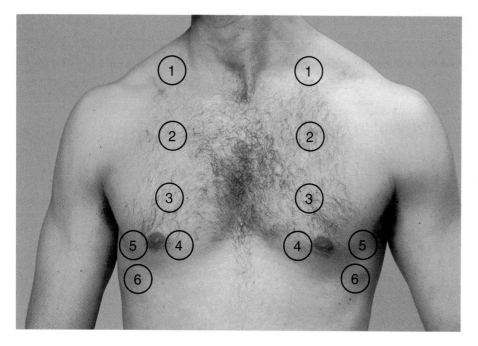

With a female client, ask her to move her breast for you. Alternately, gently displace the breast with your left hand while percussing with the right hand.

The dullness of right middle lobe, as pneumonia typically occurs behind the right breast. Unless the breast is displaced, you may miss the dull percussion note.

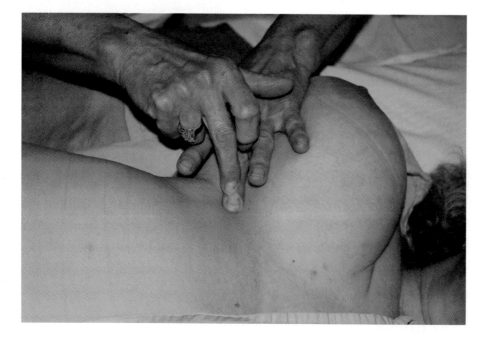

Identify and locate any area with an unexpected percussion note.

With your pleximeter finger above and parallel to the expected upper border of liver dullness, percuss in progressive steps downward in the right MCL. Identify the upper border of liver dullness. Later, during the abdominal examination, you will use this method to estimate the size of the liver. As you percuss down the chest on the left, the resonance over lung tissue usually changes to the tympany of the gastric air bubble.

Auscultation. Listen to the chest anteriorly and laterally as the client breathes with mouth open, somewhat more deeply than usual. Ask client to tell you if he or she starts to feel dizzy. Compare symmetric areas of the lungs, using the pattern suggested for percussion and extending it to adjacent areas as indicated.

Listen to the breath sounds, noting their intensity and identifying any variations from the expected vesicular breathing. Breath sounds are usually louder in the upper anterior lung fields. Bronchovesicular breath sounds may be heard over the large airways, especially on the right.

Identify any adventitious sounds, time them in the respiratory cycle, and locate them on the chest wall. Do they clear with deep breathing?

If indicated, *listen for transmitted voice sounds.*

A lung affected by COPD often displaces the upper border of the liver downward. It also lowers the level of diaphragmatic dullness posteriorly.

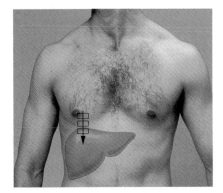

See Table 14-6, Adventitious (Added) Lung Sounds: Causes and Qualities (p. 419), and Table 14-7, Physical Findings in Selected Chest Disorders (pp. 420–421).

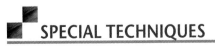

SPECIAL TECHNIQUES

Clinical Assessment of Pulmonary Function. A simple but informative way to assess breathlessness in an ambulatory client is to walk with the client down the hall or climb one flight of stairs. Observe the rate, effort, and sound of the client's breathing.

Forced Expiratory Time. This test assesses the expiratory phase of breathing, which is typically slowed in obstructive pulmonary disease. Ask the client to take a deep breath in and then breathe out as quickly and completely as possible with mouth open. Listen over the trachea with the diaphragm of a stethoscope and time the audible expiration. Try to get three consistent readings, allowing a short rest between efforts if necessary.

If the client can perform the test, a forced expiration time of 6 seconds or more suggests obstructive pulmonary disease.

Identification of a Fractured Rib. Local pain and tenderness of one or more ribs raise the question of fracture. By anteroposterior compression of the chest, you can help to distinguish a fracture from soft-tissue injury. With one hand on the sternum and the other on the thoracic spine, squeeze the chest. Is this painful? Where?

An increase in the local pain (distant from your hands) suggests rib fracture rather than just soft-tissue injury.

RECORDING AND ANALYZING FINDINGS

Information from the client history and physical examination should be precise in anatomical location, logical in order, and concise. The style in the following table contains phrases appropriate for most documentation. It is easier for the reader to quickly grasp the objective findings and their significance if they are written in the sequence of inspection, palpation, percussion, and auscultation (IPPA).

■ *Examples of Documentation for Thorax and Lungs*

Area of Assessment	Expected Findings	Unexpected Findings
Inspection of thorax	Respiratory rate regular and nonlaboured at 16 per minute. Pink skin over chest wall; scattered macules over upper posterior chest wall bilaterally. Thorax symmetrical; no retractions or use of accessory muscles. AP diameter < transverse.	Respirations shallow and irregular at 20 per minute. Audible wheeze on expiration. Retractions noted at right posterior triangle of neck. AP diameter = transverse.
Palpation of thorax	Chest expansion is upward, outward, and symmetrical. No tenderness with palpation of chest wall, anteriorly and posteriorly. Tactile fremitus equal over all lung fields and more intense in upper fields.	Decreased chest expansion of right thorax. No tenderness. Decreased tactile fremitus of left lung fields compared to right.
Percussion of lung fields	Resonant percussion note over all lung fields, including apices bilaterally. Diaphragm descends 5 cm bilaterally.	Hyperresonant note over left lung fields, with dull percussion note noted between the right 3rd and 5th intercostal spaces (ICS) at the midclavicular line (MCL). Diaphragm descends 2 cm on right and 4 cm on left.
Auscultation of lung fields	Vesicular breath sounds heard over lung periphery, anteriorly and posteriorly bilaterallly. No crackles or wheezes bilaterally.	Breath sounds distant with delayed expiratory phase and scattered expiratory wheezes over left lung fields. Inspiratory crackles heard over right lower base. E-to-A changes heard at right lower-lung field.

ANALYZING FINDINGS FROM PHYSICAL EXAMINATION AND HEALTH HISTORY

Analysis of subjective and objective data leads to formulation of nursing diagnoses and an interdisciplinary plan of care. Central to care are the unique aspects of the client and his or her input into the proposed plan. For example:

Norman Tourmay, 60 years old, arrives at a rural emergency room stating that he is having "a hard time catching my breath." You note that the client is thin, his face is ashen, and he breathes with pursed lips. Mr. Tourmay first noticed difficulty breathing about 6 months ago. He reports that in the last week "it has become much worse, and I'm coughing now." He says that he has been well all his life and takes no prescription medication. Mr. Tourmay last had a "check-up" when he worked in open-pit asbestos mines, from which he retired 5 years ago. He reports that he started smoking at age 20, used to smoke 15 cigarettes a day, but stopped smoking 10 years ago. He mentions that he has lost 7 kilograms in the last 2 months. Current vital signs are T 36.9°C, P 80, R 24 and shallow, and BP 118/72 right arm sitting. From this information, you develop the following nursing diagnosis:

Impaired gas exchange *related to difficulty breathing.*

Mr. Tourmay needs comprehensive care from a team of health professionals. He needs a complete examination (physician), chest X-ray (x-ray technician and radiologist), blood and urine tests (laboratory technician), and treatments such as oxygen, mini-nebulizer, and rebreathing exercises (respiratory therapist). A dietitian can explore how Mr. Tourmay lost 7 kilograms in 2 months and develop a dietary plan for his hospitalization and discharge to home. A pharmacist would be involved with any medications. A physical therapist can assess Mr. Tourmay's capacity for physical activities and develop an exercise plan that the client can continue after discharge.

Mr. Tourmay may need to consult a physician specializing in respiratory conditions. Registered nurses and a respiratory therapist from home care should follow up at the client's home to facilitate care and monitor progress. The client needs an assessment of his home for stairs, railings, and possible respiratory irritants. He may need equipment for respiratory treatments. How will he obtain groceries and prepare meals? Can family members assist him?

Critical Thinking Exercise

Answer the following questions about Mr. Tourmay's presentation:

- For what respiratory diseases is Mr. Tourmay at risk? (*Knowledge*)
- What constellation of history (subjective) findings is concerning? (*Comprehension*)
- How would you calculate his smoking as packs per year? (*Application*)
- What additional history questions would you want to ask? Which associated symptom(s) need additional probing? What objective signs are important to note? (*Analysis*)
- What recommendations for screening and follow-up would you suggest for Mr. Tourmay? (*Synthesis*)
- How would you evaluate the success of client teaching for Mr. Tourmay? (*Evaluation*)

Canadian Nursing Research

Bailey, P. H. (2004). The dyspnea-anxiety-dyspnea cycle—COPD clients' stories of breathliness: "It's scary when you can't breathe." *Qualitative Health Research, 14,* 760–778.

Bergerson, S. M., Cameron, S., Armstrong-Stassen, M., & Pare, K. (2006). Diverse implications of a national health crisis: A qualitative exploration of community nurses' SARS experiences. *Canadian Journal of Nursing Research, 38*(2), 42–54.

Boutin, H., Robichaud, P., Valois, P., & Labrecque, M. (2006). Impact of continuing education activity on the quality of telephone interventions by nurses in an adult asthma client base. *Journal of Nursing Care Quality, 21*(4), 335–343.

Brooks, D., Sidani, S., Graydon, J., McBride, S., Hall, L., & Wienacht, K. (2003). Evaluating the effects of music on dyspnea during exercise in individuals with chronic obstructive pulmonary disease. *Rehabilitation Nursing, 28,* 192–196.

Chalmers, K., Gupton, A., Katz, A., Hack, T., Hildes-Ripstein, E., Brown, J., et al. (2004). The description and evaluation of a longitudinal pilot study of a smoking relapse/reduction intervention for perinatal women. *Journal of Advanced Nursing, 45,* 162–171.

Cicutto, L., Conti, E., Evans, H., Lewis, R., Murphy, S., Rautiainen, K. C., et al. (2006). Creating asthma-friendly schools: A public health approach. *Journal of School Health, 76*(6), 255–258.

Egan, E., Clavarino, A., Burridge, L., Teuwen, M., & White, E. (2002). A randomized control trial of nursing–based case management for clients with chronic obstructive pulmonary disease. *Lippincott's Case Management, 7,* 170–179.

Johnson, J. L., Bottorff, J. L., Moffat, B., Ratner, P. A., Shoveller, J., & Lovato, C. Y. (2003). Tobacco dependence: Adolescents' perspectives on the need to smoke. *Social Science & Medicine, 56,* 1481–1492.

Johnson, J. L., Tucker, R. S., Ratner, P. A., Bottorff, J. L., Prkachin, K. M., Shoveller, J., et al. (2004). Sociodemographic correlates of cigarette smoking among high school students: Results from the British Columbia Youth Survey on Smoking and Health. *Canadian Journal of Public Health, 95,* 268–271.

Nurhaeni, N., Moralejo, D., & Webber, K. (2007). Identification of modifiable risk factors for acute respiratory infection in Indonesian children under 5 years of age. *Canadian Journal of Nursing Research, 39*(3), 199–201.

Ratner, P. A., Johnson, J. L., Richardson, C. G., Bottorff, J. L., Moffat, B., Mackay, M., et al. (2004). Efficacy of a smoking-cessation intervention for elective-surgical clients. *Research in Nursing & Health, 27,* 148–161.

Ross, C. J. M., Davis, T. M. A., & Hogg, D. Y. (2007). Screening and assessing adolescent asthmatics for anxiety disorders. *Clinical Nursing Research, 16*(1), 5–28.

Schultz, A. S. H., Johnson, J. L., & Bottorff, J. L. (2006). Registered nurses' perceptions on tobacco reduction: Views from Western Canada. *Canadian Journal of Nursing Research, 38*(4), 193–211.

Small, S. P., Brennan-Hunter, A. L., Best, D. G., & Solberg, S. M. (2002). Struggling to understand: The experience of nonsmoking parents with adolescents who smoke. *Qualitative Health Research, 12,* 1202–1219.

Canadian Medical and Allied Health Research

Carusone, S. B. C., Walter, S. D., Brazil, K., & Loeb, M. B. (2007). Pneumonia and lower respiratory infections in nursing home residents: Predictors of hospitalization and mortality. *Journal of the American Geriatrics Society, 55*(3), 414–419.

Faulkner, G., Taylor, A., Munro, S., Selby, P., & Gee, C. (2006). The acceptability of physical activity programming within a smoking cessation service for individuals with severe mental illness. *Client Education and Counselling, 66*(1), 123–126.

Wanyski, I., Olson, S., Brassard, P., Menzies, D., Ross, N., Behr, M., et al. (2006). Dwellings, crowding, and tuberculosis in Montreal. *Social Science & Medicine, 63*(2), 501–511.

Test Questions

1. Which of the following muscles is primarily responsible for thoracic cavity enlargement?
   a. Scalene
   b. Diaphragm
   c. Parasternal
   d. Sternomastoid

2. While inspecting the thorax, the nurse views the thorax from posterior and lateral positions to assess the:
   a. position of the trachea.
   b. curvature of the cervical spine.
   c. anteroposterior to lateral diameter.
   d. inflammation of the costochondral junction.

3. When auscultating the lungs, the nurse listens over symmetrical lung fields for:
   a. one quiet full inspiration through pursed lips.
   b. two full breaths every 10 seconds through the nose.
   c. one deep inspiration and expiration through the open mouth.
   d. two full breaths in through the mouth and out through the nose.

4. When auscultating the thorax, which breath sound is described as soft, low-pitched, and with shorter expiratory than inspiratory phase?
   a. Bronchial
   b. Tracheal
   c. Vesicular
   d. Bronchovesicular

5. When percussing the posterior lung fields, which of the following findings is **expected**?
   a. Hyperresonance over apices
   b. Dullness over the lung bases
   c. Resonance over all lung fields
   d. Tympany over 11th interspace, right scapular line

Bibliography

CITATIONS

Agency for Healthcare Research and Quality. (2005). *Helping smokers quit: A guide for nurses.* Rockville, MD: Author.

Banerji, A., Bell, A., Mills, E. L., McDonald, J., Subbarao, K., Stark, G., et al. (2001). Lower respiratory tract infections in Inuit infants on Baffin Island. *Canadian Medical Association Journal, 164*(13), 1847–1850.

Buist, M. D., Moore, G. E., Bernard, S. A., Waxman, B. P., Anderson, J. N., & Nguyen, T. V. (2002). Effects of a medical emergency team on reduction of incidence of and mortality from unexpected cardiac arrests in hospital: Preliminary study. *British Medical Journal, 324*, 1–6.

Call, S. A., Vollenwider, M. A., Hornung, C. A., Simel, D. L., & McKinney, W. P. (2005). Does this client have influenza? *Journal of the American Medical Association, 293*(8), 987–997.

Canadian Cancer Society/National Cancer Institute of Canada. (2008). *Canadian cancer statistics 2008.* Toronto, ON: Authors.

Canadian Lung Association. (2008). *Smoking and tobacco. Quitting smoking.* Retrieved March 3, 2008, from http://www.lung.ca

Cayley, W. E., Jr. (2005). Diagnosing the cause of chest pain. *American Family Physician, 72*(10), 2012–2021.

Celli, B. R., Cote, C. G., Marin, J. M., Casanova, C., Montes de Oca, M., Mendez, R. A., et al. (2004). The body-mass index, airflow obstruction, dyspnea, and exercise capacity index in chronic obstructive pulmonary disease. *New England Journal of Medicine, 350*(10), 1005–1012.

Centres for Disease Control and Prevention. (2008). *Smoking and tobacco use. Fact sheet: Cessation.* Retrieved March 11, 2009, from http://www.cdc.gov/tobacco/data_statistics/fact_sheets/cessation/cessation2.htm

Cho, S.-H., Ketefian, S., Barkauskas, V. H., & Smith, D. G. (2003). The effects of nurse staffing on adverse events, morbidity, mortality, and medical costs. *Nursing Research, 52*(2), 71–79.

Duff, B., Gardiner, G., & Barnes, M. (2007). The impact of surgical ward nurses practicing respiratory assessment on positive client outcomes. *Australian Journal of Advanced Nursing, 24*(4), 52–56.

Eder, W., Ege, M. J., & von Mutius, E. (2006). The asthma epidemic. *New England Journal of Medicine, 355*(21), 2226–2235.

Finkelstein, M. M., Jerrett, M., DeLuca, P., Finkelstein, N., Verma, D. K., Chapman, K., et al. (2003). Relation between income, air pollution and mortality: A cohort study. *Canadian Medical Association Journal, 169*(5), 397–402.

FluWatch, Public Health Agency of Canada. (n.d.). Retrieved December 2, 2007, from http://www.phac-aspc.gc.ca/fluwatch/index.html

BIBLIOGRAPHY

Goroll, A. H., & Mulley, A. G., Jr. (2006a). Chest pain. In A. H. Goroll & A. G. Mulley, Jr. (Eds.), *Primary care medicine: Office evaluation and management of the adult client* (5th ed., pp. 125–129). Philadelphia: Lippincott Williams & Wilkins.

Goroll, A. H., & Mulley, A. G., Jr. (2006b). Evaluation of subacute and chronic cough. In A. H. Goroll & A. G. Mulley, Jr. (Eds.), *Primary care medicine: Office evaluation and management of the adult client* (5th ed., pp. 320–325). Philadelphia: Lippincott Williams & Wilkins.

Heather Crowe Resource Centre. (n. d.). *Smoking cessation: 4A's program* (cat. no. 6673864857-1). Retrieved March 3, 2008, from http://esubmitit.sjpg.com/productdetail.cfm?id=6673864857%2D1

Hornick, D. B. (2007). Tuberculosis. In R. B. Wallace (Ed.), *Maxcy-Rosenau-Last public health & preventive medicine* (15th ed., pp. 248–257). New York: McGraw-Hill.

Husain, A. N., & Kumar, V. (2005). The lung. In V. Kumar, A. K. Abbas, & N. Fausto (Eds.), *Robbins and Cotran pathologic basis of disease* (p. 712). Philadelphia: Elsevier Saunders.

Kovesi, T., Gilbert, N. L., Stocco, C., Fugler, D., Dales, R. E., Guay, M., et al. (2007). Indoor air quality and the risk of lower respiratory tract infections in young Canadian Inuit children. *Canadian Medical Association Journal, 177*(2), 155–160.

Long, R., & Ellis, E. (Eds.). (2007). *Canadian tuberculosis standards* (6th ed.). Retrieved August 2, 2008, from http://www.lung.ca/cts-sct/pdf/tbstand07_e.pdf

Meyers, K. A., & Farquhar, D. R. E. (2001). Does this client have clubbing? *Journal of the American Medical Association, 286*, 341–347.

National Advisory Committee on Immunization. (2006). *Canadian immunization guide* (7th ed.). Retrieved August 1, 2008, from www.naci.gc.ca

Nicolle, L. (2007). Hygiene: What and why? *Canadian Medical Association Journal, 176*(6), 767–768.

Overfield, T. (1995). *Biologic variation in health and illness: Race, age and sex differences* (2nd ed.). Boca Raton, FL: CRC Press.

Public Health Agency of Canada. (2007). *Life and breath: Respiratory disease in Canada*. Retrieved August 2, 2008, from http://www.phac-aspc.gc.ca/publicat/2007/lbrdc-vsmrc/index-eng.php

Rigotti, N. A. (2003). Putting the research into practice. *British Medical Journal, 327*(7428), 1395–1396.

Smetana, G. W. (1999). Preoperative pulmonary evaluation. *New England Journal of Medicine, 340*(12), 937–944.

Spencer, H., & Leof, D. (1964). The innervation of the human lung. *Journal of Anatomy, 98*(4), 599–609.

Statistics Canada. (2005a). *Persons with asthma, by age and sex.* Retrieved October 5, 2007, from http://www40.statcan.ca/l01/cst01/health49a.htm

Statistics Canada. (2005b). *Smokers, by province and territory, 2005.* Retrieved October 5, 2007, from http://www40.statcan.ca/l01/cst01/health07a.htm

Tarlo, S. M. (2003). Occupational asthma: An approach to diagnosis and management. *Canadian Medical Association Journal, 168*(7), 867–871.

U.S. Public Health Service. (2009). Treating tobacco use and dependence. *Quick reference guide for clinicians*. Retrieved March 11, 2009, from http://www.surgeongeneral.gov/tobacco/tobaqrg.htm

Yildirim, A., Karakurt, C., Karademir, S., Oguz, D., Sungur, M., Oscal, B., et al. (2004). Chest pain in children. *International Pediatrics, 19*(3), 175–179.

ADDITIONAL REFERENCES

Aldington, S., & Beasley, R. (2007). Asthma exacerbations. 5. Assessment and management of severe asthma in adults in hospital. *Thorax, 62*(4), 447–458.

Bernard Bagattini, S., Bounameaux, H., Perneger, T., & Perrier, A. (2004). Suspicion of pulmonary embolism in outpatients: Nonspecific chest pain is the most frequent alternative. *Journal of Internal Medicine, 256*(2), 153–160.

Bidwell, J., & Pachner, R. W. (2005). Hemoptysis: Diagnosis and management. *American Family Physician, 72*(7), 1253–1260.

Chenille, S. D., Eikelboom, J. W., Attia, J., Miniati, M., Panju, A. A., Simel, D. L., et al. (2003). Does this client have pulmonary embolism? *Journal of the American Medical Association, 290*(20), 2849–2858.

Crapo, J. D., Glassroth, J. L., Karlinsky, J. B., & King, T. E. (Eds.). (2004). *Baum's textbook of pulmonary diseases* (7th ed.). Philadelphia: Lippincott Williams & Wilkins.

Farm Safety Association. (n.d.) *Hanta virus*. Retrieved March 2, 2008, from http://www.farmsafety.ca/factsheets/tips-e/hanta.pdf

Fleetham, J., Ayas, N., Bradley, D., Ferguson, K., Fitzpatrick, M., George, C., et al. & the CTS Sleep Disordered Breathing Committee. (2006). Canadian Thoracic Society Guidelines: Diagnosis and treatment of sleep disordered breathing in adults. *Canadian Respiratory Journal, 13*(7), 387–392.

Hogg, J. C. (2004). Pathophysiology of airflow limitation in chronic obstructive pulmonary disease. *Lancet, 364*(9435), 709–721.

Kalantir, S., Joshi, R., Lokhande, T., Singh, A., Morgan, M., Colford, J. M., Jr., et al. (2007). Accuracy and reliability of physical signs in the diagnosis of pleural effusion. *Respiratory Medicine, 101*(3), 431–438.

Kane, C., & Galanes, S. (2004). Adult respiratory disease syndrome. *Critical Care Nursing Quarterly, 27*(4), 325–335.

Lehrer, S. (2002). *Understanding lung sounds* (3rd ed.). Philadelphia: WB Saunders.

Lichtenstien, D., Goldstein, I., Mourgeon, E., Cluzel, P., Grenier, P., & Rouby, J.-J. (2004). Comparative diagnostic performances of auscultation, chest radiography, and lung ultrasonography in acute respiratory distress syndrome. *Anesthesiology, 100*(1), 9–15.

Lutfiyya, M. N., Henley, E., Chang, L. F., & Reyburn, S. W. (2006). Diagnosis and treatment of community-acquired pneumonia. *American Family Physician, 73*(3), 442–450.

O'Donnell, D. E., Aaron, S., Bourbeau, J., Hernandez, P., Marciniuk, D. D., Balter, M., et al. (2007). Canadian Thoracic Society recommendations for management of chronic obstructive pulmonary disease – 2007 update. *Canadian Respiratory Journal, 14*(Suppl. B), 5B–32B.

Pirret, A. M. (2007). The level of knowledge of respiratory physiology articulated by intensive care nurses to provide rationale for their clinical decision-making. *Intensive & Critical Care Nursing, 23*(3),145–155.

Poutanen, S. M., Low, D. E., Henry, B., Finkelstein, S., Rose, D., Green, K., et al. (2003). Identification of severe acute respiratory syndrome in Canada. *New England Journal of Medicine, 348*(20), 1995–2005.

Public Health Agency of Canada. (2008). *Tuberculosis fact sheets.* Retrieved March 2, 2008, from http://www.phac-aspc.gc.ca/tbpc-latb/fa-fi/index-eng.php

Public Health Agency of Canada. (2007). *Influenza immunization.* Retrieved March 2, 2008, from http://www.phac-aspc.gc.ca/im/2007/index-eng.html

Rennard, S. I. (2004). Looking at the client—Approaching the problem of COPD. *New England Journal of Medicine, 350*(10), 965–966.

Ross, C. J. M. (2007). Management of clients with chronic obstructive pulmonary disease. In R. A. Day, P. Paul, B. Williams, S. C. Smeltzer, & B. Bare (Eds.), *Brunner & Suddarth's textbook of medical-surgical nursing* (1st Canadian ed., pp. 572–603). Philadelphia: Lippincott Williams & Wilkins.

Ryan, B. (2005). Pneumothorax: Assessment and diagnostic testing. *Journal of Cardiovascular Nursing, 20*(4), 251–253.

Sterling, T. R., Bethel, J., Goldberg, S., Weinfurter, P., Yun, L., & Horsburgh, C. R. (2006). The scope and impact of treatment of latent tuberculosis infection in the United States and Canada. *American Journal of Respiratory Critical Care Medicine, 173*(8), 927–931.

Weinberger, S. (2004). *Principles of pulmonary medicine* (4th ed.). Philadelphia: W. B. Saunders.

Wenzel, R. P., & Fowler, A. A., III. (2006). Acute bronchitis. *New England Journal of Medicine, 355*(20), 2125–2130.

Wilson-Clark, S. D., Deeks, S. L., Gournis, E., Hay, K., Bondy, S., Kennedy, E., et al. (2006). Household transmission of SARS, 2003. *Canadian Medical Association Journal, 175*(10), 1219–1223.

CANADIAN WEB SITES AND ASSOCIATIONS

Asthma Society of Canada: http://www.asthma.ca/adults/

Canada Council for Tobacco Control (including Heather Crowe Research Centre): http://www.cctc.ca

The Canadian Best Practices Portal for Health Promotion and Chronic Disease Prevention: http://cbpp-pcpe.phac-aspc.gc.ca

Canadian Lung Association: http://www.lung.ca

Canadian Network for Asthma Care: http://www.cnac.net

Canadian Respiratory Health Professionals, c/o The Lung Association, National Office: http://www.lung.ca/about-propos/medical-medicales/respiratory-respiratoire/index_e.php

Canadian Thorax Society, c/o The Lung Association, National Office: http://www.lung.ca/cts-sct/home-accueil_e.php

Centre for Addiction & Mental Health, TEACH project: http://www.teachproject.ca

Centre for Chronic Disease Prevention and Control: http://www.phac-aspc.gc.ca/ccdpc-cpcmc/

Children's Asthma Education Centre: http://www.asthma-education.com/content/

Cystic Fibrosis Foundation (CCFF): http://www.cysticfibrosis.ca

Physicians for a Smoke Free Canada: http://www.smoke-free.ca/

INTERNATIONAL WEB SITES

American Lung Association: http://www.lungusa.org

Global Initiative for Asthma: http://www.ginasthma.com

National Heart Lung & Blood Institute: http://www.nhlbi.nih.gov/

TABLE 14-1   Dyspnea

Problem	Process	Timing
Left-Sided Heart Failure *(left ventricular failure or mitral stenosis)*	Elevated pressure in pulmonary capillary bed with transudation of fluid into interstitial spaces and alveoli, decreased compliance (increased stiffness) of the lungs, increased work of breathing	Dyspnea may progress slowly or suddenly, as in acute pulmonary edema.
Chronic Bronchitis*	Excessive mucus production in bronchi, followed by chronic obstruction of airways	Chronic productive cough followed by slowly progressive dyspnea
Chronic Obstructive Pulmonary Disease (COPD)*	Overdistention of air spaces distal to terminal bronchioles, with destruction of alveolar septa and chronic obstruction of the airways	Slowly progressive dyspnea; relatively mild cough later
Asthma	Bronchial hyperresponsiveness involving release of inflammatory mediators, increased airway secretions, and bronchoconstriction	Acute episodes, separated by symptom-free periods; nocturnal episodes common
Diffuse Interstitial Lung Diseases *(such as sarcoidosis, widespread neoplasms, asbestosis, and idiopathic pulmonary fibrosis)*	Unexpected and widespread infiltration of cells, fluid, and collagen into interstitial spaces between alveoli; many causes	Progressive dyspnea, which varies in its rate of development with the cause
Pneumonia	Inflammation of lung parenchyma from the respiratory bronchioles to the alveoli	An acute illness, timing varies with the causative agent
Spontaneous Pneumothorax	Leakage of air into pleural space through blebs on visceral pleura, with resulting partial or complete collapse of the lung	Sudden onset of dyspnea
Acute Pulmonary Embolism	Sudden occlusion of all or part of pulmonary arterial tree by a blood clot that usually originates in deep veins of legs or pelvis	Sudden onset of dyspnea
Anxiety With Hyperventilation	Overbreathing, with resultant respiratory alkalosis and fall in the partial pressure of carbon dioxide in the blood	Episodic, often recurrent

*Chronic bronchitis and *chronic obstructive pulmonary disease (COPD)* may coexist.

Factors That Aggravate	Factors That Relieve	Associated Symptoms	Setting/Environment
Exertion, lying down	Rest, sitting up, though dyspnea may become persistent	Often cough, orthopnea, paroxysmal nocturnal dyspnea; sometimes wheezing	History of heart disease or its predisposing factors
Exertion, inhaled irritants, respiratory infections	Expectoration; rest, though dyspnea may become persistent	Chronic productive cough, recurrent respiratory infections; wheezing may develop	History of smoking, air pollutants, recurrent respiratory infections
Exertion	Rest, though dyspnea may become persistent	Cough, with scant mucoid sputum	History of smoking, air pollutants, sometimes a familial deficiency in alpha$_1$-antitrypsin
Variable, including allergens, irritants, respiratory infections, exercise, and emotion	Separation from aggravating factors	Wheezing, cough, tightness in chest	Environmental and emotional conditions
Exertion	Rest, though dyspnea may become persistent	Often weakness, fatigue; cough less common than in other lung diseases	Varied; exposure to one of many substances may be causative
		Pleuritic pain, cough, sputum, fever, though not necessarily present	Varied
		Pleuritic pain, cough	Often a previously healthy young adult
		Often none; retrosternal oppressive pain if the occlusion is massive. Pleuritic pain, cough, and hemoptysis may follow an embolism if pulmonary infarction ensues. Symptoms of anxiety (see the following text).	During pregnancy, postpartum, or postoperative periods; prolonged bed rest; congestive heart failure, chronic lung disease, and fractures of hip or leg; deep venous thrombosis (often not clinically apparent)
More often occurs at rest than after exercise. An upsetting event may not be evident.	Breathing in and out of a paper or plastic bag sometimes helps the associated symptoms.	Sighing, lightheadedness, numbness, or tingling of the hands and feet, palpitations, chest pain	Other manifestations of anxiety may be present

TABLE 14-2   **Chest Pain**

Problem	Process	Location	Quality
Cardiovascular			
Angina Pectoris	Temporary myocardial ischemia, usually secondary to coronary atherosclerosis	Retrosternal or across the anterior chest, sometimes radiating to the shoulders, arms, neck, lower jaw, or upper abdomen	Pressing, squeezing, tight, heavy, occasionally burning
Myocardial Infarction	Prolonged myocardial ischemia, resulting in irreversible muscle damage or necrosis	Same as in angina	Same as in angina
Pericarditis	Irritation of parietal pleura, adjacent to the pericardium, mechanism unclear	Precordial, may radiate to the tip of the shoulder and to the neck; retrosternal	Sharp, knifelike; crushing
Dissecting Aortic Aneurysm	A splitting within the layers of the aortic wall, allowing passage of blood to dissect a channel	Anterior chest, radiating to the neck, back, or abdomen	Ripping, tearing
Pulmonary			
Tracheobronchitis	Inflammation of trachea and large bronchi	Upper sternal or on either side of the sternum	Burning
Pleural Pain	Inflammation of the parietal pleura, as in pleurisy, pneumonia, pulmonary infarction, or neoplasm	Chest wall overlying the process	Sharp, knifelike
Gastrointestinal and Other			
Reflex Esophagitis	Inflammation of the esophageal mucosa by reflux of gastric acid	Retrosternal, may radiate to the back	Burning, may be squeezing
Diffuse Esophageal Spasm	Motor dysfunction of the esophageal muscle	Retrosternal, may radiate to the back, arms, and jaw	Usually squeezing
Chest Wall Pain	Variable, often unclear	Often below the left breast or along the costal cartilages; also elsewhere	Stabbing, sticking, or dull, aching
Anxiety	Unclear	Precordial, below the left breast, or across the anterior chest	Stabbing, sticking, or dull, aching

Note: Remember that chest pain may be referred from extrathoracic structures such as the neck (arthritis) and abdomen (biliary colic, acute cholecystitis). Pleural pain may be due to abdominal conditions such as subdiaphragmatic abscess.

Severity	Timing	Factors That Aggravate	Factors That Relieve	Associated Symptoms
Mild to moderate, sometimes perceived as discomfort rather than pain	Usually 1–3 min, but up to 10 min. Prolonged episodes up to 20 min.	Exertion, especially in the cold; meals; emotional stress. May occur at rest.	Rest, nitroglycerin	Sometimes dyspnea, nausea, sweating
Often, but not always, a severe pain	20 min to several hours			Nausea, vomiting, sweating, weakness
Often severe	Persistent	Breathing, changing position, coughing, lying down, sometimes swallowing	Sitting forward may relieve it.	Of the underlying illness
Severe	Persistent			Of the underlying illness
Very severe	Abrupt onset, early peak, persistent for hours or more	Hypertension		Syncope, hemiplegia, paraplegia
Mild to moderate	Variable	Coughing		Cough
Often severe	Persistent	Breathing, coughing, movements of the trunk	Lying on the involved side may relieve it	Of the underlying illness
Mild to severe	Variable	Large meal; bending over, lying down	Antacids, sometimes belching	Sometimes regurgitation, dysphagia
Mild to severe	Variable	Swallowing of food or cold liquid; emotional stress	Sometimes nitroglycerin	Dysphagia
Variable	Fleeting to hours or days	Movement of chest, trunk, arms		Often local tenderness
Variable	Fleeting to hours or days	May follow effort, emotional stress		Breathlessness, palpitations, weakness, anxiety

TABLE 14-3   **Cough and Hemoptysis***

Problem	Cough and Sputum	Associated Symptoms and Setting
Acute Inflammation		
Laryngitis	Dry cough (without sputum), may become productive of variable amounts of sputum	An acute, fairly minor illness with hoarseness. Often associated with viral nasopharyngitis.
Tracheobronchitis	Dry cough, may become productive (as above)	An acute, often viral illness, with burning retrosternal discomfort.
Mycoplasma and Viral Pneumonias	Dry hacking cough, often becoming productive of mucoid sputum	An acute febrile illness, often with malaise, headache, and possibly dyspnea
Bacterial Pneumonias	Pneumococcal: sputum mucoid or purulent; may be blood-streaked, diffusely pinkish, or rusty	An acute illness with chills, high fever, dyspnea, and chest pain. Often preceded by acute upper respiratory infection.
	Klebsiella: similar; or sticky, red, and jellylike	Typically occurs in older men with alcoholism
Chronic Inflammation		
Postnasal Drip	Chronic cough; sputum mucoid or mucopurulent	Repeated attempts to clear the throat. Postnasal discharge may be sensed by client or seen in posterior pharynx. Associated with chronic rhinitis, with or without sinusitis.
Chronic Bronchitis	Chronic cough; sputum mucoid to purulent, may be blood-streaked or even bloody	Often long-standing cigarette smoking. Recurrent superimposed infections. Wheezing and dyspnea may develop.
Bronchiectasis	Chronic cough; sputum purulent, often copious and foul-smelling; may be blood-streaked or bloody	Recurrent bronchopulmonary infections common; sinusitis may coexist.
Pulmonary Tuberculosis	Cough dry or sputum that is mucoid or purulent; may be blood-streaked or bloody	Early, no symptoms. Later, anorexia, weight loss, fatigue, fever, and night sweats.
Lung Abscess	Sputum purulent and foul smelling; may be bloody	A febrile illness. Often poor dental hygiene and a prior episode of impaired consciousness.
Asthma	Cough, with thick mucoid sputum, especially near end of an attack	Episodic wheezing and dyspnea, but cough may occur alone. Often a history of allergy.
Gastroesophageal Reflux	Chronic cough, especially at night or early in the morning	Wheezing, especially at night (often mistaken for asthma), early morning hoarseness, and repeated attempts to clear the throat. Often a history of heartburn and regurgitation.
Neoplasm		
Cancer of the Lung	Cough dry to productive; sputum may be blood-streaked or bloody	Usually a long history of cigarette smoking. Associated manifestations are numerous.
Cardiovascular Disorders		
Left Ventricular Failure or Mitral Stenosis	Often dry, especially on exertion or at night; may progress to the pink frothy sputum of pulmonary edema or to frank hemoptysis	Dyspnea, orthopnea, paroxysmal nocturnal dyspnea
Pulmonary Emboli	Dry to productive; may be dark, bright red, or mixed with blood	Dyspnea, anxiety, chest pain, fever; factors that predispose to deep venous thrombosis
Irritating Particles, Chemicals, or Gases	Variable. There may be a latent period between exposure and symptoms.	Exposure to irritants. Eyes, nose, and throat may be affected.

*Characteristics of hemoptysis are printed in red.

| TABLE 14-4 | Deviations of the Thorax |

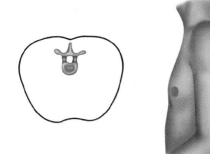
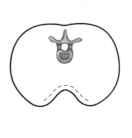
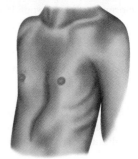

Adult

The thorax in the adult is wider than it is deep. Its lateral diameter is larger than its anteroposterior diameter.

Funnel chest (*pectus excavatum*)

Note depression in the lower portion of the sternum. Compression of the heart and great vessels may cause murmurs.

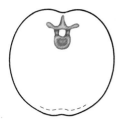
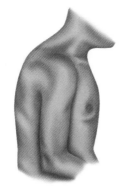

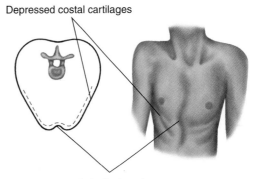

Depressed costal cartilages

Anteriorly displaced sternum

Barrel chest

There is an increased anteroposterior diameter. This shape is expected during infancy, and often accompanies aging and chronic obstructive pulmonary disease.

Pigeon chest (*pectus carinatum*)

The sternum is displaced anteriorly, increasing the anteroposterior diameter. The costal cartilages adjacent to the protruding sternum are depressed.

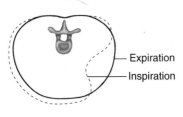

— Expiration
— Inspiration

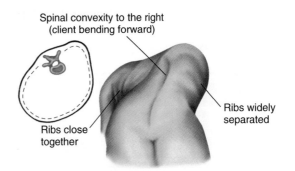

Spinal convexity to the right
(client bending forward)

Ribs widely
separated

Ribs close
together

Traumatic flail chest

Multiple rib fractures may result in paradoxical movements of the thorax. As descent of the diaphragm decreases intrathoracic pressure, on inspiration the injured area caves inward; on expiration, it moves outward.

Thoracic kyphoscoliosis

Unexpected spinal curvatures and vertebral rotation alter the chest. Distortion of the underlying lungs may make interpretation of lung findings very difficult.

The origins of breath sounds are still unclear. According to leading theories, turbulent air flow in the central airways produces the tracheal and bronchial breath sounds. As these sounds pass through the lungs to the periphery, lung tissue filters out their higher-pitched components, and only the soft and lower-pitched components reach the chest wall, where they are heard as vesicular breath sounds. It is usual that tracheal and bronchial sounds may be heard over the trachea and mainstem bronchi; vesicular breath sounds predominate throughout most of the lungs.

When lung tissue loses its air, it transmits high-pitched sounds much better. If the tracheobronchial tree is open, bronchial breath sounds may replace the usual vesicular sounds over airless areas of the lung. This change is seen in lobar pneumonia when the alveoli fill with fluid, red cells, and white cells—a process called *consolidation*. Other causes include pulmonary edema or hemorrhage. Bronchial breath sounds usually correlate with an increase in tactile fremitus and transmitted voice sounds. These findings are summarized below.

	Air-Filled Lung	Airless Lung, as in Lobar Pneumonia
	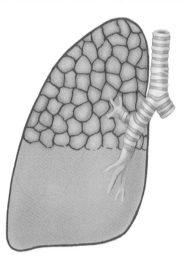	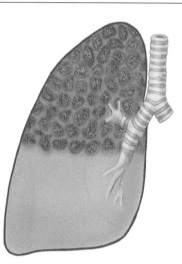
Breath sounds	Predominantly vesicular	Bronchial or bronchovesicular over the involved area
Transmitted Voice Sounds	Spoken words muffled and indistinct	Spoken words louder, clearer (*bronchophony*)
	Spoken "ee" heard as "ee"	Spoken "ee" heard as "ay" (*egophony*)
	Whispered words faint and indistinct, if heard at all	Whispered words louder, clearer (*whispered pectoriloquy*)
Tactile Fremitus	As expected	Increased

TABLE 14-6   Adventitious (Added) Lung Sounds: Causes and Qualities

Crackles Crackles have two leading explanations. (1) They result from a series of tiny explosions when small airways, deflated during expiration, pop open during inspiration. This mechanism probably explains the late inspiratory crackles of interstitial lung disease and early congestive heart failure. (2) Crackles result from air bubbles flowing through secretions or lightly closed airways during respiration. This mechanism probably explains at least some coarse crackles.

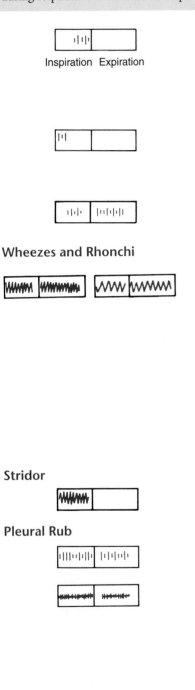

Inspiration Expiration

Late inspiratory crackles may begin in the first half of inspiration but must continue into late inspiration. They are usually fine and fairly profuse, and persist from breath to breath. These crackles appear first at the bases of the lungs, spread upward as the condition worsens, and shift to dependent regions with changes in posture. Causes include interstitial lung disease (such as fibrosis) and early congestive heart failure.

Early inspiratory crackles appear soon after the start of inspiration and do not continue into late inspiration. They are often but not always coarse and are relatively few in number. Expiratory crackles are sometimes associated. Causes include chronic bronchitis and asthma.

Midinspiratory and expiratory crackles are heard in bronchiectasis but are not specific for this diagnosis. Wheezes and rhonchi may be associated.

Wheezes and Rhonchi

Wheezes occur when air flows rapidly through bronchi that are narrowed nearly to the point of closure. They are often audible at the mouth as well as through the chest wall. Causes of wheezes that are generalized throughout the chest include asthma, chronic bronchitis, COPD, and congestive heart failure (cardiac asthma). In asthma, wheezes may be heard only in expiration or in both phases of the respiratory cycle. Rhonchi suggest secretions in the larger airways. In chronic bronchitis, wheezes and rhonchi often clear with coughing.

Occasionally in severe obstructive pulmonary disease, the client is no longer able to force enough air through the narrowed bronchi to produce wheezing. The resulting *silent chest* should raise immediate concern and not be mistaken for improvement.

A persistent localized wheeze suggests a partial obstruction of a bronchus, as by a tumour or foreign body. It may be inspiratory, expiratory, or both.

Stridor

A wheeze that is entirely or predominantly inspiratory is called *stridor*. It is often louder in the neck than over the chest wall. It indicates a partial obstruction of the larynx or trachea, and demands immediate attention.

Pleural Rub

Inflamed and roughened pleural surfaces grate against each other as they are momentarily and repeatedly delayed by increased friction. These movements produce creaking sounds known as a *pleural rub* (or pleural friction rub).

Pleural rubs resemble crackles acoustically, although they are produced by different pathologic processes. The sounds may be discrete, but sometimes are so numerous that they merge into a seemingly continuous sound. A rub is usually confined to a relatively small area of the chest wall, and typically is heard in both phases of respiration. When inflamed pleural surfaces are separated by fluid, the rub often disappears.

Mediastinal Crunch (*Hamman's Sign*)

A *mediastinal crunch* is a series of precordial crackles synchronous with the heart beat, not with respiration. Best heard in the left lateral position, it is due to mediastinal emphysema (pneumomediastinum).

TABLE 14-7   Physical Findings in Selected Chest Disorders

The red outlined boxes in this table suggest a framework for clinical assessment. Start with the three boxes under percussion note: resonant, dull, and hyperresonant. Then move from each of these to other boxes that emphasize some of the key differences among various conditions. The changes described vary with the extent and severity of the disorder. Abnormalities deep in the chest usually produce fewer signs than superficial ones, and may cause no signs at all. Use the table for the direction of typical changes, not for absolute distinctions.

Condition	Percussion Note	Trachea	Breath Sounds	Adventitious Sounds	Tactile Fremitus and Transmitted Voice Sounds
Expected The tracheobronchial tree and alveoli are clear; pleurae are thin and close together; mobility of the chest wall is unimpaired.	**Resonant**	Midline	Vesicular, except perhaps bronchovesicular and bronchial sounds over the large bronchi and trachea, respectively	None, except perhaps a few transient inspiratory crackles at the bases of the lungs	As expected
Chronic Bronchitis The bronchi are chronically inflamed, and a productive cough is present. Airway obstruction may develop.	**Resonant**	Midline	Vesicular	None; or scattered coarse *crackles* in early inspiration and perhaps expiration; or *wheezes* or *rhonchi*	As expected
Left-Sided Heart Failure (*Early*) Increased pressure in the pulmonary veins causes congestion and interstitial edema (around the alveoli); bronchial mucosa may become edematous.	**Resonant**	Midline	Vesicular	*Late inspiratory crackles* in the dependent portions of the lungs; possibly *wheezes*	As expected
Consolidation Alveoli fill with fluid or blood cells, as in pneumonia, pulmonary edema, or pulmonary hemorrhage.	**Dull** over the airless area	Midline	*Bronchial* over the involved area	*Late inspiratory crackles* over the involved area	*Increased* over the involved area, with *bronchophony*, *egophony*, and *whispered pectoriloquy*
Atelectasis (*Lobar Obstruction*) When a plug in a mainstem bronchus (as from mucus or a foreign object) obstructs air flow, affected lung tissue collapses into an airless state.	**Dull** over the airless area	May be *shifted toward involved side*	*Usually absent* when bronchial plug persists. Exceptions include right upper lobe atelectasis, where adjacent tracheal sounds may be transmitted.	None	*Its absence is usual* when the bronchial plug persists. In exceptions (e.g., right upper lobe atelectasis) may be increased

(table continues on next page)

TABLE 14-7   Physical Findings in Selected Chest Disorders *(Continued)*

Condition	Percussion Note	Trachea	Breath Sounds	Adventitious Sounds	Tactile Fremitus and Transmitted Voice Sounds
Pleural Effusion Fluid accumulates in the pleural space, separates air-filled lung from the chest wall, blocking the transmission of sound.	**Dull** to flat over the fluid	*Shifted toward opposite side* in a large effusion	*Decreased to absent,* but bronchial breath sounds may be heard near top of large effusion	None, except a *possible pleural* rub	*Decreased to absent, but may be increased* toward the top of a large effusion
Pneumothorax When air leaks into the pleural space, usually unilaterally, the lung recoils from the chest wall. Pleural air blocks transmission of sound.	**Hyperresonant** or tympanitic over the pleural air	*Shifted toward opposite side* if much air	*Decreased to absent* over the pleural air	None, except a *possible pleural* rub	*Decreased to absent* over the pleural air
Chronic Obstructive Pulmonary Disease (COPD) Slowly progressive disorder in which the distal air spaces enlarge and lungs become hyperinflated. Chronic bronchitis is often associated.	Diffusely **hyperresonant**	Midline	*Decreased to absent*	None, or the crackles, wheezes, and rhonchi of associated chronic bronchitis	*Decreased*
Asthma Widespread narrowing of the tracheobronchial tree diminishes air flow to a fluctuating degree. During attacks, air flow decreases further, and lungs hyperinflate.	**Resonant** to diffusely **hyperresonant**	Midline	*Often obscured by wheezes*	*Wheezes, possibly crackles*	*Decreased*

The Cardiovascular System

SHERI ROACH, PAT RODDICK, AND LYNN S. BICKLEY

The cardiovascular system, made up of the heart and blood vessels, has three main functions: delivering oxygen and nutrients to the body, removing metabolic waste, and maintaining adequate perfusion of organs and tissues. Consequently, its health status affects every other system in the body, in addition to overall well-being. The heart is the pump that drives circulation of blood through the pathways of the blood vessels. Blood itself transports oxygen and nutrients to cells, while removing from them waste products, such as carbon dioxide. To obtain a complete picture of a client's cardiovascular health, the nurse conducts a thorough, focused health history and uses the information gleaned to perform appropriate physical assessment of the client's heart and circulatory system.

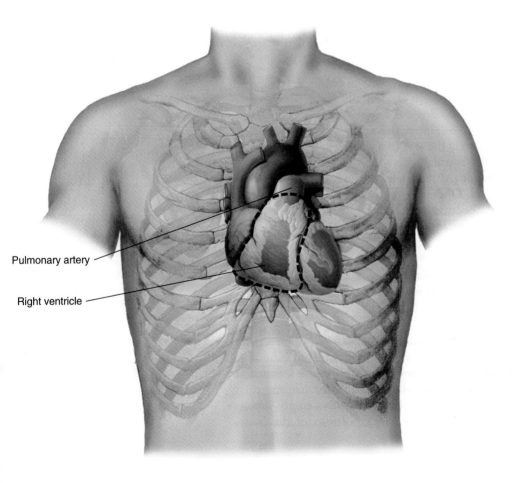

Pulmonary artery

Right ventricle

ANATOMY AND PHYSIOLOGY

To accurately assess a client's cardiovascular health, nurses need a solid understanding of cardiovascular anatomy and physiology. This includes the muscle, chambers, valves, coronary blood vessels, and electrical conduction system of the heart, and the arteries, arterioles, veins, venules, and capillaries that comprise the circulatory system. Assessment of the peripheral circulatory system is addressed in Chapter 18.

■ SURFACE PROJECTIONS OF THE HEART AND GREAT VESSELS

The heart is slightly larger than the client's clenched fist and lies behind the sternum, usually between the second rib and fifth intercostal space. It sits between the lungs and above the diaphragm in an area called the *mediastinal space*. It is helpful to visualize the underlying structures of the heart as you examine the anterior chest.

In the illustration on the previous page, note that the heart is rotated so that the *right ventricle* occupies most of the anterior cardiac surface. This chamber and the pulmonary artery form a wedgelike structure behind and to the left of the sternum, outlined in red.

The inferior border of the right ventricle lies below the junction of the sternum and the xiphoid process. The right ventricle narrows as it rises to meet the pulmonary artery at the level of the sternum. This is called the base of the heart and is located at the right and left 2nd intercostal spaces close to the sternum.

The *left ventricle* is behind the right ventricle and to the left, as outlined. Its tapered inferior tip is often termed the cardiac apex. It is clinically important because it produces the *apical impulse*, sometimes called the *point of maximal impulse*, or *PMI*. This impulse is usually found in the 5th intercostal space 7 cm to 9 cm lateral to the midsternal line. It is approximately the size of a quarter, roughly 1 cm to 2.5 cm in diameter. The apical pulse is usually easy to palpate in children and young adults, but as the anteroposterior (AP) diameter of the chest increases with age, it becomes more difficult to feel. Obesity or a thick chest wall also makes palpation of the apical pulse difficult. Because the most prominent cardiac impulse may not be apical, some authorities discourage use of the term PMI when referring to the apical pulse.

The right heart border is formed by the *right atrium*, a chamber not usually identifiable on physical examination. The *left atrium* is mostly posterior and cannot be examined directly.

Above the heart lie the great vessels. The *pulmonary artery*, which carries deoxygenated blood to the lungs, rises from the right ventricle and bifurcates into its left and right branches. The *aorta* curves upward from the left ventricle to the level of the sternal angle, where it arches backward to the left and then down. On the right, the superior vena cava and inferior vena cava empty venous blood into the right atrium from the upper and lower portions of the body, respectively.

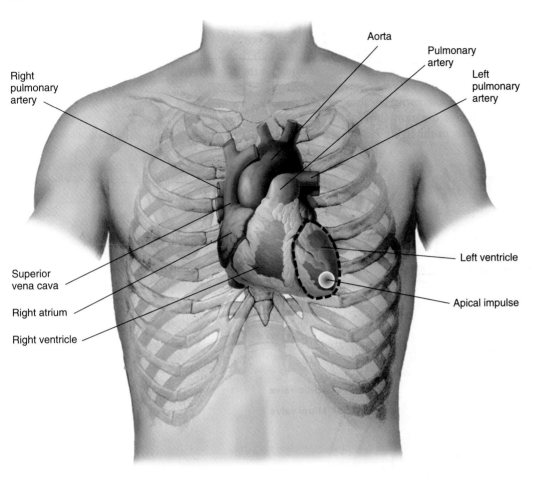

Labels: Aorta, Pulmonary artery, Left pulmonary artery, Right pulmonary artery, Left ventricle, Apical impulse, Superior vena cava, Right atrium, Right ventricle

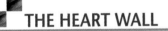

THE HEART WALL

Three layers make up the heart wall: the epicardium, myocardium, and endocardium. The *epicardium* is a thin external membrane covering the heart. The *myocardium* is a thick, muscular middle layer that makes up the bulk of the heart wall. The *endocardium* is a thin, smooth layer lining the chambers of the heart and the vessels of the circulatory system.

Cardiac muscle differs from skeletal muscle in three main ways. First, cardiac muscle cells are shorter and arranged in interlacing bundles that spiral around the heart. They cause a "wringing" effect when the heart muscle contracts, pressing blood upward and out of the ventricles. Second, cardiac muscle fibres do not operate independently like the fibres in skeletal muscle; they are interconnected by special gap junctions that conduct impulses across the whole myocardium, allowing the heart to contract as a single unit. Finally, cardiac muscle cells have a higher proportion of mitochondria (energy-producing organelles) than skeletal muscle cells. This accommodates the higher energy requirements of heart muscle.

CARDIAC CHAMBERS, VALVES, AND CIRCULATION

Circulation through the heart is shown in the following diagram, which identifies the cardiac chambers, valves, and direction of blood flow. Blood from the body's organs and tissues empties from the superior and inferior venae cavae into the right atrium, travels through the tricuspid valve to the right ventricle, and then is pushed through the pulmonic valve into the pulmonary artery. Once the blood has travelled through the lungs, it returns to the left atrium via the pulmonary veins, moves through the mitral valve into the left ventricle, and is pumped through the aortic valve into the aorta for distribution throughout the body. Because of their positions, the *tricuspid* and *mitral valves* are often called *atrioventricular valves*. The *aortic* and *pulmonic valves* are called *semilunar valves* because each of their leaflets is shaped like a half moon. Although this diagram shows all valves in an open position, they do not open simultaneously in the living heart.

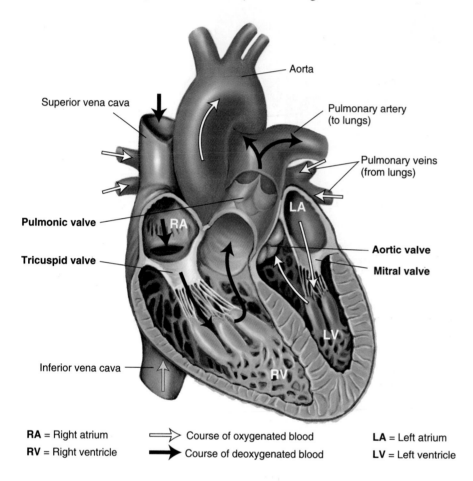

RA = Right atrium	⇒ Course of oxygenated blood	**LA** = Left atrium
RV = Right ventricle	⟹ Course of deoxygenated blood	**LV** = Left ventricle

As the heart valves close, the heart sounds arise from vibrations emanating from the leaflets, the adjacent cardiac structures, and the flow of blood. It is essential to understand the positions and movements of the valves in relation to events in the cardiac cycle.

■ EVENTS IN THE CARDIAC CYCLE

The heart serves as a pump that generates varying pressures as its chambers contract and relax. *Systole is the period of ventricular contraction.* In the following diagram, pressure in the left ventricle rises from less than 5 mm Hg in its resting state to a peak of 120 mm Hg. After the ventricle ejects much of its blood into the aorta, the pressure levels start falling down. *Diastole is the period of ventricular relaxation.* Ventricular pressure falls below 5 mm Hg, and blood flows from atrium to ventricle. Late in diastole, ventricular pressure rises slightly during the inflow of blood from atrial contraction.

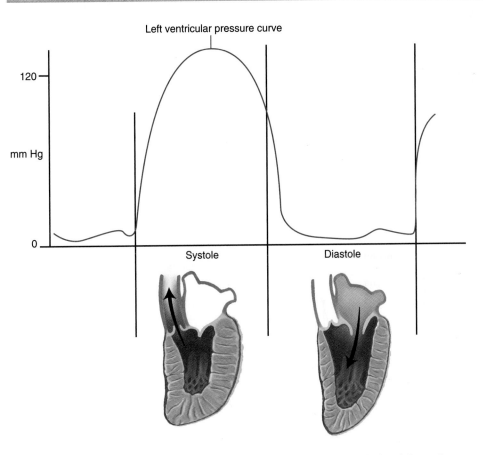

Left ventricular pressure curve

120

mm Hg

0

Systole   Diastole

Note that during *systole* the aortic valve is open, allowing ejection of blood from the left ventricle into the aorta. The mitral valve is closed, preventing blood from regurgitating back into the left atrium. In contrast, during *diastole* the aortic valve is closed, preventing regurgitation of blood from the aorta back into the left ventricle. The mitral valve is open and allows blood to flow from the left atrium into the relaxed left ventricle.

Understanding the interrelationships of the *pressure gradients* in these three chambers—left atrium, left ventricle, and aorta—together with the position and movement of the valves is fundamental to understanding heart sounds. Trace these changing pressures and sounds through one cardiac cycle. Note that during auscultation the first and second heart sounds define the duration of *systole* and *diastole*.

During *diastole*, pressure in the blood-filled left atrium slightly exceeds that in the relaxed left ventricle, and blood flows from left atrium to left ventricle across the open mitral valve. Just before the onset of ventricular systole, atrial contraction produces a slight pressure rise in both chambers.

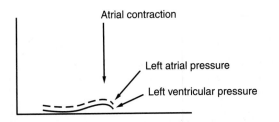

Atrial contraction

Left atrial pressure

Left ventricular pressure

During *systole*, the left ventricle starts to contract and ventricular pressure rapidly exceeds left atrial pressure, thus shutting the mitral valve. *Closure of the mitral valve produces the first heart sound, S_1.*

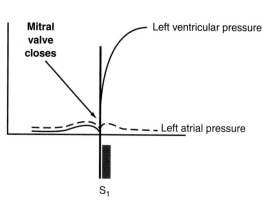

As left ventricular pressure continues to rise, it quickly exceeds the pressure in the aorta and forces the aortic valve open. In some pathologic conditions, opening of the aortic valve is accompanied by an early systolic ejection sound (Ej). *Maximal left ventricular pressure corresponds to systolic blood pressure.*

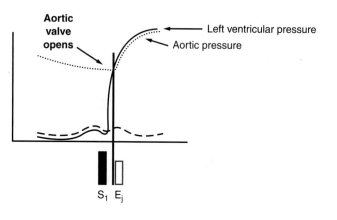

As the left ventricle ejects most of its blood, ventricular pressure begins to fall. When left ventricular pressure drops below aortic pressure, the aortic valve shuts. *Aortic valve closure produces the second heart sound, S_2, and another diastole begins.*

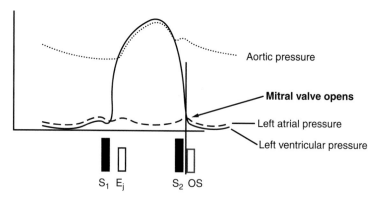

In *diastole*, left ventricular pressure continues to drop and falls below left atrial pressure. The mitral valve opens. This is usually a silent event, but may be audible as a pathologic opening snap (OS) if valve leaflet motion is restricted, as in mitral stenosis.

After the mitral valve opens, there is a period of rapid ventricular filling as blood flows early in diastole from left atrium to left ventricle. In children and young adults, a third heart sound, S_3, may arise from rapid deceleration of the column of blood against the ventricular wall. In older adults, an S_3, sometimes termed "an S_3 gallop," usually indicates a pathologic change in ventricular compliance.

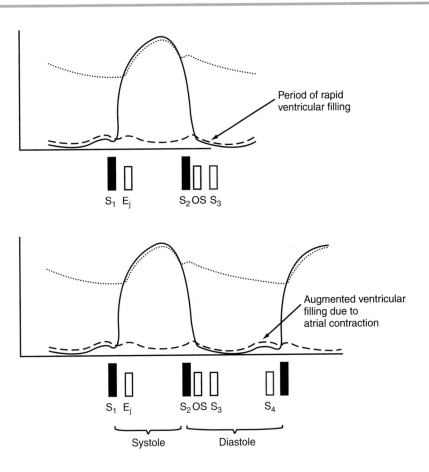

Period of rapid ventricular filling

S_1 E_j S_2 OS S_3

Finally, although not often heard in normal adults, a fourth heart sound, S_4, marks atrial contraction. It immediately precedes S_1 of the next beat, and also reflects a pathologic change in ventricular compliance.

Augmented ventricular filling due to atrial contraction

S_1 E_j S_2 OS S_3 S_4

Systole   Diastole

THE SPLITTING OF HEART SOUNDS

While these events are occurring on the left side of the heart, similar changes are occurring on the right, involving the right atrium, right ventricle, tricuspid valve, pulmonic valve, and pulmonary artery. Right ventricular and pulmonary arterial pressures are significantly lower than corresponding pressures on the left side. Furthermore, right-sided events usually occur slightly later than those on the left. Instead of a single heart sound, you may hear two discernible components, the first from left-sided aortic valve closure, or A_2, and the second from right-sided closure of the pulmonic valve, or P_2.

Consider the second heart sound and its two components, A_2 and P_2, which come from closure of the aortic and pulmonic valves, respectively. During inspiration A_2 and P_2 separate slightly and may split S_2 into its two audible components. During expiration, these two components are fused into a single sound, S_2. Splitting of the S_2 heart sound may be difficult to hear in older adults because of increased AP diameter of the chest.

HEART MURMURS

At some time over the life span, almost everyone has a heart murmur. Most murmurs occur without other cardiovascular symptoms, and may, therefore, be considered innocent deviations from the expected.

To identify murmurs accurately, you must learn to assess the chest-wall location where they are best heard, their timing in systole or diastole, and their qualities. In the section on Techniques of Examination, you will learn to integrate several characteristics, including murmur intensity, pitch, duration, and direction of radiation (see pp. 445–462).

Murmurs may also originate in large blood vessels. For example, a jugular venous hum is commonly heard in children, as is a cervical systolic murmur or bruit. The auscultation of a similar bruit in adults may indicate arterial obstruction.

RELATION OF AUSCULTATORY FINDINGS TO THE CHEST WALL

The locations on the chest wall where you hear heart sounds and murmurs help to identify the valve or chamber where they originate. Sounds and murmurs arising from the mitral valve are usually heard best at and around the cardiac apex. Those originating in the tricuspid valve are heard best at or near the lower left sternal border. Murmurs arising from the pulmonic valve are usually heard best in the 2nd and 3rd left intercostal spaces close to the sternum, but at times may also be heard at higher or lower levels, and those originating in the aortic valve may be heard anywhere from the right 2nd intercostal space to the apex. These areas overlap, as illustrated, and you will need to compare auscultatory findings with other portions of the cardiac examination to identify sounds and murmurs accurately.

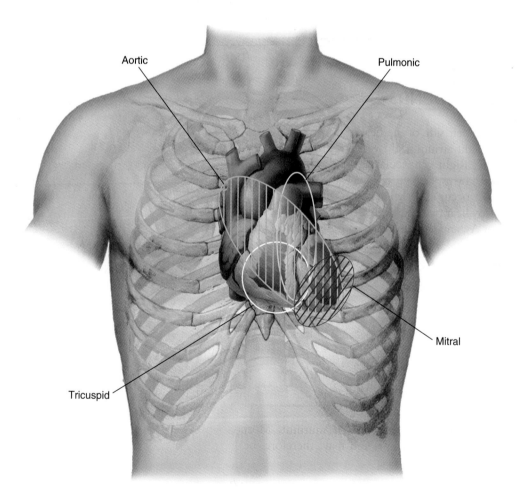

THE CONDUCTION SYSTEM

An electrical conduction system stimulates and coordinates the contraction of cardiac muscle.

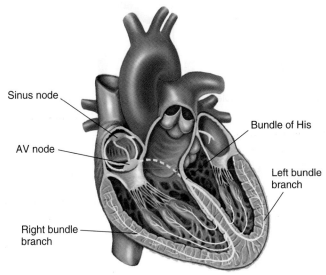

Each electrical impulse is initiated in the *sinus node*, a group of specialized cardiac cells located in the right atrium near the junction of the vena cava. The sinus node acts as the cardiac pacemaker and automatically discharges an impulse about 60 to 100 times a minute. This impulse travels through both atria to the *atrioventricular node*, a specialized group of cells located low in the atrial septum. Here the impulse is delayed before passing down the bundle of His and its branches to the ventricular myocardium. Muscular contraction follows: first the atria, then the ventricles. The expected conduction pathway is illustrated in simplified form.

The electrocardiogram, or ECG, records these events. Contraction of cardiac smooth muscle produces electrical activity, resulting in a series of waves on the ECG. The components of the *ECG* and their duration are briefly summarized here, but you will need further instruction and practice to interpret recordings from actual clients. The term *normal sinus rhythm* is used when discussing the conduction system of the heart and ECG findings. Note:

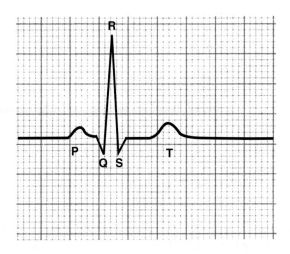

- The small *P wave* of atrial depolarization, which causes atrial contraction (duration up to 80 milliseconds; *PR interval* 120–200 milliseconds)

- The larger *QRS complex* of ventricular depolarization, which causes ventricular contraction (up to 100 milliseconds), consisting of one or more of the following:

  - The *Q wave*, a downward deflection from septal depolarization

  - The *R wave*, an upward deflection from ventricular depolarization

  - The *S wave*, a downward deflection following an R wave

- A *T wave* of ventricular repolarization, or recovery (duration relates to QRS)

The electrical impulse slightly precedes the myocardial contraction that it stimulates. The relation of electrocardiographic waves to the cardiac cycle is shown in the following diagram.

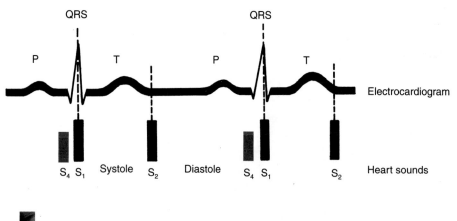

THE HEART AS A PUMP

The left and right ventricles pump blood into the systemic and pulmonary arterial trees, respectively. *Cardiac output*, the volume of blood ejected from each ventricle during 1 minute, is the product of *heart rate* and *stroke volume*. Stroke volume (the volume of blood ejected with each heartbeat) depends in turn on preload, myocardial contractility, and afterload.

Preload refers to the load that stretches the cardiac muscle before contraction. The volume of blood in the right ventricle at the end of diastole, then, constitutes its preload for the next beat. Right ventricular preload is increased by increasing venous return to the right heart. Physiologic causes include inspiration and the increased volume of blood flow from exercising muscles. The increased blood volume in a dilated right ventricle of congestive heart failure also increases preload. Causes of decreased right ventricular preload include exhalation, decreased left ventricular output, and pooling of blood in the capillary bed or the venous system.

Myocardial contractility refers to the ability of the cardiac muscle, when given a load, to shorten. Contractility increases when stimulated by action of the sympathetic nervous system, and decreases when blood flow or oxygen delivery to the myocardium is impaired.

Afterload refers to the degree of vascular resistance to ventricular contraction. Sources of resistance to left ventricular contraction include the tone in the walls of the aorta, the large arteries, and the peripheral vascular tree (primarily the small arteries and arterioles), as well as the volume of blood already in the aorta.

Pathologic increases in preload and afterload, called *volume overload* and *pressure overload*, respectively, produce changes in ventricular function that may be clinically detectable. These changes include alterations in ventricular impulses, detectable by palpation, and in usual heart sounds. Pathologic heart sounds and murmurs may also develop.

ARTERIAL PULSES AND BLOOD PRESSURE

With each contraction, the left ventricle ejects a volume of blood into the aorta and on into the arterial tree. The ensuing pressure wave moves rapidly through the arterial system, where it is felt as the *arterial pulse*. Although the pressure wave travels quickly—many times faster than the blood itself—a palpable delay between ventricular contraction and peripheral pulses makes the pulses in the arms and legs unsuitable for timing events in the cardiac cycle.

Blood pressure in the arterial system varies during the cardiac cycle, peaking in systole and falling to its lowest trough in diastole. These are the levels that are measured with the blood pressure cuff or sphygmomanometer. The difference between systolic and diastolic pressures is known as the *pulse pressure.*

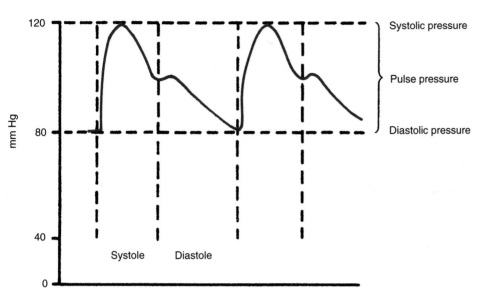

The principal factors influencing arterial pressure are as follows:

■ Left ventricular stroke volume

■ Distensibility of the aorta and the large arteries

■ Peripheral vascular resistance, particularly at the arteriolar level

■ Volume of blood in the arterial system

Changes in any of these four factors alter systolic pressure, diastolic pressure, or both. Blood pressure levels fluctuate strikingly through any 24-hour period, varying with physical activity; emotional state; pain; noise; environmental temperature; the use of coffee, tobacco, and other drugs; and even the time of day.

JUGULAR VENOUS PRESSURE

Systemic venous pressure is much lower than arterial pressure. Although venous pressure ultimately depends on left ventricular contraction, much of this force is dissipated as blood flows through the arterial tree and the capillary bed. Walls of veins contain less smooth muscle than walls of arteries. This reduces venous tone and makes veins more distensible. Other important determinants of venous pressure include blood volume and the capacity of the right heart to eject blood into the pulmonary arterial system. Cardiac disease may alter these variables, producing abnormalities in central venous pressure. For example, venous pressure falls when left ventricular output or blood volume is significantly reduced; it rises when blood backs up in the venous system, as with right-sided heart failure. These venous pressure changes are reflected in the height of the column of blood in the internal jugular veins, termed the *jugular venous pressure* or *JVP*.

Pressure in the jugular veins reflects right atrial pressure, giving clinicians an important clinical indicator of cardiac function and right heart hemodynamics. Assessing the JVP is an essential, though challenging, clinical skill. The JVP is best estimated from the internal jugular vein, usually on the *right side*, because the right internal jugular vein has a more direct anatomic channel into the right atrium (Cook & Simel, 1996).

The internal jugular veins lie deep to the sternomastoid muscles in the neck and are not directly visible, so the clinician must learn to identify the *pulsations* of the internal jugular vein that are transmitted to the surface of the neck, making sure to carefully distinguish these venous pulsations from pulsations of the carotid artery. If pulsations from the internal jugular vein cannot be identified, those of the external jugular vein can be used, but they are less reliable.

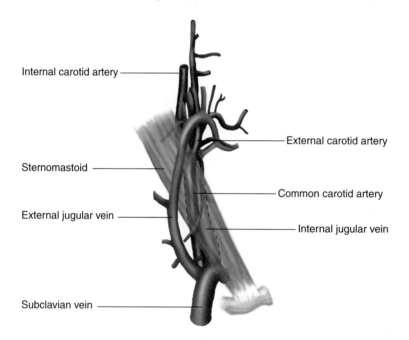

To estimate the level of the JVP, you will learn to find the *highest point of oscillation in the internal jugular vein* or, if necessary, the point above which the external jugular vein appears collapsed. The JVP is usually measured in vertical distance above the *sternal angle*, the bony ridge adjacent to the second rib where the manubrium joins the body of the sternum.

Study the following illustrations carefully. Note that regardless of the client's position, the sternal angle remains roughly 5 cm above the right atrium. In this client, however, the pressure in the internal jugular vein is somewhat elevated.

■ In *Position A*, the head of the bed is raised to the usual level, about 30°, but the JVP cannot be measured because the meniscus, or level of oscillation, is above the jaw and, therefore, not visible.

■ In *Position B*, the head of the bed is raised to 60°. The "top" of the internal jugular vein is now easily visible, so the vertical distance from the sternal angle or right atrium can now be measured.

■ In *Position C*, the client is upright and the veins are barely discernible above the clavicle, making measurement untenable.

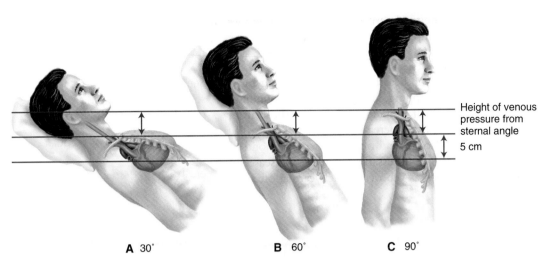

Height of venous pressure from sternal angle

5 cm

A 30°   **B** 60°   **C** 90°

Note that the height of the venous pressure as measured from the sternal angle is the *same* in all three positions, but your ability to *measure* the height of the column of venous blood, or JVP, differs according to how you position the client. Jugular venous pressure measured at more than 4 cm above the sternal angle, or more than 9 cm above the right atrium, is considered elevated. The techniques for measuring the JVP are fully described in Techniques of Examination on pp. 446–448.

The oscillations that you may see in the internal jugular veins, called jugular venous pulsations, reflect changing pressures within the right atrium. The right internal jugular vein empties more directly into the right atrium and reflects these pressure changes best.

THE HEALTH HISTORY: SUBJECTIVE DATA

Key Symptoms and Signs Reported by Client

- Chest pain
- Jaw pain
- Heartburn (pyrosis)
- Racing heart (palpitations)
- Shortness of breath (dyspnea, orthopnea, and paroxysmal nocturnal dyspnea)
- Swelling (edema)

- Fatigue
- Nausea and/or vomiting
- Heavy sweating (diaphoresis)
- Weakness
- Impending fear of death or sense of doom
- Lightheadedness
- Shoulder pain (left)

Chest pain or discomfort is one of the most important symptoms you will assess as a clinician. As you listen to the client's concerns, you must always keep serious adverse events in mind, such as *angina pectoris, myocardial infarction,* or even a *dissecting aortic aneurysm* (Goldman & Kirtane, 2003; Lee & Goldman, 2000; Snow et al., 2004). A review of the Health History section of Chapter 14, The Thorax and Lungs, which enumerates the other possible sources of chest pain, is helpful. This review is important, because symptoms such as dyspnea, wheezing, cough, and even hemoptysis (see pp. 413–417) can be cardiac as well as pulmonary in origin.

Begin the health history by asking the client general open-ended questions, such as, "Describe how you are feeling," or "Tell me about any concerns you are having

Exertional chest pain with radiation to the left side of the neck and down

about how you are feeling." Ask the client to describe his or her key sign or symptom by conducting an analysis of the symptom.

Palpitations are an unpleasant awareness of the heartbeat. When reporting these sensations, clients use various terms, such as skipping, racing, fluttering, pounding, or stopping of the heart. Palpitations may result from an irregular heartbeat, from rapid acceleration or slowing of the heart, or from increased forcefulness of cardiac contraction. Such perceptions, however, also depend on how clients respond to their own body sensations. Palpitations do not necessarily mean heart disease. In contrast, the most serious dysrhythmias, such as ventricular tachycardia, often do not produce palpitations.

the left arm in angina pectoris; sharp pain radiating into the back or into the neck in *aortic dissection*.

See Tables 15-1 and 15-2 for selected heart rates and rhythms (pp. 467–468).

Symptoms or signs of irregular heart action warrant an electrocardiogram. Only *atrial fibrillation*, which is "irregularly irregular," can be reliably identified at the bedside.

Example of Questions for Symptom/Sign Analysis—Chest Pain

- "Point to where the pain is." "Does it radiate?" "Where does it radiate?" (Location, radiating)
- "Describe your chest pain." "Is it crushing?" "Does it feel like there is something heavy on your chest?" (Quality)
- "Rate your chest pain on a scale of 0-10, with 0 being no pain and 10 being the worst pain you can imagine." "Does chest pain ever wake you up at night?" (Severity)
- "When did you start having chest pain?" "What kinds of activities bring on the pain?" (Onset)
- "Has the chest pain been present since it first started?" "How long does your chest pain last?" (Duration)
- "Have there been times that the pain seemed less?" (Constancy)

- "Is there a time of day that the pain seems worse? Or better?" (Time of day/month/year)
- "What makes the pain worse?" "Does it happen when you exert yourself?" (Aggravating factors)
- "What makes it better?" (Alleviating factors)
- "Do you have any other symptoms with your chest pain?" "Shortness of breath?" "Sweating?" "Palpitations?" "Nausea?" (Associated symptoms)
- "Have you had any recent changes in your life?" "Describe the amount of stress in your life right now." "Have you been exposed to any chemicals or other substances?" (Environmental factors)
- "How is this chest pain affecting your life?" (Significance to client)
- "What do you think may be causing your chest pain?" (Client perspective)

You may ask directly about palpitations, but if the client does not understand your question, reword it. "Are you ever aware of your heartbeat? What is it like?" Ask the client to tap out the rhythm with a hand or finger. Was it fast or slow? Regular or irregular? How long did it last? If there was an episode of rapid heartbeats, did they start and stop suddenly or gradually? (For this group of symptoms, an ECG is indicated.)

Shortness of breath is a common client concern and may represent dyspnea, orthopnea, or paroxysmal nocturnal dyspnea. *Dyspnea* is an uncomfortable awareness of breathing that is inappropriate to a given level of exertion. This concern is often made by clients with cardiac or pulmonary problems, as discussed in Chapter 14, The Thorax and Lungs, p. 381.

Orthopnea is dyspnea that occurs when the client is lying down and improves when the client sits up. Classically, it is quantified according to the number of pillows the client uses for sleeping, or by the fact that the client needs to sleep sitting up. Make sure, however, that the reason the client uses extra pillows or sleeps upright is shortness of breath when supine and not other causes.

Paroxysmal nocturnal dyspnea, or *PND*, describes episodes of sudden dyspnea and orthopnea that awaken the client from sleep, usually 1 or 2 hours after going to bed,

Clues in the history include transient skips and flip-flops (possible premature contractions); rapid regular beating of sudden onset and offset (possible paroxysmal supraventricular tachycardia); a rapid regular rate of less than 120 beats per minute, especially if starting and stopping more gradually (possible sinus tachycardia).

Orthopnea suggests *left ventricular heart failure* or *mitral stenosis*; it may also accompany obstructive lung disease.

PND suggests *left ventricular heart failure* or *mitral stenosis* and may prompting the client to sit up, stand up, or go to a window for air. There may be associated wheezing and coughing. The episode usually subsides but may recur at about the same time on subsequent nights.

Edema refers to the accumulation of excessive fluid in the interstitial tissue spaces and appears as swelling. Questions about edema are typically included in the cardiac history, but edema has many other causes, both local and general. Focus your questions on the location, timing, and setting of the swelling, and on associated symptoms. "Have you had any swelling anywhere? Where? . . . Anywhere else? When does it occur? Is it worse in the morning or at night? Do your shoes get tight?"

Continue with "Are the rings tight on your fingers? Are your eyelids puffy or swollen in the morning? Have you had to let out your belt?" Also, "Have your clothes gotten too tight around the middle?" It is useful to ask clients who retain fluid to record daily morning weights, because edema may not be obvious until several litres of extra fluid have accumulated.

be mimicked by nocturnal asthma attacks.

Dependent edema appears in the lowest body parts: the feet and lower legs when sitting, or the sacrum when bedridden. Causes may be cardiac (*congestive heart failure*), nutritional (*hypoalbuminemia*), or positional. See p. 570 in Chapter 18 for more information on edema in the legs.

Edema occurs in renal and liver disease: periorbital puffiness, tight rings in *nephritic syndrome;* enlarged waistline from ascites and *liver failure.*

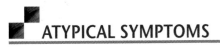

ATYPICAL SYMPTOMS

Sometimes, atypical symptoms such as pain referred to the jaw, back, or inner aspect of the upper left arm may be the only indication of a cardiovascular event. Other possible examples include heavy sweating (diaphoresis), weakness, nausea and vomiting, and a general sense of doom or fear of impending death. Older adults may describe a change in their ability to concentrate, remember things, or perform tasks such as writing a letter or balancing a chequebook. Nurses need to be aware that these changes in mentation may result from inadequate perfusion related to myocardial infarction (MI) or increasingly severe chronic heart failure.

Atypical presentations are frequent and require health care providers to investigate associated symptoms and concomitant health issues and diseases for a complete diagnostic picture. A thorough health history and focused assessment are essential nursing actions to ensure appropriate client care.

CONSIDERATIONS FOR WOMEN

The existing description of "typical" cardiac symptoms is based primarily on the experience of Caucasian, middle-aged men. Most research related to coronary heart disease (CHD) throughout the 1970s and 1980s excluded women, because CHD was not seen as a major health threat to them, and the predominant belief was that their symptoms would mirror men's (Kyker & Limacher, 2002). While chest pain remains the primary indicator of acute MI in both sexes, current research suggests women experience significantly different prodromal symptoms than men (McSweeney, Marisue, & Crane, 2001). Prodromal symptoms are those that occur intermittently within the month preceding an acute MI. The classic prodromal symptom associated with MI is angina or temporary chest pain. While recent studies show that more than 50% of men experience this classic symptom, they also show that as few as 30% of women report such chest discomfort (McSweeney et al., 2003). The most common prodromal symptoms of MI in women, ranging from mild to severe, are unusual fatigue, sleep disturbances, shortness of breath, indigestion, and anxiety (McSweeney et al., 2003). Headache and back pain also are common (Norris, Dasgupta, & Kirkland, 2006). Notably, many of the standardized screening tests in use have been developed and validated for men, but not for women (DeVon & Johnson Zerwic, 2002).

According to the Heart and Stroke Foundation of Canada (2007a), the gender-related difference in symptoms may be less pronounced than some of the literature suggests and more indicative of how men and women report symptoms rather than the symptoms themselves. Regardless, it is vital for nurses to understand these differences in their roles as health care providers and educators.

HEALTH PROMOTION

Important Topics for Health Promotion

- Prevention of cardiovascular disease and stroke
- Prevention of hypertension
- Lowering cholesterol and low-density lipoprotein (LDL)
- Metabolic syndrome
- Risk factor assessment
- Hormone replacement therapy

Despite improvements in risk factor modification, cardiovascular disease (CVD) remains the number one cause of death for Canadians and places a higher economic burden on the Canadian health care system than any other disease or injury category (Heart and Stroke Foundation of Canada, 2003). Both primary prevention in clients without CVD and secondary prevention in those with known cardiovascular events (e.g., angina, MI) remain important priorities for nurses in all health care settings. Education and support are essential to help clients prevent or contend with CVD; maintain optimal levels of blood pressure, weight, and cholesterol; and understand their relevant risk factors.

PREVENTION OF CARDIOVASCULAR DISEASE AND STROKE

Approximately 55% of all cardiovascular deaths in Canada are related to coronary artery disease (CAD), which involves *atherosclerosis* (hardening of the arteries that supply oxygenated blood to the heart muscle; Public Health Agency of Canada, 2003). CAD is also the leading cause of hospitalization in Canada. It is the leading cause of death for men 50 years or older and women 70 years or older (Heart and Stroke Foundation of Canada, 2006). Through programs such as the Cardiovascular Action Plan and the Healthy Heart Kit, Health Canada and its partners (i.e., the Heart and Stroke Foundation of Canada and Blood Pressure Canada) have placed the challenge for implementing risk factor reduction squarely on the shoulders of health practitioners. As nurses are often the primary contact for clients who access the health care system, they are in an opportune position to initiate health promotion to prevent CVD.

Despite a decrease in fatalities from CVD between 1988 and 1998, up to 40% of initial or recurring cardiovascular events, including MI, stroke, and aortic aneurysm, are fatal or disabling. Research shows that even if they survive the initial attack, up to 25% of men and 32% of women die within 1 year after MI (Tanuseputro, Manuel, Leung, Nguyen, & Johansen, 2003). It is imperative to prevent cardiovascular emergencies through early identification of risk factors and client adoption of healthy habits to counteract or control them. Risk factors for CVD vary, and include hypertension, hyperlipidemia, demographics, and lifestyle factors.

Prevention of Hypertension. In 2002, the World Health Organization (WHO) listed high blood pressure (*hypertension*) as the leading risk factor for death in North America (Blood Pressure Canada et al., 2007). Hypertension is a leading cause of death for Canadians and of health complications such as strokes, heart attacks, kidney failure, dementia, and sexual problems (Blood Pressure Canada et al., 2007). Research also shows that control of high blood pressure can prevent these problems. Medications are available for blood pressure management; however, much evidence-based research indicates clients' lifestyle choices can influence their susceptibility to hypertension, avoiding or delaying the need for pharmaceutical interventions. These choices include stopping smoking, consuming a healthy diet in accordance with Canada's Food Guide, performing regular physical activity, consuming alcohol in moderation only, reducing dietary sodium, and reducing stress (Blood Pressure Canada et al., 2007; Health Canada, 2007a).

The Canadian Hypertension Education Program (2007) outlines the following diagnostic criteria for various levels of hypertension and recommended actions for each:

- Expected blood pressure for a healthy person is approximately 120/80 mm Hg or less.

- Blood pressure with a systolic reading of 130 to 139 mm Hg, a diastolic reading of 85 to 89 mm Hg, or both is termed "high normal," and indicates a need for regular pressure monitoring as well as lifestyle modification aimed at reduction of blood pressure to a healthy level. More than half of people with high normal blood pressure who do not make appropriate lifestyle changes develop hypertension within 4 years (Canadian Hypertension Education Program, 2007). The 2007 report marked the first time recommendations focused on the significance of high normal blood pressure.

- Hypertension is diagnosed:

  - When a client's blood pressure readings are higher than 140/90 mm Hg on five visits to a health care professional

  - When a client's blood pressure readings are higher than 160/100 mm Hg on three visits to a health care professional

  - When a client's blood pressure readings are higher than 180/110 mm Hg on two visits to a health care professional over a short period

- Blood pressure above 200/120 mm Hg is extremely high and qualifies for immediate diagnosis of hypertension.

- Clients with kidney disease or diabetes are diagnosed with hypertension if their blood pressure is above 130/80 mm Hg after only two visits to a health care professional.

It is essential for nurses to understand the most current parameters, risk factors, and usual actions taken for the various levels of hypertension. Treatment often progresses from modification of lifestyle factors only, to use of a single medication in addition to lifestyle changes, to use of multiple medications with lifestyle alterations. A decrease in blood pressure of 10/5 mm Hg, achievable through lifestyle change in those with high normal pressure, decreases the chances of heart failure by 50%, stroke by 38%, heart attack by 15%, and death by 10% (Blood Pressure Canada et al., 2007). Research also shows that simple, brief interventions by health care providers can increase client adherence to lifestyle changes and compliance with prescribed medications. The need for health promotion with all clients is urgent. Appropriate and effective client education can make a potential difference to individual clients and the overall population.

Lowering Cholesterol, LDL, and VLDL. A 2003 report from the Canadian Medical Association (CMA) directly correlated high serum cholesterol levels (dyslipidemia) with CVD and provided evidence-based recommendations for management (Genest, Fodor, & McPherson, 2003). High overall levels of cholesterol present a significant risk to cardiovascular health, and low-density lipoprotein cholesterol (LDL-C) is the most significant cause of plaque buildup in blood vessels, leading to CVD and stroke (Canadian Medical Association, 2007). Very low density lipoproteins (VLDL) contain the highest amount of triglyceride, which results in increased buildup of cholesterol on the arterial walls. Increased VLDL levels and decreased high-density lipoprotein (HDL) levels contribute to atherosclerosis (Public Health Agency of Canada, 2007; WebMD, 2007) and increase the risk for heart disease and stroke (WebMD, 2007).

Dyslipidemia is generally asymptomatic and can exist undetected for many years. Routine blood tests can reveal the problem, but clients who do not undergo regular routine physical examinations may not be diagnosed before a cardiac event or stroke. Canadian guidelines recommend screening for men older than 40 years, women older than 50 years or postmenopausal, clients with diabetes, those with a strong family history of CVD, and those with risk factors, including hypertension, smoking, or abdominal obesity (Canadian Lipid Nurse Network, 2003). Screening is accomplished through a fasting lipoprotein profile that indicates levels of total and LDL cholesterol in the blood. Risk categories and target LDL-C levels are described on the previous page.

■ Risk Categories and Target Lipid Levels

Risk Category	Description	Target LDL-C
High risk	Includes: ■ Clients with established cardiovascular disease ■ Clients with chronic kidney disease ■ Adults with diabetes ■ Clients with a greater than 20% risk of death from CAD in the next 10 years	<4.5 mmol/L
Intermediate risk	Clients with 11–19% risk of death from CAD in the next 10 years	<3.5 mmol/L
Low risk	Clients with less than 10% risk of death from CAD in the next 10 years	<2.5 mmol/L

Information obtained from Genest, J. F., Fodor, G., & McPherson, R. (2003). Recommendations for the management of dyslipidemia and the prevention of cardiovascular disease. *Canadian Medical Association Journal, 169*(9), and Canadian Lipid Nurse Network. (2003). Recommendations for dyslipidemia management in Canada. Retrieved November 22, 2007, from http://lipidnurse.ca/edu_pro_managing_dyslipidemia.asp.

The "risk of death from CAD" in the previous chart is determined by a risk assessment tool developed from the internationally influential Framingham Heart

Study, done in the 1950s. The CMA endorses this tool, which calculates a person's risk of death from CAD in the next 10 years based on several factors, including blood pressure, fasting lipoprotein levels, and risks such as diabetes and obesity (http://www.americanheart.org/presenter.jhtml?identifier=3003499).

According to CMA guidelines, optimal treatment of dyslipidemia includes therapeutic lifestyle measures such as exercise, smoking cessation, and weight loss, as well as medications if deemed necessary by a physician. Pharmaceutical interventions are generally considered for clients at intermediate and high risk.

Metabolic Syndrome. Metabolic syndrome is a group of risk factors that together greatly increase a client's chance of developing CVD (Canadian Lipid Nurse Network, 2003). Clinical identification of this syndrome requires four factors: a large waist circumference (>102 cm for men, >88 cm for women), otherwise known as abdominal obesity; elevated blood pressure; high fasting blood glucose level, as determined by blood tests; and abnormal fat levels in the blood, characterized by high overall triglycerides, low levels of high-density lipoprotein cholesterol, or both (Blood Pressure Canada et al., 2007; Canadian Lipid Nurse Network, 2003). Nurses promote awareness of these factors in their clients and encourage primary prevention tactics, such as healthy lifestyle choices and screening for clients at risk.

Risk Factor Assessment. Studies show that 80% of Canadians have at least one cardiovascular risk factor (Heart and Stroke Foundation of Canada, 2003, 2006). Risk factors are classified as either uncontrollable or controllable. Uncontrollable factors are those that a client has no ability to change, such as age, sex, genetics, and race. Controllable, or modifiable, risk factors include hypertension, blood cholesterol levels, and lifestyle factors such as smoking, obesity, physical inactivity, unhealthy eating, uncontrolled diabetes, and ineffective stress management.

Health Canada in collaboration with partners (i.e., The Heart and Stroke Foundation of Canada and provincial governments) has aimed many strategies, programs, and initiatives at preventing CVD. The Canadian Heart Health Initiative, launched in 1996, is recognized worldwide as a model for significant reduction of CVD and its societal burden. Its goals are to reduce premature illness and death from heart disease, as well as the prevalence of modifiable risk factors.

Demographics. Demographic risk factors include age, sex, and genetics. Risk of developing heart disease increases with age. Men older than 45 years and postmenopausal women older than 55 years are at increased risk. Men have a higher risk of CVD than women until women go through menopause, when the risk becomes even. Genetics also play a role in susceptibility. For example, research has shown that people of First Nations, African, and South Asian descent are more likely to develop hypertension and diabetes, and therefore, CVD and stroke, than people of other backgrounds.

Family History. Risk of developing heart disease is greater if one or more immediate family members (mother, father, and siblings) have had an MI, hypertension, or high cholesterol. The risk increases if a female family member is diagnosed with or has a cardiac event before age 65 years or a male member is diagnosed with or has a cardiac event before age 55 years.

Lifestyle Factors. Modifiable lifestyle choices that influence risk for CVD include smoking, physical inactivity, uncontrolled diabetes, obesity, unhealthy eating, and unmanaged stress. The WHO rates tobacco use as the second highest risk factor for death in North America, following hypertension (Blood Pressure Canada et al., 2007). Other major risk factors for death that are also lifestyle risk factors for CVD include being overweight, lack of fruits and vegetables in the diet, and inactivity.

Smoking has several harmful effects on the heart and vasculature. Carbon monoxide binds to hemoglobin in the blood, making it more difficult for oxygen to circulate to all body tissues, and nicotine increases heart rate, both of which make the heart work harder (Canadian Health Network, 2007a). Nicotine also is a vasoconstrictor and causes increased buildup of plaque on the walls of the arteries, which leads to hypertension and can cause blood clots (Canadian Health Network, 2007a). Smoking is physically addictive, because the body craves the tar and nicotine in cigarettes; the addiction is also psychological, social, behavioural, and emotional. Within 1 year after a person stops smoking, the risk of heart disease is halved and continues to drop over time (Canadian Health Network, 2007a). Benefits from smoking cessation are not limited to the cardiovascular system, but extend to almost every system in the body, making associated health promotion efforts a priority activity for nurses. Many smoking cessation resources are available to nurses and their clients, including evidence-based information and cessation plans from the Canadian Council for Tobacco Control (2007) and the Canadian Cancer Society (2007).

Obesity, another modifiable lifestyle factor, has a major influence on cardiovascular risk. Prevalence of obesity among Canadians, as determined by a Body Mass Index (BMI) of more than 30, increases with age, peaking at 42% of those 50 to 59 years old (Tanuseputro et al., 2003). The BMI and waist circumference are the preferred measures for assessing risk of weight-related health problems. The limitations of BMI, the calculations of which are widely available in print and Internet resources such as Health Canada, are that it does not apply to pregnant or breastfeeding women, adults older than 65 years, or extremely muscular people. The BMI is useful for assessing other adults, however, and helping them set appropriate weight loss goals. The Public Health Agency of Canada (PHAC) recommends aiming for a BMI of 18.5 to 24.9 (Heart and Stroke Foundation of Canada, 2007b). People with excess weight around the abdomen (apple shape) versus around their hips (pear shape) are also at greater risk for CVD. Men should aim for a waist circumference of less than 102 cm, and women should aim for a waist circumference of less than 88 cm. The Canadian Heart and Stroke Foundation Web site has several practical recommendations of use to nurses who want to assist obese clients to attain a healthier weight.

Closely related to obesity is physical inactivity. Lack of exercise has become an epidemic in North America over the past decade. One study showed that more than half of Canadians older than 12 years are physically inactive (Health Canada, 2007b). A sedentary lifestyle is more prevalent in Canadian women than men. Research shows that 30 to 60 minutes of moderate physical activity most days lowers a person's risk of heart disease. Indications to help clients identify that they are reaching a level of exercise intensity to reap the benefits of aerobic metabolism include deep breathing, sweating in cool temperatures, and pulse rates exceeding 60% of the maximum age-adjusted heart rate (220 minus the client's age). Such physical activity does not have to happen all at once. Nurses can advise clients to add several 10-minute increments of physical activity into their lives throughout the day. Nurses and other health care providers must consider the client's existing cardiovascular, pulmonary, and musculoskeletal conditions before encouraging an exercise regimen.

An unhealthy diet is another related risk factor for CVD. Evidence-based literature recommends a heart-healthy diet rich in a variety of fruits and vegetables, whole grains, and low-fat dairy products. Based on current research, the Heart and Stroke Foundation of Canada also recommends the following:

■ Limit meat consumption and obtain protein from alternative sources such as beans, nuts, and fish.

■ Consume 25 to 30 g of fibre daily.

■ Limit fat to 20% to 35% of daily calories, and choose unsaturated fats and foods high in omega-3 fatty acids over saturated and trans fats.

■ Keep sodium consumption below 2400 mg per day (equivalent to 6 g or approximately 1 tsp of salt).

■ Keep daily alcoholic beverages to one or fewer for women and two or fewer for men (Canadian Health Network, 2007b).

Cultural Considerations

In 2007, Health Canada created and published a version of the national food guide to reflect the values, traditions, and diets of First Nations, Inuit, and Métis people. *Eating Well with Canada's Food Guide-First Nations, Inuit, and Métis* reflects the importance of both traditional and store-bought, nontraditional foods commonly available in rural and remote locations. It includes recommended servings of choices such as bannock, traditional meats, and wild game. The guide is based on scientific evidence, and addresses needs for healthy growth and development across the life span.

Canada's Food Guide to Healthy Eating, updated in 2007, offers an accessible health promotion tool for health care providers. For the first time, an adapted guide was also published with health promotion aimed at First Nations populations.

Uncontrolled diabetes mellitus presents another modifiable lifestyle risk to cardiovascular health. People with diabetes have an increased risk of hypertension, atherosclerosis, CAD, and stroke. Research shows that poor control of blood glucose levels compounds these risks (Tanuseputro et al., 2003). Nurses can help their clients with diabetes learn to monitor their blood glucose levels and to control their condition through diet, exercise, insulin administration, and oral antidiabetic medications.

The last modifiable risk factor is unmanaged stress. Researchers continue to investigate the direct link between stress and heart disease. Studies have confirmed positive correlations between stress and hypertension, dyslipidemia, and blood clots, all of which increase the risk for heart disease (Canadian Health Network, 2007c). Some stress is unavoidable, and may be positive when it drives and exhilarates a person, and stimulates the mind and body. In contrast, too much stress can take an unhealthy physical toll. Nurses help clients control their stress levels by assisting them to identify unhealthy ways of addressing stress and teaching healthy coping mechanisms. Tools are available from sources such as the Canadian Health Network (2007d) and the Canadian Mental Health Association (n.d.).

Cultural Considerations

The first Canadian primary prevention program for type 2 diabetes in a First Nations community began in 1994 in Kahnawake, an urban Mohawk community near Montreal, Quebec, with a high adult prevalence of the illness. Research findings indicated a potential correlation between Kahnawake's large proportion of overweight children and high rates of adult diabetes; thus, the program was developed for elementary school children and included a strong health promotion element, involving community health nurses. Investigations of the success of this program continue (Willows, 2005).

Hormone Replacement Therapy. A unique risk factor for CAD in older women is the postmenopausal state. As recently as 2002, the medical community believed that hormone replacement therapy (HRT; replacement of estrogen, progestin, or both), mainly used to manage menopausal symptoms, also had potential value as primary prevention of CVD. Studies have indicated, however, quite the opposite. Large randomized trials showed that women taking HRT had an increased incidence of MI and death from CAD, and increased risk for stroke and venous thromboembolism (Wathen, Feig, Feightner, Abramson, & Cheung, 2004). These adverse effects begin within the first year women take HRT and continue each subsequent year. Many trials were stopped before completion because of the health risks to the women involved. In light of this information and all the current research available at the time, the Canadian Task Force on Preventative Health Care concluded that evidence was sufficient to recommend against the use of HRT for primary prevention of CVD (Wathen et al., 2004).

The Canadian Consensus on Menopause and Osteoporosis makes two main recommendations regarding HRT with respect to CVD:

- HRT should not be used for the sole purpose of preventing cardiovascular events.

- All women should be educated on the benefits of lifestyle modifications such as smoking cessation, eating a heart-healthy diet, and maintaining ideal body weight for reducing the risk of CVD.

EMERGENCY CONCERNS

The PHAC states that Canadians wait approximately 5 hours before getting medical help for symptoms of MI. This finding is significant, because half of deaths from MI occur in the first 2 hours. It is critical to educate clients not to worry that their symptoms are a false alarm or sign of another condition. Delays in seeking medical attention cost people their lives. Currently, the Heart and Stroke Foundation of Canada recommends instructing clients if they experience any potential warning signs and symptoms of a heart attack to:

- Call 9-1-1 or the local emergency number, or get someone to call for them.

- Not to drive but to have someone drive them to a hospital or clinic.

- Stop all physical activity.

- Sit or lie down in a comfortable position.

- If taking nitroglycerine, take their usual dose.

■ Chew and swallow one adult 325 mg tablet of acetylsalicylic acid (ASA, brand name Aspirin). Or substitute two 80 mg tablets (children's ASA). Chewing is essential for getting the medication into the blood as fast as possible. Acetaminophen (e.g., Tylenol) or ibuprofen (e.g., Advil) do not work in the same way as ASA and will not help in this type of emergency.

■ Rest comfortably and wait for the ambulance to arrive.

TECHNIQUES OF EXAMINATION: OBJECTIVE DATA

CLIENT COMFORT, DIGNITY, AND SAFETY

It is essential to promote comfort and decrease anxiety for clients during all physical examination techniques. In a cardiovascular assessment, anxiety and discomfort can result in elevated blood pressure readings. For some clients, concerns about findings from assessment create anxiety and may alter results.

During cardiovascular assessment, a few simple actions can promote client comfort and safety. Provide adequate draping for women to prevent unnecessary exposure of the breasts. Place a blanket over the lower half of the body to help both male and female clients feel less exposed. Give specific instructions throughout the examination, explaining what is expected of the client. Encourage the client to breathe at a comfortable rate throughout. Perform hand hygiene, and ensure equipment such as stethoscopes are clean. Ensuring that the nurse's hands and stethoscope are both warm promotes client comfort. Finally, cardiac assessment may require several position changes. Explain the reason for them, assist the client as necessary, and ensure the client is comfortable in each position before proceeding with the examination.

As you begin the cardiovascular examination, review the blood pressure and heart rate recorded during the general survey and vital signs at the start of the physical examination. If you need to repeat these measurements, or if they have not already been done, take the time to measure the blood pressure and heart rate using optimal technique (see Chapter 6; Beevers, Lip, & O'Brien, 2001a, 2001b; Edmonds et al., 2002; McAlister & Straus, 2001; Tholl, Forstner, & Anlauf, 2004) General Survey and Vital Signs, especially pp. 140–141).

In brief, for *blood pressure*, after letting the client rest for at least 5 minutes in a quiet setting, choose a correctly sized cuff and position the client's arm at heart level, either resting on a table if seated or supported at midchest level if standing. Make sure the bladder of the cuff is centered over the brachial artery. Inflate the cuff about 30 mm Hg above the pressure at which the brachial or radial pulse disappears. As you deflate the cuff, listen first for the sounds of at least two consecutive heartbeats—these mark the *systolic* pressure. Then listen for the disappearance point of the heartbeats, which marks the *diastolic* pressure. For *heart rate*, measure the radial pulse using the pads of your index and middle fingers, or assess the apical pulse using your stethoscope (see p. 141).

Now you are ready to systematically assess the components of the cardiovascular system:

■ The jugular venous pressure and pulsations

■ The carotid upstrokes and presence or absence of bruits

- The point of maximal impulse (PMI) and any heaves, lifts, or thrills

- The first and second heart sounds, S_1 and S_2

- Presence or absence of extra heart sounds such as S_3 or S_4

- Presence or absence of any cardiac murmurs

Equipment

- Stethoscope with bell and diaphragm
- Sphygmomanometer
- Watch with second hand
- Metric rulers (two)
- Penlight
- Scale (weight and height)
- Doppler

JUGULAR VENOUS PRESSURE AND PULSATIONS

Estimating the JVP may seem difficult at first, but with practice and supervision you will find that the JVP provides valuable information about the client's volume status and cardiac function. The JVP reflects pressure in the right atrium, otherwise known as central venous pressure, and is best assessed from pulsations in the right internal jugular vein. Note, however, that the jugular veins and pulsations are difficult to see in children younger than 12 years, so they are not useful for evaluating the cardiovascular system in this age group.

To assist you in learning this portion of the cardiac examination, steps for assessing the JVP follow. As you begin your assessment, take a moment to reflect on the client's volume status and consider how you may need to alter the elevation of the head of the bed or examining table. In clients who are *hypovolemic*, you may anticipate that *the JVP will be low*, causing you to subsequently *lower the head of the bed*, sometimes even to 0°, to see the point of oscillation best. Likewise, in volume-overloaded or *hypervolemic* clients, you may anticipate that *the JVP will be high*, causing you to subsequently *raise the head of the bed*.

A hypovolemic client may have to lie flat before you see the neck veins. In contrast, when JVP is increased, an elevation up to 60° or even 90° may be required. In all these positions, the sternal angle usually remains approximately 5 cm above the right atrium, as diagrammed on p. 435.

STEPS FOR ASSESSING THE JUGULAR VENOUS PRESSURE (JVP)

- Make the client comfortable. *Raise the head slightly on a pillow* to relax the sternomastoid muscles.
- *Raise the head of the bed or examining table to about 30°. Turn the client's head slightly away from the side you are inspecting.*
- Use *tangential lighting* and examine both sides of the neck. Identify the external jugular vein on each side, then find the internal jugular venous pulsations.
- *If necessary, raise or lower the head of the bed* until you can see the oscillation point or meniscus of the internal jugular venous pulsations in the lower half of the neck.
- Focus on the *right internal jugular vein*. Look for pulsations in the suprasternal notch, between the attach-
ments of the sternomastoid muscle on the sternum and clavicle, or just posterior to the sternomastoid. The following table helps you distinguish internal jugular pulsations from those of the carotid artery.
- *Identify the highest point of pulsation in the right internal jugular vein.* Extend a long rectangular object or card horizontally from this point and a centimetre ruler vertically from the sternal angle, making an exact right angle. Measure the vertical distance in centimetres above the sternal angle where the horizontal object crosses the ruler. *This distance, measured in centimetres above the sternal angle or the right atrium, is the JVP.*

The following features help to distinguish jugular from carotid artery pulsations (Cook & Simel, 1996).

■ Distinguishing Internal Jugular and Carotid Pulsations

Internal Jugular Pulsations	Carotid Pulsations
Rarely palpable	Palpable
Soft, rapid, undulating quality, usually with two elevations and two troughs per heartbeat	A more vigourous thrust with a single outward component
Pulsations eliminated by light pressure on the vein(s) just above the sternal end of the clavicle	Pulsations not eliminated by this pressure
Level of the pulsations changes with position, dropping as the client becomes more upright	Level of the pulsations unchanged by position
Level of the pulsations usually descends with inspiration.	Level of the pulsations not affected by inspiration

Establishing the true vertical and horizontal lines to measure the JVP is difficult. Place your ruler on the sternal angle and line it up with something in the room that you know to be vertical. Then place a card or rectangular object at an exact right angle to the ruler. This constitutes your horizontal line. Move it up or down—still horizontal—so that the lower edge rests at the top of the jugular pulsations, and read the vertical distance on the ruler. Round your measurement off to the nearest centimetre.

Increased pressure suggests *right-sided congestive heart failure* or, less commonly, *constrictive pericarditis, tricuspid stenosis,* or *superior vena cava obstruction* (Aurigemma & Gaasch, 2004; Badgett, Lucey, & Muirow, 1997; Drazner et al., 2001; Jessup & Brozena, 2003; Khot, 2003; Lange & Hillis, 2004; Spodick, 2003).

In clients with obstructive lung disease, venous pressure may appear elevated on expiration only; the veins collapse on inspiration. This finding does not indicate congestive heart failure.

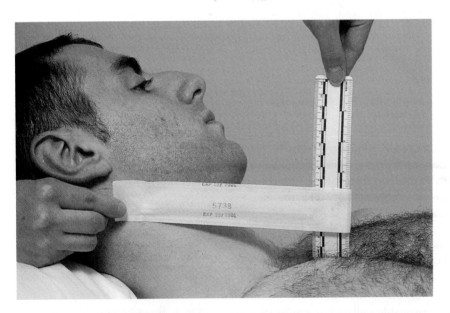

Venous pressure measured at greater than 3 cm or possibly 4 cm above the sternal angle, or more than 8 cm or 9 cm in total distance above the right atrium, is considered elevated *above expected values.*

If you cannot see pulsations in the internal jugular vein, look for them in the external jugular vein. If you see no pulsation, use *the point above which the external jugular veins appear to collapse.* Make this observation on each side of the neck. Measure the vertical distance of this point from the sternal angle.

The highest point of venous pulsations may lie below the level of the sternal angle. Under these circumstances, venous pressure is not elevated and seldom needs to be measured.

Unilateral distention of the external jugular vein is usually caused by local kinking or obstruction. Occasionally, even bilateral distention has a local cause.

Even though students may not see clinicians making these measurements very frequently in clinical settings, practicing exact techniques for measuring the JVP is important. Eventually, with experience, clinicians in cardiac care settings come to identify the JVP and estimate its height visually.

THE CAROTID PULSE

After you measure the JVP, move on to assessment of the *carotid pulse*. The carotid pulse provides valuable information about cardiac function and is especially useful for detecting stenosis or insufficiency of the aortic valve. Take the time to assess the quality of the carotid upstroke, its amplitude and contour, and presence or absence of any overlying *thrills* or *bruits*.

For irregular rhythms, see Table 15-1, Selected Heart Rates and Rhythms (p. 467), and Table 15-2, Selected Irregular Rhythms (p. 468).

To assess *amplitude and contour*, the client should be lying down with the head of the bed still elevated to about 30°. When feeling for the carotid artery, first inspect the neck for carotid pulsations. These may be visible just medial to the sternomastoid muscles. Then place your left index and middle fingers (or left thumb) on the right carotid artery in the lower third of the neck, press posteriorly, and feel for pulsations.

A tortuous and kinked carotid artery may produce a unilateral pulsatile bulge.

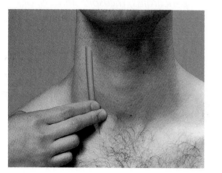
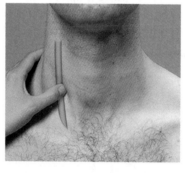

Decreased pulsations may be caused by decreased stroke volume, but may also result from local factors in the artery such as atherosclerotic narrowing or occlusion.

Press just inside the medial border of a well-relaxed sternomastoid muscle, roughly at the level of the cricoid cartilage. Avoid pressing on the *carotid sinus*, which lies at the level of the top of the thyroid cartilage. For the left carotid artery, use your right fingers or thumb. Never press both carotids at the same time. This may decrease blood flow to the brain and induce syncope.

Pressure on the carotid sinus may cause a reflex drop in pulse rate or blood pressure.

Slowly increase pressure until you feel a maximal pulsation, then slowly decrease pressure until you best sense the arterial pressure and contour. Try to assess:

■ The *amplitude of the pulse*. This correlates reasonably well with the pulse pressure.

Small, thready, or weak pulse in *cardiogenic shock; bounding* pulse in *aortic insufficiency* (see p. 449).

■ Any *variations in amplitude*, either from beat to beat or with respiration.

Pulsus alternans (see p. 461), bigeminal pulse (beat-to-beat variation); paradoxical pulse (respiratory variation).

Thrills and Bruits. During palpation of the carotid artery, you may detect humming vibrations, or *thrills*, which feel like the throat of a purring cat. Routinely, but especially in the presence of a thrill, listen over both carotid arteries with the diaphragm of your stethoscope for a *bruit*, a murmurlike sound of vascular rather than cardiac origin.

You should also listen for carotid bruits if the client is middle-aged or elderly or if you suspect cerebrovascular disease. Ask the client to hold breathing for a moment so that breath sounds do not obscure the vascular sound, then listen with the bell (Sauve et al., 1993). Heart sounds alone do not constitute a bruit.

A carotid bruit with or without a thrill in a middle-aged or older person suggests but does not prove arterial narrowing. An aortic murmur

Further examination of arterial pulses is described in Chapter 18, The Peripheral Vascular System.

The Brachial Artery.   The carotid arteries reflect aortic pulsations more accurately, but in clients with carotid obstruction, kinking, or thrills, they are unsuitable. If so, assess the pulse in the *brachial artery*, applying the techniques described previously for determining amplitude and contour.

Use the index and middle fingers or thumb of your opposite hand. Cup your hand under the client's elbow and feel for the pulse just medial to the biceps tendon. The client's arm should rest with the elbow extended, palm up. With your free hand, you may need to flex the elbow to a varying degree to get optimal muscular relaxation.

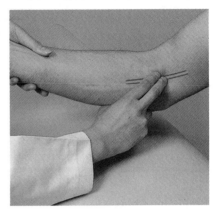

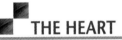
THE HEART

For most of the cardiac examination, the client should be *supine* with the upper body raised by elevating the head of the bed or table to about 30°. Two other positions are also needed: (1) *turning to the left side* and (2) *leaning forward*. These positions bring the ventricular apex and left ventricular outflow tract closer to the chest wall, enhancing detection of the PMI and aortic insufficiency. *The examiner should stand at the client's right side.*

The following table summarizes client positions and a suggested sequence for the examination.

■ *Sequence of the Cardiac Examination*

Client Position	Examination	Accentuated Findings
Supine, with the head elevated 30°	Inspect and palpate the precordium: the 2nd right and left intercostal spaces; the right ventricle; and the left ventricle, including the apical impulse (diameter, location, amplitude, duration).	
Left lateral decubitus	Palpate the apical impulse if not previously detected. Listen at the apex with the *bell* of the stethoscope.	Low-pitched extra sounds (S_3, opening snap, diastolic rumble of mitral stenosis)
Supine, with the head elevated 30°	Listen at the tricuspid area with the *bell*. Listen at all the auscultatory areas with the *diaphragm*.	
Sitting, leaning forward, after full exhalation	Listen along the left sternal border and at the apex with the *diaphragm*.	Soft decrescendo diastolic murmur of aortic insufficiency

During the cardiac examination, remember to correlate your findings with the client's JVP and carotid pulse. It is also important to identify both the anatomical location of your findings and their timing in the cardiac cycle.

■ Note the *anatomical location* of sounds in terms of intercostal spaces and their distance from the midsternal, midclavicular, or axillary lines. The midsternal line offers the most reliable zero point for measurement, but some feel that the midclavicular line accommodates the different sizes and shapes of clients.

■ Identify the *timing of impulses or sounds* in relation to the cardiac cycle. Timing of sounds is often possible through auscultation alone. In most people with regular or slow heart rates, it is easy to identify the paired heart sounds by listening through a stethoscope. S_1 is the first of these sounds, S_2 is the second, and the relatively long diastolic interval separates one pair from the next.

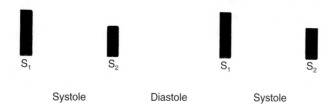

The relative intensity of these sounds may also be helpful. S_1 is usually louder than S_2 at the apex; more reliably, S_2 is usually louder than S_1 at the base.

Even experienced clinicians are sometimes uncertain about the timing of heart sounds, especially extra sounds and murmurs. "Inching" can then be helpful. Return to a place on the chest—most often the base—where it is easy to identify S_1 and S_2. Get their rhythm clearly in mind. Then inch your stethoscope down the chest in steps until you hear the new sound.

Auscultation alone, however, can be misleading. The intensities of S_1 and S_2, for example, may be different. At rapid heart rates, moreover, diastole shortens, and at about a rate of 120, the durations of systole and diastole become indistinguishable. *Use palpation of the carotid pulse or of the apical impulse to help determine whether the sound or murmur is systolic or diastolic.* Because both the carotid upstroke and the apical impulse occur in systole, right after S_1, sounds or murmurs coinciding with them are systolic and sounds or murmurs occurring after the carotid upstroke or apical impulse are diastolic.

For example, S_1 is decreased in *first-degree heart block*, and S_2 is decreased in *aortic stenosis*.

Inspection and Palpation

Overview. Careful *inspection* of the anterior chest may reveal the location of the *apical impulse* or *point of maximal impulse (PMI)*. Tangential light is best for making this observation. Use *palpation* to confirm the characteristics of the apical impulse.

Begin with general palpation of the chest wall. First palpate for heaves, lifts, or thrills using your *finger pads*. Hold them flat or obliquely on the body surface. Ventricular impulses may heave or lift your fingers. Then check for *thrills* by pressing the *ball of your hand* firmly on the chest. If subsequent auscultation reveals a loud murmur, go back and check for thrills over that area again. Be sure to assess the right ventricle by palpating the right ventricular area at the lower left sternal border and in the subxiphoid area, the pulmonary artery in the left 2nd intercostal space, and the aortic area in the right 2nd intercostal space. Review the following diagram. *Note that the "areas" designated for the left and right ventricle, the pulmonary artery, and the aorta pertain to most clients whose hearts are situated in the left chest, with expected vascular anatomy.*

Thrills may accompany loud, harsh, or rumbling murmurs as in *aortic stenosis, patent ductus arteriosus, ventricular septal defect*, and, less commonly, *mitral stenosis*. They are palpated more easily in client positions that accentuate the murmur.

On rare occasions, a client has *dextrocardia*—a heart situated on the right side. The apical impulse will then be found on the right. If

TECHNIQUES OF EXAMINATION: OBJECTIVE DATA

UNEXPECTED FINDINGS

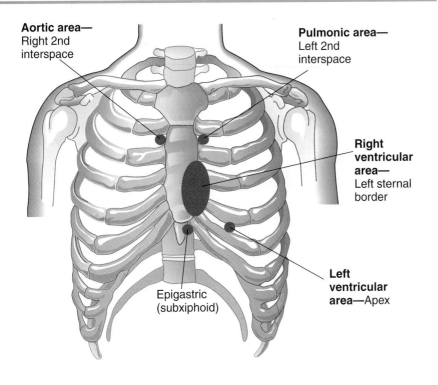

Aortic area—
Right 2nd interspace

Pulmonic area—
Left 2nd interspace

Right ventricular area—
Left sternal border

Left ventricular area—Apex

Epigastric (subxiphoid)

you cannot find an apical impulse, percuss for the dullness of heart and liver and for the tympany of the stomach. In *situs inversus*, all three of these structures are on opposite sides. A right-sided heart with a normally placed liver and stomach is usually associated with congenital heart disease.

Left Ventricular Area—The Apical Impulse or PMI. The apical impulse represents the brief early pulsation of the left ventricle as it moves anteriorly during contraction and touches the chest wall. Note that in most examinations the apical impulse is the point of maximal impulse or PMI. Some pathologic conditions, however, such as enlarged right ventricle, a dilated pulmonary artery, or an aortic aneurysm, may produce a pulsation more prominent than the apex beat.

If you cannot identify the apical impulse with the client supine, ask the client to roll partly onto the left side—this is the *left lateral decubitus* position. Palpate again using the palmar surfaces of several fingers. If you cannot find the apical impulse, ask the client to exhale fully and stop breathing for a few seconds. When examining a woman, it may be helpful to displace the left breast upward or laterally as necessary; alternatively, ask her to do this for you.

Once you have found the apical impulse, make finer assessments with your fingertips, and then with one finger.

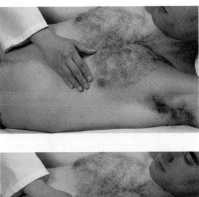

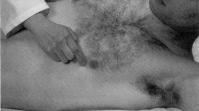

With experience, you will learn to feel the apical impulse in a high percentage of clients. Obesity, a very muscular chest wall, or an increased AP diameter of the chest, however, may make it undetectable. Some apical impulses hide behind the rib cage, despite positioning.

Now assess the location, diameter, amplitude, and duration of the apical impulse. You may wish to have the client breathe out and briefly stop breathing to check your findings.

See Table 15-3, Variations and Unexpected Findings of the Ventricular Impulses (p. 469).

■ *Location.* Try to assess location with the client *supine* because the left lateral decubitus position displaces the apical impulse to the left. Locate two points: the intercostal spaces, usually the 5th or possibly the 4th, which give the vertical location; and the distance in centimetres from the midsternal line, which gives the horizontal location. Note that even though the apical impulse falls roughly at the midclavicular line, measurements from this line are less reproducible because clinicians vary in their estimates of the midpoint of the clavicle.

The apical impulse may be displaced upward and to the left by pregnancy or a high left diaphragm.

Lateral displacement from cardiac enlargement in *congestive heart failure, cardiomyopathy, ischemic heart disease.* Displacement in deformities of the thorax and mediastinal shift.

- *Diameter.* Palpate the diameter of the apical impulse. In the supine client, it usually measures less than 2.5 cm and occupies only one intercostal space. It may feel larger in the left lateral decubitus position.

In the left lateral decubitus position, a diameter greater than 3 cm indicates left ventricular enlargement.

- *Amplitude.* Estimate the amplitude of the impulse. It is usually small and feels *brisk* and *tapping.* Some young people have an increased amplitude, or hyperkinetic impulse, especially when excited or after exercise; its duration, however, is the same.

Increased amplitude may also reflect *hyperthyroidism, severe anemia,* pressure overload of the left ventricle (e.g., *aortic stenosis*), or volume overload of the left ventricle (e.g., *mitral regurgitation*).

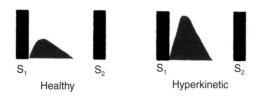

- *Duration.* Duration is the most useful characteristic of the apical impulse for identifying hypertrophy of the left ventricle. To assess duration, listen to the heart sounds as you feel the apical impulse, or watch the movement of your stethoscope as you listen at the apex. Estimate the proportion of systole occupied by the apical impulse. Usually it lasts through the first two thirds of systole, and often less, but does not continue to the second heart sound.

A sustained, high-amplitude impulse suggests left ventricular hypertrophy from pressure overload (as in hypertension). If such an impulse is displaced laterally, consider volume overload.

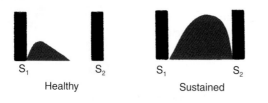

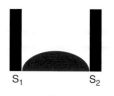

A sustained low-amplitude (hypokinetic) impulse may result from dilated cardiomyopathy.

S₃ and S₄. By inspection and palpation, you may detect ventricular movements that are synchronous with pathologic third and fourth heart sounds. For the left ventricular impulses, feel the apical beat gently with one finger. The client should lie partly on the left side, breathe out, and briefly stop breathing. By inking an X on the apex, you may be able to see these movements.

A brief middiastolic impulse indicates an S₃; an impulse just before the systolic apical beat itself indicates an S₄.

Right Ventricular Area—The Left Sternal Border in the 3rd, 4th, and 5th Intercostal spaces. The client should rest supine at 30°. Place the tips of your curved fingers in the 3rd, 4th, and 5th intercostal spaces and try to feel the systolic impulse of the right ventricle. Again, asking the client to breathe out and then briefly stop breathing improves your observation.

If an impulse is palpable, assess its location, amplitude, and duration. A brief systolic tap of low or slightly increased amplitude is sometimes felt in thin or shallow-chested people, especially when stroke volume is increased, as by anxiety.

A marked increase in amplitude with little or no change in duration occurs in chronic volume overload of the right ventricle, as from an *atrial septal defect.*

An impulse with increased amplitude and duration occurs with pressure overload of the right ventricle, as in *pulmonic stenosis* or *pulmonary hypertension.*

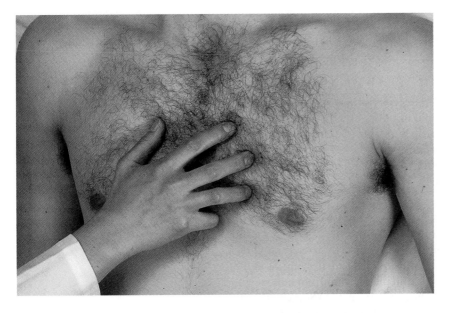

The diastolic movements of *right-sided third and fourth heart sounds* may be felt occasionally. Feel for them in the 4th and 5th left intercostal spaces. Time them by auscultation or carotid palpation.

In clients with an increased AP diameter, palpation of the *right ventricle* in the *epigastric* or *subxiphoid area* is also useful. With your hand flattened, press your index finger just under the rib cage and up toward the left shoulder and try to feel right ventricular pulsations.

In obstructive pulmonary disease, hyperinflated lung may prevent palpation of an enlarged right ventricle in the left parasternal area. The impulse is felt easily, however, high in the epigastrium where heart sounds are also often heard best.

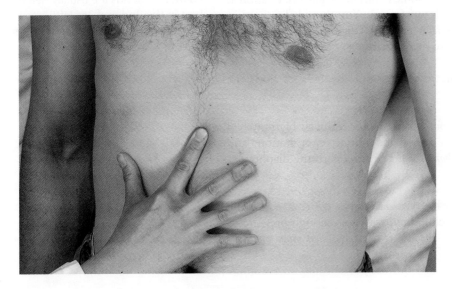

Asking the client to inhale and briefly stop breathing is helpful. The inspiratory position moves your hand well away from the pulsations of the abdominal aorta, which might otherwise be confusing. The diastolic movements of S_3 and S_4, if present, may also be felt here.

Pulmonic Area—The Left 2nd Intercostal Space.   This area overlies the *pulmonary artery*. As the client holds expiration, look and feel for an impulse and feel for possible heart sounds. In thin or shallow-chested clients, the pulsation of a pulmonary artery may sometimes be felt here, especially after exercise or with excitement.

A prominent pulsation here often accompanies dilatation or increased flow in the pulmonary artery. A palpable S_2 suggests increased pressure in the pulmonary artery (*pulmonary hypertension*).

Aortic Area—The Right 2nd Intercostal Space.   This area overlies the aortic outflow tract. Search for pulsations and palpable heart sounds.

A palpable S_2 suggests systemic *hypertension*. A pulsation here suggests a dilated or aneurysmal aorta.

Percussion.   In most cases, palpation has replaced percussion in the estimation of cardiac size. When you cannot feel the apical impulse, however, percussion may suggest where to search for it. Occasionally, percussion may be your only tool. Under these circumstances, cardiac dullness often occupies a large area. Starting well to the left on the chest, percuss from resonance toward cardiac dullness in the 3rd, 4th, 5th, and possibly 6th intercostal spaces.

A markedly dilated failing heart may have a hypokinetic apical impulse that is displaced far to the left. A large pericardial effusion may make the impulse undetectable.

Auscultation

Overview.   Auscultation of heart sounds and murmurs is a rewarding and important skill of physical examination that leads directly to several clinical diagnoses. In this section, you will learn the techniques for identifying S_1 and S_2, extra sounds in systole and diastole, and systolic and diastolic murmurs. Review the auscultatory areas on the next page with the following caveats: (1) Some authorities discourage the use of these names because murmurs of more than one origin may occur in a given area, and (2) these areas may not apply to clients with dextrocardia or anomalies of the great vessels. Also, if the heart is enlarged or displaced, your pattern of auscultation should be altered accordingly.

In a quiet room, listen to the heart with your stethoscope *in the right 2nd intercostal space* close to the sternum, *along the left sternal border* in each intercostal space from the 2nd through the 5th, and *at the apex*. Recall that the upper margins of the heart are sometimes termed the "base" of the heart. Some clinicians begin auscultation at the apex, others at the base. Either pattern is satisfactory. You should also listen in any area where you detect anything unusual in areas adjacent to murmurs to determine where they are loudest and where they radiate.

Heart sounds and murmurs that originate in the four valves are illustrated in the following diagram. Pulmonic sounds are usually heard best in the 2nd and 3rd left interspaces, but may extend further.

Know your stethoscope! It is important to understand the uses of both the diaphragm and the bell.

- *The diaphragm.* The diaphragm is better for picking up the relatively high-pitched sounds of S_1 and S_2, the murmurs of aortic and mitral regurgitation, and pericardial friction rubs. *Listen throughout the precordium* with the diaphragm, pressing it firmly against the chest.

- *The bell.* The bell is more sensitive to the low-pitched sounds of S_3 and S_4 and the murmur of mitral stenosis. Apply the bell lightly, with just enough pressure to produce an air seal with its full rim. *Use the bell at the apex, then move medially along the lower sternal border.* Resting the heel of your hand on the chest like a fulcrum may help you to maintain light pressure.

Pressing the bell firmly on the chest makes it function more like the diaphragm by stretching the underlying skin. Low-pitched sounds such as S_3 and S_4 may disappear with this technique—an observation that may help to identify them. In contrast, high-pitched sounds such as a midsystolic click, an ejection sound, or an opening snap, will persist or get louder.

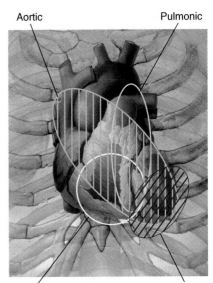

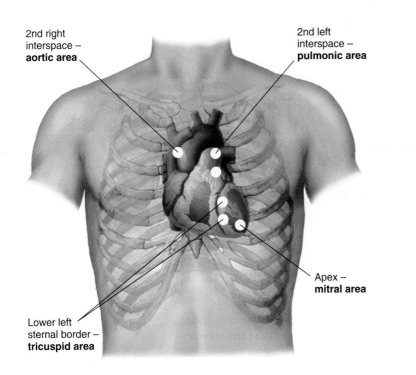

Listen to the entire precordium with the client supine. For new clients and clients needing a complete cardiac examination, use two other important positions to listen for mitral stenosis and aortic regurgitation.

■ Ask the client to *roll partly onto the left side into the left lateral decubitus position,* bringing the left ventricle close to the chest wall. Place the bell of your stethoscope lightly on the apical impulse.

This position accentuates or brings out a left-sided S_3 and S_4 and mitral murmurs, especially *mitral stenosis.* You may otherwise miss these important findings.

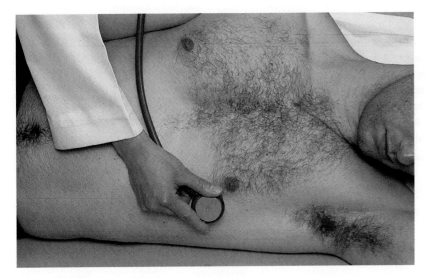

■ Ask the client to *sit up, lean forward, exhale completely, and stop breathing in expiration*. Pressing the diaphragm of your stethoscope on the chest, listen along the left sternal border and at the apex, pausing periodically so the client may breathe.

This position accentuates or brings out aortic murmurs. You may easily miss the soft diastolic murmur of *aortic regurgitation* unless you listen at this position.

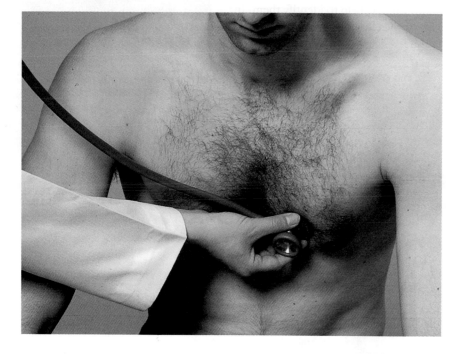

Listening for Heart Sounds. Throughout your examination, take your time at each auscultatory area. Concentrate on each of the events in the cardiac cycle listed on the next page and sounds you may hear in systole and diastole.

■ *Auscultatory Sounds*

Heart Sounds	Guides to Auscultation	
S_1	Note its intensity and any apparent splitting. Splitting that is not pathological is detectable along the lower left sternal border.	See Table 15-4, Variations in the First Heart Sound—S_1 (p. 470).
S_2	Note its intensity.	
Split S_2	Listen for splitting of this sound in the 2nd and 3rd left intercostal spaces. Ask the client to breathe quietly, and then slightly more deeply than usual. Does S_2 split into its two components, as expected? If not, ask the client to (1) breathe a little more deeply or (2) sit up. Listen again. A thick chest wall may make the pulmonic component of S_1 inaudible.	See Table 15-5, Variations in the Second Heart Sound—S_2 (p. 471). When either A_2 or P_2 is absent, as in disease of the respective valves, S_2 is persistently single.
	Width of split. How wide is the split? It is usually quite narrow.	
	Timing of split. When in the respiratory cycle do you hear the split? It is usually heard late in inspiration.	Expiratory splitting suggests an abnormality (p. XX).

(continued)

■ *Auscultatory Sounds (Continued)*

Heart Sounds	Guides to Auscultation
	Does the split disappear as it should, during exhalation? If not, listen again with the client sitting up.
Extra Sounds in Systole	Such as ejection sounds or systolic clicks
	Note their location, timing, intensity, and pitch, and the effects of respiration on the sounds.
Extra Sounds in Diastole	Such as S_3, S_4, or an opening snap
	Note the location, timing, intensity, and pitch, and the effects of respiration on the sounds. (An S_3 or S_4 in athletes is an expected finding.)
Systolic and Diastolic Murmurs	Murmurs are differentiated from heart sounds by their longer duration.

Persistent splitting results from delayed closure of the pulmonic valve or early closure of the aortic valve.

The systolic click of mitral valve prolapse is the most common of these sounds. See Table 15-6, Extra Heart Sounds in Systole (p. 472).

See Table 15-7, Extra Heart Sounds in Diastole (p. 473).

See Table 15-8, Pansystolic (Holosystolic) Murmurs (p. 474), Table 15-9, Diastolic Murmurs (p. 475) and Table 15-10, Midsystolic Murmurs (pp. 476–477).

Attributes of Heart Murmurs. If you detect a heart murmur, you must learn to identify and describe its *timing, shape, location of maximal intensity, radiation* (or transmission from this location), *intensity, pitch, and quality.*

■ *Timing.* First decide if you are hearing a *systolic murmur*, falling between S_1 and S_2, or a *diastolic murmur*, falling between S_2 and S_1. Palpating the carotid pulse as you listen can help you with timing. *Murmurs that coincide with the carotid upstroke are systolic.*

Systolic murmurs are usually *midsystolic* or *pansystolic*. Late systolic murmurs may also be heard.

Diastolic murmurs usually indicate valvular heart disease. Systolic murmurs may indicate valvular disease, but often occur when the heart valves are entirely healthy.

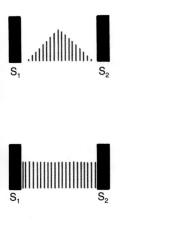

A *midsystolic murmur* begins after S_1 and stops before S_2. Brief gaps are audible between the murmur and the heart sounds. Listen carefully for the gap just before S_2. It is heard more easily and, if present, usually confirms the murmur as midsystolic, not pansystolic.

A *pansystolic (holosystolic) murmur* starts with S_1 and stops at S_2, without a gap between murmur and heart sounds.

Midsystolic murmurs most often are related to blood flow across the semilunar (aortic and pulmonic) valves. See Table 15-10, Midsystolic Murmurs (pp. 476–477).

Pansystolic murmurs often occur with regurgitant (backward) flow across the atrioventricular valves. See Table 15-8, Pansystolic (Holosystolic) Murmurs (p. 474).

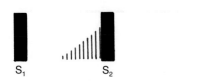

A *late systolic murmur* usually starts in mid- or late systole and persists up to S_2.

This is the murmur of mitral valve prolapse and is often, but not always, preceded by a systolic click (see p. 472).

Diastolic murmurs may be *early diastolic, middiastolic,* or *late diastolic.*

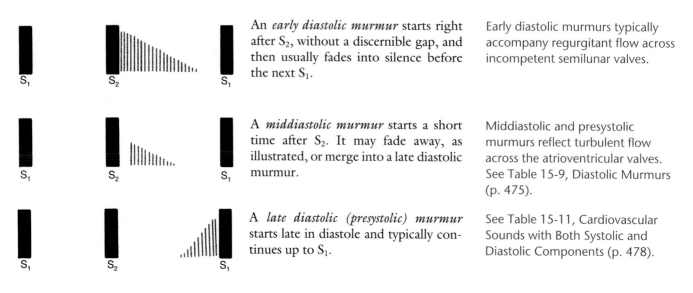

An *early diastolic murmur* starts right after S_2, without a discernible gap, and then usually fades into silence before the next S_1.

Early diastolic murmurs typically accompany regurgitant flow across incompetent semilunar valves.

A *middiastolic murmur* starts a short time after S_2. It may fade away, as illustrated, or merge into a late diastolic murmur.

Middiastolic and presystolic murmurs reflect turbulent flow across the atrioventricular valves. See Table 15-9, Diastolic Murmurs (p. 475).

A *late diastolic (presystolic) murmur* starts late in diastole and typically continues up to S_1.

See Table 15-11, Cardiovascular Sounds with Both Systolic and Diastolic Components (p. 478).

An occasional murmur, such as the murmur of a patent ductus arteriosus, starts in systole and continues without pause through S_2 into but not necessarily throughout diastole. It is then called a *continuous murmur.* Other cardiovascular sounds, such as pericardial friction rubs or venous hums, have *both systolic and diastolic components.* Observe and describe these sounds according to the characteristics used for systolic and diastolic murmurs.

- *Shape.* The shape or configuration of a murmur is determined by its intensity over time.

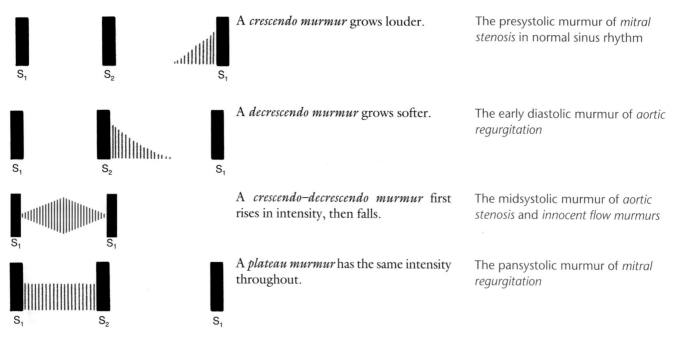

A *crescendo murmur* grows louder.

The presystolic murmur of *mitral stenosis* in normal sinus rhythm

A *decrescendo murmur* grows softer.

The early diastolic murmur of *aortic regurgitation*

A *crescendo–decrescendo murmur* first rises in intensity, then falls.

The midsystolic murmur of *aortic stenosis* and *innocent flow murmurs*

A *plateau murmur* has the same intensity throughout.

The pansystolic murmur of *mitral regurgitation*

TABLE 15-1   **Selected Heart Rates and Rhythms**

Cardiac rhythms may be classified as *regular* or *irregular*. When rhythms are irregular or rates are fast or slow, obtain an ECG to identify the origin of the beats (sinus node, AV node, atrium, or ventricle) and the pattern of conduction. Note that with AV (atrioventricular) block, arrhythmias may have a fast, normal, or slow ventricular rate.

	ECG Pattern	Usual Resting Rate
WHAT IS THE RATE?		
FAST (>100)	Sinus tachycardia	100–180
	Supraventricular (atrial or nodal) tachycardia	150–250
	Atrial flutter with a regular ventricular response	100–175
	Ventricular tachycardia	110–250
OR		
NORMAL (60–100)	Normal sinus rhythm	60–100
	Second-degree AV block	60–100
	Atrial flutter with a regular ventricular response	75–100
OR		
SLOW (<60)	Sinus bradycardia	<60
	Second-degree AV block	30–60
	Complete heart block	<40
RHYTHMIC OR SPORADIC	With early beats, atrial or nodal (supraventricular) premature contraction OR ventricular premature contractions	
	Sinus arrhythmia	See Table 15-2
OR		
TOTAL	Atrial fibrillation	
	Atrial flutter with varying block	

REGULAR

IS THE RHYTHM REGULAR OR IRREGULAR?

IRREGULAR

WHAT IS THE PATTERN OF IRREGULARITY?

TABLE 15-2   Selected Irregular Rhythms

Type of Rhythm	ECG Waves and Heart Sounds	
Atrial or Nodal Premature Contractions (*Supraventricular*)	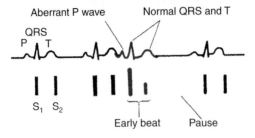 Aberrant P wave · Normal QRS and T · QRS · P · T · S$_1$ · S$_2$ · Early beat · Pause	**Rhythm.** A beat of atrial or nodal origin comes earlier than the next expected beat. A pause follows, and then the rhythm resumes. **Heart Sounds.** S$_1$ may differ in intensity from the S$_1$ of regular beats, and S$_2$ may be decreased. Both sounds are otherwise similar to those of regular beats.
Ventricular Premature Contractions	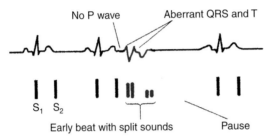 No P wave · Aberrant QRS and T · S$_1$ · S$_2$ · Early beat with split sounds · Pause	**Rhythm.** A beat of ventricular origin comes earlier than the next expected beat. A pause follows, and the rhythm resumes. **Heart Sounds.** S$_1$ may differ in intensity from the S$_1$ of the regular beats, and S$_2$ may be decreased. Both sounds are likely to be split.
Sinus Arrhythmia	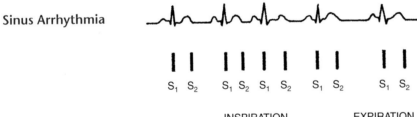 S$_1$ S$_2$ S$_1$ S$_2$ S$_1$ S$_2$ S$_1$ S$_2$ S$_1$ S$_2$ · INSPIRATION · EXPIRATION	**Rhythm.** The heart varies cyclically, usually speeding up with inspiration and slowing down with expiration. **Heart Sounds.** Regular, although S$_1$ may vary with the heart rate.
Atrial Fibrillation and Atrial Flutter with Varying AV Block	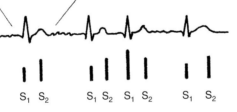 No P waves · Fibrillation waves · S$_1$ S$_2$ S$_1$ S$_2$ S$_1$ S$_2$ S$_1$ S$_2$	**Rhythm.** The ventricular rhythm is totally irregular, although short runs of the irregular ventricular rhythm may seem regular. **Heart Sounds.** S$_1$ varies in intensity.

In the healthy heart, the *left ventricular impulse* is usually the *point of maximal impulse,* or *PMI.* This brief impulse is generated by the movement of the ventricular apex against the chest wall during contraction. The *right ventricular impulse* is usually not palpable beyond infancy, and its characteristics are indeterminate. In contrast, learn the classical descriptors of the left ventricular PMI:

- *Location:* in the 4th or 5th intercostal space, ~7–10 cm lateral to the midsternal line, depending on the diameter of the chest
- *Diameter: discrete,* or ≤2 cm
- *Amplitude: brisk* and *tapping*
- *Duration:* ≤2/3 of systole

Careful examination of the ventricular impulse gives you important clues about underlying cardiovascular hemodynamics. The quality of the ventricular impulse changes as the left and right ventricles adapt to high-output states (anxiety, hyperthyroidism, and severe anemia) and to the more pathologic conditions of chronic pressure or volume overload. Note the distinguishing features of three types of ventricular impulses: the *hyperkinetic ventricular impulse* from transiently increased stroke volume—this change does not necessarily indicate heart disease; the *sustained* ventricular impulse of ventricular hypertrophy from chronic pressure load, known as *increased afterload* and the *diffuse* ventricular impulse of ventricular dilation from chronic volume overload, or *increased preload.*

	Left Ventricular Impulse			Right Ventricular Impulse		
	Hyperkinetic	*Pressure Overload*	*Volume Overload*	*Hyperkinetic*	*Pressure Overload*	*Volume Overload*
Examples of Causes	Anxiety, hyperthyroidism, severe anemia	Aortic stenosis, hypertension	Aortic or mitral regurgitation	Anxiety, hyperthyroidism, severe anemia	Pulmonic stenosis, pulmonary hypertension	Atrial septal defect
Location	4th or 5th intercostal space, 7–10 cm lateral to midsternal line	4th or 5th intercostal space, 7–10 cm lateral to midsternal line	Displaced to the left and possibly downward	3rd, 4th, or 5th left intercostal space	3rd, 4th, or 5th left intercostal space, also subxiphoid	Left sternal border, extending toward the left cardiac border, also subxiphoid
Diameter	~2 cm, though increased amplitude may make it seem larger	>2 cm	>2 cm	Not useful	Not useful	Not useful
Amplitude	More forceful tapping	More forceful tapping	*Diffuse*	Slightly more forceful	More forceful	Slightly to markedly more forceful
Duration	<2/3 systole	*Sustained* (up to S_2)	Often slightly sustained	≤2/3 systole	Sustained	≤2/3 systole to slightly sustained

TABLE 15-4   Variations in the First Heart Sound—S₁

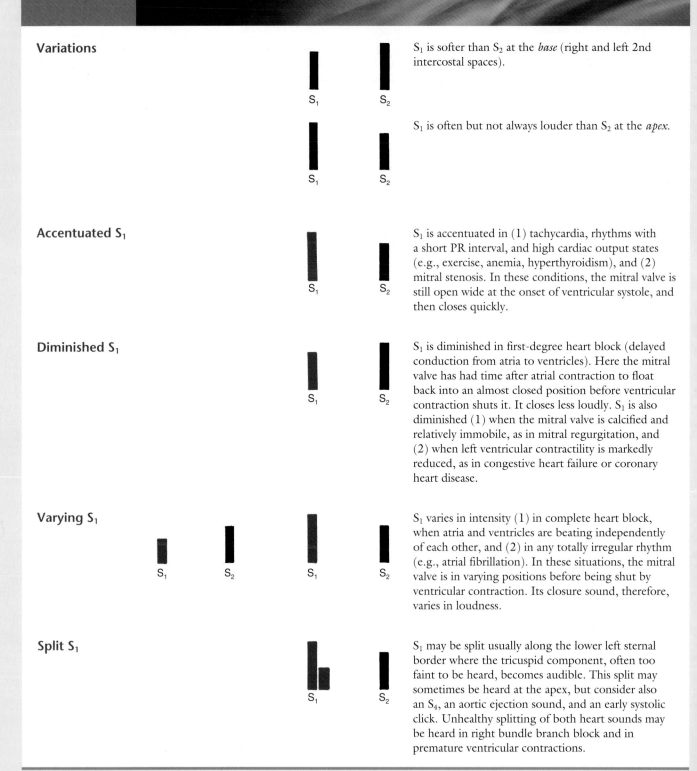

Variations

S_1 is softer than S_2 at the *base* (right and left 2nd intercostal spaces).

S_1 is often but not always louder than S_2 at the *apex*.

Accentuated S₁

S_1 is accentuated in (1) tachycardia, rhythms with a short PR interval, and high cardiac output states (e.g., exercise, anemia, hyperthyroidism), and (2) mitral stenosis. In these conditions, the mitral valve is still open wide at the onset of ventricular systole, and then closes quickly.

Diminished S₁

S_1 is diminished in first-degree heart block (delayed conduction from atria to ventricles). Here the mitral valve has had time after atrial contraction to float back into an almost closed position before ventricular contraction shuts it. It closes less loudly. S_1 is also diminished (1) when the mitral valve is calcified and relatively immobile, as in mitral regurgitation, and (2) when left ventricular contractility is markedly reduced, as in congestive heart failure or coronary heart disease.

Varying S₁

S_1 varies in intensity (1) in complete heart block, when atria and ventricles are beating independently of each other, and (2) in any totally irregular rhythm (e.g., atrial fibrillation). In these situations, the mitral valve is in varying positions before being shut by ventricular contraction. Its closure sound, therefore, varies in loudness.

Split S₁

S_1 may be split usually along the lower left sternal border where the tricuspid component, often too faint to be heard, becomes audible. This split may sometimes be heard at the apex, but consider also an S_4, an aortic ejection sound, and an early systolic click. Unhealthy splitting of both heart sounds may be heard in right bundle branch block and in premature ventricular contractions.

TABLE 15-5   Variations in the Second Heart Sound—S_2

	Inspiration	Expiration

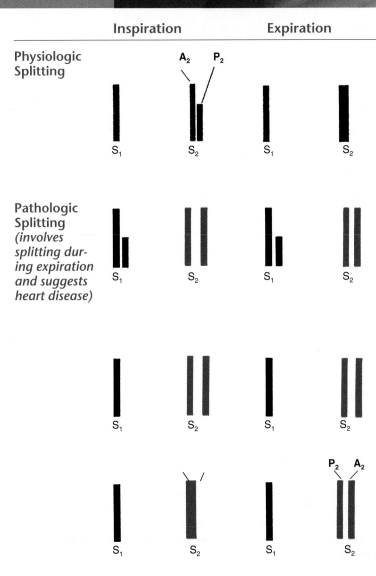

Physiologic Splitting

Listen for *physiologic splitting* of S_2 in the *2nd or 3rd left intercostal space.* The pulmonic component of S_2 is usually too faint to be heard at the apex or aortic area, where S_2 is a single sound derived from aortic valve closure alone. Expected splitting is *accentuated by inspiration* and usually *disappears on expiration.* In some clients, especially younger ones, S_2 may not become single on expiration. It may merge when the client sits up.

Pathologic Splitting *(involves splitting during expiration and suggests heart disease)*

Wide splitting of S_2 refers to an increase in the usual splitting that persists throughout the respiratory cycle. Wide splitting can be caused by delayed closure of the pulmonic valve (e.g., by pulmonic stenosis or right bundle branch block). As illustrated here, right bundle branch block also causes splitting of S_1 into its mitral and tricuspid components. Wide splitting can also be caused by early closure of the aortic valve, as in mitral regurgitation.

Fixed splitting refers to wide splitting that does not vary with respiration. It occurs in atrial septal defect and right ventricular failure.

Paradoxical or reversed splitting refers to splitting that appears on expiration and disappears on inspiration. Closure of the aortic valve is delayed so that A_2 follows P_2 in expiration. Inspiratory delay of P_2 makes the split disappear. The most common cause of paradoxical splitting is left bundle branch block.

Increased Intensity of A_2 in the Right Second Intercostal (where only A_2 can usually be heard) occurs in systemic hypertension because of the increased pressure load. It also occurs when the aortic root is dilated, probably because the aortic valve is then closer to the chest wall.

Decreased or Absent A_2 in the Right Second Intercostal is noted in calcified aortic stenosis because of valve immobility. If A_2 is inaudible, no splitting is heard.

Increased Intensity of P_2. When P_2 is equal to or louder than A_2, suspect pulmonary hypertension. Other causes include a dilated pulmonary artery and an atrial septal defect. When a split S_2 is heard widely, even at the apex and the right base, P_2 is accentuated.

Decreased or Absent P_2 is usually due to the increased anteroposterior diameter of the chest associated with aging. It can also result from pulmonic stenosis. If P_2 is inaudible, no splitting is heard.

TABLE 15-6   **Extra Heart Sounds in Systole**

There are two kinds of extra heart sounds in systole: (1) early ejection sounds, and (2) clicks, commonly heard in mid and late systole.

Early Systolic Ejection Sounds

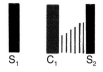

S_1 E_j S_2

Early systolic ejection sounds occur shortly after S_1, coincident with opening of the aortic and pulmonic valves. They are relatively high in pitch; have a sharp, clicking quality; and are heard better with the diaphragm of the stethoscope. An ejection sound indicates cardiovascular disease.

Listen for an *aortic ejection sound* at both the base and apex. It may be louder at the apex and usually does not vary with respiration. An aortic ejection sound may accompany a dilated aorta, or aortic valve disease from congenital stenosis or a bicuspid valve.

A *pulmonic ejection sound* is heard best in the 2nd and 3rd left intercostal spaces. When S_1, usually relatively soft in this area, appears to be loud, you may be hearing a pulmonic ejection sound. Its intensity often *decreases with inspiration*. Causes include dilatation of the pulmonary artery, pulmonary hypertension, and pulmonic stenosis.

Systolic Clicks

S_1 C_1 S_2

Systolic clicks are usually due to *mitral valve prolapse*—an unexpected systolic ballooning of part of the mitral valve into the left atrium. The clicks are usually mid- or late systolic. Prolapse of the mitral valve is a common cardiac condition, affecting about 5% of the general population. There is equal prevalence in men and women.

The click is usually single, but you may hear more than one, usually *at or medial to the apex*, but also *at the lower left sternal border*. It is high-pitched, so listen with the diaphragm. The click is often followed by a late systolic murmur from mitral regurgitation—a flow of blood from left ventricle to left atrium. The murmur usually crescendos up to S_2. Auscultatory findings are notably variable. Most clients have only a click, some have only a murmur, and some have both. Systolic clicks may also be of extracardial or mediastinal origin.

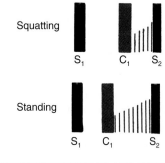

Squatting

S_1 C_1 S_2

Standing

S_1 C_1 S_2

Findings vary from time to time and often change with body position. Several positions are recommended to identify the syndrome: supine, seated, squatting, and standing. *Squatting delays the click and murmur; standing moves them closer to S_1.*

TABLE 15-7   Extra Heart Sounds in Diastole

Opening Snap

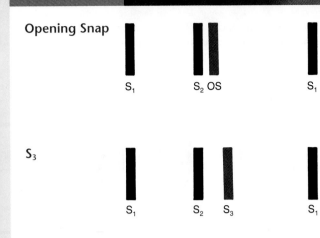

The *opening snap* is a very early diastolic sound usually produced by the opening of a *stenotic mitral valve*. It is heard best just medial to the apex and along the lower left sternal border. When it is loud, an opening snap radiates to the apex and to the pulmonic area, where it may be mistaken for the pulmonic component of a split S_2. Its high pitch and snapping quality help to distinguish it from an S_2. It is heard better with the diaphragm.

S_3

You will detect *physiologic* S_3 frequently in children and in young adults to the age of 35 or 40. It is common during the last trimester of pregnancy. Occurring early in diastole during rapid ventricular filling, it is later than an opening snap, dull and low in pitch, and heard best at the apex in the left lateral decubitus position. The bell of the stethoscope should be used with very light pressure.

A *pathologic* S_3 or *ventricular gallop* sounds just like a physiologic S_3. An S_3 in a person over age 40 (possibly a little older in women) is almost certainly pathologic. Causes include decreased myocardial contractility, congestive heart failure, and volume overloading of a ventricle, as in mitral or tricuspid regurgitation. A *left-sided* S_3 is heard typically at the apex in the left lateral decubitus position. A *right-sided* S_3 is usually heard along the lower left sternal border or below the xiphoid with the client supine, and is louder on inspiration. The term *gallop* comes from the cadence of three heart sounds, especially at rapid heart rates, and sounds like "Kentucky."

S_4

An S_4 (*atrial sound* or *atrial gallop*) occurs just before S_1. It is dull, low in pitch, and heard better with the bell. An S_4 is heard occasionally in an apparently healthy person, especially in trained athletes and older age groups. More commonly, it is due to increased resistance to ventricular filling following atrial contraction. This increased resistance is related to decreased compliance (increased stiffness) of the ventricular myocardium.

Causes of a left-sided S_4 include hypertensive heart disease, coronary artery disease, aortic stenosis, and cardiomyopathy. A *left-sided* S_4 is heard best at the apex in the left lateral position; it may sound like "Tennessee." The less common *right-sided* S_4 is heard along the lower left sternal border or below the xiphoid. It often gets louder with inspiration. Causes of a right-sided S_4 include pulmonary hypertension and pulmonic stenosis.

An S_4 may also be associated with delayed conduction between atria and ventricles. This delay separates the usually faint atrial sound from the louder S_1 and makes it audible. An S_4 is never heard in the absence of atrial contraction, which occurs with atrial fibrillation.

Occasionally, a client has both an S_3 and an S_4, producing a *quadruple rhythm* of four heart sounds. At rapid heart rates, the S_3 and S_4 may merge into one loud extra heart sound, called a *summation gallop*.

TABLE 15-8   **Pansystolic (Holosystolic) Murmurs**

Pansystolic (holosystolic) murmurs are pathologic, arising from blood flow from a chamber with high pressure to one of lower pressure, through a valve or other structure that should be closed. The murmur begins immediately with S_1 and continues up to S_2.

	Mitral Regurgitation[a]	**Tricuspid Regurgitation**	**Ventricular Septal Defect**
	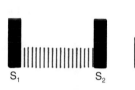	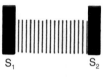	
Murmur	*Location.* Apex	*Location.* Lower left sternal border	*Location.* 3rd, 4th, and 5th left intercostal spaces
	Radiation. To the left maxilla, less often to the left sternal border	*Radiation.* To the right of the sternum, to the xiphoid area, and perhaps to the left midclavicular line, but not into the maxilla	*Radiation.* Often wide
	Intensity. Soft to loud; if loud, associated with an apical thrill	*Intensity.* Variable	*Intensity.* Often very loud, with a thrill
	Pitch. Medium to high	*Pitch.* Medium	*Pitch.* High, holosystolic
	Quality. Harsh, holosystolic	*Quality.* Blowing, holosystolic	*Quality.* Often harsh
	Aids. Unlike tricuspid regurgitation, it does not become louder in inspiration.	*Aids.* Unlike mitral regurgitation, the intensity may increase slightly with inspiration.	
Associated Findings	S_1 is often decreased.	The right ventricular impulse is increased in amplitude and may be *sustained*.	A_2 may be obscured by the loud murmur.
	An apical S_3 reflects volume overload on the left ventricle.		
	The apical impulse is increased in amplitude and may be *sustained*.	An S_3 may be audible along the lower left sternal border. The jugular venous pressure is often elevated, and large *v* waves may be seen in the jugular veins.	Findings vary with the severity of the defect and with associated lesions.
Mechanism	When the *mitral valve fails to close fully in systole*, blood regurgitates from left ventricle to left atrium, causing a murmur. This leakage creates volume overload on the left ventricle, with subsequent dilatation and hypertrophy. Several structural abnormalities cause this condition, and findings may vary accordingly.	When the *tricuspid valve fails to close fully in systole*, blood regurgitates from right ventricle to right atrium, producing a murmur. The most common cause is right ventricular failure and dilatation, with resulting enlargement of the tricuspid orifice. Either pulmonary hypertension or left ventricular failure is the usual initiating cause.	A ventricular septal defect is a congenital abnormality in which *blood flows from the relatively high-pressure left ventricle into the low-pressure right ventricle through a hole*. The defect may be accompanied by other abnormalities, but an uncomplicated lesion is described here.

[a]Pierard & Lancellotti, 2004.

TABLE 15-9   **Diastolic Murmurs**

Diastolic murmurs almost always indicate heart disease. There are two basic types. *Early decrescendo diastolic murmurs* signify regurgitant flow through an incompetent semilunar valve, more commonly the aortic. *Rumbling diastolic murmurs in mid- or late diastole* suggest stenosis of an atrioventricular valve, usually the mitral.

	Aortic Regurgitation[a]	Mitral Stenosis
Murmur	*Location.* 2nd to 4th left intercostal spaces	*Location.* Usually limited to the apex
	Radiation. If loud, to the apex, perhaps to the right sternal border	*Radiation.* Little or none
	Intensity. Grade 1–3	*Intensity.* Grade 1–4
	Pitch. High. *Use the diaphragm.*	*Pitch.* Decrescendo low-pitched rumble. *Use the bell.*
	Quality. Blowing decrescendo; may be mistaken for breath sounds	
	Aids. The murmur is heard best with the *client sitting, leaning forward*, with breath held after exhalation.	*Aids.* Placing the bell exactly on the apical impulse, turning the client into a *left lateral position*, and mild exercise all help to make the murmur audible. It is heard better in exhalation.
Associated Findings	An ejection sound may be present.	S_1 is accentuated and may be palpable at the apex.
	An S_3 or S_4, if present, suggests severe regurgitation.	An opening snap (OS) often follows S_2 and initiates the murmur.
	Progressive changes in the apical impulse include increased amplitude, displacement laterally and downward, widened diameter, and increased duration.	If pulmonary hypertension develops, P_2 is accentuated, and the right ventricular impulse becomes palpable.
	The pulse pressure increases, and *arterial pulses are often large and bounding.* A midsystolic flow murmur or an Austin Flint murmur suggests large regurgitant flow.	Mitral regurgitation and aortic valve disease may be associated with mitral stenosis.
Mechanism	The leaflets of the aortic valve fail to close completely during diastole, and blood regurgitates from the aorta back into the left ventricle. Volume overload on the left ventricle results. Two other murmurs may be associated: (1) a midsystolic murmur from the resulting increased forward flow across the aortic valve, and (2) a mitral diastolic (*Austin Flint*) murmur, attributed to diastolic impingement of the regurgitant flow on the anterior leaflet of the mitral valve.	When the leaflets of the mitral valve thicken, stiffen, and become distorted from the effects of rheumatic fever, the *mitral valve fails to open sufficiently in diastole.* The resulting murmur has two components: (1) middiastolic (during rapid ventricular filling), and (2) presystolic (during atrial contraction). The latter disappears if atrial fibrillation develops, leaving only a middiastolic rumble.

[a]Babu, Kymes, & Fryer, 2003; Enriquez-Serano & Tajik, 2004.

TABLE 15-10   **Midsystolic Murmurs**

Midsystolic ejection murmurs are the most common kind of heart murmur. They may be (1) *innocent*—without any detectable physiologic or structural abnormality; (2) *physiologic*—from physiologic changes in body metabolism; or (3) *pathologic*—arising from a structural abnormality in the heart or great vessels (Etchells, Bell, & Robb., 1997; Lembo et al., 1988). Midsystolic murmurs tend to peak near midsystole and usually stop before S_2. The crescendo–decrescendo or "diamond" shape is not always audible, but the gap between the murmur and S_2 helps to distinguish midsystolic from pansystolic murmurs.

	Innocent Murmurs	**Physiologic Murmurs**
Murmur	*Location*. 2nd to 4th left intercostal spaces between the left sternal border and the apex *Radiation*. Little *Intensity*. Grade 1–2, possibly 3 *Pitch*. Soft to medium *Quality*. Variable *Aids*. Usually decreases or disappears on sitting	Similar to innocent murmurs
Associated Findings	None: expected splitting, no ejection sounds, no diastolic murmurs, and no palpable evidence of ventricular enlargement. Occasionally, both an innocent murmur and another kind of murmur are present.	Possible signs of a likely cause
Mechanism	Innocent murmurs result from turbulent blood flow, probably generated by ventricular ejection of blood into the aorta from the left and occasionally the right ventricle. Very common in children and young adults—may also be heard in older people. There is no underlying cardiovascular disease.	Turbulence due to a temporary increase in blood flow in predisposing conditions such as anemia, pregnancy, fever, and hyperthyroidism.

[a]Etchells, Glenns, Shadowitz, Bell, & Siu, 1998.

Pathologic Murmurs

Aortic Stenosis[a]	*Hypertrophic Cardiomyopathy*	*Pulmonic Stenosis*

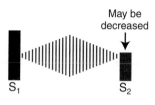

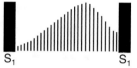

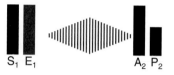

Location. Right 2nd intercostal space

Radiation. Often to the carotids, down the left sternal border, even to the apex

Intensity. Sometimes soft but often loud, with a thrill

Pitch. Medium, harsh; crescendo–decrescendo may be higher at the apex

Quality. Often harsh; may be more musical at the apex

Aids. Heard best with the client sitting and leaning forward

A_2 decreases as aortic stenosis worsens. A_2 may be delayed and merge with P_2 single S_2 on expiration or paradoxical S_2 split. Carotid upstroke may be *delayed* with slow rise and small amplitude. Hypertrophied left ventricle may *sustained* apical impulse and an S_4 from decreased compliance.

Significant aortic valve stenosis impairs blood flow across the valve, causing turbulence, and increases left ventricular afterload. Causes are congenital, rheumatic, and degenerative; findings may differ with each cause. Other conditions mimic aortic stenosis without obstructing flow: *aortic sclerosis,* a stiffening of aortic valve leaflets associated with aging; a *bicuspid aortic valve,* a congenital condition that may not be recognized until adulthood; *a dilated aorta,* as in arteriosclerosis, syphilis, or Marfa's syndrome; *pathologically increased flow across the aortic valve* during systole, as in aortic regurgitation.

Location. 3rd and 4th left intercostal spaces

Radiation. Down the left sternal border to the apex, possibly to the base, but not to the neck

Intensity. Variable

Pitch. Medium

Quality. Harsh

Aids. Decreases with squatting, increases with straining down from Valsalva

An S_3 may be present. An S_4 is often present at the apex (unlike mitral regurgitation). The apical impulse may be *sustained* and have two palpable components. The carotid pulse rises *quickly,* unlike the pulse in aortic stenosis.

Massive ventricular hypertrophy is associated with unusually rapid ejection of blood from the left ventricle during systole. Outflow tract obstruction to flow may coexist. Accompanying distortion of the mitral valve may cause mitral regurgitation.

Location. 2nd and 3rd left intercostal spaces

Radiation. If loud, toward the left shoulder and neck

Intensity. Soft to loud; if loud, associated with a thrill

Pitch. Medium; crescendo–decrescendo

Quality. Often harsh

In severe stenosis, S_2 is widely split, and P_2 is diminished or inaudible. An early pulmonic ejection sound is common. May hear a right-sided S_4. Right ventricular impulse often increased in amplitude and *sustained.*

Pulmonic valve stenosis impairs flow across the valve, increasing right ventricular afterload. Congenital and usually found in children. In an *atrial septal defect,* the systolic murmur from pathologically increased flow across the pulmonic valve may mimic pulmonic stenosis.

Some cardiovascular sounds extend beyond one phase of the cardiac cycle. Three examples, further described here, are as follows: (1) a *venous hum,* a benign sound produced by turbulence of blood in the jugular veins—common in children; (2) a *pericardial friction rub,* produced by inflammation of the pericardial sac; and (3) *patent ductus arteriosus,* a congenital abnormality in which an open channel persists between aorta and pulmonary artery. *Continuous murmurs* begin in systole and extend through S_2 into all or part of diastole, as in *patent ductus arteriosus.*

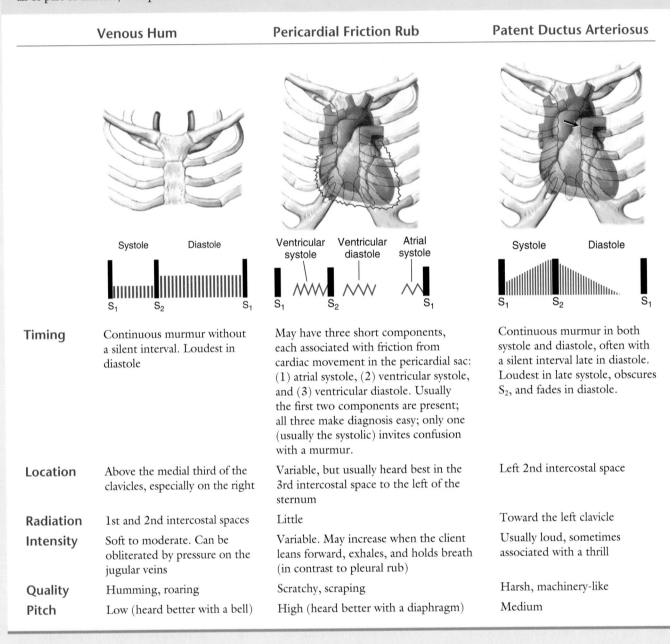

	Venous Hum	**Pericardial Friction Rub**	**Patent Ductus Arteriosus**
Timing	Continuous murmur without a silent interval. Loudest in diastole	May have three short components, each associated with friction from cardiac movement in the pericardial sac: (1) atrial systole, (2) ventricular systole, and (3) ventricular diastole. Usually the first two components are present; all three make diagnosis easy; only one (usually the systolic) invites confusion with a murmur.	Continuous murmur in both systole and diastole, often with a silent interval late in diastole. Loudest in late systole, obscures S_2, and fades in diastole.
Location	Above the medial third of the clavicles, especially on the right	Variable, but usually heard best in the 3rd intercostal space to the left of the sternum	Left 2nd intercostal space
Radiation	1st and 2nd intercostal spaces	Little	Toward the left clavicle
Intensity	Soft to moderate. Can be obliterated by pressure on the jugular veins	Variable. May increase when the client leans forward, exhales, and holds breath (in contrast to pleural rub)	Usually loud, sometimes associated with a thrill
Quality	Humming, roaring	Scratchy, scraping	Harsh, machinery-like
Pitch	Low (heard better with a bell)	High (heard better with a diaphragm)	Medium

16

The Breasts and Axillae

RENE A. DAY AND LYNN S. BICKLEY

In many cultures, the female breasts represent nurturing of infants, sexuality, and femininity. The male breasts represent "strength, fitness, and masculinity" (Estes, 2006, p. 414). Clients of either sex may be uncomfortable talking about their breasts and especially having their breasts exposed for an examination. When faced with a diagnosis of breast cancer, female and male clients fear loss of sexual attractiveness, loss of a significant other, disfigurement, and death.

Nurses in many settings have teaching opportunities about breast health, the Know Your Breasts (KYB) approach (Canadian Cancer Society, 2009a) (formerly Breast Self-Examination, BSE), screening tests, and risk factors for cancer to both sexes. Also, nurses provide support for clients undergoing diagnostic procedures, surgery, and treatment for breast conditions (e.g., cancer, enhancement, reduction). In settings such as long-term care, nurses should take responsibility for assisting residents with the KYB approach.

ANATOMY AND PHYSIOLOGY

THE FEMALE BREASTS

The female breasts lie against the anterior thoracic wall, extending from the clavicle and 2nd rib down to the 6th rib, and from the sternum across to the midaxillary line.

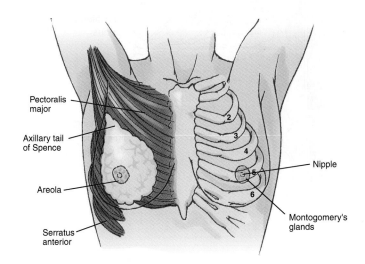

The breasts overlie the pectoralis major and at its inferior margin, the serratus anterior muscles.

To describe clinical findings, each breast is divided into four quadrants based on horizontal and vertical lines crossing at the nipple. An axillary tail of breast tissue (tail of Spence) extends into the axilla and toward the anterior axillary fold. Alternatively, findings can be localized as the time on the face of a clock (e.g., 3 o'clock) and the distance in centimetres from the nipple.

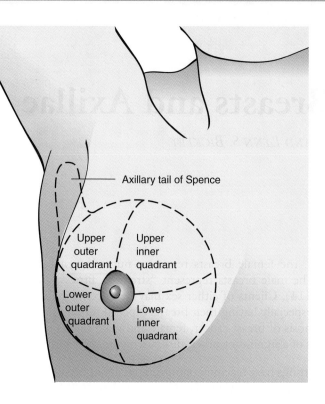

The breasts are hormonally sensitive tissue, responsive to the changes of monthly cycling and aging. *Glandular tissue*, namely secretory tubuloalveolar glands and ducts, forms 15 to 20 septated *lobes* radiating around the nipple. Within each lobe are many smaller *lobules*. These drain into milk-producing ducts and sinuses that open onto the surface of the *areola*, or nipple. *Fibrous connective tissue* provides structural support in the form of fibrous bands or suspensory ligaments connected to both the skin and the underlying fascia. *Adipose tissue*, or fat, surrounds each breast, predominantly in the superficial and peripheral areas. The proportions of these components vary with age, the general state of nutrition, pregnancy, use of hormones, and other factors.

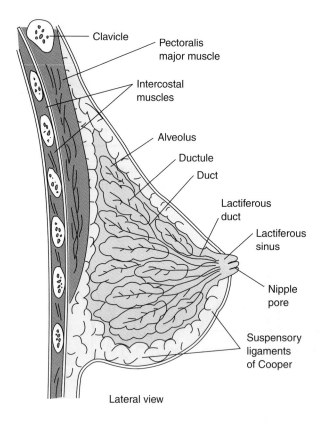

The surface of the areola has small, rounded elevations formed by sebaceous glands, sweat glands, and accessory areolar glands. A few hairs are often seen on the areola.

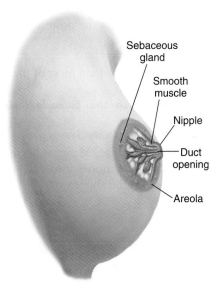

Both the nipple and the areola are well supplied with smooth muscle that contracts to express milk from the ductal system during breast feeding. Rich sensory innervation, especially in the nipple, triggers "milk letdown" following neurohormonal stimulation from infant sucking. Tactile stimulation of the area, including the breast examination, makes the nipples smaller, firmer, and more erect, whereas the areolae pucker and wrinkle. These smooth muscle reflexes are expected findings and should not be mistaken for signs of breast disease.

The adult breast may be soft, but it often feels granular, nodular, or lumpy. This uneven texture is a usual finding and is often bilateral, and may be evident throughout the breasts or only in parts of them. (For breast changes during adolescence, see Chapter 22; for pregnancy, see p. 857; and for aging, see p. 894.)

Occasionally, one or more extra or supernumerary nipples are located along the "milk line," illustrated on the right. Only a small nipple and areola are usually present, often mistaken for a common mole. There may be underlying glandular tissue. An extra nipple has no pathologic significance. Supernumerary nipples are more common in women of African descent.

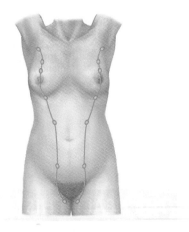

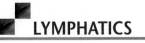
THE MALE BREASTS

Up until puberty, female and male breasts are the same. Each *male breast* consists chiefly of a small nipple and areola. These overlie a thin disc of undeveloped breast tissue that may not be distinguishable clinically from the surrounding tissues. A firm button of breast tissue 2 cm or more in diameter has been described in roughly one of three adult men. The limits of what is expected have not yet been clearly established.

LYMPHATICS

Lymph from each breast drains mainly toward the respective axilla. Of the axillary lymph nodes, the *central nodes* are most frequently palpable. They lie along the chest wall, usually high in the axilla and midway between the anterior and posterior axillary folds. Into them drain channels from three other groups of lymph nodes, which are seldom palpable:

■ *Pectoral nodes—anterior*, located along the lower border of the pectoralis major inside the anterior axillary fold. These nodes drain the anterior chest wall and much of the breast.

■ *Subscapular nodes—posterior*, located along the lateral border of the scapula; palpated deep in the posterior axillary fold. They drain the posterior chest wall and a portion of the arm.

■ *Lateral nodes*—located *along the upper humerus*. They drain most of the arm.

Lymph drains from the central axillary nodes to the *infraclavicular* and *supraclavicular* nodes.

Not all the lymphatics of the breasts drain into the axillae. Malignant cells from a breast cancer may spread directly to the infraclavicular nodes into deep channels within the chest (toward the opposite breast) or into the abdomen.

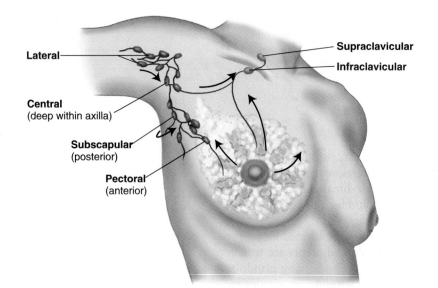

THE HEALTH HISTORY: SUBJECTIVE DATA

Key Symptoms and Signs Reported by Client

- ■ Reddened and warm breast skin
- ■ Rash/ulceration
- ■ Breast pain or discomfort
- ■ Nipple discharge
- ■ Changes in breast shape
- ■ Dimpling of breast skin
- ■ Breast lump or mass

The health history related to the breasts can pose challenges for both the client and the nurse. The client may feel embarrassed to discuss his or her breasts and often is fearful that a serious abnormality will be found. Nursing students and new graduates may also feel embarrassed, anxious, and uncertain about how to ask the client very personal questions. A useful strategy for nurses is to first focus on their own anxiety management. Doing so will increase their ability to approach clients in a calm and caring manner. Excellent communication skills are required. It is helpful to acknowledge that by coming in for a breast examination, the client is taking an important step in managing his or her own health (Estes, 2006).

Begin with an open-ended question such as "Tell me about any concerns you have about your breasts." If the client reports a concern, ask for further details (see Examples of Questions for Symptom Analysis—Breast Lump, below).

Reddened and Warm Breast Skin, Rash, or Ulceration.

The client may indicate a concern about skin changes such as reddened breast skin that is warm to the touch, a rash (often on the underside of the breast), or an ulceration on the breast or nipple. The presence of these signs alerts the nurse to wear gloves during the physical examination.

Skin conditions of the breast may indicate bacterial infection or the presence of yeast (*Candida albicans*). Ulceration of the nipple may be *Paget's disease of the breast.*

Breast Pain.

Discomfort, tenderness, or pain in the breasts (mastalgia) are symptoms often mentioned by clients. Collect additional information related to location in the breasts and the time in the menstrual cycle when the symptoms occur. Premenstrual breast enlargement and tenderness are common signs and symptoms. Santen and Mansel (2005) report that 40% of breast pain has a musculoskeletal cause such as pain over the costochondrial junctions (costochondritis) or is referred from arthritis in the neck. If pain is limited to a definitive area and is described as "burning" or "knife-like," it is likely coming from the chest wall.

Cysts in the breast tissue increase in size and in degree of tenderness in the premenstrual phase from increased fluid retention. Mastalgia is caused by fibrocystic breast changes, congestion during lactation, infection, or advanced breast cancer.

Nipple Discharge.

Clients are concerned about discharge from their nipples. Is the discharge coming from one or both breasts? It is important to determine when the discharge occurs. If it appears only after squeezing the nipple, it is considered physiologic. If the discharge is spontaneous (seen on the underwear or night clothes without local stimulation), ask about its colour, consistency, and quantity. While discharge may be "viscous, watery, serosanguineous, grossly bloody, clear, blue-black or green" (Santen & Mansel, 2005, p. 208), only the presence of blood (or occult blood) requires further investigation.

Galactorrhea, milky bilateral discharge, may reflect pregnancy or prolactin or other hormonal imbalance. Spontaneous persistent nonlactational discharge that is bloody and unilateral (from one duct) is pathological and suggests local breast disease from *papilloma* or a possible breast cancer, which occurs in 5% of women, particularly those who are older (Murad, Contesso, & Mouriesse, 1982).

Breast Shape and Dimpling of Breast Skin.

Other client concerns relate to changes in breast shape and dimpling of breast skin. These changes may suggest breast cancer.

See Table 16-1, Visible Signs of Breast Cancer, p. 508.

If the client reports a breast lump or mass, collect pertinent information using a symptom analysis. See the following box.

Example of Questions for Symptom Analysis—Breast Lump

- "Which breast has the lump?" "Is there more than one lump?" "Show me where the lump is in your breast." (*Location, radiating*)
- "Describe what the lump is like." "Is the lump painful?" (*Quality*)
- "Describe the size of the breast lump." (*Severity*)
- "When did you first notice the lump?" "How did you first notice the lump?" (*Onset*)
- "Has the lump been present since you first noticed it?" (*Duration*)
- "Has the lump changed in any way since you first noticed it?" (*Constancy*)
- "Is there a time of the month (e.g., before your menstrual period) when the lump feels different in size?" "Or different in terms of pain/discomfort?" (*Time of day/month/year*)
- "Has anything made the lump larger?" "Or more painful?" (*Aggravating factors*)
- "Does anything make the lump smaller?" "Or less painful? (*Alleviating factors*)
- "What other symptoms have you noticed?" "Any nipple discharge?" "Is the nipple pulled inward (retraction)?" "Any enlargement of the breast?" "Are the lymph nodes in your axillae (armpit) tender?" (*Associated symptoms*)

(continued)

- "Have you recently changed anything in your home?" "Or in your work environment?" "Have you recently been eating different foods?" "Any change in amount of food?" "How much red meat (beef, pork, lamb) have you eaten weekly over the past 3 years?" "Have you recently changed the types of beverages you drink?" "Or the amounts you drink?" "Have you taken any new medication (including over-the-counter drugs)?" "Have you taken any hormones?" "Have you been exposed to pesticides?" "Have you had any injury to your breast/chest?" (*Environmental factors*)
- "Tell me how this lump is affecting your life." (*Significance to client*)
- "What do you think is happening?" (*Client perspective*)

HEALTH PROMOTION

Important Topics for Health Promotion

- Breast size
- Breast support
- Risk factors for benign breast disorders
- Risk factors for benign breast disorders
- Risk factors for breast cancer
- Breast cancer screening
  - Know Your Breasts (KYB) approach
  - Clinical breast examination (CBE)
  - Mammography
  - Magnetic resonance imaging (MRI)

BREAST SIZE

Women may have concerns that their breasts are too small or are too large. Consideration of surgical intervention needs thorough discussion and examination with nurses and other members of the interdisciplinary team. Augmentation mammoplasty (enlarging the breasts with implants) is the most common surgery performed by U.S. plastic surgeons (American Society of Plastic Surgeons, 2009). One concern from an assessment viewpoint is that having implants makes KYB and clinical breast examinations (CBEs) and mammograms more difficult to interpret. Researchers found that while the mortality rate for women in Ontario and Quebec having breast implants was lower than for those having other cosmetic procedures, what was of concern was the higher suicide rates for both those with implants and those with other cosmetic surgery. Further study related to assessing risk factors for suicide for women having cosmetic surgery is needed (Villeneuve et al., 2006).

Women with very large breasts (*macromastia*) reach the decision for reduction mammoplasty for many reasons: neck and shoulder pain, changes in curvature of the spine, fatigue, breast pain, difficulties with KYB, poor posture from the weight of the breasts and attempts to make the breasts appear less conspicuous, challenges to find clothes that fit, and the embarrassment of people staring at their breasts. Breast feeding is still possible for approximately half of women following reduction mammoplasty (Chow, 2007). Canadian women were assessed prior to having a reduction mammoplasty and at 6 and 21.5 months following surgery. Researchers found significant and sustained improvement on four measurements: 7 of 8 health status domains improved, decreased symptoms, increased self-esteem, and weight loss and lower Body Mass Index (BMI) scores (O'Blenes et al., 2006).

BREAST SUPPORT

Women now recognize the need to wear a supportive bra or sports bra, particularly during exercise. A bra decreases discomfort and helps to preserve the tissue elasticity of the breasts. For women 30 to 50 years old with fibrocystic breast changes, wearing a supportive bra day and night for the week before the menstrual period may offer pain relief (Chow, 2007). Older women find that a supportive bra helps relieve discomfort from sagging breasts (D'Amico & Barbarito, 2007).

BENIGN BREAST DISORDERS (BBD)

Although many more women seek care for BBD than for cancer, interest has generally been limited to the possible relationship between BBD and later development of breast cancer (Courtillot et al., 2005). The term *benign breast disorders* encompasses several masses related to different components of the breasts. Because some forms of BBD are asymptomatic, actual incidence of BBD is unknown. It is known that as age increases, the frequency of BBD decreases and cancer rates increase (Houssami & Dixon, 2006). Awareness of changes in breast structures across the life span leads to better understanding of BBD. The Aberrations of Normal Development and Involution (ANDI) classification of BBD includes usual processes, aberrations of expected changes, and diseases.

Stage	Usual Process	Aberration	Disease
Early reproductive (15–25 years)	Lobular development	Fibroadenoma	Giant fibroadenoma > 5 cm in diameter Multiple fibroadenomas 3 to 5 lesions in 1 breast
Mature reproductive (25–40 years)	Cyclical changes during each menstrual cycle	Cyclical mastalgia Nodularity	Incapacitating mastalgia
Involution (35–55 years)	Lobular involution	Macrocysts Sclerosing lesions	Periductal mastitis
	Epithelial turnover	Simple epithelial hyperplasia	Epithelial hyperplasia with atypia

Adapted from Hughes, L. E., Mansel, R. E., & Webster, D. J. (1987). Aberrations of normal development and involution (ANDI): A new perspective on pathogenesis and nomenclature of benign breast disorders. *Lancet, 2*(8571), 1316–1319.

ANDI (Aberrations of Normal Development and Involution) Classification.
Between 15 and 25 years, the main activity in the breast is adding lobular structures to the ductal system. The repeated changes of menstruation and pregnancy in women in the age group of 15 to 50 years provide opportunities for minor aberrations to occur. An added risk is an overlap of approximately 20 years with involution, which occurs between the age of 35 and 55 years and results in replacement of hormone-responsive connective tissue in the lobules with fibrous tissues. After menopause, few ducts and lobular structures remain in the breasts.

Disorders of Development: Fibroadenomas.
Because these benign masses arise from the lobules, they occur mainly in women aged 15 to 25 years. Incidence of fibroadenomas identified from autopsy results was in the range of 15% to 23% (Hughes, Mansel, & Webster, 1987). Fibroadenomas, usually 1 cm to 2 cm in diameter, are smooth, round, firm, and highly mobile. Diagnosis in women younger than 35 years of age is by ultrasound. Fine needle aspiration biopsy or core needle biopsy is required if the client is older than 25 years. Women with

fibroadenomas and no family history of breast cancer have no increased risk of developing breast cancer (Courtillot et al., 2005).

 Cultural Considerations

In Saudi Arabia, which has a large population of young women, incidence of fibroadenoma was 21.1%. Another 16.2% had pathological conditions associated with lactation (Amr et al., 1995).

Disorders of Cyclical Change: Mastalgia and Nodularity.
Most women experience discomfort and nodularity with the premenstrual enlargement and postmenstrual involution of the breasts with each menstrual cycle. Discomfort and nodularity may be from increased estrogen secretion from the ovaries and lack of sufficient progesterone production (Courtillot et al., 2005). Approximately 50% of women have palpable lumps or nodularity. Painful nodularity lasting longer than 1 week of the cycle and not resolved by onset of menses is considered outside of the range of expected discomfort. Severe or incapacitating mastalgia is considered a first step of BBD and is linked to subsequent cancer (Goodwin et al., 1995; Plu-Bureau et al., 1992). Mammography or ultrasound is only required if nodularity is present.

Disorders of Involution: Cyst Formation and Fibrous Change.
Cysts and fibrous changes (formerly called fibrocystic disease) occur mainly in the middle and later reproductive phases. The term now used is "fibrocystic changes," because 50% to 60% of women with lumpy breasts or breasts with nondiscrete nodules do not have breast disease and are not at increased risk of breast cancer (Santen & Mansel, 2005). The incidence of cysts increases starting at about 35 years of age, with most occurring between the ages 40 and 50 years. In cohort studies using biopsy results, fibrocystic changes before the age of 65 years occurred in 8.8% of women (Goehring & Morabia, 1997). Cysts generally disappear after menopause, unless the client takes hormone therapy. Cysts are not related to the menstrual cycle in terms of pain or size, and nipple discharge is unusual. On palpation, cysts feel like a smooth, tense structure against the chest wall and may seem to be attached to the breast tissue. Diagnosis includes ultrasound, complete needle aspiration of the cyst, and cytology only if the fluid is blood-stained (indicates presence of an associated carcinoma).

Assessment of Breast Masses or Lumps.
A "triple" assessment is required. In the CBE, breasts are examined within 5 to 7 days after the onset of menstruation to approximately Day 13 (before ovulation occurs) for two consecutive months. A woman's age and the physical characteristics of the mass provide some clues to its origin. The second assessment is imaging: ultrasound for women aged 25 to 35 years; mammograms for women older than 35 years; magnetic resonance imaging (MRI) for women aged more than 30 years with BRCA1 or BRCA2 genes, strong family history of breast cancer, or who have dense breasts. The third step is fine needle aspiration of the lump or a core needle biopsy.

Risk Factors for BBD.
Younger women are at increased risk for BBD. By menopause the risk for BBD is low unless a woman is taking hormone therapy, which increases the risk for BBD (Rohan & Miller, 1999). Women with gene mutations of BRCA1 or BRCA2 have a higher frequency of multiple benign breast masses (Hoogerbrugge et al., 2003). Women taking tamoxifen (an anti-estrogen drug) to prevent breast cancer had reduced risk for BBD (Tan-Chiu et al., 2003). Researchers in China identified high level of education, high BMI, high intake of dairy products, and depression as risk factors for BBD, while long-term contraception was a protective factor (Li et al., 2005). In Quebec, researchers noted

that breast pain and having more than 12 years of education were the best predictors of fibrocystic breast changes, while use of oral contraceptives, cholesterol intake of 300 mg/day or more, and more than 10% of calories from fat had a protective effect (Vobecky et al., 1993).

■ *Palpable Masses of the Breast*

Age	Common Lesion	Characteristics
15–25	Fibroadenoma	Usually fine, round, mobile, nontender
25–50	Cysts	Usually soft to firm, round, mobile; often tender
	Fibrocystic changes	Nodular, ropelike
	Cancer	Irregular, stellate, (star-shaped) firm, not clearly delineated from surrounding tissue
Over 50	Cancer until proven otherwise	As above
Pregnancy/lactation	Lactating adenomas, cysts, cancer, and mastitis	As above / Tough and doughy, tender

Source: Adapted from Schultz, M. Z., Ward, B. A., & Reiss, M. Breast diseases. In J. Noble, H. L. Greene, W. Levinson, et al. (Eds.), *Primary Care Medicine*, 2nd ed. St. Louis, Mosby, 1996. See also Venet, L., Strax, P., Venet, W., et al. Adequacies and inadequacies of breast examinations by physicians in mass screenings. *Cancer, 28*(6):1546–1551, 1971.

BREAST CANCER

Incidence of Breast Cancer. Breast cancer is the most common cause of death from cancer in women worldwide (Anderson, 2006). More than 1.1 million women are diagnosed with breast cancer every year (Anderson, 2006). In 2000, more than half of all breast cancer cases in the world occurred in high-income countries (International Agency for Research on Cancer, World Health Organization, 2002). The exception was Japan, which had a low incidence rate.

Cultural Considerations

Caucasian women older than 40 years have rates of breast cancer higher than for any other racial or ethnic group (D'Amico & Barbarito, 2007). Incidence of breast cancer is low in women in Saudi Arabia, Japan, and Singapore (Weber & Kelley, 2007). In Saudi Arabia, the mean age for ductal carcinoma was 47.1 years versus 54 years in Western countries (Amr et al., 1995). In Jordan, 62% of breast cancers in women are diagnosed before age 53 years (Petro-Nustas, Norton, & al-Masarweh, 2002). For women in Ghana, complete surgical removal of a breast lump is the only acceptable treatment. Risk of cancer increases, especially after the age of 30 years (Ohene-Yeboah, 2005).

Estimates are that 1 in 9 women in Canada will develop breast cancer during her lifetime, and one in 27 will die of the disease. In 2008, more than 22,000 Canadian women were diagnosed with and 5300 died from breast cancer. New diagnoses of breast cancer in 2008 were more than double those of lung cancer among Canadian women. On a positive note, the incidence of breast cancer in women in Canada has been stable since 1993, and the rate of death has decreased by 2.7% each year to the lowest it has been since 1950 (Canadian Cancer Society/National Cancer Institute of Canada, 2008). The risk of being diagnosed with breast cancer increases until the age of 59 years and then decreases, while the risk of dying from breast cancer increases with age.

■ Age Distribution of Breast Cancer Cases and Deaths in Canadian Women		
Age (Years)	**Breast Cancer Cases**	**Breast Cancer Deaths**
<29	<1%	<1%
30–39	4%	2%
40–49	16%	9%
50–59	28%	18%
60–69	24%	19%
70–79	17%	22%
80+	12%	31%

Source: Canadian Cancer Society/National Cancer Institute of Canada, 2007.

In 2008, 170 Canadian men were diagnosed with and 50 died from breast cancer (Canadian Cancer Society/National Cancer Institute of Canada, 2008). Breast cancer in men accounts for approximately 1% of all cases and is usually diagnosed between 60 and 70 years. Breast cancer rates for men have increased in the last 25 years. Possible contributors may include increased carcinogens in the environment, increased awareness (which leads to increased diagnosis), and the increasing rate of obesity (Ontario Ministry of Health Promotion, 2007). Men rarely report concerns about a breast mass. Consequently, men are diagnosed with breast cancer at an older age than women (67 years for men vs. 62 years for women) and at a later stage of the disease (with metastases; Ontario Ministry of Health Promotion, 2007). However, survival rates are similar for both men and women and depend on how early the cancer is diagnosed (Ontario Ministry of Health Promotion, 2007).

Alberta nurse researchers interviewed men with breast cancer. The men were concerned with the lack of awareness of male breast cancer, not just by the public, but also by health professionals. Also, men were stressed by their cancer diagnosis, had body-image concerns, experienced role strain, and noted a lack of information about male breast cancer. Because the men were not interested in traditional support groups, further research is needed into what supports would be beneficial (Pituskin et al., 2007).

Risk Factors for Breast Cancer in Men.
Risk factors include increasing age, excess estrogen, low testosterone levels, testicular disorders such as infection and injury, exposure to radiation in childhood, strong family history of breast cancer in female relatives (particularly mother and sister), and alteration of the BRCA2 gene. Excess estrogen can result from gynecomastia (excess growth of male mammary tissue), Klinefelter's syndrome (abnormal chromosome pattern of XXY rather than XY), cirrhosis, and increased circulating estrogen related to increased body fat (obesity; National Cancer Institute, 2006).

Nurses and interdisciplinary health care team members have a role to play in raising awareness that men get breast cancer and need to seek help as soon as they note breast signs and symptoms. Men with risk factors should be offered instructions about the KYB approach. Mammograms are not used for screening for breast cancer in men, but are used for diagnosis once a mass is found.

Risk Factors for Breast Cancer in Women.
The cause of breast cancer is not known, but the primary risk factors include being female and aging.

Women coming to Canada from areas where the rate of breast cancer is low may be unaware that their rate of cancer will increase to match that of Canadian women. For example, incidence patterns for cancer in Indo-Canadian women were different from those from India and were more similar to those of the general population of British Columbia where they resided (Hislop et al., 2007, p. 107). When an immigrant woman develops breast cancer, her community may not believe the diagnosis, leaving the woman without support.

In developing countries, women delayed seeking care for palpable breast lumps until other symptoms such as "pain, weakness, and malodorous fungating lesions" occurred (Meneses & Yarbro, 2007, p. 107). For example, in Saudi Arabia, many women presented with large tumours, skin, and/or nipple involvement, and 61.7% had metastasis to axillary lymph nodes (Amr et al., 1995). Some women delayed treatment because the stigma of breast cancer might affect a daughter's marriage. For others, the family made the decision whether to have treatment or not based on resources.

Men of African descent and Jewish men with a European background have increased rates of breast cancer (INFO Breast Cancer, 2006).

Cultural Considerations

In a study of South Asian women living in western Canada, nurse researchers identified five beliefs about the cause of cancer: (1) physical damage to the breast; (2) "can catch it" and spread it to others; (3) negative lifestyle ("bring it on yourself"); (4) is in the "hands of others" through careless words, curses, or divine power; and (5) passed down in the family (Johnson et al., 1999, p. 243).

For *screening of asymptomatic women*, target risk factors, including family history. Other risk factors for breast cancer include previous breast cancer and a family history of ovarian cancer (Canadian Cancer Society, 2009b). The clinician and individual client should review demographic data, family history, reproductive history, and any prior history of proliferative breast disease, especially if a biopsy has shown atypical hyperplasia or lobular carcinoma in situ. Several models help establish the female client's risk of breast cancer. The Breast Cancer Risk Assessment Tool of the National Cancer Institute (http://www.cancer.gov/bcrisktool) and the Gail model are among the most widely used (Gail & Benichou, 1994; Gail et al., 1989).

■ Summary of Breast Cancer Risk Factors

Factor	Relative Risk (%)
Family History	
First-degree relative with breast cancer	1.2–3.0
Premenopausal	3.1
Premenopausal and bilateral	8.5–9.0
Postmenopausal	1.5
Postmenopausal and bilateral	4.0–5.4
BRCA1/BRCA2 genes	3.0–7.0
Menstrual History	
Age at menarche <12	1.3
Age at menopause >55	1.5–2.0
Pregnancy	
First live birth from ages 25–29	1.5
First live birth after age 30	1.9
First live birth after age 35	2.0–3.0
Nulliparous	3.0
Breast Conditions and Diseases	
Nonproliferative disease	1.0
Proliferative disease	1.9
Proliferative with atypical hyperplasia	4.4
Lobular carcinoma in situ	6.9–12.0
Breast density on mammography	1.8–6.0

Adapted from Bilmoria, M. M., & Morrow, M. The woman at increased risk for breast cancer: evaluation and management strategies. *CA Cancer Journal for Clinicians, 45*(5):263, 1995, and from Clemons, M., & Goss, P. Estrogen and the risk of breast cancer. *New England Journal of Medicine, 344*(4):276–285, 2001.

However, the Gail model does not include risk factors such as the degree of breast density, plasma levels of free estradiol, bone density, weight gain after menopause, and waist-to-hip ratio (Santen & Mansel, 2005).

Demographic Factors—Age, Education, and Income.

Approximately 80% of breast cancers occur in women older than 50 years, and more than 53% in women older than 60 years. Higher education and income levels appear to double the risk for breast cancer, possibly because of differences in age at first birth and parity. In 2001, mortality rates for First Nation women on reserves in Canada as well as those off reserves in British Columbia and Alberta were 11.2 per 100,000 of population versus 25 per 100,000 of population for all other Canadian women (Health Canada, 2005). Older First Nations women in Ontario preferred Web-based material that included health attitudes and behaviours of First Nations women and their breast cancer risk (Friedman & Hoffman-Goetz, 2007).

Family History.

The relative risks for breast cancer (risk relative to a person without a given risk factor) associated with menarche and menopause, age at first pregnancy, and breast conditions and diseases is summarized in the previous table. Risk for familial breast cancer has two patterns: family history of breast cancer and genetic predisposition. First-degree relatives, namely, a mother or sister with breast cancer, establish a "positive family history." Within this group, menopausal status and extent of disease play key roles. Having a first-degree relative with premenopausal breast cancer confers highest risk. Even when a mother or sister has bilateral breast cancer, the probability of breast cancer is only 25% (U.S. Preventive Services Task Force, 1996).

Inherited disease in women carrying the breast cancer susceptibility genes *BRCA1* and *BRCA2* accounts for 5% to 10% of breast cancers (Canadian Cancer Society, 2009c). When present, these autosomal-dominant genes pose a risk for cancer of 50% in women younger than 50 years and 80% in women older than 65 years. Red flags for these mutations include multiple relatives with breast cancer, ovarian cancer, or both; a woman with more than one primary cancer (e.g., bilateral disease or combined breast and ovarian); and vertical transmission through two or more generations.

Researchers examined the options used to prevent cancer by women in Western Canada, Ontario, and Quebec who were previously diagnosed with BRCA1 and BRCA2 mutations. These options were surgery—removal of both breasts (mastectomy) and removal of both ovaries (oophorectomy)—and chemoprevention with tamoxifen or raloxifene. Approximately two-thirds of the Quebec women took no preventative option, compared with one-third of Western Canadian and Ontario women. More Western Canadians (67%) had bilateral oophorectomies and bilateral mastectomies (46%). Ontario had the highest participation (16%) in using tamoxifen or raloxifene. Further research is needed to understand whether these differences involved the information provided by nurses and other interdisciplinary providers (Metcalfe et al., 2007).

Researchers identified IKBKE as a human breast cancer oncogene that is "amplified and overexpressed" in a significant number of human breast tumours and plays a role in the transformation of mammary cells (Boehm et al., 2007). Some breast cancer cells require IKBKE to proliferate and survive. This suggests that treatments could be developed to specifically target IKBKE.

Breast density is now recognized as a significant risk factor for breast cancer, accounting for 16% to 30% of cases. Family history and the known genes account for a much smaller number of breast cancers (Boyd et al., 2007).

Menstrual History and Pregnancy.   Early menarche (before 12 years), delayed menopause (after 50 to 55 years), and first live birth after 35 years, each raise the risk for breast cancer two-fold to three-fold. These factors, especially when combined, relate to duration of breast tissue exposure to stimulation from unopposed estrogen (Clemons & Goss, 2001).

Breast Conditions and Diseases.   BBD with biopsy findings of atypical hyperplasia or lobular carcinoma in situ carries significantly increased relative risks—4.4 and 6.9 to 12.0, respectively.

Other Factors.   Additional factors include previous radiation to the chest for treatment of Hodgkin's lymphoma, number of breast biopsies (even if results were negative for breast cancer), and recent migration from a region with a low rate for breast cancer, such as China.

Lifestyle Issues.   Use of alcohol daily, weight gain of 20 kg or more after menopause (Santen & Mansel, 2005), and high-fat diet are risk factors for breast cancer. A 2007 study in the United Kingdom found that for postmenopausal women, eating as little as 57 gm of red meat (beef, lamb, and pork) daily was a significant risk for breast cancer. Postmenopausal women eating larger amounts (103 gm) of processed meats (sausage, bacon, and ham) had an increased risk of breast cancer. Premenopausal women with the highest intake of meat also had increased risk for breast cancer (Taylor et al., 2007). Using the same population, researchers found that in premenopausal women, total fibre intake protected against breast cancer. Cereal fibre was most protective, while fruit fibre may potentially be protective. No significant relationship existed between fibre intake and breast cancer in postmenopausal women (Cade et al., 2007).

In a study of healthy postmenopausal women aged 55 years and older, the group taking 1400 to 1500 mg of calcium and 1000 International Units (IU) of vitamin D_3 (cholecalciferol) daily had a 77% relative cancer reduction compared to the placebo group. The calcium-only group (1400–1500 mg daily) had a 41% relative risk reduction (Lappe et al., 2007). Based on this study and others, the Canadian Cancer Society now recommends that adult Canadians take 1000 IU of vitamin D_3 daily, particularly during the fall and winter, to help prevent breast, colorectal, and prostate cancers. An upper limit of 2000 IU of vitamin D_3 allows room to obtain vitamin D from food sources such as milk, multivitamins, and the sun (Canadian Cancer Society, 2009d).

In 2005, 80% of women with breast cancer living in Ontario used complementary or alternative medicine (CAM), with 41% specifically using CAM to manage breast cancer. CAM included self-medication with products such as green tea, vitamins C and E, and flaxseed, and visits to CAM practitioners. Use of both products and CAM practitioner visits increased significantly since 1998 (Boon, Olatunde, & Zick, 2007). Nurses need to be informed about CAM and to ask clients about their use of CAM.

Considering occupational risks, women from Windsor, Ontario, with breast cancer were nearly three times more likely to have worked in farming. For those who also subsequently worked either in automotive-related manufacturing or health care, the risks were even greater (Brophy et al., 2006).

Breast Cancer Screening.   For women with average risk, the Canadian Cancer Society (2009a) recommends a KYB approach, CBE by a health professional annually, and mammograms every 2 years for women 50 to 69 years.

Cultural Considerations

Immigrant women from some cultures were raised to avoid looking at or touching their breasts. They may not follow a KYB approach, see a health professional for CBE, or have mammograms.

Language can be a barrier. The Canadian Cancer Society (2009e) has information on cancer in languages other than English.

In some immigrant groups, the husband controls the wife's access to health care. One provincial breast-screening centre worked with multicultural health brokers to provide programs for husbands to increase their understanding of breast cancer risk in women and the need for examinations and mammography. Educational programs can be offered to immigrant women's groups in community settings other than clinics.

Know Your Breasts (KYB). Although not validated as a method for detecting breast cancer, recent guidelines support KYB as a means of promoting health awareness. Most breast cancers are found by women themselves by accident (Kearney & Murray, 2006). Nurses recognize cultural and personal beliefs and know that some women may not feel comfortable touching their breasts. Nurses have a role to play in discussing KYB practices (e.g., when to do KYB, what to do if a lump is found) and in teaching techniques.

Others may be afraid to think about breast cancer. A successful health promotion project was the Train-the-Trainer (TTT) International Breast Health Program developed by Meneses and Yarbro (2007). The goal was to prepare nurses with the knowledge and skills needed to teach BSE; perform CBE; and provide treatment, education, and support groups. The programs were "grounded in the cultural beliefs and practices of the target population" and provided new ways to meet the worldwide burden of breast cancer (Meneses & Yarbro, 2007, p. 106). Thirty-two nurses from 20 countries educated more than 900 health care providers who provided care to more than 1400 clients.

Cultural Considerations

If a country has a basic health care system (few resources), the focus should be educating women to do BSE to detect lumps. In countries with more resources, the focus is on CBE for women in at-risk groups (outreach and education), followed by ultrasound or mammography for those with breast lumps (Eniu et al., 2006).

Clinical Breast Examination (CBE). These examinations are used primarily to screen for breast cancer in women with no symptoms. The *sensitivity* of CBE, estimated at 54%, is the frequency that breast cancer is found in clients who have it (Barton, Harris, & Fletcher, 1999). Sensitivity increases under the following conditions:

■ Examiners use a standardized examination method.

■ The duration of the examination is longer—sensitivity increased to 69% in the Canadian National Screening Study when examiners spent 5 to 10 minutes examining the breasts (Baines, Miller, & Bassett, 1989).

■ The size of the lump is larger (14% sensitivity for 3-mm mass vs. 79% sensitivity for a 1-cm mass; Campbell et al., 1991).

■ The degree of hardness of the lump increases.

■ The age of the client increases—more sensitive if the client is in her 50s (as breast tissue become less dense and more fatty) than in her 40s (Baines & Miller, 1997).

Sensitivity decreases if the client's breasts are lumpy or if she has large breasts. CBE can, however, detect breast cancers that mammography misses.

Specificity is the frequency with which CBE is negative for cancer in women who do not have it (estimated at 94%; Barton et al., 1999). Of note, the CBE has a high rate of false-positive results (identifies cancer when it is not present) and an even higher rate of false-negative results (identifies masses as not cancerous when, in fact, they are). This last situation raises serious concerns about the psychological effects on the women involved (Barton et al., 1999).

Mammograms. Since 2003, every Canadian province and territory (except Nunavut) has had a program of biennial mammography screening of asymptomatic women (aged 50–69 years) with no history of breast cancer (Canadian Cancer Society/National Cancer Institute of Canada, 2006). Despite a goal of 70% participation, 34% has been reached. However, the actual number of women screened is higher because women also access other accredited Canadian Association of Radiologists' clinics. Reported barriers to screening include not having a regular physician, living in rural areas, less education, and being Asian-born (Canadian Cancer Society/National Cancer Institute of Canada, 2006).

Women choosing to do KYB are encouraged to report any new breast symptoms. Intervals for mammography between the ages 40 and 50, however, are subject to controversy. Mammography is less accurate in glandular and dense breasts, especially when stimulated by higher estrogen levels before menopause, contributing to varying estimates of benefit. Breast density decreases approximately 1% per year (Boyd et al., 2007). However, British Columbia researchers reported that mammographic screening in women in the age group of 40 to 79 years reduced subsequent mortality rates from breast cancer (Coldman et al., 2007).

> Risk factors for breast cancer include previous breast cancer, an affected mother or sister, biopsy showing atypical hyperplasia, density of breast tissue, increasing age, early menarche, late menopause, late or no pregnancies, and previous radiation to the chest wall.

Women younger than 50 and older than 69 years should consult their health care providers about a schedule for mammograms. Mammography can detect breast masses less than 1 cm, which is before they are palpable. False negatives, however, occur in 5% to 10% of all mammograms (Chow, 2007). For women at increased risk due to their family history, clinicians advise starting screening 10 years before the date of onset of cancer in the client's relative. For example, if the client's mother was diagnosed with breast cancer at 48 years, then the client should begin screening at 38 years (Hartmann et al., 1999). For women at increased risk, many clinicians advise initiating screening mammograms between 30 and 40 years, then every 2 to 3 years until 50 years. For women 50 to 69 years, annual mammography and CBE are widely recommended (U.S. Preventive Services Task Force, 1996).

After 70 years, the benefits of mammography are less well defined, but may continue to be important, particularly with clients who have risk factors and long-term exposure to hormone therapy. In older clients, it is easier to detect cancer using CBE (the breasts have more fatty tissue but fewer duct and lobular structures). Older women may not see themselves at risk for cancer and may be resistant to the idea of mammograms (White, Urban, & Taylor, 1993).

Magnetic Resonance Imaging (MRI). Pediconi et al., (2007) recommend that all women with newly diagnosed breast cancer in one breast should undergo MRI to pick up potential cancer missed by mammograms of the other breast (mammograms may miss these cancers in 3% of cases). MRI is also recommended for women aged 30 years or older with a mutation of BRCA1 or BRCA2 genes, treated for Hodgkin's disease, or with a strong family history (two or more close relatives with breast or ovarian cancer or a close relative with breast cancer before 50 years; Saslow et al., 2007). MRIs show increased or unusual blood flow in breast tissue, an early sign of breast cancer not picked up by mammography, and are better at identifying cancer in women with dense breasts.

EMERGENCY CONCERNS

Two breast infections, mastitis and lactational abscess, can be emergencies. *Mastitis* is an infection of breast tissue, most common in women who are nursing (2–3 weeks following childbirth). The cause can be the transfer of microorganisms from the client's hands to the breast, infection from the breast-feeding infant (oral, eye, or skin), or blood-borne organisms. Infection in the breast ducts progresses and results in milk being trapped in several lobules. The client may report a dull pain over the affected area and purulent, serous, or bloody nipple discharge, which should be cultured. Treatment includes 7 to 10 days of a broad-spectrum antibiotic, hot compresses, a snug bra for support, rest, hydration, and careful personal hygiene (Chow, 2007).

Untreated mastitis can progress to *lactational abscess* as the body tries to wall off the infection. The breast becomes tender, red, and painful, with purulent nipple drainage. Fever, chills, delirium, and tachycardia are other possible symptoms. Treatment at this point is incision and drainage of the abscess. Severe infection can destroy the duct structure of the breast, resulting in no milk being produced from it after a subsequent pregnancy (Northrup, 1994).

TECHNIQUES OF EXAMINATION: OBJECTIVE DATA

THE FEMALE BREASTS

The CBE is an important component of women's health care: It enhances detection of breast cancers that mammography may miss and provides an opportunity to demonstrate the KYB approach to the client. Clinical investigation has shown, however, that variations in examiner experience and technique affect the value of the CBE. Nurses are advised to adopt a more standardized approach, especially for palpation, and to use a systemic and thorough search pattern, varying palpation pressure, and a circular motion with the finger pads (Barton et al., 1999). These techniques will be discussed in more detail in the following pages. Inspection is routinely recommended, but its value in breast cancer detection is less well studied.

PROMOTING CLIENT COMFORT, DIGNITY, AND SAFETY

Ensure that there is complete privacy before beginning the examination. A warm room is helpful. Assist the client to sitting and supine positions as required.

As you begin the examination of the breasts, be aware that women and girls may feel apprehensive. Be reassuring and adopt a courteous and gentle approach. Before you begin, let the client know that you are about to examine her breasts.

An adequate inspection requires full exposure of the chest, but later in the examination, cover one breast while you are palpating the other. Because breasts tend to swell and become more nodular before menses as a result of increasing estrogen stimulation, the best time for examination is 5 to 7 days *after* the onset of menstruation. Nodules appearing during the premenstrual phase should be reevaluated at this later time.

Equipment

- Examination gown
- Small pillow or towel
- Sheet for draping
- Metric tape measure
- Gloves if drainage or open sores/rash present

INSPECTION

Inspect the breasts and nipples with the client in the sitting position and disrobed to the waist. A thorough examination of the breasts includes careful inspection (from anterior and lateral views) for skin changes, symmetry, contours, and retraction in four views—arms at sides, arms over head, arms pressed against hips, and leaning forward. When examining an adolescent girl, assess her breast development according to Tanner's sex maturity ratings described on page 00.

Arms at Sides. Note the following clinical features:

- The *appearance of the skin*, including colour

  Redness may be from local infection or inflammatory carcinoma.

- Thickening of the skin and unusually prominent pores, which may accompany lymphatic obstruction

  Thickening and prominent pores suggest breast cancer.

- The *size and symmetry of the breasts.* Some difference in the size of the breasts, including the areolae, is common (left breast is often larger than the right) and is usually expected, as shown in the following photograph.

- The *contour of the breasts.* Look for changes such as masses, dimpling, or flattening. Compare one side with the other.

  Flattening of the usually convex breast suggests cancer. See Table 16-1, Visible Signs of Breast Cancer (p. 508).

- The *characteristics of the nipples,* including *size and shape, direction* in which they point, any *rashes* or *ulceration,* or any *discharge.*

  Asymmetry of directions in which nipples point suggests an underlying cancer. Rash or ulceration in Paget's disease of the breast (see p. 508).

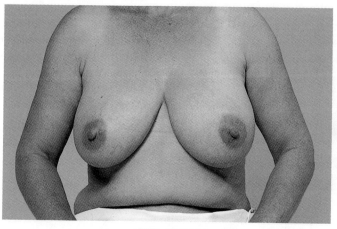

ARMS AT SIDES

Occasionally, the shape of the nipple is *inverted*, or depressed below the areolar surface. It may be enveloped by folds of areolar skin, as illustrated. Long-standing inversion is a usual variant of no clinical consequence, except for possible difficulty when breast feeding.

Recent or fixed flattening or depression of the nipple suggests nipple retraction. A retracted nipple may also be broadened and thickened, suggesting an underlying cancer.

Arms Over Head, Hands Pressed Against Hips, Leaning Forward.

To bring out dimpling or retraction that may otherwise be invisible, ask the client to raise her arms over her head. Then have her press her hands against her hips or press her hands together above or below her breasts to contract the pectoral muscles. Inspect the breast contours carefully in each position. If the breasts are large or pendulous, it may be useful to have the client stand and lean forward, supported by the back of the chair or the examiner's hands.

Ask the client to lift her breasts, then inspect for rashes, and excoriations (intertrigo) caused by friction of skin surfaces, moisture, and warmth.

Burning, itching, moisture, and redness progressing to erosion fissures. More common in women with large breasts, obesity, and diabetes mellitus.

Dimpling or retraction of the breasts in these positions suggests an underlying cancer. When a cancer or its associated fibrous strands are attached to both the skin and the fascia overlying the pectoral muscles, pectoral contraction can draw the skin inward, causing dimpling.

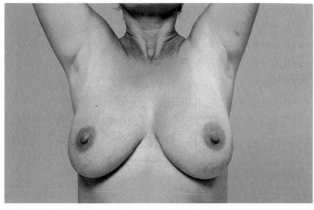

ARMS OVER HEAD

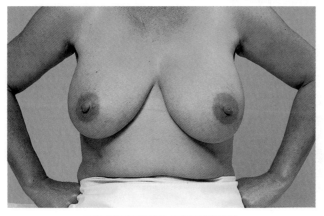

HANDS PRESSED AGAINST HIPS

Occasionally, these signs may be associated with benign lesions such as posttraumatic fat necrosis or mammary duct ectasia, but they must always be further evaluated.

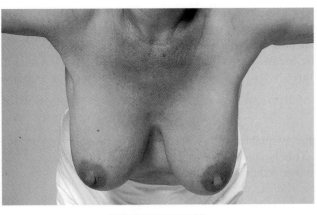

LEANING FORWARD

This position may reveal an asymmetry of the breast or nipple not otherwise visible. Retraction of the nipple and areola suggests an underlying cancer. See Table 16-1, Visible Signs of Breast Cancer (p. 508).

PALPATION

The Breasts.   If the client has large pendulous breasts, inspect her shoulders for indentations from bra straps and ask about pain in breasts, shoulders, neck, or back. Check for changes in the curvature of the spine (Chapter 19). Then complete the bimanual palpation while she is in the sitting position, leaning forward. Place your nondominant hand under her breast and your dominant hand near the top of the breast. Palpate the breast between your two hands, using finger pads, working in semicircles downward toward the nipple. Repeat on the other breast. By bringing the breast tissue away from the chest wall, the examiner may feel masses that are not palpable in the supine position. This manoeuvre also helps to differentiate breast pain from chest-wall pain.

Palpation is best performed when the breast tissue is flattened. The client should be supine. Plan to palpate a rectangular area extending from the clavicle to the inframammary fold or bra line (3 cm below the breast), and from the midsternal line to the posterior axillary line and well into the axilla for the tail of the breast (tail of Spence).

A thorough examination will take at least 3 minutes for each breast. Use the *fingerpads* of the 2nd, 3rd, and 4th fingers, keeping the fingers flat. Flex only at the wrist. The Canadian Cancer Society recommends a *horizontal* pattern, and this approach will be highlighted. In contrast, the American Cancer Society (2006) recommends a *vertical strip pattern* over the concentric circle and spoke approaches as the best-validated technique for detecting breast masses (Barton et al., 1999). Both the horizontal and vertical methods are systematic approaches to ensure that all breast tissue is examined.

When pressing deeply on the breast, you may mistake a rib for a hard breast mass.

The upper outer quadrant of each breast and the axillary tail of Spence require careful examination because most of the glandular tissue and 50% of all breast cancers are located there (Gest & Schlesinger, 1995). To examine the breast have the client supine with the pillow removed from under the head. If the breasts are large, place a small pillow under the shoulder on the side to be examined. This will help to shift the breast tissue medially and distribute it more evenly over the chest wall. Ask the client to move her arm slightly away from the chest on the side being examined to relax the pectoral muscle. Begin palpation below the clavicle and move in straight lines back and forth across the chest, continuing to make small circles while maintaining contact with the skin. Move the hand down one finger width for each row. Carefully palpating the rectangular area ensures examination of glandular tissue, the areola area, the nipple, and the tail of Spence. Squeezing the nipple to check for discharge is not part of a regular screening examination as it is not a "useful prognostic sign of cancer" (Gulay et al., 1994).

Nodules in the tail of the breast are sometimes mistaken for enlarged axillary lymph nodes (and vice versa).

Thickening of the nipple or skin and loss of elasticity suggest an underlying cancer.

■ *Consistency* of the tissues. Consistency varies widely, depending in part on the relative proportions of firmer glandular tissue and soft fat. Physiologic nodularity may be present, increasing before menses. There may be a firm transverse ridge of compressed tissue along the lower margin of the breast, especially in large breasts. This is the inframammary ridge, not a tumour.

Tender cords suggest *mammary duct ectasia*, a benign but sometimes painful condition of dilated ducts with surrounding inflammation, sometimes with associated masses.

■ *Tenderness*, as in premenstrual fullness

■ *Nodules*. Palpate carefully for any lump or mass that is qualitatively different from or larger than the rest of the breast tissue. This is sometimes called a dominant mass and may reflect a pathologic change that requires evaluation by mammogram, aspiration, or biopsy. Assess and describe the characteristics of any nodule:

See Table 16-2, Common Breast Masses (p. 509).

Location—by quadrant or clock, with centimetres from the nipple
Size—in centimetres
Shape—round or cystic, disc-like, or irregular in contour
Consistency—soft, firm, or hard
Delimitation—well-circumscribed or not
Tenderness—present or not, location
Mobility—in relation to the skin, pectoral fascia, and chest wall. Gently move the breast near the mass and watch for dimpling.

Hard, irregular, poorly circumscribed nodules fixed to the skin or underlying tissues strongly suggest cancer.

Cysts, inflamed areas; some cancers may be tender.

Next, try to move the mass itself while the client relaxes her arm and then while she presses her hand against her hip.

A mobile mass that becomes fixed when the arm relaxes is attached to the ribs and intercostal muscles; if fixed when the hand is pressed against the hip, it is attached to the pectoral fascia.

THE MALE BREASTS

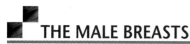

Because men have less fatty tissue in their breasts than women, it is easier to detect abnormalities through inspection and palpation (Canadian Cancer Society, 2009f). The examination of the male breasts will take less time but is important. Ask about breast or chest-wall pain and nipple discharge. *Inspect the nipple, areola, and breast* for nodules, swelling, redness, dimpled or retracted breast tissue, nipple discharge, and ulceration. *Palpate the areola and breast tissue* for nodules and increased warmth. If the breast appears enlarged, distinguish between the soft fatty enlargement of obesity and the firm disc of glandular enlargement called *gynecomastia*.

Gynecomastia is attributed to an imbalance of estrogens and androgens, sometimes drug-related. A hard, irregular, eccentric, or ulcerating nodule is not gynecomastia and suggests breast cancer.

Heat, redness, and swelling may indicate *inflammatory breast cancer*. *Infiltrating ductal cancer* is the most common type of cancer in men.

THE AXILLAE

Although the axillae may be examined with the client lying down, a sitting position is preferable.

INSPECTION

Inspect the skin of each axilla, noting evidence of the following:

■ Rash

Deodorant and other rashes

■ Infection

Sweat gland infection (*hidradenitis suppurativa*)

■ Unusual pigmentation

Deeply pigmented, velvety axillary skin suggests *acanthosis nigricans*—one form is associated with internal malignancy.

PALPATION

If signs of infection are present, wear gloves for palpation. Assist the client to dry the axillae. To examine the left axilla, ask the client to relax with the left arm down. Help by supporting the left wrist or hand with your left hand. Cup together the fingers of your right hand and reach as high as you can toward the apex of the axilla. Warn the client that this may feel uncomfortable. Your fingers should lie directly behind the pectoral muscles, pointing toward the midclavicle. Now press your fingers in toward the chest wall and slide them downward, trying to feel the *central nodes* (3–4 nodes) against the chest wall. Of the axillary nodes, these are the most often palpable. One or more soft, small (<1 cm), nontender nodes are frequently felt.

Enlarged axillary nodes from infection of the hand or arm, recent immunizations or skin tests in the arm, or part of a generalized lymphadenopathy. Check the epitrochlear nodes and other groups of lymph nodes.

Use your left hand to examine the right axilla.

Nodes that are large (≥1 cm) and firm or hard, matted together, or fixed to the skin or to underlying tissues suggest malignant involvement.

■ *Pectoral or anterior nodes* (4 or 5 nodes)—grasp the anterior axillary fold between your thumb and fingers, and with your finger pads, palpate inside the border of the pectoral muscle.

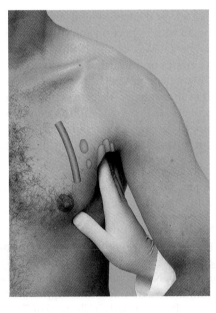

■ *Lateral nodes* (4–6 nodes)—from high in the axilla, feel along the upper humerus.

■ *Subscapular or posterior* (6 or 7 nodes) *nodes*—step behind the client (or turn your hand) and, with your finger pads, feel inside the muscle of the posterior axillary fold.

Also, feel for *infraclavicular nodes* (below the clavicle) (6–12 nodes) and reexamine the *supraclavicular nodes* (above the clavicle) (6–12 nodes).

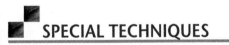

SPECIAL TECHNIQUES

Assessment of Spontaneous Nipple Discharge. If there is a history of spontaneous nipple discharge, try to determine its origin by compressing the areola with your index finger, placed in radial positions around the nipple. Watch for discharge appearing through one of the duct openings on the nipple's surface. Note the colour, consistency, and quantity of any discharge and the exact location where it appears. Take a culture of the discharge.

Milky discharge unrelated to a prior pregnancy and lactation is called *nonpuerperal galactorrhea*. Leading causes are hormonal and pharmacologic.

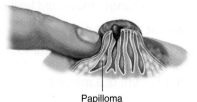

Papilloma

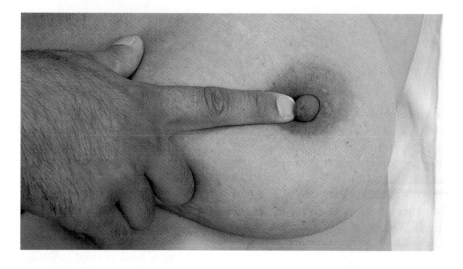

A nonmilky unilateral discharge suggests local breast disease. The causative lesion is usually benign, but may be malignant, especially in elderly women. A benign intraductal papilloma is shown above in its usual subareolar location. Note the drop of blood exuding from a duct opening.

Examination of the Client Who Has Had a Mastectomy.

The woman with a mastectomy warrants special care on examination. She may be embarrassed about the appearance of her surgical incision and anxious about the examination of the remaining breast. Begin with inspection and palpation of the breast and axillae of the unaffected side (Barkauskas et al., 1998). Inspect the mastectomy scar and axilla carefully for any masses or unusual nodularity. Note any change in colour or signs of inflammation. Lymphedema may be present in the axilla and upper arm from impaired lymph drainage after surgery. Palpate gently along the scar—these tissues may be unusually sensitive. Use a circular motion with two or three fingers. Pay special attention to the upper outer quadrant and axilla. Note any enlargement of the lymph nodes or signs of inflammation or infection. Encourage the client to consider the KYB approach.

It is especially important to carefully palpate the breast tissue and incision lines of women with breast augmentation, reconstruction, or reduction.

Masses, nodularity, and change in colour or inflammation, especially in the incision line, suggest recurrence of breast cancer.

Instructions for the KYB Approach.

Any setting visit is a time to ask if the client is interested in learning the KYB approach. A high proportion of breast masses are detected by women examining their own breasts. Although BSE has not been shown to reduce breast cancer mortality, the KYB approach is inexpensive and may promote stronger health awareness and more active self-care. Approximately 25% to 30% of women were reported to do BSE regularly (Chow, 2007). It is important to talk with women about why they do not do BSE on a regular basis and then to incorporate their information into teaching sessions (Day et al., 2007). For early detection of breast cancer, the KYB is most useful when coupled with regular breast examination by an experienced clinician and mammography. The BSE is best timed just after menses, when hormonal stimulation of breast tissue is low.

THE KNOW YOUR BREASTS (KYB) APPROACH

Take charge of your breast health. This starts with knowing your breasts so that you are more likely to notice changes that could lead to problems.

About the KYB Approach

KYB is different from mammography and clinical breast examination (CBE). KYB is done by you, standing in front of a mirror and lying down, looking at and feeling your breasts, under your arms, and chest. The best time for KYB is 5 to 13 days after your period starts. If you no longer menstruate, select any day.

Changes to Look For

KYB will help you see and feel changes in your breasts. First you need to learn what is usual for your breasts. They may usually feel a bit lumpy. Check for any new

(Continued)

THE KNOW YOUR BREASTS (KYB) APPROACH (Continued)

place they feel thicker or harder than the rest of your breast. If your breasts are large, they may fold over on your chest and feel like a firm ridge. Lift them up to check the skin underneath.

The KYB Approach

Stand in front of a mirror:

- With your arms at your sides, look in the mirror at your breasts.
  - Slowly turn from side to side.
  - Check for changes in size and shape from last time you looked.
  - Check for rashes or puckers in the skin.
  - Look for any discharge from your nipples.
- Raise your arms above your head. Keep looking in the mirror.
- Put your hands behind your ears.
  - Look at your breasts and under your arms.
  - Lean forward and look at your breasts.
  - Check for any changes from last KYB check.
- Place hands on hips, pressing firmly
  - Check for any changes from last KYB check.
- Feel your breasts with your fingers. Some women do this in the shower because soap makes it easier to move their hand over the breast. Do this step for each breast. Using a horizontal pattern to guide you, make small circles.

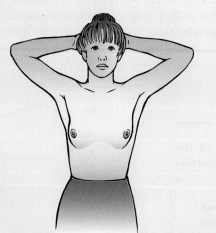

Stay standing. Using the opposite hand to each breast.

- Hold the fingers of your hand together.
- Keep your fingers stiff and your hand flat.
- Do not cup your hand.

Source: Adapted from the Canadian Cancer Society, 2009a.

- Use the pads of your fingers, not the tips.
- Make small circles in straight lines starting just below the collarbone.

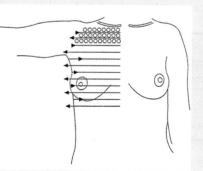

- Go slowly all the way across the breast area.
- Maintain constant contact with and pressure on your skin.
- Move your fingers down one finger width.
- Repeat the small circles back and forth across your breast.
- Bend your wrist to go over the curve of your breast.
- Make sure you feel over the nipple.
- Keep moving down until you are below your breast. You may need to make many circles to check your whole breast.
- Check under your arm.
  - Relax your arm by your side.
  - Slide your other hand under that arm and make small circles like you did over your breasts.
  - Repeat for other arm.

Lying down:

- Lie on your back, on a firm surface.
- Put one hand behind your head.
- Keep the fingers of your other hand together.
- Check both breasts again, using the pads of your fingers and bending your wrist to cover the curves of your breasts.
- Switch hands and do the other breast.

What To Do If You Feel a Change

Most of the time, changes women find in their breasts are not cancer. The only way to know that a lump or any other change is not cancer is to have your doctor check it as soon as possible.

RECORDING AND ANALYZING FINDINGS

Documentation of the information obtained through the client history and the physical examination of the breasts and axillae needs to be thorough, accurate, and clear for all members of the interdisciplinary team to ensure that comprehensive and appropriate care can be planned and implemented for the client.

■ *Examples of Documentation for Breasts and Axillae*

Area of Assessment	Expected Findings	Unexpected Findings
Breast	Pendulous bilaterally. Left breast is slightly larger than right. Colour similar to body. Firm, smooth, no tenderness bilaterally. No masses or lesions; no signs of dimpling, retraction, or *peau d'orange* skin bilaterally.	Venous pattern is asymmetrical, more prominent on right breast. A 2.0 cm mass palpated in upper outer quadrant of right breast, 3.0 cm from nipple. Mass is firm, irregular shape with no definite border, nontender, fixed to adjacent structures. No lesions or signs of dimpling, retraction, or *peau d'orange* skin visible bilaterally. No masses palpable in left breast.
Nipples	Everted bilaterally, point upward and laterally. No cracks, rashes, or discharge noted bilaterally.	Right nipple inverted for 1 month. Left is everted. Nipples are reddened but not cracked. No discharge bilaterally.
Areolae	Darker in colour than breasts. No rashes noted bilaterally.	Redness, scaly appearance on right areola. No change in colour, no rashes noted on left areola.
Axillae	Skin clear, intact bilaterally. No palpable axillary, infraclavicular, or supraclavicular nodes bilaterally. No tenderness bilaterally.	Red rash over both axillae, with slight itchiness reported (used new deodorant yesterday). A 2.0 cm firm mobile central node palpable over left chest wall. No tenderness over the node or elsewhere in the axillae. No other axillary nodes or infraclavicular or supraclavicular nodes were palpable bilaterally.

■ ANALYZING FINDINGS FROM HEALTH HISTORY AND PHYSICAL EXAMINATION

Following documentation of findings, the nurse completes an analysis of the information from the health history and examination findings to identify *nursing diagnoses* and to plan an *interdisciplinary approach*. For example:

Mrs. McKay, a 61-year-old high school English teacher, presents at the clinic. "I found another lump in my left breast. I have such a bad family history. Will it be cancer this time?" She has a history of three previous negative biopsies at ages 39, 41, and 44 years. Mrs. McKay's mother was diagnosed with breast cancer at 60 years and died from it at 63 years. Mrs. McKay's two older sisters were diagnosed with breast cancer in their 50s and died from the cancer. Her younger sister was diagnosed with breast cancer at 45 years, had a recurrence in the remaining breast at 55 years, and is currently doing well. Mrs. McKay has three daughters (30, 33, and 41 years).

Findings include height (1.6 metres); weight (90 kg), BMI 35; BP 160/90 (right arm, sitting position); pulse 102. There is a round, firm, nontender mass in the upper outer quadrant of the left breast, 1.5 cm from the nipple. Borders are not clear; it is not fixed to adjacent structures. Axillary, infraclavicular, and supraclavicular lymph nodes are not enlarged.

From this information, you develop the following nursing diagnosis:

Fear *related to breast lump and family history of breast cancer*

Many interdisciplinary health care team members may become involved in Mrs. MacKay's care. A physician immediately needs to evaluate the breast lump. A technician and radiologist will be involved with mammography of both breasts; other diagnostic tests include ultrasound, needle biopsy, and MRI. Given her family history, Mrs. McKay may need to see a geneticist to test for the BRCA1 and BRCA2 gene mutations.

If the lump is not cancerous, Mrs. McKay may still want to meet with a surgeon to discuss prophylactic or risk-reduction mastectomy. If a diagnosis of breast cancer is made, the client will need to see a surgeon to discuss operative intervention. An oncologist would be consulted at this point about additional postoperative treatments. Mrs. McKay may benefit from meeting breast cancer survivors through the Canadian Cancer Society Reach to Recovery Program. She may consult a plastic surgeon at or following surgery about breast reconstruction. If axillary nodes are removed during surgery, a physiotherapist will help with exercises to prevent/reduce lymphedema. After surgery, Mrs. McKay might attend a support group, often led by a clinical psychologist. Mrs. McKay's daughters need risk assessment for breast cancer. Over the longer term, Mrs. McKay should see a dietitian for weight reduction and meal planning. Throughout the process of diagnosis, treatment, and recovery, nurses are involved with assessment, monitoring, teaching, and providing care and support.

Critical Thinking Exercise

Answer the following questions about Mrs. McKay.

- What age group of women are most at risk for breast cancer? (*Knowledge*)
- Why is cancer in the upper outer quadrant of the breast so high risk? (*Comprehension*)
- How can you distinguish between Mrs. McKay's breast signs and symptoms and those for breast cancer or a benign breast mass? (*Application*)
- What lifestyle factors might be contributing to Mrs. McKay's risk for breast cancer? (*Analysis*)
- What recommendations for screening and follow-up would you suggest for Mrs. McKay and her daughters? (*Synthesis*)
- How would you evaluate the success of client teaching for Mrs. McKay? (*Evaluation*)

Canadian Nursing Research

Bottorff, J. L., McCullum, M., Balneaves, L. G., Esplen, M. J., Carroll, J., Kelly, M., et al. (2005a). Establishing roles in genetic nursing: Interviews with Canadian nurses. *Canadian Journal of Nursing Research, 37*(4), 96–115.

Bottorff, J. L., McCullum, M., Balneaves, L. G., Esplen, M. J., Carroll, J. C., Kelly, M., et al. (2005b). Canadian nursing in the genomic era: A call for leadership. *Canadian Journal of Nursing Leadership, 18*(2), 56–72.

Esplen, M. J., Hunter, J., Leszcz, M., Warner, E., Narod, S., Metcalfe, K., et al. (2004). A multicenter study of supportive-expressive group therapy for women with BRCA1/BRCA2 mutations. *Cancer, 101*(10), 2327–2340.

Hilton, B. A., Crawford, J. A., & Tarko, M. A. (2000). Men's perspectives on individual and family coping with their wives' breast cancer and chemotherapy. *Western Journal of Nursing Research, 22*(4), 438–459.

Johnson, J. L., Bottorff, J. L., Balneaves, L. G., Grewal, S., Bhagat, R., Hilton, B. A., et al. (1999). South Asian women's' views on the causes of breast cancer: Images and explanations. *Patient Education and Counseling, 37*(3), 243–254.

Metcalfe, K. A., Esplen, M. J., Goel, V., & Narod, S. A. (2004). Psychosocial functioning in women who have undergone bilateral prophylactic mastectomy. *Psycho-Oncology, 13*(1), 14–25.

Metcalfe, K. A., Esplen, M. J., Goel, V., & Narod, S. A. (2005). Predictors of quality of life in women with a bilateral prophylactic mastectomy. *Breast Journal, 11*(1), 65–69.

Pituskin, E., Williams, B., Au, H.-J., & Martin-McDonald, K. (2007). Experiences of men with breast cancer: A qualitative study. *The Journal of Men's Health & Gender, 4*(1), 44–51.

International Nursing Research

Meneses, K. D., & Yarbro, C. H. (2007). Cultural perspectives of international breast health and breast cancer education. *Journal of Nursing Scholarship, 39*(2), 105–112.

Petro-Nustas, W., Norton, M. E., & al-Masarweh, I. (2002). Risk factors for breast cancer in Jordanian women. *Journal of Nursing Scholarship, 34*(1), 19–25.

Test Questions

1. Screening measures for breast cancer include all of the following **except:**
   a. breast x-rays.
   b. mammography.
   c. Know Your Breasts approach.
   d. clinical breast examination.

2. The nurse reviews factors related to which of the following areas to assess risk of breast cancer?
   a. Family history, age, occupation
   b. Age, family history, reproductive history
   c. Lifestyle, occupation, exposure to hazardous chemicals
   d. Exposure to hazardous chemicals, lifestyle, reproductive history

3. The four major axillary node groups are the:
   a. anterior, subscapular, lateral, central.
   b. central, anterior, posterior, infraclavicular.
   c. infraclavicular, epitrochlear, lateral, pectoral.
   d. pectoral, epitrochlear, subscapular, supraclavicular.

4. When palpating the female breast for masses, the nurse distinguishes which of the following characteristics as a potentially cancerous mass?
   a. Single, firm, fixed nodule
   b. Multiple, round, mobile nodules
   c. Multiple, soft, nontender nodules
   d. Single, tender, well-delineated nodule

5. When inspecting the nipples, which of the following findings is unexpected?
   a. Bilateral retraction
   b. Long-standing inversion
   c. Supernumerary nipples
   d. Downward point of the nipples

Bibliography

CITATIONS

American Cancer Society. (2006). *Can breast cancer be found early?* Retrieved April 2, 2007, from http://www.cancer.org/docroot/CRI/content/CRI_2_4_3X_Can_breast_cancer_be_found_early_5.asp

American Society of Plastic Surgeons. (2009). *National Clearinghouse of Plastic Surgery Statistics. Procedural statistics trends 2000—2007.* Retrieved March 11, 2009, from http://www.plasticsurgery.org/Media/Press_Kits/Procedural_Statistics.html

Amr, S. S., Sa'di, A. R. M., Ilahi, F., & Sheikh, S. S. (1995). The spectrum of breast diseases in Saudi Arab females: A 26 year pathological survey at Dhahran Health Centre. *Annals of Saudi Medicine, 15*(2), 125–132.

Anderson, B. O. (2006). Breast healthcare and cancer control in limited-resource countries: A framework for change. *Nature Clinical Practice Oncology, 3*(1), 4–5.

Baines, C. J., & Miller, A. B. (1997). Mammography versus clinical examination of the breasts. *Journal of the National Cancer Institute. Monographs, 22,* 125–129.

Baines, C. J., Miller, A. B., & Bassett, A. A. (1989). Physical examination. Its role as a single screening modality in the Canadian National Breast Screening Study. *Cancer, 63*(9), 1816–1822.

Barkauskas, V. H., Stoltenberg-Allen, K., Baumann, L. C., & Darling-Fisher, C. (1998). *Health & physical assessment* (2nd ed.). St. Louis, MO: Mosby-Year Book.

Barton, M. B., Harris, R., & Fletcher, S. (1999). Does this client have breast cancer? The screening clinical breast examination: Should it be done? How? *Journal of the American Medical Association, 282*(13), 1270–1280.

Boehm, J. S., Zhao, J. J., Yao, J., Kim, S. Y., Firestein, R., Dunn, I. F., et al. (2007). Intergrative genomic approaches identify *IKBKE* as a breast cancer oncogene. *Cell, 129*(6), 1065–1079.

Boon, H. S., Olatunde, F., & Zick, S. M. (2007). Trends in complementary/alternative medicine use by breast cancer survivors: Comparing survey data from 1998 and 2005. *BMC Women's Health, 7,* Article 4.

Boyd, N. F., Guo, H., Martin, L. J., Sun, L., Stone, J., Fishell, E., et al. (2007). Mammographic density and the risk and detection of breast cancer. *New England Journal of Medicine, 356*(3), 227–236.

Brophy, J. T., Keith, M. M., Gorey, K. M., Luginaah, I., Laukkanen, E., Hellyer, D., Reinhartz, A., et al. (2006). Occupation and breast cancer: A Canadian case-control study. *Annals of the New York Academy of Sciences, 1076,* 765–777.

Cade, J. E., Burley, V. J., Greenwood, D. C., & The UK Women's Cohort Study Steering Group. (2007). Dietary fibre and risk of breast cancer in the UK women's cohort study. *International Journal of Epidemiology, 36*(20), 431–438.

Campbell, H. S., Fletcher, S. W., Pilgrim, C. A., Morgan, T. M., & Lin, S. (1991). Improving physicians' and nurses' clinical breast examination: A randomized controlled trial. *American Journal of Preventive Medicine, 7*(1), 1–8.

Canadian Cancer Society. (2009a). *Know your breasts.* Retrieved March 22, 2009, from http://www.cancer.ca/canada-wide/prevention/get%20screened/know%20your%20breasts.aspx?sc_lang=en

Canadian Cancer Society. (2009b). *Causes of breast cancer*. Retrieved March 22, 2009, from http://www.cancer.ca/Canada-wide/About%20cancer/Types%20of%20cancer/Causes%20of%20breast%20cancer.aspx?sc_lang=en

Canadian Cancer Society. (2009c). *Canadian Cancer Encyclopedia. Risk factors for breast cancer*. Retrieved March 22, 2009, from http://info.cancer.ca/E/CCE/cceexplorer.asp?tocid=10

Canadian Cancer Society. (2009d). *Vitamin D*. Retrieved March 11, 2009, from http://www.cancer.ca/canada-wide/prevention/use%20sunsense/vitamin%20d.aspx

Canadian Cancer Society. (2009e). *Cancer information in other languages*. Retrieved March 22, 2009, from http://www.cancer.ca/Canada-wide/About%20cancer/Other%20languages.aspx?sc_lang=en

Canadian Cancer Society. (2009f). *Breast cancer in men*. Retrieved March 22, 2009, from http://www.cancer.ca/Canada-wide/About%20cancer/Types%20of%20cancer/Breast%20cancer%20in%20men.aspx?sc_lang=en

Canadian Cancer Society/National Cancer Institute of Canada. (2006). *Canadian cancer statistics 2006*. Toronto, ON: Author.

Canadian Cancer Society/National Cancer Institute of Canada. (2007). *Canadian cancer statistics 2007*. Toronto, ON: Author.

Canadian Cancer Society/National Cancer Institute of Canada. (2008). *Canadian cancer statistics 2008*. Toronto, ON: Author.

Chow, J. (2007). Assessment and management of clients with breast disorders. In R. A. Day, P. Paul, B. Williams, S. C. Smeltzer, & B. Bare (Eds.), *Brunner & Suddarth's textbook of medical-surgical nursing* (1st Canadian ed., pp. 1700–1738). Philadelphia: Lippincott Williams & Wilkins.

Clemons, M., & Goss, P. (2001). Estrogen and the risk of breast cancer. *New England Journal of Medicine, 344*(4), 276–285.

Coldman, A., Phillips, N., Warren, L., & Kan, L. (2007). Breast cancer mortality after screening mammography in British Columbia women. *International Journal of Cancer, 120*(5), 1076–1080.

Courtillot, C., Plu-Bureau, G., Binart, N., Balleyguier, C., Sigal-Zafrani, B., Goffin, V., et al. (2005). Benign breast diseases. *Journal of Mammary Gland Biology & Neoplasia, 10*(4), 325–335.

D'Amico, D., & Barbarito, C. (2007). *Health & physical assessment in nursing*. Upper Saddle River, NJ: Pearson Education.

Eniu, A., Carlson, R. W., Aziz, Z., Bines, J., Hortobagyi, G. N., Bese, N. S., et al. (2006). Breast cancer in limited-resource countries: Treatment and allocation of resources. *Breast Journal, 12*(Suppl. 1), S38–S53.

Estes, M. E. Z. (2006). *Health assessment and physical examination* (3rd ed.). Clifton Park, NY: Thomson Delmar Learning.

Friedman, D. B., & Hoffman-Goetz, L. (2007). Assessing cultural sensitivity of breast cancer information for older aboriginal women. *Journal of Cancer Education, 22*(2), 112–118.

Gail, M. H., & Benichou, J. (1994). Validation studies on a model for breast cancer risk (editorial). *Journal of the National Cancer Institute, 86*, 573–575.

Gail, M. H., Brinton, L. A., Byar, D. P., Corle, D. K., Green, S. B., & Schairer, C. (1989). Projecting individual probabilities of developing breast cancer for white females who are being examined annually. *Journal of the National Cancer Institute, 81*, 1879–1886.

Gest, T. R., & Schlesinger, J. (1995). *MedCharts anatomy*. New York: ILOC.

Goehring, C., & Morabia, A. (1997). Epidemiology of benign breast disease, with special attention to histologic types. *Epidemiologic Reviews, 19*(2), 310–327.

Goodwin, P. J., DeBoer, G., Clark, R. M., Catton, P., Redwood, S., Hood, N., et al. (1995). Cyclical mastopathy and premenopausal breast cancer risk. Results of a case-control study. *Breast Cancer Research and Treatment, 33*(1), 63–73.

Gulay, H., Bora, S., Kilicturgay, S., Hamaloglu, E., & Goksel, H. A. (1994). Management of nipple discharge. *Journal of the American College of Surgeons, 178*(5), 471–474.

Hartmann, L. C., Schaid, D. J., Woods, J. E., Crotty, T. P., Myers, J. L., Arnold, P. G., et al. (1999). Efficacy of bilateral prophylactic mastectomy in women with a family history of breast cancer. *New England Journal of Medicine, 340*(2), 77–84.

Health Canada. (2005). *First Nations comparable health indicators*. Retrieved March 22, 2009, from http://www.hc-sc.gc.ca/fniah-spnia/diseases-maladies/2005-01_health-sante_indicat-eng.php

Hislop, T. G., Bajdik, C. D., Saroa, S. R., Yeole, B. B., & Barroetavena, M. C. (2007). Cancer incidence in Indians from three areas: Delhi and Mumbai, India, and British Columbia, Canada. *Journal of Immigrant & Minority Health, 9*(3), 221–227.

Hoogerbrugge, N., Bult, P., de Widt-Levert, L. M., Beex, L. V., Kiemeney, L. A., Ligtenberg, M. J., et al. (2003). High prevalence of premalignant lesions in prophylactically removed breasts from women at hereditary risk for breast cancer. *Journal of Clinical Oncology, 21*(1), 41–45.

Houssami, N., & Dixon, J. M. (2006). Diagnosis and management of benign breast disease in older women. *Geriatrics and Aging, 9*(9), 600–606.

Hughes, L. E., Mansel, R. E., & Webster, D. J. (1987). Aberrations of normal development and involution (ANDI): A new perspective on pathogenesis and nomenclature of benign breast disorders. *Lancet, 2*(8571), 1316–1319.

INFO Breast Cancer. (2006). *Male breast cancer*. Retrieved April 2, 2007, from http://www.infobreastcancer.ca/malebc.htm

International Agency for Research on Cancer, World Health Organization. (2002). Breast cancer and screening. In *IARC handbooks of cancer prevention, volume 7: Breast cancer screening*. Geneva, Switzerland: IARC Press.

Johnson, J. L., Bottorff, J. L., Balneaves, L. G., Grewal, S., Bhagat, R., Hilton, B. A., et al. (1999). South Asian women's views on the causes of breast cancer: Images and explanations. *Patient Education and Counselling, 37*(3), 243–254.

Kearney, A. J., & Murray, M. (2006). Commentary—Evidence against breast self examination is not conclusive: What policymakers and health professionals need to know. *Journal of Public Health Policy, 27*(3), 282–292.

Lappe, J. M., Travers-Gustafson, D., Davies, K. M., Recker, R. R., & Heaney, R. P. (2007). Vitamin D and calcium supplementation reduces cancer risk: Results of a randomized trial. *American Journal of Clinical Nutrition, 85*(6), 1586–1591.

Li, J., Wang, M.-S., Huang, J., Yao, M.-X., Yu, Z.-H., & Liang, Y.-Q. (2005). Risk factors of breast cancer in the patients with breast diseases. *Zhongguo Linchuang Kangfu, 9*(2), 158–159.

MacMillan, K. (2008). Nurses' knowledge helps clients make informed choices. *Canadian Nurse, 104*(2), 5.

Meneses, K. D., & Yarbro, C. H. (2007). Cultural perspectives of international breast health and breast cancer education. *Journal of Nursing Scholarship, 39*(2), 105–112.

Metcalfe, K. A., Ghadirian, P., Roaen, B., Foulkes, W., Kim-Sing, C., Eisen, A., et al. (2007). Variation in rates of uptake of preventive options by Canadian women carrying the *BRCA1* or *BRCA2* genetic mutation. *Open Medicine, 1*(2).

Murad, T. M., Contesso, G., & Mouriesse, H. (1982). Nipple discharge from the breast. *Annals of Surgery, 195*(3), 259–264.

National Cancer Institute. (2006). *Male breast cancer (PDQ®): Treatment.* Retrieved April 2, 2007, from http://www.cancer.gov/cancertopics/pdq/treatment/malebreast/Patient

National Cancer Institute. (2007). *Breast cancer risk assessment tool.* Retrieved March 23, 2007, from http://www.cancer.gov/bcrisktool/

Northrup, C. (1994). *Women's bodies, women's wisdom.* New York: Bantam Books.

O'Blenes, C. A. E., Delbridge, C. L., Miller, B. J., Pantelis, A., & Morris, S. F. (2006). Prospective study of outcomes after reduction mammoplasty: Long-term follow-up. *Plastic & Reconstructive Surgery, 117*(2), 351–358.

Ohene-Yeboah, M. O. K. (2005). An audit of excised breast lumps in Ghanaian women. *West African Journal of Medicine, 24*(3), 252–255.

Pediconi, F., Catalano, C., Roselli, A., Padula, S., Altomari, F., Moriconi, E., et al. (2007). Contrast-enhanced MR mammography for evaluation of the contralateral breast in clients with diagnosed unilateral breast cancer or high-risk lesions. *Radiology, 243*(3), 670–680.

Petro-Nustas, W., Norton, M. E., & al-Masarweh, I. (2002). Risk factors for breast cancer in Jordanian women. *Journal of Nursing Scholarship, 34*(1), 19–25.

Pituskin, E., Williams, B., Au, H., & Martin-McDonald, K. (2007). Experiences of men with breast cancer: A qualitative study. *The Journal of Men's Health & Gender, 4*(1), 44–51.

Plu-Bureau, G., Thalabard, J. C., Sitruk-Ware, R., Asselain, B., & Mauvais-Jarvis, P. (1992). Cyclical mastalgia as a marker of breast cancer susceptibility: Results of a case-control study among French women. *British Journal of Cancer, 65*(6), 945–949.

Rohan, T. E., & Miller, A. B. (1999). Hormone replacement therapy and risk of benign proliferative epithelial disorders of the breast. *European Journal of Cancer Prevention, 8*(2), 123–130.

Santen, R. J., & Mansel, R. (2005). Benign breast disorders. *New England Journal of Medicine, 353*(3), 275–285.

Saslow, D., Boetes, C., Burke, W., Harms, S., Leach, M. O., Lehman, C. D., et al. (2007). American Cancer Society guidelines for breast screening with MRI as an adjunct to mammography. *CA: A Cancer Journal for Clinicians, 57*(2), 75–89.

Tan-Chiu, E., Wang, J., Costantino, J. P., Paik, S., Butch, C., Wickerham, D. L., et al. (2003). Effects of tamoxifen on benign breast disease in women at high risk for breast cancer. *Journal of the National Cancer Institute, 95*(4), 302–307.

Taylor, E. F., Burley, V. J., Greenwood, D. C., & Cade, J. E. (2007). Meat consumption and risk of breast cancer in the UK women's cohort study. *British Journal of Cancer, 96*(7), 1139–1146.

U.S. Preventive Services Task Force. (1996). Screening for breast cancer. In *Guide to clinical preventive services* (2nd ed., pp. 73–87). Baltimore: Williams & Wilkins.

Villeneuve, P. J., Holowaty, E. J., Brisson, J., Xie, L., Ugnat, A.-M., Latulippe, L., et al. (2006). Mortality among Canadian women with cosmetic breast implants. *American Journal of Epidemiology, 164*(4), 334–341.

Vobecky, J., Simard, A., Vobecky, J. S., Ghadirian, P., Lamothe-Guay, M., & Falardeau, M. (1993). Nutritional profile of women with fibrocystic breast disease. *International Journal of Epidemiology, 22*(6), 989–999.

Weber, J., & Kelley, J. (2007). *Health assessment in nursing* (3rd ed.). Philadelphia: Lippincott Williams & Wilkins.

White, E., Urban, N., & Taylor, V. (1993). Mammography utilization, public health impact, and cost-effectiveness in the United States. *Annual Review of Public Health, 14*, 605–633.

ADDITIONAL RESOURCES

Bland, K. I., Vezerdis, M. P., & Copeland, E. M. (2005). Breast. In F. C. Brunicardi & S. I. Schwartz (Eds.), *Schwartz's principles of surgery* (8th ed.). New York: McGraw-Hill, Medical Pub. Division.

Chlebowski, R. T., Hentrix, S. L., Langer, R. D., Stefanick, M. L., Gass, M., Lane, D., et al. (2003). Influence of estrogen plus progestin on breast cancer and mammography in healthy postmenopausal women: The Women's Health Initiative Randomized Trial. *Journal of the American Medical Association, 289*(24), 3243–3253.

English, J. C., III, Middleton, C., Patterson, J. W., & Slingluff, C. L. (2000). Cancer of the male breast. *International Journal of Dermatology, 39*(12), 881–886.

Giordano, S. H., Cohen, D. S., & Buzdar, A. U. (2004). Breast carcinoma in men: A population-based study. *Cancer, 101*(1), 51–57.

Harris, J. R., Morrow, M., & Bonadonna, G. (2004). Cancer of the breast. In V. T. DeVita, S. Hellman, & S. A. Rosenberg (Eds.), *Cancer principles & practice of oncology* (7th ed.). Philadelphia: Lippincott Williams & Wilkins.

Woodward, V., & Webb, C. (2001). Women's anxieties surrounding breast disorders: A systematic review of the literature. *Journal of Advanced Nursing, 33*(1), 29–41.

Yarbrough, S. S., & Braden, C. J. (2001). Utility of health belief model as a guide for explaining or predicting breast cancer screening behaviours. *Journal of Advanced Nursing, 33*(5), 677–688.

ASSOCIATIONS AND WEB SITES

Canadian Cancer Encyclopedia: http://info.cancer.ca/E/CCE/cceexplorer.asp?tocid=10

NCI Breast Cancer Risk Assessment tool: http://www.cancer.gov/bcrisktool/

WHO Breast Cancer and Screening: http://www.emro.who.int/ncd/publications/breastcancerscreening.pdf

Canadian Association of Nurses in Oncology: http://www.cano-acio.ca

Canadian Breast Cancer Foundation: http://www.cbcf.org

Canadian Breast Cancer Network (CBCN): http://www.cbcn.ca

Canadian Breast Cancer Research Alliance: http://www.breast.cancer.ca

Canadian Cancer Society: www.cancer.ca

Saunders-Matthey Cancer Prevention Coalition: http://www.stopcancer.org

TABLE 16-1   **Visible Signs of Breast Cancer**

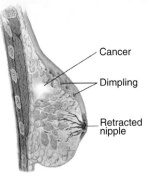

Retraction Signs

As breast cancer advances, it causes fibrosis (scar tissue). Shortening of this tissue produces dimpling, changes in contour, and retraction or deviation of the nipple. Other causes of retraction include fat necrosis and mammary duct ectasia.

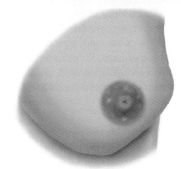

Unusual Contours

Look for any variation in the usual convexity of each breast, and compare one side with the other. Special positioning may again be useful. Shown here is marked flattening of the lower outer quadrant of the left breast.

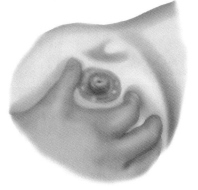

Skin Dimpling

Look for this sign with the client's arm at rest, during special positioning, and on moving or compressing the breast, as illustrated here.

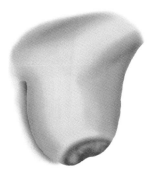

Nipple Retraction and Deviation

A retracted nipple is flattened or pulled inward, as illustrated here. It may also be broadened and feels thickened. When involvement is radially asymmetric, the nipple may deviate or point in a different direction from its counterpart, typically toward the underlying cancer.

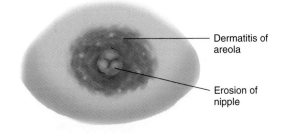

Edema of the Skin

Edema of the skin is produced by lymphatic blockage. It appears as thickened skin with enlarged pores—the so-called *peau d'orange* (orange peel) *sign*. It is often seen first in the lower portion of the breast or areola.

Paget's Disease of the Nipple

This is an uncommon form of breast cancer that usually starts as a scaly, eczema-like lesion. The skin may also weep, crust, or erode. A breast mass may be present. Suspect Paget's disease in any persisting dermatitis of the nipple and areola.

TABLE 16-2   Common Breast Masses

The three most common kinds of breast masses are *fibroadenoma* (a benign tumour), *cysts*, and *breast cancer*. The clinical characteristics of these masses are listed below. However, any breast mass should be carefully evaluated and usually warrants further investigation by ultrasound, aspiration, mammography, magnetic resonance imaging (MRI), or biopsy. The masses depicted below are rather large, for purposes of illustration. Ideally, breast cancer should be identified early, when the mass is small. *Fibrocystic changes*, not illustrated, are also commonly palpable as nodular, ropelike densities in women ages 25–50. They may be tender or painful. They are considered benign and are not viewed as a risk factor for breast cancer unless there is a family history of breast cancer.

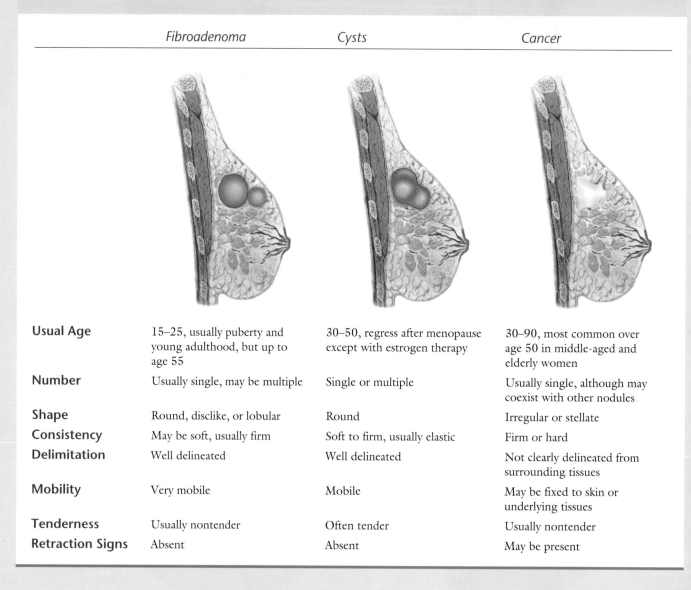

	Fibroadenoma	*Cysts*	*Cancer*
Usual Age	15–25, usually puberty and young adulthood, but up to age 55	30–50, regress after menopause except with estrogen therapy	30–90, most common over age 50 in middle-aged and elderly women
Number	Usually single, may be multiple	Single or multiple	Usually single, although may coexist with other nodules
Shape	Round, disclike, or lobular	Round	Irregular or stellate
Consistency	May be soft, usually firm	Soft to firm, usually elastic	Firm or hard
Delimitation	Well delineated	Well delineated	Not clearly delineated from surrounding tissues
Mobility	Very mobile	Mobile	May be fixed to skin or underlying tissues
Tenderness	Usually nontender	Often tender	Usually nontender
Retraction Signs	Absent	Absent	May be present

The Abdomen

Nicole Harder, D. Lynn Skillen, and Lynn S. Bickley

Assessing the abdominal region can be challenging. It is important for nurses to determine from the health history and physical examination if the concerns of clients are related to the gastrointestinal or urinary tract; to the cardiovascular, respiratory, hematologic, endocrine, reproductive, musculoskeletal, or neurologic system; or to psychogenic causes. This complexity requires thoughtful history taking, sound understanding of abdominal structures and their functions, and methodical, systematic physical examination.

ANATOMY AND PHYSIOLOGY

The abdomen is a single large cavity that extends from the diaphragm to the pelvic outlet. It contains vital body organs: the adrenal glands, aorta, bladder, gallbladder, iliac arteries, kidneys, large and small intestines, liver, pancreas, spleen, and stomach. Anteriorly, the abdomen is defined by the costal margins, xiphoid process, abdominal muscles (rectus abdominis, external abdominal oblique), inguinal ligaments, and symphysis pubis. Posteriorly, the boundaries include the 11th and 12th thoracic ribs, lumbar spine, iliac crests, and muscles (latissimus dorsi, paravertebral, external abdominal oblique).

Visualize or palpate the landmarks of the abdominal wall and pelvis, as illustrated. The rectus abdominis muscles become more prominent when the client raises the head and shoulders from the supine position.

For descriptive purposes, the abdomen is often divided by imaginary lines cross-

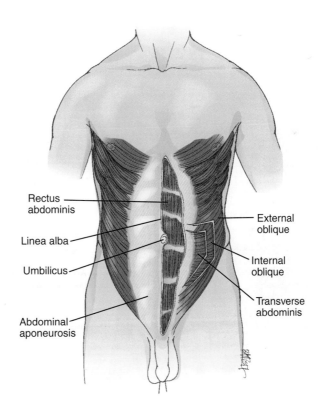

ing at the umbilicus, forming the right upper, right lower, left upper, and left lower quadrants. Another system divides the abdomen into nine sections. Terms for three of them are commonly used: epigastric, umbilical, and hypogastric or suprapubic.

When examining the abdomen, you may be able to feel several structures. The sigmoid *colon* is frequently palpable as a firm, narrow tube in the left lower quadrant, whereas the cecum and part of the ascending colon form a softer, wider tube in the right lower quadrant. Portions of the transverse and descending colon may also be palpable. None of these structures should be mistaken for a tumour. Although the healthy *liver* often extends down just below the right costal margin, its soft consistency makes it difficult to feel through the abdominal wall. The lower margin of the liver, the liver edge, is often palpable. Also, in the right upper quadrant, but usually at a deeper level, lies the lower pole of the right kidney. It is occasionally palpable, especially in thin people with relaxed abdominal muscles. Pulsations of the *abdominal aorta* are frequently visible and usually palpable in the upper abdomen, whereas the pulsations of the *iliac arteries* may sometimes be felt in the lower quadrants.

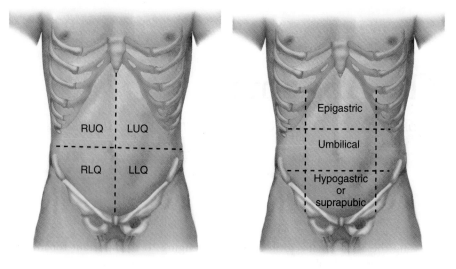

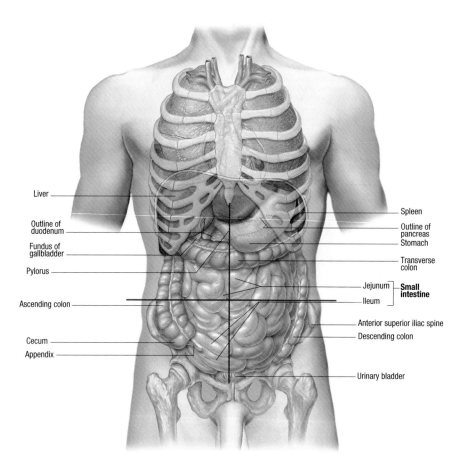

The abdominal cavity extends up under the rib cage to the dome of the diaphragm. In this protected location, beyond the reach of the palpating hand, are much of the liver and *stomach,* and all of the healthy spleen. The *spleen* lies against the diaphragm at the level of the 9th, 10th, and 11th ribs, mostly posterior to the left midaxillary line. It is lateral, posterior to, and behind the stomach, and just superior to the left kidney. The tip of the healthy spleen is palpable below the left costal margin in a small percentage of adults.

Most of the *gallbladder* lies deep inside the liver and cannot be distinguished from it clinically. The *duodenum* and *pancreas* lie deep in the upper abdomen, where they are not usually palpable.

A distended *bladder* may be palpable above the symphysis pubis. The bladder accommodates roughly 300 mL of urine filtered by the kidneys into the renal pelvis and the ureters. Expansion of the bladder stimulates contraction of its smooth muscle, the *detrusor muscle*, at relatively low pressures. Rising pressure in the bladder triggers the conscious urge to void.

Increased intraurethral pressure can overcome rising pressures in the bladder and prevent incontinence. Intraurethral pressure is related to such factors as smooth muscle tone in the internal urethral sphincter, the thickness of the urethral mucosa, and, in women, sufficient support to the bladder and proximal urethra from pelvic muscles and ligaments to maintain proper anatomical relationships. Striated muscle around the urethra can also contract voluntarily to interrupt voiding.

Neuroregulatory control of the bladder functions at several levels. In infants, the bladder empties by reflex mechanisms in the sacral spinal cord. Voluntary control of the bladder depends on higher centres in the brain and on motor and sensory pathways between the brain and the reflex arcs of the sacral spinal cord. When voiding is inconvenient, higher centres in the brain can inhibit detrusor contractions until the capacity of the bladder, approximately 400 to 500 mL, is exceeded. The integrity of the sacral nerves that innervate the bladder can be tested by assessing perirectal and perineal sensation in the S2, S3, and S4 dermatomes (see p. 694).

Other structures sometimes palpable in the lower abdomen include the *uterus* enlarged by pregnancy or fibroids, which may also rise above the symphysis pubis, and the *sacral promontory*, the anterior edge of the first sacral vertebra. Until you are familiar with this structure, you may mistake its stony hard outlines for a tumour. Another stony hard lump that can sometimes mislead you, and may occasionally alarm a client, is the *xiphoid process*.

The *kidneys* are posterior organs. The ribs protect their upper portions. The *costovertebral angle*—the angle formed by the lower border of the 12th rib and the transverse processes of the upper lumbar vertebrae—defines the region to assess for kidney tenderness.

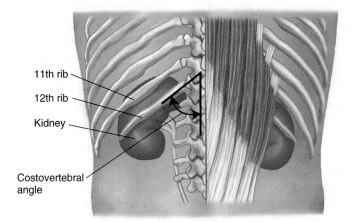

11th rib

12th rib

Kidney

Costovertebral angle

THE HEALTH HISTORY

Key Signs and Symptoms Reported by Client

Gastrointestinal Disorders
- Indigestion
- Lack or loss of appetite (anorexia)
- Nausea, vomiting, or bloody vomit (hematemesis)
- Changes in weight
- Abdominal pain
- Difficulty swallowing (dysphagia), pain with swallowing (odynophagia)
- Change in bowel movements, bloating, excessive gas
- Constipation or diarrhea
- Yellowing of skin and eyes (jaundice)

Urinary and Renal Disorders
- Pain in lower abdomen (suprapubic)

- Pain with urination (dysuria); urgency or frequency of urination
- Decreased urine stream in males, hesitancy in starting urine stream
- Increased amount of urine with voiding (polyuria)
- Urination at night (nocturia)
- Loss of control of urine (urinary incontinence)
- Change in colour of urine, blood in urine (hematuria)
- Flank or back (kidney) pain
- Severe flank, back, and/or lower abdominal pain (ureteral colic)

Nurses encounter a wide variety of gastrointestinal and urinary concerns in clinical practice. Careful interviewing leads to the underlying disorder.

Begin the health history interview with broad opening questions, such as "What can I help you with today?" or "What concerns have you come about today?" Open-ended questions allow clients to express themselves freely. If a client reports a symptom or sign, you first complete an analysis of the symptom/sign before continuing with more of the health history.

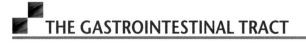

THE GASTROINTESTINAL TRACT

Indigestion. "How is your *appetite*?" is a good starting question and may lead to other important areas, such as *indigestion, anorexia, nausea, vomiting,* and changes in weight. Clients often report *indigestion,* and that refers to distress associated with eating, but they use the term for many different symptoms. Find out just what the client means.

Possible causes include the following:

- *Heartburn,* or a sense of burning or warmth that is retrosternal and may radiate from the epigastrium to the neck. It usually originates in the esophagus. If persistent, especially in the epigastric area, it may raise the question of heart disease. Some clients with coronary artery disease describe their pain as burning, "like indigestion." Pay special attention to what brings on and relieves the discomfort. Is it precipitated by exertion and relieved by rest, suggesting angina, or is it related to meals and made worse during or after eating, suggesting gastroesophageal reflux?

Heartburn suggests gastric acid reflux into the esophagus, often precipitated by a heavy meal, lying down, or bending forward, as well as by ingesting alcohol, citrus juices, or aspirin. If chronic, consider reflux esophagitis.

See Table 15-1, Selected Heart Rates and Rhythms, p. 467.

- *Excessive gas,* especially with frequent belching, abdominal bloating or distention, or *flatus,* the passage of gas by rectum, usually about 600 mL per day. Find out if these symptoms are associated with eating specific foods. Ask if symptoms are related to ingestion of milk or milk products.

Belching, but not bloating or excess flatus, is normally seen in *aerophagia,* or swallowing air.

Also consider legumes and other gas-producing foods, intestinal lactase deficiency, and irritable bowel syndrome.

■ Unpleasant *abdominal fullness* after meals of usual size, or *early satiety*, the inability to eat a full meal.

Consider high-fat meal, diabetic gastroparesis, anticholinergic drugs, gastric outlet obstruction, gastric cancer; early satiety in hepatitis.

Anorexia, Nausea, Vomiting, Hematemesis.

Anorexia is a loss or lack of appetite. Find out if it arises from intolerance to certain foods, reluctance to eat because of anticipated discomfort, difficulty chewing or swallowing, or concerns over body image. *Nausea*, often described as "feeling sick to my stomach," may progress to retching or vomiting. *Retching* describes the spasmodic movements of the chest and diaphragm that precede and culminate in *vomiting*, the forceful expulsion of gastric contents out through the mouth.

Anorexia, nausea, and vomiting occur in many gastrointestinal disorders, as well as in infectious diseases.

Vomiting is associated with pain, pregnancy, diabetic ketoacidosis, adrenal insufficiency, hypercalcemia, uremia, liver disease, emotional states, and adverse drug reactions. Vomiting is induced, but without nausea, in anorexia/bulimia nervosa.

Some clients may not actually vomit, but raise esophageal or gastric contents without nausea or retching; this is called *regurgitation*.

Regurgitation occurs in esophageal narrowing from stricture or cancer, as well as in incompetent gastroesophageal sphincter.

Ask about any emesis or regurgitated material and inspect it yourself, if possible. What colour is it? What does the vomitus smell like? How much has there been? Ask specifically if it contains any blood, and try to determine how much. You may have to help the client with the amount—a teaspoon? Two teaspoons? A cupful?

Fecal odour in small bowel obstruction or gastrocolic fistula

Gastric juice is clear or mucoid. Small amounts of yellowish or greenish bile are common and have no special significance. Brownish or blackish emesis with a "coffee-grounds" appearance suggests blood altered by gastric acid. Coffee-grounds emesis or red blood is termed *hematemesis*.

Hematemesis occurs in duodenal or peptic ulcer, esophageal or gastric varices, and gastritis.

Do the client's symptoms suggest any complications of vomiting such as *aspiration* into the lungs, seen in elderly, debilitated, impaired, or obtunded clients? Is there dehydration or electrolyte imbalance from prolonged vomiting, or significant loss of blood? Is the client voiding expected quantities? Reporting dry lips and mucosa?

Suspect aspiration if tachycardia, dyspnea, central cyanosis, hypertension. Symptoms of blood loss such as lightheadedness or syncope depend on the rate and volume of bleeding and rarely appear until blood loss exceeds 500 mL.

Changes in Weight.

Weight gain in the abdomen may indicate an unexpected accumulation of body fluid in the form of ascites (see Table 17-9). Another factor for increased abdominal girth is abdominal fat related to an energy-expenditure imbalance between caloric intake and output. *Weight loss* may be related to anorexia, dieting, dysphagia, early pregnancy, vomiting, malabsorption of nutrients from the gastrointestinal tract, loss of nutrients through urine or feces, or increased metabolic requirements. It may also be related to malnutrition.

Abdominal Pain.

Abdominal pain has several possible mechanisms and clinical patterns and warrants careful clinical assessment. See Chapter 7, Pain Assessment. Be familiar with threek broad categories of abdominal pain:

See Table 17-1, Abdominal Pain (p. 547)

- *Visceral pain* occurs when hollow abdominal organs such as the intestine or biliary tree contract unusually forcefully or are distended or stretched. Solid organs such as the liver can also become painful when their capsules are stretched. Visceral pain may be difficult to localize. It is typically palpable near the midline at levels that vary according to the structure involved, as illustrated below.

Visceral pain varies in quality and may be gnawing, burning, cramping, or aching. When it becomes severe, it may be associated with sweating, pallor, nausea, vomiting, and restlessness.

Visceral pain in the right upper quadrant from liver distention against its capsule in alcoholic hepatitis.

Visceral (generalized) periumbilical pain occurs in early acute appendicitis from distention of the inflamed appendix, which gradually changes to parietal (localized) pain in the right lower quadrant from inflammation of the adjacent parietal peritoneum.

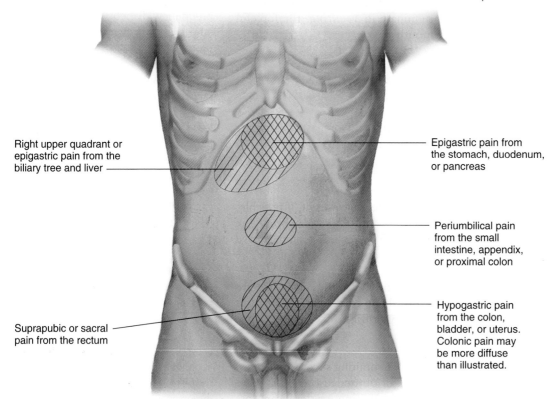

Right upper quadrant or epigastric pain from the biliary tree and liver

Epigastric pain from the stomach, duodenum, or pancreas

Periumbilical pain from the small intestine, appendix, or proximal colon

Hypogastric pain from the colon, bladder, or uterus. Colonic pain may be more diffuse than illustrated.

Suprapubic or sacral pain from the rectum

TYPES OF VISCERAL PAIN

- *Parietal pain* originates in the parietal peritoneum and is caused by inflammation. It is a steady aching pain that is usually more severe than visceral pain and more precisely localized over the involved structure. It is typically aggravated by movement or coughing. Clients with this type of pain usually prefer to lie still.

- *Referred pain* is felt in more distant sites, which are innervated at approximately the same spinal levels as the disordered structure. Referred pain often develops as the initial pain becomes more intense and thus seems to radiate or travel from the initial site. It may be felt superficially or deeply but is usually well localized.

Pain of duodenal or pancreatic origin may be referred to the back; pain from the biliary tree, to the right shoulder or the right posterior chest.

Pain may also be referred to the abdomen from the chest, spine, or pelvis, thus complicating the assessment of abdominal pain.

Pain from *pleurisy* or *acute myocardial infarction* may be referred to the upper abdomen.

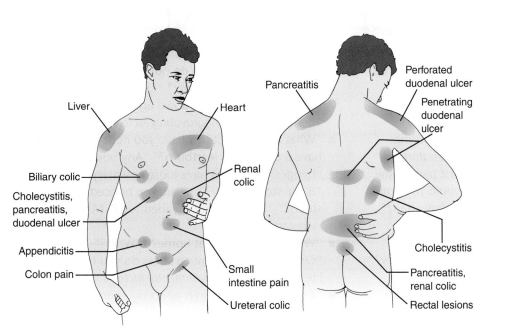

Ask clients to *point to the location of pain* and *describe the abdominal pain in their own words*. If clothes interfere, repeat the question during the physical examination. You need to pursue important details: "Where does the pain start?" "Does it radiate or travel anywhere?" "What is the pain like?" If the client has trouble describing the pain, give some words to help stimulate descriptions, such as "Is it aching?" "Burning?" "Gnawing?"

You need to ask, "How severe is the pain?" "How would you rate it on a scale of 0 (no pain) to 10 (worst pain)?" Find out if it is bearable or interferes with the client's usual activities. Does it make the client lie down? The description of the *severity (intensity or quantity)* of the pain may tell you something about the client's responses to pain and its effects on the client's life, but it is not consistently helpful in assessing the cause of pain. Sensitivity to abdominal pain varies widely and tends to diminish in older clients, especially those in or beyond their 70s; this masks acute abdominal problems.

Determine the *aggravating* and *alleviating factors*, with special reference to meals, antacids, alcohol, medications (including aspirin, aspirin-like drugs, and any over-the-counter drugs), emotional factors, and body position or movement. Also, is the pain related to defecation, urination, menstruation, or intercourse? You need to ask about any *associated symptoms*, such as fever or chills, and their sequence.

Environmental factors may contribute to the pain. Inquire about events or changes in the client's life. Ask about the *significance of the pain* in the client's life. "What do you think is causing your pain?" (*Client perspective*). The client's answers may provide valuable insights to incorporate into your response to the situation. It is important to ask this question last so that the client's perspective does not limit your questioning about symptom characteristics.

Cramping, colicky pain is often related to peristalsis.

Citrus fruits may aggravate the pain of reflux esophagitis; lactase deficiency is possible if abdominal discomfort is linked to milk ingestion.

Examples of Questions for Symptom Analysis: Right Upper Quadrant (RUQ) Pain

- "Where do you feel the pain?" "How big is the area of pain?" "Is it limited to a small area?" "Show me." (*Location*)
- "Does the RUQ pain go anywhere else?" "Do you feel pain in your right shoulder?" (*Radiation*)
- "What is the pain like?" For example, "Is it gripping?" "Colicky?" "Crampy?" (*Quality/nature*)
- "On a scale of 0 (no pain) to 10 (worst pain), how would you rate your pain?" "How would you compare your pain to other pain that you have had?" (*Quantity/intensity*)
- "When did the pain start?" (*Onset*)
- "Did it start suddenly or did it come on gradually?" "Is it related to eating? Drinking? Activity?" (*Timing*)
- "How long does the pain last?" (*Duration*)
- "Does it come and go?" "Or is it constant?" (*Frequency*)
- "What makes the pain better?" "What helps to ease the pain?" (*Alleviating factors*)

- "What makes the pain worse?" "Did you eat anything recently that you do not usually consume?" "Drink anything different?" "Does alcohol aggravate the pain?" "Does lying down aggravate the pain?" "Bending over?" (*Aggravating factors*)
- "What other symptoms have you noticed?" "Do you have a cough?" "Heartburn?" "Any bowel changes?" "Do you have loose or watery stools?" "Is the stool bloody?" "Have you noticed floating stools?" "Fever?" "Lightheadedness?" (*Associated symptoms*)
- "What is happening at home?" "Work?" "School?" "Or leisure?" "How much stress do you have in your life right now?" (*Environmental factors*)
- "Tell me how the pain is affecting your life." (*Significance to client*)
- "What do you think is causing your pain?" (*Client perspective*)

Dysphagia and/or Odynophagia. Less commonly, clients may report difficulty swallowing, or *dysphagia*, the sense that food or liquid is sticking, hesitating, or "won't go down right." Dysphagia may result from esophageal disorders or from difficulty transferring food from the mouth to the esophagus. The sensation of a lump in the throat or in the retrosternal area, unassociated with swallowing, is not true dysphagia.

For types of dysphagia, see Table 17-2, Dysphagia, p. 548.

Ask the client to point to where the dysphagia occurs and describe with what types of food it occurs. Does it occur with relatively solid foods such as meat, with softer foods such as ground meat and mashed potatoes, or with hot or cold liquids? Has the pattern changed?

Pointing to the throat suggests a transfer or esophageal disorder; pointing to the chest suggests an esophageal disorder.

Establish the timing. When did it start? Is it intermittent or persistent? Is it progressing? If so, over what period? What are the associated symptoms and medical conditions?

Dysphagia with solid food in mechanical narrowing of the esophagus; dysphagia related to both solids and liquids suggests a disorder of esophageal motility.

Odynophagia, or pain on swallowing, may occur in two forms. A sharp, burning pain suggests mucosal inflammation, whereas a squeezing, cramping pain suggests a muscular cause. Odynophagia may accompany dysphagia, but either symptom may occur independently.

Mucosal inflammation in reflux esophagitis or infection from *Candida*, herpes virus, or cytomegalovirus.

Change in Bowel Function. With respect to the lower gastrointestinal tract, you will frequently need to assess *bowel function*. Start with open-ended questions: "Describe your bowel movements." "How frequent are they?" "Do you have any difficulties?" "Have you noticed any change in your bowel habits?" Frequency of bowel movements typically ranges from about three times a day to twice a week. A change in pattern within these limits, however, may be significant for an individual client.

Constipation or Diarrhea. Clients vary widely in their views of constipation and diarrhea. Be sure to clarify what the client means by these terms. For example, is *constipation* a decrease in frequency of bowel movements? The passage of hard and perhaps painful stools? The need to strain unusually? A sense of incomplete defecation or pressure in the rectum? Ask if the client actually looks at the stool. If yes, what does the stool look like in terms of colour and bulk? What remedies has the client tried? What is the daily fibre intake? Do medications, stress, unrealistic ideas about routine bowel habits, or time and setting allotted for defecation play a role? Occasionally, there is complete constipation with no passage of either feces or gas, or *obstipation*.

See Table 17-3, Constipation (p. 549) and Table 17-4, Diarrhea (pp. 550–551).

Thin pencil-like stool in an obstructing "apple-core" lesion of the sigmoid colon.

Obstipation in *intestinal obstruction.*

Inquire about the colour of the stools and ask about any *black tarry stools*, suggesting *melena*, or *red blood in the stools*, known as *hematochezia*. If either condition is present, find out how long and how often. If the blood is red, how much is there? Is it pure blood mixed with stool or on the surface of the stool? Is there blood on the toilet paper?

See Table 17-5, Black and Bloody Stools, p. 552.

Blood on the stool surface and on toilet paper in *hemorrhoids.*

Diarrhea is an excessive frequency in the passage of stools that are usually unformed or watery. Ask about size, frequency, and volume. Are the stools bulky or small? How many episodes of diarrhea occur each day?

Consistently large diarrheal stools are often observed in small-bowel or proximal-colon disorders; small frequent stools with urgency of defecation are noted in left colon or rectal disorders.

Ask for descriptive terms. Are the stools greasy or oily? Frothy? Foul smelling? Floating on the surface because of excessive gas, making them difficult to flush? Accompanied by mucus, pus, or blood?

Mucus, pus, or blood occur in infectious diseases. Large yellowish or grey greasy foul-smelling stools, sometimes frothy or floating, in *steatorrhea*, or fatty stools—seen in malabsorption.

Assess the course of diarrhea over time. Is it acute, chronic, or recurrent? Or is your client experiencing the first acute episode of a chronic or recurrent illness? Look into other factors as well. Does the diarrhea awaken the client at night? What seem to be the aggravating or relieving factors? Does the client get relief from a bowel movement, or is there an intense urge with straining but little or no result, known as *tenesmus*? What is the setting? Does it entail travel, stress, or a new medication? Do family members or companions have similar symptoms? Are there associated symptoms?

Nocturnal diarrhea suggests a pathophysiologic cause.

Relief after passing feces or gas suggests left colon or rectal disorders; *tenesmus* in rectal conditions near the anal sphincter.

Jaundice. In some clients, you will notice *jaundice* or *icterus*, the yellowish discoloration of the skin and sclerae from increased levels of bilirubin, a bile pigment derived chiefly from the breakdown of hemoglobin. Usually the hepatocytes conjugate (or combine) unconjugated bilirubin with other substances to make the bile water soluble, and then excrete it into the bile. The bile passes through the cystic duct into the common bile duct, which also drains the extrahepatic ducts from the liver. More distally, the common bile duct and the pancreatic ducts empty into the duodenum at the ampulla of Vater. Mechanisms of jaundice include the following:

■ Increased production of bilirubin

■ Decreased uptake of bilirubin by the hepatocytes

■ Decreased ability of the liver to conjugate bilirubin

Predominantly unconjugated bilirubin from the first three mechanisms, as in *hemolytic anemia* (increased production) and *Gilbert's syndrome.*

■ Decreased excretion of bilirubin into the bile, resulting in absorption of *conjugated* bilirubin back into the blood.

Impaired excretion of conjugated bilirubin in *viral hepatitis, cirrhosis, primary biliary cirrhosis,* drug-induced cholestasis, as from oral contraceptives, methyl testosterone, chlorpromazine.

Intrahepatic jaundice can be *hepatocellular,* from damage to the hepatocytes, or *cholestatic,* from impaired excretion as a result of damaged hepatocytes or intrahepatic bile ducts. *Extrahepatic* jaundice arises from obstruction of the extrahepatic bile ducts, most commonly the cystic and common bile ducts.

Obstruction of the common bile duct is caused by gallstones or *pancreatic carcinoma.*

As you assess the client with jaundice, pay special attention to the associated symptoms and the setting in which the illness occurred. What was the *colour of the urine* as the client became ill? When the level of conjugated bilirubin increases in the blood, it may be excreted into the urine, turning the urine a dark yellowish brown or tea colour. Unconjugated bilirubin is not water soluble, so it is not excreted into urine.

Dark urine from bilirubin indicates impaired excretion of bilirubin into the gastrointestinal tract.

Ask also about the *colour of the stools.* When excretion of bile into the intestine is completely obstructed, the stools become grey or light coloured, or *acholic,* without bile.

Acholic stools occur briefly in *viral hepatitis,* common in obstructive jaundice.

Does the skin itch without other obvious explanation? Is there associated pain? What is its pattern? Has it been recurrent in the past?

Itching occurs in cholestatic or obstructive jaundice, and pain could be due to a distended liver capsule, *biliary cholic, or pancreatic cancer.*

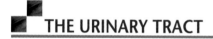

THE URINARY TRACT

General questions for a urinary history include: "Do you have any difficulty passing your urine?" "How often do you go?" "Do you have to get up at night? How often?" "How much urine do you pass at a time?" "Is there any pain or burning?" "Do you ever have trouble getting to the toilet in time?" "Do you ever leak any urine? Or wet yourself involuntarily? Do you sense when the bladder is full and when voiding occurs?"

See Table 17-6, Frequency, Nocturia, and Polyuria (p. 553).

Involuntary voiding or lack of awareness suggests cognitive or neurosensory deficits.

Ask women if sudden coughing, sneezing, or laughing makes them lose urine. Roughly half of young women report this experience even before bearing children. Occasional leakage is not necessarily significant. Ask older men, "Do you have trouble starting your stream?" "Do you have to stand close to the toilet to void?" "Is there a change in the force or size of your stream, or straining to void?" "Do you hesitate or stop in the middle of voiding?" "Is there dribbling when you're through? Do you have a feeling of not emptying your bladder?"

Stress incontinence from decreased intraurethral pressure common in men with partial bladder outlet obstruction from *benign prostatic hyperplasia;* it is also seen with *urethral stricture.*

Suprapubic Pain.   Disorders in the urinary tract may cause pain in either the abdomen or the back. Bladder disorders may cause *suprapubic pain.* In *bladder infection,* pain in the lower abdomen is typically dull, and felt as pressure. In sudden overdistention of the bladder, pain is often agonizing; in contrast, chronic bladder distention is usually painless.

Pain of sudden overdistention in acute urinary retention.

Dysuria, Urgency, or Frequency.   Infection or irritation of either the bladder or urethra often provokes several symptoms. Frequently, there is *pain on urination,* usually felt as a burning sensation. Some clinicians refer to this as *dysuria,* whereas others reserve the term dysuria for difficulty voiding. Women may report internal urethral discomfort, sometimes described as a pressure, or an external burning from the flow of urine across irritated or inflamed labia. Men typically feel

Painful urination occurs with cystitis or urethritis. Also consider bladder stones, foreign bodies, tumours; also *acute prostatitis.* In women, internal burning in urethritis, external burning in *vulvovaginitis.*

a burning sensation proximal to the glans penis. In contrast, *prostatic pain* is felt in the perineum and occasionally in the rectum.

Other associated symptoms are common. Urinary *urgency* is an unusually intense and immediate desire to void, sometimes leading to involuntary voiding or *urge incontinence*. Urinary *frequency*, or abnormally frequent voiding, may occur. Ask about any related fever or chills, blood in the urine, or any pain in the abdomen, flank, or back (see illustration on p. 520). Men with partial obstruction to urinary outflow often report *hesitancy* in starting the urine stream, *straining to void, reduced calibre and force of the urinary stream, inability to fully empty the bladder*, or *dribbling* as voiding is completed.

Polyuria or Nocturia.
Three additional terms describe important alterations in the pattern of urination. *Polyuria* refers to a significant increase in 24-hour urine volume, roughly defined as exceeding 3 litres. It should be distinguished from urinary frequency, which can involve voiding in high amounts, seen in polyuria, or in small amounts, as in infection. Nocturia refers to urinary frequency at night, sometimes defined as awakening the client more than once; urine volumes may be large or small. Clarify any change in nocturnal voiding patterns and the number of trips to the bathroom.

Urinary Incontinence.
Involuntary loss of urine may become socially embarrassing and create problems for hygiene and skin integrity. Urinary incontinence is an important health problem that affects more than 3.3 million Canadians, many of them older adults (Canadian Continence Foundation, 2007). When a client reports incontinence, you need to consider the four broad incontinence categories when asking your questions, although a client may have a combination of causes (see Table 17-7, Urinary Incontinence). To differentiate, pay attention to precipitating factors; timing; amount of leakage; voluntary inhibition; presence of urgency, frequency, or nocturia; and spontaneous remissions. Consider the effects of drugs prescribed for other reasons. Is there a sensation of difficulty emptying the bladder or of bladder fullness after voiding? Are there symptoms of infections? (See Symptom Analysis Box p. 520.) A required multidisciplinary approach to management may involve nurses, family physicians, urologists, gynecologists, geriatricians, physiotherapists, pharmacists, social workers, and home care workers.

As described earlier, bladder control involves complex neuroregulatory and motor mechanisms (see p. 511). A number of central or peripheral nerve lesions may affect routine voiding. Can the client sense when the bladder is full? And when voiding occurs?

In addition, the client's functional status may significantly affect voiding behaviours even when the urinary tract is intact. Is the client mobile? Alert? Able to respond to voiding cues and reach the bathroom? Is alertness or voiding affected by medications?

Hematuria.
Blood in the urine, or *hematuria*, is an important cause for concern. When visible to the naked eye, it is called *gross hematuria*. The urine may appear frankly bloody. Blood may be detected only during microscopic urinalysis; this condition is known as *microscopic hematuria*. Smaller amounts of blood may tinge the urine with a pinkish or brownish cast. In women, be sure to distinguish menstrual blood from hematuria. If the urine is reddish, ask about ingestion of beets or medications that might discolour the urine. Test the urine with a dipstick and microscopic examination before you settle on the term hematuria.

Urgency is observed in bladder infection or irritation. In men, painful urination without frequency or urgency suggests urethritis.

Unexpectedly high renal production of urine occurs in polyuria. Frequency without polyuria during the day or night in bladder disorder or impairment to flow at or below the bladder neck.

See Table 17-7, Urinary Incontinence (p. 554).

Stress incontinence occurs with increased intra-abdominal pressure from decreased contractility of urethral sphincter or poor support of bladder neck. *Urge incontinence,* the state in which one is unable to hold the urine, results from detrusor overactivity. *Overflow incontinence,* when the bladder cannot be emptied until bladder pressure exceeds urethral pressure, occurs from anatomical obstruction by prostatic hypertrophy or stricture, as well as neurogenic abnormalities.

Functional incontinence results from impaired cognition, musculoskeletal problems, immobility.

Painful and bloody urination occurs in hemorrhagic cystitis.

Kidney or Flank Pain; Ureteral Colic.

Disorders of the urinary tract may also cause *kidney pain*, often reported as *flank pain* at or below the posterior costal margin near the costovertebral angle. It may radiate anteriorly toward the umbilicus. Kidney pain is a visceral pain usually produced by distention of the renal capsule and typically dull, aching, and steady. *Ureteral pain* is dramatically different. It is usually severe and colicky, originating at the costovertebral angle and radiating around the trunk into the lower quadrant of the abdomen, or possibly into the upper thigh and testicle or labium. Ureteral pain results from sudden distention of the ureter and associated distention of the renal pelvis. Ask about any associated fever chills, hematuria, nausea, or vomiting.

Kidney pain occurs in *acute pyelonephritis.*

Renal or ureteral colic is caused by sudden obstruction of a ureter, as by urinary stones or blood clots.

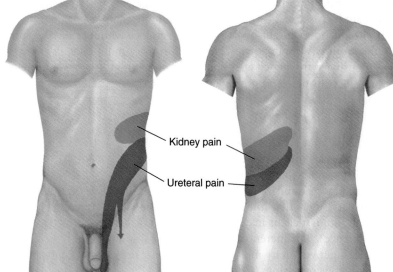

Kidney pain

Ureteral pain

Examples of Questions for Symptom Analysis: Urinary Incontinence

- "Does the urine seem to come from the usual place?" "Is it coming further back?" (*Location*)
- "Do you ever find urine on your clothing, but are unaware of when the leakage occurred?" "Does the leakage require that you wear pads?" "Is there any odour to your leakage?" "Any colour?" "To what extent can you control it?" "Does it hurt when you urinate?" "Sting?" "Burn?" "Does the urge to urinate wake you?" (*Quality/nature*)
- "Is leakage accompanied by a sudden and strong urge to void?" "How much leakage do you experience?" "To what extent is your clothing wet?" "How many pads do you use?" (*Quantity/intensity*)
- "Do you ever leak urine when you have a strong urge on the way to the bathroom?" "When did the leakage problem begin?" (*Onset*)
- "How often do you have to change pads or underwear?" "How often do you leak?" (*Frequency*)
- "Is this a problem during the day?" "During the night?" (*Timing*)

- "What else have you noticed when you have a leakage problem?" (*Associated symptoms*)
- "What makes the leakage worse?" "Do you leak if you sneeze?" "During sexual intercourse?" (*Aggravating factors*)
- "Is there anything you do that decreases the amount of leakage?" (*Alleviating factors*)
- "Has anything changed recently in your home?" "Work?" "Other activities?" "Has anything happened in your life that might be related to this?" "How accessible are toilet facilities?" "Are you lifting heavy objects more often?" "Have you had any recent stressors in your life that have made the problem worse?" (*Environmental factors*)
- "How has this affected your life?" (*Significance to client*)
- "What do you think is the cause?" (*Client perspective*)

HEALTH PROMOTION

Important Topics for Health Promotion

- Digestive health (fibre, fluid, and nutrient intake)
- Constipation and diarrhea
- Screening for alcohol and substance abuse
- Risk factors for hepatitis A, B, and C
- Vaccination for hepatitis A and B

- Risk factors and screening for colorectal cancer
- Risk factors and teaching for bowel disorders
- Risk factors for pancreatic cancer
- Risk factors and teaching for bladder disorders, kidney disease, and renal calculi

THE GASTROINTESTINAL TRACT

Digestive health is an important topic for health promotion because digestive diseases create the highest economic burden for the Canadian health care system, will increase with Canada's aging population, and have a long history of being under-researched as a result of insufficient funding (Beck, 2001). Nurses promote digestive health by encouraging clients to maintain a healthy body weight; ensure adequate fluid intake; exercise regularly; avoid excessive caffeine, alcohol, and saturated fatty foods; and follow Canada's Food Guide for a nutritious, balanced, and high-fibre diet (see Chapter 8).

To help clients avoid *constipation* or *diarrhea*, nurses consider the risk factors for each condition and reinforce choices that promote digestive health. Risk factors for *constipation* are numerous. They include client medications, such as opioids for chronic pain, iron supplements, antacids with aluminum, tranquilizers, antihypertensives, antidepressants, and anticholinergics. When assessing risk, nurses consider a client's personal history of hemorrhoids or fissures, irritable bowel syndrome (IBS), diverticular disease, and cancer of the bowel; they also consider the possibility of lead poisoning. They evaluate the history for endocrine, metabolic, neurologic, and muscular conditions. Nurses are alert to clients who are inactive, stressed, weak, and inattentive to body signals for defecation. Prevention focuses on encouraging a daily high-fibre intake of 25 mg for women and 38 mg for men, adequate fluid intake, physical activity, and a diet rich in fruits and vegetables (Dieticians of Canada, 2007).

Risk factors for *diarrhea* are related to client use of laxatives, stool softeners, antibiotics, antacids, thyroid hormone, and chemotherapeutics. Risk is also associated with travel, endocrine or metabolic conditions, AIDS, infections, malabsorption disorders, lax anal sphincter, and intestinal conditions. Nurses counsel clients about staying healthy while travelling and palliative measures such as avoiding caffeine, fat, and high-fibre foods; using rehydration measures and following a liquid diet; and changing to a bland diet once diarrhea subsides. Screening includes stool tests for ova and parasites, pathogens, food residues, occult blood, and fat. Prevention focuses on identifying potential causes of diarrhea for counselling and advising appropriately to ensure hydration and electrolyte stability.

"*Good health begins with good digestive health*" is a slogan of the Canadian Digestive Health Foundation. Nurses are aware of the common digestive disorders in Canadians to carry out primary and secondary prevention when counselling clients about digestive health.

Irritable bowel syndrome (IBS), a functional disorder involving intestinal motility, affects one out of six healthy people. It is more common in women, although it also affects men. Risk factors for IBS include psychosocial factors (stress, anxiety, or depression), alcohol and caffeine intake, tobacco use, high fat intake, and irritating foods such as spicy or fried foods. Nurses ensure that clients understand how to prevent or control the associated constipation, diarrhea, or bloating by identifying the foods that irritate, maintaining a high-fibre diet, using stress-reduction measures, exercising, eating regularly, and avoiding fluid intake with meals. Screening involves ruling out structural conditions and other colon diseases.

Inflammatory bowel disease (IBD) encompasses Crohn's disease and ulcerative colitis. In 2007, researchers identified three genes that pose risks for Crohn's disease and a gene associated with ulcerative colitis. A positive family history and ethnicity, especially Ashkenazi Jewish heritage, are implicated. The Canadian Society of Intestinal Research (2008a) estimates that IBD affects 13% to 20% of Canadians. More than 150,000 Canadians suffer from IBD (Nabalamba et al., 2004). Approximately 10,000 new cases per year occur in Canada (Canadian Society of Intestinal Research, 2008b). Nurses consider the family history and personal symptoms for early identification of clients with IBD. Although research results suggest directions for developing therapies, prevention is not yet a possibility. Nurses assist clients to adhere to management plans and minimize the inflammatory processes.

Liver disease may be acute or chronic. A nutritious diet with adequate protein, fat, carbohydrates, and calories assists the liver to regenerate cells. It is important for nurses to promote liver health by counselling clients regarding factors leading to preventable liver disease. Liver conditions are most commonly related to viral infections (hepatitis), workplace and environmental toxins, obesity, autoimmune disorders, genetics, and alcohol and drug misuse.

Hepatitis A, B, and C are the most common viral infections in the liver. All three types are preventable through lifestyle practices; types A and B are preventable through vaccination. All three may be asymptomatic, creating difficulties for assessing the incidence among Canadians.

Hepatitis A is transmitted by the fecal-oral route and prevented by a vaccine and personal hygiene. In 2003, 396 cases were reported in Canada (Public Health Agency of Canada [PHAC], 2007a). Risk factors include anal sexual intercourse, travel to countries with endemic hepatitis A, inadequate access to sanitation and potable water, exposures in residential institutions, and lower standards of hygiene associated with illicit drug use. Vaccination is recommended for travellers, food handlers, military personnel, child care givers, Aboriginals, health care workers, injection drug users, and homosexual clients.

Hepatitis B has been decreasing in recent years because of vaccination. No national data are available on chronic infection in Canadians, but estimates are that fewer than 5% have been infected in the past, and that fewer than 1% are carriers (PHAC, 2003). Risk factors are unprotected sexual contact; intravenous drug use and needle sharing; sharps injuries; bite wounds; migration from regions such as Africa, the Middle East, and Southeast Asia; and transmission from mother to child. Screening with blood tests is required for people at high risk and pregnant women. Vaccination is recommended for all young adults, people at risk for sexually transmitted infections, travellers, recipients of blood products (such as in hemodialysis), and health care workers.

Hepatitis C is the most prevalent form world-wide and noted for its chronicity. In Canada, it is a major cause of chronic liver disease and an important threat to public health. Incidence rates are higher in cities such as Calgary, Edmonton, and Vancouver, and in the provinces of British Columbia and New Brunswick. Risk factors include unprotected sex, injection drug use, maternal infection with hepatitis C, body piercing, hemodialysis, tattooing, and being a recipient of blood transfusion before 1990, when no screening test for hepatitis C in blood donations was available. In Canada, hepatitis C compensation programs are available for the years in which infection occurred because of the blood system (PHAC, 2007). Other potential risks include drug snorting, acupuncture, workplace exposure to blood, and incarceration (Wu et al., 2006). Approximately 20% of affected clients develop cirrhosis, which may lead to liver cancer and end-stage liver disease requiring transplantation. Without a vaccine for hepatitis C, prevention by nurses needs to focus on identifying those at risk for infection, especially drug users 15 to 39 years old, and opportune counselling to infected clients about treatment successes.

Prevention of hepatitis A and B requires advocacy for vaccination, personal hygiene, and safe lifestyle choices.

Alcohol misuse is associated with the development of liver cirrhosis. Alcohol intake, tobacco use, and hypertension are the three top factors influencing the burden of disease in Canada. In April 2007, the National Alcohol Strategy Working Group (NASWG) released the National Framework for Action to Reduce the Harms Associated with Alcohol and Other Drugs and Substances in Canada. Its underlying premise is to develop a culture of moderation in Canada to assist people to evaluate their drinking decisions. Canada ranks 43rd out of 185 countries for adult alcohol consumption. More than 3 million Canadians (approximately 14%) are considered high-risk drinkers (NASWG, 2007). At-risk populations include those who are young, elderly, Aboriginal, pregnant, or homeless.

Three commonly used screening tests for alcohol use are available to nurses. The CAGE test consists of four questions that are easy to remember when assessing for alcohol abuse and dependence (see Chapter 3, p. 74). The MAST instrument uses more specific questions geared toward a younger population (Bowman & Gerber, 2006). The third is the World Health Organization Alcohol Use Disorders Identification Test (AUDIT), which was developed as a simple method for screening excessive drinking (Babor et al., 2001). According to the Canadian Community Health Survey, five or more drinks on a single occasion constitute heavy drinking (Tjepkema, 2004). Nurses need to be familiar with the application of the screening tests and with 12 risky drinking practices identified by the NASWG. Prevention of alcohol abuse starts with their sensitive questioning about drinking patterns, contexts, and reasons. Nurses provide facts from the guidelines for standard drink size, number of drinks per day for men (2) and women (1), and maximum number of drinks per week (see Chapters 3 and 8). They discuss the effects of alcohol consumption with their clients.

In 2004, 35% of cases of *gallbladder disease* in Canadians was attributed to obesity (Luo et al., 2007). Gallbladder disease includes inflammation, gallstone formation, and cancer. Gallbladder cancer is rare in Canadians, but linked with a positive family history. The most common disorder that affects 10% of Canadians is the development of stones from cholesterol or pigment. At highest risk are Canadians older than 40 years, female, or Aboriginal. Risk factors include diabetes, pregnancy, obesity, frequent or rapid weight alterations, and use of oral contraceptives, hormone-replacement therapy, or cholesterol-reducing therapy. Prevention includes controlling modifiable risk factors; following Canada's Food Guide; limiting intake of alcohol, caffeine, and refined sugar; consuming a moderate amount of healthful fat; and avoiding desserts, snacks, meats, and high-fat dairy products (e.g., whole milk, ice cream).

Colorectal cancer is the third most common cancer in Canadian men and women (Health Canada, 2007). Estimates were that 21,500 Canadians would be diagnosed with colorectal cancer in 2008, and 8900 would die from it (Canadian Cancer Society, National Cancer Institute of Canada, Statistics Canada, Provincial/ Territorial Cancer Registries, & Public Health Agency of Canada [The Partners], 2008). Although death rates per 100,000 of a standard age distribution have declined steadily, the number diagnosed has continued to increase. Every week on average, 400 Canadians are diagnosed with the disease and 167 die from it (Health Canada, 2007). Risk factors associated with colorectal cancer include age 50 years or older; history of polyps or prior colorectal cancer; IBD; positive family history; personal history of ovarian, endometrial, or breast cancer; type 2 diabetes mellitus; obesity; lack of exercise; smoking; and an unhealthy diet (Giovannucci & Michaud, 2007; Health Canada, 2007). Two inherited syndromes (familial adenomatous polyposis and nonpolyposis colorectal cancer) uncommonly affect younger adults. A high intake of nondairy fat and red meat, and low intake of fibre, fruits, and vegetables create risk for polyp development and subsequent cancer. Alcohol, beer in particular, may increase the risk (Health Canada, 2007). Evidence suggests that adequate intake of calcium and folic acid, and diets high in fibre can reduce polyp formation and malignancy (Colorectal Cancer Association of Canada, 2008; The Partners, 2007). Health care providers may also recommend the prophylactic use of nonsteroidal anti-inflammatory drugs (NSAIDs).

Screening by digital rectal examination and regular fecal occult blood test (FOBT) can reduce death rates by 15% to 33% in Canadians 50 to 74 years (Health Canada, 2007). Some authorities recommend an annual FOBT in Canadians older than 50 years. Further screening may be done by flexible sigmoidoscopy or colonoscopy. Canadian provinces are in the process of establishing opportunistic screening programs for colorectal cancer. Regular screening can diagnose the condition at an early stage, when it is more treatable.

Pancreatic cancer increases worldwide with age, male gender, and black and Jewish genetics. In Canada, estimates were that more women (1850) than men (1750) would be diagnosed and die with the disease in 2007 (The Partners, 2007). A genetic predisposition has been discovered in 3% to 5% of all cases of pancreatic cancer (Chappuis et al., 2001). Obesity has a positive association with the disease. A BMI greater than 30 has been related to increased rates in men, but decreased rates in women (Nothlings et al., 2007). Long-standing type 2 diabetes mellitus increases the risk by 50% (Giovannucci & Michaud, 2007). A strong positive association exists between smoking and pancreatic cancer (Giovannucci & Michaud, 2007; Hassan et al., 2006). Mortality from chronic pancreatitis increases with diabetes and smoking. Nkondjock and colleagues (2005) suggest that a high intake of fruits and vegetables may reduce the risk in Canadian men. To identify the disease in early stages, better screening methods need to be developed.

THE URINARY TRACT

Bladder conditions are very common in women. As many as 20% of all Canadian women suffer from a bladder infection in any given year. Anatomic differences subject women much more frequently than men to cystitis. The shorter female urethra and its proximity to the rectum and vagina create the conditions for development of acute bacterial infections of the bladder lining (*common* cystitis, a urinary tract infection [UTI]). *Interstitial* cystitis is a chronic inflammation between the bladder muscle and the lining, and is characterized by the absence of bacteria. Men with prostate enlargement and difficulty emptying the bladder of urine may also report symptoms of cystitis. Elderly men and women are more prone to UTIs because of catheterization, retention of urine, or reduced fluid intake in an attempt to manage urinary incontinence (see Table 17-6 Frequency, Nocturia, and Polyuria, and Chapter 25). Risk factors for UTIs in women include inadequate genital hygiene, frequent sexual intercourse, high number of sexual partners, use of spermicides or diaphragms for birth control, catheter use, and menopause, which lowers estrogen levels. Women and men with diabetes are both at higher risk for UTIs. Except for higher rates in women, risk factors for interstitial cystitis are poorly understood.

Screening methods include urinalysis, cystoscopy, urine culture, and diagnostic imaging to assess the structures of the urinary tract. Prevention of UTIs is enhanced if clients' fluid intake is at least 30 to 40 mL per kilogram of body weight and includes unsweetened pure cranberry juice. Such juice is high in vitamin C and hippuric acid, which prevents bacteria from adhering to the bladder wall. An adequate substitute for this intake of juice is cranberry-extract capsules (one 500 mg capsule equals 250–300 mL of juice and has 50% more fibre). Prevention includes women's personal hygiene practices of wiping from front to back, voiding before and after sexual intercourse, and voiding every 2 hours during the day. Interstitial cystitis is subject to dietary control and lifestyle changes. Avoidance of alcohol, spices, acidic foods, artificial sweeteners, and caffeine, and limiting the number of sexual partners reduce the irritation of the bladder.

Bladder cancer is more common in men than women. The Canadian Cancer Society and its partners (2008) estimated that 5100 men and 1700 women would develop bladder cancer in 2008, and that a total of 1800 people would die from it. In men, bladder cancer is the fourth most common form, after prostate, lung, and colorectal cancer. Although some people develop bladder cancer without exposure to known risk factors, several factors increase the chances of developing it. Examples include age older than 50 years, male gender, smoking, and exposure to particular chemicals in the manufacture of dyes, paints, textiles, leathers, and rubber products (Mayo Clinic, 2008). Arsenic in drinking water systems, abuse of some analgesics, genetic background, and previous bladder cancer also create risk (Canadian Cancer Society, 2008). Caucasians are more prone to bladder cancer than Latin Americans, blacks, or Asians. Aboriginals in Canada, despite smoking rates that are double the Canadian average, have lower rates of bladder cancer; however, these findings may simply reflect the long latency period of the disease (Marrett & Chaudhry, 2003). A personal or family history of bladder cancer increases the risk of developing the disease. If hereditary nonpolyposis colorectal cancer is in the family, it can create risk for developing cancer in the urinary system.

Kidney disease is life-threatening and frequently leads to incurable kidney failure. By 2001, more than 14,000 Canadians were suffering from end-stage kidney disease that required dialysis, and 4000 were needing kidney transplants (Kidney Research Centre, 2007). Risk factors for kidney disease include high blood pressure, diabetes, smoking, obesity, family history, age 65 years or older, and certain ethnic and genetic backgrounds, including Aboriginal and Asian ancestry (Northern Alberta & The Territories Branch, Kidney Foundation of Canada, 2008). In First Nations communities, type 2 diabetes is 3 to 5 times higher than in the general population, and rates among the Inuit are increasing (Health Canada, 2007). As the number of Canadians with risk factors increases, so does the rate of kidney disease. Exposure to lead and other heavy metals in the workplace creates risk, as does failure to adhere to a medication plan. Smoking increases renal vascular disease. Among the Inuit, smoking rates are four times the national average (Inuit Tapiriit Kanatami, 2007). Screening for kidney disease includes diagnostic imaging. Family history of polycystic kidney disease is a factor in disease development.

Elevated rates of *kidney cancer* have been found in First Nations people despite their generally lower cancer rates (Marrett & Chaudhry, 2003). Diet, obesity, and limited physical activity are implicated, but not environmental factors. For overall Canada, estimates were that kidney cancer would develop in 2700 men and 1750 women in

2008. The most common type is renal cell carcinoma, which is strongly linked with obesity as a risk factor (The Partners, 2008). Other risk factors include tobacco use, polycystic kidney disease, unopposed estrogen therapy, and occupational exposure to heavy metals, asbestos, and petroleum products (Degler, 2007). A positive family history is rare. Screening includes urinalysis, radiography, ultrasonography, and diagnostic imaging.

Kidney stones (renal calculi), which occur in 1 out of 20 Canadians, usually develop in the kidneys or ureters, and are more common in Caucasian genetic background and men. Development is associated with decreased urine volume; increased excretion of substances such as calcium, oxalate, urate, cystine, xanthine, and phosphate; or intake of water with a high mineral content. An inherited condition that produces stones (malabsorption of cystine) is rare; however, nurses should still carefully review each client's family history for it. Avoiding stone recurrence is important: one preventive measure is to ensure a daily urine output of at least 2 L. A positive family history may suggest that learned dietary habits are a risk factor. Stone analysis provides direction for dietary precautions, which may involve limiting intake of animal protein to 60 grams per day, and avoiding nitrogen, sodium, and foods with high oxalate content such as rhubarb, strawberries, and spinach. Clients should avoid dehydration by maintaining a high fluid intake, especially in warm weather and while exercising. Screening for stones occurs with urinalysis for hematuria, radiography, intravenous pyelography, and tomography.

■ EMERGENCY CONCERNS

Direct trauma to the abdomen requires immediate attention. A ruptured organ (e.g., spleen, bladder) requires emergency assessment and treatment. Its contents can spill into the abdominal cavity where they may contribute to *peritonitis*. This severe generalized inflammation of the serous membranes that line the abdominal cavity and its organs represents another medical emergency.

All cases of abdominal pain require prompt and careful assessment of the abdominal region to identify life-threatening conditions that may derive from not only intra-abdominal causes, but also extra-abdominal origins. Ruptures, perforations, severe infections, infarctions, obstructions, occlusions, dissections, and incarcerations underlie emergency concerns that all present with abdominal pain *in addition to* other symptoms or signs. Rarely is abdominal pain alone, *without any other signs or symptoms*, emergent (Seller, 2007).

Intra-abdominal emergencies are related primarily to gastrointestinal, urinary, or hematologic systems, or to peritonitis. When abdominal pain is associated with distention, rebound tenderness, rigidity, extreme restlessness, or stillness, referral to a surgical facility is essential. Intra-abdominal emergencies include dissecting abdominal aortic aneurysm (characterized by mottled skin below the waist, pulsating epigastric mass, and mid-back pain), perforated peptic ulcer, appendicitis, renal colic, sepsis, ureteral obstruction, large and small bowel obstruction, mesenteric artery occlusion, acute pancreatitis, and peritonitis. Incarcerated hernias, testicular torsion, and priapism are addressed in Chapter 21, ovarian torsion in Chapter 22, and ectopic pregnancies in Chapter 24.

Black tarry stools (melena), frank blood in the stool, emesis with a fecal odour, yellowing of the skin, dark urine or gross hematuria, inability to void, pruritus, and prolonged nausea and vomiting should be assessed promptly.

Extra-abdominal emergencies (cardiovascular and respiratory systems) are detected because of referred pain to the upper abdomen (myocardial infarction, pneumothorax).

TECHNIQUES OF EXAMINATION: OBJECTIVE DATA

◼ PROMOTING CLIENT COMFORT, DIGNITY, AND SAFETY

A skilled abdominal examination requires a relaxed client, good lighting, and full exposure of the abdomen from above the xiphoid process to the symphysis pubis. Position the supine client with his or her knees slightly flexed to facilitate relaxation of the abdominal muscles for all aspects of the examination, especially palpation. Drape the breasts and genitalia, leaving a thin margin of pubic hair and both inguinal areas visible. Examine any areas of pain or discomfort last.

TIPS FOR ENHANCING EXAMINATION OF THE ABDOMEN

- Check that the client has an empty bladder.
- Make the client comfortable in the supine position, with a pillow under the head and perhaps another under the knees. Slide your hand under the low back to see if the client is relaxed and lying flat on the table.
- Ask the client to keep the arms at the sides or folded across the chest. If the arms are above the head, the abdominal wall stretches and tightens, making palpation difficult.
- Before you begin palpation, ask the client to point to any areas of pain and examine these areas last.
- Warm your hands and stethoscope. To warm your hands, rub them together or place them under hot water. You can also palpate through the client's gown to absorb warmth from the client's body before exposing the abdomen.
- Approach the client calmly and avoid quick unexpected movements. *Watch the client's face for any signs of pain or discomfort.* Make sure you avoid long fingernails.
- Distract the client, if necessary, with conversation or questions. If the client is frightened or ticklish, begin palpation with the client's hand under yours. After a few moments, slip your hand underneath to palpate directly.

An arched back thrusts the abdomen forward and tightens the abdominal muscles.

Equipment

- Ruler
- Felt marking pen
- Alcohol wipes
- Disposable gloves (in case of lesions or exudates)
- Penlight
- Stethoscope

◼ THE ABDOMEN

Inspection. Starting from your usual standing position at the right side of the bed or examining table, inspect the abdomen. As you look at the contour of the abdomen, watch for peristalsis. It is helpful to sit or bend down so that you can view the abdomen tangentially and horizontally. Tangential lighting may assist visualization.

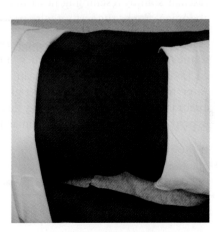

Inspect the surface, contours, and movements of the abdomen, including the following:

■ *The skin*. Note the following:

Scars. Describe or diagram their location.

Striae. Old silver striae or stretch marks are expected.

Pink–purple striae of *Cushing's syndrome.*

Dilated veins. A few small veins may be visible.

Dilated veins of *hepatic cirrhosis* or of *inferior vena cava obstruction* may be seen.

Rashes and lesions

■ *The umbilicus*. Observe its contour and location and any inflammation or bulges suggesting a hernia.

See Table 17-8, Localized Bulges in the Abdominal Wall (p. 556).

■ *The contour of the abdomen*

Is it flat, rounded, protuberant, or scaphoid (markedly concave or hollowed)?

See Table 17-9, Protuberant Abdomens (p. 557).

Do the flanks bulge or are there local bulges? Survey the inguinal and femoral area.

Bulging flanks of *ascites*; suprapubic bulge of a distended bladder or pregnant uterus, and hernias.

Is the abdomen symmetric?

Asymmetry from an enlarged organ or mass.

Are there visible organs or masses? Look for an enlarged liver or spleen that has descended below the rib cage.

Lower abdominal mass of an ovarian or a uterine tumour.

■ *Peristalsis*. Observe for several minutes if you suspect intestinal obstruction. Peristalsis may be visible and expected in very thin people.

Increased peristaltic waves of *intestinal obstruction.*

■ *Pulsations*. The aortic pulsation is frequently visible in the epigastrium.

Increased pulsation may be due to an *aortic aneurysm* or *increased pulse pressure.*

Auscultation.   Auscultation provides important information about bowel motility. *Listen to the abdomen before performing percussion or palpation because these manoeuvres may alter the frequency of bowel sounds.* Practice auscultation until you are thoroughly familiar with variations in bowel sounds and can detect changes suggestive of inflammation or obstruction. Auscultation may also reveal *bruits*, or vascular sounds resembling heart murmurs, over the aorta or other arteries in the abdomen. Bruits suggest vascular occlusive disease.

Bowel sounds may be altered in diarrhea, intestinal obstruction, *paralytic ileus*, and *peritonitis.*

Place the diaphragm of your stethoscope gently on the abdomen. Listen for bowel sounds and note their frequency and character. Expected sounds consist of clicks and gurgles, occurring at an estimated frequency of 5 to 34 per minute. After timing the sounds in the right lower quadrant, listen in the other three quadrants. Occasionally you may hear *borborygmi*—long prolonged gurgles of hyperperistalsis—the familiar "stomach growling."

See Table 17-10, Sounds in the Abdomen (p. 558).

If the client has high blood pressure, listen in the epigastrium and in each upper quadrant for *bruits*. Later in the examination, when the client sits up, listen also in the costovertebral angles. Epigastric bruits confined to systole may be heard.

A bruit in one of these areas that has both systolic and diastolic components strongly suggests *renal artery stenosis* as the cause of hypertension.

Listen for bruits over the aorta, iliac arteries, and femoral arteries. Bruits confined to systole are relatively common, and do not necessarily signify occlusive disease.

Listening points for bruits in these vessels are in the following illustration. Listen over the liver and spleen for *friction rubs*.

Bruits with both systolic and diastolic components suggest the turbulent blood flow of *partial arterial occlusion* or *arterial insufficiency*.

See Table 17-10, Sounds in the Abdomen (p. 558).

Friction rubs in liver tumour, gonococcal infection around the liver, splenic infarction.

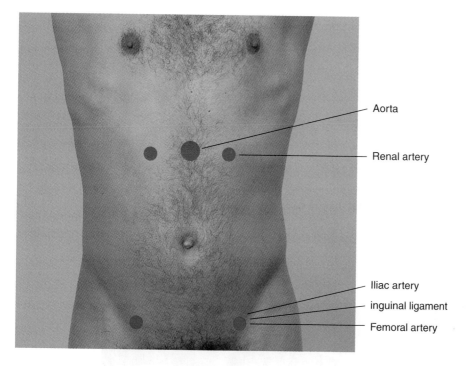

Aorta

Renal artery

Iliac artery

inguinal ligament

Femoral artery

Percussion.
Percussion helps you to assess the amount and distribution of gas in the abdomen, identify possible masses that are solid or fluid filled, and discover tender areas. Its use in estimating the size of the liver and spleen is described later.

Percuss the abdomen lightly in all four quadrants to assess the distribution of *tympany* and *dullness*. Tympany usually predominates because of gas in the gastrointestinal tract, but scattered areas of dullness from fluid and feces are also typical. You will usually find liver dullness and tympany over the gastric bubble and splenic flexure of the colon.

■ Note any large dull areas that might indicate an underlying mass or enlarged organ. This observation will guide your palpation.

■ On each side of a protuberant abdomen, note where abdominal tympany changes to the dullness of solid posterior structures.

A protuberant abdomen that is tympanitic throughout suggests *intestinal obstruction*. See Table 17-9, Protuberant Abdomens (p. 557).

In *situs inversus* (rare), organs are reversed: the air bubble is found on the right, and liver dullness on the left.

Pregnant uterus, ovarian tumour, distended bladder, large liver or spleen, or fecal impaction.

Dullness in both flanks requires further assessment for ascites (see p. 537).

Palpation
Light Palpation.
Feeling the abdomen gently is especially helpful for identifying abdominal tenderness, muscular resistance, and some superficial organs and masses. It also serves to reassure and relax the client.

Keeping your hand and forearm on a horizontal plane, with fingers together and flat on the abdominal surface, palpate the abdomen with a light, gentle, dipping motion.

When moving your hand from place to place, raise it just off the skin. Moving smoothly, feel in all quadrants and watch the client's face.

Identify any superficial organs or masses and any area of tenderness or increased resistance to your hand. If resistance is present, try to distinguish voluntary guarding from involuntary muscular spasm. To do this:

■ Try all the relaxing methods you know (see p. 527).

■ Feel for the relaxation of abdominal muscles that usually accompanies exhalation.

■ Ask the client to mouth-breathe with jaw dropped open.

Voluntary guarding often decreases with these manoeuvres.

> Involuntary rigidity (muscular spasm) typically persists despite these manoeuvres. It indicates *peritoneal inflammation.*

Deep Palpation.   This is generally required to delineate abdominal masses. Again using the palmar surfaces of your fingers, feel in all four quadrants. Identify any masses and note their location, size, shape, consistency, tenderness, pulsations, and any mobility with respiration or with the examining hand. Correlate your palpable findings with their percussion notes.

> Abdominal masses may be categorized in several ways: physiologic (pregnant uterus), inflammatory (diverticulitis of the colon), vascular (an aneurysm of the abdominal aorta), neoplastic (carcinoma of the colon), or obstructive (a distended bladder or dilated loop of bowel).

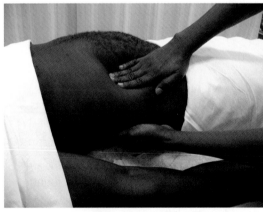

LIGHT PALPATION

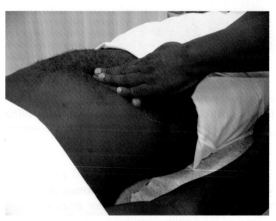

TWO-HANDED DEEP PALPATION

Assessment for Peritoneal Inflammation.   Abdominal pain and tenderness, especially when associated with muscular spasm, suggest inflammation of the parietal peritoneum. Localize the pain as accurately as possible. First, even before palpation, *ask the client to cough* and determine where the cough produces pain. Then, *palpate gently with one finger* to map the tender area. Pain produced by light percussion has similar localizing value. These gentle manoeuvres may be all you need to establish an area of peritoneal inflammation.

> Abdominal pain when coughing or with light percussion suggests peritoneal inflammation. See Table 17-11, Tender Abdomens (pp. 559–560).

If not, look for *rebound tenderness.* Press down with your fingers firmly and slowly, and then withdraw them quickly. Watch and listen to the client for signs of pain. Ask the client "Which hurts more, when I press or let go?" Have the client locate the pain exactly. Pain induced or increased by quick withdrawal constitutes *rebound tenderness* caused by rapid movement of an inflamed peritoneum.

> Rebound tenderness suggests peritoneal inflammation. If tenderness is felt elsewhere than where you were trying to elicit rebound, that area may be the real source of the problem.

Cultural Considerations

The Inuit language of Inuktitut has no question format. Questions are asked as positive sentences *with a rising inflection at the end*. "You are having more pain with pressure?" and "You are having more pain . . . when I let go?" Always watch the Inuit client's face for a nonverbal response or listen for "Ah – AH."

Avoid using negative questions with any clients, especially those who speak English as a second language. For example, if you ask "You are not having pain now?" the client will answer "Yes" or will raise eyebrows to indicate "Correct, I am not having pain now."

THE LIVER

Because the rib cage shelters most of the liver, assessment is difficult. Liver size and shape can be estimated by percussion and perhaps palpation; the palpating hand helps you to evaluate its surface, consistency, and tenderness.

Percussion.   Identify the *upper border of liver dullness* in the midclavicular line. Lightly percuss from lung resonance down toward liver dullness. Gently displace a woman's breast as necessary to be sure that you start in a resonant area. The course of percussion in the following illustration.

Starting at a level below the umbilicus (in an area of tympany, not dullness), lightly percuss upward toward the liver. Ascertain the *lower border of liver dullness* in the midclavicular line. Next, measure the vertical span of liver dullness in the right midclavicular line.

The span of liver dullness is *increased* when the liver is enlarged.

The span of liver dullness is *decreased* when the liver is small or when free air is present below the diaphragm, as from a *perforated hollow viscus.* Serial observations may show a decreasing span of dullness with resolution of *hepatitis* or *congestive heart failure* or, less commonly, with progression of *fulminant hepatitis.*

Liver dullness may be displaced downward by the low diaphragm of *chronic obstructive pulmonary disease.* Span, however, remains as expected.

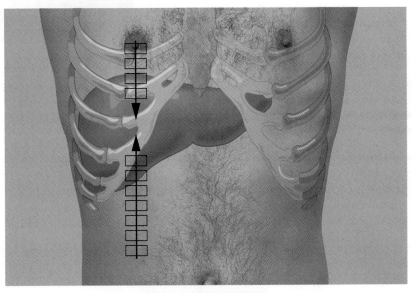

PERCUSSING LIVER SPANS

Now measure in centimetres the distance between your two points—the vertical span of liver dullness. Expected liver spans, shown in the figure, are generally greater in men than in women, in tall people than in short. If the liver seems to be enlarged, outline the lower edge by percussing in other areas such as the midsternal line.

Dullness of a right pleural effusion or consolidated lung, if adjacent to liver dullness, may falsely *increase* the estimate of liver size.

Gas in the colon may produce tympany in the right upper quadrant, obscure liver dullness, and falsely *decrease* the estimate of liver size.

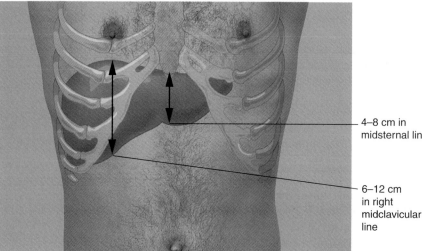

4–8 cm in midsternal line

6–12 cm in right midclavicular line

EXPECTED LIVER SPANS

Although percussion is probably the most accurate clinical method for estimating the vertical size of the liver, it typically leads to underestimation.

Palpation. In preparation for palpation, determine the lowest point of liver descent. Instruct the client to take a deep breath and percuss upward to dullness.

Place your left hand behind the client, parallel to and supporting the right 11th and 12th ribs and adjacent soft tissues below. Remind the client to relax on your hand if necessary. By pressing your left hand forward, the client's liver may be felt more easily by your other hand.

Place your right hand on the client's right abdomen lateral to the rectus muscle, with your fingertips well below the lower border of liver dullness on deep inspiration. Some examiners like to point their fingers up toward the client's head, whereas others prefer a somewhat more oblique position parallel to the costal margin (see figure). In either case, press gently in and up.

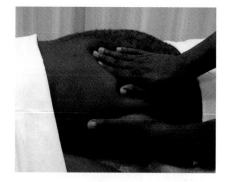

Ask the client to take a deep breath. Try to feel the liver edge as it comes down to meet your fingertips. If you feel it, lighten the pressure of your palpating hand slightly so that the liver can slip under your finger pads and you can feel its anterior surface. Note any tenderness. If palpable at all, the liver edge is usually soft, sharp, and regular, with a smooth surface. The healthy liver may be slightly tender.

Firmness or hardness of the liver, bluntness or rounding of its edge, and irregularity of its contour suggest an unexpected finding of the liver.

On inspiration, the liver is palpable about 3 cm below the right costal margin in the midclavicular line. Some people breathe more with their chests than with their diaphragms. It may be helpful to encourage such a client to "breathe with the abdomen," thus bringing the liver, as well as the spleen and kidneys, into a palpable position during inspiration.

An obstructed, distended gallbladder may form an oval mass below the edge of the liver, merging with it. It is dull to percussion.

In order to feel the liver, you may have to alter your pressure according to the thickness and resistance of the abdominal wall. If you cannot feel it, move your palpating hand closer to the costal margin and try again.

The edge of an enlarged liver may be missed by starting palpation too high in the abdomen.

Try to trace the liver edge both laterally and medially. Palpation through the rectus muscles, however, is especially difficult. Describe or sketch the liver edge, and measure its distance from the right costal margin in the midclavicular line.

See Table 17-12, Liver Enlargement: Apparent and Real (p. 561).

◼ THE SPLEEN

When a spleen enlarges, it expands anteriorly, downward, and medially, often replacing the tympany of stomach and colon with the dullness of a solid organ. It then becomes palpable below the costal margin. Percussion cannot confirm splenic enlargement, but can raise your suspicions of it. Palpation can confirm the enlargement, but often misses large spleens that do not descend below the costal margin.

Percussion.   Two techniques may help you to detect *splenomegaly*, an enlarged spleen:

- ◼ *Percuss the left lower anterior chest wall* between the 6th rib, anterior axillary line, and costal margin, an area termed *Traube's space*. As you percuss along the routes suggested by the arrows in the following figures, note the lateral extent of tympany.

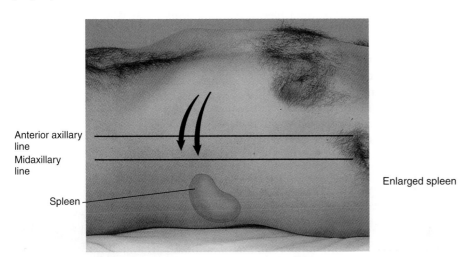

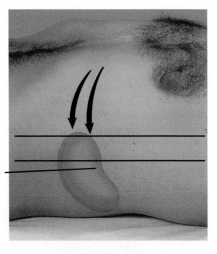

This is variable, but if tympany is prominent, especially laterally, splenomegaly is not likely. The expected dullness of a spleen is usually hidden within the dullness of other posterior tissues.

Fluid or solids in the stomach or colon may also cause dullness in Traube's space.

- ◼ *Check for a splenic percussion sign.* Percuss the lowest interspace in the left anterior axillary line, as in the following figure. This area is usually tympanitic. Then ask the client to take a deep breath, and percuss again. The percussion note usually remains tympanitic.

A change in percussion note from tympany to dullness on inspiration suggests splenic enlargement. This is a *positive splenic percussion sign*.

If either or both of these tests are positive, pay extra attention to palpation of the spleen.

The splenic percussion sign may also be positive when the spleen is not enlarged.

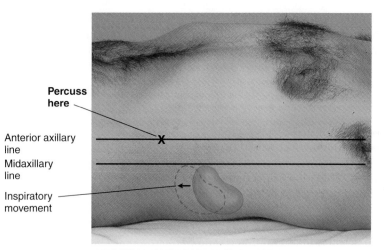

Percuss
here

Anterior axillary
line

Midaxillary
line

Inspiratory
movement

NEGATIVE SPLENIC PERCUSSION SIGN

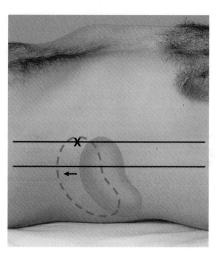

POSITIVE SPLENIC PERCUSSION SIGN

Palpation. With your left hand, reach over and around the client to support and press forward the lower left rib cage and adjacent soft tissue. With your right hand below the left costal margin, press in toward the spleen. Begin palpation low enough so that you are below a possibly enlarged spleen. (If your hand is close to the costal margin, moreover, it is not sufficiently mobile to reach up under the rib cage.) Ask the client to take a deep breath. Try to feel the tip or edge of the spleen as it comes down to meet your fingertips. Note any tenderness, assess the splenic contour, and measure the distance between the spleen's lowest point and the left costal margin. In a small percentage of adults, the tip of the spleen is usually palpable. Causes include a low, flat diaphragm, as in chronic obstructive pulmonary disease, and a deep inspiratory descent of the diaphragm.

An enlarged spleen may be missed if the examiner starts too high in the abdomen to feel the lower edge.

A palpable spleen tip, though not necessarily unexpected, may indicate splenic enlargement. The spleen tip below is just palpable the left costal margin.

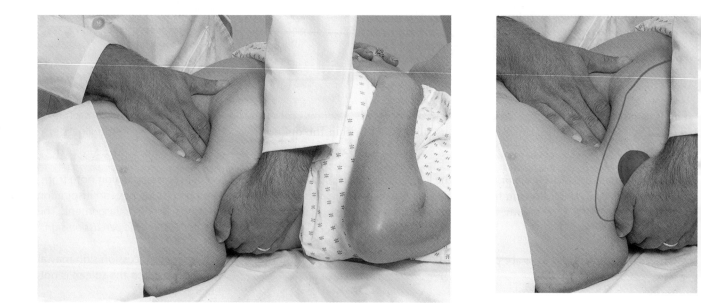

THE KIDNEYS

Palpation. Although kidneys are not usually palpable, you should learn and practise the techniques for examination. Detecting an enlarged kidney may prove to be very important.

Palpation of the Left Kidney.
Reach across to the client's left side. Place your left hand behind the client just below and parallel to the 12th rib, with your fingertips just reaching the costovertebral angle. Lift, trying to displace the kidney anteriorly. Place your right hand gently in the left upper quadrant, lateral to the rectus muscle. Ask the client to take a deep breath. At the peak of inspiration, press your right hand firmly and deeply into the left upper quadrant, just below the costal margin, and try to palpate the kidney between your two hands. Ask the client to breathe out and then to stop breathing briefly. Slowly release the pressure of your right hand, feeling at the same time for the kidney to slide back into its expiratory position. A left kidney is rarely palpable. If the kidney is palpable, describe its size, contour, and any tenderness.

Palpation of the Right Kidney.
To palpate the right kidney, use your left hand to lift from in back, and your right hand to feel deep in the right upper quadrant. Proceed as before.

A right kidney may be palpable, especially in thin, well-relaxed women. It may or may not be slightly tender. The client is usually aware of palpation and release. Occasionally, a right kidney is located more anteriorly than usual and then must be distinguished from the liver. The edge of the liver, if palpable, tends to be sharper and to extend farther medially and laterally. It cannot be captured. The lower pole of the kidney is rounded.

A left flank mass (see the solid line on photo on previous page) may represent marked *splenomegaly* or an enlarged left kidney. Suspect *splenomegaly* if notch is palpated on medial border, edge extends beyond the midline, percussion is dull, and your fingers can probe medial and lateral borders but not between the mass and the costal margin. Confirm findings with further evaluation.

Attributes favouring an *enlarged kidney* over an enlarged spleen include preservation of tympany in the left upper quadrant and the ability to probe with your fingers between the mass and the costal margin, but not deep to its medial and lower borders.

Causes of kidney enlargement include hydronephrosis, cysts, and tumours. Bilateral enlargement suggests polycystic disease.

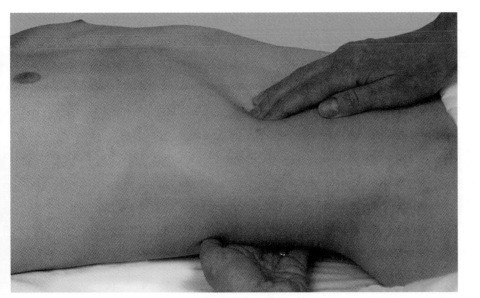

Assessing Kidney Tenderness. You may note tenderness when examining the abdomen, but also search for it at each costovertebral angle. Pressure from your fingertips may be enough to elicit tenderness, but if not, use fist percussion. Place the ball of one hand in the costovertebral angle and strike it with the ulnar surface of your fist. Use enough force to cause a perceptible but painless jar or thud in your client. To save the client needless exertion, integrate this assessment with your examination of the back (see p. 88).

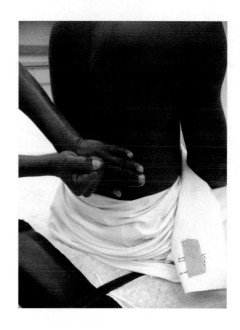

Pain with pressure or fist percussion suggests *pyelonephritis* but may also have a musculoskeletal cause.

THE BLADDER

The bladder usually cannot be examined unless it is distended superior to the symphysis pubis. Use percussion to check for dullness and to determine how high the bladder rises. Percussion is more comfortable than palpation for the client with bladder distention. On palpation, the dome of the distended bladder feels smooth and round. Check for tenderness.

Bladder distention results from outlet obstruction due to *urethral stricture, prostatic hyperplasia,* as well as from medications and neurologic disorders such as *stroke, multiple sclerosis.*

Suprapubic tenderness occurs in *bladder infection.*

THE AORTA

Press firmly deep in the upper abdomen, slightly to the left of the midline, and identify the aortic pulsations. In people older than age 50, try to assess the width of the aorta by pressing deeply in the upper abdomen with one hand on each side of the aorta, as illustrated. In this age group, the aorta is expected to be not more than 3.0 cm wide (average 2.5 cm). This measurement does not include the thickness of the abdominal wall. Try to distinguish an anterior aortic pulsation from a widened horizontal pulsation over 3.0 cm wide. The ease of feeling aortic pulsations varies greatly with the thickness of the abdominal wall and with the anteroposterior diameter of the abdomen.

In an older person, a periumbilical or upper abdominal mass with expansile pulsations suggests an *aortic aneurysm.*

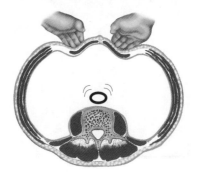
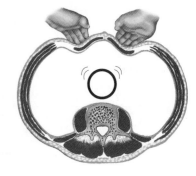

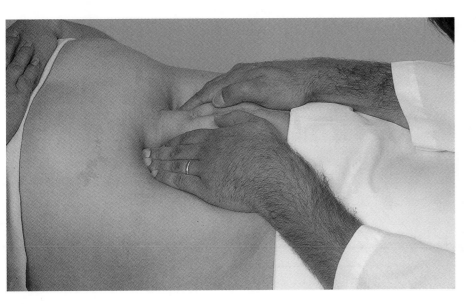

An *aortic aneurysm* is a pathologic dilatation of the aorta, usually due to arteriosclerosis. A merely tortuous abdominal aorta, however, may be difficult to distinguish from an aneurysm on clinical grounds.

Although an aneurysm is usually painless, pain may herald its most dreaded and frequent complication—rupture of the aorta.

Apparent enlargement of the aorta requires assessment by ultrasound.

◼ SPECIAL TECHNIQUES

ASSESSMENT TECHNIQUES FOR:

- Ascites
- Suspected splenomegaly
- Appendicitis
- Ventral hernia
- Acute cholecystitis
- Mass in abdominal wall
- Suspected liver enlargement or tenderness

Assessing Possible Ascites. A protuberant abdomen with bulging flanks suggests the possibility of ascitic fluid. Because ascitic fluid characteristically sinks with gravity, whereas gas-filled loops of bowel float to the top, percussion gives a dull note in dependent areas of the abdomen. Look for such a pattern by percussing outward in several directions from the central area of tympany. Map the border between tympany and dullness.

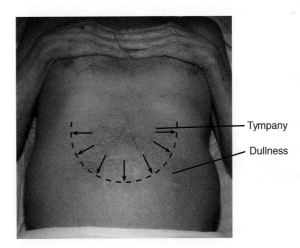

Two further techniques help to confirm ascites, although both signs may be misleading.

- *Test for shifting dullness.* After mapping the borders of tympany and dullness, ask the client to turn onto one side. Percuss and mark the borders again. In a person without ascites, the borders between tympany and dullness usually stay relatively constant.

In ascites, dullness shifts to the more dependent side, whereas tympany shifts to the top.

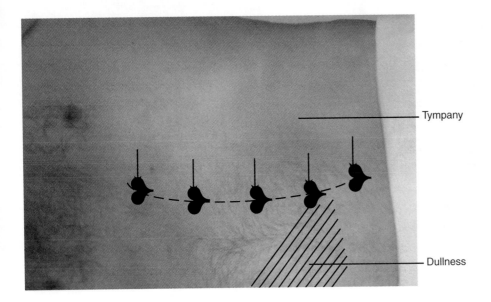

- *Test for a fluid wave.* Ask the client or an assistant to press the edges of both hands firmly down the midline of the abdomen. This pressure helps to stop the transmission of a wave through fat. While you tap one flank sharply with your fingertips, feel on the opposite flank for an impulse transmitted through the fluid. Unfortunately, this sign is often negative until ascites is obvious, and it is sometimes positive in people without ascites.

An easily palpable impulse suggests ascites.

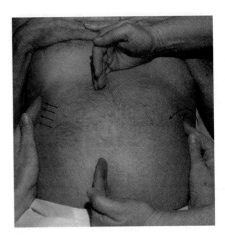

Identifying an Organ or a Mass in an Ascitic Abdomen. Try to *ballotte* the organ or mass, exemplified here by an enlarged liver. Straighten and stiffen the fingers of one hand together, place them on the abdominal surface, and make a brief jabbing movement directly toward the anticipated structure. This quick movement often displaces the fluid so that your fingertips can briefly touch the surface of the structure through the abdominal wall.

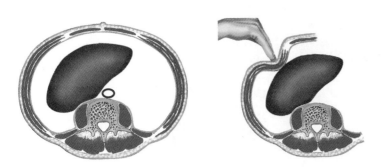

Assessing Possible Appendicitis

- Ask the client to point to where the pain began and where it is now. Ask the client to cough. Determine whether and where pain results.

The pain of appendicitis classically begins near the umbilicus, then shifts to the right lower quadrant, where coughing increases it. Older clients report this pattern less frequently than younger ones.

■ Search carefully for an area of local tenderness.

Localized tenderness anywhere in the right lower quadrant, even in the right flank, may indicate appendicitis.

■ Feel for muscular rigidity.

Early voluntary guarding may be replaced by involuntary muscular rigidity.

■ *Perform a rectal examination and, in women, a pelvic examination.* These manoeuvres may not help you to detect an inflamed appendix, but they may help to identify an inflamed appendix atypically located within the pelvic cavity. They may also suggest other causes of the abdominal pain.

Right-sided rectal tenderness may be caused by, for example, inflamed adnexa or an inflamed seminal vesicle, as well as by an inflamed appendix.

Additional techniques are sometimes helpful:

■ Check the tender area for rebound tenderness. (If other signs are typically positive, you can save the client unnecessary pain by omitting this test.)

Rebound tenderness suggests peritoneal inflammation, as from appendicitis.

■ Check for *Rovsing's sign* and for referred rebound tenderness. Press deeply and evenly in the *left* lower quadrant. Then quickly withdraw your fingers.

Pain in the *right* lower quadrant during *left*-sided pressure suggests appendicitis (a positive Rovsing's sign). So does right lower quadrant pain on quick withdrawal (*referred rebound tenderness*).

■ Look for a *psoas sign*. Place your hand just above the client's right knee and ask the client to raise that thigh against your hand. Alternatively, ask the client to turn onto the left side. Then extend the client's right leg at the hip. Flexion of the leg at the hip makes the psoas muscle contract; extension stretches it.

Increased abdominal pain on either manoeuvre constitutes a *positive psoas* sign, suggesting irritation of the psoas muscle by an inflamed appendix.

■ Look for an *obturator sign*. Flex the client's right thigh at the hip, with the knee bent, and rotate the leg internally at the hip. This manoeuvre stretches the internal obturator muscle. (Internal rotation of the hip is described on p. 650.)

Right hypogastric pain constitutes a positive obturator sign, suggesting irritation of the obturator muscle by an inflamed appendix.

■ Test for *cutaneous hyperesthesia*. At a series of points down the abdominal wall, gently pick up a fold of skin between your thumb and index finger, without pinching it. This manoeuvre should not typically be painful.

Localized pain with this manoeuvre, in all or part of the right lower quadrant, may accompany appendicitis.

Assessing Possible Acute Cholecystitis.

When right upper quadrant pain and tenderness suggest acute cholecystitis, look for *Murphy's sign*. Hook your left thumb or the fingers of your right hand under the costal margin at the point where the lateral border of the rectus muscle intersects with the costal margin. Alternatively, if the liver is enlarged, hook your thumb or fingers under the liver edge at a comparable point below. Ask the client to take a deep breath. Watch the client breathing and note the degree of tenderness.

A sharp increase in tenderness with a sudden stop in inspiratory effort constitutes a *positive Murphy's sign* of *acute cholecystitis*. Hepatic tenderness may also increase with this manoeuvre, but usually to a lesser degree.

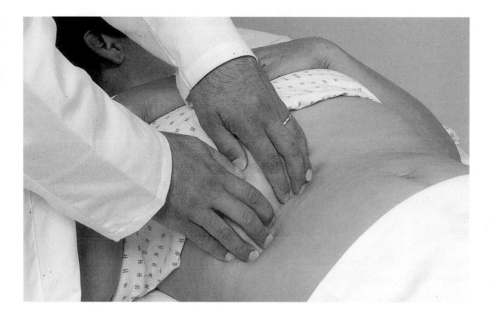
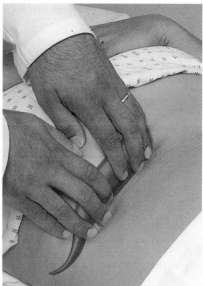

Suspected Liver Enlargement or Tenderness. The "hooking technique" may be helpful, especially when the client is obese. Stand to the right of the client's chest. Place both hands, side by side, on the right abdomen below the border of liver dullness. Press in with your fingers and up toward the costal margin. Ask the client to take a deep breath. The liver edge, shown in the following illustration, is palpable with the fingerpads of both hands.

Assessing Tenderness of a Nonpalpable Liver. Place your left hand flat on the lower right rib cage and then gently strike your hand with the ulnar surface of your right fist. Ask the client to compare the sensation with that produced by a similar strike on the left side.

Tenderness over the liver suggests inflammation, as in *hepatitis,* or congestion, as in *heart failure.*

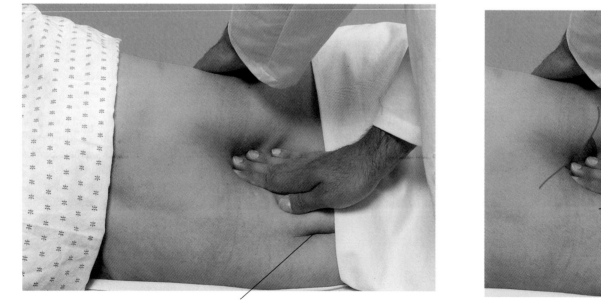

Umbilicus

Suspected Splenomegaly. Have the client lie on the right side with legs somewhat flexed at hips and knees. In this position, gravity may bring an enlarged spleen forward and to the right into a palpable location.

The enlarged spleen is palpable about 2 cm below the left costal margin on deep inspiration.

Assessing Ventral Hernias. Ventral hernias are hernias in the abdominal wall exclusive of groin hernias. If you suspect but do not see an umbilical or incisional hernia, ask the client to raise head and shoulders off the table.

The bulge of a hernia will usually appear with this action (see p. 556).

Inguinal and femoral hernias are discussed in the next chapter. They can give rise to important abdominal problems and must not be overlooked.

The cause of intestinal obstruction or peritonitis may be missed by overlooking a strangulated femoral hernia.

Mass in the Abdominal Wall

To Distinguish an Abdominal Mass From a Mass in the Abdominal Wall. An occasional mass is in the abdominal wall rather than inside the abdominal cavity. Ask the client either to raise the head and shoulders or to strain down, thus tightening the abdominal muscles. Feel for the mass again.

A mass in the abdominal wall remains palpable; an intra-abdominal mass is obscured by muscular contraction.

RECORDING AND ANALYZING FINDINGS

Documentation of the information obtained from the client's health history and physical examination of the abdomen must be thorough, accurate, and clear for all members of the interdisciplinary team. Follow the principles of documentation to ensure the planning and implementation of comprehensive and appropriate care for the client.

■ *Examples of Documentation for Abdomen Assessment*

Area of Assessment	Expected Findings	Unexpected Findings
Abdomen		
Skin	No scars, old silver striae bilaterally	Pink-purple striae, purpura lower quadrants, purplish blue echymosis left upper quadrant
Contour	Flat, symmetric, faint aortic pulsations upper left quadrant	Rounded, asymmetric, localized bulge right lower quadrant, marked aortic pulsations left of midline, upper quadrant
Auscultation—four quadrants	Approximately 20 clicks and gurgles per minute in right lower quadrant, borborygmi upper quadrants, occasional clicks in left lower quadrant	Bruit left of midline in upper quadrant, absent bowel sounds, friction rub over liver
Percussion—four quadrants	Predominantly tympany, some dullness, all quadrants	Dullness over right and left upper quadrants
Palpation—four quadrants	Relaxed, nontender, soft all quadrants	Firm, boardlike, involuntary rigidity, rebound tenderness right midquadrant
Liver	Liver span 8 cm right midclavicular line, nontender, soft smooth edge 1 cm inferior to right costal margin	Liver span 14 cm right midclavicular line, hard, rounded, irregular liver contour palpated 7 cm inferior to costal margin
Spleen	Tympany over Traube's space, tympany on inspiration in lowest left anterior axillary interspace, nonpalpable	Dullness in Traube's space, tender, palpable tip 1 cm inferior to left costal margin
Kidneys	Right and left nonpalpable, nontender bilaterally to fist percussion	Left CVA tenderness to finger pressure, palpable left kidney

(continued)

■ *Examples of Documentation for Abdomen Assessment (Continued)*

Area of Assessment	Expected Findings	Unexpected Findings
Bladder	Percussed at level of symphysis pubis, nonpalpable	Percussed 3 cm superior to symphysis pubis, suprapubic tenderness
Aorta	2.5–3 cm wide, anterior pulsation	Over 3 cm wide, lateral pulsation
Appendix	Not identifiable	Localized pain right lower mid quadrant, muscle rigidity, rebound tenderness, positive psoas sign, positive obturator sign
Gallbladder	Nonpalpable, nontender right upper quadrant	Positive Murphy's sign

◤ ANALYZING FINDINGS FROM PHYSICAL EXAMINATION AND HEALTH HISTORY

After documenting findings, it is important to analyze the information from the health history and physical examination to determine one or more nursing diagnoses and plan an interdisciplinary approach. For example:

Mrs. Black, 47 years old, presents to the clinic with complaints of steady, aching pain in her right upper quadrant, fever, and "pain in my back." Her BMI is 33, and she was recently diagnosed with hypertension. She reports that pain is worse after eating high-fat meals and that she ate deep-fried fish and chips earlier today. During examination, the nurse detects dullness and tenderness to percussion in the right upper quadrant and a positive Murphy's sign. This information influences the following nursing diagnoses:

- ■ *Pain potentially related to inflammatory (infectious) process of the gallbladder*

- ■ *Imbalanced nutrition: More than body requirements*

An interdisciplinary approach ensures comprehensive care for Mrs. Black. The registered nurse monitors vital signs and fluid balance, assesses psychosocial issues, provides analgesia, establishes intravenous fluid and electrolyte replacement, and ensures that the client takes nothing by mouth. A gastroenterologist performs a complete abdominal assessment, including diagnostic tests. A registered dietitian assesses Mrs. Black's dietary intake and knowledge of nutrition, a fitness expert explores exercise goals, and the pharmacist provides information about appropriate medications to treat Mrs. Black conservatively.

After a treatment plan is established, Mrs. Black needs continued follow-up with her dietitian, nurse, and family physician to ensure that she understands and follows an appropriate diet and exercise regimen, support systems are in place, and the team is assessing concerning symptoms opportunely.

Critical Thinking Exercises

Answer the following questions about Mrs. Black.

- ■ What observation is associated with a positive Murphy's sign? (*Knowledge*)
- ■ Distinguish between hepatic tenderness and gallbladder tenderness. (*Comprehension*)
- ■ Relate diet and exercise regimen to the overall health status of Mrs. Black. (*Application*)

- ■ How does a diet and exercise regimen specifically affect gallbladder problems? What elements in particular in the diet would contribute to pain? Why? (*Analysis*)
- ■ When Mrs. Black's acute pain has been resolved, what recommendations do you expect the dietitian, nurse, and physician to make in their follow-up appointments? (*Synthesis*)
- ■ How you would evaluate the success of client teaching for Mrs. Black? (*Evaluation*)

Canadian Research

Canadian Centre on Substance Abuse. (2005). *Canadian addictions survey.* Ottawa, ON: Author.

Daniel, M., & Cargo, M. D. (2004). Association between smoking, insulin resistance and beta-cell function in a Northwestern First Nation. *Diabetic Medicine, 21*(2), 188–193.

Hilsden, R. J., McGregor, E., Murray, A., Khoja, S., & Bryant, H. (2005). Colorectal cancer screening: Practices and attitudes of gastroenterologists, internists and surgeons. *Canadian Journal of Surgery, 48*(6), 434–440.

Hunter, K. F., Moore, K. N., Cody, D. J., et al. (2005). *The Cochrane Library, 2.* ID#CD001843.

Moore, K. N., Day, R. A., & Albers, M. (2002). Pathogenesis of urinary tract infections: A review. *Journal of Clinical Nursing, 11*(5), 568–574.

Moore, K. N., & Jensen, L. (2000). Testing the Incontinence Impact Questionnaire (IIQ – 7) with men after radical prostatectomy. *Journal of Wound, Ostomy and Continence Nursing, 27*(6), 304–312.

Pan, S. Y., Johnson, K. C., Ugnat, A.-M., Wen, S. W., & Mao, Y. (2004). Association of obesity and cancer risk in Canada. *American Journal of Epidemiology, 159*(3), 259–268.

Panaccione, R., Fedorak, R. N., Aumais, G., Bernstein, C. N., Bitton, A., Croitoru, K., et al. (2004) Canadian Association of Gastroenterology clinical practice guidelines: The use of infliximab in Crohn's disease. *Canadian Journal of Gastroenterology, 18*(8), 503–508.

Trolli, P., A., Conwell, D. L., & Zuccaro, G. Jr. (2001). Pancreatic enzyme therapy and nutritional status of outclients with chronic pancreatitis. *Gastroenterology Nursing, 24*(2), 84–87.

Villeneuve, P. J., Johnson, K. C., Mao, Y., et al. (2004). Environmental tobacco smoke and the risk of pancreatic cancer: Findings from a Canadian population-based case-control study. *Canadian Journal of Public Health, 95*(1), 32–37.

Wu, J. X., Wu, J., Wong, T., et al. (2006). Enhanced surveillance of newly acquired hepatitis C virus infection in Canada, 1998 to 2004. *Scandinavian Journal of Infectious Diseases, 38*(6), 482–489.

Test Questions

1. When assessing risk of colon cancer, which of the following health history components are most important for the nurse to obtain?
   a. Family history, dietary habits
   b. Dietary habits, social patterns
   c. Past medical history, family history
   d. Social patterns, past medical history

2. When visualizing the structures of the abdominal cavity, which of the following would the nurse expect to be in the right upper quadrant (RUQ)?
   a. Right kidney, ascending colon, liver
   b. Right ovary, pancreas, sigmoid colon
   c. Right ovary, descending colon, spleen
   d. Right kidney, transverse colon, inguinal ligament

3. When inspecting the abdomen, which of the following client positions facilitates correct examination technique?
   a. Sitting with hands on hips
   b. Trendelenberg, with hands over head
   c. Semi-Fowler's with pillows under head and knees
   d. Supine with arms at sides or folded across chest

4. The nurse percusses the lowest interspace in the left anterior axillary line, asks the client to take a deep breath, and percusses again. The nurse is assessing for:
   a. kidney tenderness.
   b. splenic percussion sign.
   c. diaphragmatic displacement.
   d. tenderness of a nonpalpable liver.

5. When assessing the abdomen, the nurse auscultates before percussing because:
   a. auscultation will identify any painful regions.
   b. percussion may alter the character of bowel sounds.
   c. percussion may alter the frequency of bowel sounds.
   d. percussion and palpation may increase the frequency of bruits.

Bibliography

CITATIONS

Babor, T. F., Higgins-Biddle, J. C., Saunders, J. B., & Monteiro, M. G. (2001). *AUDIT: The alcohol use disorders identification test* (2nd ed.). Geneva, Switzerland: World Health Organization.

Beck, I. T. (2001). Disproportion of economic impact, research achievements and research support in digestive diseases in Canada. *Clin Invest Med, 24*(1), 12–36.

Bowman, P., & Gerber, S. (2006). Alcohol in the older population, part 2: MAST you speak the truth in an AUDIT or are you too CAGE-y? *The Case Manager, 17*(6), 48–53, 59.

Canadian Cancer Society. (2008). *Causes of bladder cancer.* Retrieved April 19, 2008, from http://www.cancer.ca/ccs/internet/standard/0,3182,33172_10175_272631_langId-en,00.html

Canadian Cancer Society, National Cancer Institute of Canada, Statistic Canada, Provincial/Territorial Cancer Registries, & Public Health Agency of Canada. (2008). *Canadian cancer statistics 2008.* Retrieved March 15, 2009, from http://www.cancer.ca/Canada-wide/About%20cancer/Cancer%20statistics/

Canadian Continence Foundation. (2007). *Welcome.* Retrieved July 30, 2007, from http://www.continence-fdn.ca

Canadian Society of Intestinal Research. (2008a). *Irritable bowel syndrome.* Retrieved April 18, 2008, from http://www.badgut.com/index.php?contentFile=ibs&title=Irritable%20Bowel%20Syndrome

Canadian Society of Intestinal Research. (2008b). *Frequently asked questions about IBD.* Retrieved April 18, 2008, from http://www.badgut.com/index.php?contentFile=ibd_faq&title=Inflammatory%20Bowel%2

Chappuis, P. O., Ghadirian, P., & Foulkes, W. D. (2001). The role of genetic factors in the etiology of pancreatic adenocarcinoma: An update. *Cancer Investigation, 19*, 65–75.

Colorectal Cancer Association of Canada. (2008). *Just the facts: Prevention.* Retrieved April 18, 2008, from http://www.colorectal-cancer.ca/en/just-the-facts/prevention/

Degler, M. A. (2007). Assessment of renal and urinary tract function. In R. A. Day, P. Paul, B. Williams, S. C. Smeltzer, & B. Bare (Eds.), *Brunner and Suddarth's textbook of medical-surgical nursing: First Canadian edition* (pp. 1254–1275). Philadelphia: Lippincott Williams & Wilkins.

Dietitians of Canada. (2007). *Tips: Food and nutrient advice/recommendations.* Retrieved August 24, 2007, from http://www.dietitians.ca/public/content/eat_well_live_well/english/faqs_tips_facts/dc_tips/

Giovannucci, D., & Michaud, D. (2007). The role of obesity and related metabolic disturbances in cancers of the colon, prostate, and pancreas. *Gastroenterology, 132*(6), 2208–2225.

Hassan, M. M., Abbruzzese, J. L., Bondy, M. L., et al. (2007). Passive smoking and the use of noncigarette tobacco products in association with risk for pancreatic cancer: A case-control study. *Cancer, 109*(12), 2547–2556.

Health Canada. (2007). *Diseases and health conditions.* Retrieved August 10, 2007, from http://www.hc-sc.gc.ca/fnih-spni/diseases-maladies/index_e.html

Inuit Tapiriit Kanatama. (2008). *Inuit statistical profile.* Retrieved March 15, 2009, from http://www.itk.ca/

Kidney Research Centre. (2007). *Grand opening of the Kidney Research Centre.* Retrieved April 18, 2008, from http://www.ohri.ca/newsroom/newsstory.asp?ID=83

Luo, W., Morrison, H., de Groh, M., et al. (2007). The burden of adult obesity in Canada. *Chronic Diseases in Canada, 27*(4), 135–144.

Marrett, L. D., & Chaudhry, M. (2003). Cancer incidence and mortality in Ontario First Nations, 1968–1991 (Canada). *Cancer Causes and Control, 14*, 259–268.

Mayo Clinic. (2008). *Bladder cancer.* Retrieved April 19, 2008, from http://www.mayoclinic.com/health/bladder-cancer/DS00177/DSECTION=4

Nabalamba, A., Bernstein, C. N., & Seko, C. (2004). Inflammatory bowel disease-Hospitalization. *Health Reports, 15*(4).

National Alcohol Strategy Working Group. (2007). *Reducing alcohol related harm in Canada: Toward a culture of moderation.* Ottawa, ON: Canadian Centre on Substance Abuse.

Nkondjock, A., Krewski, D., Johnson, K. C., & Ghadirian, P. (2005). Dietary patterns and risk of pancreatic cancer. *International Journal of Cancer, 114*(5), 817–823.

Northern Alberta & The Territories Branch, The Kidney Foundation of Canada. (2008). *Kidney health: Prevention of kidney disease.* Retrieved April 19, 2008, from http://www.kidney.ab.ca/health/index.html

Nothlings, U., Wilkens, L. R., Murphy, S. P., Hankin, J. H., Henderson, B. E., & Kolonel, L. N. (2007). Body mass index and physical activity as risk factors for pancreatic cancer: The Multiethnic Cohort Study. *Cancer Causes & Control, 18*(2), 165–175.

Public Health Agency of Canada. (2007a). *Vaccine-preventable diseases: Hepatitis A.* Retrieved April 19, 2008, from http://www.phac-aspc.gc.ca/im/vpd-mev/hepatitis-a-eng.php

Public Health Agency of Canada. (2007b). *Compensation.* Retrieved August 26, 2007, from http//www.phac-aspc.gc.ca/hepc/comp-index_e.html

Public Health Agency of Canada. (2003). *Vaccine preventable diseases.* Retrieved March 15, 2009, from http://www.phac-aspc.gc.ca/im/vpd-mev/index-eng.php

Seller, R. H. (2007). *Differential diagnosis of common complaints* (5th ed.). Philadelphia: Saunders/Elsevier.

Tjepkema, M. (2004). Alcohol and illicit drug dependence. *Supplement to Health Reports, 15*, 9–63. Statistics Canada Catalogue 82-003.

Wu, J. X., Wu, J., Wong, T., et al. (2006). Enhanced surveillance of newly acquired hepatitis C virus infection in Canada, 1998 to 2004. *Scandinavian Journal of Infectious Diseases, 38*(6), 482–489.

ADDITIONAL RESOURCES

Bradley, K., Bush, K., Mcdonell, M., Malone, T., & Fihn, S. (1998). Screening for problem drinking: Comparison of CAGE and AUDIT. *Journal of General Internal Medicine, 13*(6), 379–388.

Public Health Agency of Canada. (2006). *Canadian immunization guide* (7th ed.). Retrieved August 26, 2007, from http://www.phac-aspc.gc.ca/publicat/cig-gci/index.html

Roy, E., Haley, N., Leclerc, P., Boivin, J., Cédras, L., & Vincelette, J. (2001). Risk factors for hepatitis C virus infection among street youths. *Canadian Medical Association Journal, 165*(5), 557–560.

Swanson, G., Skelly, J., Hutchison, B., & Kaczorowski, J. (2002). Urinary incontinence in Canada. *Canadian Family Physician, 48,* 86–92.

CANADIAN ASSOCIATIONS AND WEB SITES

Canadian Association for Enterostomal Therapy: http://www.caet.ca

Canadian Coalition for Immunization Awareness & Promotion: http://www.immunize.cpha.ca

Canadian Centre on Substance Abuse: http://www.ccsa.ca/ccsa

Canadian Continence Foundation: http://www.continence-fdn.ca

Canadian Digestive Health Foundation: http://www.CDHF.ca

Canadian Gastroenterological Association: http://www.cag-acg.org/

Canadian Interstitial Cystitis Association: http://www.orw.ca

Canadian Interstitial Cystitis Support Groups: http://www.canadaic.com/supportgroups.html

Canadian Liver Foundation: http://www.liver.ca

Canadian Society of Intestinal Research: http://www.badgut.com

Canadian Society of Nephrology: http://csnscn.ca

Canadian Urology Association: http://www.cua.org

Crohn's and Colitis Foundation of Canada: http://www.ccfc.ca

Colorectal Cancer Association of Canada: http://www.ccac-accc.ca

Colorectal Cancer Screening Initiative Foundation: http://www.screencolons.ca

NutritionLink Services Society: http://www.dialadietitian.org

Dietitians of Canada: http://www.dietitians.ca

Hepatitis Information Network: http://www.hepnet.com

Kidney Foundation of Canada: http://www.kidney.ca

National Cancer Institute of Canada: http://www.ncic.cancer.ca

United Ostomy Association of Canada: http://www.ostomycanada.ca

Urology Nurses of Canada: http://www.unc.org

TABLE 17-1   Abdominal Pain

Problem	Process	Location	Quality
Peptic Ulcer and Dyspepsia *(These disorders cannot be reliably differentiated by symptoms and signs.)*	Peptic ulcer refers to a demonstrable ulcer, usually in the duodenum or stomach. Dyspepsia causes similar symptoms but no ulceration. Infection by *Helicobacter pylori* is often present.	Epigastric, may radiate to the back	Variable: gnawing, burning, boring, aching, pressing, or hungerlike
Cancer of the Stomach	A malignant neoplasm	Epigastric	Variable
Acute Pancreatitis	An acute inflammation of the pancreas	Epigastric, may radiate to the back or other parts of the abdomen; may be poorly localized	Usually steady
Chronic Pancreatitis	Fibrosis of the pancreas secondary to recurrent inflammation	Epigastric, radiating through to the back	Steady, deep
Cancer of the Pancreas	A malignant neoplasm	Epigastric and in either upper quadrant; often radiates to the back	Steady, deep
Biliary Colic	Sudden obstruction of the cystic duct or common bile duct by a gallstone	Epigastric or right upper quadrant; may radiate to the right scapula and shoulder	Steady, aching; *not* colicky
Acute Cholecystitis	Inflammation of the gallbladder, usually from obstruction of the cystic duct by a gallstone	Right upper quadrant or upper abdominal; may radiate to the right scapular area	Steady, aching
Acute Diverticulitis	Acute inflammation of a colonic diverticulum, a saclike mucosal outpouching through the colonic muscle	Left lower quadrant	May be cramping at first, but becomes steady
Acute Appendicitis	Acute inflammation of the appendix with distention or obstruction	<ul><li>Poorly localized periumbilical pain, followed usually by</li></ul><ul><li>*Right lower quadrant* pain</li></ul>	<ul><li>Mild but increasing, possibly cramping</li><li>Steady and more severe</li></ul>
Acute Mechanical Intestinal Obstruction	Obstruction of the bowel lumen, most commonly caused by (1) adhesions or hernias (small bowel), or (2) cancer or diverticulitis (colon)	<ul><li>*Small bowel:* periumbilical or upper abdominal</li><li>*Colon:* lower abdominal or generalized</li></ul>	<ul><li>Cramping</li><li>Cramping</li></ul>
Mesenteric Ischemia	Blood supply to the bowel and mesentery blocked from thrombosis or embolus (acute arterial occlusion), or reduced from hypoperfusion	May be periumbilical at first, then diffuse	Cramping at first, then steady

Timing	Factors That May Aggravate	Factors That May Relieve	Associated Symptoms and Setting
Intermittent. Duodenal ulcer is more likely than gastric ulcer or dyspepsia to cause pain that (1) wakes the client at night, and (2) occurs intermittently over a few weeks, then disappears for months, and then recurs.	Variable	Food and antacids may bring relief, but not necessarily in any of these disorders and least commonly in gastric ulcer.	Nausea, vomiting, belching, bloating; heartburn (more common in duodenal ulcer), weight loss (more common in gastric ulcer). Dyspepsia is more common in the young (20–29 yrs), gastric ulcer in those over 50 yrs, and duodenal ulcer in those from 30 to 60 yrs.
The history of pain is typically shorter than in peptic ulcer. The pain is persistent and slowly progressive.	Often food	*Not* relieved by food or antacids	Anorexia, nausea, early satiety, weight loss, and sometimes bleeding. Most common in ages 50–70.
Acute onset, persistent pain	Lying supine	Leaning forward with trunk flexed	Nausea, vomiting, abdominal distention, fever. Often a history of previous attacks and alcohol abuse or gallstones.
Chronic or recurrent course	Alcohol, heavy or fatty meals	Possibly leaning forward with trunk flexed; often intractable	Symptoms of decreased pancreatic function may appear: diarrhea with fatty stools (steatorrhea) and diabetes mellitus.
Persistent pain; relentlessly progressive illness		Possibly leaning forward with trunk flexed; often intractable	Anorexia, nausea, vomiting, weight loss, and jaundice. Emotional symptoms, including depression.
Rapid onset over a few minutes, lasts one to several hours and subsides gradually. Often recurrent.			Anorexia, nausea, vomiting, restlessness.
Gradual onset; course longer than in biliary colic	Jarring, deep breathing		Anorexia, nausea, vomiting, fever.
Often a gradual onset			Fever, constipation. There may be initial brief diarrhea.
■ Lasts roughly 4–6 hr ■ Depends on intervention	■ Movement or cough	■ If it subsides temporarily, suspect perforation of the appendix.	Anorexia, nausea, possibly vomiting, which typically follow the onset of pain; low fever.
■ Paroxysmal; may decrease as bowel mobility is impaired ■ Paroxysmal, though typically milder			■ Vomiting of bile and mucus (high obstruction) or fecal material (low obstruction). Obstipation develops. ■ Obstipation early. Vomiting late if at all. Prior symptoms of underlying cause.
Usually abrupt in onset, then persistent			Vomiting, diarrhea (sometimes bloody), constipation, shock

TABLE 17-2   **Dysphagia**

Process and Problem	Timing	Factors That Aggravate	Factors That Relieve	Associated Symptoms and Conditions
Transfer Dysphagia, *due to motor disorders affecting the pharyngeal muscles*	Acute or gradual onset and a variable course, depending on the underlying disorder	Attempts to start the swallowing process		Aspiration into the lungs or regurgitation into the nose with attempts to swallow. Neurologic evidence of stroke, bulbar palsy, or other neuromuscular conditions
Esophageal Dysphagia				
Mechanical Narrowing				
■ Mucosal rings and webs	Intermittent	Solid foods	Regurgitation of the bolus of food	Usually none
■ Esophageal stricture	Intermittent, may become slowly progressive	Solid foods	Regurgitation of the bolus of food	A long history of heartburn and regurgitation
■ Esophageal cancer	May be intermittent at first; progressive over months	Solid foods, with progression to liquids	Regurgitation of the bolus of food	Pain in the chest and back and weight loss, especially late in the course of illness
Motor Disorders				
■ Diffuse esophageal spasm	Intermittent	Solids or liquids	Manoeuvres described below; sometimes nitroglycerin	Chest pain that mimics angina pectoris or myocardial infarction and lasts minutes to hours; possibly heartburn
■ Scleroderma	Intermittent, may progress slowly	Solids or liquids	Repeated swallowing, movements such as straightening the back, raising the arms, or a Valsalva manoeuvre (straining down against a closed glottis)	Heartburn; other manifestations of scleroderma
■ Achalasia	Intermittent, may progress	Solids or liquids		Regurgitation, often at night when lying down, with nocturnal cough; possibly chest pain

TABLE 17-3   Constipation

Problem	Process	Associated Symptoms and Setting
Life Activities and Habits		
Inadequate Time or Setting for the Defecation Reflex	Ignoring the sensation of a full rectum inhibits the defecation reflex.	Hectic schedules, unfamiliar surroundings, bed rest
False Expectations of Bowel Habits	Expectations of "regularity" or more frequent stools than a person's norm	Beliefs, treatments, and advertisements that promote the use of laxatives
Diet Deficient in Fibre	Decreased fecal bulk	Other factors such as debilitation and constipating drugs may contribute.
Irritable Bowel Syndrome	A common disorder of bowel motility	Small, hard stools, often with mucus. Periods of diarrhea. Cramping abdominal pain. Stress may aggravate.
Mechanical Obstruction		
Cancer of the Rectum or Sigmoid Colon	Progressive narrowing of the bowel lumen	Change in bowel habits; often diarrhea, abdominal pain, and bleeding. In rectal cancer, tenesmus and pencil-shaped stools.
Fecal Impaction	A large, firm, immovable fecal mass, most often in the rectum	Rectal fullness, abdominal pain, and diarrhea around the impaction. Common in debilitated, bedridden, and often elderly clients.
Other Obstructing Lesions (such as diverticulitis, volvulus, intussusception, or hernia)	Narrowing or complete obstruction of the bowel	Colicky abdominal pain, abdominal distention, and in intussusception, often "currant jelly" stools (red blood and mucus)
Painful Anal Lesions	Pain may cause spasm of the external sphincter and voluntary inhibition of the defecation reflex.	Anal fissures, painful hemorrhoids, perirectal abscesses
Drugs	A variety of mechanisms	Opiates (especially codeine), anticholinergics, antacids containing calcium or aluminum, and many others
Depression	A disorder of mood	Fatigue, feelings of depression, and other somatic symptoms
Neurologic Disorders	Interference with the autonomic innervation of the bowel	Spinal cord injuries, multiple sclerosis, Hirschsprung's disease, and other conditions
Metabolic Conditions	Interference with bowel motility	Pregnancy, hypothyroidism, hypercalcemia

TABLE 17-4 **Diarrhea**

Problem	Process	Characteristics of Stool
Acute Diarrhea *Secretory Infections*	Infection by viruses, preformed bacterial toxins (such as *Staphylococcus aureus, Clostridium perfringens*, toxigenic *Escherichia coli, Vibrio cholerae*), cryptosporidium, *Giardia lamblia*, Clostridium difficile	Watery, without blood, pus, or mucus
Inflammatory Infections	Colonization or invasion of intestinal mucosa (nontyphoid *Salmonella, Shigella, Yersinia, Campylobacter*, enteropathic *E. coli, Entamoeba histolytica*)	Loose to watery, often with blood, pus, or mucus
Drug-Induced Diarrhea	Action of many drugs, such as magnesium-containing antacids, antibiotics, antineoplastic agents, and laxatives	Loose to watery
Chronic Diarrhea *Diarrheal Syndromes* ■ Irritable bowel syndrome	A disorder of bowel motility with alternating diarrhea and constipation	Loose; may show mucus but no blood. Small, hard stools with constipation.
■ Cancer of the sigmoid colon	Partial obstruction by a malignant neoplasm	May be blood-streaked
Inflammatory Bowel Disease ■ Ulcerative colitis	Inflammation of the mucosa and submucosa of the rectum and colon with ulceration; cause unknown	Soft to watery, often containing blood
■ Crohn's disease of the small bowel (regional enteritis) or colon (granulomatous colitis)	Chronic inflammation of the bowel wall, typically involving the terminal ileum and/or proximal colon	Small, soft to loose or watery, usually free of gross blood (enteritis) or with less bleeding than ulcerative colitis (colitis)
Voluminous Diarrheas ■ Malabsorption syndromes	Defective absorption of fat, including fat-soluble vitamins, with steatorrhea (excessive excretion of fat) as in pancreatic insufficiency, bile salt deficiency, bacterial overgrowth	Typically bulky, soft, light yellow to grey, mushy, greasy or oily, and sometimes frothy; particularly foul-smelling; usually floats in the toilet
■ Osmotic diarrheas Lactose intolerance	Deficiency in intestinal lactase	Watery diarrhea of large volume
Abuse of osmotic purgatives	Laxative habit, often surreptitious	Watery diarrhea of large volume
■ Secretory diarrheas from bacterial infection, secreting villous adenoma, fat or bile salt malabsorption, hormone-mediated conditions (gastrin in Zollinger–Ellison syndrome, vasoactive intestinal peptide [VIP])	Variable	Watery diarrhea of large volume

Timing	Associated Symptoms	Setting, Persons at Risk
Duration of a few days, possibly longer. Lactase deficiency may lead to a longer course.	Nausea, vomiting, periumbilical cramping pain. Temperature normal or slightly elevated.	Often travel, a common food source, or an epidemic
An acute illness of varying duration	Lower abdominal cramping pain and often rectal urgency, tenesmus, fever	Travel, contaminated food or water. Men and women who have had frequent anal intercourse.
Acute, recurrent, or chronic	Possibly nausea; usually little if any pain	Prescribed or over-the-counter medications
Often worse in the morning. Diarrhea rarely wakes the client at night.	Crampy lower abdominal pain, abdominal distention, flatulence, nausea, constipation	Young and middle-aged adults, especially women
Variable	Change in usual bowel habits, crampy lower abdominal pain, constipation	Middle-aged and older adults, especially older than 55 yrs
Onset ranges from insidious to acute. Typically recurrent, may be persistent. Diarrhea may wake the client at night.	Crampy lower or generalized abdominal pain, anorexia, weakness, fever	Often young people
Insidious onset, chronic or recurrent. Diarrhea may wake the client at night.	Crampy periumbilical or right lower quadrant (enteritis) or diffuse (colitis) pain, with anorexia, low fever, and/or weight loss. Perianal or perirectal abscesses and fistulas.	Often young people, especially in the late teens, but also those in the middle years. More common in people of Jewish descent.
Onset of illness typically insidious	Anorexia, weight loss, fatigue, abdominal distention, often crampy lower abdominal pain. Symptoms of nutritional deficiencies such as bleeding (vitamin K), bone pain and fractures (vitamin D), glossitis (vitamin B), and edema (protein).	Variable, depending on cause
Follows the ingestion of milk and milk products; is relieved by fasting	Crampy abdominal pain, abdominal distention, flatulence	Afro-Canadians, Asians, Aboriginals
Variable	Often none	Persons with anorexia nervosa or bulimia nervosa
Variable	Weight loss, dehydration, nausea, vomiting, and cramping abdominal pain	Variable depending on cause

TABLE 17-5 **Black and Bloody Stools**

Problem	Selected Causes	Associated Symptoms and Setting
Melena Melena refers to the passage of black, tarry (sticky and shiny) stools. Tests for occult blood are positive. Melena signifies the loss of at least 60 mL of blood into the gastrointestinal tract (less in infants and children), usually from the esophagus, stomach, or duodenum. Less commonly, when intestinal transit is slow, the blood may originate in the jejunum, ileum, or ascending colon. In infants, melena may result from swallowing blood during the birth process.	Peptic ulcer	Often, but not necessarily, a history of epigastric pain
	Gastritis or stress ulcers	Recent ingestion of alcohol, aspirin, or other anti-inflammatory drugs; recent bodily trauma, severe burns, surgery, or increased intracranial pressure
	Esophageal or gastric varices	Cirrhosis of the liver or other cause of portal hypertension
	Reflux esophagitis	History of heartburn
	Mallory-Weiss tear, a mucosal tear in the esophagus from retching and vomiting	Retching, vomiting, often recent ingestion of alcohol
Black, Nonsticky Stools Black stools may result from other causes and then usually give negative results when tested for occult blood. (Ingestion of iron or other substances, however, may cause a positive test result in the absence of blood.) These stools have no pathologic significance.	Ingestion of iron, bismuth salts as in Pepto-Bismol, licorice, or even commercial chocolate cookies	
Red Blood in the Stools Red blood usually originates in the colon, rectum, or anus, and much less frequently in the jejunum or ileum. Upper gastrointestinal hemorrhage, however, may also cause red stools. The amount of blood lost is then usually large (more than a litre). Transit time through the intestinal tract is accordingly rapid, giving insufficient time for the blood to turn black.	Cancer of the colon	Often a change in bowel habits
	Benign polyps of the colon	Often no other symptoms
	Diverticula of the colon	Often no other symptoms
	Inflammatory conditions of the colon and rectum	
	▪ Ulcerative colitis, Crohn's disease	See Table 17-4, Diarrhea.
	▪ Infectious dysenteries	See Table 17-4, Diarrhea.
	▪ Proctitis (various causes) in men or women who have had frequent anal intercourse	Rectal urgency, tenesmus
	Ischemic colitis	Lower abdominal pain and sometimes fever or shock in persons older than 50 yrs
	Hemorrhoids	Blood on the toilet paper, on the surface of the stool, or dripping into the toilet
	Anal fissure	Blood on the toilet paper or on the surface of the stool; anal pain
Reddish but Nonbloody Stools	Ingestion of beets	Pink urine, which usually precedes the reddish stool

TABLE 17-6   Frequency, Nocturia, and Polyuria

Problem	Mechanisms	Selected Causes	Associated Symptoms
Frequency	Decreased capacity of the bladder		
	■ Increased bladder sensitivity to stretch because of inflammation	*Infection*, stones, tumour, or foreign body in the bladder	Burning on urination, urinary urgency, sometimes gross hematuria
	■ Decreased elasticity of the bladder wall	Infiltration by scar tissue or tumour	Symptoms of associated inflammation (see above) are common.
	■ Decreased cortical inhibition of bladder contractions	Motor disorders of the central nervous system, such as a stroke	Urinary urgency; neurologic symptoms such as weakness and paralysis
	Impaired emptying of the bladder, with residual urine in the bladder		
	■ Partial mechanical obstruction of the bladder neck or proximal urethra	Most commonly, benign prostatic hyperplasia; also urethral stricture and other obstructive lesions of the bladder or prostate	Prior obstructive symptoms: hesitancy in starting the urinary stream, straining to void, reduced size and force of the stream, and dribbling during or at the end of urination
	■ Loss of peripheral nerve supply to the bladder	Neurologic disease affecting the sacral nerves or nerve roots, e.g., diabetic neuropathy	Weakness or sensory defects
Nocturia			
With High Volumes	Most types of polyuria (see p. 519)		
	Decreased concentrating ability of the kidney with loss of the typical decrease in nocturnal urinary output	Chronic renal insufficiency from various diseases	Possibly other symptoms of renal insufficiency
	Excessive fluid intake before bedtime	Habit, especially involving alcohol and coffee	
	Fluid-retaining, edematous states Dependent edema accumulates during the day and is excreted when the client lies down at night.	Congestive heart failure, nephrotic syndrome, hepatic cirrhosis with ascites, chronic venous insufficiency	Edema and other symptoms of the underlying disorder. Urinary output during the day may be reduced as fluid reaccumulates in the body. See Table 18-1, Some Peripheral Causes of Edema.
With Low Volumes	Frequency Voiding while up at night without a real urge, a "pseudo-frequency"	Insomnia	Variable
Polyuria	Deficiency of antidiuretic hormone (diabetes insipidus)	A disorder of the posterior pituitary and hypothalamus	Thirst and polydipsia, often severe and persistent; nocturia
	Renal unresponsiveness to antidiuretic hormone (nephrogenic diabetes insipidus)	A number of kidney diseases, including hypercalcemic and hypokalemic nephropathy; drug toxicity, e.g., from lithium	Thirst and polydipsia, often severe and persistent; nocturia
	Solute diuresis		
	■ Electrolytes, such as sodium salts	Large saline infusions, potent diuretics, certain kidney diseases	Variable
	■ Nonelectrolytes, such as glucose	Uncontrolled diabetes mellitus	Thirst, polydipsia, and nocturia
	Excessive water intake	Primary polydipsia	Polydipsia tends to be episodic. Thirst may not be present. Nocturia is usually absent.

TABLE 17-7   Urinary Incontinence*

Problem	Mechanisms
Stress Incontinence The urethral sphincter is weakened so that transient increases in intra-abdominal pressure raise the bladder pressure to levels that exceed urethral resistance.	In women, most often a weakness of the pelvic floor with inadequate muscular support of the bladder and proximal urethra and a change in the angle between the bladder and the urethra. Suggested causes include childbirth and surgery. Local conditions affecting the internal urethral sphincter, such as postmenopausal atrophy of the mucosa and urethral infection, may also contribute. In men, stress incontinence may follow prostatic surgery.
Urge Incontinence Detrusor contractions are stronger than usual and overcome urethral resistance. The bladder is typically *small*.	■ Decreased cortical inhibition of detrusor contractions, as by strokes, brain tumours, dementia, and lesions of the spinal cord above the sacral level ■ Hyperexcitability of sensory pathways, as in bladder infections, tumours, and fecal impaction ■ Deconditioning of voiding reflexes, as in frequent voluntary voiding at low bladder volumes
Overflow Incontinence Detrusor contractions are insufficient to overcome urethral resistance. The bladder is typically *large*, even after an effort to void.	■ Obstruction of the bladder outlet, as by benign prostatic hyperplasia or tumour ■ Weakness of the detrusor muscle associated with peripheral nerve disease at the sacral level ■ Impaired bladder sensation that interrupts the reflex arc, as from diabetic neuropathy
Functional Incontinence This is a functional inability to get to the toilet in time because of impaired health or environmental conditions.	Problems in mobility resulting from weakness, arthritis, poor vision, or other conditions. Environmental factors such as an unfamiliar setting, distant bathroom facilities, bed rails, or physical restraints.
Incontinence Secondary to Medications Drugs may contribute to any type of incontinence listed.	Sedatives, tranquilizers, anticholinergics, sympathetic blockers, and potent diuretics

*Clients may have more than one kind of incontinence.

Symptoms	Physical Signs
Momentary leakage of small amounts of urine concurrent with stresses such as coughing, laughing, and sneezing while the person is in an upright position. A desire to urinate is not associated with pure stress incontinence.	The bladder is not detected on abdominal examination. Stress incontinence may be demonstrable, especially if the client is examined before voiding and in a standing position. Atrophic vaginitis may be evident.
Incontinence preceded by an urge to void. The volume tends to be moderate. Urgency Frequency and nocturia with small to moderate volumes If acute inflammation is present, pain on urination Possibly "pseudo-stress incontinence"—voiding 10–20 sec after stresses such as a change of position, going up or down stairs, and possibly coughing, laughing, or sneezing	The bladder is not detectable on abdominal examination. When cortical inhibition is decreased, mental deficits or motor signs of central nervous system disease are often, though not necessarily, present. When sensory pathways are hyperexcitable, signs of local pelvic problems or a fecal impaction may be present.
A continuous dripping or dribbling incontinence Decreased force of the urinary stream Prior symptoms of partial urinary obstruction or other symptoms of peripheral nerve disease may be present.	An enlarged bladder is often found on abdominal examination and may be tender. Other possible signs include prostatic enlargement, motor signs of peripheral nerve disease, a decrease in sensation including perineal sensation, and diminished to absent reflexes.
Incontinence on the way to the toilet or only in the early morning	The bladder is not detectable on physical examination. Look for physical or environmental clues to the likely cause.
Variable. A careful history and chart review are important.	Variable

TABLE 17-8   Localized Bulges in the Abdominal Wall

Localized bulges in the abdominal wall include *ventral hernias* (defects in the wall through which tissue protrudes) and subcutaneous tumours such as *lipomas*. The more common ventral hernias are umbilical, incisional, and epigastric. Hernias and a rectus diastasis usually become more evident when the client raises head and shoulders from a supine position.

Umbilical Hernia

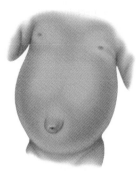

INFANT

A protrusion through a defective umbilical ring is most common in infants but also occurs in adults. In infants, but not in adults, it usually closes spontaneously within 1–2 yrs.

Diastasis Recti

Separation of the two rectus abdominis muscles, through which abdominal contents form a midline ridge when the client raises head and shoulders. Often is seen in repeated pregnancies, obesity, and chronic lung disease. It has no clinical consequences.

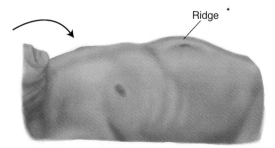

Ridge

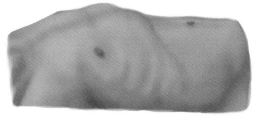

Incisional Hernia

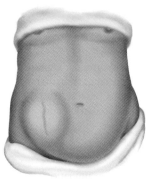

This is a protrusion through an operative scar. Palpate to detect the length and width of the defect in the abdominal wall. A small defect, through which a large hernia has passed, has a greater risk for complications than a large defect.

Epigastric Hernia

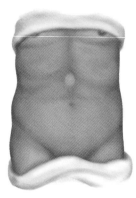

A small midline protrusion through a defect in the linea alba occurs between the xiphoid process and the umbilicus. With the client's head and shoulders raised (or with the client standing), run your fingerpad down the linea alba to feel it.

Lipoma

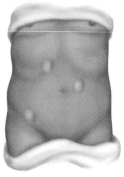

Common, benign, fatty tumours usually occur in the subcutaneous tissues almost anywhere in the body, including the abdominal wall. Small or large, they are usually soft and often lobulated. Press your finger down on the edge of a lipoma. The tumour typically slips out from under it.

TABLE 17-9   **Protuberant Abdomens**

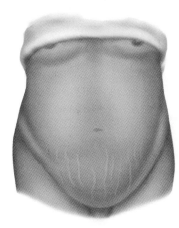

Fat

Fat is the most common cause of a protuberant abdomen. Fat thickens the abdominal wall, the mesentery, and omentum. The umbilicus may appear sunken. A *pannus*, or apron of fatty tissue, may extend below the inguinal ligaments. Lift it to look for inflammation in the skin folds or even for a hidden hernia.

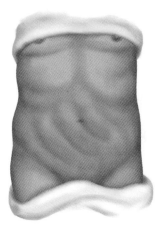

Gas

Gaseous distention may be localized or generalized. It causes a tympanitic percussion note. Increased intestinal gas production from certain foods may cause mild distention. More serious are intestinal obstruction and adynamic (paralytic) ileus. Note the location of the distention. Distention becomes more marked in colonic than in small bowel obstruction.

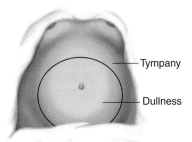

Tumour

A large, solid tumour, usually rising out of the pelvis, is dull to percussion. Air-filled bowel is displaced to the periphery. Causes include ovarian tumours and uterine myomata. Occasionally a markedly distended bladder may be mistaken for such a tumour.

Pregnancy

Pregnancy is a common cause of a pelvic "mass." Listen for the fetal heart (see p. 878).

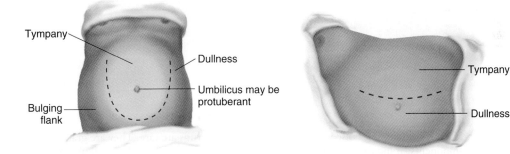

Ascitic Fluid

Ascitic fluid seeks the lowest point in the abdomen, producing bulging flanks that are dull to percussion. The umbilicus may protrude. Turn the client onto one side to detect the shift in position of the fluid level (shifting dullness). (See pp. 537–538 for the assessment of ascites.)

TABLE 17-10   **Sounds in the Abdomen**

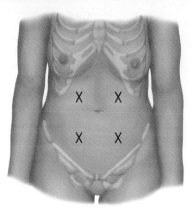

Bowel Sounds

Bowel sounds may be:

- *Increased*, as from diarrhea or *early intestinal obstruction*
- *Decreased*, then absent, as in *adynamic ileus and peritonitis.* Before deciding that bowel sounds are absent, sit down and listen where shown for 2 min or even longer.

High-pitched tinkling sounds suggest intestinal fluid and air under tension in a dilated bowel. *Rushes of high-pitched sounds* coinciding with an abdominal cramp indicate intestinal obstruction.

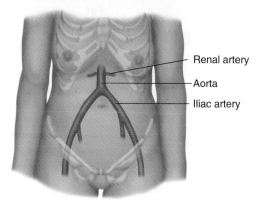

Bruits

A *hepatic bruit* suggests carcinoma of the liver or alcoholic hepatitis. *Arterial bruits* with both systolic and diastolic components suggest partial occlusion of the aorta or large arteries. Partial occlusion of a renal artery may explain hypertension.

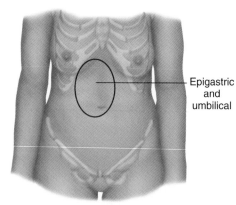

Venous Hum

A venous hum is rare. It is a soft humming noise with both systolic and diastolic components. It indicates increased collateral circulation between portal and systemic venous systems, as in hepatic cirrhosis.

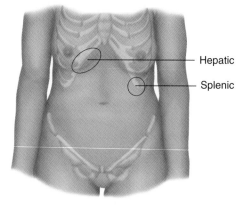

Friction Rubs

Friction rubs are rare. They are grating sounds with respiratory variation. They indicate inflammation of the peritoneal surface of an organ, as from a liver tumour, chlamydial or gonococcal perihepatitis, recent liver biopsy, or splenic infarct. When a systolic bruit accompanies a hepatic friction rub, suspect carcinoma of the liver.

TABLE 17-11   Tender Abdomens

Abdominal Wall Tenderness

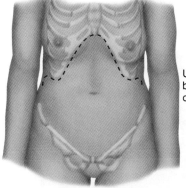

Superficial tender area

Deep tender area

Tenderness may originate in the abdominal wall. When the client raises head and shoulders, this tenderness persists, whereas tenderness from a deeper lesion (protected by the tightened muscles) decreases.

Visceral Tenderness

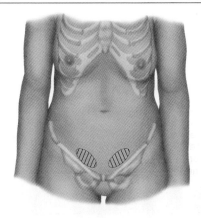

Enlarged liver

Aorta

Cecum

Usual or spastic sigmoid colon

The structures shown may be tender to deep palpation. Usually the discomfort is dull with no muscular rigidity or rebound tenderness. A reassuring explanation to the client may prove quite helpful.

Tenderness From Disease in the Chest and Pelvis

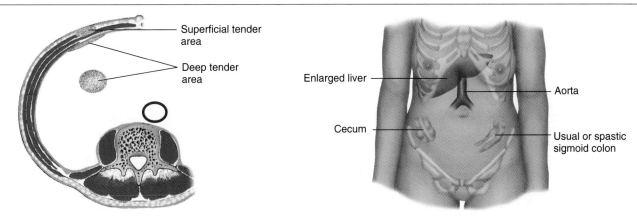

Unilateral or bilateral, upper or lower abdomen

Acute Pleurisy

Abdominal pain and tenderness may result from acute pleural inflammation. When unilateral, it may mimic acute cholecystitis or appendicitis. Rebound tenderness and rigidity are less common; chest signs are usually present.

Acute Salpingitis

Frequently bilateral, the tenderness of acute salpingitis (inflammation of the fallopian tubes) is usually maximal just above the inguinal ligaments. Rebound tenderness and rigidity may be present. On pelvic examination, motion of the uterus causes pain.

(table continues on next page)

TABLE 17-11   **Tender Abdomens** *(Continued)*

Tenderness of Peritoneal Inflammation

Tenderness associated with peritoneal inflammation is more severe than visceral tenderness. Muscular rigidity and rebound tenderness are frequently, but not necessarily, present. Generalized peritonitis causes exquisite tenderness throughout the abdomen, together with boardlike muscular rigidity. Local causes of peritoneal inflammation include:

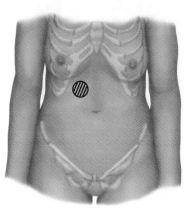

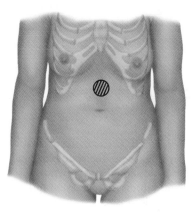

Acute Cholecystitis

Signs are maximal in the right upper quadrant. Check for Murphy's sign (see p. 539).

Acute Pancreatitis

In acute pancreatitis, epigastric tenderness and rebound tenderness are usually present, but the abdominal wall may be soft.

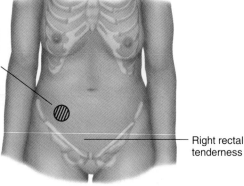

At the two-thirds point on a line joining the umbilicus and the anterior superior iliac spine

Right rectal tenderness

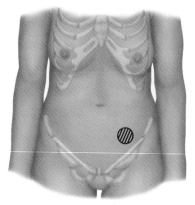

Acute Appendicitis

Right lower quadrant signs are typical of acute appendicitis, but may be absent early in the course. The typical area of tenderness is illustrated. Explore other portions of the right lower quadrant as well as the right flank.

Acute Diverticulitis

Acute diverticulitis most often involves the sigmoid colon and then resembles a left-sided appendicitis.

TABLE 17-12   **Liver Enlargement: Apparent and Real**

A palpable liver does not necessarily indicate hepatomegaly (an enlarged liver), but more often results from a change in consistency—from the expected softness to an unexpected firmness or hardness, as in cirrhosis. Clinical estimates of liver size should be based on both percussion and palpation, although even these techniques are far from perfect.

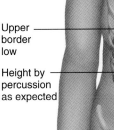

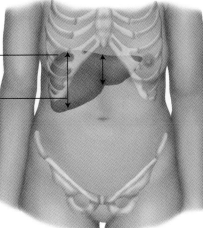

Upper border low

Height by percussion as expected

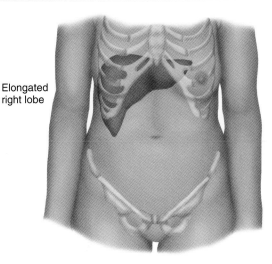

Elongated right lobe

Downward Displacement of the Liver by a Low Diaphragm

This finding is common when the diaphragm is low (e.g., in emphysema). The liver edge may be readily palpable well below the costal margin. Percussion, however, reveals a low upper edge also, and the vertical span of the liver is within expected measurements.

Expected Variations in Liver Shape

In some people, especially those with a lanky build, the liver tends to be somewhat elongated so that its right lobe is easily palpable as it projects downward toward the iliac crest. Such an elongation, sometimes called *Riedel's lobe*, represents a variation in shape, not an increase in liver volume or size. This variant illustrates the basic limitations of assessing liver size. Examiners can only estimate the upper and lower borders of an organ that has three dimensions and differing shapes. Some error is unavoidable.

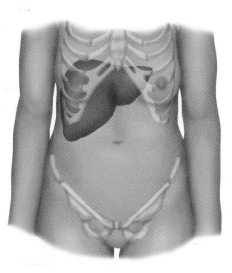

Smooth Large Liver

Cirrhosis may produce an enlarged liver with a firm *nontender* edge. The liver is not always enlarged in this condition, however, and many other diseases may produce similar findings. An enlarged liver with a smooth *tender* edge suggests inflammation, as in hepatitis, or venous congestion, as in right-sided heart failure.

Irregular Large Liver

An enlarged liver that is firm or hard and has an irregular edge or surface suggests malignancy. There may be one or more nodules. The liver may or may not be tender.

The Peripheral Vascular System

DANA EDGE, RENE A. DAY, AND LYNN S. BICKLEY

The focus of this chapter is circulation in the periphery, notably the arms and legs. Discussion includes the arteries, veins, interconnecting capillary bed, lymphatic system with its lymph nodes, and fascia compartments.

Peripheral and central circulations rely upon the integrity of arterial and venous vasculature. Gaseous and chemical exchange occurs at the capillary level, and the vital function of the cardiovascular system is compromised if diffusion cannot occur. Assessment of the peripheral vascular system provides essential clues to the internal functioning of vessels, as well as the oxygenation of surrounding tissues.

Nurses in many settings have opportunities to assess peripheral circulation. By promoting healthy practices, nurses can assist clients to reduce risks for or severity of peripheral vascular disease. In some emergencies, the nurse's assessment, decision making, and actions may save a limb and even a life.

Peripheral vascular health predicts other cardiovascular events, such as coronary heart disease (CHD) and stroke (Golomb, Dang, & Criqui, 2006; see Chapter 15). Arteries, carrying blood away from the heart, are distinguished from veins by relatively thicker, muscular walls with more smooth muscle and elastic fibres. This permits greater contractility compared to veins. The vein walls are typically thinner and cannot tolerate stretching or distortion as well as arteries; typically, veins contain valves, which prevent backward (regurgitated) flow in the low-pressure venous system.

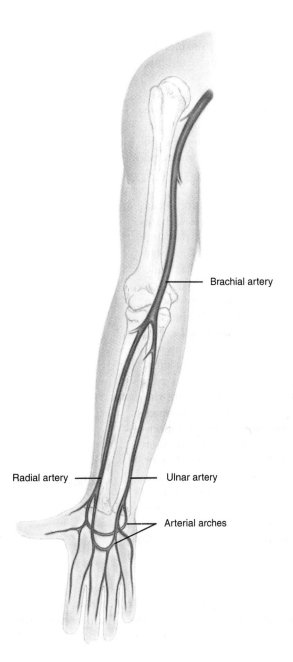

Brachial artery

Radial artery — — Ulnar artery

Arterial arches

ANATOMY AND PHYSIOLOGY

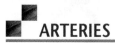

ARTERIES

Arterial pulses are palpable when an artery lies close to the body surface. In the arms, there are two or sometimes three such locations. Pulsations of the *brachial artery* can be felt in and above the bend of the elbow, just medial to the biceps tendon and muscle. The brachial artery divides into the radial and ulnar arteries. *Radial artery* pulsations can be felt on the flexor surface of the wrist laterally. Medially, pulsations of the *ulnar artery* may be palpable, but overlying tissues frequently obscure them.

The radial and ulnar arteries are interconnected by two vascular arches within the hand. Circulation to the hand and fingers is thereby doubly protected against possible arterial occlusion.

In the legs, arterial pulsations can usually be felt in four places. Those of the *femoral artery* are palpable below the inguinal ligament, midway between the anterior superior iliac spine and the symphysis pubis. The femoral artery travels downward deep within the thigh, passes medially behind the femur, and becomes the *popliteal artery*. Popliteal pulsations can be felt in the tissues behind the knee. Below the knee, the popliteal artery divides into two branches that both continue to the foot. There the anterior branch becomes the *dorsalis pedis artery*. Its pulsations are palpable on the dorsum of the foot just lateral to the extensor tendon of the big toe. The posterior branch, the *posterior tibial artery*, can be felt as it passes behind the medial malleolus of the ankle. Like the hand, the foot is protected by an interconnecting arch between its two chief arterial branches.

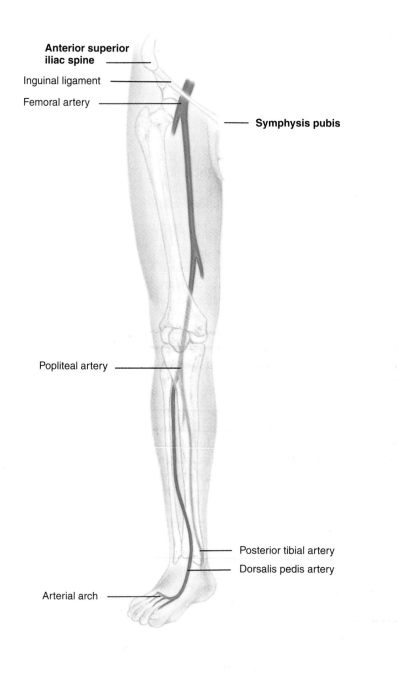

The *peroneal artery*, while not commonly assessed, can be used when measuring the ankle–brachial index (ABI) if the systolic pressure of the dorsalis pedis and posterior tibial arteries cannot be measured. The peroneal arteries are also sites for plaque formation and blockage in peripheral arterial disease (PAD).

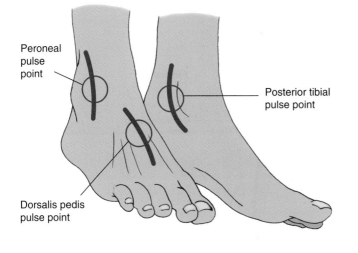

Peroneal
pulse
point

Posterior tibial
pulse point

Dorsalis pedis
pulse point

VEINS

The veins from the arms, together with those from the upper trunk and the head and neck, drain into the superior vena cava and on into the right atrium. Veins from the legs and the lower trunk drain upward into the inferior vena cava. Because the leg veins are especially susceptible to dysfunction, they warrant special attention.

The *deep veins* of the legs carry approximately 90% of the venous return from the lower extremities. They are well supported by surrounding tissues.

In contrast, the *superficial veins* are located subcutaneously and are supported relatively poorly. The superficial veins include (1) the *great saphenous vein*, which originates on the dorsum of the foot, passes just in front of the medial malleolus, and then continues up the medial aspect of the leg to join the femoral vein of the deep venous system, below the inguinal ligament; and (2) the *small saphenous vein*, which begins at the side of the foot and passes upward along the back of the leg to join the deep system in the popliteal space. Anestomotic veins connect the two saphenous veins superficially and, when dilated, are readily visible. In addition, *communicating*, or *perforating*, *veins* connect the saphenous system with the deep venous system.

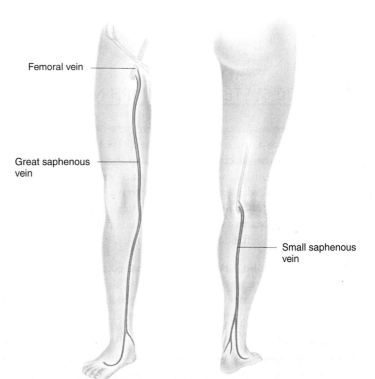

Femoral vein

Great saphenous
vein

Small saphenous
vein

Deep, superficial, and communicating veins all have one-way valves. These allow venous blood to flow from the superficial to the deep system and toward the heart, but not in the opposite directions. Muscular activity contributes importantly to venous blood flow. As calf muscles contract in walking, for example, blood is squeezed upward against gravity, and competent valves keep it from pooling and falling back.

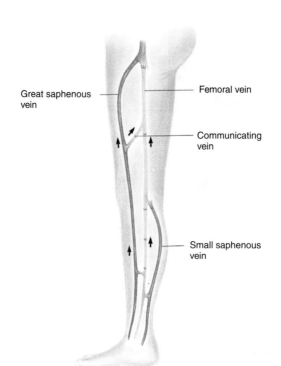

THE LYMPHATIC SYSTEM AND LYMPH NODES

The lymphatic system comprises an extensive vascular network that drains lymph fluid (resembles plasma but has a much lower concentration of proteins) from body tissues and returns it to the venous circulation. The system starts peripherally as blind lymphatic capillaries, continues centrally as thin vascular channels, and converges into collecting ducts, which finally empty into major veins at the base of the neck. The smaller *right lymphatic duct* drains the right side of the body superior to the diaphragm; the larger *thoracic duct* on the left drains the entire body inferior to the diaphragm, as well as the left side of the upper body.

Lymph nodes are small oval, round, or kidney bean–shaped organs surrounded by a connective tissue capsule. They vary in size according to body location. Some lymph nodes, such as the preauriculars, are typically very small, if palpable at all. The inguinal nodes, in contrast, are relatively large, often 1 cm in diameter and occasionally even 2 cm in adults.

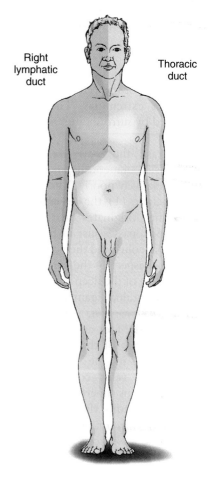

In addition to its vascular functions, the lymphatic system filters and purifies lymph in the lymph nodes before the fluid returns to the venous system. Cells within the lymph nodes engulf debris and pathogens as the fluid passes by. Antigens removed in this process are presented to lymphocytes, serving as an early warning system and the first step in the activation of an immune response (Martini, 2001). With overwhelming infection or the migration of tumour cells, the lymphatic capillaries provide little resistance; in such instances, the lymphatic channels serve as an important pathway for the spread of disease (Schoen, 2005).

Only the superficial lymph nodes are accessible to physical examination. These include the following nodes:

- In the head and neck: preauricular, posterior auricular, submandibular, submental, superficial cervical, deep cervical chain, and posterior cervical

- Above the clavicle: supraclavicular

- Below the clavicle: infraclavicular

- Axilla: central, pectoral, lateral, subscapular

- In the arms: epitochlear

- In the legs: superficial inguinal nodes, which are made up of the horizontal group and the vertical group

Recall that the axillary lymph nodes drain most of the arm. Lymphatics from the ulnar surface of the forearm and hand, the little and ring fingers, and the adjacent surface of the middle finger, however, drain first into the *epitrochlear nodes*. These are located on the medial surface of the arm approximately 3 cm above the elbow. Lymphatics from the rest of the arm drain mostly into the axillary nodes. A few drain directly into the infraclavicular nodes.

The lymphatics of the lower limb, following the venous supply, consist of both deep and superficial systems. Only the superficial nodes are palpable. The *superficial inguinal nodes* include two groups. The *horizontal group* lies in a chain high in the anterior thigh below the inguinal ligament. It drains the superficial portions of the lower abdomen and buttock, the external genitalia (but not the testes), the anal canal and perianal area, and the lower vagina.

The *vertical group* clusters near the upper part of the saphenous vein and drains a corresponding region of the leg. In contrast, lymphatics from the portion of leg drained by the small saphenous vein (the heel and outer aspect of the foot) join the deep system at the level of the popliteal space. Lesions in this area, therefore, are not usually associated with palpable inguinal lymph nodes.

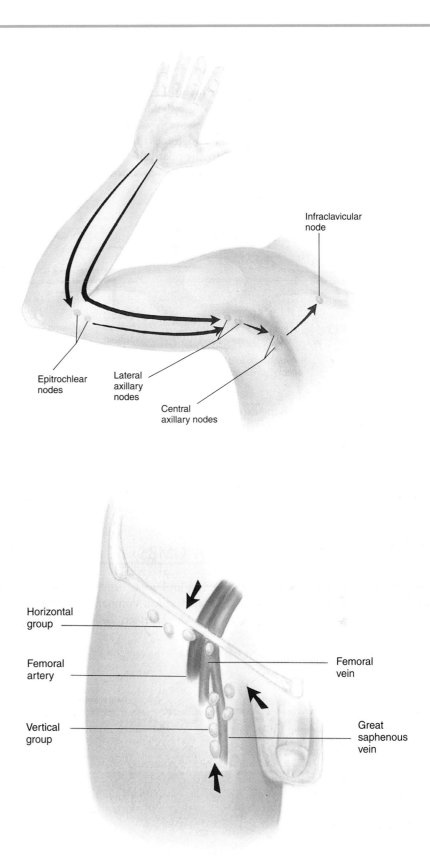

FLUID EXCHANGE AND THE CAPILLARY BED

Blood circulates from arteries to veins through the capillary bed. Here fluids diffuse across the capillary membrane, maintaining a dynamic equilibrium between the vascular and interstitial spaces. Blood pressure (*hydrostatic pressure*) within the capillary bed, especially near the arteriolar end, forces fluid out into the tissue spaces. In effecting this movement, it is aided by the relatively weak osmotic attraction of proteins within the tissues (*interstitial colloid oncotic pressure*) and is opposed by the hydrostatic pressure of the tissues.

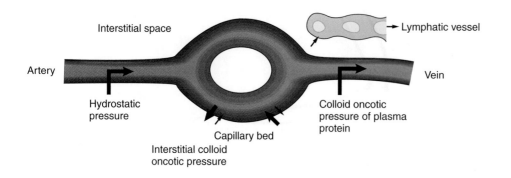

As blood continues through the capillary bed toward the venous end, its hydrostatic pressure falls, and another force gains dominance. This is the *colloid oncotic pressure of plasma proteins*, which pulls fluid back into the vascular.

Lymphatic obstruction or disturbances in hydrostatic or osmotic forces can disrupt this equilibrium. The most common clinical result is increased interstitial fluid, known as edema (see Table 18-2, Some Peripheral Causes of Edema).

FASCIA COMPARTMENT OF LIMBS

The fibrous, bandlike membranes covering and separating muscles are known as *fascia*. The human body contains 46 anatomical compartments/areas where fascia enclose blood vessels, nerves, and muscles (Altizer, 2006). Of these, 36 are

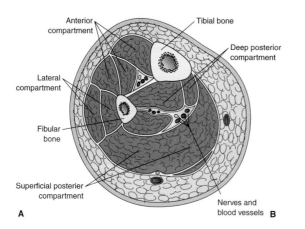

Cross-section of the middle lower third of the left leg, illustrating the four compartments with their associated peripheral nerves. (From Mubarak SJ, Owen CA. Double-Incision Fasciotomy of the Leg for Decompression in Compartment Syndromes. J Bone Joint Surg 1977;59-A:184.)

found in the upper and lower limbs. Any increase in pressure within a compartment can compromise vascular perfusion and lymphatic flow, resulting in *compartment syndrome*.

THE HEALTH HISTORY: SUBJECTIVE DATA

Key Symptoms and Signs Reported by Client

- Numbness or tingling sensation in hands, fingers, feet, or toes
- Colour changes in fingertips or toes, especially in cold weather
- Pain in arms, hands, legs, or feet
- Change in temperature of hands or feet
- Swelling of arms, hands, calves, legs, or feet
- Swelling with redness or tenderness
- Pale hands or feet
- Hair loss from feet, legs

See Table 18-1, Painful Peripheral Vascular Disorders and Their Mimics, pp. 594–595.

Early changes in vascular function often are subtle. People with vascular symptoms or disease may not voice concerns until the problem has become advanced (Bonham, 2006; Sieggreen, 2006; White, 2007). Therefore, a systematic approach to gathering subjective data from clients will lessen the likelihood of missing important cues. Poor perfusion of oxygen into the tissues results in alterations in skin integrity, colour, temperature, and hair growth. Nourishment to nerves may be altered, resulting in numbness or pain in the extremities. Pain may arise from the skin, peripheral vascular system, musculoskeletal system, or nervous system. In addition, visceral pain may be referred to the extremities, such as the pain of myocardial infarction that radiates to the left arm or cervical arthritis that radiates to the shoulder.

Atherosclerosis can cause symptomatic limb ischemia with exertion; distinguish this from *spinal stenosis*, which produces leg pain with exertion that may be reduced by leaning forward (stretching the spinal cord in the narrowed vertebral canal) and less readily relieved by rest.

Start with the symptoms and signs that the client reports. Then ask open-ended questions: "How are your legs? Your arms? Shoulders?" To elicit symptoms of *arterial peripheral vascular disease* in the legs, inquire about *intermittent claudication*, which is exercise-induced pain that is absent at rest, makes the client stop exertion, and is relieved within about 10 minutes. Ask, "Have you ever had any cramplike pain in your calves when you walk? Or exercise?" and "How far can you walk without stopping to rest?" Also, "Does the pain get better with rest?" These questions clarify what makes the client stop and how quickly the pain is relieved. Ask also about *coldness, numbness,* or *pallor* in the legs and feet or *loss of hair* over the anterior tibial surfaces (shin). Does the client have a history of varicose veins? Or any swollen glands? If the client reports any limitations or concerns, explore the nature of the symptom/sign thoroughly, using a Symptom Analysis framework.

Hair loss over the anterior tibiae occurs with decreased arterial perfusion, "Dry" or brown-black ulcers from gangrene may ensue.

Less than 20% of affected clients have the classic symptoms of external calf pain relieved with rest.

Etiology of common leg cramps and "restless legs" is not well understood (National Institute of Neurological Disorders and Stroke, 2007). Leg cramps sometimes arise from hypokalaemia induced by diuretic use.

Given that many clients with PAD have few symptoms, it is important to address existing risk factors. Assess the client's history of tobacco use. Ask if the client has hypertension, diabetes, or hyperlipidemia. In addition, is there any client or family history of myocardial infarction, angina, or stroke? Such individuals warrant further evaluation, even if they do not report symptoms in the extremities. Finally, inquire about current medications, use of herbal medicines, general fitness, and exercise tolerance (Baker, Murali-Krishnan, & Fowler, 2005).

Ginkgo biloba L. (also known as ginkyo, kew tree, yin guo) is used for peripheral arterial disease (PAD). The extract is known to contain ginkgolides, which reduce the clotting time of blood; clients should avoid taking gingko and aspirin (ASA) (Libster, 2002).

Examples of Questions for Symptom Analysis—Lower Leg Swelling (Edema)

- "Tell me where you notice the swelling." "Are both legs swollen?" (*Location*)
- "Describe how your leg(s) feel(s)." (*Quality*)
- "How has the swelling affected your activities?" "Can you wear shoes?" "Any problems with clothing fitting too tight?" (*Quantity/severity*)
- "When did you first notice the swelling?" "Did the swelling start suddenly?" "Or gradually?" "Is there a time of day when the swelling seems worse?" (*Timing*)
- "What were you doing when you first noticed the swelling?" (*Setting*)
- "Describe to me what makes the swelling worse." "Do you take medicine for high blood pressure?" Which drugs?" (*Aggravating factors*)
- "What makes the swelling better?" "What have you tried to reduce the swelling?" (*Alleviating factors*)
- "What other symptoms or signs have you noticed?" "Have you had any shortness of breath?" "Have you had any redness with the swelling?" "Or pain with the swelling?" (*Associated symptoms*)
- "What type of work do you do?" "How much of your day are you standing?" "How much of your day are you sitting?" "Do you have rest periods when you could put your feet up higher than your heart?" "How often do you travel by air?" "Or by car?" "Tell me about the exercise you get in a typical day." "How many flights of stairs do you climb each day (counting work and home)?" "What do you do for leisure activities?" (*Environmental factors*)
- "How is the swelling affecting your life?" "And the things you enjoy doing?" (*Significance to the client*)
- "What do you think might be happening with your legs?" (*Client's perspective*)

To elicit symptoms of arterial spasm in the fingers or toes, ask, "Do your fingertips ever change colour in cold weather or when you handle cold objects?" "What colour changes do you notice?" "What about your toes?"

Digital ischemic changes of blanching, followed by cyanosis, then rubor with cold exposure and rewarming occur in *Raynaud's phenomenon* or *disease*.

There may be symptoms of *venous peripheral vascular disease*, such as *swelling of the feet and legs*. Ask about any ulcers on the lower legs, often near the ankles.

Hyperpigmentation, edema, and possible cyanosis, especially when legs are dependent, occur with *venous stasis ulcers*.

The redness, swelling, and tenderness of local inflammation are seen in some vascular disorders and in other conditions that mimic them. In contrast, relatively brief leg cramps that commonly occur at night in otherwise healthy people do not indicate a circulatory problem, and cold hands and feet are so common in healthy people that they have relatively little predictive value.

Inflammation may be from *cellulitis, superficial thrombophlebitis,* and *erythema nodosum*.

HEALTH PROMOTION

Important Topics for Health Promotion

- Alterations in arterial circulation
- Use of the ABI for PAD screening
- Alterations in venous circulation
- Reduction of risk factors for peripheral vascular disease (PVD)

ALTERATIONS IN ARTERIAL CIRCULATION

Peripheral arterial disease (PAD) generally refers to atherosclerotic occlusion of lower-extremity arteries. *Atherosclerosis* (hardening of arteries) occurs when cholesterol and scar tissue accumulate to form plaque inside an artery, causing blockage. It most commonly affects the femoral and popliteal arteries, followed by the tibial and peroneal arteries.

PAD affects 1,000,000 Canadians, is most common in men and women older than 50 years, and occurs in 12% to 20% of Canadians aged 65 years or older (Toronto Endovascular Centre, 2007). Current and rapidly increasing obesity levels contribute to the growing prevalence of PAD (Golledge et al., 2007; Shields & Tjepkema, 2006). In 2004, atherosclerosis caused 2154 Canadian deaths, representing 45% of all circulatory-related cases (Statistics Canada, 2007). Arterial insufficiency is responsible for 20% of all ankle/foot ulcers (Gloviczki & Yao, 2001).

Cultural Considerations

PAD varies greatly among populations; U.S. 2000 census estimates showed African Americans had the highest rates and Asian American men the lowest (Allison et al., 2007). Genetic variation has not been fully explored and may be partly attributable to inflammatory marker differences (e.g., C-reactive protein; Anand et al., 2006). While PAD is typically more prevalent in men, women may have more asymptomatic disease (Higgins & Higgins, 2003).

Most clients have no or nonspecific leg symptoms, such as aching, cramping, numbness, tingling, and fatigue. The classic triad for intermittent claudication is as follows: (1) exercise-induced calf pain, (2) pain causes stoppage of exercise, (3) relief of pain within 10 minutes may occur in less than 20% of affected clients (McDermott et al., 2001; White, 2007). Pain increases with walking uphill or climbing stairs. Decreased blood flow may lead to small, round, deep, nonhealing ulcers on the soles, tips of and webs between toes, ankles (especially medially), outer side of fifth toes, and pressure points or injury sites (Cantwell-Gab, 2008). As PAD progresses, foot and toe pain increases and occurs even with rest. Findings in the lower limbs include the following:

- Cool temperature

- Shiny and thin skin

- Loss of hair from toes and feet

- Absent or mild edema

- Pale colour on elevation; dusky red colour when dependent

- Pulses that may not be palpable (Olson & Treat-Jacobson, 2004)

Eventually changes lead to gangrene and amputation. See Table 18-3, Chronic Insufficiency of Arteries and Veins, p. 597 for a comparison of chronic arterial insufficiency and chronic venous insufficiency.

Aortoiliac occlusive disease is a specific type of PAD. The aorta divides at the umbilicus into two iliac arteries and then to femoral arteries that go down to the toes. Walking causes intermittent claudication with pain in the thighs and buttocks.

Foot and toe pain occurs even on rest. Men may also have erectile dysfunction. Femoral pulses may be decreased or absent. As disease progresses, muscles weaken, and the limb is cold, numb to touch, and very painful. Ulcers on toes, heels, and lower legs lead to gangrene. Once signs and symptoms are this severe, leg arteries may be blocked at several locations.

Risk Factor Assessment.   Those with current or past tobacco use, diabetes, hypertension, hyperlipidemia, or cardiovascular or cerebrovascular disease are at increased risk for atherosclerotic PAD. Family history of cardiovascular disease, diabetes, or hyperlipidemia requires thorough inquiry and potential investigation. Evidence that asymptomatic PAD is a predictor of coronary artery disease (CAD) and cerebrovascular disease (CBVD) has led to calls for more vigourous screening of asymptomatic at-risk clients, particularly those older than 50 years (Bonham, 2006; Goff et al., 2007; Golomb et al., 2006; Sieggreen, 2006; Toronto Endovascular Centre, 2007; White, 2007).

Screening and Maintenance.   Nurses can use the ankle-brachial index (ABI) to detect asymptomatic or subclinical PAD (Bonham, 2006). As arteries narrow, systolic pressure below the involved area decreases. The ABI is the ratio of ankle systolic blood pressure (BP) to arm systolic BP. The procedure for determining ABI follows:

1. Have the client rest in the supine position for 5 minutes.

2. Choose the correct BP cuff for the arms and ankles: width of the cuff bladder should be "at least 40% and length at least 80% of the limb circumference" (Cantwell-Gab, 2008, p. 827).

3. Arms: To measure systolic BP of the brachial artery, place the BP cuff around the right upper arm. Place the Doppler ultrasonography (8-MHz probe) at a 45° to 60° angle over the brachial artery. A "whooshing" sound is the brachial pulse. Pump the BP cuff 20 to 30 mm Hg higher than when the sound was heard. Deflate at 2 mm Hg/sec. Identify when the sound is heard, which is systolic BP for the right arm. Repeat procedure on left arm.

4. Ankles: Place the BP cuff above the right malleolus and the Doppler over the posterior tibial artery, then the dorsalis pedis artery. Record systolic BP of each artery. Repeat on the left ankle. If unable to determine the pressures of the posterior tibial or dorsalis pedis, apply the Doppler over the peroneal artery (see p. 564).

5. Determine the **higher** value of the right and left brachial systolic BPs. For example:

    Right brachial systolic pressure = 150 mm Hg

    Left brachial systolic pressure = 120 mm Hg

    Select 150 mm Hg to use for brachial pressure in calculating the ABI.

6. Determine the **higher** value of the posterior tibial and dorsalis pedis systolic pressures on the right side. For example:

    Right posterior tibial systolic pressure = 60 mm Hg

    Right dorsalis pedis systolic pressure = 50 mm Hg

    Select 60 mm Hg for the right ankle pressure.

7. Determine the **higher** value of the posterior tibial and dorsalis pedis systolic pressures on the left side. For example:

Left posterior tibial systolic pressure = 100 mm Hg

Left dorsalis pedis systolic pressure = 110 mm Hg

Select 110 mm Hg for the left ankle pressure.

8. To calculate the ABI, divide the ankle pressure by the brachial pressure:

Right side: 60/150 = 0.40

Left side: 110/150 = 0.73

Usually systolic ankle pressure is similar to or slightly higher than that of the arm, giving an ABI of about 1.0. Recheck any arterial pressure 40 mm Hg or less—it may be venous instead of arterial pressure. Always record the size of the BP cuff used for the arms and ankles. ABI categories are as follows:

- 0.90–1.30: expected value

- 0.41–0.90: mild to moderate PAD, usually with symptoms of claudication

- 0.00–0.40: severe PAD with critical leg ischemia

In the previous example, the right-side ABI (0.40) suggests severe PAD with critical leg ischemia, while the left-side ABI (0.73) suggests mild to moderate PAD, usually with symptoms of claudication. The ABI has a reported sensitivity of 90% (those with angiographically determined PAD) and a specificity of 95% (test is negative in those without the disease) (Criqui, 2001).

Severity of PVD closely parallels risk for myocardial infarction, ischemic stroke, and death from vascular causes. Clients with the lowest ABIs have a 20% to 25% annual risk for death (Hirsh et al., 2001).

Work is in progress in the United States to establish a national program of exercise therapy to reduce claudication symptoms. The goal of the 12-week program of supervised treadmill exercise and atherosclerosis risk reduction is to improve quality of life and to prolong lives for clients with claudication (Society for Vascular Medicine and Biology, 2007).

Specific Prevention. Exercise, a healthy diet low in saturated fat, not smoking, desirable body mass index (BMI), control of blood glucose level if diabetic, and blood pressure control are associated with prevention of atherosclerosis (McDermott et al., 2006; Warburton, Nicol, & Bredin, 2006; White, 2007). For clients, nurses:

- Assess for risk factors for atherosclerosis.

- Provide education about control and management of diabetes and hypertension; tobacco cessation; reduced alcohol use; a diet high in protein, vitamins C and A, and zinc for wound healing; and regular exercise.

- Offer instruction on foot care (inspecting daily with a mirror for injury, pressure points, or ulcers; daily washing and drying; wearing cotton socks; wearing shoes, not sandals; avoiding scratching or rubbing; and careful cutting of toenails). The goal is to keep the feet clean and dry. Clients with limited vision, dexterity, or both require referral to foot care nurses or podiatrists.

- Provide information about positioning to increase circulation to feet and to reduce pain (have legs in a slightly dependent position).

- Teach about appropriate exercises (may refer to physiotherapists).

- Teach to immediately report nonhealing sores on toes, feet, or lateral ankles.

VARICOSE VEINS AND CHRONIC VENOUS INSUFFICIENCY

Varicose veins (varicosities) are superficial veins (primarily in the legs) that have become dilated and tortuous. Blood pools (venous stasis) due to a lack of calf-muscle activity and eventually incompetent valves in the veins. Incidence is approximately 15% of Canadians and increases with age; varicose veins affect primarily women (Noon, 2007).

Cultural Considerations

Prevalence is lower for African Americans (1–3%) than Caucasians (10–18%). African Americans have fewer valves in the external iliac veins but considerably more in the lower leg (Overfield, 1995).

Signs and symptoms range from initial concerns about appearance, to dull aching, muscle cramps, and fatigue of the legs, to ankle edema, feeling of heaviness in the legs, and leg cramps at night. Eventually deep leg veins become involved with signs and symptoms of chronic venous insufficiency:

- Pain in legs is aching, especially if legs are in a dependent position.

- Edema becomes marked.

- Pulses in legs are present but difficult to palpate because of edema.

- Skin of the lower legs becomes pigmented as the rupture of small surface blood vessels leads to petechiae and brownish discolouration; it also becomes thickened.

- Ulcers develop on the lower third of the leg, particularly on the medial sides of the ankles; may become infected; and are difficult to heal. (About 75% of leg ulcers are from chronic venous insufficiency; Gloviczki & Yao, 2001)

- Gangrene does not develop (Noon, 2007).

Risk Factor Assessment. People in occupations requiring prolonged standing (e.g., nurses, teachers, surgeons, salespeople, hair stylists) are at highest risk. Risk factors also include long periods of inactivity, such as bed rest, sitting (especially with legs crossed at thighs), pregnancy, inactive lifestyle, and family history.

Screening and Maintenance. Assessment includes mapping of the veins (p. 588), evaluation of venous valves (Trendelenburg test, p. 588), and a duplex ultrasound scan to test for the severity of valvular reflux.

Specific Prevention. Prevention includes less standing; less sitting, with getting up and walking every hour; daily walking (1.5–3.0 km); leg exercises while sitting and standing; use of elastic compression stockings; and elevating feet above heart level several times a day.

EMERGENCY CONCERNS

Onset of acute extremity pain requires immediate assessment. This includes thorough symptom analysis and simultaneous examination of the extremity for pulses and "CSMT" (Colour, Sensation, Movement, and Temperature).

If a pulse is not palpable at the most distal location in the limb, the nurse assesses the next most proximal pulse and continues medially (toward the body) until a pulse is detected. In the leg, the sequence is pedal (dorsalis pedis, posterior tibial, and peroneal), popliteal, and femoral. In the arm, the sequence is radial and ulnar, then brachial. A Doppler ultrasound device is useful. If a pulse cannot be located, the nurse immediately notifies an appropriate health care provider to initiate further assessment and treatment and to continue with ongoing monitoring (Morgan, 2005; Morrison, 2006).

Failure to check pulses or thoroughly assess a client's concerns has led to disastrous consequences for both clients and providers. Two Canadian lawsuits (*MacDonald vs. York County, Badger vs. Surkan et al.*), adjudicated nearly 40 years ago, highlight the seriousness of proper assessment of circulatory status, as well as the obligation to communicate findings to the health care team (Philpott, 1985). In both situations, casts had been applied to fractured lower legs; lack of communication and proper assessment led to compartment syndrome and subsequent limb amputation. In *MacDonald vs. York County*, the Supreme Court of Canada observed that "any person who has even the most elementary knowledge of first aid, or of the human anatomy including even a school child of fairly tender years knows that circulatory impairment is a very serious matter and that time is of the essence" (Philpott, 1985, p. 91). Nurses and other health care professionals are held to a higher standard of knowledge and care than expected of an average citizen.

Client situations that predispose to serious vascular compromise, and are frequently encountered by nurses, include arterial occlusion, compartment syndrome, deep venous thrombosis (DVT), and pulmonary emboli.

Arterial Occlusion: Thrombosis and Embolus. A thrombus (clot) or an embolus (clot that has broken away from its original site) may block arteries. Thrombi form from injury to arterial walls, such as with insertion or removal of cardiac catheters, fractures, crushing injuries, and penetrating wounds. Thrombi are more frequent in clients with existing ischemic symptoms.

An easy way to remember how to assess for signs and symptoms of acute arterial occlusion in an extremity includes the six Ps: *pain* is acute and severe, *pallor* (when an extremity may have a mottled appearance), *pulselessness, polar* sensation (cold to touch), *paresthesia* (burning, tingling, numbness), and *paralysis* (Dillon, 2007). Onset is rapid, with the part of the extremity below the occlusion being considerably colder and paler than that above the occlusion. Lack of a pulse and quality of pain help distinguish arterial occlusion from compartment syndrome.

Compartment Syndrome. This problem most commonly involves a leg muscle. A key symptom is "deep, throbbing, unrelenting pain" not relieved by usual measures of elevating or lowering the leg, or analgesics (Friesen & Larsen, 2007). Pain results from reduced size of the muscle compartment from outside or internal pressure. External pressure on the enclosing fascia is caused by a cast or dressing that is too tight. Internal pressure is caused by increased muscle compartment contents from edema, hemorrhage from fractures or crush injuries, or both. A muscle accessible to palpation will feel enlarged and "hard" to the touch. Increased pressure inside the compartment results in decreased microcirculation, which leads to anoxia and necrosis of nerves, then muscle. As a result, paresthesia (burning or tingling and numbness) precedes paralysis. Damage can be permanent if anoxia continues more than 6 hours (Friesen & Larsen, 2007). See Table 18-4 (p. 598) Internal and External Causes of Compartment Syndrome.

DVT or Venous Thromboembolism.

The deep veins in the lower extremity run parallel to the arteries and have the same names. DVT (clot in a deep vein) occurs in 50,000 Canadians each year (Ottawa Health Research Institute, 2006). For travellers, DVT can occur 4 to 15 days after flying (Mendis, Yach, & Alwan, 2002). One study found that 42.8% of clients who developed DVT had been hospitalized in the preceding 3 months. More DVTs were diagnosed in the 3 months after discharge than during hospitalization (Spencer, Lessard, Emery, Reed, & Goldberg, 2007).

Following a DVT, some clients develop postthrombotic syndrome (PTS) in which the affected leg remains edematous and painful. They are at increased risk for varicosities, hyperpigmentation, and venous ulcers (Kahn, Elman, Rodger, & Wells, 2003). Wearing class II elastic compression stockings may significantly reduce the risk of PST (Brandjes et al., 1997).

Risk Factor Assessment.

While the specific cause of DVT is not known, three factors (Virchow's triad) are prerequisites for clot formation: (1) blood stasis (venous stasis), (2) injury to the vein wall, and (3) increased coagulation. Two of the three factors are needed for thrombus formation (Noon, 2007).

RISK FACTORS FOR DEEP VEIN THROMBOSIS

Venous Stasis

- Bed rest (reduces blood flow to the legs by at least 50%)
- Prolonged immobility
- Anesthesia
- Surgery (especially total hip replacement)
- Spinal cord injury
- Travel of more than 4 hours (by plane, train, bus, or car), especially if the person is shorter than 163 cm or taller than 193 cm (Public Health Agency of Canada, 2006; World Health Organization, 2007)
- Heart failure and shock
- Obesity
- History of varicose veins
- Decreased ankle joint mobility (reduces the calf muscle pump and motion for walking and climbing stairs; Pieper, Templin, Birk, & Kirsner, 2007)
- Age (older than 65 years)
- Pregnancy (clot often occurs in femoral veins from fetal pressure)

Damage to Vein Wall

- Direct trauma, including leg fractures
- Surgery (of abdomen and pelvis; clients with cancer)
- Diseases of veins
- Chemical irritation of veins (upper extremities: from IV medications, solutions, illicit IV drug use)
- Internal trauma to veins (central venous catheters; pacemaker leads; illicit IV drug use involving the groin, legs, and feet)
- Effort thrombosis (especially upper extremities)—repetitive motion injuries in tennis players, swimmers, and construction workers

Altered Blood Coagulation

- Oral contraception
- Hormone therapy
- Previous blood clot
- Family history of internal clotting problems
- Presence of Factor V Leiden (Horne & McCloskey, 2006)
- Presence of congenital proteins C and S

Source: Adapted from Noon, J. (2007). Cardiovascular, circulatory and hematologic function. In R. A. Day, P. Paul, B. Williams, S. M. Smeltzer, & B. Bare (Eds.), *Brunner & Suddarth's textbook of medical-surgical nursing* (1st Canadian ed., pp. 846–847). Philadelphia: Lippincott Williams & Wilkins.

Screening and Maintenance. Signs and symptoms of DVT are often nonspecific. Assessment includes measuring leg circumference at intervals from ankle to thigh bilaterally for edema, feeling for increased skin temperature especially over ankles and calves, and gently palpating for pain.

Specific Prevention. In Canada, March is DVT Awareness Month. The goal in preventing DVT is to avoid anything that causes venous stasis and to increase muscle activity of the legs.

- Avoid tight clothing at waist, groin, and upper legs.

- Avoid long periods of sitting, especially with legs crossed at thighs; dorsiflex and plantar flex feet every hour; walk for 10 minutes, every 1 to 2 hours.

- Avoid long periods of standing; while standing, go up on toes, and then up on heels; walk around every hour.

- Aim to walk 1.5 to 3.0 kilometres per day.

- Walk up stairs rather than taking an elevator.

- Go swimming, a useful non-weight-bearing exercise.

- Elevate legs above heart level for periods each day.

- Maintain appropriate weight for height.

- Wear elastic compression stockings daily. These come in knee-high and thigh-high sizes for men and women, and as pantyhose. A prescription and fitting are required for Class I, II, or III levels. Stockings exert pressure, which narrows the diameter of veins and allows valves to close, decreasing blood pooling. Stocking pressure is always highest in feet and ankles, lower over calves, and lowest over thighs. For example, the pressures for Class I compression stockings are 20 to 30 mm Hg at feet and ankles, 15 to 20 mm Hg in lower calves, 12 to 18 mm Hg in upper calves, and 5 to 10 mm Hg over thighs (Vein Institute of Toronto and Medical Aesthetic Clinic, 2008). Clients should don stockings as soon as possible after getting out of bed.

Kahn et al. (2003) reported that 34 Canadian thrombosis physicians ordered knee-high rather than mid- or full-thigh stockings for 70% of clients. This reflects confidence that knee-high stockings are effective and easier and cooler to wear. In this study, 91% of clients purchased the stockings and 87% reported wearing them daily, which was higher than the physicians' expected rate of 50% compliance. If the DVT was proximal rather than distal, clients reported greater reduction in pain and swelling, and that their legs were "completely" or "a lot better." While the stockings were expensive (over $100.00), severity of symptoms and disease and expected effectiveness were more important in client decision making. Nurses should ensure that all clients who have had DVT receive a prescription for elastic compression stockings, along with teaching about why they are necessary and how to put them on.

Additional Precautions for Travellers. The goal is to prevent compression, narrowing, or blockage of deep veins (from long periods of sitting), which results in more blood pooling in legs and less returning to the heart.

- If a person is shorter than 163 cm, place a small carry-on bag under the seat in front as a foot rest (Transport Canada, 2007). This prevents kinking and compression of popliteal veins when legs dangle (Mendis et al., 2002).

- If the person is taller than 193 cm, keep the space under the seat in front free of luggage to allow room to stretch the legs (Transport Canada, 2007).

- Avoid alcohol or sedatives, which increase the likelihood of immobility.

- Avoid tight clothes.

- Wear elastic compression stockings or special travel socks.

- Do leg exercises; walk around every 1 to 2 hours for 10 minutes, if possible.

- Keep well hydrated with water and juice (Mendis et al., 2002).

Pulmonary Embolus (PE).   PE occurs when an embolus breaks free (often from deep veins in the pelvis and legs), travels through the blood, and lodges in a pulmonary blood vessel. The embolus can also be air, fat, amniotic fluid, or septic fluid. This situation is life threatening if the PE blocks circulation to a large enough section. The most frequent symptom is shortness of breath (dyspnea); the most frequent sign is rapid respiratory rate (tachypnea; Goldhaber, 2004). Other findings are chest pain that worsens with deep breaths, rapid heart rate, sweating, faintness, bloody sputum, and narrowed pulse pressure. Quick assessment and intervention are critical, because a second PE could be fatal. A single PE occurs in 100 people per 100,000. Death can occur within 1 hour of onset of symptoms (Noon, 2007); approximately 15% of clients die within 48 hours (White, 2003). Survivors may have heart damage, dyspnea, and pulmonary hypertension.

Risk Factor Assessment.
A key nursing role is to identify high-risk clients and to decrease risks for all clients (Ross, 2007). PE is the leading cause of maternal deaths, because risk is six times greater during pregnancy. Clients having surgery for cancer have a three times higher risk for PE. Fatal PE is the most common preventable cause of hospital deaths in North America. Clients who have had a PE with previous surgery are at increased risk with future surgeries. Presence of a DVT is a definite risk factor. Other risks are blood stasis, venous injury, predisposition to clot formation, hypercoagulability, heart failure, chronic lung disease, diabetes, increasing age, and obesity. Sometimes a PE occurs in apparently healthy individuals.

Screening and Maintenance.
Consider the following (Noon, 2007):

- Signs and symptoms of DVT in the legs

- Chest x-ray to exclude other conditions

- ECG, arterial blood gases, and peripheral vascular studies

- Ventilation-profusion scan—the test of choice (if a mismatch of ventilation and profusion occurs, PE is probable)

- Pulmonary angiography—this gold standard is used if other test findings are not conclusive. Contrast media is injected into client's arteries. Nevertheless, this test will not identify PE in up to 20% of clients with PE.

Specific Prevention.
Take measures to prevent DVT. Examples include active leg exercises; deep breathing and coughing; frequent turning; early ambulation; elastic compression stockings; travel precautions; and understanding of the need to continue anticoagulant therapy, how to prevent bruising and deal with bleeding, and signs/symptoms of potential DVT.

TECHNIQUES OF EXAMINATION: OBJECTIVE DATA

■ PROMOTING CLIENT COMFORT, DIGNITY, AND SAFETY

Accurate peripheral vascular assessment requires a warm room and warm examiner hands. Prepare the client by describing the examination. Begin with the client sitting and facing you, with a drape of a half-sheet or bath blanket over the client's lower extremities. Ensure that he or she is comfortable. Wash your hands thoroughly and then proceed with examination of the arms. When examining the legs, first assist the client into a supine position and reposition the drape over the legs. Throughout the examination, provide ongoing explanation and attend to the client's comfort level. Use of an assistant may be advisable when examining femoral pulses and superficial inguinal lymph nodes if the client is the opposite sex of the examiner.

■ INITIAL SURVEY OF THE PERIPHERAL VASCULAR SYSTEM

Begin with inspection of the overall appearance of the client. Does it coincide with stated age? Or does the client appear younger or older than reported? Are signs of discomfort or pain present (e.g., grimacing, diaphoresis)? Are outward cues of potential peripheral vascular risk factors present, based on observation of weight, skin colour, and condition?

Compare temperature of each extremity bilaterally. Are there noticeable differences in skin colour, skin texture, lesions, hair distribution, or limb circumference or size? If the client presents with a concern in one extremity, examine the unaffected limb first. Explain that you will look at the affected area/limb last; otherwise, the client may question whether you have truly listened to his or her concerns.

Equipment
■ Half-sheet or bath blanket ■ Tape measure ■ Gloves, if skin lesions present ■ Doppler ultrasonography device

■ EXAMINATION OF THE ARMS

Inspection. *Inspect both arms* from the fingertips to the shoulders. Note:

■ Their size, symmetry, and any swelling

Lymphedema of the arm and hand may follow axillary node dissection and radiation therapy.

■ The venous pattern

Prominent veins in an edematous arm suggest venous obstruction.

■ The colour of the skin and nail beds and the texture of the skin

Palpate the pulses in order to assess the arterial circulation.

■ *The femoral pulse.* Press deeply, below the inguinal ligament and about midway between the anterior superior iliac spine and the symphysis pubis. As in deep abdominal palpation, the use of two hands, one on top of the other, may facilitate this examination, especially in clients who are obese.

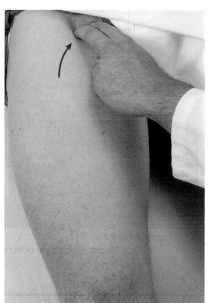

A diminished or absent pulse indicates partial or complete occlusion proximally; for example, at the aortic or iliac level, all pulses distal to the occlusion are typically affected. Chronic arterial occlusion, usually from atherosclerosis, causes *intermittent claudication* (p. 571), postural colour changes (p.587), and trophic changes in the skin (p. 597).

An exaggerated, widened femoral pulse suggests a femoral aneurysm, a pathologic dilatation of the artery.

■ *The popliteal pulse.* The client's knee should be somewhat flexed, the leg relaxed. Place the fingertips of both hands so that they just meet in the midline behind the knee and press them deeply into the popliteal fossa. The popliteal pulse is often more difficult to find than other pulses. It is deeper and feels more diffuse.

An exaggerated, widened popliteal pulse suggests an aneurysm of the popliteal artery. Neither popliteal nor femoral aneurysms are common. They are usually due to atherosclerosis, and occur primarily in men older than age 50.

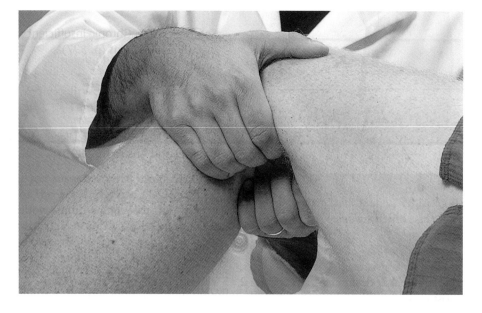

If you cannot feel the popliteal pulse with this approach, try with the client prone. Flex the client's knee to about 90°, let the lower leg relax against your shoulder or upper arm, and press your two thumbs deeply into the popliteal fossa.

Atherosclerosis (arteriosclerosis obliterans) most commonly obstructs arterial circulation in the thigh. The femoral pulse is then present, the popliteal decreased or absent.

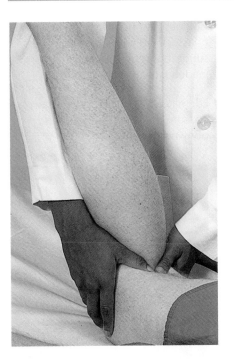
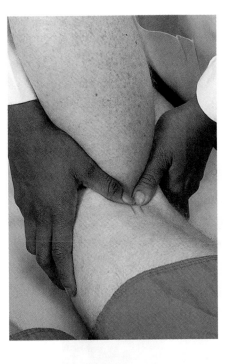

■ *The dorsalis pedis pulse.* Feel the dorsum of the foot (not the ankle) just lateral to the extensor tendon of the great toe. If you cannot feel a pulse, explore the dorsum of the foot more laterally.

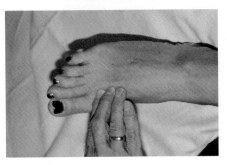

The dorsalis pedis artery may be congenitally absent in 8% to 10% of the population (Sieggreen, 2006) or may branch higher in the ankle. Search for a pulse more laterally.

■ *The posterior tibial pulse.* Curve your fingers behind and slightly below the medial malleolus of the ankle. (This pulse may be hard to feel if fatty tissue or edema is present at the ankle.)

Decreased or absent pedal pulses (assuming a warm environment) with femoral and popliteal pulses present suggest occlusive disease in the lower popliteal artery or its branches—a pattern often associated with diabetes mellitus.

Tips on feeling difficult pulses: (1) Position your own body and examining hand comfortably; awkward positions decrease your tactile sensitivity. (2) Place your hand properly and linger there, varying the pressure of your fingers to pick up a weak pulsation. If unsuccessful, then explore the area deliberately. (3) Do not confuse the client's pulse with your own pulsating fingertips. If you are unsure, count your own heart rate and compare it with the client's. The rates are usually different. Your carotid pulse is convenient for this comparison.

Sudden arterial occlusion, as from embolism or thrombosis, causes pain and numbness or tingling. The limb distal to the occlusion becomes cold, pale, and pulseless. Emergency treatment is required. If collateral circulation is good, only numbness and coolness may result.

Note the temperature of the feet and legs with the backs of your fingers. Compare one side with the other. Bilateral coldness is most often due to a cold environment or anxiety.

Coldness, especially when unilateral or associated with other signs, suggests arterial insufficiency from inadequate arterial circulation.

Look for edema. Compare one foot and leg with the other, noting their relative size and the prominence of veins, tendons, and bones.

Edema causes swelling that may obscure the veins, tendons, and bony prominences.

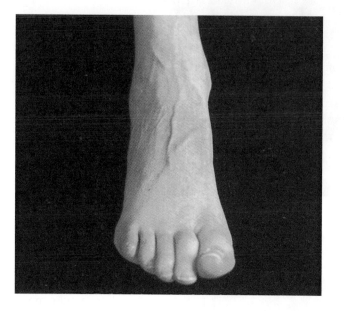

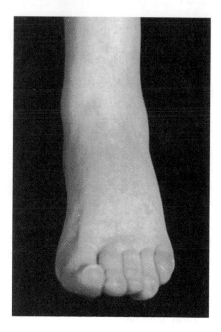

See Table 18-2, Some Peripheral Causes of Edema (p. 598).

See Table 18-6, Description of Edema Characteristics and Grading, p. 600.

Check for pitting edema. Press firmly but gently with your thumb for at least 5 seconds (1) over the dorsum of each foot, (2) behind each medial malleolus, and (3) over the shins. Look for *pitting*—a depression caused by pressure from your thumb. Usually there is none. The severity of edema is graded on a 4-point scale, from *slight* to *very marked*.

Shown below is 3+ pitting edema.

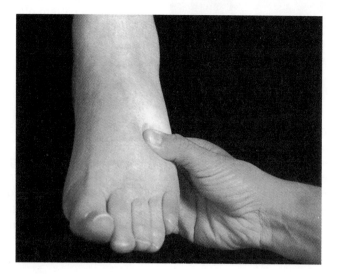

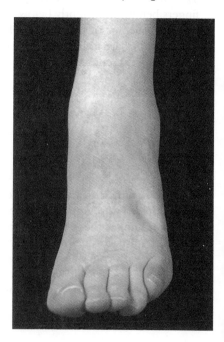

If you suspect edema, *measurement of the legs* may help you to identify it and to follow its course. With a flexible tape, measure (1) the forefoot, (2) the smallest possible circumference above the ankle, (3) the largest circumference at the calf, and (4) the midthigh, a measured distance above the patella with the knee extended. Compare one side with the other. A difference of more than 1 cm just above the ankle or 2 cm at the calf is unusual in most people and suggests edema.

Conditions such as muscular atrophy can also cause different circumferences in the legs.

If edema is present, look for possible causes in the peripheral vascular system. These include (1) recent DVT, (2) chronic venous insufficiency due to previous DVT or to incompetence of the venous valves, and (3) lymphedema. Note the extent of the swelling. How far up the leg does it go?

In *deep venous thrombosis*, the extent of edema suggests the location of the occlusion: the calf when the lower leg or the ankle is swollen, the iliofemoral veins when the entire leg is swollen.

Is the swelling unilateral or bilateral? Are the veins unusually prominent?

Venous distention suggests a venous cause of edema.

Try to identify any venous tenderness that may accompany DVT. Palpate the groin just medial to the femoral pulse for tenderness of the femoral vein. Next, with the client's leg flexed at the knee and relaxed, palpate the calf. With your finger pads, gently compress the calf muscles against the tibia, and search for any tenderness or cords. DVT, however, may have no demonstrable signs, and diagnosis often depends on high clinical suspicion and other testing.

A painful, pale swollen leg, together with tenderness in the groin over the femoral vein, suggests deep *iliofemoral thrombosis*. Only half of clients with *deep venous thrombosis* in the calf have tenderness and cords deep in the calf. Calf tenderness is nonspecific, however, and may be present without thrombosis.

Note the *colour of the skin*.

- Is there a local area of redness? If so, note its temperature, and gently try to feel the firm cord of a thrombosed vein in the area. The calf is most often involved.

Local swelling, redness, warmth, and a subcutaneous cord suggest *superficial thrombophlebitis*.

- Are there brownish areas near the ankles?

A brownish colour or ulcers just above the ankle suggest *chronic venous insufficiency*.

- Note any ulcers in the skin. Where are they?
- Feel the thickness of the skin.

Thickened brawny skin occurs in lymphedema and advanced venous insufficiency.

Ask the client to stand, and *inspect the saphenous system for varicosities*. The standing posture allows any varicosities to fill with blood and makes them visible. You can easily miss them when the client is in a supine position. Feel for any varicosities, noting any signs of thrombophlebitis.

◩ SPECIAL TECHNIQUES

Evaluating the Arterial Supply to the Hand.
If you suspect arterial insufficiency in the arm or hand, try to feel the *ulnar pulse* as well as the radial and brachial pulses. Feel for it deeply on the flexor surface of the wrist medially. Partially flexing the client's wrist may help you. The pulse of an intact ulnar artery, however, may not be palpable.

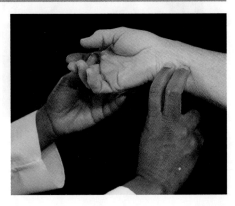

Varicose veins are dilated and tortuous. Their walls may feel somewhat thickened. Many varicose veins can be seen in the leg on p. 588.

The *Allen test* gives further information. This test is also useful to ensure the patency of the ulnar artery before puncturing the radial artery for blood samples. The client should rest with hands in lap, palms up.

Ask the client to make a tight fist with one hand, and then compress both radial and ulnar arteries firmly between your thumbs and fingers.

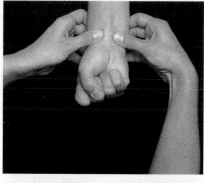

Arterial occlusive disease is much less common in the arms than in the legs. Absent or diminished pulses at the wrist in acute embolic occlusion and in *Buerger's disease*, or thromboangiitis obliterans.

Next, ask the client to open the hand into a relaxed slightly flexed position. The palm is pale.

Extending the hand fully may cause pallor and a falsely positive test.

Release your pressure over the ulnar artery. If the ulnar artery is patent, the palm flushes within about 3 to 5 seconds.

Persisting pallor indicates occlusion of the ulnar artery or its distal branches.

Patency of the radial artery may be tested by releasing the radial artery while still compressing the ulnar.

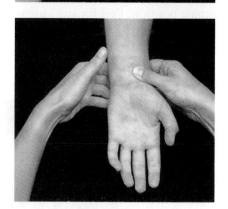

Postural Colour Changes of Chronic Arterial Insufficiency. If pain or diminished pulses suggest arterial insufficiency, look for postural colour changes. Raise both legs, as shown at the right, to about 60° until maximal pallor of the feet develops—usually within a minute. In light-skinned persons, either maintenance of usual colour, as seen in this right foot, or slight pallor is expected.

Marked pallor on elevation suggests *arterial insufficiency*.

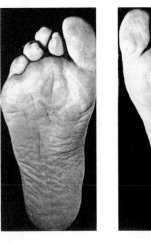

Then ask the client to sit up with legs dangling down. Compare both feet, noting the time required for the following:

- Return of pinkness to the skin, usually about 10 seconds or less

- Filling of the veins of the feet and ankles, usually about 15 seconds

This right foot has expected colour and the veins on the foot have filled. These usual responses suggest an adequate circulation.

The foot in the following figure is still pale, and the veins are just starting to fill—signs of arterial insufficiency.

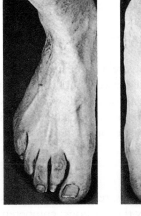

Look for any unusual *rubor* (dusky redness) to replace the pallor of the dependent foot. Rubor may take a minute or more to appear.

Usual responses accompanied by diminished arterial pulses suggest that a good collateral circulation has developed around an arterial occlusion.

Colour changes may be difficult to see in darker-skinned persons. Inspect the soles of the feet for these changes, and use tangential lighting to see the veins.

Persisting rubor on dependency suggests arterial insufficiency (see p. 599). When veins are incompetent, dependent rubor and the timing of colour return and venous filling are not reliable tests of arterial insufficiency.

Source of foot photos: Kappert A, Winsor T: Diagnosis of Peripheral Vascular Disease. Philadelphia: FA Davis, 1972.

Mapping Varicose Veins. You can map out the course and connections of varicose veins by transmitting pressure waves along the blood-filled veins. With the client standing, place your palpating fingers gently on a vein and, with your other hand below it, compress the vein sharply. Feel for a pressure wave transmitted to the fingers of your upper hand. A palpable pressure wave indicates that the two parts of the vein are connected.

A wave may also be transmitted downward, but not as easily.

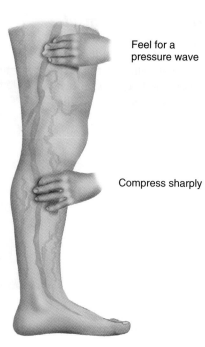

Feel for a pressure wave

Compress sharply

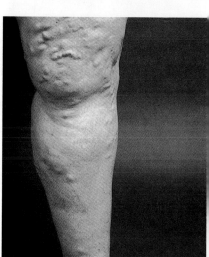

Evaluating the Competency of Venous Valves. By the *retrograde filling (Trendelenburg) test*, you can assess the valvular competency in both the communicating veins and the saphenous system. Start with the client supine. Elevate one leg to about 90° to empty it of venous blood.

Next, occlude the great saphenous vein in the upper thigh by manual compression, using enough pressure to occlude this vein but not the deeper vessels. Ask the client to stand. While you keep the vein occluded, watch for venous filling in the leg. Usually the saphenous vein fills from below, taking about 35 seconds as blood flows through the capillary bed into the venous system.

Rapid filling of the superficial veins while the saphenous vein is occluded indicates incompetent valves in the communicating veins. Blood flows quickly in a retrograde direction from the deep to the saphenous system.

After the client stands for 20 seconds, release the compression, and look for sudden additional venous filling. Usually there is none; competent valves in the saphenous vein block retrograde flow. Slow venous filling continues.

Sudden additional filling of superficial veins after release of compression indicates incompetent valves in the saphenous vein.

When both steps of this test are as expected, the response is termed negative–negative. Negative–positive and positive–negative responses may also occur.

When the results of both steps are unexpected the test is positive–positive.

RECORDING AND ANALYZING FINDINGS

Information from the client history and physical examination should be precise in anatomical setting, logical in order, and concise. The following style is appropriate for most documentation. It is easiest for the reader to quickly grasp objective findings written in the sequence of inspection, palpation, percussion, and auscultation (IPPA).

■ *Examples of Peripheral Vascular Documentation*

Area of Assessment	Expected Findings	Unexpected Findings
Inspection of arms	Skin over upper extremities pink with fine macular lesions over forearms bilaterally. Arms symmetrical in size, without edema.	Skin erythemateous over right ring finger, extending 15 cm into right forearm. Lower and upper right arm edematous compared to left.
Inspection of legs	Pink lower extremities bilaterally, without lesions, varicosities, or stasis. Equal hair distribution bilaterally.	Lower left leg pale, below the knee, with noticeable hair loss compared to right leg. Rubor when left leg dependent. No edema or ulceration bilaterally.
Palpation of arms	Arms warm and dry to touch. Skinfold on both hands returns to original position in < 1 second. No lymphadenopathy noted at epitrochlear fossa bilaterally.	Right hand and forearm hot to touch; palpable edema at wrist (2+). Two mobile, tender, 1 cm nodes palpable at right epitrochlear fossa.
Palpation of legs	Legs warm and dry to touch bilaterally. Calves supple and nontender bilaterally. Several 1 cm nontender, superficial inguinal nodes (horizontal group) palpated bilaterally.	Left leg cool to touch below the knee compared to right leg. Skin appears thin and dry over left lower leg. No palpable edema bilaterally.
Peripheral pulses	Brachial, radial, femoral, posterior tibial, and dorsalis pedis pulses are 2+ and symmetric. Unable to palpate the popliteal pulses bilaterally.	Brachial, radial, femoral pulses symmetric and 2+. Right popliteal, posterior tibial, dorsalis pedis pulses 2+. Left popliteal 1+, with absent left posterior tibial and dorsalis pedis pulses.
Auscultation for bruits	No femoral or renal bruits bilaterally.	Bruit over left femoral artery but not over right. No bruits over renal arteries.

◢ ANALYZING FINDINGS FROM PHYSICAL EXAMINATION AND HEALTH HISTORY

Analysis of subjective and objective data leads to the formulation of nursing diagnoses and a plan for interprofessional care, central to which are the unique aspects of the client and his or her input. For example:

Mrs. Maria Giovanni, 70 years old, works as a cashier in her family's grocery. For 8 weeks, she has been treating an ulcer on her right lower leg with petroleum jelly, and has continued standing for 10 hours a day at work. Aching and heaviness in her leg and increased size of the ulcer caused her to see her family physician, who has referred Mrs. Giovanni to home care and has told her she is not to work until the ulcer has healed.

When the nurse arrives, Mrs. Giovanni is resting with legs elevated. The client reports she is very worried about the ulcer. Physical findings are as follows:

- *Blood pressure: 185/100, right arm, sitting*

- *Heart rate: 102*

- *Peripheral pulses: femoral, popliteal, posterior tibial, and dorsalis pedis present and equal (+2) bilaterally*

- *Edema: 2+ left leg, 3+ right leg*

- *BMI: 40*

The nurse carefully removes the dressing covering the ulcer and takes a swab from the ulcer bed for culture and sensitivity. He then photographs the ulcer and sends the image via telehealth to a wound care nurse expert, who then advises methods for cleaning the ulcer and applying dressings. From this information, the home care nurse develops the following nursing diagnosis:

Impaired skin integrity *related to vascular insufficiency*

Comprehensive care includes duplex ultrasound, arteriography, and venogram with x-ray and ultrasound technicians. A dietician is consulted about adequate nutrition for wound healing (high protein, vitamins C and A, iron, zinc) and weight reduction. A physical therapist assists with leg exercises and eventually will work with Mrs. Giovanni to improve physical mobility and on strategies to avoid trauma to her legs. An occupational therapist can provide diversional activities while Mrs. Giovanni is immobilized, and assistance with obtaining a special floor mat for her return to work. A health care consultant will measure Mrs. Giovanni for elastic compression stockings. The nurse monitors the healing process and the client's understanding of the health education, and apprises the family physician of the client's progress. If the ulcer does not heal, a plastic surgeon may be consulted about surgery to close the wound.

Critical Thinking Exercise

Answer the following questions about Mrs. Giovanni:

- What pathophysiology underlies development of venous leg ulcers? (*Knowledge*)
- How would you distinguish between the signs and symptoms of a venous ulcer or an arterial ulcer? (*Comprehension*)
- What would you teach Mrs. Giovanni about ways to promote healing of her leg ulcer? (*Application*)
- What lifestyle factors might be contributing to the leg ulcer? (*Analysis*)
- What recommendations for screening and follow-up would you suggest for Mrs. Giovanni? (*Synthesis*)
- How would you evaluate the success of client teaching? (*Evaluation*)

Canadian Research

Al-Omran, M., Lindsay, T., Major, J., Jawas, A., Leiter, L. A., & Verma, S. (2006). Perceptions of Canadian vascular surgeons toward pharmacological risk reduction in clients with peripheral arterial disease. *Annals of Vascular Surgery, 20*(5), 555–563.

Chambers, L. W., Kaczorowski, J., Dolovich, L., Karwalajtys, T., Hall, H. L., McDonough, B., et al. (2005). A community-based program for cardiovascular health awareness. *Canadian Journal of Public Health, 96*(4), 294–298.

Hanley, A. J. G., Harris, S. B., Mamakeesick, M., Goodwin, K., Fiddler, E., Hegele, R. A., et al. (2003). Complications of type 2 diabetes among Aboriginal Canadians: Increasing the understanding of prevalence and risk factors. *Canadian Journal of Diabetes, 27*(4), 455–463.

Harrison, M. B., Graham, I. D., Lorimer, K., Friedberg, E., Pierscianowski, T., & Brandys, T. (2005). Leg-ulcer care in the community, before and after implementation of an evidence-based service. *Canadian Medical Association Journal, 172*(11), 1447–1452.

Nemeth, K. A., Harrison, M. B., Graham, I. D., & Burke, S. (2003). Pain in pure and mixed aetiology venous leg ulcers: A three-phase prevalence study. *Journal of Wound Care, 12*(9), 336–340.

Nemeth, K. A., Harrison, M. B., Graham, I. D., & Burke, S. (2004). Understanding venous leg ulcer pain: Results of a longitudinal study. *Ostomy Wound Management, 50*(1), 34–46.

Virani, S., Strong, D., Tennant, M., Greve, M., Young, H., Shade, S., et al. (2006). Rationale and Implementation of the SLICK Project: Screening for Limb, I-Eye, Cardiovascular and Kidney (SLICK) complications in individuals with type 2 diabetes in Alberta's First Nations communities. *Canadian Journal of Public Health, 97*(3), 241–247.

Xiong, L. M. D. P., Jang, K. P., Montplaisir, K., Levchencho, J., Thibodeau, A., Gaspar, P., et al. (2007). Canadian restless legs syndrome twin study. *Neurology, 68*(19), 1631–1633.

Test Questions

1. Which of the following is an essential topic when discussing risk factors for peripheral arterial disease with a client?
   a. Exercise tolerance
   b. Prevention of varicose veins
   c. Extent of tobacco use and exposure
   d. Significance of cardiac dysrhythmias

2. During the health history interview, the client reports exercise-induced calf pain. Typically, the pain should be relieved in
   a. 15 minutes after sitting down.
   b. 5 minutes if legs are elevated.
   c. 10 minutes after exercise is stopped.
   d. 20 minutes of rest with legs dependent.

3. A finding on palpation that suggests venous insufficiency is
   a. cool lower legs and feet.
   b. ulcerations on toes of left foot.
   c. diminished sensations over dorsum of right foot.
   d. diminished dorsalis pedis pulse in an edematous foot.

4. If palpable, superficial inguinal nodes are expected to be
   a. fixed, tender, and 2.5 cm in diameter.
   b. discrete, tender, and 2 cm in diameter.
   c. nontender, mobile, and 1 cm in diameter.
   d. fixed, nontender, and 1.5 cm in diameter.

5. A client at risk for PVD should be screened by which of the following tests?
   a. Ankle–brachial index
   b. Doppler testing of femoral arteries
   c. Bilateral vascular claudication assessment
   d. Angiogram of femoral and popliteal arteries

Bibliography

CITATIONS

Allison, M. A., Ho, E., Denenberg, J. O., Langer, R. D., Newman, A. B., Fabsitz, R. R., et al. (2007). Ethnic-specific prevalence of peripheral arterial disease in the United States. *American Journal of Preventive Medicine, 32*(4), 328–333.

Altizer, L. (2006). Compartment syndrome. *Orthopaedic Nursing, 23*(6), 391–396.

Anand, S. S., Razak, F., Yi, Q., Davis, B., Jacobs, R., Vuksan, V., et al. (2006). C-reactive protein as a screening test for cardiovascular risk in a multiethnic population. *Arteriosclerosis, Thrombosis & Vascular Biology, 24*(8), 1509–1515.

Baker, N., Murali-Krishnan, S., & Fowler, D. (2005). A user's guide to foot screening. Part 2: Peripheral arterial disease... second of a series of three. *Diabetic Foot, 8*(2), 58, 60, 62, 64, 66, 68, 70.

Bonham, P. A. (2006). Get the LEAD out: Noninvasive assessment for lower extremity arterial disease using ankle brachial index and toe brachial index measurements. *Journal of Wound Ostomy and Continence Nursing, 33*, 30–41.

Brandjes, D. P. M., Buller, H. R., Heijboer, H., Hulsman, M. V., de Rijk, M., & Jagt, H. (1997). Randomized trial of effect of compression stockings in clients with symptomatic proximal-vein thrombosis. *Lancet, 349*, 759–762.

Cantwell-Gab, K. (2008). Assessment and management of clients with vascular disorders and problems of peripheral circulation. In S. C. Smeltzer, B. G. Bare, J. L. Hinkle, & K. H. Cheever (Eds.), *Brunner & Suddarth's textbook of medical-surgical nursing* (11th ed., pp. 974–1019). Philadelphia: Lippincott Williams & Wilkins.

Criqui, M. (2001). Systematic atherosclerosis risk and the mandate for intervention in atherosclerotic peripheral disease. *American Journal of Cardiology, 88*(Suppl.), 43J–47J.

Dillon, P. M. (2007). *Nursing health assessment: Clinical pocket guide* (2nd ed.). Philadelphia: F. A. Davis.

Friesen, B., & Larsen, L. (2007). Management of clients with musculoskeletal traumas. In R. A. Day, P. Paul, B. Williams, S. C. Smeltzer, & B. Bare (Eds.), *Brunner & Suddarth's textbook of medical-surgical nursing* (1st Canadian ed., pp. 2095–2096). Philadelphia: Lippincott Williams & Wilkins.

Gloviczki, P., & Yao, J. T. (2001). *Handbook of venous disorders— Guidelines of the American Venus Forum* (2nd ed.). New York: Oxford University Press.

Goff, D. C., Jr., Brass, L., Braun, L. T., Croft, J. B., Fowkes, F. G. R., Hong, Y., et al. (2007). Essential features of a surveillance system to support the prevention and management of heart disease and stroke: A scientific statement from the American Heart Association Councils on Epidemiology and Prevention, Stroke, and Cardiovascular Nursing and the Interdisciplinary Working Groups on Quality of Care and Outcomes Research and Atherosclerotic Peripheral Vascular Disease. *Circulation, 115*(1), 127–155.

Goldhaber, S. Z. (2004). Pulmonary embolism. *Lancet, 363* (9417), 1295–1305.

Golledge, J., Leicht, A., Crowther, R. G., Clancy, P., Spinks, W. L., & Quigley, F. (2007). Association of obesity and metabolic syndrome with the severity and outcome of intermittent claudication. *Journal of Vascular Surgery, 45*, 40–46.

Golomb, B. A., Dang, T. T., & Criqui, M. H. (2006). Peripheral arterial disease: Morbidity and mortality implications. *Circulation, 114*, 688–699.

Higgins, J. P., & Higgins, J. A. (2003). Epidemiology of peripheral arterial disease in women. *Journal of Epidemiology, 13*(1), 1–14.

Hirsh, A. T., Criqui, M. H., Treat-Jacobson, D., Regensteiner, J. G., Creager, M. A., Olin, J. W., et al. (2001). Peripheral arterial disease: Detection, awareness, and treatment in primary care. *Journal of the American Medical Association, 286*(11), 1317–1324.

Horne, M. K., & McCloskey, D. J. (2006). Factor V Leiden as a common genetic risk factor for venous thromboembolism. *Journal of Nursing Scholarship, 38*(1), 19–25.

Kahn, S. R., Elman, E., Rodger, M. A., & Wells, P. S. (2003). Use of elastic compression stockings after deep vein thrombosis: A comparison of practices and perceptions of thrombosis physicians and clients. *Journal of Thrombosis and Haemostasis, 1*(6), 500–506.

Kesteven, P. L. J. (2000). Traveller's thrombosis. *Thorax, 55*(Suppl. 1), 532–536.

Libster, M. (2002). *Delmar's integrative herb guide for nurses* (pp. 763–770). Albany, NY: Delmar, Thomson Learning.

Martini, F. H. (2001). *Fundamentals of anatomy & physiology* (5th ed., pp. 751–796). Upper Saddle River, NJ: Prentice Hall.

McDermott, M. M., Greenland, P., Liu, K., Guralnik, J. M., Criqui, M. H., Dolan, N. C., et al. (2001). Leg symptoms in peripheral arterial disease: Associated clinical characteristics and functional impairment. *Journal of the American Medical Association, 286*, 1599–1606.

McDermott, M. M., Liu, K., Ferucci, L., Criqui, M. H., Greenland, P., Guralnik, J. M., et al. (2006). Physical performance in peripheral arterial disease: A slower rate of decline in clients who walk more. *Annals of Internal Medicine, 144*(1), 10–21.

Mendis, S., Yach, D., & Alwan, A. (2002). Air travel and venous thromboembolism. *Bulletin of the World Health Organization, 80*(5), 403–406.

Morgan, E. (2005). When critical limb ischemia strikes. *Nursing, 35*(8), 32cc1–32cc3.

Morrison, R. (2006). Venous thromboembolism: Scope of the problem and the nurse's role in risk assessment and prevention. *Journal of Vascular Nursing, 24*, 82–90.

National Institute of Neurological Disorders and Stroke, National Institutes of Health. (2007) *Restless legs syndrome fact sheet.* Retrieved June 25, 2007, from http://www.ninds.nih.gov/disorders/restless_legs/detail_restless_legs.htm

Noon, J. (2007). Assessment and management of clients with vascular disorders and problems of peripheral circulation. In R. A. Day, P. Paul, B. Williams, S. C. Smeltzer, & B. Bare (Eds.), *Brunner & Suddarth's textbook of medical-surgical nursing* (1st Canadian ed., pp. 819–851). Philadelphia: Lippincott Williams & Wilkins.

Olson, K. W. P., & Treat-Jacobson, D. (2004). Symptoms of peripheral arterial disease: A critical review. *Journal of Vascular Nursing, 22*(3), 72–77.

Ottawa Health Research Institute. (2006). *Monthly focus— Thrombosis researchers lead revolution in diagnosing and treating deadly blood clots.* Retrieved September 29, 2008, from http://www.ohri.ca/monthly_focus.asp?ID=40

Overfield, T. (1995). *Biologic variation in health and illness: Race, age and sex differences* (2nd ed.). Boca Raton, FL: CRC Press.

Philpott, M. (1985). *Legal liability & the nursing process* (pp. 90–93). Toronto, ON: W. B. Saunders, Canada Ltd.

Pieper, B., Templin, T. N., Birk, T. J., & Kirsner, R. S. (2007). Effects of injection-drug injury on ankle mobility and chronic venous disorders. *Journal of Nursing Scholarship, 39*(4), 312–318.

Public Health Agency of Canada. (2006). International note: Travel by air and health considerations. *Canada Communicable Disease Report, 32*(01), Ottawa, ON: Author. Retrieved March 10, 2008, from http://www.phac-aspc.gc.ca/publicat/ccdr-rmtc/06vol32/dr3201ea.html

Ross, C. J. M. (2007). Management of clients with chest and lower respiratory tract disorders. In R. A. Day, P. Paul, B. Williams, S. C. Smeltzer, & B. Bare (Eds.), *Brunner & Suddarth's textbook of medical-surgical nursing* (1st Canadian ed., pp. 552–556). Philadelphia: Lippincott Williams & Wilkins.

Schoen, F. J. (2005). Blood vessels. In V. Kumar, A. K. Abbas, & N. Fausto (Eds.), *Robbins and Cotran pathologic basis of disease* (pp. 511–554). Philadelphia: Elsevier Saunders.

Shields, M., & Tjepkema, M. (2006). Trends in adult obesity. *Health Reports, 17*(3), 53–59.

Sieggreen, M. (2006). A contemporary approach to peripheral arterial disease. *The Nurse Practitioner, 31*(7), 15–18, 23–25.

Society for Vascular Medicine and Biology (SVMB). (2007). *CPT code published for PAD vascular rehabilitation.* Retrieved March 13, 2008, from http://www.svmb.org/CPTCode.html

Spencer, F. A., Lessard, D., Emery, C., Reed, G., & Goldberg, R. J. (2007). Venous thromboembolism in the outclient setting. *Archives of Internal Medicine, 167*(14), 1471–1475.

Statistics Canada. (2007). *CANSIM Table 102-0529, Death by cause, Chapter IX: Diseases of circulatory system (I00 to I99), age group and sex, Canada, annual (2004).* Retrieved September 16, 2007, from http://cansim2.statcan.ca/cgi-win/cnsmcgi.pgm?Lang=E&ArrayId=1020529&Array_Pick=1&RootDir=CII/&ResultTemplate=CII\CII___

The Vein Institute of Toronto and Medical Aesthetic Clinic. (2008). *Medical compression stockings.* Retrieved March 18, 2009, from http://www.theveininstitute.com/stockings.php

Toronto Endovascular Centre. (2007). *Peripheral artery occlusive disease (PAD) and claudication.* Retrieved March 10, 2008, from http://www.torontoendovascularcentre.com/pat/pad_background.html

Transport Canada. (2007). *Deep vein thrombosis.* Retrieved March 13, 2008, from http://www.tc.gc.ca/CivilAviation/commerce/CabinSafety/DVT.htm

Warburton, D. E. R., Nicol, C. W., & Bredin, S. S. D. (2006). Health benefits of physical activity: The evidence. *Canadian Medical Association Journal, 174*(6), 801–809.

White, C. (2007). Intermittent claudication. *New England Journal of Medicine, 356*, 1241–1250.

White, R. H. (2003). Epidemiology of venous thromboembolism. *Circulation, 1107*, 14–18.

World Health Organization. (2007). *Exercise legs on long journeys, WHO advises.* Retrieved March 13, 2008, from http://www.cbc.ca/health/story/2007/06/28/dvt-travel.html

ADDITIONAL REFERENCES

Bates, S. M., & Giosberg, J. S. (2004). Treatment of deep-vein thrombosis. *New England Journal of Medicine, 351*(3), 268–276.

The Coalition to Prevent Deep-Vein Thrombosis. (2007). *Risk assessment tool: Are you at risk for a DVT blood clot?* Retrieved March 13, 2008, from http://www.preventdvt.org/docs/pdf/DVTRiskAssessmentTool.pdf

Falagas, M. E., & Vergidis, P. I. (2005). Narrative review: Diseases that masquerade as infectious cellulitis. *Annals of Internal Medicine, 142*(1), 47–55.

Vascular Disease Foundation. (2007). *Deep vein thrombosis (DVT).* Retrieved March 13, 2008, from http://www.vdf.org/pdfs/VDFOnePage_DVT_000.pdf

Wigley, F. M. (2002). Raynaud's phenomenon. *New England Journal of Medicine, 347*(13), 1001–1008.

BIBLIOGRAPHY

CANADIAN RESOURCES AND WEB SITES

Canadian Cardiovascular Society: http://www.ccs.ca

Canadian Council of Cardiovascular Nurses: http://www.cccn.ca

Canadian Hypertension Society: www.hypertension.ca/chs

The Canadian Best Practices Portal for Health Promotion and Chronic Disease Prevention: http://cbpp-pcpe.phac-aspc.gc.ca

Heart and Stroke Foundation of Canada: http://ww1.heartandstroke.ca

Ottawa Health Research Institute: http://www.ohri.ca/home.asp

Physical Activity Guide, Public Health Agency of Canada: http://www.phac-aspc.gc.ca/pau-uap/paguide/index.html

The Thrombosis Interest Group of Canada: http://www.tigc.org/

The Vein Institute of Toronto and Medical Aesthetic Clinic: http://www.theveininstitute.com/

Toronto Endovascular Centre: http://www.torontoendovascularcentre.com/

INTERNATIONAL WEB SITES

American Heart Association: http://www.americanheart.org

National Heart, Lung, and Blood Institute: http://www.nhlbi.nih.gov

Society for Vascular Medicine: http://www.svmb.org/

The Coalition to Prevent Deep-Vein Thrombosis: http://www.preventdvt.org

Vascular Disease Foundation: http://www.vdf.org/

TABLE 18-1 **Painful Peripheral Vascular Disorders and Their Mimics**

Problem	Process	Location of Pain
Arterial Disorders		
Atherosclerosis (arteriosclerosis obliterans)		
■ Intermittent claudication	Episodic muscular ischemia induced by exercise, due to obstruction of large or medium-sized arteries by atherosclerosis	Usually the calf, but also may be in the buttock, hip, thigh, or foot, depending on the level of obstruction
■ Rest pain	Ischemia even at rest	Distal pain, in the toes or forefoot
Acute Arterial Occlusion	Embolism or thrombosis, possibly superimposed on arteriosclerosis obliterans	Distal pain, usually involving the foot and leg
Raynaud's Disease and Phenomenon	*Raynaud's disease:* Episodic spasm of the small arteries and arterioles; no vascular occlusion *Raynaud's phenomenon:* Syndrome is secondary to other conditions such as collagen vascular disease, arterial occlusion, trauma, drugs	Distal portions of one or more fingers. Pain is usually not prominent unless fingertip ulcers develop. Numbness and tingling are common.
Venous Disorders		
Superficial Thrombophlebitis	Clot formation and acute inflammation in a superficial vein	Pain in a local area along the course of a superficial vein, most often in the saphenous system
Deep Venous Thrombosis	Clot formation in a deep vein	Pain, if present, is usually in the calf, but the process more often is painless.
Chronic Venous Insufficiency (deep)	Chronic venous engorgement secondary to venous occlusion or incompetency of venous valves	Diffuse aching of the leg(s)
Thromboangiitis Obliterans (Buerger's disease)	Inflammatory and thrombotic occlusions of small arteries and also of veins, occurring in smokers	■ Intermittent claudication, particularly in the arch of the foot ■ Rest pain in the fingers or toes
Acute Lymphangitis	Acute bacterial infection (usually streptococcal) spreading up the lymphatic channels from a portal of entry such as an injured area or an ulcer	An arm or a leg
Mimics*		
Acute Cellulitis	Acute bacterial infection of the skin and subcutaneous tissues	Arms, legs, or elsewhere
Erythema Nodosum	Subcutaneous inflammatory lesions associated with a variety of systemic conditions such as pregnancy, sarcoidosis, tuberculosis, and streptococcal infections	Anterior surfaces of both lower legs

* Mistaken primarily for acute superficial thrombophlebitis.

Timing	Factors That Aggravate	Factors That Relieve	Associated Manifestations
Fairly brief; pain usually forces the client to rest	Exercise such as walking	Rest usually stops the pain in 1–3 min.	Local fatigue, numbness, diminished pulses, often signs of arterial insufficiency (see p. 597)
Persistent, often worse at night	Elevation of the feet, as in bed	Sitting with legs dependent	Numbness, tingling, trophic signs, and colour changes of arterial insufficiency (see p. 587)
Sudden onset; associated symptoms may occur without pain			Coldness, numbness, weakness, absent distal pulses
Relatively brief (minutes) but recurrent	Exposure to cold, emotional upset	Warm environment	Colour changes in the distal fingers: severe pallor (essential for the diagnosis) followed by cyanosis and then redness
An acute episode lasting days or longer			Local redness, swelling, tenderness, a palpable cord, possibly fever
Often hard to determine because of lack of symptoms			Possibly swelling of the foot and calf and local calf tenderness; often nothing
Chronic, increasing as the day wears on	Prolonged standing	Elevation of the leg(s)	Chronic edema, pigmentation, possibly ulceration (see p. 599)
■ Fairly brief but recurrent ■ Chronic, persistent, may be worse at night	■ Exercise	■ Rest ■ Permanent cessation of smoking helps both kinds of pain	Distal coldness, sweating, numbness, and cyanosis; ulceration and gangrene at the tips of fingers or toes; migratory thrombophlebitis
An acute episode lasting days or longer			Red streak(s) on the skin, with tenderness; enlarged, tender lymph nodes; and fever
An acute episode lasting days or longer			A local area of diffuse swelling, redness, and tenderness with enlarged, tender lymph nodes and fever; no palpable cord
Pain associated with a series of lesions over several weeks			Raised, red, tender swellings recurring in crops; often malaise, joint pains, and fever

TABLE 18-2   Some Peripheral Causes of Edema

Approximately one-third of total body water is extracellular, or outside the body's cells. Approximately 25% of extracellular fluid is plasma; the remainder is interstitial fluid. At the arteriolar end of the capillaries, *hydrostatic pressure* in the blood vessels and *colloid oncotic pressure* in the interstitium cause fluid to move into the tissues; at the venous end of the capillaries and in the lymphatics, hydrostatic pressure in the interstitium and the colloid oncotic pressure of plasma proteins cause fluid to return to the vascular compartment. Several clinical conditions disrupt this balance, resulting in *edema*, or a clinically evident accumulation of interstitial fluid. Not depicted below is capillary leak syndrome, in which protein leaks into the interstitial space, seen in burns, angioedema, snake bites, and allergic reactions.

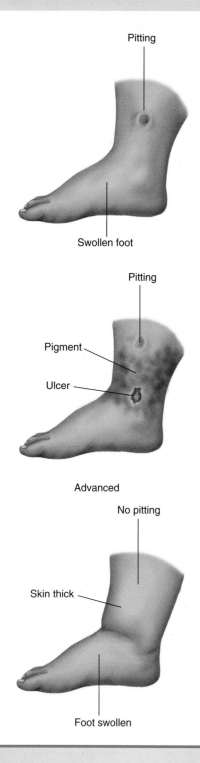

Pitting Edema

Edema is soft, bilateral, with pitting on pressure, and including the feet. There is no skin thickening, ulceration, or pigmentation. Pitting edema results when legs are dependent in cases of prolonged standing or sitting, which leads to increased hydrostatic pressure in the veins and capillaries; congestive heart failure leading to decreased cardiac output; increased hydrostatic pressure in the veins or capillaries; nephrotic syndrome, cirrhosis, or malnutrition leading to low albumin and decreased intravascular colloid oncotic pressure; and drug use.

Chronic Venous Insufficiency

Edema is soft, with pitting on pressure; it may progress to brawny (hard). Skin may be thickened, especially near the ankle. Ulceration, pigmentation, and edema in the feet are common, occasionally in a bilateral presentation. Examples include chronic obstruction or valvular incompetence of the deep veins.

Lymphedema

Edema is soft in the early stages, then becomes indurated, hard, and nonpitting. Skin is markedly thickened; ulceration is rare. There is no pigmentation. Edema is found in the feet and toes, often bilaterally. Lymphedema develops in cases of lymph channels obstructed by tumour, fibrosis, or inflammation, as well as in the arms in cases of axillary node dissection and radiation.

TABLE 18-3   **Chronic Insufficiency of Arteries and Veins**

Chronic Arterial Insufficiency *(Advanced)*

Chronic Venous Insufficiency *(Advanced)*

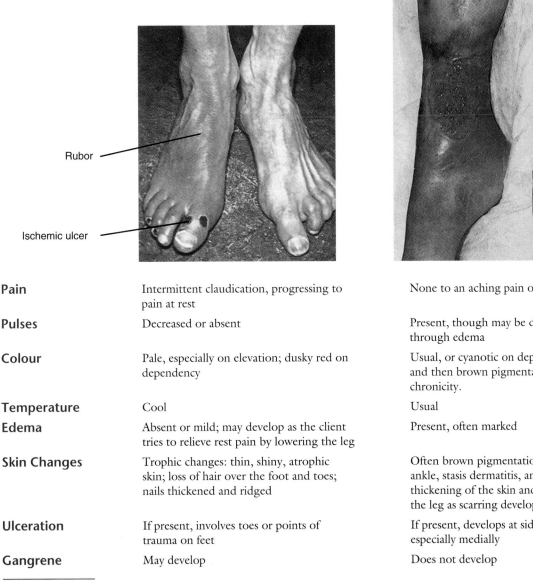

Rubor

Ischemic ulcer

	Chronic Arterial Insufficiency (Advanced)	Chronic Venous Insufficiency (Advanced)
Pain	Intermittent claudication, progressing to pain at rest	None to an aching pain on dependency
Pulses	Decreased or absent	Present, though may be difficult to feel through edema
Colour	Pale, especially on elevation; dusky red on dependency	Usual, or cyanotic on dependency. Petechiae and then brown pigmentation appear with chronicity.
Temperature	Cool	Usual
Edema	Absent or mild; may develop as the client tries to relieve rest pain by lowering the leg	Present, often marked
Skin Changes	Trophic changes: thin, shiny, atrophic skin; loss of hair over the foot and toes; nails thickened and ridged	Often brown pigmentation around the ankle, stasis dermatitis, and possible thickening of the skin and narrowing of the leg as scarring develops
Ulceration	If present, involves toes or points of trauma on feet	If present, develops at sides of ankle, especially medially
Gangrene	May develop	Does not develop

Photo sources: Arterial Insufficiency—Kappert, A., & Winsor, T. Diagnosis of Peripheral Vascular Disease. Philadelphia: FA Davis, 1972; Venous Insufficiency—Marks, R. Skin Disease in Old Age. Philadelphia: JB Lippincott, 1987.

TABLE 18-4   Internal and External Causes of Compartment Syndrome

	Acute Compartment Syndrome	Chronic Compartment Syndrome	Crush Syndrome
Internal Source	■ Edema ■ Bleeding ■ Contusions ■ Fractures ■ Burns ■ Inactivity after surgery ■ Infiltrated IV sites	■ Exercise ■ Increased muscle volume ■ History of previous fracture, casting, or extremity surgery	

External Source	■ Tight dressing or cast
	■ Braces
	■ Traction
	■ Surgical positioning
	■ Pneumatic antishock garments
	■ Automatic blood pressure devices
	■ Burn eschar
			■ Crush injury with muscle infarction. Examples:
			  ■ Trapped under heavy equipment or fallen objects
			  ■ Overdose, with extremity under body
			  ■ Wringer-type injury

Symptoms and Signs	■ Increasing pain out of proportion to etiology ■ Deep, unrelenting, throbbing and localized pain ■ Pain with passive stretch ■ Paresthesias (burning, tingling) ■ Taut skin ■ Muscle feels edematous and hard ■ Sensation deficit (hypoesthesia) ■ Motor weakness ■ Usual occurrence 6–8 h after injury	■ Positive history of exercise ■ Limb tightness, aching ■ Point tenderness over muscle ■ Rare to have neurological deficits ■ Usually resolved with rest	■ Deep pain ■ Severe edema ■ Taut skin ■ Vesicles, bulla with erythema ■ Hypovolemia ■ Hyperkalemia

Adapted from Altizer, 2006 and Friesen & Larsen, 2007.

TABLE 18-5   Common Ulcers of the Feet and Ankles

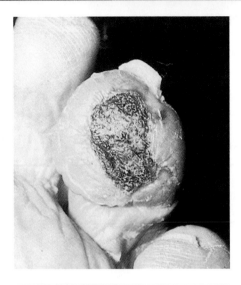

Arterial Insufficiency

This condition occurs in the toes, feet, or possibly in areas of trauma (e.g., the shins). Surrounding skin shows no callus or excess pigment, although it may be atrophic. Pain often is severe unless neuropathy masks it. Gangrene may be associated, along with decreased pulses, trophic changes, foot pallor on elevation, and dusky rubor on dependency.

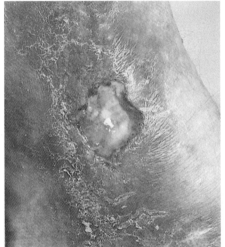

Chronic Venous Insufficiency

This condition appears on the inner or sometimes outer ankle. Surrounding skin is pigmented and sometimes fibrotic. Pain is not severe, with no gangrene. Associated signs include edema, pigmentation, stasis dermatitis, and possibly cyanosis of the foot on dependency.

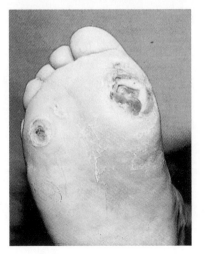

Neuropathic Ulcer

This condition develops in pressure points of areas with diminished sensation (e.g., with diabetic polyneuropathy). Surrounding skin is calloused. There is no pain, which sometimes results in the ulcer going unnoticed. In uncomplicated cases, there is no gangrene. Associated signs include decreased sensation and absent ankle jerks.

Photo source: Marks, R. *Skin Disease in Old Age*. Philadelphia: JB Lippincott, 1987.

Description	Depression Depth	Time for Pitting to Disappear	Grade
Slight pitting	2 mm	Disappears rapidly	1+
Deeper pitting	4 mm	10–15 sec	2+
Visible swelling of extremity	6 mm	More than 1 min	3+
Grossly swollen extremity	8 mm	Up to 2–3 min	4+

Adapted from Dillon, P. M. (2007). *Nursing Health Assessment: Clinical Pocket Guide* (2nd ed., p. 180). Philadelphia: F. A. Davis.

The Musculoskeletal System

Sheri Roach, Pat Roddick, and Lynn S. Bickley

ASSESSING THE MUSCULOSKELETAL SYSTEM

Composed of bones, joints, and muscles, the musculoskeletal system serves several purposes in the body. Physical assessment often is focused on the structure, support, and movement this system provides, but other functions include protection of internal organs, production of red blood cells (*hematopoiesis*), and storage of calcium and phosphorus in the bones. Musculoskeletal disorders (MSDs) are common throughout the lifespan, and a complete musculoskeletal assessment allows nurses to identify risk factors, unexpected findings, or dysfunction early, and to plan appropriate health promotion, teaching, and interventions.

GUIDE TO ORGANIZATION OF THIS CHAPTER

Musculoskeletal issues and disorders are leading causes of health care visits in Canada (Murphy et al., 2006). For example, statistics show that 80% of Canadian adults have at least one episode of back pain in their lives (Schultz & Kopec, 2003), and almost all Canadians have some degree of osteoarthritis by 70 years (Public Health Agency of Canada [PHAC], 2006). This chapter serves to help strengthen your approach and examination skills as you master assessment of common conditions of the joints.

This chapter presents the structure and function of the major joints and their connecting bony structures, muscles, and soft tissues. Because of the specialized nature of joint assessment, the organization of the chapter is a unique departure from other regional examination chapters in this book. Physical assessment of joint concerns requires both visualization and thorough knowledge of surface landmarks and underlying anatomy. To help students pair their knowledge of each joint's structure and function with its related methods of examination, the Anatomy and Physiology and Techniques of Examination for each joint *are combined*. The format of the chapter is as follows:

FORMAT OF THIS CHAPTER

- Structure and Function of Joints
- The Health History
- Health Promotion
- Examination of Specific Joints: Anatomy and Physiology and Related Techniques of Examination. To promote a systematic approach to the examination of the musculoskeletal system, the sections on p. 616 follow a "head-to-toe" sequence, beginning with the jaw and joints of the upper extremities, then proceeding to the spine and hip and the joints of the lower extremities:
  - Temporomandibular Joint
  - Shoulder
  - Elbow
  - Wrist and Hand
  - Spine
  - Hip
  - Knee and Lower Leg
  - Ankle and Foot

For each of these joints there are subsections on *Joint Overview, Bony Structures and Joints, Muscle Groups and Additional Structures,* and *Techniques of Examination.*

- The *Joint Overview* is designed to orient you to the distinguishing anatomical and functional characteristics of each joint. As you study the subsequent subsections, practice identifying the important surface landmarks on yourself or a fellow student.
- Then turn to *Techniques of Examination* to learn the fundamental steps for examining that joint—inspection, palpation of bony landmarks and soft-tissue structures, assessment of range of motion (or the directions of joint movement), and techniques to test the joint's function and stability. Mastering these techniques is one of the challenges of successful examination of the musculoskeletal system and will require both supervision and practice. These techniques are increasingly important to identifying unexpected findings and planning health promotion activities.

STRUCTURE AND FUNCTION OF JOINTS

It is helpful to begin by reviewing some anatomical terminology.

- *Articular structures* include the joint capsule and articular cartilage, the synovium and synovial fluid, intra-articular ligaments, and juxta-articular bone.

- *Nonarticular structures* include periarticular ligaments, tendons, bursae, muscle, fascia, bone, nerve, and overlying skin.

- *Ligaments* are ropelike bundles of collagen fibres that connect bone to bone.

- *Tendons* are collagen fibres connecting muscle to bone. Another type of collagen matrix forms the *cartilage* that overlies bony surfaces.

- *Bursae* are pouches of synovial fluid that cushion the movement of tendons and muscles over bone or other joint structures.

To understand joint function, study the various types of joints and how they articulate, or interconnect, and the role of bursae in easing joint movement.

TYPES OF JOINTS

There are three primary types of joint articulation—synovial, cartilaginous, and fibrous—allowing varying degrees of joint movement.

■ *Joints*

Type of Joint	Extent of Movement	Example
Synovial	Freely movable	Knee, shoulder
Cartilaginous	Slightly movable	Vertebral bodies of the spine
Fibrous	Immovable	Skull sutures

Synovial Joints. The bones do not touch each other, and the joint articulations are *freely moveable*. The bones are covered by *articular cartilage* and separated by a *synovial cavity* that cushions joint movement, as shown. A *synovial membrane* lines the synovial cavity and secretes a small amount of viscous lubricating fluid—the *synovial fluid*. The membrane is attached at the margins of the articular cartilage and pouched or folded to accommodate joint movement. Surrounding the synovial membrane is a fibrous *joint capsule*, which is strengthened by ligaments extending from bone to bone.

Cartilaginous Joints. These joints, such as those between vertebrae and the symphysis pubis, are *slightly moveable*. Fibrocartilaginous discs separate the bony surfaces. At the center of each disc is the *nucleus pulposus*, fibrocartilaginous material that serves as a cushion or shock absorber between bony surfaces.

Fibrous Joints. In these joints, such as the sutures of the skull, intervening layers of fibrous tissue or cartilage hold the bones together. The bones are almost in direct contact, which allows *no appreciable movement*.

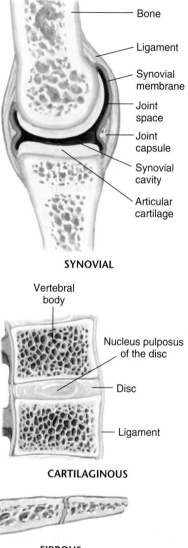

SYNOVIAL

CARTILAGINOUS

FIBROUS

STRUCTURE OF SYNOVIAL JOINTS

As you learn about the examination of the musculoskeletal system, think about how the anatomy of the joint relates to its movement.

■ Synovial Joints

Type of Joint	Articular Shape	Movement	Example
Spheroidal (ball and socket)	Convex surface in concave cavity	Wide-ranging flexion, extension, abduction, adduction, rotation, circumduction	Shoulder, hip
Hinge	Flat, planar	Motion in one plane; flexion, extension	Interphalangeal joints of hand and foot; elbow
Condylar	Convex or concave	Movement of two articulating surfaces not dissociable	Knee; temporo-mandibular joint

Many of the joints we examine are *synovial*, or movable, *joints*. The shape of the articulating surfaces of synovial joints determines the direction and extent of joint motion.

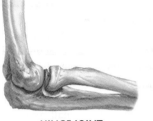

HINGE JOINT

- *Spheroidal joints* have a ball-and-socket configuration—a rounded, convex surface articulating with a cuplike cavity, allowing a wide range of rotatory movement, as in the shoulder and hip.

**SPHEROIDAL JOINT
(BALL AND SOCKET)**

- *Hinge joints* are flat, planar, or slightly curved, allowing only a gliding motion in a single plane, as in flexion and extension of the elbow.

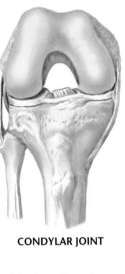

- In *condylar joints*, such as the knee, the articulating surfaces are convex or concave, termed condyles.

CONDYLAR JOINT

Bursae.   Easing joint action are *bursae*, roughly disc-shaped synovial sacs that allow adjacent muscles or muscles and tendons to glide over each other during movement. They lie between the skin and the convex surface of a bone or joint (as in the prepatellar bursa of the knee, p. 652) or in areas where tendons or muscles rub against bone, ligaments, or other tendons or muscles (as in the subacromial bursa of the shoulder, p. 623).

Knowledge of the underlying joint anatomy and movement will help you assess joints subjected to trauma. Your knowledge of the soft-tissue structures, ligaments, tendons, and bursae will help you evaluate the changes of aging, as well as arthritis.

THE HEALTH HISTORY: SUBJECTIVE DATA

Key Symptoms and Signs Reported by Clients

- Back pain
- Neck pain
- Joint pain
- Swollen, warm joints
- Joint pain in association with other symptoms (fever, chills, rash, anorexia, weight loss)

- Weakness
- Muscle pain
- Joint stiffness
- Decreased mobility
- Bruising

A thorough and accurate health history or, at the very least, a focused health history directed at the musculoskeletal system is an essential starting point for assessment. Pain, weakness, and stiffness are three of the most common concerns of clients seeking assistance for musculoskeletal issues. In addition to collecting the usual elements of symptom analysis, the following three tips will guide your subsequent examination and nursing diagnoses:

- Ask the client to point to the area of pain, stiffness, or weakness. This helps to establish the location.

- Clarify and record the mechanism of injury, if applicable, particularly if there is a history of trauma.

- Determine whether pain is localized or diffuse, acute or chronic, and inflammatory or noninflammatory.

Begin the health history with general open-ended questions such as, "Tell me how you are feeling" or "Describe any concerns you have about how you are feeling." To gain more comprehensive information about the sign or symptom, conduct an analysis of it.

BACK PAIN

You may wish to begin with "Any pains in your back?" because *backache* is the most common and widespread disorder of the musculoskeletal system. Use your health history interview to develop a clear picture of the issue, especially its location. Establish whether the pain is on the midline, in the area of the vertebrae, or off the midline. If the pain radiates into the legs or feet, ask about any associated numbness, tingling, or weakness.

See Table 19-1, Low Back Pain, p. 670.

Causes of *midline back pain* include musculoskeletal strain, vertebral collapse, disc herniation, or spinal cord metastases. *Pain of the midline* may arise from sacroiliitis, trochanteric bursitis, sciatica, or arthritis in the hips.

NECK PAIN

Neck pain is also common, especially after trauma. Approach it in the same manner. For both neck and back pain, be especially alert for symptoms such as weakness, loss of sensation, or loss of bladder or bowel function.

See Table 19-2, Pains in the Neck, p. 671.

Motor or sensory deficits, loss of bladder or bowel function in spinal cord compression at S2–S4

JOINT PAIN

To pursue other MSDs ask, "Do you have any pains in your joints?"

Joint pain may be *localized, diffuse, or systemic*. Ask the client to *point to the pain*. If the joint pain is localized and involves only one joint, it is *monoarticular*. Pain originating in the small joints of the hands and feet is more sharply localized than that from the larger joints. Pain from the hip joint is especially deceptive. Although it is typically felt in the groin or buttock, it is sometimes felt in the anterior thigh or partly or solely in the knee.

Pain in one joint suggests trauma, monoarticular arthritis, possible tendonitis, or bursitis. Hip pain near the greater trochanter suggests *trochanteric bursitis*.

More diffuse joint pain may be *polyarticular*, involving several joints. Ask whether the pain involves one joint or several joints. If polyarticular, what is the pattern of involvement—migrating from joint to joint or steadily spreading from one joint to multiple joint involvement? Is the involvement symmetric, affecting similar joints on both sides of the body?

Migratory pattern of spread in *rheumatic fever* or *gonococcal arthritis*; progressive additive pattern with symmetric involvement typically in *rheumatoid arthritis*

Note that joint pain may also be *nonarticular*, involving bones, muscles, and tissues around the joint such as the tendons, bursae, or even overlying skin. Generalized "aches and pains" are called *myalgias* if in muscles and *arthralgias* if there is pain but no evidence of arthritis.

Problems in tissues around joints include inflammation of bursae (*bursitis*), tendons (*tendonitis*), or tendon sheaths (*tenosynovitis*); also *sprains* from stretching or tearing of ligaments.

Assess the chronicity, quality, and severity of the joint symptoms. *Timing* is especially important. Did the pain or discomfort develop rapidly over the course of a few hours or insidiously over weeks or even months? Has the pain progressed slowly or fluctuated? With periods of improvement? And worsening? How long has the pain lasted? What is it like over the course of a day—in the morning and as the day wears on?

Severe pain of rapid onset in a swollen joint in the absence of trauma seen in *acute septic arthritis* or *gout*. In children consider *osteomyelitis* in bone contiguous to a joint.

If more rapid in onset, how did the pain arise? Was there an acute injury? Or overuse from repetitive motion of the same part of the body? If the pain comes from trauma, what was the *mechanism of injury* or the series of events that caused the joint pain? Further, what aggravates pain? What relieves the pain? What are the effects of exercise, rest, and treatment?

See Table 19-3, Patterns of Pain in and Around the Joints, pp. 672–673.

Try to determine whether the problem is *inflammatory* or *noninflammatory*. Is there *tenderness*? *Warmth*? Or *redness*? These features are best assessed on examination, but clients can sometimes guide you to points of tenderness. Ask about systemic symptoms such as fever or chills.

Fever, chills, warmth, redness in *septic arthritis;* also consider *gout* or possible *rheumatic fever.*

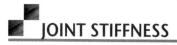

JOINT STIFFNESS

Additional symptoms can help you decide if the pain is *articular* in origin, such as *swelling*, *stiffness*, or *decreased range of motion*. Localize any *swelling* as accurately as possible. If *stiffness* is present, it may be difficult to assess because people use the term differently. In the context of musculoskeletal issues, stiffness refers to a perceived tightness or resistance to movement, the opposite of feeling limber. It is often associated with discomfort or pain. If the client does not report stiffness spontaneously, ask about it and try to calculate its duration. Find out when the client gets up in the morning and when the joints feel the most limber.

Pain, swelling, loss of active and passive motion, "locking," deformity in *articular joint pain,* loss of active but not passive motion, tenderness outside the joint, absence of deformity often in *nonarticular pain* Stiffness and limited motion after inactivity, sometimes called *gelling,* in degenerative joint disease but usually lasts only a few minutes; stiffness lasting ≥30 minutes in rheumatoid arthritis and other inflammatory arthritides. Stiffness also with *fibromyalgia* and *polymyalgia rheumatica (PMR).*

To assess *limitations of motion*, ask about changes in level of activity because of problems with the involved joint. When relevant, inquire specifically about the client's ability to walk, stand, lean over, sit up, rise from a sitting position, climb, pinch, grasp, turn a page, open a door handle or jar, and care for bodily needs such as combing hair, brushing teeth, eating, dressing, and bathing.

JOINT PAIN ASSOCIATED WITH OTHER SYMPTOMS

Some problems originating in the joints have *systemic* features such as fever, chills, rash, anorexia, weight loss, and weakness.

Generalized symptoms are common in *rheumatoid arthritis, systemic lupus erythematosus (SLE), PMR,* and other inflammatory arthritides. High fever and chills suggest an infectious cause.

Other joint disorders may be linked to *organ systems outside the musculoskeletal system*. Symptoms elsewhere in the body can give important clues to these conditions. Be alert to symptoms such as the following:

- *Skin conditions*

  - A butterfly rash on the cheeks

Systemic lupus erythematosus

- The scaly rash and pitted nails of psoriasis

Psoriatic arthritis

- A few papules, pustules, or vesicles on reddened bases, located on the distal extremities

Gonococcal arthritis

- An expanding erythematous patch early in an illness

Lyme disease

- Hives

Serum sickness, drug reaction

- Erosions or scale on the penis and crusted scaling papules on the soles and palms

Reiter's syndrome, which also includes arthritis, urethritis, and uveitis

- The maculopapular rash of rubella

Arthritis of *rubella*

- Clubbing of the fingernails (see p. 277)

Hypertrophic osteoarthropathy

- Red, burning, and itchy eyes (*conjunctivitis*)

Reiter's syndrome, Behcet's syndrome (Sakane et al., 1999)

- Preceding *sore throat*

Acute rheumatic fever or *gonococcal arthritis*

- *Diarrhea, abdominal pain, cramping*

Arthritis with *ulcerative colitis, regional enteritis, scleroderma*

- Symptoms of *urethritis*

Reiter's syndrome or possibly *gonococcal arthritis*

- Mental status change, facial or other weakness, stiff neck

Lyme disease with central nervous system involvement

MUSCLE PAIN

Muscle pain often feels like cramping or soreness. Healthy people experience muscle soreness after unusually strenuous muscular exertion; such symptoms tend to peak at approximately the second day after exertion. In the acute stage, pain indicates tissue damage; however, chronic muscle pain may persist in the absence of detectable trauma (The Canadian Chiropractic Association, 1996).

Mild paralysis (paresis) in *multiple sclerosis* (Multiple Sclerosis in Newfoundland & Labrador, 2006) or fluctuating weakness of muscle groups in *myasthenia gravis* (Myasthenia Gravis Association of BC, 2008). Muscle weakness caused by chronic use of corticosteroids.

MUSCLE WEAKNESS

Muscle weakness may be associated with injury or certain diseases. It can migrate from one muscle to another or between muscle groups. Identifying whether weakness is related to proximal or distal muscle groups also may be helpful. Proximal weakness often is related to *myopathy* (a disease in the muscle tissue), while distal weakness is more often the result of *neuropathy* (a disease of the nervous system). Muscular weakness in the proximal arm muscles may manifest as difficulty lifting objects or combing hair, while muscular weakness in the distal arm muscles often presents as difficulty dressing or turning doorknobs.

Example Questions for Symptom Analysis—Decreased Joint Mobility

- "Which joint(s) are you having difficulty moving?" "Please point to the area(s)?" (*Location, radiating*)
- "What movements are difficult for you?" "Describe what the movement feels like." (*Quality*)
- "Please tell me how much movement you have with the joint(s)." "On a scale of 0 to 10 with 0 being no movement and 10 being easy, free movement, how would you rate your mobility of this joint?" (*Quantity/severity*)
- "Did it start suddenly? Gradually?" "Did a particular event cause the decrease in mobility?" (*Onset*) "How long has it been difficult moving this joint?" (*Duration*) "Is there a time of day that it (joint mobility) is worse? Better?" (*Time of day/month/year*)
- "What makes the movement worse?" (*Aggravating factors*)
- "What makes it (joint mobility) better?" (*Alleviating factors*)

- "How does exercise affect your ability to move the joint(s)?" (*Aggravating/alleviating factors*)
- "Have you noticed any other symptoms? Swelling? Chills? Fever?" "Do you have pain associated with your difficulty moving the joint(s)?" "Describe the pain to me." (*Associated symptoms*)
- "How would you describe your work in terms of being physically demanding" "Are there particular motions you perform several times a day?" "Do you play any sports?" "What kind of stress is in your life right now?" (*Environmental factors*)
- "How is this affecting your daily life?" (*Significance to client*)
- "What do you think is happening?" (*Client perspective*)

HEALTH PROMOTION

Important Topics for Health Promotion

- Prevention of back injury
- Prevention of osteoporosis
- Health promotion related to osteoarthritis
- Prevention of falls
- Risk factor assessment
- Screening
- Emergency concerns

Musculoskeletal health is becoming a prominent global issue. In 2003, the World Health Organization (WHO) published *The Burden of Musculoskeletal Disease at the Start of the New Millennium*, a report focused on the growing effects of international musculoskeletal health. The report states that musculoskeletal injuries are the most common cause of disability in the developed world and have enormous social and economic consequences that will increase proportionately with the aging populations of these countries. The WHO report also identifies that the growing success of treating communicable diseases and reducing childhood mortality in developing countries, combined with an increase in traffic-related accidents, is causing more musculoskeletal injuries and conditions in these countries.

In Canada, diseases and injuries of the musculoskeletal system significantly affect the health of its people. Statistics Canada documented the effects of musculoskeletal pain, reduced physical functioning, and fatigue on Canadians' activities of daily living, including social and work commitments. Research has linked musculoskeletal dysfunction to emotional problems, including anxiety and depression (Murphy et al., 2006). As such, it is important to review the more common musculoskeletal health issues that nurses may address through health promotion. These include prevention of back injury, osteoporosis, osteoarthritis, and falls, as well as demographic risk factors, workplace and lifestyle contributors, screening, and emergency concerns.

PREVENTION OF BACK INJURY

Almost two-thirds of Canadians have at least one episode of back pain in their lives (Statistics Canada, 2006). Of those, this pain disables 1 in 50 (Statistics Canada, 2006). Back pain can occur at any point along the spine and may manifest as soreness, muscle tension, stiffness, tingling, burning, or weakness in the legs or feet (The Arthritis Society, 2007a). When discomfort originates in the cervical region of the spine, it is usually described as neck pain, but neck pain will be grouped with back pain. Back pain is classified as acute or chronic. Acute back pain lasts weeks or less, while chronic pain is classified as lasting longer than 3 months (The Arthritis Society, 2007a).

Stress on the muscles and ligaments that support the vertebrae often causes back pain, which most commonly affects the lumbar region, because this region tends to carry more weight than other areas of the spine (The Arthritis Society, 2007a). One of the most vulnerable parts of the skeleton is L5-S1, where the sacral vertebra makes a sharp posterior angle. Back pain also can originate in bone, intervertebral discs, and nerves. Men and women experience back pain with equal frequency, and it occurs most commonly in people 30 to 50 years (National Institute for Neurological Disorders and Stroke, 2003). Acute back pain sometimes may be attributed directly to a single cause, such as trauma, improper lifting, illness, or disease. More commonly, however, no specific precipitating event can be identified, especially with chronic back pain (Hicks et al., 2002).

Research shows that the insidious causes of back pain are largely preventable. Poor posture is the most common cause of back pain, with other major contributors including lack of exercise, excess body weight, and emotional stress (The Arthritis Society of Canada, 2007a). All these issues fall into the realm of health promotion teaching by nurses and other health practitioners. Client education about the importance of keeping a neutral head position, holding shoulders in alignment, and maintaining the natural curvature of the spine can contribute to the prevention of back pain and injury (The College of Family Physicians of Canada, 2007). Education about lifting strategies and biomechanics of injury is prudent for clients who do repetitive lifting, such as nurses, heavy-machinery operators, and construction workers. For occupational back pain, increasing graded physical activity and behavioural counselling show promise in improving functional status and return to work (Stahl et al., 2004).

PREVENTION OF OSTEOPOROSIS

Osteoporosis is a disease characterized by decreased bone strength, which leads to bone fragility and risk of fracture (Osteoporosis Canada, 2007a). Bone strength reflects two elements: bone density, which is the interaction between bone mass, new bone formation, and bone resorption by the body; and bone quality, which refers to the physical structure of the bone. The WHO (2003) uses bone density to define osteoporosis. A 10% decrease in bone density is associated with a 20% increase in risk for fracture.

Osteoporosis can strike at any age; however, it is most common in older adults. In Canada, one in four women and one in eight men have osteoporosis (Osteoporosis

Canada, 2007a). Osteoporosis is insidious, meaning that no symptoms precede a fracture (Osteoporosis Canada, 2007b). When osteoporosis has weakened bones, a forceful sneeze or simple movements like bending over to lift a bag of groceries can result in broken bones (Osteoporosis Canada, 2007b). The most common fractures associated with osteoporosis are vertebral compression fractures, followed by fractures of the hip and wrist (Osteoporosis Canada, 2007c; Siminoski, 2005). More than 1.6 million hip fractures occur in Canada each year, which equals approximately one every 20 seconds (The Bone Wellness Centre, 2007). In Canada, 70% of hip fractures are attributed to osteoporosis, and 20% of these fractures are fatal (Osteoporosis Canada, 2007c). Of the survivors, 50% have a permanent disability (Osteoporosis Canada, 2007c).

Awareness of risk factors and efforts to slow bone loss can reduce a client's risk of osteoporosis. Key nonmodifiable risk factors include age more than 50 years, postmenopausal status for women, prior fractures, history of falls, and family history of fragility fractures (Osteoporosis Canada, 2007a). The most significant risk factor for osteoporosis-related fractures is low bone mineral density (Osteoporosis Canada, 2007a). While it may not be possible to prevent low bone mineral density altogether, attending to modifiable risk factors may slow bone loss. Modifiable risk factors include poor nutrition, lack of physical activity, use of alcohol and tobacco, and being overweight (Osteoporosis Canada, 2007d). Use of certain medications, for example, corticosteroids, can also contribute to osteoporosis (Osteoporosis Canada, 2007a), but cessation may be undesirable, depending on the client's other health issues.

Research findings over the past several years are conflicting related to the effects of caffeine intake on bone health. Currently, Osteoporosis Canada's position is that the healthy adult population is not at risk of adverse effects from caffeine on bone health if they limit intake to 400 mg/day (500–750 mL of coffee), as recommended by Canada's Food Guide (Health Canada, 2007a). If a client is drinking more than four cups of coffee daily, he or she should add a glass of milk for each cup of coffee (Osteoporosis Canada, 2007e).

Vitamin D. Vitamin D and calcium are important dietary elements related to bone health because they inhibit bone resorption. Vitamin D_3 (cholecalciferol) is necessary for healthy muscles and to prevent osteoporosis and forms of cancer such as breast, colorectal, and prostate (Canadian Cancer Society, 2007). Vitamin D prevents osteoporosis by increasing calcium absorption from 30% to 80% (Osteoporosis Canada, 2007f). One glass (250 mL) of fortified milk provides approximately 100 IU of vitamin D (Osteoporosis Canada, 2007f). Both sodium (salt) (mostly from food) and caffeine (mostly from coffee and colas) contribute to calcium loss from the body in the urine (Osteoporosis Canada, 2007e).

While skin can synthesize vitamin D_3 from sunlight (ultraviolet exposure [UVB]), Canada's northern location means that from October to March, the sun's rays are too low and not strong enough for synthesis. Use of sunscreen also reduces natural production of vitamin D. Currently there is no consensus on the daily recommended supplemental amount of vitamin D. Some recommendations are as follows:

- 400 IU for adults older than 50 years (Health Canada, 2007b)

- 400 IU for Canadians 19 to 50 years (Osteoporosis Canada, 2007f)

- 800 IU for Canadians older than 50 years (Osteoporosis Canada, 2007f)

- 1000 IU for all adults during fall and winter months (Canadian Cancer Society, 2007)

Calcium. Excellent sources of calcium are foods such as milk, cheese, and yogurt that contain high amounts of calcium that can be easily absorbed. Calcium has been added to some soy beverages and orange juices. Other sources include vegetables, canned salmon and sardines (fish with bones), and meat alternatives (beans and lentils) (Osteoporosis Canada, 2007g).

Information about the amount of daily calcium required is conflicting. Osteoporosis Canada (2007e) suggests 1300 mg/day for people 9 to 18 years, 1000 mg/day for those 19 to 50 years, and 1500 mg/day for those older than 50 years. Health Canada (2007b) recommends 3-plus servings of milk and alternatives daily for clients 9 to 18 years (900 to 1200 mg of calcium); 2 servings daily for those 19 to 50 years (600 mg of calcium); and 2 servings daily for people older than 50 years (900 mg of calcium). One serving equals 250 mL (1 cup) of milk, 175 g (3/4 cup) of yogurt, or 50 g (1.5 oz) of cheese. Note that one serving of milk (250 mL) contains 300 mg of calcium (Osteoporosis Canada, 2007e).

Another compelling element of health promotion related to the musculoskeletal system is the implication of bone growth in childhood on future health. Ninety percent of skeletal growth occurs by age 17 years, and peak bone mass occurs by age 16 years in females and age 20 years in males (Osteoporosis Canada, 2007g). Without adequate nutrition and physical activity, the quality of this bone is lacking, leaving clients more prone to osteoporosis (Bone Health and Fracture Prevention Steering Committee [BHFPSC], 2001). As well, research shows approximately half of Canadian girls are on reduced-calorie diets, making it difficult for them to obtain the calcium and vitamin D necessary for healthy bone development. Studies in the United States estimate that only 10% of girls and 25% of boys ingest appropriate amounts of calcium in their diets (BHFPSC, 2001). Therefore, osteoporosis has been called a pediatric disease with serious geriatric consequences.

HEALTH PROMOTION RELATED TO OSTEOARTHRITIS

Arthritis is a blanket term for more than 100 different conditions ranging from relatively mild single-joint problems (e.g., tendonitis, bursitis), to crippling systemic diseases (e.g., rheumatoid arthritis). All types involve some form of inflammation of the joints (The Arthritis Society, 2007b). Nearly one in every six Canadians older than 15 years has arthritis, and almost two-thirds of arthritis sufferers are younger than 65 years, making this a significant problem for this population (Health Canada, 2003).

Osteoarthritis is the most common form of arthritis (Health Canada, 2003). It causes pain, stiffness, and reduced movement of the affected joints, eventually affecting physical ability and quality of life (Osteoporosis Canada, 2007b). While osteoarthritis, which involves destruction of the cartilage that protects the ends of the bones and damage to the underlying bone, cannot truly be prevented because it develops naturally in aging joints, clients can take several steps to slow the degenerative process (Obesity Canada, 2001). For example, maintaining a healthy weight is an effective way to slow the development of osteoarthritis. Obesity Canada reports that overweight people develop osteoarthritis at a much younger age (Obesity Canada, 2001). While weight loss will not prevent osteoarthritis, it will relieve joint pain and may slow the progression of the disease by decreasing the pressure placed on joints. The most commonly replaced joints as a result of osteoarthritis are knees and hips (Osteoporosis Canada, 2007d). Additionally, osteoarthritis develops more commonly in overused or injured joints (Osteoporosis Canada, 2007b). Health promotion can raise awareness that occupation-related or recreational sports-related overuse of particular joints can contribute to osteoarthritis.

At the other end of the spectrum, inactivity can also contribute to osteoarthritis, which is another topic for nurses to target in health promotion efforts with clients.

FALL PREVENTION

Unintentional falls account for more than half of all hospital injury admissions in Canada (Mirolla, 2004). A 2004 Canadian report showed that adults older than 65 years account for 48% of all fractures and dislocations of the lower limbs and 27% of all fractures and dislocations of the upper limbs (Mirolla, 2004). The fall-related injury rate is nine times greater among seniors than among those younger than 65 years (PHAC, 2005a).

Concern about falls among Canada's senior citizen population and related health issues gained attention throughout the 1990s (PHAC, 2005b). Fall prevention has become a major movement in health promotion across Canada, led by a joint effort between Health Canada and Veterans Affairs Canada (PHAC, 2005b). The magnitude of the problem is reflected in the 300% increase in publications from 1985 to 2005 about falls among older adults (Close, 2005). The PHAC (2005b) lists several risk factors for falls in four categories:

1. Biological and Medical Risk Factors

   - Muscle weakness/reduced physical fitness
   - Advanced age
   - Gender
   - Impaired control of balance and gait
   - Vision changes
   - Chronic disease or conditions (e.g., arthritis, stroke, Parkinson's disease, hypotension)
   - Physical disabilities
   - Acute illness (in relation to the symptoms of disease and the loss in bone density from even short periods of inactivity)
   - Cognitive impairment
   - Depression

2. Behavioural Risk Factors

   - History of previous falls (increases the risk of repeat falls threefold)
   - Risk-taking behaviours (e.g., standing on unsteady chairs, not using prescribed mobility devices)
   - Certain medications and polypharmacy
   - Excessive consumption of alcohol
   - Choice of footwear and clothing
   - Inactivity and inadequate nutrition
   - Fear of falling (can lead to reduction of activities needed to maintain confidence, strength, and balance, as well as to maladaptive changes in balance control such as stiffening)

3. Environmental Risk Factors

- Stairs (especially those without uniform risers, handrails, or gripping surface)

- Elements around home or in long-term care facilities (e.g., throw rugs, low furniture, lack of grab bars in bathrooms)

- Factors in the public environment (e.g., cracked/uneven sidewalks, poor lighting)

- Assistive devices that are not properly maintained (e.g., worn cane tips, dysfunctional locking mechanisms on wheelchairs or walkers)

4. Socioeconomic Risk Factors

- Income

- Education

- Housing

- Social connectedness

The socioeconomic factors listed are well-established determinants of health that have been shown to increase risk of chronic health conditions, which in turn have been shown to increase risk for falls. Little is known regarding the direct correlation between these factors and falls in seniors. A 2005 study by the Registered Nurses Association of Ontario found that financial strain was a predictor of injurious falls. A 2004 report from the British Columbia Ministry of Health Planning extrapolated that while the contribution of social and economic factors to falls is poorly understood, contributing factors may include muscle weakness or ill health resulting from an inability to access or read printed resources on strategies for preventing falls.

RISK FACTOR ASSESSMENT

Musculoskeletal disorders (MSDs) are the most prevalent category of chronic conditions in Canada, and the second most expensive, behind circulatory diseases (Mirolla, 2004). Comprehensive review of nurses' roles in caring for clients with MSDs includes attention to both uncontrollable and controllable risk factors. Uncontrollable risk factors, those the client cannot change, include age, gender, ethnic background, and heredity. Controllable, or modifiable, risk factors include lifestyle factors such as inactivity, excess weight, and poor nutrition. Low body weight is the single best predictor of low bone density, and bone density at the femoral neck is the best predictor of subsequent hip fracture (Margolis et al., 2000).

Demographics. Demographic risk factors include age, gender, and race. Age-related research shows clients deal with similar musculoskeletal issues across the lifespan, in varying degrees or with different causes at different stages. For example, falls are the second leading cause of injury-related hospitalization for Canadians of all ages (PHAC, 2005a). While those older than 80 years are most likely to fall and be injured (PHAC, 2005b), a Safe Kids Canada report showed that most hospitalizations in clients 14 years and younger were related to falls (Safe Kids Canada, 2006). Fortunately, the same report shows that over the decade from 1993 to 2003, the number of childhood injuries decreased as the result of a three-pronged approach to health promotion: (1) education, such as through public awareness campaigns about protective sports equipment; (2) environmental changes, such as building safer playgrounds; and (3) enforcement of laws or standards, such as bicycle helmet education.

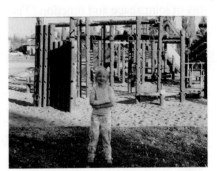

🌐 Cultural Considerations

In 2001, a First Nations research nurse coordinated a joint research project between the University of Manitoba and Assembly of Manitoba Chiefs to gather data about bone health and high fracture rates in First Nations women. The First Nations Bone Health Study showed that average bone density was significantly lower in First Nations women than in Caucasian women, and that First Nations women have lower levels of vitamin D (needed to absorb calcium in the body) than Caucasian women (Leslie, 2004). Other Canadian research has shown that both First Nations men and women had double the risk for fractures than other racial groups, with even higher risk for wrist, skull, and facial fractures (Leslie et al., 2004). While skull and facial fracture rates were high among young men and generally attributed to violence, all other fractures were more prevalent in older women, and mirrored the pattern seen in osteoporosis (Leslie et al., 2004).

Gender is the second demographic risk factor for MSDs. Women fall more often, and thereby sustain more injuries, than men (PHAC, 2005b). Dietitians of Canada issued a statement that osteoporosis is reaching "epidemic proportions" in North American women (Affenito & Kerstetter, 1999). The danger is further increased for postmenopausal women, who often suffer accelerated bone loss once their estrogen levels decline (PHAC, 2005b). In contrast, men have a higher frequency of work-related musculoskeletal injuries (Smith & Mustard, 2004) and increased incidence of some diseases, such as ankylosing spondylitis (The Arthritis Society, 2007c).

Ethnic background, a third demographic risk factor, also plays a role in susceptibility to MSDs. For example, people of African genetic background tend to have greater bone density, while those of Chinese and Irish background tend to have lower-than-average bone density (Purnell & Paulanka, 2003). Another example is dwarfism syndrome, which is found in nearly all Amish communities (Purnell & Paulanka, 2003).

Family History. Family history of certain disorders of the musculoskeletal system, such as rheumatoid arthritis, osteoporosis, and bone cancer, increases a client's chances of having these conditions (Health Canada, 2005).

Lifestyle Factors. Risk factors for MSDs are largely modifiable. Four important lifestyle risk factors for which clients may require education and support are physical inactivity, obesity, poor nutrition, and smoking.

Physical inactivity, the first modifiable risk factor, is problematic because muscles and connective tissues degenerate and weaken when they are not used, leading to loss of joint shape and function (The Arthritis Society, 2007b). A panel of geriatric specialists and orthopaedic surgeons found muscle weakness and reduced physical activity to be the most important risk factor for falls, increasing risk by four to five times (PHAC, 2005a). Nurses can help clients understand the necessity of physical activity and recommend both weight-bearing and muscle-building exercises to help build and maintain healthy bones and muscles. Low-impact exercises such as swimming, walking, water aerobics, and stationary cycling are suggestions for clients who experience pain with higher-impact activities. These options minimize pain while building or maintaining strength and flexibility (The Arthritis Society, 2007b).

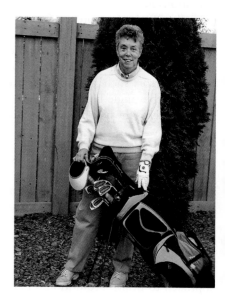

Obesity is a second major modifiable risk factor for MSDs. Research shows that even at a slightly elevated Body Mass Index, Canadians have a significantly higher risk of arthritis, back pain, activity limitations, and repetitive strain injury (Colman, 2000). Staying within the parameters of one's recommended Body Mass Index helps to prevent musculoskeletal injury by decreasing stress on the joints (The Arthritis Society, 2007b).

Poor nutrition is the third important lifestyle-related risk factor. As previously mentioned in the discussion on osteoporosis, nutritional choices early in life can have direct consequences later in life for bone health.

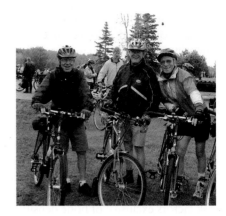

Smoking, which affects every human tissue, is a fourth risk factor for MSDs. Research has shown a positive correlation between smoking and development of osteoporosis, hip fractures, low back pain, and rheumatoid arthritis (Clough, 2007). Studies also show that smoking reduces blood supply to the bones and that nicotine slows the production of bone-forming cells and impairs absorption of calcium (Clough, 2007). Researchers also believe that smoking increases risk for exercise-related injury. Some studies show that tears to the rotator cuff are twice as large in smokers as in nonsmokers (Clough, 2007). Smokers also have increased incidence of overuse injuries such as tendonitis and bursitis, and increased likelihood of traumatic injuries such as strains and fractures (Clough, 2007).

Occupational Risk Factors. The Centre of Research Expertise for the Prevention of Musculoskeletal Disorders states that four factors contribute to workplace injuries: use of force, awkward posture, repetition, and long duration (Occupational Health and Safety Council of Ontario, 2007). Any one of these in excess can cause injury on its own—for example, lifting a heavy box, even if the correct lifting technique is used. Any task that combines two or more of the four factors increases the worker's risk of musculoskeletal injury. Workers who perform forceful and repetitive activities over a sustained period are at higher risk; however, the use of force is not necessary for an MSD to develop (Premji, 2007). Work-related psychosocial factors such as monotony, lack of job control, lack of role clarity, and limited social support also contribute to the development of MSDs (Premji, 2007).

Distinct differences between the incidence and nature of workplace-related MSDs exist for men and women. While U.S. studies show that two-thirds of all work-related injuries and illnesses involving days away from work occur to men, Health Canada reports that health care workers, most of whom are women, have a higher incidence of MSDs than other occupational groups and the general population (Office of Nursing Policy, Health Canada, 2004). Additionally, female workers account for more than 60% of all work-related cases of repetitive strain injuries, carpal tunnel syndrome, and tendonitis (Premji, 2007). Women are more likely than men to have work areas that are poorly adapted to their size and shape, especially in nontraditional jobs (Premji, 2007). Finally, women are less likely than men to be promoted out of positions that present higher risks for MSDs (Torgen & Kilbom, 2000). Awareness of these facts can help nurses provide relevant education, support, and advocacy for both male and female clients in the workforce to prevent MSDs.

SCREENING

Osteoporosis is the only MSD for which screening is recommended at this time. The most recent clinical practice guideline of the Osteoporosis Society of Canada recommended the assessment of all postmenopausal women, and men older than 50 years, for risk factors of osteoporosis (Brown & Josse, 2002). While several factors can contribute to osteoporosis, the most important predictive factors are low bone density combined with age, fracture history, various drug treatments, weight loss, and physical fitness. These suggestions, however, may be adopted at the discretion of various health care decision makers. For example, the British Columbia Ministry of Health (2005) recommends bone mineral density measurement only when the results are likely to alter client care and the client meets specific risk factor guidelines.

Another recently developed screening tool is the Fracture Risk Assessment Tool (FRAX) created by the WHO. This tool combines assessment of risk factors with bone mineral density to predict the 10-year probability that a client will have a major osteoporotic fracture (i.e., spine, forearm, hip, shoulder) (Kanis, n.d.). The FRAX is available at http://www.shef.ac.uk/FRAX/index.htm. Adaptations that focus on risk factors exclusive of bone density are also available.

EMERGENCY CONCERNS

The nurse refers any client with a suspected fracture to a physician for assessment and potential treatment. While recent research shows that the risk of infection when clients wait more than 48 hours for reparative surgery does not increase as dramatically as previously believed, these clients are still at increased risk of morbidity and mortality from pain, disability, and inconvenience (McGregor & Atwood, 2007). Thus, Canadian guidelines maintain that hip fracture correction, in particular, should occur within 24 hours of injury, barring medical contraindication.

Osteoporotic spinal fractures are not always easily diagnosed. The nurse should advise clients who have sudden, severe back pain or pain that follows bending or twisting to seek immediate medical attention if they have been previously diagnosed with osteoporosis (Osteoporosis Canada, 2007h).

If trauma to the spine is suspected following an injury, continued movement of the cervical spine can cause further damage. For example, a fracture or dislocation of the spine without neurologic damage can progress to a much more complex situation involving irreversible neurological injury if the spine is not immediately stabilized.

EXAMINATION OF SPECIFIC JOINTS: ANATOMY AND PHYSIOLOGY AND TECHNIQUES OF EXAMINATION

PROMOTING CLIENT COMFORT, DIGNITY, AND SAFETY

During musculoskeletal assessment, a few simple actions can promote client comfort and safety. The nurse must provide adequate draping to prevent unnecessary exposure and to keep the client from feeling chilled. Giving specific instructions throughout the examination will help the client understand what is expected of him or her. Perform hand hygiene, and clean any shared equipment thoroughly. Musculoskeletal assessment will require movement and changes in position. Explain the reasons for position changes, and assist the client as necessary, ensuring he or she is comfortable and secure in the new position before continuing with the examination.

Important Areas of Examination for Each of the Major Joints

- Inspection for joint symmetry, alignment, bony deformities
- Inspection and palpation of surrounding tissues for skin changes, nodules, muscle atrophy, crepitus
- Range of motion and manoeuvres to test joint function and stability, integrity of ligaments, tendons, bursae, especially if pain or trauma
- Assessment of inflammation or arthritis, especially swelling, warmth, tenderness, redness

Equipment

- Tape measure
- Felt marker
- Goniometer (to measure joint angles)

During the interview you have evaluated the client's ability to carry out normal activities of daily living. Keep these abilities in mind during your physical examination.

In your initial survey of the client you have assessed general appearance, body proportions, and ease of movement. Now, as you apply techniques of examination to the musculoskeletal system, visualize the underlying anatomy and recall the key elements of the history—for example, the mechanism of injury, if there is trauma, or the time course of symptoms and limitations in function in arthritis.

Your examination should be systematic. It should include inspection, palpation of bony landmarks as well as related joint and soft-tissue structures, assessment of range of motion, and *special manoeuvres* to test specific movements. Recall that the anatomical shape of each joint determines its range of motion (American College of Rheumatology Ad Hoc Committee on Clinical Guidelines, 1996).

TIPS FOR SUCCESSFUL EXAMINATION OF THE MUSCULOSKELETAL SYSTEM

- During inspection, look for *symmetry* of involvement. Is there a symmetric change in joints on both sides of the body, or is the change only in one or two joints?

  Also note any *joint deformities* or *malalignment of bones*.

- Use inspection and palpation to assess the *surrounding tissues*, noting skin changes, subcutaneous nodules, and muscle atrophy. Note any *crepitus*, an audible or palpable crunching during movement of tendons or ligaments over bone. This may occur in healthy joints but is more significant when associated with symptoms or signs.

(Continued)

Acute involvement of only one joint suggests trauma, septic arthritis, and gout. *Rheumatoid arthritis* typically involves several joints, symmetrically distributed (Arnett et al., 1988; Goldring, 2000; Lee & Weinblatt, 2001).

Dupuytren's contracture (p. 678), bowlegs, or knock-knees

Subcutaneous nodules in rheumatoid arthritis or rheumatic fever; effusions in trauma; crepitus over inflamed joints, in osteoarthritis, or inflamed tendon sheaths

TIPS FOR SUCCESSFUL EXAMINATION OF THE MUSCULOSKELETAL SYSTEM (Continued)

- Testing range of motion and manoeuvres (described for each joint) may demonstrate *limitations in range of motion* or increased mobility and joint instability from excess mobility of joint ligaments, called *ligamentous laxity*.

- Finally, testing *muscle strength* may aid in the assessment of joint function (for these techniques, see Chapter 20).

Be especially alert to *signs of inflammation and arthritis.*

- *Swelling.* Palpable swelling may involve (1) the synovial membrane, which can feel boggy or doughy; (2) effusion from excess synovial fluid within the joint space; or (3) soft-tissue structures such as bursae, tendons, and tendon sheaths.

- *Warmth.* Use the backs of your fingers to compare the involved joint with its unaffected contralateral joint, or with nearby tissues if both joints are involved.
- *Tenderness.* Try to identify the specific anatomical structure that is tender. Trauma may also cause tenderness.

- *Redness.* Redness of the overlying skin is the *least* common sign of inflammation near the joints.

Decreased range of motion in arthritis, inflammation of tissues around a joint, fibrosis in or around a joint, or bony fixation (*ankylosis*). Ligamentous laxity of the ACL in knee trauma.

Muscle atrophy or weakness in *rheumatoid arthritis*

Palpable bogginess or doughiness of the synovial membrane indicates *synovitis,* which is often accompanied by effusion. Palpable joint fluid in effusion, tenderness over the tendon sheaths in *tendonitis*

Arthritis, tendonitis, bursitis, osteomyelitis

Tenderness and warmth over a thickened synovium may suggest arthritis or infection.

Redness over a tender joint suggests septic or gouty arthritis, or possibly *rheumatoid arthritis.*

If the person has painful joints, move the person gently. Clients may move more comfortably by themselves. Let them show you how they manage. If joint trauma is present, consider an x-ray before attempting movement.

The detail needed for examining the musculoskeletal system may vary widely. This section presents examination techniques for both comprehensive and targeted assessment of joint function. Clients with extensive or severe musculoskeletal problems will require more time.

TEMPOROMANDIBULAR JOINT

OVERVIEW, BONY STRUCTURES, AND JOINTS

The temporomandibular joint is the most active joint in the body, opening and closing up to 2000 times a day. It is formed by the fossa and articular tubercle of the temporal bone and the condyle of the mandible. It lies midway between the external acoustic meatus and the zygomatic arch.

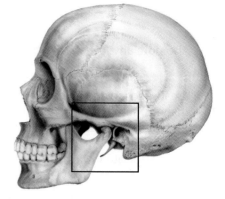

A fibrocartilaginous disc cushions the action of the condyle of the mandible against the synovial membrane and capsule of the articulating surfaces of the temporal bone. Hence, it is a condylar synovial joint.

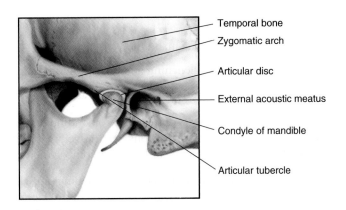

- Temporal bone
- Zygomatic arch
- Articular disc
- External acoustic meatus
- Condyle of mandible
- Articular tubercle

MUSCLE GROUPS AND ADDITIONAL STRUCTURES

The principal muscles opening the mouth are the *external pterygoids.* Closing the mouth are the muscles innervated by Cranial Nerve V, the trigeminal nerve (see p. 688)—the *masseter,* the *temporalis,* and the *internal pterygoids.*

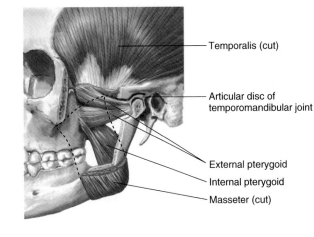

- Temporalis (cut)
- Articular disc of temporomandibular joint
- External pterygoid
- Internal pterygoid
- Masseter (cut)

TECHNIQUES OF EXAMINATION

Inspection and Palpation. Inspect the face for symmetry. Inspect the temporomandibular joint for swelling or redness. Swelling may appear as a rounded bulge approximately 0.5 cm anterior to the external auditory meatus.

Facial asymmetry associated with *TMJ syndrome,* or unilateral chronic pain with chewing, jaw clenching, or teeth grinding, often associated with stress (may also present as headache)

Swelling, tenderness, and decreased range of motion in inflammation or arthritis

Dislocation of the TMJ may be seen in trauma.

To locate and palpate the joint, place the tips of your index fingers just in front of the tragus of each ear and ask the client to open his or her mouth. The fingertips should drop into the joint spaces as the mouth opens. Check for smooth range of motion; note any swelling or tenderness. Snapping or clicking may be felt or heard in healthy people.

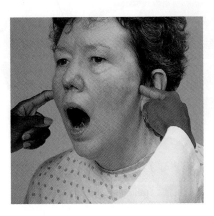

Palpable crepitus or clicking in poor occlusion, meniscus injury, or synovial swelling from trauma

Also palpate the muscles of mastication:

- The *masseters*, externally, at the angle of the mandible

- The *temporal muscles*, externally, during clenching and relaxation of the jaw

- The *pterygoid muscles*, internally, between the tonsillar pillars at the mandible

Range of Motion and Manoeuvres. The temporomandibular joint has glide and hinge motions in its upper and lower portions, respectively. Grinding or chewing consists primarily of gliding movements in the upper compartments.

Range of motion is threefold: ask the client to demonstrate opening and closing, protrusion and retraction (by jutting the jaw forward), and lateral, or side-to-side, motion. As the mouth is opened wide, three fingers can be inserted between the incisors. During protrusion of the jaw, the bottom teeth can be placed in front of the upper teeth.

THE SHOULDER

OVERVIEW

The shoulder is distinguished by wide-ranging movement in all directions. The humerus virtually dangles from the scapula, suspended from the shallow glenoid fossa by the joint capsule, the intra-articular capsular ligaments, the glenoid labrum, and a meshwork of muscles and tendons. The shoulder derives its mobility from a complex interconnected structure of four joints, three large bones, and three principal muscle groups, often referred to as the *shoulder girdle*. The clavicle and acromion stabilize the shoulder girdle, allowing the humerus to swing out and away from the body, giving the shoulder its remarkable range of motion.

BONY STRUCTURES

The bony structures of the shoulder include the humerus, the clavicle, and the scapula. The scapula is anchored to the axial skeleton only by the sternoclavicular joint and inserting muscles, often called the *scapulothoracic articulation* because it is not a true joint.

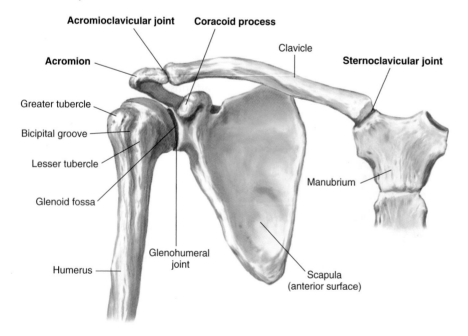

Identify the manubrium, the sternoclavicular joint, and the clavicle. With your fingers, trace the clavicle laterally. Now, from behind, follow the bony spine of the scapula laterally and upward until it becomes the *acromion*, the summit of the shoulder. Its upper surface is rough and slightly convex.

■ Identify the anterior tip of the acromion (**A**), and mark it with ink. With your index finger on top of the acromion, just behind its tip, press medially to find the slightly elevated ridge that marks the distal end of the clavicle at the *acromioclavicular joint* (shown by the arrow).

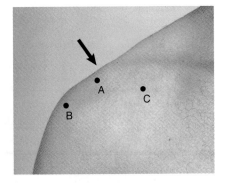

■ Move your finger laterally and down a short step to the next bony prominence, the *greater tubercle of the humerus* (**B**). Mark this with ink.

■ Now sweep your finger medially until you feel a large bony prominence, the *coracoid process* of the scapula (**C**). Mark this also.

These three points—the tip of the acromion, the greater tubercle of the humerus, and the coracoid process—orient you to the anatomy of the shoulder.

JOINTS

Three different joints articulate at the shoulder:

■ The *glenohumeral joint*. In this joint, the head of the humerus articulates with the shallow glenoid fossa of the scapula. This joint is deeply situated and not usually palpable. It is a ball-and-socket joint, allowing the arm its wide arc of movement—flexion, extension, abduction (movement away from the trunk), adduction (movement toward the trunk), rotation, and circumduction.

■ The *sternoclavicular joint*. The convex medial end of the clavicle articulates with the concave hollow in the upper sternum.

■ The *acromioclavicular joint*. The lateral end of the clavicle articulates with the acromion process of the scapula.

MUSCLE GROUPS

Three groups of muscles attach at the shoulder:

The Scapulohumeral Group. This group extends from the scapula to the humerus and includes the muscles inserting directly on the humerus, known as "*SITS muscles*" of the rotator cuff:

■ *Supraspinatus*—runs above the glenohumeral joint; inserts on the greater tubercle

- *Infraspinatus* and *teres minor*—cross the glenohumeral joint posteriorly; insert on the greater tubercle

- *Subscapularis* (not illustrated)—originates on the anterior surface of the scapula and crosses the joint anteriorly; inserts on the lesser tubercle.

The scapulohumeral group rotates the shoulder laterally (the *rotator cuff*) and depresses and rotates the head of the humerus. (See p. 626 for discussion of rotator cuff injuries.)

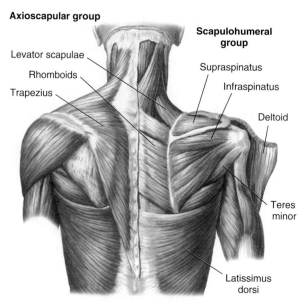

Axioscapular group

Scapulohumeral group

Levator scapulae
Rhomboids
Trapezius
Supraspinatus
Infraspinatus
Deltoid
Teres minor
Latissimus dorsi

Posterior view
AXIOSCAPULAR GROUP (PULLS SHOULDER BACKWARD)

The Axioscapular Group.
This group attaches the trunk to the scapula and includes the trapezius, rhomboids, serratus anterior, and levator scapulae. These muscles rotate the scapula.

The Axiohumeral Group.
This group attaches the trunk to the humerus and includes the pectoralis major and minor and the latissimus dorsi. These muscles produce internal rotation of the shoulder.

The biceps and triceps, which connect the scapula to the bones of the forearm, are also involved in shoulder movement, particularly abduction.

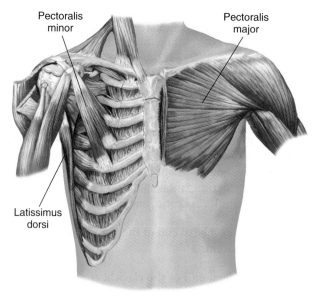

Pectoralis minor
Pectoralis major
Latissimus dorsi

Anterior view
AXIOHUMERAL GROUP (ROTATES SHOULDER INTERNALLY)

ADDITIONAL STRUCTURES

Also important to shoulder movement are the *articular capsule and bursae*. Surrounding the glenohumeral joint is a fibrous articular capsule formed by the tendon insertions of the rotator cuff and other capsular muscles. The loose fit of the capsule allows the shoulder bones to separate, and contributes to the shoulder's wide range of movement. The capsule is lined by a synovial membrane with two outpouchings—the *subscapular bursa* and the *synovial sheath of the tendon of the long head of the biceps*.

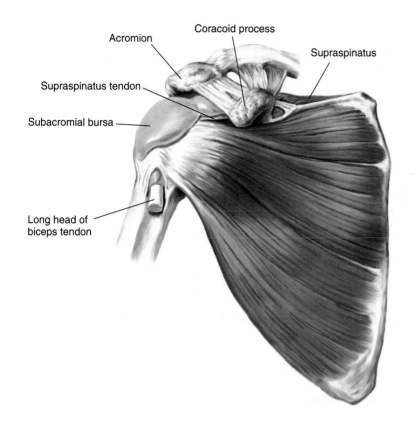

To locate the biceps tendon, rotate your arm externally and find the tendinous cord that runs just medial to the greater tubercle. Roll it under your fingers. This is the tendon of the long head of the biceps. It runs in the bicipital groove between the greater and lesser tubercles.

The principal bursa of the shoulder is the *subacromial bursa*, positioned between the acromion and the head of the humerus and overlying the supraspinatus tendon. Abduction of the shoulder compresses this bursa. Usually the supraspinatus tendon and the subacromial bursa are not palpable. However, if the bursal surfaces are inflamed (subacromial bursitis), there may be tenderness just below the tip of the acromion, pain with abduction and rotation, and loss of smooth movement.

TECHNIQUES OF EXAMINATION

Inspection. Observe the shoulder and shoulder girdle anteriorly, and inspect the scapulae and related muscles posteriorly. Note any swelling, deformity, muscle atrophy or fasciculations (fine tremors of the muscles), or unexpected positioning.

Scoliosis may cause elevation of one shoulder. With *anterior dislocation of the shoulder,* the rounded lateral aspect of the shoulder appears flattened (Liume et al., 2004; Woodward & Best, 2000a).

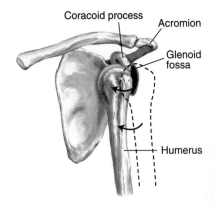

Coracoid process
Acromion
Glenoid fossa
Humerus

ANTERIOR DISLOCATION OF HUMERUS

Look for swelling of the joint capsule anteriorly or a bulge in the subacromial bursa under the deltoid muscle. Survey the entire upper extremity for colour change, skin alteration, or unusual bony contours.

A significant amount of synovial fluid is needed before the joint capsule appears distended.

Palpation.   If there is a history of shoulder pain, ask the client to point to the painful area. The location of the pain provides clues to its origin:

See Table 19-4, Painful Shoulders (pp. 674–675)

■ Top of the shoulder, radiating toward the neck—acromioclavicular joint

■ Lateral aspect of the shoulder, radiating toward the deltoid insertion—rotator cuff

■ Anterior shoulder—bicipital tendon

Now identify the bony landmarks of the shoulder and then palpate the area of pain. Locate the *acromion process* and press medially to locate the distal tip of the clavicle at the *acromioclavicular joint.* Palpate laterally and down a short step to the greater tubercle of the humerus, and then press medially to locate the *coracoid process* of the scapula. Next, palpate the painful area and identify the structures involved.

Range of Motion and Manoeuvres.   The six motions of the shoulder girdle are flexion, extension, abduction, adduction, and internal and external rotation.

Restricted range of motion in *bursitis, capsulitis, rotator cuff tears* or *sprains, or tendonitis.*

Watch for smooth, fluid movement as you stand in front of the client and ask the client to:

1. raise *(abduct)* the arms to shoulder level (90°) with palms facing down (tests pure glenohumeral motion)

2. raise the arms to a vertical position above the head with the palms facing each other (tests scapulothoracic motion for 60°, and combined glenohumeral and scapulothoracic motion during adduction for the final 30°)

3. place both hands behind the neck, with elbows out to the side (tests *external rotation* and *abduction*)

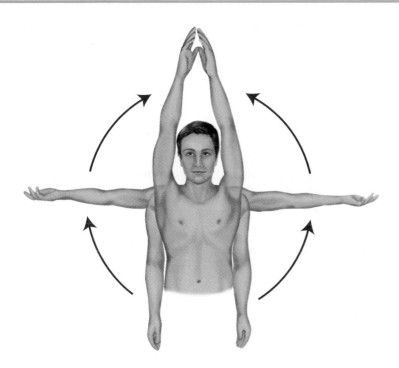

4. place both hands behind the small of the back (tests *internal rotation* and *adduction*).

Placing your hand on the shoulder during these movements allows you to detect any crepitus.

The examination of the shoulder often requires selective evaluation of the acromioclavicular joint, the subacromial and subdeltoid bursae, the rotator cuff, the bicipital groove and tendon, and the articular capsule and synovial membrane of the glenohumeral joint (Burkhardt, 2000). Techniques for examining these structures are described in the following pages.

Crepitus during movement suggests osteoarthritis.

■ Techniques for Examining the Shoulder

Structure	Technique	
Acromioclavicular Joint	Palpate and compare both joints for swelling or tenderness. Adduct the client's arm across the chest, sometimes called the *"crossover test."*	

(continued)

Localized tenderness or pain with adduction suggests inflammation or arthritis of the acromioclavicular joint. See Table 19-4, Painful Shoulders (pp. 674–675).

■ Techniques for Examining the Shoulder (Continued)

Structure	Technique
Subacromial and Subdeltoid Bursae	Passively extend the shoulder by lifting the elbow posteriorly. This exposes the bursa anterior to the acromion. Palpate carefully over the subacromial and subdeltoid bursae. 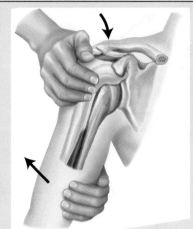

Localized tenderness arises from *subacromial* or *subdeltoid bursitis*, degenerative changes, or calcific deposits in the rotator cuff.

Swelling suggests a *bursal tear* with communication into the articular cavity.

Overall Shoulder Rotation	Ask the client to touch the opposite scapula using the two motions shown below (the Apley scratch test).

Difficulty with these motions suggests rotator cuff disorder.

Tests abduction and external rotation.

Tests adduction and internal rotation

Rotator Cuff	With the client's arm hanging at the side, palpate the three "SITS" muscles that insert on the greater tuberosity of the humerus. (The fourth muscle, the subscapularis, inserts anteriorly and is not palpable.) ■ **Supraspinatus** directly under the acromion ■ **Infraspinatus**—posterior to supraspinatus ■ **Teres minor**—posterior and inferior to the supraspinatus

Tenderness over the "SITS" muscle insertions and inability to lift the arm above shoulder level are seen in sprains, tears, and tendon rupture of the rotator cuff, most commonly the *supraspinatus*. See Table 19-4, Painful Shoulders (pp. 674–675).

(continued)

▪Techniques for Examining the Shoulder (Continued)

Structure	Technique	
	Passively extend the shoulder by lifting the elbow posteriorly. This manoeuvre also moves the rotator cuff out from under the acromion. Palpate the rounded SITS muscle insertions near the greater tuberosity of the humerus.	Subacromial bursa Rotator cuff

Check the *"drop-arm" sign*. Ask the client to fully abduct the arm to shoulder level (or up to 90°) and lower it slowly. (Note that abduction above shoulder level, from 90° to 120°, reflects action of the deltoid muscle.)

If the client is unable to hold the arm fully abducted at shoulder level, the "drop arm" test is positive, indicating a tear in the rotator cuff.

See also Bicipital Tendonitis in Table 19-4 Painful Shoulders (pp. 674–675).

Bicipital Groove and Tendon

Rotate the arm and forearm externally and locate the biceps muscle distally near the elbow. Track the muscle and its tendon proximally into the bicipital groove along the anterior aspect of the humerus. As you check for tendon tenderness, rolling the tendon under the fingertips may be helpful.

PALPATION OF THE BICIPITAL GROOVE AND TENDON

Finally, hold the client's elbow against the body with the forearm flexed at a right angle. Ask the client to supinate the forearm against resistance.

Tenderness or pain against resistance occurs with tenosynovitis of the bicipital tendon sheath, tendonitis, or biceps tendon rupture.

Articular Capsule, Synovial Membrane, and Glenohumeral Joint

The fibrous articular capsule and the broad flat tendons of the rotator cuff are so closely associated that they must be examined simultaneously. Swelling in the capsule and synovial membrane is often best detected by looking down on the shoulder from above. Palpate the capsule and synovial membrane beneath the anterior and posterior acromion.

Tenderness and effusion suggest synovitis of the glenohumeral joint. If the margins of the capsule and synovial membrane are palpable, a moderate to large effusion is present. Minimal degrees of synovitis at the glenohumeral joint cannot be detected on palpation.

Source: **Woodward & Best, 2000b.**

The following manoeuvres test individual muscles of the shoulder girdle and help localize pain. Note that medial rotation against resistance also tests the pectoralis major, teres major, and latissimus dorsi. Additional evaluation of muscle strength; sensation over the neck, shoulder, and arm; and upper extremity reflexes is often warranted to complete your assessment (see Chapter 20).

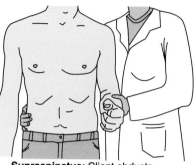

Supraspinatus: Client abducts against resistance.

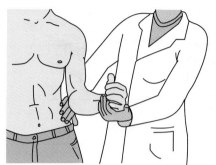

Subscapularis: Client rotates forearm medially against resistance.

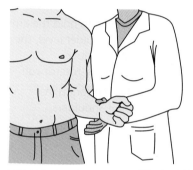

Infraspinatus, teres minor: Client rotates forearm laterally against resistance.

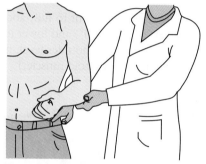

Thoracohumeral group: Client adducts forearm against resistance.

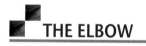

THE ELBOW

OVERVIEW, BONY STRUCTURES, AND JOINTS

The elbow helps position the hand in space and stabilizes the lever action of the forearm. The elbow joint is formed by the humerus and the two bones of the forearm, the radius and the ulna. Identify the medial and lateral epicondyles of the humerus and the olecranon process of the ulna.

These bones have three articulations: the *humeroulnar joint*, the *radiohumeral joint*, and the *radioulnar joint*. All three share a large common articular cavity and an extensive synovial lining.

MUSCLE GROUPS AND ADDITIONAL STRUCTURES

Muscles traversing the elbow include the *biceps* and *brachioradialis* (flexion), the *triceps* (extension), the *pronator teres* (pronation), and the *supinator* (supination).

Note the location of the *olecranon bursa* between the olecranon process and the skin. The bursa is not usually palpable, but swells and becomes tender when inflamed. The *ulnar nerve* runs posteriorly in the ulnar groove between the medial epicondyle and the olecranon process. On the ventral forearm, the *median nerve* is just medial to the brachial artery.

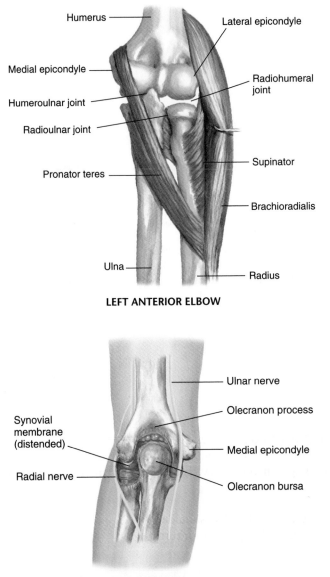

Humerus

Lateral epicondyle

Medial epicondyle

Radiohumeral joint

Humeroulnar joint

Radioulnar joint

Supinator

Pronator teres

Brachioradialis

Ulna

Radius

LEFT ANTERIOR ELBOW

Ulnar nerve

Olecranon process

Synovial membrane (distended)

Medial epicondyle

Radial nerve

Olecranon bursa

LEFT POSTERIOR ELBOW

TECHNIQUES OF EXAMINATION

Inspection and Palpation.
Support the client's forearm with your opposite hand so the elbow is flexed to about 70°. Identify the medial and lateral epicondyles and the olecranon process of the ulna. Inspect the contours of the elbow, including the extensor surface of the ulna and the olecranon process. Note any nodules or swelling.

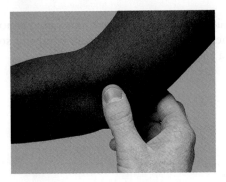

See Table 19-5, Swollen or Tender Elbows (p. 676).

Swelling over the olecranon process in olecranon bursitis; inflammation or synovial fluid in arthritis.

Palpate the olecranon process, and press on the epicondyles for tenderness. Note any displacement of the olecranon.

Tenderness in *lateral epicondylitis* (tennis elbow) and less commonly in *medial epicondylitis* (pitcher's or golfer's elbow)

The olecranon is displaced posteriorly in *posterior dislocation of the elbow* and *supracondylar fracture.*

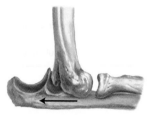

POSTERIOR DISLOCATION OF THE ELBOW

Palpate the grooves between the epicondyles and the olecranon, noting any tenderness, swelling, or thickening. The synovium is most accessible to examination between the olecranon and the epicondyles. (Usually neither synovium nor bursa is palpable.) The sensitive ulnar nerve can be felt posteriorly between the olecranon process and the medial epicondyle.

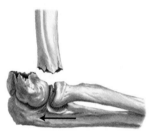

SUPRACONDYLAR FRACTURE OF THE ELBOW

Range of Motion and Manoeuvres. Range of motion includes *flexion* and *extension* at the elbow and *pronation* and *supination* of the forearm. To test flexion and extension, ask the client to bend and straighten the elbow. Elbow extension reduces intra-articular volume.

Full elbow extension makes intra-articular process, effusion, or hemarthrosis unlikely.

With the client's arms at the sides and elbows flexed to minimize shoulder movement, ask the client to *supinate*, or turn up the palms, and to *pronate*, or turn the palms down.

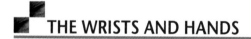

THE WRISTS AND HANDS

OVERVIEW

The wrist and hands form a complex unit of small, highly active joints used almost continuously during waking hours. There is little protection from overlying soft tissue, increasing vulnerability to trauma and disability.

BONY STRUCTURES

The wrist includes the distal radius and ulna and eight small carpal bones. At the wrist, identify the bony tips of the radius and the ulna.

The carpal bones lie distal to the wrist joint within each hand. Identify the carpal bones, each of the five metacarpals, and the proximal, middle, and distal phalanges. Note that the thumb lacks a middle phalanx.

JOINTS

The numerous joints of the wrist and hand lend unusual dexterity to the hands.

■ *Wrist joints.* The wrist joints include the *radiocarpal* or *wrist joint,* the *distal radioulnar joint,* and the *intercarpal joints.* The joint capsule, articular disc, and synovial membrane of the wrist join the radius to the ulna and to the proximal carpal bones. On the dorsum of the wrist, locate the groove of the *radiocarpal joint,* which provides most of the flexion and extension at the wrist because the ulna does not articulate directly with the carpal bones.

■ *Hand joints.* The joints of the hand include the *metacarpophalangeal joints* (MCPs), the *proximal interphalangeal joints* (PIPs), and the *distal interphalangeal joints* (DIPs). Flex the hand and find the groove marking the MCP joint of each finger. It is distal to the knuckle and is best felt on either side of the extensor tendon.

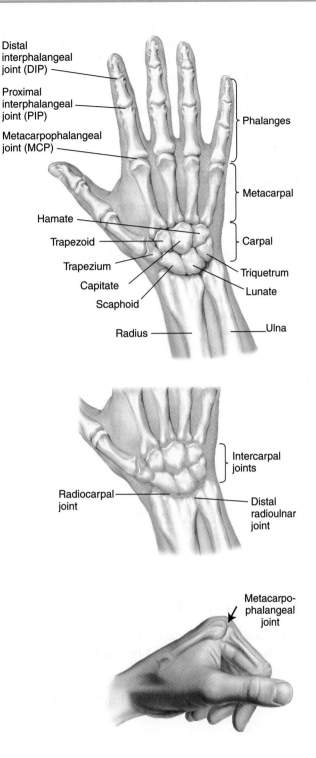

MUSCLE GROUPS

Wrist flexion arises from the two carpal muscles located on the radial and ulnar surfaces. Three muscles, two radial and one ulnar, provide wrist extension. Supination and pronation result from muscle contraction in the forearm.

The thumb is powered by three muscles that form the thenar eminence and provide flexion, abduction, and opposition. The muscles of extension are at the base of the thumb along the radial margin. Movement in the digits depends on action of the flexor and extensor tendons of muscles in the forearm and wrist.

The intrinsic muscles of the hand attaching to the metacarpal bones are involved in flexion *(lumbricals)*, abduction *(dorsal interossei)*, and adduction *(palmar interossei)* of the fingers.

ADDITIONAL STRUCTURES

Soft-tissue structures, especially tendons and tendon sheaths, are extremely important in the wrist and hand. Six extensor tendons and two flexor tendons pass across the wrist and hand to insert on the fingers. Through much of their course these tendons travel in tunnel-like sheaths, generally palpable only when swollen or inflamed.

Be familiar with the structures in the *carpal tunnel*, a channel beneath the palmar surface of the wrist and proximal hand. The canal contains the sheath and flexor tendons of the forearm muscles and the *median nerve*.

Holding the tendons and tendon sheath in place is a transverse ligament, the *flexor retinaculum*. The median nerve lies between the flexor retinaculum and the tendon sheath. It provides sensation to the palm and the palmar surface of most of the thumb, the second and third digits, and half of the fourth digit. It also innervates the thumb muscles of flexion, abduction, and opposition.

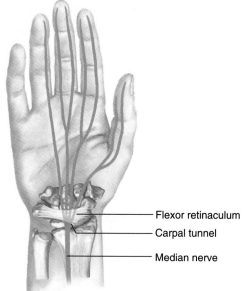

— Flexor retinaculum
— Carpal tunnel
— Median nerve

TECHNIQUES OF EXAMINATION

Inspection. Observe the position of the hands in motion to see if movements are smooth and natural. At rest, the fingers should be slightly flexed and aligned almost in parallel.

Inspect the palmar and dorsal surfaces of the wrist and hand carefully for swelling over the joints.

Note any deformities of the wrist, hand, or finger bones, as well as any angulation from radial or ulnar deviation.

Guarded movement suggests injury; finger misalignment seen in flexor tendon damage.

Diffuse swelling in arthritis or infection; local swelling from cystic ganglion. See Table 19-6, Arthritis in the Hands (p. 677) and Table 19-7, Swellings and Deformities of the Hands (p. 678).

In *osteoarthritis*, Heberden's nodes at the DIP joints, Bouchard's nodes at the PIP joints. In *rheumatoid arthritis*, symmetric deformity in the PIP, MCP, and wrist joints, with ulnar deviation.

Observe the contours of the palm, namely the thenar and hypothenar eminences.

Thenar atrophy in median nerve compression from *carpal tunnel syndrome;* hypothenar atrophy in *ulnar nerve compression.*

Note any thickening of the flexor tendons or flexion contractures in the fingers.

Flexion contractures in the ring, fifth, and third fingers, or *Dupuytren's contractures,* arise from thickening of the palmar fascia (see p. 679).

Palpation. At the wrist, palpate the distal radius and ulna on the lateral and medial surfaces. Palpate the groove of each wrist joint with your thumbs on the dorsum of the wrist, your fingers beneath it. Note any swelling, bogginess, or tenderness.

Tenderness over the distal radius in *Colles' fracture.* Any tenderness or bony step-offs are suspicious for fracture.

Swelling and/or tenderness suggests *rheumatoid arthritis* if bilateral and of several weeks' duration.

Palpate the radial styloid bone and the *anatomical snuffbox,* a hollowed depression just distal to the radial styloid process formed by the abductor and extensor muscles of the thumb. The "snuffbox" becomes more visible with lateral extension of the thumb away from the hand.

Tenderness over the extensor and abductor tendons of the thumb at the radial styloid in *De Quervain's tenosynovitis* and *gonococcal tenosynovitis.* See Table 19-8, Tendon Sheath and Palmar Space Infections; Felons (p. 679).

Tenderness over the "snuffbox" in *scaphoid fracture,* the most common injury of the carpal bones. Poor blood supply puts the scaphoid bone at risk for *avascular necrosis.*

Palpate the eight carpal bones lying distal to the wrist joint, and then each of the five metacarpals and the proximal, middle, and distal phalanges.

Palpate any other area where you suspect an abnormality.

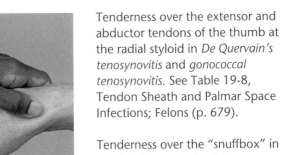

Compress the MCP joints by squeezing the hand from each side between the thumb and fingers. Alternatively, use your thumb to palpate each MCP joint just distal to and on each side of the knuckle as your index finger feels the head of the metacarpal in the palm. Note any swelling, bogginess, or tenderness.

Synovitis in the MCPs is painful with this pressure—a point to remember when shaking hands.
The MCPs are often boggy or tender in *rheumatoid arthritis* (but rarely involved in osteoarthritis). Pain with compression also in *posttraumatic arthritis.*

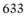

Now examine the fingers and thumb. Palpate the medial and lateral aspects of each PIP joint between your thumb and index finger, again checking for swelling, bogginess, bony enlargement, or tenderness.

PIP changes seen in *rheumatoid arthritis,* Bouchard's nodes in *osteoarthritis.* Pain at the base of the thumb in first *carpometacarpal arthritis.*

Hard dorsolateral nodules on the DIP joints, or *Heberden's nodes,* common in osteoarthritis; DIP joint involvement in *psoriatic arthritis*

Using the same techniques, examine the DIP joints.

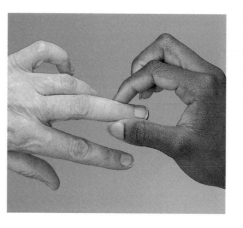

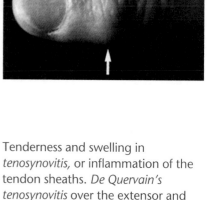

In any area of swelling or inflammation, palpate along the tendons inserting on the thumb and fingers.

Tenderness and swelling in *tenosynovitis,* or inflammation of the tendon sheaths. *De Quervain's tenosynovitis* over the extensor and abductor tendons of the thumb as they cross the radial styloid. See Table 19-8, Tendon Sheath and Palmar Space Infections; Felons (p. 679).

Range of Motion and Manoeuvres. Now assess range of motion for the wrists, fingers, and thumbs.

Conditions that impair range of motion include *arthritis, tenosynovitis, Dupuytren's contracture.* See Table 19-7, Swelling and Deformities of the Hands (p. 678).

Wrists. At the wrist, test flexion, extension, and ulnar and radial deviation.

■ *Flexion.* With the client's forearm stabilized, place the wrist in extension and put your fingertips in the client's palm. Ask the client to flex the wrist against gravity, then against graded resistance.

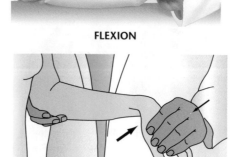

FLEXION

■ *Extension.* With the client's forearm stabilized, place the wrist in flexion and put your hand on the client's dorsal metacarpals. Ask the client to extend the wrist against gravity, then against graded resistance.

EXTENSION

■ *Ulnar and radial deviation.* With palms down, ask the client to move the wrists laterally and medially.

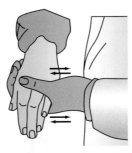

ULNAR AND RADIAL DEVIATION

Make an approximate test of *grip strength* by asking the client to grasp your second and third finger. This manoeuvre tests function of the intrinsic muscles and joints of the hand, the joints of the wrist, and the flexor tendons and muscles of the forearm. (Use a dynometer for more accurate measurements.)

Wrist pain and grip weakness in *de Quervain's tenosynovitis.* Decreased grip strength in *arthritis, carpal tunnel syndrome,* epicondylitis, and *cervical radiculopathy* (Anderson, 2004).

GRIP STRENGTH

Fingers. Test flexion, extension, abduction, and adduction of the fingers:

■ *Flexion and extension.* Ask the client to make a tight fist with each hand, thumb across the knuckles, and then extend and spread the fingers. The fingers should close and open smoothly and easily. At the MCPs, the fingers may extend beyond the neutral position. This manoeuvre also tests overall thumb function. Also test flexion and extension at the PIP and DIP joints.

Impaired hand movement in arthritis, trigger finger, Dupuytren's contracture

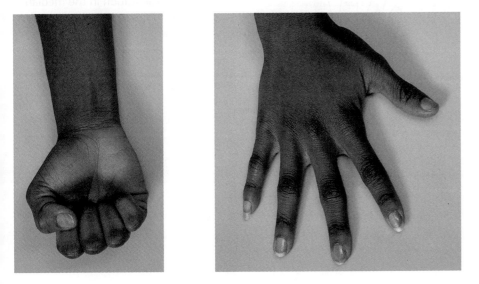

■ *Abduction and adduction.* Ask the client to spread the fingers apart (abduction) and back together (adduction). Check for smooth, coordinated movement.

Thumbs. At the thumb, assess flexion, extension, abduction, adduction, and opposition. Ask the client to move the thumb across the palm and touch the base of the 5th finger to test flexion, and then to move the thumb back across the palm and away from the fingers to test extension.

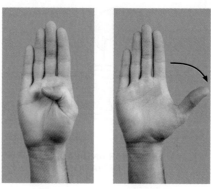

FLEXION **EXTENSION**

Next, ask the client to place the fingers and thumb in the neutral position with the palm up, then have the client move the thumb anteriorly away from the palm to assess abduction and back down for adduction. To test opposition, or movements of the thumb across the palm, ask the client to touch the thumb to each of the other fingertips.

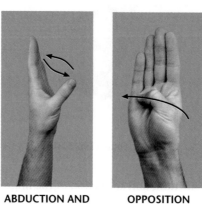

ABDUCTION AND **OPPOSITION**
ADDUCTION

Test sensation in the fingers only along the lateral and medial surfaces to isolate any alterations in the digital nerves. Test median, ulnar, and radial nerve function by checking sensation as follows:

- Pulp of the index finger—median nerve

- Pulp of the 5th finger—ulnar nerve

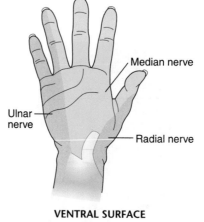

Median nerve

Ulnar nerve

Radial nerve

VENTRAL SURFACE

Decreased sensation in the median nerve distribution in carpal tunnel syndrome.

■ Dorsal web space of the thumb and index finger—radial nerve

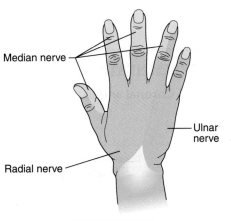

DORSAL SURFACE

THE SPINE

OVERVIEW

The vertebral column, or spine, is the central supporting structure of the trunk and back. Note the *concave curves* of the cervical and lumbar spine and the *convex curves* of the thoracic and sacrococcygeal spine. These curves help distribute upper body weight to the pelvis and lower extremities and cushion the concussive impact of walking or running.

The complex mechanics of the back reflect the coordinated action of:

■ The vertebrae and intervertebral discs

■ An interconnecting system of ligaments between anterior vertebrae and posterior vertebrae, ligaments between the spinous processes, and ligaments between the lamina of two adjacent vertebrae

■ Large superficial muscles, deeper intrinsic muscles, and muscles of the abdominal wall

Viewing the client from behind, identify the following landmarks:

1. Spinous processes, usually more prominent at C7 and T1 and more evident on forward flexion

2. Paravertebral muscles on either side of the midline

3. Scapulae

4. Iliac crests

5. Posterior superior iliac spines, usually marked by skin dimples.

A line drawn above the posterior iliac crests crosses the spinous process of L4.

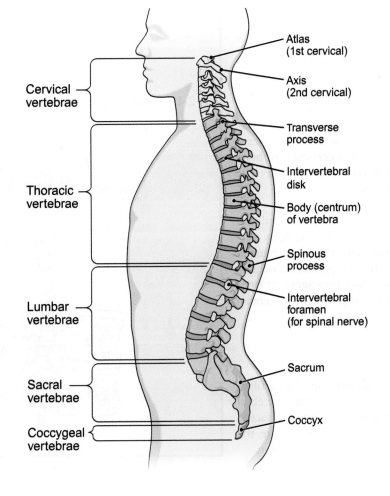

BONY STRUCTURES

The vertebral column contains 24 vertebrae stacked on the sacrum and coccyx. A typical vertebra contains sites for joint articulations, weight bearing, and muscle attachments, as well as foramina for the spinal nerve roots and peripheral nerves. Anteriorly, the *vertebral body* supports weight bearing. The posterior *vertebral arch* encloses the spinal cord. Review the location of the vertebral processes and foramina, with particular attention to:

■ The *spinous process* projecting posteriorly in the midline and the two transverse processes at the junction of the *pedicle* and the *lamina*. Muscles attach at these processes.

■ The *articular processes*—two on each side of the vertebra, one facing up and one facing down, at the junction of the pedicles and laminae, often called *articular facets*.

■ The *vertebral foramen*, which encloses the spinal cord, the *intervertebral foramen*, formed by the inferior and superior articulating process of adjacent vertebrae, creating a channel for the spinal nerve roots; and in the cervical vertebrae, the *transverse foramen* for the vertebral artery.

The proximity of the spinal cord and spinal nerve roots to their bony vertebral casing and the intervertebral discs makes them especially vulnerable to disc herniation, impingement from degenerative changes in the vertebrae, and trauma.

JOINTS

The spine has slightly movable cartilaginous joints between the vertebral bodies and between the articular facets. Between the vertebral bodies are the *intervertebral discs*, each consisting

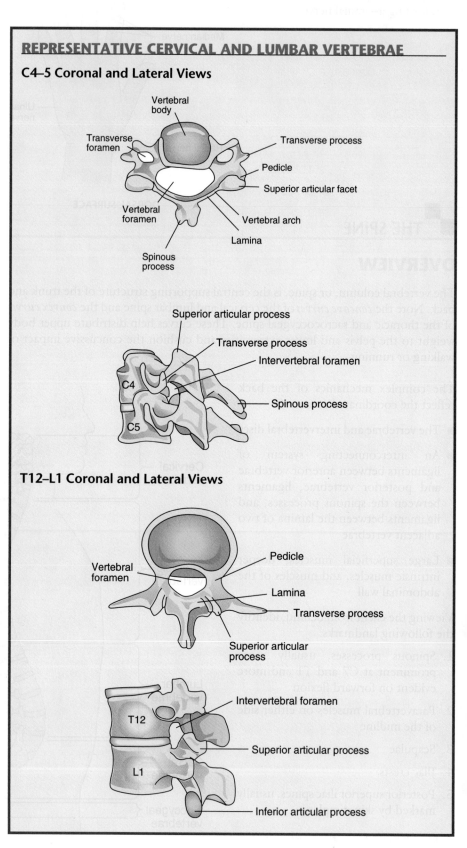

REPRESENTATIVE CERVICAL AND LUMBAR VERTEBRAE

C4–5 Coronal and Lateral Views

Vertebral body

Transverse foramen

Transverse process

Pedicle

Superior articular facet

Vertebral foramen

Vertebral arch

Lamina

Spinous process

Superior articular process

Transverse process

Intervertebral foramen

C4

Spinous process

C5

T12–L1 Coronal and Lateral Views

Vertebral foramen

Pedicle

Lamina

Transverse process

Superior articular process

Intervertebral foramen

T12

Superior articular process

L1

Inferior articular process

of a soft mucoid central core, the *nucleus pulposus*, rimmed by the tough fibrous tissue of the *annulus fibrosis*. The intervertebral discs cushion movement between vertebrae and allow the vertebral column to curve, flex, and bend. The flexibility of the spine is largely determined by the angle of the articular facet joints relative to the plane of the vertebral body, and varies at different levels of the spine. Note that the vertebral column angles sharply posterior at the *lumbosacral junction* and becomes immovable. The mechanical stress at this angulation contributes to the risk for disc herniation and subluxation, or slippage, of L5 on S1.

MUSCLE GROUPS

The *trapezius* and *latissimus dorsi* form the large outer layer of muscles attaching to each side of the spine. They overlie two deeper muscle layers—a layer attaching to the head, neck, and spinous processes (*splenius capitis*, *splenius cervicis*, and *sacrospinalis*) and a layer of smaller intrinsic muscles between vertebrae. Muscles attaching to the anterior surface of the vertebrae, including the *psoas* muscle and muscles of the abdominal wall, assist with flexion.

The muscles moving the neck and lower vertebral column are briefly described in the following table.

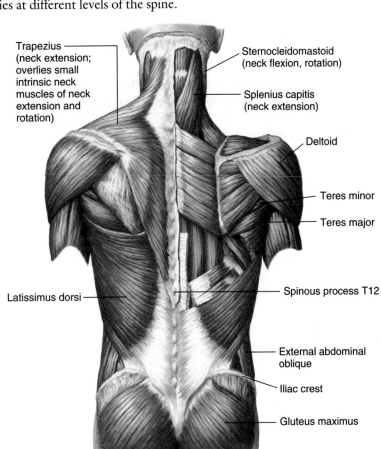

Trapezius (neck extension; overlies small intrinsic neck muscles of neck extension and rotation)

Latissimus dorsi

Sternocleidomastoid (neck flexion, rotation)

Splenius capitis (neck extension)

Deltoid

Teres minor

Teres major

Spinous process T12

External abdominal oblique

Iliac crest

Gluteus maximus

■ *Muscles of the Neck and Lower Vertebrae*

Movement	Principal Muscle Group
Cervical Spine (neck)	
Flexion	Sternocleidomastoid, scalene, and prevertebral muscles
Extension	Splenius, trapezius, small intrinsic neck muscles
Rotation	Sternocleidomastoid, small intrinsic neck muscles
Lateral bending	Scalene and small intrinsic neck muscles
Lumbar Spine	
Flexion	Psoas major, psoas minor, quadratus lumborum; abdominal muscles such as the internal and external obliques and rectus abdominis, attaching to the anterior vertebrae
Extension	Intrinsic muscles of the back, sacrospinalis
Rotation	Abdominal muscles, intrinsic muscles of the back
Lateral bending	Abdominal muscles, intrinsic muscles of the back

TECHNIQUES OF EXAMINATION

Inspection. Begin by observing the client's posture, including the position of both the neck and trunk, when entering the room.

Assess the client for erect position of the head, smooth, coordinated neck movement, and ease of gait.

Neck stiffness signals arthritis, muscle strain, or other underlying pathology that should be pursued.

Drape or gown the client to expose the entire back for complete inspection. If possible, the client should be upright in the natural standing position—with feet together and arms hanging at the sides. The head should be midline in the same plane as the sacrum, and the shoulders and pelvis should be level.

Lateral deviation and rotation of the head suggests *torticollis*, from contraction of the sternocleidomastoid muscle.

Inspect the client from the side. Evaluate the spinal curvatures.

Palpation. From a sitting or standing position, palpate the *spinous processes* of each vertebra with your thumb.

Tenderness suggests fracture or dislocation if preceded by trauma, underlying infection, or arthritis.

In the neck, also palpate the *facet joints* that lie between the cervical vertebrae about 2.5 cm lateral to the spinous processes of C2–C7. These joints lie deep to the trapezius muscle and may not be palpable unless the neck muscles are relaxed.

Tenderness in arthritis, especially at the facet joints between C5 and C6

Check the lower lumbar area carefully for any vertebral "step-offs," and determine if a spinous process seems unusually prominent (or recessed) in relation to the one above it. Identify any tenderness.

Step-offs in *spondylolisthesis*, or forward slippage of one vertebra, which may compress the spinal cord. Vertebral tenderness is suspicious for fracture or infection.

Palpate the sacroiliac joint, often identified by the dimple overlying the posterior superior iliac spine.

Tenderness over the sacroiliac joint in sacroiliitis. *Ankylosing spondylitis* may produce sacroiliac tenderness.

You may wish to percuss the spine for tenderness by thumping, but not too roughly, with the ulnar surface of your fist.

Pain on percussion may arise from *osteoporosis, infection,* or *malignancy.*

Inspect and palpate the paravertebral muscles for tenderness and spasm. Muscles in spasm feel firm and knotted and may be visible.

Spasm occurs in degenerative and inflammatory processes of muscles, prolonged contraction from abnormal posture, or anxiety.

With the hip flexed and the client lying on the opposite side, palpate the sciatic nerve, the largest nerve in the body, consisting of nerve roots from L4, L5, S1, S2, and S3. The nerve lies midway between the greater trochanter and the ischial tuberosity as it leaves the pelvis through the sciatic notch.

Sciatic nerve tenderness suggests a herniated disc or mass lesion impinging on the contributing nerve roots.

■ *Inspection of the Spine*

View of Client	Focus of Inspection	
From the side	Cervical, thoracic, and lumbar curves.	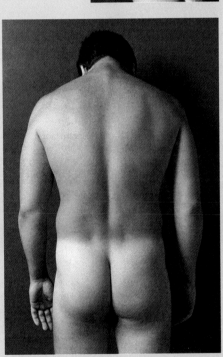 Cervical concavity Thoracic convexity Lumbar concavity
From behind	Upright spinal column (an imaginary line should fall from C7 through the gluteal cleft) Alignment of the shoulders, the iliac crests, and the skin creases below the buttocks (gluteal folds)	
	Skin markings, tags, or masses	

Increased *thoracic kyphosis* occurs with aging. In children a correctable structural deformity should be pursued.

In *scoliosis*, there is lateral and rotatory curvature of the spine to bring the head back to midline. Scoliosis often becomes evident during adolescence, before symptoms appear.

Unequal shoulder heights seen in: scoliosis; Sprengel's deformity of the scapula (from the attachment of an extra bone or band between the upper scapula and C7); in "winging" of the scapula (from loss of innervation of the serratus anterior muscle by the long thoracic nerve); and in contralateral weakness of the trapezius.

Unequal heights of the iliac crests, or *pelvic tilt,* suggest unequal lengths of the legs and disappear when a block is placed under the short leg and foot. Scoliosis and hip abduction or adduction may also cause a pelvic tilt. "Listing" of the trunk to one side is seen with a herniated lumbar disc.

Birthmarks, port-wine stains, hairy patches, and lipomas often overlie bony defects such as *spina bifida.*

Café-au-lait spots (discoloured patches of skin), skin tags, and fibrous tumours in *neurofibromatosis*

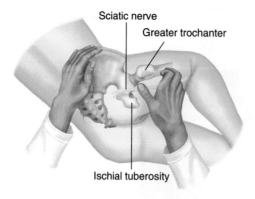

Sciatic nerve
Greater trochanter
Ischial tuberosity

Palpate for tenderness any other areas that are suggested by the client's symptoms. Recall that low back pain warrants careful assessment for cord compression, the most serious cause of pain, because of risk for paralysis of the affected limb.

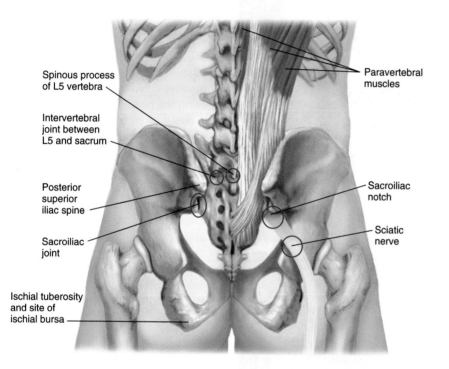

Spinous process of L5 vertebra

Intervertebral joint between L5 and sacrum

Posterior superior iliac spine

Sacroiliac joint

Ischial tuberosity and site of ischial bursa

Paravertebral muscles

Sacroiliac notch

Sciatic nerve

Herniated intervertebral discs, most common between L5 and S1 or between L4 and L5, may produce tenderness of the spinous processes, the intervertebral joints, the paravertebral muscles, the sacrosciatic notch, and the sciatic nerve.

Rheumatoid arthritis may also cause tenderness of the intervertebral joints.

Remember that tenderness in the costovertebral angles may signify kidney infection rather than a musculoskeletal problem.

See Table 19-1, Low Back Pain (p. 670).

Range of Motion and Manoeuvres. The neck is the most mobile portion of the spine, remarkable for its seven fragile vertebrae supporting the 5- to 7-kg head. Flexion and extension occur primarily between the skull and C1 (the atlas), rotation at C1–C2 (the axis), and lateral bending at C2–C7.

Ask the client to perform the following manoeuvres, and check for smooth, coordinated motion:

- *Flexion*. Touch the chin to the chest.

- *Extension*. Look up at the ceiling.

Limitations in range of motion can arise from stiffness from arthritis, pain from trauma, or muscle spasm such as *torticollis*.

It is important to assess any concerns or findings of neck, shoulder, or arm pain or numbness for possible cervical cord or nerve root compression. See Table 19-2, Pains in the Neck (p. 671).

■ *Rotation*. Turn the head to each side, looking directly over the shoulder.

■ *Lateral bending*. Tilt the head, touching each ear to the corresponding shoulder.

Tenderness, loss of sensation, or impaired movement warrants careful neurologic testing of the neck and upper extremities.

Now assess range of motion in the spinal column.

■ *Flexion*. Ask the client to bend forward to touch the toes (flexion). Note the smoothness and symmetry of movement, the range of motion, and the curve in the lumbar area. As flexion proceeds, the lumbar concavity should flatten out.

Tenderness at C1-C2 in *rheumatoid arthritis* suggests possible risk for subluxation and high cervical cord compression.

Deformity of the thorax on forward bending in *scoliosis*.

Persistence of lumbar lordosis suggests muscle spasm or *ankylosing spondylitis*.

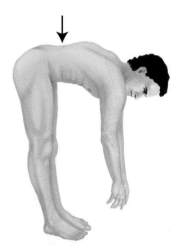

You may wish to measure the degree of flexion of the spine with the client standing and bending forward. Mark the spine at the lumbosacral junction, then 10 cm above and 5 cm below this point. A 4-cm increase between the two upper marks is usually seen. The distance between the lower two marks should be unchanged.

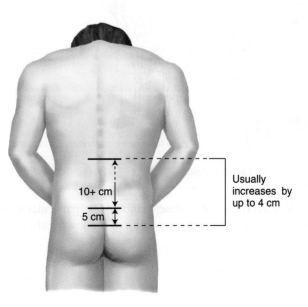

- *Extension*. Place your hand on the posterior superior iliac spine, with your fingers pointing toward the midline, and ask the client to bend backward as far as possible.

- *Rotation*. Stabilize the pelvis by placing one hand on the client's hip and the other on the opposite shoulder. Then rotate the trunk by pulling the shoulder and then the hip posteriorly. Repeat these manoeuvres for the opposite side.

- *Lateral bending*. Again stabilize the pelvis by placing your hand on the client's hip. Ask the client to lean to both sides as far as possible.

Decreased spinal mobility in *osteoarthritis* and *ankylosing spondylitis,* among other conditions (Haywood et al., 2004)

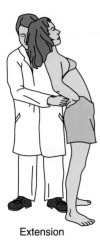

Extension

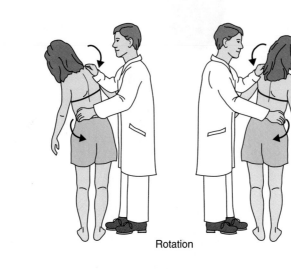

Rotation

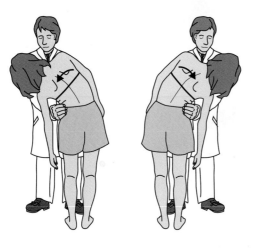

Lateral bending

As with the neck, pain or tenderness with these manoeuvres, particularly with radiation into the leg, warrants careful neurologic testing of the lower extremities.

Underlying cord or nerve root compression should be considered. Note that arthritis or infection in the hip, rectum, or pelvis may cause symptoms in the lumbar spine. See Table 19-1, Low Back Pain (p. 670).

◼ THE HIP

OVERVIEW

The hip joint is deeply embedded in the pelvis, and is notable for its strength, stability, and wide range of motion. The stability of the hip joint, so essential for weight bearing, arises from the deep fit of the head of the femur into the *acetabulum*, its strong fibrous articular capsule, and the powerful muscles crossing the joint and inserting below the femoral head, providing leverage for movement of the femur.

BONY STRUCTURES AND JOINTS

The hip joint lies below the middle third of the inguinal ligament, but in a deeper plane. It is a ball-and-socket joint—note how the rounded head of the femur articulates with the cuplike cavity of the acetabulum. Because of its overlying muscles and depth, it is not readily palpable. Review the bones of the pelvis—the *acetabulum*, the *ilium*, and the *ischium*—and the connection inferiorly at the *symphysis pubis* and posteriorly with the sacroiliac bone.

On the *anterior aspect* of the hip, identify the *iliac crest* at the upper margin of the pelvis at the level of L4. Follow the downward anterior curve and locate the *iliac tubercle*, marking the widest point of the crest, and continue tracking downward to the *anterior superior iliac spine*. Place your thumbs on the anterior superior spines and move your fingers downward from the iliac tubercles to the *greater trochanter* of the femur. Then move your thumbs medially and obliquely to the *pubic symphysis*, which lies at the same level as the greater trochanter.

On the *posterior aspect* of the hip, locate the *posterior superior iliac spine* directly underneath the visible dimples just above the buttocks. Placing your left thumb and index finger over the posterior superior iliac spine, next, locate the *greater trochanter* laterally with your fingers at the level of the gluteal fold, and place your thumb medially on the *ischial tuberosity*. The *sacroiliac joint* is not always palpable. Note that an imaginary line between the posterior superior iliac spines crosses the joint at S2.

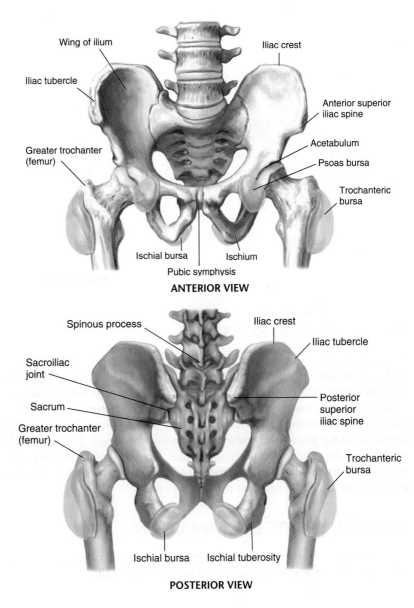

ANTERIOR VIEW

Wing of ilium · Iliac tubercle · Greater trochanter (femur) · Ischial bursa · Pubic symphysis · Iliac crest · Anterior superior iliac spine · Acetabulum · Psoas bursa · Trochanteric bursa · Ischium

POSTERIOR VIEW

Spinous process · Sacroiliac joint · Sacrum · Greater trochanter (femur) · Iliac crest · Iliac tubercle · Posterior superior iliac spine · Trochanteric bursa · Ischial bursa · Ischial tuberosity

MUSCLE GROUPS

Four powerful muscle groups move the hip. Picture these groups as you examine clients, and remember that to move the femur or any bone in a given direction, the proximal and distal muscle insertions must *extend across the joint line*.

The *flexor group* lies anteriorly and flexes the thigh. The primary hip flexor is the *iliopsoas*, extending from above the iliac crest to the lesser trochanter. The *extensor group* lies posteriorly and extends the thigh. The *gluteus maximus* is the primary extensor of the hip. It forms a band crossing from its origin along the medial pelvis to its insertion below the trochanter.

The *adductor group* is medial and swings the thigh toward the body. The muscles in this group arise from the rami of the pubis and ischium and insert on the posteromedial aspect of the femur. The *abductor group* is lateral, extending from the iliac crest to the head of the femur, and moves the thigh away from the body. This group includes the *gluteus medius* and *minimus*. These muscles help stabilize the pelvis during the stance phase of gait.

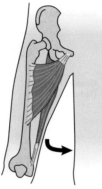

Iliopsoas

Gluteus maximus

Flexor group

Extensor group

Adductor group

Abductor group

ADDITIONAL STRUCTURES

A strong dense articular capsule, extending from the acetabulum to the femoral neck, encases and strengthens the hip joint, reinforced by three overlying ligaments and lined with synovial membrane. There are three principal bursae at the hip. Anterior to the joint is the psoas (also termed *iliopectineal* or *iliopsoas*) *bursa*, overlying the articular capsule and the psoas muscle. Find the bony prominence lateral to the hip joint—the *greater trochanter* of the femur. The large multilocular *trochanteric bursa* lies on its posterior surface. The *ischial* (or *ischiogluteal*) *bursa*—not always present—lies under the *ischeal tuberosity* on which a person sits. Note its proximity to the sciatic nerve, as shown on p. 642.

TECHNIQUES OF EXAMINATION

Inspection. Inspection of the hip begins with careful observation of the client's gait on entering the room. Observe the two phases of gait:

■ *Stance*—when the foot is on the ground and bears weight (60% of the walking cycle)

Most problems appear during the weight-bearing stance phase.

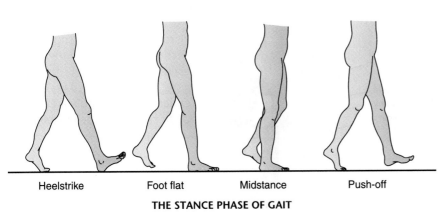

| Heelstrike | Foot flat | Midstance | Push-off |

THE STANCE PHASE OF GAIT

■ *Swing*—when the foot moves forward and does not bear weight (40% of the cycle)

Observe the gait for the width of the base, the shift of the pelvis, and flexion of the knee. The width of the base should be 5 to 10 cm from heel to heel. Expected gait has a smooth, continuous rhythm, achieved in part by contraction of the abductors of the weight-bearing limb. Abductor contraction stabilizes the pelvis and helps maintain balance, raising the opposite hip. The knee should be flexed throughout the stance phase, except when the heel strikes the ground to counteract motion at the ankle.

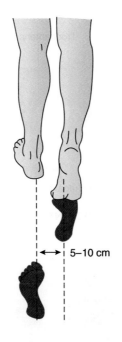

5–10 cm

A wide base suggests cerebellar disease or foot problems.

Hip dislocation, arthritis, or abductor weakness can cause the pelvis to drop on the opposite side, producing a waddling gait.

Lack of knee flexion interrupts the smooth pattern of gait.

Observe the lumbar portion of the spine for slight lordosis and, with the client supine, assess the length of the legs for symmetry. (To measure leg length, see Special Techniques, p. 663.)

Loss of lordosis may reflect *paravertebral spasm*; excess lordosis suggests a *flexion deformity* of the hip.

Changes in leg length are seen in abduction or adduction deformities and scoliosis. Leg shortening and external rotation suggest *hip fracture*.

Inspect the anterior and posterior surfaces of the hip for any areas of muscle atrophy or bruising.

Palpation. Review the surface landmarks of the hip. On the *anterior surface* locate the *iliac crest*, the *iliac tubercle*, and the *anterior superior iliac spine*. On the *posterior surface* identify the *posterior superior iliac spine*, the *greater trochanter*, the *ischial tuberosity*, and the *sciatic nerve*.

With the client supine, ask the client to place the heel of the leg being examined on the opposite knee. Then palpate along the *inguinal ligament*, which extends from the anterior superior iliac spine to the pubic tubercle. The femoral nerve, artery, and vein bisect the overlying inguinal ligament; lymph nodes lie medially. The mnemonic **NAVEL** may help you remember the lateral-to-medial sequence of **N**erve—**A**rtery—**V**ein— **E**mpty space—**L**ymph node.

If the hip is painful, palpate the *(psoas) bursa* below the inguinal ligament but on a deeper plane.

With the client resting on one side and the hip flexed and internally rotated, palpate the *trochanteric bursa* lying over the greater trochanter. Usually, the *ischiogluteal bursa*, over the ischial tub-erosity, is not palpable unless inflamed.

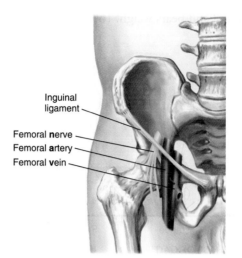

Inguinal ligament

Femoral **nerve**
Femoral **artery**
Femoral **vein**

Bulges along the ligament may suggest an *inguinal hernia* or, on occasion, an *aneurysm*.

Enlarged lymph nodes suggest infection in the lower extremity or pelvis.

Tenderness in the groin area may be due to *synovitis* of the hip joint, *bursitis*, or possibly *psoas abscess*.

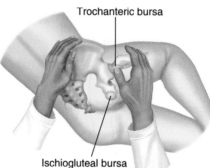

Trochanteric bursa

Ischiogluteal bursa

TROCHANTERIC BURSA

Focal tenderness over the trochanter in *trochanteric bursitis*. Tenderness over the posterolateral surface of the greater trochanter in localized tendonitis or muscle spasm from referred hip pain.

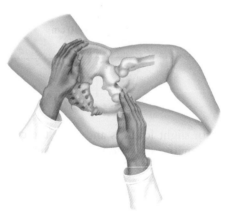

ISCHIOGLUTEAL BURSA

Tenderness in *ischiogluteal bursitis* or "weaver's bottom"—because of the adjacent sciatic nerve, this may mimic sciatica.

Range of Motion and Manoeuvres. Motions at the hip include *flexion*, *extension*, *abduction*, *adduction*, and *rotation*. Note that the hip can flex farther when the knee is also flexed. The direction of rotation at the hip while the knee is flexed may be confusing at first: when the lower leg swings laterally, the femur rotates internally. It is the motion of the femur at the hip joint that identifies these movements.

■ *Flexion*. With the client supine, place your hand under the client's lumbar spine. Ask the client to bend each knee in turn up to the chest and pull it firmly against the abdomen. Note when the back touches your hand, indicating usual flattening of the lumbar lordosis—further flexion must arise from the hip joint itself.

In *flexion deformity of the hip,* as the opposite hip is flexed (with the thigh against the chest), the affected hip does not allow full leg extension, and the affected thigh appears flexed.

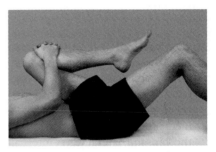

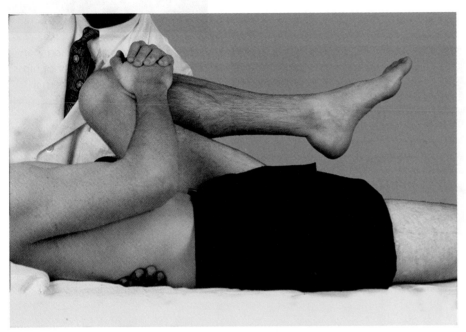

HIP FLEXION AND FLATTENING OF LUMBAR LORDOSIS

As the thigh is held against the abdomen, observe the degree of flexion at the hip and knee. Usually, the anterior portion of the thigh can almost touch the chest wall. Note whether the opposite thigh remains fully extended, resting on the table.

Flexion deformity may be masked by an increase, rather than flattening, in lumbar lordosis and an anterior pelvic tilt.

■ *Extension*. With the client lying face down, extend the thigh toward you in a posterior direction. Alternatively, carefully position the supine client near the edge of the table and extend the leg posteriorly.

■ *Abduction*. Stabilize the pelvis by pressing down on the opposite anterior superior iliac spine with one hand. With the other hand, grasp the ankle and abduct the extended leg until you feel the iliac spine move. This movement marks the limit of hip abduction.

Restricted abduction is common in hip *osteoarthritis*.

Alternatively, stand at the foot of the table, grasp both ankles, and spread them maximally, abducting both extended legs at the hips. This method provides easy comparison of two sides when movements are restricted, but it is impractical when range of motion is full.

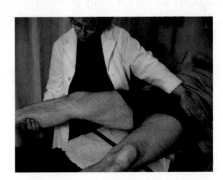

■ *Adduction.* With the client supine, stabilize the pelvis, hold one ankle, and move the leg medially across the body and over the opposite extremity.

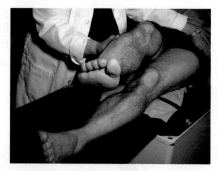

■ *External and internal rotation.* Flex the leg to 90° at hip and knee, stabilize the thigh with one hand, grasp the ankle with the other, and swing the lower leg—medially for external rotation at the hip and laterally for internal rotation.

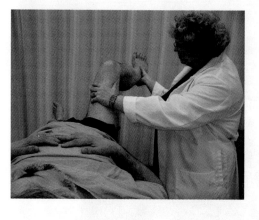

Restriction of internal rotation is an especially sensitive indicator of hip disease such as arthritis. External rotation is also often restricted.

THE KNEE

OVERVIEW

The knee joint is the largest joint in the body. It is a hinge joint involving three bones: the femur, the tibia, and the patella (or knee cap), with three articular surfaces, two between the femur and the tibia and one between the femur and the patella. Note how the two rounded condyles of the femur rest on the relatively flat tibial plateau. There is no inherent stability in the knee joint itself, making it dependent on ligaments to hold its articulating bones in place. This feature, in addition to the lever action of the femur on the tibia and lack of padding from fat or muscle, makes the knee highly vulnerable to injury.

BONY STRUCTURES

Landmarks in and around the knee will orient you to this complicated joint. Bring your fingertips firmly down the medial surface of the thigh along a line analogous to the inner seam of a pant leg. Your fingers will run up against an abrupt bony prominence, the *adductor tubercle*. Just below this is the *medial epicondyle*. The *lateral epicondyle* is comparably situated on the other side.

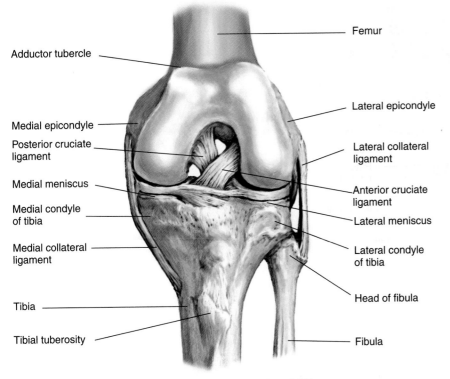

ANTERIOR ASPECT OF THE KNEE

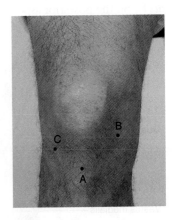

Identify the flat medial surface of the tibia—the shin. Follow its anterior border upward to the *tibial tuberosity* (**A**). Mark this point with a dot of ink. Now follow the medial border of the tibia upward until it merges into a bony prominence—the *medial condyle* of the tibia (**B**). This is somewhat higher than the tibial tuberosity. In a comparable location on the other side of the knee, find a similar prominence—the *lateral condyle* (**C**). Mark both condyles with ink. On the lateral surface of the knee, somewhat below the level of the lateral tibial condyle, find the head of the fibula.

The *patella* rests on the anterior articulating surface of the femur, midway between the epicondyles, embedded in the tendon of the quadriceps muscle. This tendon continues below the knee joint as the *patellar tendon* and inserts on the tibial tuberosity.

JOINTS

Two condylar *tibiofemoral joints* are formed by the convex curves of the medial and lateral condyles of the femur as they articulate with the concave condyles of the tibia. The third articular surface is the *patellofemoral joint*. The patella slides in a groove on the anterior aspect of the distal femur, called the *trochlear groove*, during flexion and extension of the knee.

With the knee flexed about 90°, you can press your thumbs—one on each side of the patellar tendon—into the groove of the tibiofemoral joint. Note that the patella lies just above this joint line. As you press your thumbs downward, you can feel the edge of the tibial plateau, the upper surface of the tibia. Follow it medially, then laterally, until you are stopped by the converging femur and tibia. By moving your thumbs upward toward the midline to the top of the patella, you can follow the articulating surface of the femur and identify the margins of the joint.

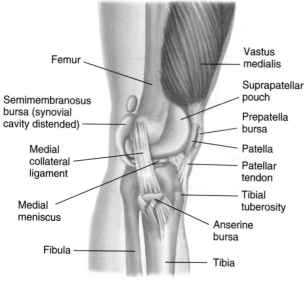

LEFT KNEE—MEDIAL VIEW

MUSCLE GROUPS

Powerful muscles move and support the knee. The *quadriceps femoris* extends the leg, covering the anterior, medial, and lateral aspects of the thigh. The *hamstring muscles* lie on the posterior aspect of the thigh and flex the knee.

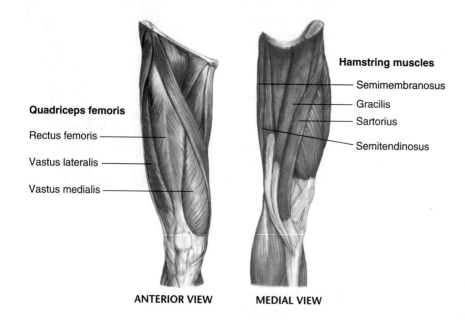

ANTERIOR VIEW   **MEDIAL VIEW**

ADDITIONAL STRUCTURES

Two important pairs of ligaments, the collateral ligaments and the cruciate ligaments, and the menisci provide stability to the knee (see pp. 651 and 654).

■ The *medial collateral ligament* (MCL), not easily palpable, is a broad flat ligament connecting the medial condyles of the femur and the tibia. To locate the anatomical region of the MCL, move your fingers medially and posteriorly along the joint line, and then palpate along the ligament from its origin to insertion.

- The *lateral collateral ligament* (LCL) connects the lateral femoral condyle and the head of the fibula. To feel the LCL, cross one leg so the ankle rests on the opposite knee and find the firm cord that runs from the lateral epicondyle of the femur to the head of the fibula. The MCL and LCL provide medial and lateral stability to the knee.

- The *anterior cruciate ligament* (ACL) crosses obliquely from the lateral femoral condyle to the medial tibia, preventing the tibia from sliding forward on the femur.

- The *posterior cruciate ligament* (PCL) crosses from the lateral tibia and lateral meniscus to the medial femoral condyle, preventing the tibia from slipping backward on the femur. Because these ligaments lie within the knee joint, they are not palpable. They are nonetheless crucial to the anteroposterior stability of the knee.

- The *medial and lateral menisci* cushion the action of the femur on the tibia. These crescent-shaped fibrocartilaginous discs add a cuplike surface to the otherwise flat tibial plateau. Palpate the *medial meniscus* by pressing on the medial soft-tissue depression along the upper edge of the tibial plateau. Place the knee in slight flexion and palpate the *lateral meniscus* along the lateral joint line.

Observe the concavities that are usually evident at each side of the patella and also above it. Occupying these areas is the synovial cavity of the knee, the largest joint cavity in the body. This cavity includes an extension 6 cm above the upper border of the patella, lying upward and deep to the quadriceps muscle—the *suprapatellar pouch*. The joint cavity covers the anterior, medial, and lateral surfaces of the knee, as well as the condyles of the femur and tibia posteriorly. Although the synovium is not usually detectable, these areas may become swollen and tender when the joint is inflamed.

Several bursae lie near the knee. The *prepatellar bursa* lies between the patella and the overlying skin. The *anserine bursa* lies 2 to 5 cm below the knee joint on the medial surface, proximal and medial to the attachments of the medial hamstring muscles on the proximal tibia. It cannot be palpated due to these overlying tendons. Now identify the large *semimembranosus bursa* that communicates with the joint cavity, also on the posterior and medial surfaces of the knee.

TECHNIQUES OF EXAMINATION

Inspection.   Observe the gait for a smooth, rhythmic flow as the client enters the room. The knee should be extended at heel strike and flexed at all other phases of swing and stance.

Check the alignment and contours of the knees. Observe any atrophy of the quadriceps muscles.

Look for loss of the hollows around the patella, a sign of swelling in the knee joint and suprapatellar pouch; note any other swelling in or around the knee.

Palpation.   Ask the client to sit on the edge of the examining table with the knees in flexion. In this position, bony landmarks are more visible, and the muscles, tendons, and ligaments are more relaxed, making them easier to palpate.

Stumbling or pushing the knee into extension with the hand during heel strike suggests *quadriceps weakness.*

Bowlegs (*genu varum*) and knock-knees (*genu valgum*) are common; flexion contracture (inability to extend fully) in limb paralysis.

Swelling over the patella suggests *prepatellar bursitis.* Swelling over the tibial tubercle suggests *infrapatellar* or, if more medial, *anserine bursitis.*

First, review the important bony landmarks of the knee. Facing the knee, place your thumbs in the soft-tissue depressions on either side of the *patellar tendon*. On the medial aspect, move your thumb upward, then downward, and identify the *medial femoral condyle* and the upper margin of the *medial tibial plateau*. Trace the patellar tendon distally to the *tibial tubercle*. The *adductor tubercle* is posterior to the *medial femoral condyle*.

Lateral to the patellar tendon, identify the *lateral femoral condyle* and the *lateral tibial plateau*. The medial and lateral femoral *epicondyles* are lateral to the condyles, with the knee in flexion. Locate the *patella*.

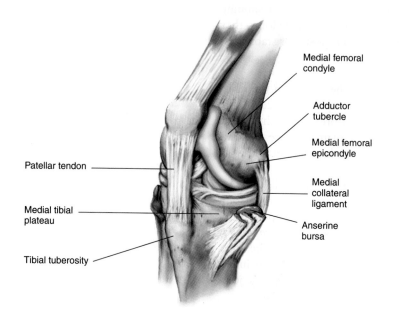

Palpate the ligaments, the borders of the menisci, and the bursae of the knee, paying special attention to any areas of tenderness. Pain is a common complaint in knee problems, and localizing the structure causing pain is important for accurate evaluation.

In the *patellofemoral compartment*, palpate the patellar tendon and ask the client to extend the leg to make sure the tendon is intact.

Tenderness over the tendon or inability to extend the leg suggests a partial or complete tear of the patellar tendon.

With the client supine and the knee extended, compress the patella against the underlying femur. Ask the client to tighten the quadriceps as the patella moves distally in the trochlear groove. Check for a smooth sliding motion (the *patellofemoral grinding test*).

Pain and crepitus suggest roughening of the patellar undersurface that articulates with the femur. Similar pain may occur with climbing stairs or getting up from a chair.

Pain with compression and with patellar movement during quadriceps contraction suggests *chondromalacia*, or degenerative patella (the patellofemoral syndrome).

Now assess the *medial and lateral compartments* of the *tibiofemoral joint*. Flex the client's knee to about 90°. The client's foot should rest on the examining table. Palpate the MCL between the medial femoral epicondyle and the femur; then palpate the cordlike LCL between the lateral femoral epicondyle and the fibular head.

Palpate the *medial and lateral menisci* along the medial and lateral joint lines. It is easier to palpate the medial meniscus if the tibia is internally rotated. Note any swelling or tenderness.

Note any irregular bony ridges along the joint margins.

Try to feel any thickening or swelling in the suprapatellar pouch and along the sides of the patella. Start 10 cm above the superior border of the patella (well above the pouch) and feel the soft tissues between your thumb and fingers. Move your hand distally in progressive steps, trying to identify the pouch. Continue your palpation along the sides of the patella. Note any tenderness or warmth greater than in the surrounding tissues.

MCL tenderness after injury is suspicious for an MCL tear. (The LCL is less subject to injury.)

Tenderness from tears following injury is more common in the medial meniscus.

Tender bony ridges along the joint margins may be felt in osteoarthritis (Altman et al., 1986; Cibere et al., 2004)

Swelling above and adjacent to the patella suggests synovial thickening or effusion in the knee joint.

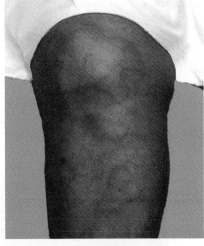

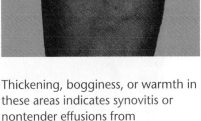

Thickening, bogginess, or warmth in these areas indicates synovitis or nontender effusions from osteoarthritis.

Check three other bursae for bogginess or swelling. Palpate the *prepatellar bursa* and over the *anserine bursa* on the posteromedial side of the knee between the MCL and the tendons inserting on the medial tibial and plateau. On the posterior surface, with the leg extended, check the medial aspect of the popliteal fossa.

Prepatellar bursitis ("housemaid's knee") from excessive kneeling. *Anserine bursitis* from running, valgus knee deformity, fibromyalgias, osteoarthritis. A *popliteal or "baker's" cyst* from distention of the gastrocnemius semimembranosus bursa.

Three further tests will help you detect fluid in the knee joint.

- The *Bulge Sign (for minor effusions)*. With the knee extended, place the left hand above the knee and apply pressure on the suprapatellar pouch, displacing or "milking" fluid downward. Stroke downward on the medial aspect of the knee and apply pressure to force fluid into the lateral area. Tap the knee just behind the lateral margin of the patella with the right hand.

A fluid wave or bulge on the medial side between the patella and the femur is considered a positive bulge sign consistent with an effusion.

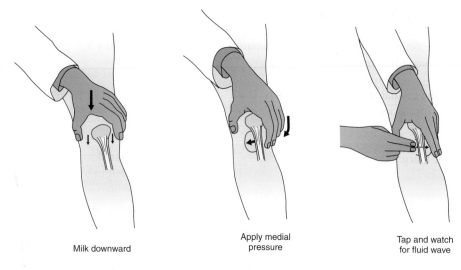

Milk downward   Apply medial   Tap and watch
                       pressure   for fluid wave

■ The *Balloon Sign (for major effusions)*. Place the thumb and index finger of your right hand on each side of the patella; with the left hand, compress the suprapatellar pouch against the femur. Feel for fluid entering (or ballooning into) the spaces next to the patella under your right thumb and index finger.

When the knee joint contains a large effusion, suprapatellar compression ejects fluid into the spaces adjacent to the patella. A palpable fluid wave signifies a positive "balloon sign." A returning fluid wave into the suprapatellar pouch confirms an effusion.

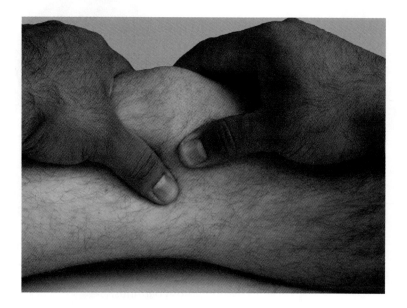

■ *Ballotting the patella*. To assess large effusions, you can also compress the suprapatellar pouch and "ballotte" or push the patella sharply against the femur. Watch for fluid returning to the suprapatellar pouch.

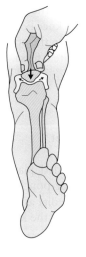

Palpable fluid returning into the pouch further confirms the presence of a large effusion.

A palpable patellar click with compression may also occur, but yields more false positives.

Range of Motion and Manoeuvres.

The principal movements of the knee are flexion, extension, and internal and external rotation. Ask the client to flex and extend the knee while sitting. To check internal and external rotation, instruct the client to rotate the foot medially and laterally. Knee flexion and extension can also be assessed by asking the client to squat and stand up—provide support if needed to maintain balance.

You will often need to test ligamentous stability and integrity of the menisci, particularly when there is a history of trauma or palpable tenderness (Jackson, O'Malley, & Kroenke, 2003; Solomon et al., 2001). Always examine both knees and compare findings.

Crepitus uteri flexion and extension in osteoarthritis (Altman et al., 1986; Cibere et al., 2004)

■ Techniques for Examining the Knee

Structure	Manoeuvre
Medial collateral ligament (MCL)	**Abduction (or Valgus) Stress Test.** With the client supine and the knee slightly flexed, move the thigh about 30° laterally to the side of the table. Place one hand against the lateral knee to stabilize the femur and the other hand around the medial ankle. Push medially against the knee and pull laterally at the ankle to open the knee joint on the medial side (*valgus stress*).
Lateral collateral ligament (LCL)	**Adduction (or Varus) Stress Test.** Now, with the thigh and knee in the same position, change your position so you can place one hand against the medial surface of the knee and the other around the lateral ankle. Push medially against the knee and pull laterally at the ankle to open the knee joint on the lateral side (*varus stress*).
Anterior cruciate ligament (ACL)	**Anterior Drawer Sign.** With the client supine, hips flexed and knees flexed to 90° and feet flat on the table, cup your hands around the knee with the thumbs on the medial and lateral joint line and the fingers on the medial and lateral insertions of the hamstrings. Draw the tibia forward and observe if it slides forward (like a drawer) from under the femur. Compare the degree of forward movement with that of the opposite knee.

Pain or a gap in the medial joint line points to ligamentous laxity and a partial tear of the *medial collateral ligament*. Most injuries are on the medial side.

Pain or a gap in the lateral joint line points to ligamentous laxity and a partial tear of the *lateral collateral ligament*.

A few degrees of forward movement are usual if equally present on the opposite side.

A forward jerk showing the contours of the upper tibia is a *positive anterior drawer sign* and suggests a tear of the *ACL*.

(continued)

■ Techniques for Examining the Knee (Continued)

Structure	Manoeuvre
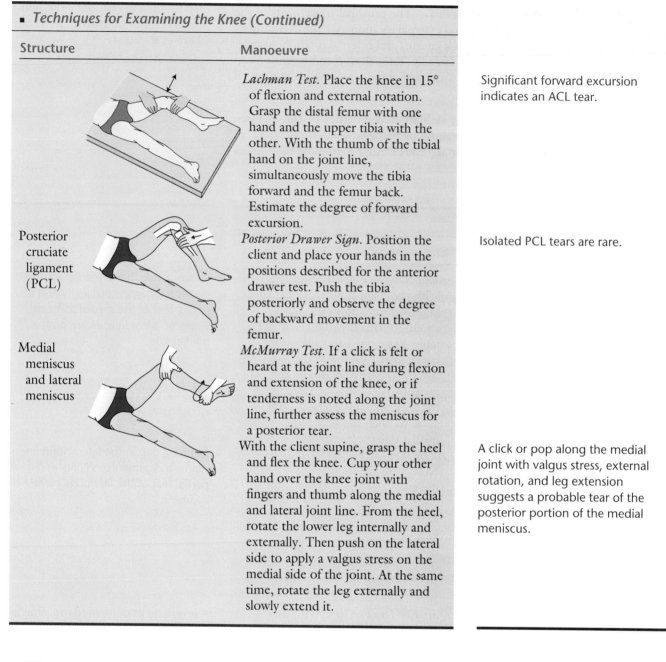	*Lachman Test*. Place the knee in 15° of flexion and external rotation. Grasp the distal femur with one hand and the upper tibia with the other. With the thumb of the tibial hand on the joint line, simultaneously move the tibia forward and the femur back. Estimate the degree of forward excursion.
Posterior cruciate ligament (PCL)	*Posterior Drawer Sign*. Position the client and place your hands in the positions described for the anterior drawer test. Push the tibia posteriorly and observe the degree of backward movement in the femur.
Medial meniscus and lateral meniscus	*McMurray Test*. If a click is felt or heard at the joint line during flexion and extension of the knee, or if tenderness is noted along the joint line, further assess the meniscus for a posterior tear. With the client supine, grasp the heel and flex the knee. Cup your other hand over the knee joint with fingers and thumb along the medial and lateral joint line. From the heel, rotate the lower leg internally and externally. Then push on the lateral side to apply a valgus stress on the medial side of the joint. At the same time, rotate the leg externally and slowly extend it.

Significant forward excursion indicates an ACL tear.

Isolated PCL tears are rare.

A click or pop along the medial joint with valgus stress, external rotation, and leg extension suggests a probable tear of the posterior portion of the medial meniscus.

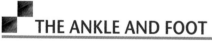

THE ANKLE AND FOOT

OVERVIEW

The total weight of the body is transmitted through the ankle to the foot. The ankle and foot must balance the body and absorb the impact of the heel strike and gait. Despite thick padding along the toes, sole, and heel and stabilizing ligaments at the ankles, the ankle and foot are frequent sites of sprain and bony injury.

BONY STRUCTURES AND JOINTS

The ankle is a hinge joint formed by the *tibia*, the *fibula*, and the *talus*. The tibia and fibula act as a mortise, stabilizing the joint while bracing the talus like an inverted cup.

The principal joints of the ankle are the *tibiotalar joint*, between the tibia and the talus, and the *subtalar (talocalcaneal) joint*.

Note the principal landmarks of the ankle: the *medial malleolus*, the bony prominence at the distal end of the tibia, and the *lateral malleolus*, at the distal end of the fibula. Lodged under the talus and jutting posteriorly is the *calcaneus*, or heel.

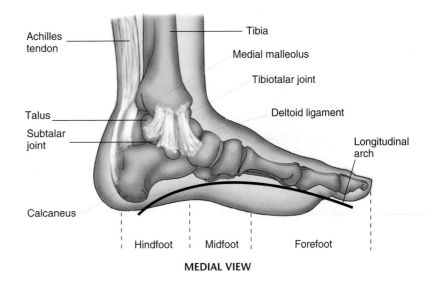

MEDIAL VIEW

An imaginary line, the *longitudinal arch*, spans the foot, extending from the calcaneus of the hind foot along the tarsal bones of the midfoot (see cuneiforms, navicular, and cuboid bones below) to the forefoot metatarsals and toes. The *heads of the metatarsals* are palpable in the ball of the foot. In the forefoot, identify the *metatarsophalangeal joints*, proximal to the webs of the toes, and the *proximal and distal interphalangeal joints* of the toes.

MUSCLE GROUPS AND ADDITIONAL STRUCTURES

Movement at the ankle joint is limited to dorsiflexion and plantar flexion. *Plantar flexion* is powered by the gastrocnemius, the posterior tibial muscle, and the toe flexors. Their tendons run behind the malleoli. The *dorsiflexors* include the anterior tibial muscle and the toe extensors. They lie prominently on the anterior surface, or dorsum, of the ankle, anterior to the malleoli.

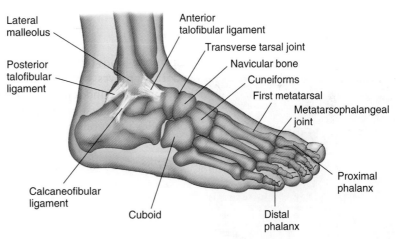

LATERAL VIEW

Ligaments extend from each malleolus onto the foot. Medially, the triangle-shaped *deltoid ligament* fans out from the inferior surface of the medial malleolus to the talus and proximal tarsal bones, protecting against stress from eversion (ankle bows inward). The three ligaments on the lateral side are less substantial, with higher risk for injury: the *anterior talofibular ligament*—most at risk in injury from inversion (ankle bows outward) injuries; the *calcaneofibular ligament*, and the *posterior talofibular ligament*. The strong Achilles tendon inserts on the heel posteriorly. The plantar fascia inserts on the medial tubercle of the calcaneus.

TECHNIQUES OF EXAMINATION

Inspection. Observe all surfaces of the ankles and feet, noting any deformities, nodules, or swellings, and any calluses or corns.

See Table 19-9, Unexpected Findings of the Feet (p. 680) and Table 19-10, Unexpected Findings of the Toes and Soles (p. 681).

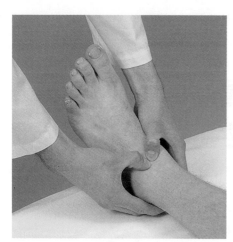

Palpation. With your thumbs, palpate the anterior aspect of each *ankle joint*, noting any bogginess, swelling, or tenderness.

Localized tenderness in arthritis, ligamentous injury, or infection of the ankle

Feel along the *Achilles tendon* for nodules and tenderness.

Rheumatoid nodules; tenderness in Achilles tendonitis, bursitis, or partial tear from trauma

Palpate the heel, especially the posterior and inferior calcaneus, and the plantar fascia for tenderness.

Bone spurs may be present on the calcaneus. Focal heel pain on palpation of the plantar fascia suggests *plantar fasciitis;* seen in prolonged standing or heel-strike exercise, also in rheumatoid arthritis, gout (Buchbinder, 2004; Young et al., 2001).

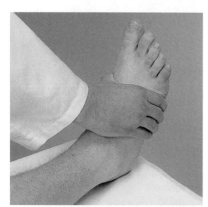

Palpate the *metatarsophalangeal joints* for tenderness. Compress the forefoot between the thumb and fingers. Exert pressure just proximal to the heads of the 1st and 5th metatarsals.

Tenderness on compression is an early sign of *rheumatoid arthritis.* Acute inflammation of the first metatarsophalangeal joint is associated with gout.

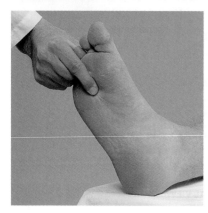

Palpate the heads of the five metatarsals and the grooves between them with your thumb and index finger. Place your thumb on the dorsum of the foot and your index finger on the plantar surface.

Pain and tenderness, called *metatarsalgia,* seen in trauma, arthritis, vascular compromise

Tenderness over the 3rd and 4th metatarsal heads on the plantar surface in Morton's neuroma (see p. 680)

Range of Motion and Manoeuvres. Range of motion at the ankle includes *flexion* and *extension at the ankle (tibiotalar) joint* and, *in the foot, inversion* and *eversion* at the subtalar and transverse tarsal joints.

■ *The ankle (tibiotalar) joint.* Dorsiflex and plantar-flex the foot at the ankle.

- *The subtalar (talocalcaneal) joint.* Stabilize the ankle with one hand, grasp the heel with the other, and invert and evert the foot.

- *The transverse tarsal joint.* Stabilize the heel and invert and evert the forefoot.

Pain during movements of the ankle and the foot helps to localize possible arthritis.

An arthritic joint is frequently painful when moved in any direction, whereas a ligamentous sprain produces maximal pain when the ligament is stretched. For example, in a common form of sprained ankle, inversion and plantar flexion of the foot cause pain, whereas eversion and plantar flexion are relatively pain-free.

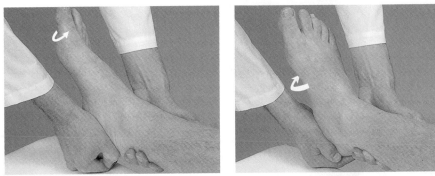

INVERSION   **EVERSION**

- *The metatarsophalangeal joints.* Flex the toes in relation to the feet.

■ SPECIAL TECHNIQUES

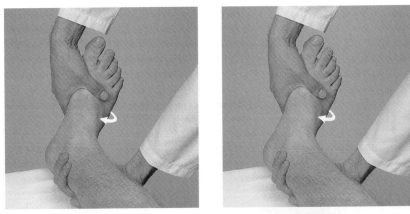

INVERSION   **EVERSION**

FOR CARPAL TUNNEL SYNDROME

Pain and numbness on the ventral surface of the first three digits of the hand (but not in the palm), especially at night, suggest median nerve compression in the carpal tunnel, which lies between the carpal bones dorsally and a ventral band of more superficial fascia, the *flexor retinaculum.*

Onset often related to repetitive motion with wrists flexed (e.g., keyboard use, mail sorting), pregnancy, rheumatoid arthritis, diabetes, hypothyroidism.

Appropriate symptoms and objective loss of sensation on the ventral surface of the hand in the distribution of the median nerve (see p. 629), and *weak abduction of the thumb* on muscle strength testing are the most helpful for making the diagnosis (D'Arcy & McGee, 2000). Two additional clinical tests are also used—when positive, Tinel's test appears more likely to be confirmed by further diagnostic testing (Katz & Simmons, 2002).

Thenar atrophy may also be present.

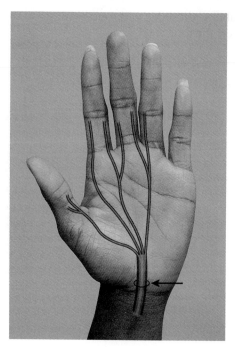

Thumb Abduction. Ask the client to raise the thumb perpendicular to the palm as you apply downward pressure on the distal phalanx. (This manoeuvre reliably tests the strength of the abductor pollicis brevis, which is innervated only by the median nerve.)

Tinel's Sign. With your finger, percuss lightly over the course of the median nerve in the carpal tunnel at the spot indicated by the arrow.

Tingling or electric sensations in the distribution of the median nerve constitute a positive test, suggesting *carpal tunnel syndrome.*

Phalen's Test. Hold the client's wrists in acute flexion for 60 seconds. Alternatively, ask the client to press the backs of both hands together to form right angles. These manoeuvres compress the median nerve.

If numbness and tingling develop over the distribution of the median nerve (e.g., the palmar surface of the thumb, and the index, middle, and part of the ring fingers), the sign is positive, suggesting *carpal tunnel syndrome.*

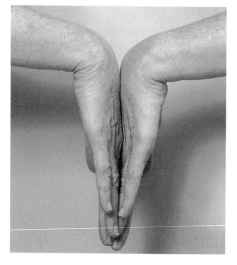

FOR LOW BACK PAIN WITH RADIATION INTO THE LEG

If the client has noted low back pain that radiates down the leg, check straight leg-raising on each side in turn. The client should lie supine. Raise the client's relaxed and straightened leg until pain occurs. Then, dorsiflex the foot.

Record the degree of elevation at which pain occurs, the quality and distribution of the pain, and the effects of dorsiflexion. Tightness and mild discomfort in the hamstrings with these manoeuvres are common and do not indicate radicular pain.

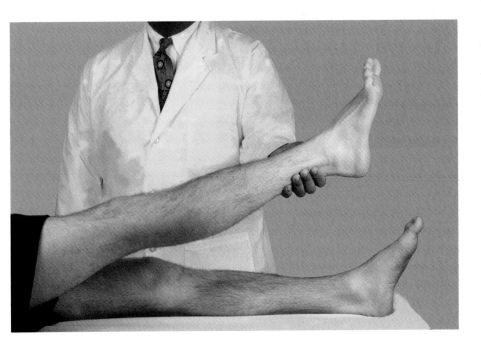

Examine the client neurologically, focusing on the motor and sensory function and the reflexes at the lumbosacral levels. These are outlined in the next chapter.

See Table 19-1, Low Back Pain (p. 670).

MEASURING THE LENGTH OF LEGS

If you suspect that the client's legs are unequal in length, measure them. Get the client relaxed in the supine position and symmetrically aligned with legs extended. With a tape, measure the distance between the anterior superior iliac spine and the medial malleolus. The tape should cross the knee on its medial side.

Unequal leg length may explain a scoliosis.

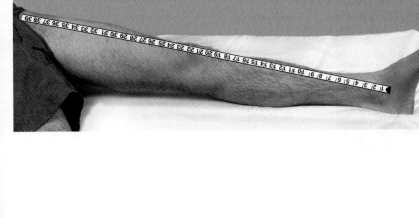

DESCRIBING LIMITED MOTION OF A JOINT

Although measurement of motion is seldom necessary, limitations can be described in degrees. Pocket goniometers are available for this purpose. In the two examples shown here, the red lines indicate the range of the client's movement, and the black lines suggest the expected range.

Observations may be described in several ways. The numbers in parentheses are suitably abbreviated recordings.

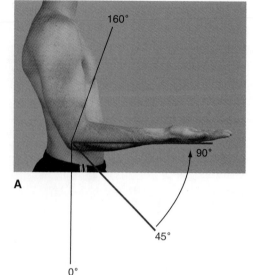

A

A. The elbow flexes from 45° to 90° (45° 90°),

OR

The elbow has a flexion deformity of 45° and can be flexed farther to 90° (45° 90°).

B. Supination at elbow = 30° (0° 30°)

Pronation at elbow = 45° (0° 45°)

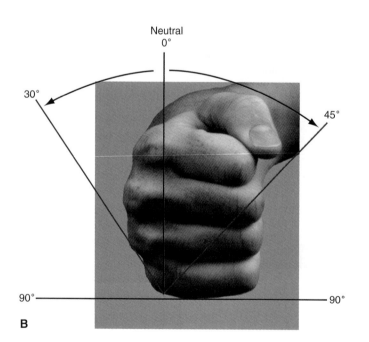

B

RECORDING AND ANALYZING FINDINGS

RECORDING AND ANALYZING FINDINGS

■ Examples of Documentation for Musculoskeletal System

Area of Assessment	Expected Findings	Unexpected Findings
Spine	Intact curvature of cervical, thoracic, and lumbar spine noted; full, smooth range of motion in cervical and lumbar spine; upper and lower extremities symmetrical	Accentuated thoracic curve (kyphosis); accentuated lumbar curve (lordosis); shoulders asymmetrical
Posture	Head erect and midline; client sits upright in chair	Rigid, stooped posture with head hanging forward
Gait	Smooth, even gait with arms swinging in opposition	Bilateral foot drop with external hip rotation; shuffling gait
Joints	Full range of motion in all joints; no swelling or deformity	Pain rated 4/10 with flexion and extension of right hip; moderate crepitus noted; tenderness over medial meniscus
Muscle Strength	Strength rated 5/5; active motion against resistance for all muscle groups	Strength rated 2/5 for all muscle groups; passive range of motion performed on lower extremities.

ANALYZING FINDINGS FROM PHYSICAL EXAMINATION AND HEALTH HISTORY

Once the nurse has collected and documented assessment data, he or she should use the information gathered to formulate a nursing diagnosis and plan of care. For example:

Sarah Rogers, a 35-year-old registered nurse, presents at a clinic with a sore back. She works on an orthopaedic unit at the local hospital, and reports: "I'm on my feet all day long, moving clients around, lifting and transferring. It's exhausting." Sarah says she injured her back 5 years ago when a client fell during a transfer. She was off work for 2 months and went to physiotherapy for almost 1 year after the incident. Sarah's current back pain is such that she has stopped going to the gym. She has been taking ibuprofen and acetaminophen for the pain, but says she thinks she needs "something stronger."

While gathering Sarah's health history, the nurse notes that her pain is located at the midline of her lower back and radiates into her legs. Using this information, the nurse develops the following nursing diagnoses:

Impaired physical mobility *and **acute pain** related to back injury*

Upon meeting Sarah, the nurse at the clinic would collect a detailed health history and perform a focused assessment of her musculoskeletal system. The history should include, in addition to a comprehensive assessment, questions about elements of her lifestyle and job that could have precipitated her back pain. Comprehensive care for Sarah includes examination by a physician specializing in orthopaedic injuries and a physical therapist. Further diagnostic tests for Sarah include x-rays and possible MRI.

Critical Thinking Exercise

Answer the following questions about Sarah Rogers:

- What are some possible causes of Sarah's back pain? (*Knowledge*)
- What additional questions would you ask to clarify her symptoms? (*Comprehension*)
- What lifestyle or work factors might be contributing to Sarah's back pain? What changes might the nurse suggest? (*Analysis*)
- What physical signs would you look for? (*Application*)
- What recommendations for follow-up would you suggest to Sarah? (*Synthesis*)
- How would you evaluate Sarah's understanding of any teaching you do? (*Evaluation*)

Canadian Research

Leslie, B. (2004). High fracture risk in Canadian First Nations. *Bone and Joint Decade Canada: Osteoporosis Issue,* *2*(2), 9.

Naylor, P. J., Macdonald, H. M., Reed, K. E., & McKay, H. A. (2006). Action Schools! BC: A socio-ecological approach to modifying chronic disease risk factors in elementary school children. *Preventing Chronic Disease,* *3*(2), A60.

Petit, M., Macdonald, H. M., & McKay, H. A. (2006). Growing bones: How important is exercise? *Current Opinion in Orthopaedics 17,* 431–437.

Test Questions

1. Risk factors in the following area are most readily changed to reduce the potential for falls and fractures:
   a. Social
   b. Cognitive
   c. Physiological
   d. Environmental

2. Which of the following risk factors for osteoporosis is the best predictor of low bone density?
   a. Smoking
   b. Low body weight
   c. Estrogen deficiency
   d. Prior vertebral fracture

3. When assessing the upper extremities, the nurse instructs the client to put the hands behind the neck with elbows pointing laterally. This positioning facilitates assessment of which of the following functions?
   a. Elbow flexion
   b. Internal rotation of the shoulder
   c. Muscle strength of the deltoids
   d. External rotation of the shoulders

4. Assessment of a client's ankle joint includes palpation along the Achilles tendon to look for
   a. Tension and strength
   b. Atrophy and flexibility
   c. Bogginess and calluses
   d. Tenderness and nodules

5. As the client lies supine, the nurse grasps the ankles and manipulates the legs to assess the range of motion of the hips. Which of the following findings is unexpected?
   a. Internal rotation, bilaterally
   b. External rotation, bilaterally
   c. Maximum abduction of the extended leg is 15 degrees
   d. One leg crosses over the other by 15 degrees of midline

Bibliography

CITATIONS

Affenito, S. G., & Kerstetter, J. (1999). Women's health and nutrition: Position of Dietitians of Canada and The American Dietetic Association. *Canadian Journal of Dietetic Practice and Research, 60,* 85–100.

Altman, R., Asch, E., Bloch, D., et al. (1986). Development of criteria for the classification and reporting of osteoarthritis. Classification of osteoarthritis of the knee. *Arthritis and Rheumatology, 29*(8), 1039–1049.

American College of Rheumatology Ad Hoc Committee on Clinical Guidelines. (1996). Guidelines for the initial evaluation of the adult client with acute musculoskeletal symptoms. *Arthritis and Rheumatology, 39*(1), 1–8.

Anderson, B. C. (2004). *Office orthopedics for primary care: Diagnosis and treatment* (2nd ed.). Philadelphia: W. B. Saunders.

Arnett, F. C., Edworthy, S. M., Bloch, D. A., et al. (1988). The American Rheumatism Association 1987 revised criteria for the classification of rheumatoid arthritis. *Arthritis and Rheumatology, 31,* 315–324.

Atlas, S. J., & Deyo, R. A. (2001). Evaluating and managing acute low back pain in the primary care setting. *Journal of General Internal Medicine, 16*(2), 120–131.

Bone Health and Fracture Prevention Steering Committee. (2001). A provincial strategy for bone health and fracture prevention. *British Columbia Ministry of Health and Ministry Responsible for*

Seniors. Retrieved April 8, 2008, from http://www.health.gov. bc.ca/whb/publications/bonehealthprovstr.pdf

British Columbia Ministry of Health. (2005). Bone density measurement in women. Retrieved April 17, 2008, from http://www.health.gov.bc.ca/gpac/guideline_bone_density.html

British Columbia Ministry of Health Planning. (2004). *Prevention of falls and injuries among the elderly: A special report from the Office of the Provincial Health Officer.* Office of the Provincial Health Officer. Retrieved April 6, 2008, from http://www.healthservices.gov.bc.ca/library/publications/year/2004/falls.pdf

Brown, J. P., & Josse, R. J. (2002). 2002 clinical practice guidelines for the diagnosis and management of osteoporosis in Canada. *Canadian Medical Association Journal, 167*(10 Suppl).

Buchbinder, R. (2004). Plantar fasciitis. *New England Journal of Medicine, 350*(21), 2159–2166.

Burkhardt, S. S. (2000). A 26-year-old woman with shoulder pain. *Journal of the American Medical Association, 284*(12), 1559–1567.

Canadian Cancer Society. (2007). *Vitamin D.* Retrieved June 11, 2008, from http://www.cancer.ca/ccs/internet/standard/0,3182,3172_1176359459__langId-en,00.html

Cibere, J., Bellamy, N., Thorne, A., et al. (2004). Reliability of the knee examination in osteoarthritis. *Arthritis and Rheumatology, 50*(2), 458–468.

Close, J. C. (2005). Prevention of falls: A time to translate evidence into practice. *Age and Ageing, 34*(2), 98–100.

Clough, M. (2007). Smoking and musculoskeletal health. *American Academy of Orthopaedic Surgeons.* Retrieved April 18, 2008, from http://orthoinfo.aaos.org/topic.cfm?topic=A00192&webid=1702&clientpage=patient_info2.cfm

Colman, R. (2000). Cost of obesity in Alberta. *GPIAtlantic.* Retrieved April 17, 2008, from http://www.gpiatlantic.org/pdf/health/obesity/ab-obesity.pdf

D'Arcy, C. A., & McGee, S. (2000). Does this client have carpal tunnel syndrome? The rational clinical examination. *Journal of the American Medical Association, 283*(23), 3110–3117.

Goldenberg, D. L., Burckhardt, C., & Crofford, L. (2004). Management of fibromyalgia syndrome. *Journal of the American Medical Association, 292*(19), 2388–2395.

Goldring, S. R. (2000). A 55-year-old woman with rheumatoid arthritis. *Journal of the American Medical Association, 283*(4), 524–529.

Haywood, K. L., Garratt, A. M., Jordan, K., et al. (2004). Spinal mobility in ankylosing spondylitis: Reliability, validity and responsiveness. *Rheumatology, 43*, 750–757.

Health Canada. (2007a). *It's your health: Caffeine.* Retrieved April 7, 2008, from http://www.hc-sc.gc.ca/iyh-vsv/food-aliment/caffeine_e.html

Health Canada. (2007b). *Eating well with Canada's Food Guide.* Ottawa, ON: Author.

Health Canada. (2005). *Assessment of the musculoskeletal system. Clinical practice guidelines for nurses in primary care.* Retrieved April 17, 2008, from http://www.hc-sc.gc.ca/fnih-spni/pubs/nursing-infirm/2000_clin-guide/chap_07a_e.html

Health Canada. (2003). *Arthritis in Canada. An ongoing challenge.* Cat. # H39-4/14-2003E. Retrieved April 10, 2008, from http://www.acreu.ca/pdf/Arthritis_in_Canada.pdf

Hicks, G. S., Duddleston, D. N., Russell, L. D., Holman, H. E., Shepherd, J. M., & Brown, A. (2002). Low back pain. *The American Journal of the Medical Sciences, 324*(4), 207–211.

Jackson, J. L., O'Malley, P. G., & Kroenke, K. (2003). Evaluation of acute knee pain in primary care. *Annals of Internal Medicine, 139*(7), 575–588.

Kanis, J. A. (n. d.). *FRAX: WHO fracture risk assessment tool.* World Health Organization Collaborating Centre for Metabolic Bone Diseases. Retrieved March 15, 2008, from http://www.shef.ac.uk/FRAX/index.htm

Katz, J. N., & Simmons, B. P. (2002). Carpal tunnel syndrome. *New England Journal of Medicine, 346*(23), 1807–1811.

Lee, D. M., & Weinblatt, M. E. (2001). Rheumatoid arthritis. *Lancet, 358*, 903–911.

Leslie, B. (2004). High fracture risk in Canadian First Nations. *Bone and Joint Decade Canada: Osteoporosis Issue, 2*(2), 9.

Leslie, W. D., Derksen, S., Metge, C., Lix, L. M., Salamon, E. A., Wood Steiman, P., et al. (2004). Fracture risk among First Nations people: A retrospective matched cohort study. *Canadian Medical Association Journal, 171*(8).

Levanthal, L. J. (1999). Management of fibromyalgia. *Annals of Internal Medicine, 131*(11), 850–858.

Liume, J. J., Verhagen, A. P., Meidema, H. S., et al. (2004). Does this client have an instability of the shoulder or a labrum lesion? The rational clinical examination. *Journal of the American Medical Association, 292*, 1989–1999.

Margolis, K. L., Ensrud, K. E., Schreiner, P. J., et al. (2000). Body size and risk for clinical fractures in older women. *Annals of Internal Medicine, 133*(2), 123–127.

McGregor, M., & Atwood, C. V. (2007). Wait times at the MUHC No:3 fracture management. *Centre Universitaire de santé McGill.* Retrieved March 30, 2008, from http://www.mcgill.ca/files/tau/Wait_Time_Fractures_May2007_Final.pdf

Mirolla, M. (2004). *The cost of chronic disease in Canada.* Retrieved April 6, 2008, from http://www.gpiatlantic.org/pdf/health/chroniccanada.pdf

Multiple Sclerosis in Newfoundland & Labrador. (2006). *Multiple sclerosis symptoms—weakness.* Retrieved March 15, 2008, from http://www.mi.mun.ca/users/ldunphy/msnewfoundland/weakness.htm

Murphy, K. A., Spence, S. T., McIntosh, C. N., & Connor Gorber, S. K. (2006). *Health state descriptions for Canadians: Musculoskeletal diseases.* [Statistics Canada, Catalogueue 82-619-MIE2006303]. Retrieved March 11, 2008, from http://www.statcan.ca/english/research/82-619-MIE/82-619-MIE2006003.pdf

Myasthenia Gravis Association of BC. (2008). *Facts about autoimmune Myasthenia Gravis for clients and families.* Retrieved March 15, 2008, from http://www.myastheniagravis.ca/id7.html

National Institute for Neurological Disorders and Stroke. (2003). *Low back pain fact sheet.* Retrieved April 6, 2008, from http://www.ninds.nih.gov/disorders/backpain/detail_backpain.htm

Obesity Canada. (2001). *Musculoskeletal problems.* Retrieved April 7, 2008, from http://www.obesitycanada.com/musculoskeletal.php

Occupational Health and Safety Council of Ontario. (2007). *MSD prevention toolbox.* Retrieved March 18, 2007, from http://www.iapa.on.ca/documents/MSD_2006%20_Prevention_Toolbox.pdf

Office of Nursing Policy, Health Canada. (2004). *Trends in workplace injuries, illnesses, and policies in healthcare across Canada.* Retrieved April 6, 2008, from http://www.hc-sc.gc.ca/hcs-sss/pubs/nurs-infirm/2004-hwi-ipmst/index-eng.php

Osteoporosis Canada. (2007a). *What is osteoporosis?* Retrieved March 16, 2008, from http://www.osteoporosis.ca/english/About%20Osteoporosis/what-is/default.asp?s=1

Osteoporosis Canada. (2007b). *Osteoporosis and osteoarthritis.* Retrieved March 16, 2008, from http://www.osteoporosis.ca/english/about%20osteoporosis/osteoarthritis/default.asp?s=1

Osteoporosis Canada. (2007c). *Osteoporosis and osteoarthritis: Symptoms.* Retrieved March 16, 2008, from http://www.osteoporosis.ca/english/About%20Osteoporosis/Osteoarthritis/symptoms/default.asp?s=1

Osteoporosis Canada. (2007d). *Osteoporosis and osteoarthritis: Treatment.* Retrieved March 16, 2008, from http://www.osteoporosis.ca/english/About%20Osteoporosis/Osteoarthritis/treatment/default.asp?s=1

Osteoporosis Canada. (2007e). *About osteoporosis—How much calcium do we need?* Retrieved July 4, 2008, from http://www.osteoporosis.ca/english/About%20Osteoporosis/Nutrition/Calcium%20Requirements/default.asp?s=1

Osteoporosis Canada. (2007f). *About osteoporosis—Vitamin D: A key factor in good calcium absorption.* Retrieved July 4, 2008, from http://www.osteoporosis.ca/english/about%20osteoporosis/nutrition/vitamin%20d/default.asp?s=1

Osteoporosis Canada. (2007g). *25 facts about osteoporosis.* Retrieved April 8, 2008, from http://www.osteoporosis.ca/english/Media%20Room/Background/2007_25facts/default.asp?s=1

Osteoporosis Canada. (2007h). *If you fracture.* Retrieved March 30, 2008, from http://www.osteoporosis.ca/english/About%20Osteoporosis/Living-well/if-you-fracture/default.asp?s=1

Premji, S. (2007). A call to action: Women's health at work & musculoskeletal disorders. *The Canadian Women's Health Network.* Retrieved April 6, 2008, from http://www.cwhn.ca/resources/workplace/msd.html

Public Health Agency of Canada. (2005a). *Report on seniors' falls in Canada.* Retrieved April 6, 2008, from http://www.phac-aspc.gc.ca/seniors-aines/pubs/seniors_falls/index.htm

Public Health Agency of Canada. (2005b). *Osteoporosis info sheet for seniors.* Retrieved April 17, 2008, from http://www.phac-aspc.gc.ca/seniors-aines/pubs/info_sheets/osteoporosis/osteo_e.htm

Public Health Agency of Canada. (2006). *Aging and seniors: Arthritis.* Retrieved March 11, 2008, from http://www.phac-aspc.gc.ca/seniors-aines/pubs/info_sheets/arthritis/arthritis_e.htm

Purnell, L. D., & Paulanka, B. J. (2003). *Transcultural healthcare: A culturally competent approach* (2nd ed.). Philadelphia: F.A. Davis.

Registered Nurses Association of Ontario. (2005). *Prevention of falls and fall injuries in the older adult.* Retrieved April 6, 2008, from http://www.rnao.org/Storage/12/617_BPG_Falls_rev05.pdf

Safe Kids Canada. (2006). *Child & youth unintentional injury: 10 years in review 1994–2003.* Retrieved April 9, 2008, from http://www.ccsd.ca/pccy/2006/pdf/skc_injuries.pdf

Sakane, T., Talenko, M., Suzuki, N., et al. (1999). Behcet's disease. *New England Journal of Medicine, 341*(17), 1284–1291.

Schultz, S. E., & Kopec, J. A. (2003). Impact of chronic conditions. *Health Reports, 14*(4), 41–53.

Siminoski, K. (2005). Vertebral compression fractures: Practical tips for effective assessment. *Osteoporosis Update, 9*(1), 4–5.

Smith, P., & Mustard, C. (2004). *Examining the associations between physical work demands and work injury rates for men and women in Ontario 1990–2000.* Institute for Work and Health. Retrieved April 17, 2008, from http://www.iwh.on.ca/archive/pdfs/psmith.pdf

Solomon, D. H., Simel, D. L., Bates, D. W., et al. (2001). Does this client have a torn meniscus or ligament of the knee? Value of the physical examination. The rational physical examination. *Journal of the American Medical Association, 286,* 1610–1620.

Stahl, J. B., Hlobil, H., Twoisk, J. W. R., et al. (2004). Graded activity for low back pain in occupational health care. *Annals of Internal Medicine, 140*(2), 77–84.

Statistics Canada. (2006). *Back pain.* Retrieved April 6, 2008, from http://www.statcan.ca/english/research/82-619-MIE/2006003/backpain.htm

The Arthritis Society. (2007a). *Chronic back injury.* Retrieved March 16, 2008, from http://www.arthritis.ca/types%20of%20arthritis/chronicback/default.asp?s=1

The Arthritis Society. (2007b). *Introduction to arthritis.* Retrieved March 16, 2008, from http://www.arthritis.ca/types%20of%20arthritis/default.asp?s=1

The Arthritis Society. (2007c). *Ankylosing spondylitis.* Retrieved April 17, 2008, from http://www.arthritis.ca/types%20of%20arthritis/as/default.asp?s=1

The Bone Wellness Centre. (2007). *What is osteoporosis?* Retrieved April 7, 2008, from http://www.bonewellness.com/osteoporosis.php

The Canadian Chiropractic Association. (1996). *Glenerin guidelines: Chiropractic clinical practice guidelines.* Retrieved March 15, 2008, from http://www.ccachiro.org/client/cca/cca.nsf/web/Glenerin%20Guidelines?OpenDocument

The College of Family Physicians of Canada. (2007). *Low back pain—Tips on pain relief and prevention.* Retrieved April 6, 2008, from http://www.cfpc.ca/English/cfpc/programs/client%20education/low%20back%20pain/default.asp?s=1

Torgen, M., & Kilbom, A. (2000). Physical workload between 1970 and 1993 – did it change? *Scandinavian Journal of Work and Environmental Health, 26*(2), 161–168

Wolfe, F., Smythe, H. A., Yunus, M. B., et al. (1990). The American College of Rheumatology 1990 Criteria for the Classification of Fibromyalgia. Report of the Multicentre Criteria Committee. *Arthritis and Rheumatology, 33*(2), 160–172.

Woodward, T. W., & Best, T. M. (2000a). The painful shoulder. Part I. Clinical evaluation. *American Family Physician, 61*(10), 3079–3088.

Woodward, T. W., & Best, T. M. (2000b). The painful shoulder. Part II. Acute and chronic disorders. *American Family Physician, 61*(11), 3291–3300.

World Health Organization. (2003). *The burden of musculoskeletal conditions at the start of the new millennium.* Retrieved March 18, 2008, from http://whqlibdoc.who.int/trs/WHO_TRS_919.pdf

Young, C. C., Rutherford, D. S., & Niedfeldt, M. W. (2001). Treatment of plantar fasciitis. *American Family Physician, 63,* 467–474, 477–478.

ADDITIONAL REFERENCES

Deyo, R. A., Rainville, J., & Kent, D. L. (1992). What can the history and physical examination tell us about low back pain? *Journal of the American Medical Association, 268*(6), 760–765.

BIBLIOGRAPHY

Greene, W. B., American Academy of Orthopaedic Surgeons, American Academy of Pediatrics. (2001). *Essentials of musculoskeletal care* (2nd ed.). Rosemont, IL: American Academy of Orthopaedic Surgeons.

Harris, E. D., & Kelley, W. N. (2005). *Kelley's textbook of rheumatology* (7th ed.). Philadelphia: Elsevier Saunders.

Hoppenfeld, S., & Hutton, R. (1976). *Physical examination of the spine and extremities.* New York: Appleton-Century-Crofts.

Koopman, W. J., & Moreland, L. W. (2005). *Arthritis and allied conditions: A textbook of rheumatology* (15th ed.). Philadelphia: Lippincott Williams & Wilkins.

Lew, D. P., & Waldvogel, F. A. (1997). Osteomyelitis. *New England Journal of Medicine, 336*(14), 999–1007.

Murrell, G. A. C., & Walton, J. R. (2001). Diagnosis of rotator cuff tears. *Lancet, 357*(9258), 769–770.

CANADIAN ASSOCIATIONS, WEB SITES, AND RESOURCES

Institute of Musculoskeletal Health and Arthritis: http://www.cihr-irsc.gc.ca/e/193.html

The Arthritis Society: http://www.arthritis.ca

The Bone and Joint Decade Canada: http://www.bjdcanada.org/

Canadian Orthopaedic Association: http://www.coa-aco.org

Canadian Orthopaedic Nurses Association: http://www.cona-nurse.org

Osteoporosis Canada: http://www.osteoporosis.ca

TABLE 19-1   **Low Back Pain**

Patterns	Possible Causes	Possible Physical Signs
Mechanical Low Back Pain		
Acute, often recurrent, or possibly chronic aching pain in the lumbosacral area, possibly radiating into the posterior thighs but not below the knees. Often precipitated or aggravated by moving, lifting, or twisting motions and relieved by rest. Spinal movement typically limited by pain. Common from the teenage years through the 40s.	Causes cannot usually be proven; include intervertebral disc disease, congenital disorders of the spine, such as spondylolisthesis, in older women or people on long-term corticosteroid therapy, osteoporosis complicated by a collapsed vertebra.	Local tenderness, muscle spasm, pain on movement of the back, and loss of the usual lumbar lordosis, but no motor or sensory loss or reflex abnormalities. In osteoporosis there may be a thoracic kyphosis, percussion tenderness over a spinous process, or fractures elsewhere such as in the thoracic spine or in a hip.
Radicular Low Back Pain		
A radicular nerve root pain, usually superimposed on low back pain. The sciatic pain is shooting and radiates down one or both legs, usually to below the knee(s) in a dermatomal distribution, often with associated numbness and tingling and possibly local weakness. The pain is usually worsened by spinal movement such as bending and by sneezing, coughing, or straining (Atlas & Deyo, 2001).	A herniated intervertebral disc with compression or traction of nerve root(s) is the most common cause in persons ≤ age 50. Nerve roots of L5 or S1 are most often affected. Spinal cord tumours or abscesses are much less common and tend to affect more nerve roots, producing more neurologic deficits.	Pain on straight leg-raising (see p. 663), tenderness of the sciatic nerve, loss of sensation in a dermatomal distribution, local muscular weakness and atrophy, and decreased to absent reflex(es), especially affecting the ankle jerks. Dermatomal signs and reflex changes may be absent when only a single root is affected.
Back and Leg Pain From Lumbar Spinal Stenosis		
Pseudoclaudication is a pain in the back or legs that worsens with walking and improves with flexing of the spine, as by sitting or bending forward.	Lumbar stenosis, or a combination of degenerative disc disease and osteoarthritis, which narrows the spinal canal and impinges on the spinal nerves, often after age 60.	Posture may become flexed forward, with motor weakness and hyporeflexia in the lower extremities.
Chronic Persistent Low Back Stiffness	Ankylosing spondylitis, a chronic inflammatory polyarthritis, most common in young men	Loss of the usual lumbar lordosis, muscle spasm, and limitation of anterior and lateral flexion
	Diffuse idiopathic skeletal hyperostosis (DISH), which affects middle-aged and older men	Flexion and immobility of the spine
Aching Nocturnal Back Pain, Unrelieved by Rest	Consider *metastatic malignancy* in the spine from cancer of the prostate, breast, lung, thyroid, and kidney, and multiple myeloma.	Variable with the source. Local bone tenderness may be present.
Back Pain Referred From the Abdomen or Pelvis		
Usually a deep, aching pain; the level varies with the source	Peptic ulcer, pancreatitis, pancreatic cancer, chronic prostatitis, endometriosis, dissecting aortic aneurysm, retroperitoneal tumour, and other causes	Spinal movements are not painful and range of motion is not affected. Look for signs of the primary disorder.

TABLE 19-2   Pains in the Neck

Patterns	Possible Causes	Possible Physical Signs
"Simple Stiff Neck"		
Acute, episodic, localized pain in the neck, often appearing on awakening and lasting 1–4 days. No dermatomal radiation	Mechanisms are not understood.	Local muscular tenderness and pain from certain movements
Aching Neck		
A persistent dull aching in the back of the neck, often spreading to the occiput. Common from postural strain, as in prolonged typing or studying; may also accompany tension and depression.	Poorly understood; may be related to sustained muscle contraction	Local muscular tenderness. When areas of pain and tenderness are also present elsewhere in the body, consider the fibromyalgia syndrome (see Table 19-3, Patterns of Pain in and Around the Joints).
"Cervical Sprain"		
Acute and often recurrent neck pains, which are often more severe and last longer than simple stiff neck. There may be a precipitating factor such as a whiplash injury, heavy lifting, or a sudden movement, but there is no dermatomal radiation.	Poorly understood	Local tenderness and pain on movement
Neck Pain With Dermatomal Radiation		
Neck pain as in cervical sprain, but with radiation of the pain to the shoulder, back, or arm in a dermatomal distribution. This radicular pain is typically sharp, burning, or tingling in quality.	Compression of one or more nerve roots caused by either a herniated cervical disc or degenerative disease of the intervertebral discs with bony spurring*	Muscle tenderness and spasm; limited range of neck motion; increase in pain on coughing or straining; and possible sensory loss, weakness, muscular atrophy, and decreased reflexes in the areas involved
Neck Pain From Possible Compression of the Cervical Spinal Cord		
Associated here is weakness or paralysis of the legs, often with a decrease in or loss of sensation. These symptoms may occur in addition to the radicular symptoms or by themselves. Neck pain may be mild or even absent.	Compression of the spinal cord in the neck caused by either a herniated cervical disc or degenerative disease of the intervertebral discs with bony spurring. Trauma may also be the cause.*	Limited range of motion in the neck, weakness or paralysis in the legs of the central nervous system type, Babinski responses, loss of position and vibration sense in the legs, and, less commonly, loss of pain and temperature sensation. Radicular signs in the arms may also be present.

*Tumours or abscesses of the cervical spinal cord, though less common, should also be considered.

Problem	Process	Common Locations	Pattern of Spread	Onset	Progression and Duration
Rheumatoid Arthritis	Chronic inflammation of *synovial membranes* with secondary erosion of adjacent cartilage and bone, and damage to ligaments and tendons	Hands (proximal interphalangeal and metacarpophalangeal joints), feet (metatarsophalangeal joints), wrists, knees, elbows, ankles	Symmetrically additive; progresses to other joints while persisting in the initial ones	Usually insidious	Often chronic, with remissions and exacerbations
Osteoarthritis (*degenerative joint disease*)	Degeneration and progressive loss of cartilage within the joints, damage to underlying bone, and formation of new bone at the margins of the cartilage	Knees, hips, hands (distal, sometimes proximal interphalangeal joints), cervical and lumbar spine, and wrists (first carpometacarpal joint); also joints previously injured or diseased	Additive; however, only one joint may be involved.	Usually insidious	Slowly progressive, with temporary exacerbations after periods of overuse
Gouty Arthritis					
Acute Gout	An inflammatory reaction to microcrystals of sodium urate	Base of the big toe (the first metatarsophalangeal joint), the instep or dorsum of feet, the ankles, knees, and elbows	Early attacks are usually confined to one joint.	Sudden, often at night, often after injury, surgery, fasting, or excessive food or alcohol intake	Occasional isolated attacks lasting days up to 2 weeks; they may get more frequent and severe, with persisting symptoms.
Chronic Tophaceous Gout	Multiple local accumulations of sodium urate in the joints and other tissues (tophi), with or without inflammation	Feet, ankles, wrists, fingers, and elbows	Additive, not so symmetric as rheumatoid arthritis	Gradual development of chronicity with repeated attacks	Chronic symptoms with acute exacerbations
Polymyalgia Rheumatica	A disease of unclear nature in people older than 50, especially women; may be associated with giant cell arteritis	Muscles of the hip girdle and shoulder girdle; symmetric		Insidious or abrupt, even appearing overnight	Chronic but ultimately self-limiting
Fibromyalgia[a] Syndrome	Widespread musculoskeletal pain and tender points. May accompany other diseases. Mechanisms unclear.	"All over," but especially in the neck, shoulders, hands, low back, and knees	Shifts unpredictably or worsens in response to immobility, excessive use, or chilling	Variable	Chronic, with "ups and downs"

[a]The vagueness of these characteristics is in itself a clue to fibromyalgia syndrome.

Associated Symptoms

Swelling	Redness, Warmth, and Tenderness	Stiffness	Limitation of Motion	Generalized Symptoms
Frequent swelling of synovial tissue in joints or tendon sheaths; also subcutaneous nodules	Tender, often warm, but seldom red	Prominent, often for an hour or more in the mornings, also after inactivity	Often develops	Weakness, fatigue, weight loss, and low fever are common.
Small effusions in the joints may be present, especially in the knees; also bony enlargement.	Possibly tender, seldom warm, and rarely red	Frequent but brief (usually 5–10 min), in the morning and after inactivity	Often develops	Usually absent
Present, within and around the involved joint	Exquisitely tender, hot, and red	Not evident	Motion is limited primarily by pain.	Fever may be present.
Present, as tophi, in joints, bursae, and subcutaneous tissues	Tenderness, warmth, and redness may be present during exacerbations.	Present	Present	Possibly fever; client may also develop symptoms of renal failure and renal stones.
None	Muscles often tender, but not warm or red	Prominent, especially in the morning	Usually none	Malaise, a sense of depression, possibly anorexia, weight loss, and fever, but no true weakness
None	Multiple specific and symmetric tender "trigger points," often not recognized until the examination	Present, especially in the morning	Absent, though stiffness is greater at the extremes of movement	A disturbance of sleep, usually associated with morning fatigue

TABLE 19-4 | **Painful Shoulders**

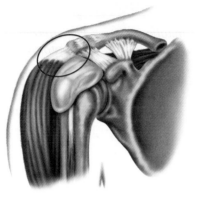

Rotator Cuff Tendonitis

Repeated shoulder motion, as in throwing or swimming, can cause edema and hemorrhage followed by inflammation, most commonly involving the supraspinatus tendon. Acute, recurrent, or chronic pain may result, often aggravated by activity. Clients may report sharp catches of pain, grating, and weakness when lifting the arm overhead. When the supraspinatus tendon is involved, tenderness is maximal just below the tip of the acromion. Typically, clients are athletically active.

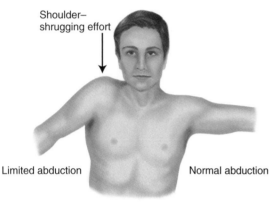

Shoulder–shrugging effort

Limited abduction   Normal abduction

Rotator Cuff Tears

When the arm is raised in forward flexion, the rotator cuff may impinge against the undersurface of the acromion and the coracoacromial ligament. Injury from a fall or repeated impingement may weaken the rotator cuff, causing a partial or complete tear, usually after age 40. Weakness, atrophy of the supraspinatus and infraspinatus muscles, pain, and tenderness may ensue. In a complete tear of the supraspinatus tendon (illustrated), active abduction and forward flexion at the glenohumeral joint is severely impaired, producing a characteristic shrugging of the shoulder and a positive "drop arm" test (see p. 627).

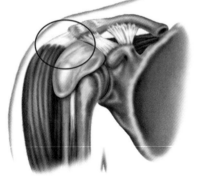

Calcific Tendonitis

Calcific tendonitis refers to a degenerative process in the tendon associated with the deposition of calcium salts. Usually involves the supraspinatus tendon. Acute, disabling attacks of shoulder pain may occur, usually in clients older than 30 years and more often in women. The arm is held close to the side, and all motions are severely limited by pain. Tenderness is maximal below the tip of the acromion. The subacromial bursa, which overlies the supraspinatus tendon, may be inflamed. Chronic, less severe pain may also occur.

(table continues on next page)

TABLE 19-4   **Painful Shoulders** *(Continued)*

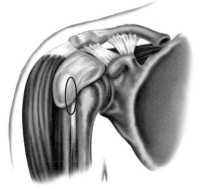

Bicipital Tendonitis

Inflammation of the long head of the biceps tendon and its sheath causes anterior shoulder pain that may resemble rotator cuff tendonitis and may coexist with it. Often this is a sign of shoulder instability. This tendon, like the cuff, may suffer impingement injury. Tenderness is maximal in the bicipital groove. By externally rotating and abducting the arm, you can more easily separate this area from the subacromial tenderness of supraspinatus tendonitis. With the client's arm at the side, elbow flexed to 90°, ask the client to supinate the forearm against your resistance. Increased pain in the bicipital groove confirms this condition.

Acromioclavicular Arthritis

Acromioclavicular arthritis is not a common cause of shoulder pain. When present, it usually is the result of direct injury to the shoulder girdle with resulting degenerative changes. Tenderness is localized over the acromioclavicular joint. Although motion in the glenohumeral joint is not painful in acromioclavicular arthritis, as it is in many other painful conditions of the shoulder, movements of the scapula, such as shoulder shrugging, are.

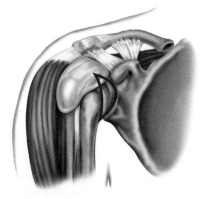

Adhesive Capsulitis (Frozen Shoulder)

Adhesive capsulitis refers to a mysterious fibrosis of the glenohumeral joint capsule, manifested by diffuse, dull, aching pain in the shoulder and progressive restriction of active and passive range of motion, but usually no localized tenderness. The condition is usually unilateral and occurs in people aged 50 to 70. There is often an antecedent painful disorder of the shoulder or possibly another condition (such as myocardial infarction) that has decreased shoulder movements. The course is chronic, lasting months to years, but the disorder often resolves spontaneously, at least partially.

Source: Woodward & Best, 2000a, 2000b.

TABLE 19-5 Swollen or Tender Elbows

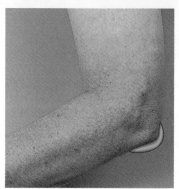

Olecranon
bursitis

Olecranon Bursitis

Swelling and inflammation of the olecranon bursa may result from trauma or may be associated with rheumatoid or gouty arthritis. The swelling is superficial to the olecranon process.

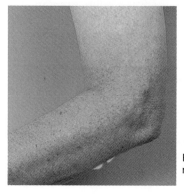

Rheumatoid
nodules

Rheumatoid Nodules

Subcutaneous nodules may develop at pressure points along the extensor surface of the ulna in clients with rheumatoid arthritis or acute rheumatic fever. They are firm and nontender, and are not attached to the overlying skin. They may or may not be attached to the underlying periosteum. Although they may develop in the area of the olecranon bursa, they often occur more distally.

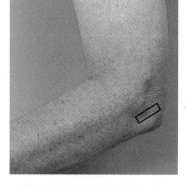

Arthritis

Arthritis of the Elbow

Synovial inflammation or fluid is best felt in the grooves between the olecranon process and the epicondyles on either side. Palpate for a boggy, soft, or fluctuant swelling and for tenderness.

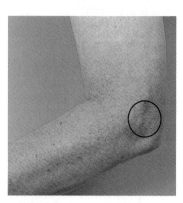

Epicondylitis

Epicondylitis

Lateral epicondylitis (tennis elbow) follows repetitive extension of the wrist or pronation–supination of the forearm. Pain and tenderness develop at the lateral epicondyle and possibly in the extensor muscles close to it. When the client tries to extend the wrist against resistance, pain increases.

Medial epicondylitis (pitcher's, golfer's, or Little League elbow) follows repetitive wrist flexion, as in throwing. Tenderness is maximal at the medial epicondyle. Wrist flexion against resistance increases the pain.

TABLE 19-6   Arthritis in the Hands

Acute Rheumatoid Arthritis

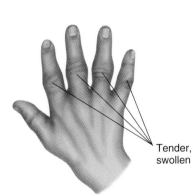

Tender, painful, stiff joints in rheumatoid arthritis, usually with symmetric involvement on both sides of the body. The proximal interphalangeal, metacarpophalangeal, and wrist joints are the most frequently affected. Note the fusiform or spindle-shaped swelling of the proximal interphalangeal joints in acute disease.

Chronic Rheumatoid Arthritis

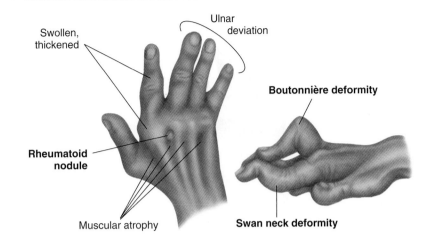

In chronic disease, note the swelling and thickening of the metacarpophalangeal and proximal interphalangeal joints. Range of motion becomes limited, and fingers may deviate toward the ulnar side. The interosseous muscles atrophy. The fingers may show "swan neck" deformities (hyperextension of the proximal interphalangeal joints with fixed flexion of the distal interphalangeal joints). Less common is a boutonnière deformity (persistent flexion of the proximal interphalangeal joint with hyperextension of the distal interphalangeal joint). Rheumatoid nodules seen in the acute or chronic stage.

Osteoarthritis (*Degenerative Joint Disease*)

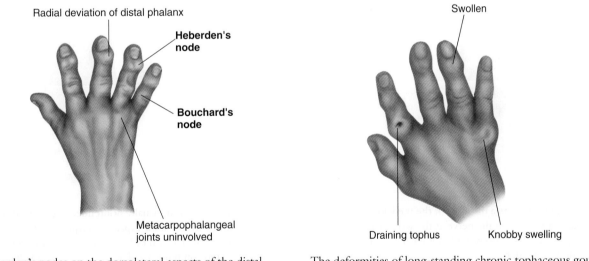

Heberden's nodes on the dorsolateral aspects of the distal interphalangeal joints from bony overgrowth of osteoarthritis. Usually hard and painless, they affect the middle-aged or elderly; often associated with arthritic changes in other joints. Flexion and deviation deformities may develop. Bouchard's nodes on the proximal interphalangeal joints are less common. The metacarpophalangeal joints are spared.

Chronic Tophaceous Gout

The deformities of long-standing chronic tophaceous gout can mimic rheumatoid arthritis and osteoarthritis. Joint involvement is usually not as symmetric as in rheumatoid arthritis. Acute inflammation may be present. Knobby swellings around the joints ulcerate and discharge white chalklike urates.

TABLE 19-7 **Swellings and Deformities of the Hands**

Dupuytren's Contracture

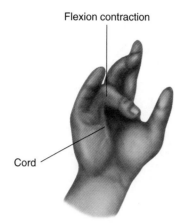

Flexion contraction

Cord

The first sign of a Dupuytren's contracture is a thickened plaque overlying the flexor tendon of the ring finger and possibly the little finger at the level of the distal palmar crease. Subsequently, the skin in this area puckers, and a thickened fibrotic cord develops between palm and finger. Flexion contracture of the fingers may gradually ensue.

Trigger Finger

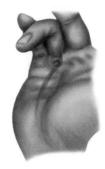

Caused by a painless nodule in a flexor tendon in the palm, near the head of the metacarpal. The nodule is too big to enter easily into the tendon sheath during extension of the fingers from a flexed position. With extra effort or assistance, the finger extends and flexes with a palpable and audible snap as the nodule pops into the tendon sheath. Watch and listen as the client flexes and extends the fingers, and feel for both the nodule and the snap.

Thenar Atrophy

Usual hypothenar eminence

Flattened thenar eminence

Thenar atrophy suggests a disorder of the median nerve or its components. Pressure on the nerve at the wrist is a common cause (carpal tunnel syndrome). Hypothenar atrophy suggests an ulnar nerve disorder.

Ganglion

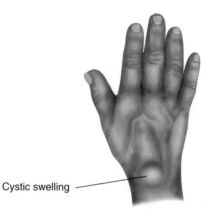

Cystic swelling

Ganglia are cystic, round, usually nontender swellings located along tendon sheaths or joint capsules, frequently at the dorsum of the wrist. Flexion of the wrist makes ganglia more prominent; extension tends to obscure them. Ganglia may also develop elsewhere on the hands, wrists, ankles, and feet.

TABLE 19-8	Tendon Sheath and Palmar Space Infections; Felons

Acute Tenosynovitis

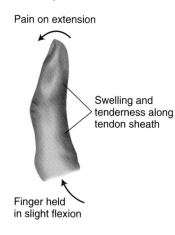

Pain on extension

Swelling and
tenderness along
tendon sheath

Finger held
in slight flexion

Infection of the flexor tendon sheaths (acute tenosynovitis) may follow local injury, even when trivial in nature. Unlike arthritis, tenderness and swelling develop not in the joint but along the course of the tendon sheath, from the distal phalanx to the level of the metacarpophalangeal joint. The finger is held in slight flexion; finger extension is very painful.

Acute Tenosynovitis and Thenar Space Involvement

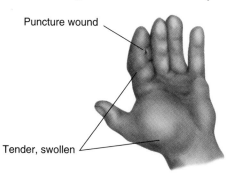

Puncture wound

Tender, swollen

If the infection progresses, it may extend from the tendon sheath into the adjacent fascial spaces within the palm. Infections of the index finger and thenar space are illustrated. Early diagnosis and treatment are important.

Felon

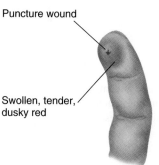

Puncture wound

Swollen, tender,
dusky red

Injury to the fingertip may result in infection in the enclosed fascial spaces of the finger pad. Severe pain, localized tenderness, swelling, and dusky redness are characteristic. Early diagnosis and treatment are important.

TABLE 19-9   **Unexpected Findings of the Feet**

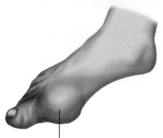

Hot, red, tender, swollen

Acute Gouty Arthritis

The metatarsophalangeal joint of the great toe may be the first joint involved in acute gouty arthritis. It is characterized by a very painful and tender, hot, dusky red swelling that extends beyond the margin of the joint. It is easily mistaken for a cellulitis. Acute gout may also involve the dorsum of the foot.

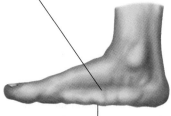

Medial border becomes convex

Sole touches floor

Flat Feet

Signs of flat feet may be apparent only when the client stands, or they may become permanent. The longitudinal arch flattens so that the sole approaches or touches the floor. The usual concavity on the medial side of the foot becomes convex. Tenderness may be present from the medial malleolus down along the medial-plantar surface of the foot. Swelling may develop anterior to the malleoli. Inspect the shoes for excess wear on the inner side of the soles and heels.

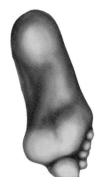

Hallux Valgus

In hallux valgus, the great toe is unusually abducted in relation to the first metatarsal, which itself is deviated medially. The head of the first metatarsal may enlarge on its medial side, and a bursa may form at the pressure point. This bursa may become inflamed.

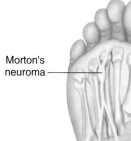

Morton's neuroma

Morton's Neuroma

Tenderness over the plantar surface, third and fourth metatarsal heads, from probable entrapment of the medial and lateral plantar nerves. Symptoms include hyperesthesia, numbness, aching, and burning from the metatarsal heads into the third and fourth toes.

TABLE 19-10	Unexpected Findings of the Toes and Soles

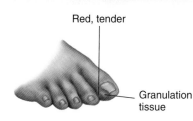

Red, tender

Granulation tissue

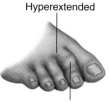

Hyperextended

Flexed

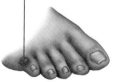

Red, thickened

Ingrown Toenail

The sharp edge of a toenail may dig into and injure the lateral nail fold, resulting in inflammation and infection. A tender, reddened, overhanging nail fold, sometimes with granulation tissue and purulent discharge, results. The great toe is most often affected.

Hammer Toe

Most commonly involving the second toe, a hammer toe is characterized by hyperextension at the metatarso-phalangeal joint with flexion at the proximal interphalangeal joint. A corn frequently develops at the pressure point over the proximal interphalangeal joint.

Corn

A corn is a painful conical thickening of skin that results from recurrent pressure on normally thin skin. The apex of the cone points inward and causes pain. Corns characteristically occur over bony prominences (e.g., the fifth toe). When located in moist areas (e.g., at pressure points between the fourth and fifth toes), they are called soft corns.

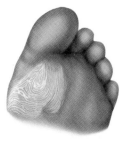

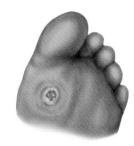

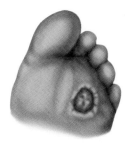

Callus

Like a corn, a callus is an area of greatly thickened skin that develops in a region of recurrent pressure. Unlike a corn, however, a callus involves skin that is usually thick, such as the sole, and is usually painless. If a callus is painful, suspect an underlying plantar wart.

Plantar Wart

A plantar wart is a common wart (verruca vulgaris) located in the thickened skin of the sole. It may look somewhat like a callus or even be covered by one. Look for the characteristic small dark spots that give a stippled appearance to a wart. Skin lines usually stop at the wart's edge.

Neuropathic Ulcer

When pain sensation is diminished or absent (as in diabetic neuropathy, for example), neuropathic ulcers may develop at pressure points on the feet. Although often deep, infected, and indolent, they are painless. Callus formation about the ulcer is diagnostically helpful. Like the ulcer itself, it results from chronic pressure.

The Nervous System

MARJORIE C. ANDERSON AND LYNN S. BICKLEY

Assessment of the nervous system may intimidate many nurses, given that this complex system controls thought processing, speech, sensory perceptions, and motor functions. In fact, all body functions and regions are under the control of the nervous system. Nurses need to comprehend the voluntary and autonomic responses of the nervous system to internal and external stimuli. During history taking, attention to subtle unexpected changes in a client's sensory and motor patterns alerts the nurse to assess related physical manifestations. During examination of the eyes, ears, and head and neck (see Chapters 11–13), nurses assess sensory and motor functions of the cranial nerves. During mental status assessment (see Chapter 9), nurses examine level of consciousness, orientation, thought processing, speech production, and language comprehension. This chapter focuses on examination of cranial nerve function, motor and sensory systems, and reflexes.

ANATOMY AND PHYSIOLOGY

The nervous system, in conjunction with the endocrine system, has the major responsibility for maintaining body homeostasis. The nervous system controls mental processing and emotions, sensory perceptions, skeletal and involuntary muscles, and some glandular activities. The two major divisions are the central and peripheral nervous systems. The *central nervous system* (CNS) consists of the brain and spinal cord. The *peripheral nervous system* (PNS) consists of 12 pairs of cranial nerves and 31 pairs of spinal and peripheral nerves.

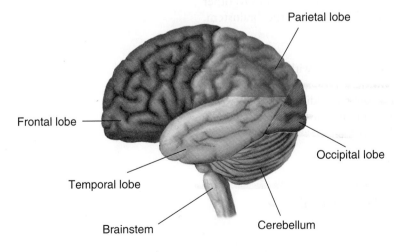

LEFT LATERAL VIEW OF THE BRAIN

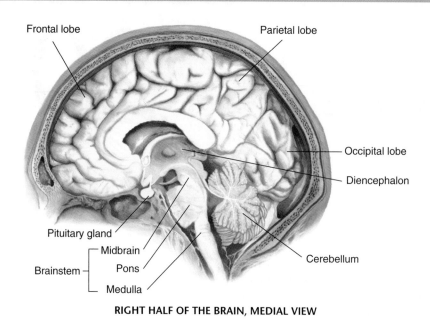

Frontal lobe

Parietal lobe

Occipital lobe

Diencephalon

Pituitary gland

Midbrain

Pons

Medulla

Brainstem

Cerebellum

RIGHT HALF OF THE BRAIN, MEDIAL VIEW

CENTRAL NERVOUS SYSTEM

THE BRAIN

The brain lies within the cranium and is protected by the skull and three *meningeal layers*. The dura mater, a tough fibrous layer, lines the skull, while the pia mater, a thin, fragile vascular layer, adheres to the many gyri and grooves of the brain itself. Between these two layers, but adjacent to the dura, lies the arachnoid, a highly vascular layer. Between the arachnoid and pia mater is the subarachnoid space, which contains cerebral spinal fluid (CSF) produced by the choroid plexus within the lining of the fourth ventricle. The CSF circulates in the subarachnoid space around the brain and spinal cord, cushioning and nourishing both. The CSF is absorbed through arachnoid villi that project into the venous sinus, which lies between the arachnoid and dura mater.

The brain is a vast network of interconnecting *neurons* (nerve cells). Neurons consist of cell bodies with *dendrites*—the several branching processes that extend outward from the cell body—and *axons*—single long fibres that conduct impulses to other parts of the nervous system. The four regions of the brain are the brainstem, cerebellum, diencephalon, and cerebrum.

The *brainstem*, located at the base of the brain, is continuous with the spinal cord and consists of the medulla, pons, and midbrain. Both sensory and motor pathways travel via the brainstem to the spinal cord or cerebrum. In addition, all but two of the cranial nerves (olfactory and optic) arise from the brainstem. Within the medulla are centres that regulate respiratory and cardiac functions, and centres for vomiting and coughing.

The *cerebellum* lies at the base of the cerebrum. It facilitates smooth coordinated body movements and helps maintain body position upright in space.

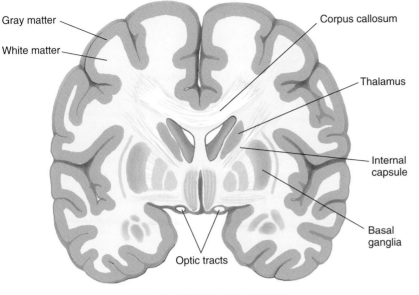

Gray matter

White matter

Corpus callosum

Thalamus

Internal capsule

Basal ganglia

Optic tracts

CORONAL SECTION OF THE BRAIN

The *diencephalon* (forebrain) contains the thalamus and hypothalamus. The *thalamus* screens all incoming sensory impulses and relays them to the cerebral cortex. The *hypothalamus* maintains homeostasis by regulating bodily functions, including temperature, heart rate, blood pressure, food intake, thirst, and urine output. The hypothalamus also plays a role in emotional behaviours such as anger and sexual drive, and secretes hormones that act directly on the pituitary gland.

The *cerebrum* is divided into right and left hemispheres and contains the largest mass of brain tissue. Each hemisphere is subdivided into frontal, parietal, temporal, and occipital lobes, as shown in the previous illustration. The corpus callosum connects and enables communication between the two hemispheres. Cerebral tissue appears grey or white in cross-section. *Grey matter* consists of aggregations of neuronal cell bodies. It rims the surfaces of the cerebral hemispheres, forming the cerebral cortex. *White matter* consists of neuronal axons coated with myelin. The myelin sheaths, which create the colour of the white matter, allow nerve impulses to travel more rapidly.

Deep in the cerebral white matter lie additional nuclei (clusters) of grey matter—the *basal ganglia*. These ganglia affect movement in several ways, including maintaining purposeful motor movements and sustaining upright posture. In the coronal section of the brain can be seen the *internal capsule*, a collection of myelinated axons that converge from all parts of the motor cortex carrying motor impulses to the brainstem.

Consciousness depends on the interaction between intact cerebral hemispheres and the *reticular activating (arousal) system* (RAS). The reticular formation, a network of interconnecting neurons located in the diencephalon and upper brainstem, receives, integrates, and forwards sensory input to the RAS. The RAS, through fibres that spread throughout the cerebral hemispheres, controls the overall level of cortical alertness (consciousness and attention).

THE SPINAL CORD

The spinal cord is a cylindrical mass of nerve tissue encased within the bony vertebral column, extending from the medulla to the first or second lumbar vertebra. It contains sensory and motor nerve pathways that enter and exit through posterior and anterior nerve roots, respectively. The spinal cord also mediates reflex activity of the deep tendon reflexes from the spinal nerves. As noted earlier, it is protected by and continuous with the same three meningeal layers and CSF as the brain.

The spinal cord is divided into five segments: cervical, from C1 to C8; thoracic, from T1 to T12; lumbar, from L1 to L5; sacral, from S1 to S5; and coccygeal.

Note that the spinal cord is not as long as the vertebral canal. The lumbar and sacral roots travel the longest intraspinal distance and fan out like a horse's tail at L1 to L2, giving rise to the term *cauda equina*. To avoid injury to the spinal cord, most lumbar punctures are performed at the L2 to L4 vertebral interspace.

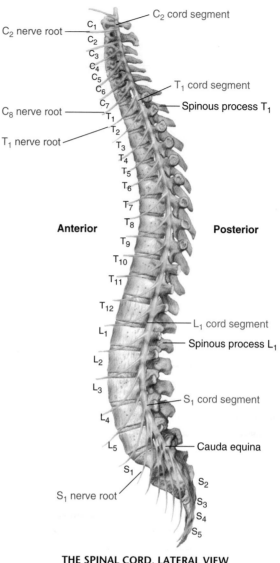

THE SPINAL CORD, LATERAL VIEW

PERIPHERAL NERVOUS SYSTEM

THE CRANIAL NERVES

Twelve pairs of special nerves called *cranial nerves* play important roles in neurologic function and control. View the inferior surface of the brain for actual locations of the cranial nerves.

Cranial Nerve Pairs	Origin of Fibres
I Olfactory	Nasal olfactory epithelium
II Optic	Retina
III Oculomotor	Midbrain
IV Trochlear	Midbrain
V Trigeminal	Pons
	(continued)

Cranial Nerve Pairs	Origin of Fibres
VI Abducens	Pons
VII Facial	Pons
VIII Acoustic	Inner ear
IX Glossopharyngeal	Midbrain
X Vagus	Medulla
XI Spinal accessory	Medulla
XII Hypoglossal	Medulla

Functions of the cranial nerves (CN) most relevant to physical examination are summarized in the following table.

■ Cranial Nerves

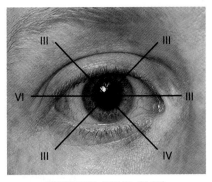

RIGHT EYE (CN III, IV, VI)

No.	Name	Function
I	Olfactory	Sense of smell
II	Optic	Vision
III	Oculomotor	Pupillary constriction, opening the eye, and most extraocular movements
IV	Trochlear	Downward, inward movement of the eye
V	Abducens	Lateral movement of the eye
VI	Trigeminal	*Motor*—temporal and masseter muscles (jaw clenching), also lateral movement of the jaw *Sensory*—facial. The nerve has three divisions: (1) ophthalmic, (2) maxillary, and (3) mandibular.

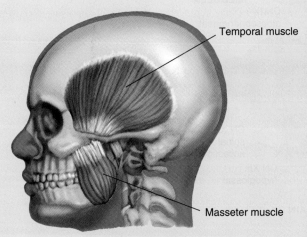

Temporal muscle

Masseter muscle

CN V—MOTOR

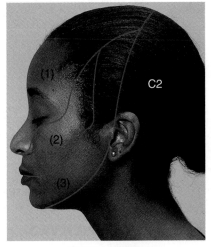

CN V—SENSORY

VII	Facial	*Motor*—facial movements, including those of facial expression, closing the eye, and closing the mouth *Sensory*—taste for salty, sweet, sour, and bitter substances on the anterior two thirds of the tongue

(continued)

▪ Cranial Nerves (Continued)

No.	Name	Function
VIII	Acoustic	Hearing (cochlear division) and balance (vestibular division)
IX	Glossopharyngeal	*Motor*—pharynx *Sensory*—posterior portions of the eardrum and ear canal, the pharynx, and the posterior tongue, including taste (salty, sweet, sour, bitter)
X	Vagus	*Motor*—palate, pharynx, and larynx *Sensory*—pharynx, larynx, and carotid sinus
XI	Spinal accessory	*Motor*—the sternomastoid and upper portion of the trapezius
XII	Hypoglossal	*Motor*—tongue

Sternomastoid muscle

Trapezius muscle

CN XI—MOTOR

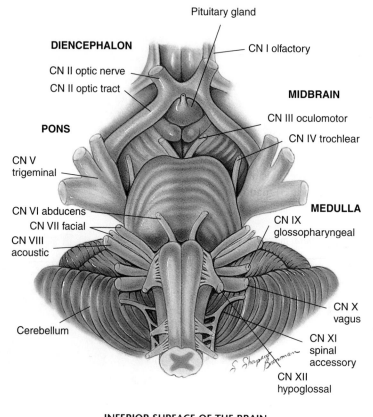

INFERIOR SURFACE OF THE BRAIN

THE SPINAL NERVES

In addition to cranial nerves, the PNS includes spinal nerves that carry impulses to and from the cord. Thirty-one pairs of nerves emerge from the spinal cord: 8 cervical, 12 thoracic, 5 lumbar, 5 sacral, and 1 coccygeal. Each nerve has an anterior (ventral) root containing motor fibres, and a posterior (dorsal) root containing sensory fibres. The anterior and posterior roots merge to form a short *spinal nerve*. Spinal nerve fibres comingle with similar fibres from other levels to form *peripheral nerves*. Most peripheral nerves contain both *sensory* (afferent) and *motor* (efferent) fibres.

Like the brain, the spinal cord contains both grey matter and white matter. Nuclei of grey matter, which are aggregations of nerve cell bodies, are surrounded by white tracts of nerve fibres connecting the brain to the PNS. Note the butterfly appearance of the grey-matter nuclei, with anterior and posterior horns.

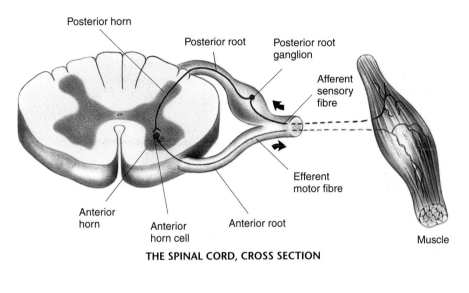

THE SPINAL CORD, CROSS SECTION

SPINAL REFLEXES

DEEP TENDON RESPONSES

The deep tendon or muscle stretch reflexes are relayed over structures of both the central and peripheral nervous systems. Recall that a *reflex* is an involuntary stereotypical response that may involve as few as two neurons, one afferent (sensory) and one efferent (motor), across a single synapse. The deep tendon reflexes in the arms and legs are such monosynaptic reflexes. They illustrate the simplest unit of sensory and motor function. (Other reflexes are polysynaptic, involving interneurons interposed between sensory and motor neurons.)

To elicit a deep tendon reflex, briskly tap the tendon of a partially stretched muscle. For the reflex to fire, all five components of the reflex must be intact: sensory nerve fibres, spinal cord synapse, motor nerve fibres, neuromuscular junction, and muscle fibres. Tapping the tendon activates special sensory fibres in the partially stretched muscle, triggering a sensory impulse that travels to the spinal cord via a peripheral nerve. The stimulated sensory fibre synapses directly with the anterior horn cell innervating the same muscle. When the impulse crosses the neuromuscular junction, the muscle suddenly contracts, completing the reflex arc.

Because each deep tendon reflex involves specific spinal segments, together with their sensory and motor fibres, an unexpected reflex can help you to locate a pathologic lesion. Learn the segmental levels of the deep tendon reflexes. You can remember them easily by their numerical sequence in ascending order from ankle to triceps: S1—L2, 3, 4,—C5, 6, 7.

Ankle reflex	Sacral 1 primarily
Knee reflex	Lumbar 2, 3, 4
Supinator (brachioradialis) reflex	Cervical 5, 6
Biceps reflex	Cervical 5, 6
Triceps reflex	Cervical 6, 7

SUPERFICIAL (CUTANEOUS) REFLEXES

Reflexes may be initiated by stimulating skin as well as muscle. Stroking the skin of the abdomen, for example, produces a localized muscular twitch. These superficial (cutaneous) reflexes and their corresponding spinal segments include the following:

Corneal reflex	Cranial nerves 5, 7
Abdominal reflexes	
Upper	Thoracic 8, 9, 10
Lower	Thoracic 10, 11, 12
Plantar responses	Lumbar 5, Sacral 1

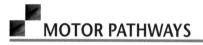

MOTOR PATHWAYS

Motor pathways contain upper motor neurons, synapses in the brainstem or spinal cord, and lower motor neurons. Nerve cell bodies or *upper motor neurons* lie in the primary motor cortex of the cerebral cortex and in several brainstem nuclei; their axons synapse with motor nuclei in the brainstem (for cranial nerves) and in the spinal cord (for spinal nerves). *Lower motor neurons* have cell bodies in the anterior horn of (anterior horn cells). Their axons transmit impulses through the anterior roots and spinal nerves into peripheral nerves, terminating at the neuromuscular junction.

Three kinds of motor pathways impinge on the anterior horn cells: the corticospinal tract, the basal ganglia system, and the cerebellar system. There are additional pathways originating in the brainstem that mediate flexor and extensor tone in limb movement and posture, most notable in coma (see Table 20-11, p. 758).

THE PRINCIPAL MOTOR PATHWAYS

■ The *corticospinal (pyramidal) tract.* The corticospinal tracts mediate voluntary movement and integrate skilled, complicated, or delicate movements by stimulating selected muscular actions and inhibiting others. They also carry impulses that inhibit *muscle tone,* the slight tension maintained by intact muscle even when relaxed. The corticospinal tracts originate in the primary cortex of the brain and travel through the internal capsule into the lower medulla, where they form an anatomical structure resembling a pyramid. There, most of these fibres cross to the opposite or *contralateral* side of the medulla, continue downward, and synapse with anterior horn cells or with intermediate neurons. Tracts synapsing in the brainstem with motor nuclei of the cranial nerves are termed *corticobulbar.*

The *extrapyramidal tracts* include the *basal ganglia system* and *cerebellar system*. The exceedingly complex basal ganglia system consists of motor pathways among the cerebral cortex, basal ganglia, brainstem, and spinal cord. The *cerebellar system* receives both sensory and motor input. Neither system acts directly on motor efferent fibres; they each indirectly modify output originating from the cerebral motor cortex. The basal ganglia system inhibits muscle tone, while the cerebellar system enhances it. The cerebellar system coordinates and refines skilled voluntary motor movements initiated by the motor cortex and helps to maintain balance and to control eye movements. Basal nuclei help to coordinate slow, sustained movements related to posture. Both are used for motor memory making. Actions such as walking, swimming, and playing the piano can become virtually automatic.

All of these higher motor pathways affect movement only through the lower motor neuron systems—sometimes called the final common pathway. Any movement, whether initiated voluntarily in the cortex, "automatically" in the basal ganglia, or reflexly in the sensory receptors, must ultimately be translated into action via the anterior horn cells. A lesion in any of these areas will affect movement or reflex activity.

When a corticospinal tract is damaged or destroyed, its functions are reduced or lost below the level of injury. *When upper motor neuron systems are damaged above the crossover of its tracts in the medulla, motor impairment develops on the opposite or contralateral side. In damage below the crossover, motor impairment occurs on the same or ipsilateral side of the body.* The affected limb becomes weak or paralyzed, and skilled, complicated, or delicate movements are performed especially poorly when compared with gross movements.

In upper motor neuron lesions, muscle tone is increased and deep tendon reflexes are exaggerated because suppression from upper motor neurons is no longer present. Damage to the lower motor neuron systems causes ipsilateral weakness and paralysis, but in this case, muscle tone and reflexes are decreased or absent.

Disease of the basal ganglia system or cerebellar system does not cause paralysis, but can be disabling. Damage to the basal ganglia system produces changes in muscle tone (most often an increase), disturbances in posture and gait, a slowness or lack of spontaneous and automatic movements termed *bradykinesia*, and a variety of involuntary movements. Cerebellar damage impairs coordination, gait, and equilibrium and decreases muscle tone.

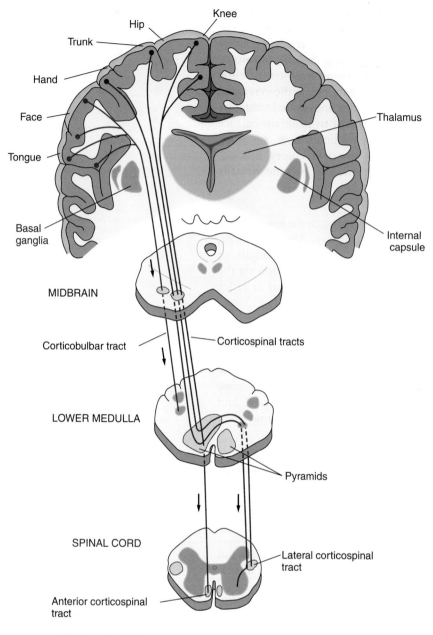

MOTOR PATHWAYS: CORTICOSPINAL AND CORTICOBULBAR TRACTS

SENSORY PATHWAYS

Sensory impulses not only participate in reflex activity, as previously described, but also give rise to conscious sensation, calibrate body position in space, and help regulate internal autonomic functions like blood pressure, heart rate, and respiration.

A complex system of sensory receptors relays impulses from skin, mucous membranes, muscles, tendons, and viscera. Sensory receptors and their afferent peripheral nerves registering sensations such as pain, temperature, position, and touch pass through the posterior roots and enter the spinal cord. Once inside the cord, sensory impulses reach the sensory cortex of the brain via one of the two pathways: the spinothalamic tracts or the posterior columns.

Within one or two spinal segments from their entry into the cord, fibres conducting the sensations of *pain* and *temperature* pass into the posterior horn of the spinal cord and synapse with secondary sensory neurons. Fibres conducting *crude touch*—a sensation perceived as light touch but without accurate localization—also pass into the posterior horn and synapse with secondary neurons. The secondary neurons then cross to the opposite side and pass upward in the *spinothalamic tract* into the thalamus.

Fibres conducting the sensations of *position* and *vibration* pass directly into the *posterior columns* of the cord and travel upward to the medulla, together with fibres transmitting *fine touch*—touch that is accurately localized and finely discriminating. These fibres synapse in the medulla with secondary sensory neurons. Fibres projecting from secondary neurons cross to the opposite side at the medullary level and continue on to the thalamus.

At the *thalamic level*, the general quality of sensation is perceived (e.g., pain, cold, pleasant, and unpleasant), but fine distinctions are not made. For full perception, a third group of sensory neurons sends impulses from the thalamus to the *sensory cortex* of the brain. Here stimuli are localized and higher-order discriminations are made.

Lesions at different points in the sensory pathways produce different kinds of sensory loss. Patterns of sensory loss, together with their associated motor findings, help you to identify where the causative lesions might be. A lesion in the sensory cortex may not impair the perception of pain, touch, and position, for example, but does impair finer discrimination. A person so affected cannot appreciate the size, shape, or texture of an object by feeling it and, therefore, cannot identify it. Loss of position and vibration sense with preservation of other sensations points to disease of the posterior columns, whereas loss of all sensations from the waist down, together with paralysis and hyperactive reflexes in the legs, indicates transection of the spinal cord (see Table 20-11, p. 758). Crude and light touch are often preserved despite partial damage to the cord because impulses originating on one side of the body travel up both sides of the cord.

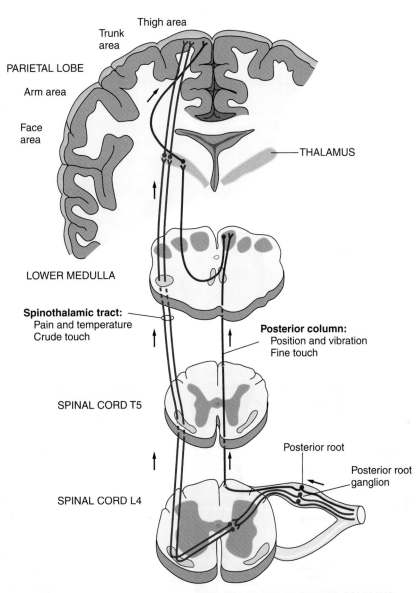

SENSORY PATHWAYS: SPINOTHALAMIC TRACT AND POSTERIOR COLUMNS

DERMATOMES

A knowledge of *dermatomes* also aids in localizing neurologic lesions. *A dermatome is the band of skin innervated by the sensory root of a single spinal nerve.* Dermatome patterns are mapped in the next two figures. Their levels are considerably more variable than the diagrams suggest, and dermatomes overlap each other. The sensory nerves from each side of the body overlap slightly across the midline. The distribution of a few key peripheral nerves is shown in the inserts on the left.

Do not try to memorize all the dermatomes. It is useful, however, to remember the locations of some, such as those shaded in green on the right side of the diagrams.

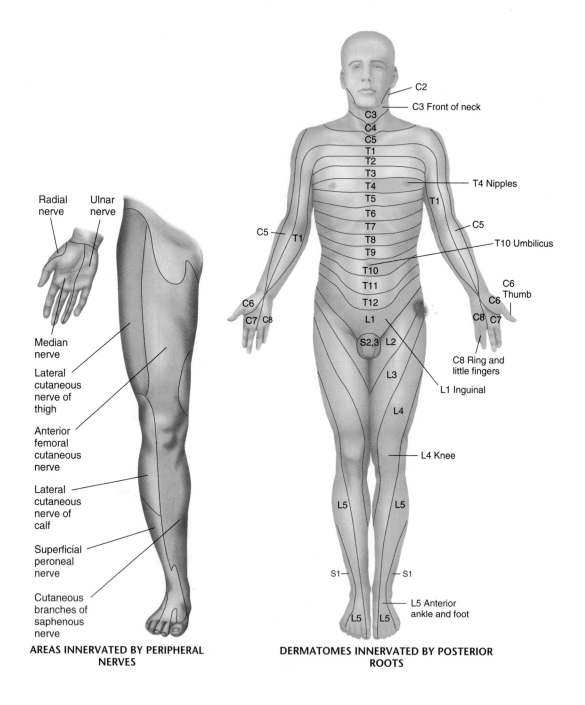

AREAS INNERVATED BY PERIPHERAL NERVES

DERMATOMES INNERVATED BY POSTERIOR ROOTS

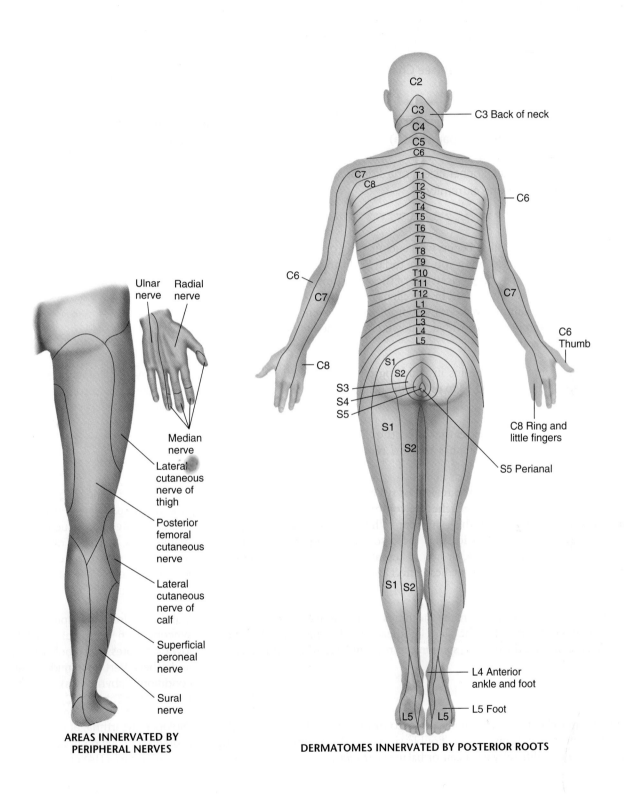

C2

C3 — C3 Back of neck
C4
C5
C6

C7
C8

T1
T2
T3
T4
T5
T6
T7
T8
T9
T10
T11
T12
L1
L2
L3
L4
L5

C6 — C6

C6
C7

C7

C6
Thumb

C6
C7

C8

S1
S2
S3
S4
S5

C8

S1

S2

C8 Ring and
little fingers

S5 Perianal

S1 S2

L4 Anterior
ankle and foot

L5 Foot

L5 L5

Ulnar
nerve

Radial
nerve

Median
nerve

Lateral
cutaneous
nerve of
thigh

Posterior
femoral
cutaneous
nerve

Lateral
cutaneous
nerve of
calf

Superficial
peroneal
nerve

Sural
nerve

**AREAS INNERVATED BY
PERIPHERAL NERVES**

DERMATOMES INNERVATED BY POSTERIOR ROOTS

THE HEALTH HISTORY: SUBJECTIVE DATA

Key Symptoms and Signs Reported by Client

- Sudden vision or hearing changes (see Chapters 12 and 13)
- Headache
- Dizziness or vertigo
- Numbness or loss of sensation (paresthesia)
- Pins and needles or tingling
- Muscle weakness (paresis): generalized, one side of body (hemiparesis), or one extremity

- Loss of consciousness, fainting (syncope), or feeling faint (near syncope)
- Convulsions (seizures)
- Tremors or involuntary movements
- Slurring of speech (dysarthria)
- Difficulty swallowing (dysphagia)

The health history interview often begins with encouraging open-ended questions, such as: "What health concerns bring you here today?" If the concerns involve the nervous system, the client may have voiced one of the symptoms documented in the previous box. Each symptom expressed by the client warrants a complete symptom analysis that includes asking how the symptom affects the client's work life and personal life. Partial examples are provided, followed by a complete example for the symptoms of numbness and tingling.

Two of the most common symptoms in neurologic disorders are *headache* and *dizziness*. Turn to Chapters 11 and 13 to review the health history pertinent to these symptoms.

See Table-11-1 Primary Headaches and Table 11-3, Secondary Headaches.

If headaches are frequent, ask whether they affect the client's work life. Also inquire about what interventions the client has tried to relieve the headache and their outcomes.

Occasionally, questioning during the review of systems reveals a history of head trauma including concussion. As headaches are common sequelae to head injury, it is important to inquire regarding this symptom. While conducting the symptom analysis (see p. 282), be sure to identify the associated symptoms of nausea, vomiting, visual changes, weakness, or loss of sensation. Ask whether coughing, sneezing, or sudden movements of the head affect the headache.

Subarachnoid hemorrhage may evoke "the worst headache of my life." Dull headache affected by such manoeuvres, especially on awakening and recurring in the same location, is seen with mass lesions such as a brain tumour.

The symptom of *dizziness* can have many meanings. You will need to elicit exactly what the client has experienced. Is the client lightheaded or feeling faint? Or is there *vertigo*, a perception that the room is spinning or rotating? Has the client fallen?

Lightheadedness in palpitations, near syncope from vasovagal stimulation, low blood pressure, febrile illness, and others. Vertigo in middle-ear conditions (labyrinthitis), brainstem tumour. See Table 20-2, p. 742.

Especially in older clients, are any medications contributing to the dizziness? Are there any associated symptoms, such as double vision (*diplopia*) difficulty forming words (*dysarthric*), or difficulty with gait or balance (*ataxia*)?

Diplopia, dysarthria, ataxia in posterior circulation *transient ischemic attack* (TIA) or *stroke*

Weakness or paralysis in transient ischemic attack or stroke; focal weakness may arise from ischemic, vascular, or mass lesions in the central nervous system; also from peripheral nervous system disorders, neuromuscular disorders, or the muscles themselves. See Table 20-7, pp. 751–753.

For weakness without lightheadedness, try to distinguish between *proximal* and *distal weakness*. For proximal weakness, ask about combing hair, trying to reach something on a high shelf, or difficulty getting up out of a chair or taking a high step up. Does the weakness increase with repeated effort and improve after rest? Are there associated sensory or other symptoms? For distal weakness in the arms, inquire about hand movements such as opening a jar or can, or using hand tools such as scissors, pliers, or a screwdriver. For distal weakness in the legs, ask about frequent tripping.

Bilateral proximal weakness as in myopathy. Bilateral, predominantly distal weakness in polyneuropathy. Weakness made worse with repeated effort and improved with rest suggests myasthenia gravis.

See Table 20-7, Disorders of the Central and Peripheral Nervous Systems.

Find out whether the client has had any *loss of sensation*. Ask whether there has been any *numbness*, but clarify its meaning and location. Has there been loss of sensation in conjunction with clumsy movements or altered sensations such as tingling or pins and needles? Those peculiar sensations without an obvious stimulus are called *paresthesias*. They also occur commonly when an arm or leg "goes to sleep" following compression of a nerve and may be described as tingling, prickling, or feelings of warmth, coldness, or pressure. *Dysesthesias* are distorted sensations in response to a stimulus and may last longer than the stimulus itself. For example, a person may perceive a light touch or pinprick as a burning or tingling sensation that is irritating or unpleasant and may be described as painful. *Pain* may arise from neurologic causes, but is usually reported with symptoms of other body systems, such as the head and neck or the musculoskeletal system.

Loss of sensation, paresthesias, and dysesthesias in central lesions in the brain and spinal cord, as well as disorders of peripheral sensory roots and nerves; paresthesias in the hands and around the mouth in hyperventilation. Burning pain in painful sensory neuropathy.

"Have you ever fainted or passed out?" leads the discussion to any *loss of consciousness*. It is important to begin by exploring what the client means by loss of consciousness. Did the client black out completely, or could voices be heard throughout the episode, indicating some consciousness? Be sure to use descriptive terms carefully and precisely. *Syncope* is the sudden but temporary loss of consciousness that occurs with decreased blood flow to the brain, commonly described as *fainting*. Symptoms of feeling faint, lightheaded, or weak, but without actual loss of consciousness, are called *near syncope* or *presyncope*.

See Table 20-1, Syncope and Similar Disorders, p. 741.

Get as complete and unbiased a description of the event as you can. What brought on the episode? Were there any warning symptoms? Was the client standing, sitting, or lying down when the episode began? How long did it last? Could voices be heard while passing out and coming to? How rapidly did the client recover? In retrospect, were onset and offset slow or fast?

Young people with emotional stress and warning symptoms of flushing, warmth, or nausea may have *vasodepressor (or vasovagal) syncope* of slow onset, slow offset. *Cardiac syncope* from arrhythmias, more common in older clients, often with sudden onset, sudden offset.

Muscle *weakness* is another common symptom that requires detailed exploration. Probe for exactly how the weakness is affecting the client. Determine whether the client cannot move a part or side of the body (*paralysis*). Did the weakness start slowly or suddenly? Has it progressed? If so, how and where? What areas of the body are now involved: an extremity, one side, both sides? What movements are affected? Walking? Dressing? Is speech impaired (*dysphasia*)? Is swallowing difficult (*dysphagia*)?

A *seizure* is a paroxysmal disorder caused by sudden excessive electrical discharge in the cerebral cortex or its underlying structures. Seizures can be of several types. Depending on the type, there may or may not be loss of consciousness. With some types of seizures, there may be unusual feelings, thought processes, and sensations, including smells, as well as unusual movements. Asking, "Have you ever had any seizures or 'spells'?" or "Any fits or convulsions?" can open the discussion. As with syncope, aim for a full and complete description, including precipitating

See Table 20-2, Seizure Disorders, pp. 742–743.

circumstances, warnings, symptoms, and behaviour and feelings both during the attack and afterward. Ask about age at onset, frequency, any change in frequency or symptom pattern, and use of medications. Is there any history of prior head injury or other conditions that may be causally related?

Tremors and other *involuntary movements* occur with or without additional neurologic manifestations. Ask about any trembling, shakiness, or body movements that the client seems unable to control.

See Table 20-3, Tremors and Involuntary Movements, pp. 744–745. Tremor, rigidity, and bradykinesia in Parkinson's disease.

Distinct from these symptoms is an almost indescribable *restlessness of the legs* that typically develops at rest and is accompanied by an urge to move about. Walking gives relief.

The common but often overlooked restless legs syndrome, usually benign

---

EXAMPLES OF QUESTIONS FOR SYMPTOM ANALYSIS—NUMBNESS AND TINGLING IN LEGS

- "Where do you have this sensation of numbness?" "One or both legs?" (*Location*)
- "Can you point to where the numbness ends in each leg?" (*Location/radiation*)
- "You describe this area as being 'numb.' Could other words also describe the sensation?" "Cold?" "Gone to sleep?" "Would you describe the sensation as tingling?" "Pins and needles?" "Prickling? Stinging? Crawling?" (*Quality/nature*)
- "Has the area of numbness extended, or become larger over time?" "Can you feel pressure?" "Cold, hot, or pain over the area?" (*Severity/quantity/intensity*)
- "When did you first notice the numbness?" "The tingling?" "Did the tingling occur before or after the numbness started?" "Did they occur at the same time?" (*Timing—Onset*)
- "Has the sensation ever gone away?" "If so, how long ago?" "When did the numbness come back?" "How long has the numbness persisted?" (*Timing—Duration*)
- "How often in the past year has the numbness gone away and returned?" (*Timing—Frequency*)
- "Does the intensity of the numbness change throughout the day?" "Is the tingling more noticeable at night?" (*Timing—Time of day*)
- "Does any action or position increase the intensity of the numbness or tingling?" (*Aggravating factors*)
- "What helps to lessen the numbness, the tingling, or both?" "A warm bath?" "Elevating the legs?" (*Alleviating factors*)
- "Have you noticed any other symptoms?" "Besides the numbness and tingling, have you noticed any pain with the tingling?" "Do you feel unusually cool at times?" "Do you have any back pain or pain down the leg at any time?" (*Associated symptoms*)
- "Can you think of anything that could contribute to these sensations?" "Anything at home?" "In your work environment?" "Leisure activities?" "For example, do you work with solvents or other chemicals? Do heavy lifting?" (*Environmental factors*)
- "Tell me how this numbness in your legs has affected your lifestyle at work, at home, during leisure pursuits." (*Significance to the client*)
- "What do you think might be causing the numbness and tingling you are experiencing?" (*Client perspective*)

HEALTH PROMOTION

Important Topics for Health Promotion

- Risk factors for and prevention of cerebrovascular disease—transient ischemic attacks (TIAs) and stroke (brain attack)
- Risk factors for and prevention of head injury (brain trauma)
- Risk factors for and prevention of spinal cord injuries
- Prevention of exposure to neurotoxins such as lead, mercury, pesticides
- Reduction of risk factors for infections such as meningitis and encephalitis
- Reduction of risk factors for peripheral neuropathies
- Reduction of risk factors for seizure activity
- Maintenance of brain health throughout life

SPECIFIC PREVENTION FOR SPECIFIC DISEASES AND DISORDERS

Cerebrovascular diseases caused more than 16,000 deaths in Canada in 2005 (Statistics Canada, 2008) and are the third leading cause of death in this country. They are a significant cause of neurological morbidity, often resulting in a continuing need for assistance with activities of daily living. A significant number of people with cerebrovascular disease first experience a *transient ischemic attack* (TIA): sudden loss of motor and/or sensory function on one side of the face, body, or both; difficulty speaking or understanding; or a change in visual perception in one or both eyes. Usually lasting 5 to 10 minutes, the TIA is followed by complete recovery of function. Nurses recognize TIA as a warning sign for stroke (brain attack or cerebrovascular accident [CVA]) and advise clients to seek medical attention without delay. Because there is a 10% to 20% risk for stroke to follow TIA within 1 month, prompt follow-up is essential and can be lifesaving (Agyeman et al., 2006; Giles, Flossman, & Rothwell, 2006).

Stroke has occurred if the neurological deficit lasts longer than 24 hours. Approximately 85% of strokes result from atherothrombosis secondary to atherosclerosis (ischemic stroke) or a released embolus that travels from the heart or an atherosclerotic vessel to lodge in a distal cranial artery (embolic stroke). Infarction of cranial tissue results distal to the occluded artery. The remaining 15% are hemorrhagic strokes, often heralded by a severe headache from rupture of a cerebral aneurysm into the subarachnoid space or intracerebral tissue (Kasper & Harrison, 2005; Heart and Stroke Foundation of Canada, 2008). Nonmodifiable risk factors include age (older than 55 years), gender (male > female), ethnicity (First Nations, African, or Asian genetic background), family history of cerebrovascular disease, and previous stroke (Heart and Stroke Foundation of Canada, 2008). Nurses cannot effect change in these risk factors, but can identify clients at increased risk for stroke.

Nurses advocate for management of modifiable risk factors by strongly recommending the following measures:

- Controlling serum glucose level (in clients with diabetes mellitus)
- Maintaining blood pressure of 130/85 or less (in clients with hypertension)
- Lowering elevated serum cholesterol level
- Treating atrial fibrillation
- Ceasing tobacco smoking and illicit drug use
- Eating a low-fat and high-fibre diet
- Limiting alcohol intake to two drinks per day
- Engaging in regular aerobic exercise
- Controlling weight

Sources: Mouradian et al., 2005; Qureshi, Suri, Guterman, & Hopkins, 2001; Young & Hachinski, 2003.

Hypertension is the most significant risk factor to control (Campbell, Petrella, & Kaczorowski, 2006; Qureshi, Suri, Kirmani, Divani, & Mohammad, 2005; Seshadri et al., 2006). A diet rich in cereal, grains, fruits, and vegetables, with a modest intake of omega-3 fatty acids in nuts and fish, and low intakes of salt and animal and dairy saturated fats has been linked to reduced risk of stroke (Adams & Standridge, 2006; He, Nowson, & MacGregor, 2006; Hu, 2003). Some clients, especially older women, may benefit from antiplatelet agents such as aspirin (Ridker et al., 2005).

Traumatic head injuries were responsible for more than 16,800 hospital admissions and 1368 deaths in Canada from 2003 to 2004 (Canadian Institute of Health Information [CIHI], 2006). The leading cause for hospitalizing people with head injuries is falls, which include work injuries, sport injuries (e.g., diving), motor vehicle collisions, and physical assaults. Head injuries from falls are more common in children, youth, and older adults, while motor vehicle collisions are more frequent in people 20 to 29 years. Moderate to severe head injuries frequently have significant physical, cognitive, social, and emotional consequences for survivors (Duff, 2002; Van Neste-Kenny, 2003). *Spinal cord injuries* frequently occur in conjunction with head injuries. In Canada, the incidence of spinal cord injuries is approximately 900 per year; an estimated 36,000 people currently live with the condition (Canadian Paraplegic Association, 2008). The specialized care associated with the long-term morbidity found with many people with head and spinal cord injuries is often costly to the health care system and to family members.

Nurses play a vital role in the prevention of head and spinal cord injuries. It is well known that the use of seat belts and motorcycle helmets contributes to a decrease in mortality from head and spinal cord injuries and that drinking and driving contribute to serious motor vehicle collisions.

Nurses can support initiatives that advocate for the following:

- Abstinence from drugs and alcohol if driving
- Seat belt use by all passengers in a moving vehicle
- Helmet use when riding a bicycle or motorcycle, skiing, horseback riding
- Fall prevention programs for the elderly (Dryden et al., 2003; Pickett, Campos-Benitez, Keller, & Duggal, 2006; Stewart, Girotti, Nikore, & Williamson, 2003)
- Properly installed car seats of the correct size for children
- Use of booster seats for children up to 8 years
- Supervision of young children at play in certain environments such as a park with climbing apparatus

---

The prevalence of *Parkinson's disease* (PD) in Canada is difficult to determine because documentation is available only through billing. Estimates are that PD is the second most common progressive neurodegenerative disorder in Canada, currently affecting approximately 100,000 people (Parkinson Society of Canada, 2008). Nurses assess for gradual onset (usually beginning after 60 years), unilateral resting tremors that increase with stress, rigidity in muscle tone, postural instability, and bradykinesia. The cause is unknown, but current research points to the possible combination of genetic factors and environmental exposure to viral infections and neurotoxins in herbicides and pesticides (Guttman, Kish, & Furukawa, 2003; Kumar et al., 2004). Nurses advocate for the use of personal protective equipment for workers who must be exposed to herbicides and pesticides.

Multiple sclerosis (MS) is a neurodegenerative disease caused by demyelination of nerves within the CNS. It may be an autoimmune disease that develops in genetically susceptible people who have lived prior to their mid-teens in temperate climates, especially southern Canada, Northern United States, Europe, and Australia (Noseworthy, Lucchinetti, Rodrigues, & Weinshenker, 2000; Willer et al., 2005). An estimated 55,000 to 75,000 Canadians live with MS, one of the highest prevalence rates in the world. Approximately 1000 new cases are diagnosed yearly (Multiple Sclerosis Society of Canada [MSSC], n.d.). Interestingly, a small group of Canadian aboriginals of Algonquin background have been diagnosed with MS (Mirsattari et al., 2001). Onset is usually between 15 and 40 years and is 3 times as common in females as in males of Northern European background (MSSC). Nurses must be alert for various combinations of visual disturbances, loss of balance, muscle stiffness, speech articulation problems, and fatigue in young adults when no obvious cause can be identified. Screening is achieved through MRI to observe demyelinated nerves within the CNS. Nurses encourage early diagnosis and treatment, which may achieve remission and decrease neurological deficits.

Unfortunately, the possibility of *lead poisoning* continues. The developing brains of children are especially vulnerable, resulting in deficits in cognitive and language development as well as slowed growth. Adults experience neurological changes that include headache, peripheral motor neuropathy, and deficits in short-term memory. Public health and occupational health nurses are alert for children's toys contaminated with lead paint, workers exposed to lead during demolition work and paint removal, and welders, potters, and metal smelter workers who may be exposed to lead at work sites (BC HealthGuide, 2007). Longstanding exposure to *mercury* vapour or the ingestion of mercury, a neurotoxin, can cause memory loss, tremors, and changes in visual-motor coordination. Public health and occupational health nurses must be alert to signs and symptoms of exposure. Nurses may advise clients that levels of mercury in [wild] salmon, cod, shrimp, and canned light tuna are considered so low that they need not restrict consumption (Erstad & Henley, 2007).

Ingestion of more than 1 to 2 *alcohol* drinks per day is ill-advised because alcohol is a neurotoxin. Even one drink may disturb sleep patterns. After several drinks, alcohol relaxes muscles in the pharynx, contributing to snoring, poor judgement, and impaired balance and motor coordination. Excessive long-time ingestion, often accompanied by thiamine deficiency, is implicated in the development of peripheral neuropathy, cerebellar degeneration, Wernicke's syndrome (ataxia and encephalopathy), and Korsakoff's syndrome (alcohol-induced persistent amnesic disorder). Nurses understand that alcohol abuse significantly increases the risk of injuries in operating automobiles, Skidoos, aircraft, and moving machinery. They advise clients not to use alcohol as a sedative and to limit intake if sleep apnea is a health concern (Kasper & Harrison, 2005; Spencer, 2005).

Peripheral neuropathy refers to peripheral nerve disorders from any cause, but commonly diabetes or prolonged entrapment of the ulnar or median nerves. Clients with *diabetic peripheral neuropathy* describe loss of sensation as well as sensations of tingling, prickling, burning, and pain in the feet that progress upward in a stocking-like fashion. Typically, hyperglycemia is long-standing. Nurses encourage clients with diabetes to decrease their risk of developing peripheral neuropathies by maintaining optimal serum blood glucose levels, reporting symptoms as soon as they occur, and practising vigilant foot care (Kasper & Harrison, 2005; Wieman, 2005).

The client's *ulnar nerve* may become damaged by entrapment at the elbow or by prolonged pressure on the base of the palm through use of hand tools or bicycle riding. The *median nerve* may become damaged through excessive repetitive use of the wrist, often in the workplace, resulting in carpal tunnel syndrome. In problems with both the ulnar and median nerves, weakness in the small hand muscles is observed. Nurses need to provide clients with ways to decrease their risks. For example, an ergonomic assessment of a work station may provide insights for subsequent change to alleviate causation of repetitive strain (Kasper & Harrison, 2005).

Bell's palsy, unilateral paralysis of the facial nerve (CN VII), results in loss of motor control of facial muscles on the affected side. Inability to raise both eyebrows distinguishes Bell's palsy from a stroke (see Table 20-5) when this function is maintained. The condition is usually of unknown cause and self-limiting, but nurses encourage prompt medical attention for medication that prevents sequelae.

Trigeminal neuralgia (tic douloureux) is characterized by excruciating paroxysms of pain of unknown origin in the lips, gums, cheeks, or chin upon stimulation of the maxillary and mandibular branches of the trigeminal nerve (CN V). Very rarely does trigeminal neuralgia affect the distribution of the ophthalmic division. The condition occurs most often in middle-aged and elderly people. Nurses assist clients to determine what stimuli trigger the pain and discuss options for long-term pain management (Kasper & Harrison, 2005).

Several infectious diseases can cause neurological deficits in adults and children. Vaccination of children with inactivated *poliovirus* (IPV) has essentially eradicated this disease in Canada. It remains endemic in India, Pakistan, Nepal, Afghanistan, Indonesia, and much of East and West Africa, where its effects on people are still seen. Nurses advise clients traveling to these countries to have a one-time booster of IPV 6 to 8 weeks prior to their travel (Canadian Immunization Guide, 2006).

Meningitis is caused by a bacteria or virus, with symptoms of fever, headache, and nuchal (neck) rigidity. For *bacterial* meningitis, the most common causative organism is *Streptococcus pneumoniae*, with *Neisseria meningitides* a close second. Risk factors for *S. pneumoniae* meningitis include pneumococcal pneumonia, acute or chronic otitis media, and head trauma with basilar skull fracture. Immune-compromised people, when the nasopharynx is colonized with *N. meningitides*, are at risk for developing meningitis. Prevention of meningococcal infections through vaccination with meningoccal C conjugate vaccine is recommended in Canada for adults and children. Nurses recommend the quadravalent meningococcal polysac-charde vaccine for military personnel and travelers to sub-Saharan Africa (Canadian Immunization Guide, 2006). Since the introduction of *H. influenzae* type b (Hib) conjugate vaccine, this cause of meningitis is seen primarily in unvaccinated people.

Typically occurring during the summer months, *viral* (aseptic) meningitis and encephalitis are caused in 80% of cases by an enterovirus or arbovirus. Transmission of enterovirus is by the fecal–oral route; transmission of the arbovirus is by ticks (e.g., tick-borne relapsing fever) or mosquitoes (e.g., West Nile viral infections, equine encephalitis). Infected ticks also transmit Lyme disease (by Lyme borreliosis) and Rocky Mountain Spotted Fever (by *Rockettsia rockettsii*; Dworkin, Shoemaker, Fritz, Dowell, & Anderson, 2002; Health Canada, 2007; Health Canada and Public Health Agency of Canada, 2007). Herpes simplex viruses (HSVs) types 1 and 2 cause meningitis and encephalitis in the remaining 20% of cases. Nurses can teach prevention of the transmission of enterovirus (hand washing), the arbovirus and tick-borne diseases (appropriate use of DEET-containing insect repellents and protective clothing), and HSV-2 infections (condoms). Immunization is available if an adult tests seronegative for varicella-zoster virus, the cause of chicken pox and later *shingles* (herpes zoster). Shingles occurs in people previously infected with the varicella-zoster virus. Nurses are alert to painful eruption of vesicles in a dermatome, a particular concern when the eye is involved. They encourage clients to seek immediate treatment with an antiviral medication (Kasper & Harrison, 2005).

Seizures result from a sudden excessive and simultaneous electrical discharge of an aggregate of cerebral neurons that results in full-body convulsive activity (generalized tonic–clonic [grand mal]), localized seizure activity, or subclinical seizures (petit mal—brief loss of consciousness without loss of postural control). After a seizure, the nurse advises the client to seek medical intervention as soon as possible. Approximately 15,500 new cases of epilepsy are diagnosed yearly in Canada. Causes include head trauma of any type, brain tumours, stroke, fevers and infection, metabolic disturbances, drug and alcohol withdrawal, and age older than 65 years; the cause also may be unknown (Epilepsy Canada, 2005). Nurses advocate for prevention of causative factors such as head injuries through sports, work hazards, and driving; they also promote occupational safety programs that include the use of protective head gear and seat belts. Nurses are aware that cultural stigma against epilepsy persists and can best be combated through education. Because uncontrolled seizures and driving pose obvious safety hazards, nurses support the restriction of driving privileges after seizure activity. Nurses must report all first incidents of adult epilepsy to the Ministry of Transport. When the person is seizure-free (on or off medications) for a restricted period, he or she may resume driving (Epilepsy Canada, 2005).

Brain health is a relatively new concept. Research studies increasingly reveal that lifestyle choices can positively affect the health of the brain, including cognitive functioning. Evidence from several studies seems to demonstrate that regular aerobic exercise and a diet high in omega-3 fatty acids and vitamins B_9 and B_{12} may have a protective effect against cognitive decline and dementia (Gillette et al., 2007; Johnson & Schaefer, 2006; Larson et al., 2006; Schaefer et al., 2006; van Gelder, Tijhuis, Kalmijn, & Kromhout, 2007). Also, studies have shown that cognitive training effectively slows decline in performing instrumental activities of daily living (Willis et al., 2006). Research studies provide nurses with evidence to endorse a lifestyle with regular aerobic exercise; diet rich in whole grains, fruits, vegetables, and omega-3 fatty acids; and mental activity for slowing cognitive decline.

EMERGENCY CONCERNS

STROKE AND TRANSIENT ISCHEMIC ATTACK

A person should receive immediate emergency intervention with the onset of symptoms of stroke, even if symptoms prove to be transient. Transportation by ambulance is preferred to facilitate quick transfer to a stroke unit, determination of the type of stroke, and early intervention (Agyeman et al., 2006). While observing for ability and symmetry, the nurse asks the client to raise both arms above the head, speak a simple sentence, smile, and stick out the tongue. Administration of tissue-plasminogen activator (t-PA) within 3 hours may improve the outcome of ischemic stroke (Heart and Stroke Foundation of Canada, 2008).

HEAD AND SPINAL CORD INJURY

A potential head or spinal cord injury requires immediate treatment with correct immobilization to prevent further damage to the brain or spine. At the scene, nurses protect victims from unnecessary movement, ensure a patent airway, and initiate emergency services. *Concussion* is the immediate, but transient, loss of consciousness associated with blunt trauma to the head; nurses teach that clients require observation over 24 hours for a change in level of conscious necessitating referral for follow-up. Clients must be taken to the hospital emergency department if they have difficulty awakening or speaking, vomiting, confusion, or lateralizing signs (i.e., asymmetrical findings for left and right sides).

SEIZURE ACTIVITY

During an observed seizure, nurses protect the client by easing him or her to the floor, removing dangerous objects in the immediate environment, loosening restrictive clothing, ensuring a patent airway, and placing the client in the "recovery position" following the seizure. Throughout the seizure, nurses observe the client closely to enable accurate reporting of the sequence of the seizure activity.

TECHNIQUES OF EXAMINATION: OBJECTIVE DATA

PROMOTING CLIENT COMFORT, DIGNITY, AND SAFETY

A full examination of the nervous system involves all regions of the body. For efficiency and client comfort, nurses may perform it in conjunction with other systems or regions. For example, while examining the head and neck, a nurse may test the client's cranial nerves. While assessing the musculoskeletal or peripheral vascular systems of the lower extremities, a nurse may examine sensory and motor functions. Such approaches minimize unnecessary movement by the client and require fewer changes in draping.

If the major focus of the assessment is the nervous system, adequate draping for warmth and coverage yet full exposure of the head, neck, arms, and legs in turn ensures client comfort and dignity. Usually, clients are seated for cranial nerve testing and examination of motor, sensory, and reflex function of the upper extremities. Nurses prefer that clients lie down for examining the lower extremities, but ask them to stand for testing coordination and strength in the legs, and gait. Some tests require clients to close their eyes while lying, sitting, and standing. It is imperative that nurses protect clients from loss of position or balance that could lead to injury.

Important Areas of Examination

- Cranial Nerves I through XII
- Motor system: muscle bulk, tone, and strength; coordination, gait, and stance
- Sensory system: pain and temperature, position and vibration, light touch, discrimination
- Deep tendon, abdominal, and plantar reflexes

Now return to the three important questions that govern the neurologic examination:

- Is the mental status intact? See Chapter 9.

- Are right-sided and left-sided findings symmetric?

- If the findings are asymmetric or otherwise unexpected, does the causative lesion lie in the CNS or the PNS?

In this section, you will learn the techniques for a practical and reasonably comprehensive examination of the nervous system. It is important to master the techniques for a thorough examination. At first these techniques may seem difficult, but with practice, dedication, and supervision, you will come to feel comfortable evaluating neurologic symptoms and disease. You should be active in your learning and ask your instructors or even a neuroscience nurse practitioner to review your skills.

The detail of an appropriate neurologic examination varies widely. As you gain experience, you will find that in healthy people, your examination will come to be relatively brief. When you detect unexpected findings, your examination will become more comprehensive. Be aware that neurologists may use many other techniques in specific situations.

Organize your thinking into categories: (1) mental status, speech, and language; (2) cranial nerves; (3) the motor system; (4) the sensory system; and (5) reflexes. If your findings are unexpected, begin to group them into patterns of central or peripheral disorders.

> **Equipment**
>
> - Reflex hammer
> - Splintered tongue blades and intact cotton swabs
> - 128 Hz tuning fork
> - Cotton ball made into a fine wisp
> - At least two familiar objects (e.g., coin, safety pin)
> - At least two familiar odours (e.g., cloves, lemon extract)
> - Two test tubes, one filled with hot water, the other with ice water

THE CRANIAL NERVES

The examination of the cranial nerves (CNs) can be summarized as follows:

I. Smell

II. Visual acuity, visual fields, and ocular fundi

II, III. Pupillary reactions

III, IV, VI. Extraocular movements

V. Corneal reflex, facial sensation, and jaw movements

VII. Facial movements

VIII. Hearing and balance

IX, X. Swallowing and rise of the palate, gag reflex

V, VII, X, XII. Voice and speech

XI. Shoulder and neck movements

XII. Tongue symmetry and position

Cranial Nerve I—Olfactory. Test the *sense of smell* by presenting the client with familiar and nonirritating odours. First, ensure that that each nasal passage is open by compressing one side of the nose and asking the client to sniff through the other. The client should then close both eyes. Occlude one nostril and test smell in the other with such substances as cloves, coffee, soap, or vanilla. Ask whether the client smells anything and, if so, what. Test the other side. A person can be expected to perceive odour on each side and can often identify it.

Loss of smell has many causes, including nasal disease, head trauma, smoking, ageing, and the use of cocaine. It may be congenital.

Cranial Nerve II—Optic. Test *visual acuity* (see p. 310).

Inspect the *optic fundi* with your ophthalmoscope, paying special attention to the optic discs (see p. 317).

Optic atrophy, papilledema

Screen the visual fields by confrontation (see p. 311). Occasionally—in a client who has had a CVA, for example—screening indicates a visual field defect, such as a homonymous hemianopsia, which you cannot confirm by testing one eye at a time. This screening observation, nevertheless, is significant. See Table 12-4 on p. 329.

These findings suggest visual *extinction*, a subtle impairment detectable only when testing both eyes simultaneously. It suggests a lesion in the parietal cortex.

Cranial Nerves II and III—Optic and Oculomotor. Inspect the size and shape of the pupils, and compare one side with the other. Test the *pupillary reactions to light;* if these are unusual, examine the *near reaction* (see p. 304).

See Table 12-6, Variations, p. 331.

Cranial Nerves III, IV, and VI—Oculomotor, Trochlear, and Abducens.

Test the *extraocular movements* in the six cardinal directions of gaze, and look for loss of conjugate movements in any of the six directions. Check convergence of the eyes. Identify any nystagmus, noting the direction of gaze in which it appears, the plane in which movements occur (horizontal, vertical, rotary, or mixed), and the direction of the quick and slow components.

Look for *ptosis* (drooping of the upper eyelids). A slight difference in the width of the palpebral fissures may be noted in about one-third of all people.

Cranial Nerve V—Trigeminal

Motor. While palpating the temporal and masseter muscles in turn, ask the client to clench his or her teeth. Note the strength of muscle contraction. It should be strong (5/5) and equal.

See Table 12-7, Dysconjugate Gaze, p. 332.

See Table 20-4, Nystagmus, pp. 746–747.

Ptosis in 3rd nerve palsy, Horner's syndrome (ptosis, meiosis, anhidrosis), myasthenia gravis

Weak or absent contraction of the temporal and masseter muscles on one side suggests a lesion of CNV. Bilateral weakness may result from peripheral or central involvement. When the client has no teeth, this test may be difficult to interpret.

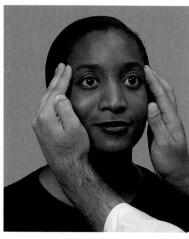

PALPATING TEMPORAL MUSCLES

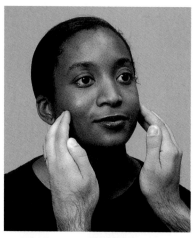

PALPATING MASSETER MUSCLES

Sensory. After explaining what you plan to do, test the forehead, cheeks, and jaw on each side in turn for *pain sensation*. Suggested areas are indicated by the circles. The client's eyes should be closed. Use a splintered tongue blade (1) to test each of the six areas, comparing sides, and (2) to test for veracity, occasionally substituting the blunt end for the point as a stimulus. Ask the client to report whether it is "sharp" or "dull" and to compare sides. Expect responses to be accurate.

If your findings are unexpected, *assess temperature sensation*. Two test tubes, filled with hot and ice-cold water, are the traditional stimuli. A tuning fork may also be used. It usually feels cool. If you are near running water, the fork is easily made colder or warm. Dry it before use. Touch the skin and ask the client to identify "hot" or "cold."

Then test for *light touch*, using a fine wisp of cotton. Ask the client to respond whenever you touch the skin. Vary your rhythm as you test the six sites. Expect accurate responses.

Unilateral decrease in or loss of facial sensation suggests a lesion of CNV or of interconnecting higher sensory pathways. Such a sensory loss may also be associated with a conversion reaction.

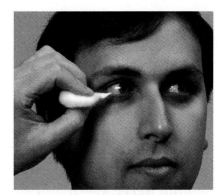

Note: To avoid transmitting infection, use a new object with each client. You can create a sharp wood splinter by breaking a tongue blade or a cotton-tipped applicator. The cotton end of the swab or the blunt end of the tongue blade can also be used as the dull stimulus.

Test *the corneal reflex.* Ask the client to look up and away from you. Approaching from the other side, out of the client's line of vision, and avoiding the eyelashes; touch the cornea (not the sclera) lightly with a fine wisp of cotton. If the client is apprehensive, touching the conjunctiva first may allay fear.

Look for blinking of the eyes, the expected reaction to this stimulus. (The sensory limb of this reflex is carried in CN V, the motor response in CN VII.) Use of contact lenses frequently diminishes or abolishes this reflex.

Absence of blinking suggests a lesion of CN V. A lesion of CN VII (innervates the muscles that close the eyes) may also impair this reflex.

Cranial Nerve VII—Facial.
Inspect the face, both at rest and during conversation with the client. Note any asymmetry (e.g., of the nasolabial folds), and observe any tics or other unusual movements.

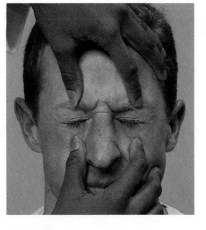

Ask the client to:

1. Raise both eyebrows

2. Frown

3. Close both eyes tightly so that you cannot open them. Test muscular strength by trying to open them, as illustrated.

4. Show both upper and lower teeth

5. Smile

6. Puff out both cheeks

Note any weakness or asymmetry. Expect movements to be relatively symmetrical. Some individuals are born with slight facial asymmetry; for example, the smile may appear "lopsided."

Flattening of the nasolabial fold and drooping of the lower eyelid suggest facial weakness.

A peripheral injury to CN VII, as in Bell's palsy, affects both the upper and the lower face; a central lesion affects mainly the lower face. See Table 20-5, Types of Facial Paralysis, pp. 748–749.

In unilateral facial paralysis, the mouth droops on the paralyzed side when the client smiles or grimaces.

Cranial Nerve VIII—Acoustic.
Assess *hearing.* Test auditory acuity (p. 357). Expect clients to readily identify whispered words. If hearing loss is present, (1) test for *lateralization,* and (2) compare *air and bone conduction* (see p. 357).

Specific tests of *vestibular function* are seldom included in the usual neurologic examination. Consult textbooks of neurology or otolaryngology as the need arises.

See Table 13-4, Patterns of Hearing Loss, p. 371.

Nystagmus may indicate vestibular dysfunction. See Table 20-4, Nystagmus, pp. 746–747.

Cranial Nerves IX and X—Glossopharyngeal and Vagus.
Listen to the client's *voice.* Is it hoarse, or does it have a nasal quality? Expect clear and articulate vocalization.

Is there difficulty in swallowing?

Hoarseness in vocal cord paralysis; a nasal voice in paralysis of the palate

Pharyngeal or palatal weakness

Ask the client to say "ah" or to yawn as you watch the *movements of the soft palate and the pharynx*. Expect the soft palate to rise symmetrically, the uvula to remain midline, and each side of the posterior pharynx to move medially, like a curtain. The slightly curved uvula seen occasionally in a healthy person should not be mistaken for a uvula deviated by a lesion of CN X.

The palate fails to rise with a bilateral lesion of the vagus nerve. In unilateral paralysis, one side of the palate fails to rise and, together with the uvula, is pulled toward the unaffected side.

Warn the client that you are going to test the *gag reflex*. Stimulate the back of the throat lightly on each side in turn and note the gag reflex. It may be symmetrically diminished or absent in some healthy people.

Unilateral absence of this reflex suggests a lesion of CN IX, perhaps CN X.

Cranial Nerve XI—Spinal Accessory.

From behind, look for atrophy or fasciculations in the trapezius muscles, and compare one side with the other. Ask the client to shrug both shoulders upward against your hands. Note the strength and contraction of the trapezii.

Weakness with atrophy and fasciculations indicates a peripheral nerve disorder. When the trapezius is paralyzed, the shoulder droops, and the scapula is displaced downward and laterally.

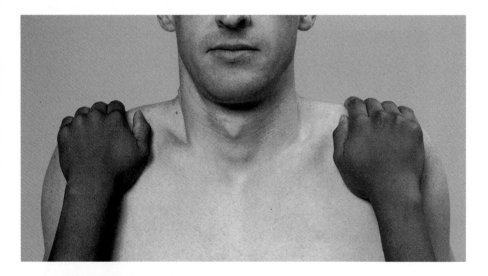

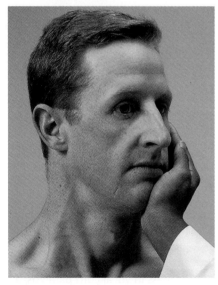

Ask the client turn his or her head to each side against your hand. Observe the contraction of the opposite sternomastoid and note the force of the movement against your hand. Expect movement of the sternomastoid muscles to be equally strong (5/5).

A supine client with bilateral weakness of the sternomastoids has difficulty raising the head off the pillow.

Cranial Nerve XII—Hypoglossal.

Listen to the articulation of the client words. This depends on Cranial Nerves V, VII, and X as well as XII. Inspect the client's tongue as it lies on the floor of the mouth. Be alert to any atrophy or *fasciculations* (fine, flickering, irregular movements in small groups of muscle fibres). Some coarser restless movements are often an expected finding. Then, with the client's tongue protruded, look for asymmetry, atrophy, or deviation from the midline. Ask the client to move the tongue from side to side and note the symmetry of the movement. In ambiguous cases, ask the client to push the tongue against the inside of each cheek in turn as you palpate externally for strength. Expect protrusion of the tongue to be midline and movement and strength bilaterally equal.

For poor articulation, or *dysarthria,* see Table 9-1, Disorders of Speech, p. 238. Atrophy and fasciculations in *amyotrophic lateral sclerosis, polio*

In a unilateral cortical lesion, the protruded tongue deviates transiently in a direction away from the side of the cortical lesion. That is, toward the side of muscle weakness.

◼ THE MOTOR SYSTEM

INSPECTION AND PALPATION

As you assess the motor system, focus on body position, involuntary movements, characteristics of the muscles (bulk, tone, and strength), and coordination. These components are described in sequence in the following sections. You may either use this sequence or check each component in the arms, legs, and trunk in turn. If you observe unexpected movements or muscle characteristics, identify the muscle(s) involved. Think about whether the unexpected movement or characteristic is central or peripheral in origin, and begin to learn which nerves innervate the affected muscles.

Body Position. Observe the client's body position during movement and at rest.

Unusual body positions alert you to neurologic deficits such as paralysis.

Involuntary Movements. Watch for involuntary movements such as tremors, tics, or fasciculations. Note their location, quality, rate, rhythm, and amplitude, and their relation to posture, activity, fatigue, emotion, and other factors.

See Table 20-3, Tremors and Involuntary Movements, pp. 744–745.

Muscle Bulk. Compare the size and contours of muscles. Do the muscles look flat or concave, suggesting atrophy? If so, is the process unilateral or bilateral? Is it proximal or distal?

When looking for atrophy, pay particular attention to the hands, shoulders, and thighs. The thenar and hypothenar eminences should be full and convex, and the spaces between the metacarpals, where the dorsal interosseous muscles lie, should be full or only slightly depressed. Atrophy of hand muscles, an anticipated age-related change, is shown on the right.

Muscular *atrophy* refers to a loss of muscle bulk (wasting). It results from diseases of the peripheral nervous system such as diabetic neuropathy, as well as diseases of the muscles themselves. *Hypertrophy* refers to an increase in bulk with proportionate strength, whereas increased bulk with diminished strength is called *pseudohypertrophy* (seen in the Duchenne form of muscular dystrophy).

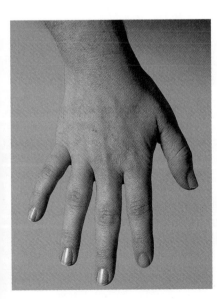

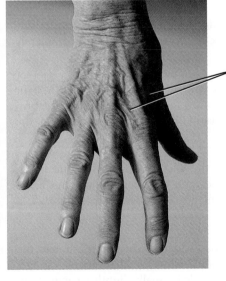

Atrophy

Flattening of the thenar and hypothenar eminences and furrowing between the metacarpals suggest atrophy. Localized atrophy of the thenar and hypothenar eminences suggests damage to the median and ulnar nerves, respectively.

Hand of a 44-year-old woman   Hand of an 84-year-old woman

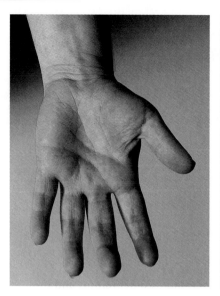 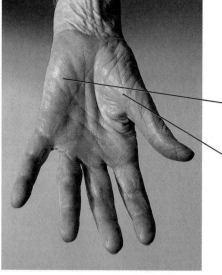

Hypothenar eminence

Flattening of the thenar eminence due to mild atrophy

Hand of a 44-year-old woman   Hand of an 84-year-old woman

Other causes of muscular atrophy include motor neuron diseases, disuse of the muscles, rheumatoid arthritis, and protein–calorie malnutrition.

Be alert for fasciculations in atrophic muscles. If absent, tap on the muscle with a reflex hammer to try to stimulate them.

Fasciculations suggest lower motor neuron disease as a cause of atrophy.

Muscle Tone. When a viable muscle with an intact nerve supply is relaxed voluntarily, it maintains a slight residual tension known as muscle tone. This can be assessed best by feeling the muscle's resistance to passive stretch. Persuade the client to relax. Take one hand with yours and, while supporting the elbow, flex and extend the client's fingers, wrist, and elbow, and put the shoulder through a moderate range of motion. With practice, these actions can be combined into a single smooth movement. On each side note muscle tone—the resistance offer to your movements. Tense clients may show increased resistance. You will learn the feel of the expected resistance only with repeated practice.

Decreased resistance suggests disease of the peripheral nervous system, cerebellar disease, or the acute stages of spinal cord injury. See Table 20-6, Disorders of Muscle Tone, p. 750.

If you suspect decreased resistance, hold the forearm and shake the hand loosely back and forth. Expect the hand to move back and forth freely but not completely floppy.

Marked floppiness indicates *hypotonic* or flaccid muscles.

If resistance is increased, determine whether it varies as you move the limb or whether it persists throughout the range of movement and in both directions, for example, during both flexion and extension. Feel for any jerkiness in the resistance.

Increased resistance that varies, commonly worse at the extremes of the range, is called *spasticity*. Resistance that persists throughout the range and in both directions is called *lead-pipe rigidity*, as observed in Parkinson's disease.

To assess muscle tone in the legs, support the client's thigh with one hand, grasp the foot with the other, and flex and extend the client's knee and ankle on each side. Note the resistance to your movements. Slight residual tension should be felt.

Muscle Strength. Healthy individuals vary widely in their strength, and the expected standard, while admittedly rough, should allow for such variables as age, sex, and muscular training. A person's dominant side is usually slightly stronger than the other side. Keep this difference in mind when you compare sides.

Test muscle strength by asking the client to move actively against your resistance or to resist your movement. Remember that a muscle is strongest when shortest, and weakest when longest.

If the muscles are too weak to overcome resistance, test them against gravity alone or with gravity eliminated. When the forearm rests in a pronated position, for example, extension at the wrist can be tested against gravity alone. When the forearm is midway between pronation and supination, extension and flexion at the wrist can be tested with gravity eliminated. Finally, if the client fails to move the body part, watch or feel for weak muscular contraction.

See Table 20-7, Disorders of the Central and Peripheral Nervous Systems, pp. 751–753.

SCALE FOR GRADING MUSCLE STRENGTH

Muscle strength is graded on a 0–5 scale:
0—No muscular contraction detected
1—A barely detectable flicker or trace of contraction
2—Active movement of the body part with gravity eliminated
3—Active movement against gravity
4—Active movement against gravity and some resistance
5—Active movement against full resistance without evident fatigue.
 This is expected muscle strength.

More experienced clinicians make further distinctions by using plus or minus signs toward the stronger end of this scale. Thus 4+ indicates good but not full strength, while 5− means a trace of weakness.

Methods for testing the major muscle groups are described in the following paragraphs. The spinal root innervations and the muscles affected are shown in parentheses. To localize lesions in the spinal cord or the PNS more precisely, additional testing may be necessary. For these specialized methods, refer to texts of neurology.

Test flexion (C5, C6—biceps) *and extension* (C6, C7, C8—triceps) *at the elbow.* Ask the client to flex the arm at the elbow and then pull and push against the resistance offered by your hand.

Impaired strength is called weakness, or *paresis*. Absence of strength is called paralysis, or *plegia*. Hemiparesis refers to weakness of one half of the body; *hemiplegia* to paralysis of one half of the body. *Paraplegia* means paralysis of the legs; *quadriplegia*, paralysis of all four limbs.

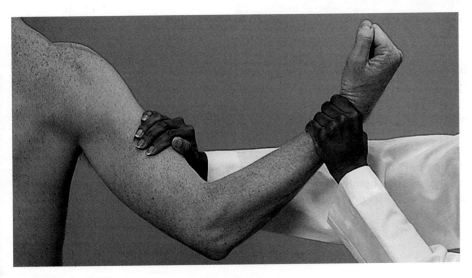

FLEXION AT ELBOW

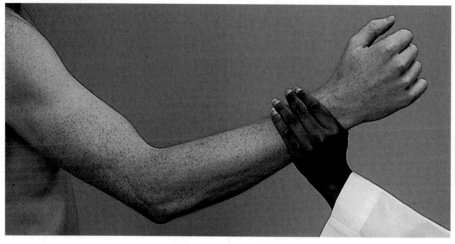

EXTENSION AT ELBOW

Both extension and flexion at the elbow should be equally strong (5/5), though the dominant may be slightly stronger.

Test extension at the wrist (C6, C7, C8, radial nerve). Ask the client to make a fist with slight extension at the wrist and resist your pulling it down.

Weakness of extension is seen in peripheral nerve disease such as radial nerve damage and in central nervous system disease–producing hemiplegia, as in stroke or multiple sclerosis.

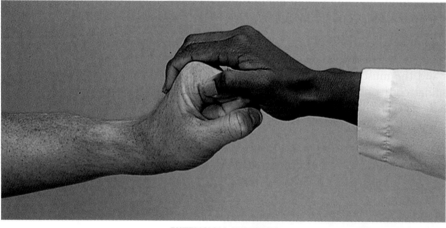

EXTENSION AT WRIST

Test flexion at the wrist (C6, C7, C8, radial nerve). Ask the client to make a fist with slight flexion at the wrist and resist your pulling it up.

Expect equally strong (5/5) muscle movements for extension and flexion.

Test the grip (C7, C8, T1). Ask the client to squeeze two of your fingers as hard as possible and not let them go (to avoid getting hurt by hard squeezes, place your own middle finger on top of your index finger). You should expect difficulty in removing your fingers from the client's grip. Testing both grips simultaneously with arms extended or in the lap facilitates comparison.

A weak grip may be due to either central or peripheral nervous system disease. It may also result from painful disorders of the hands.

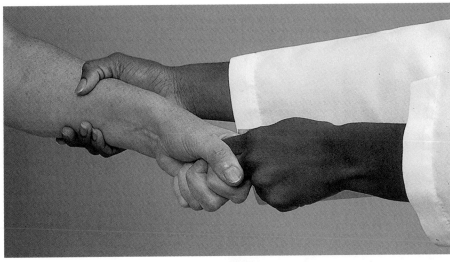

TEST OF GRIP

Test finger abduction (C8, T1, ulnar nerve). Position the client's hand with palm down and fingers spread. Instructing the client not to let you move the fingers, try to force them together. Strong resistance is expected bilaterally.

Weak finger abduction in ulnar nerve disorders

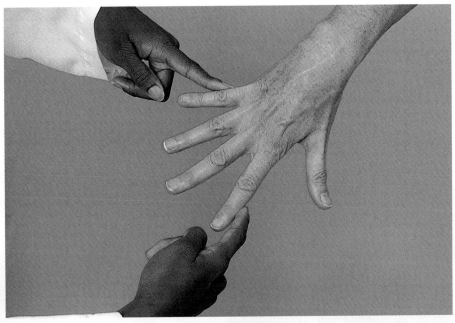

FINGER ABDUCTION

Test opposition of the thumb (C8, T1, median nerve). The client should try to touch the tip of the little finger with the thumb, against your resistance. You should expect strong pressure against your finger bilaterally.

Weak opposition of the thumb in median nerve disorders such as carpal tunnel syndrome

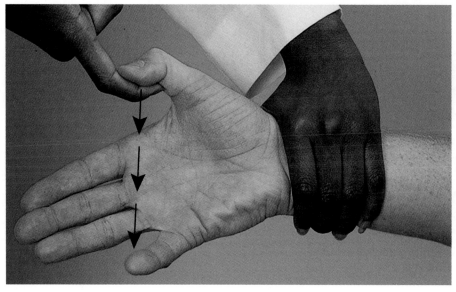

OPPOSITION OF THE THUMB

Assessment of *muscle strength of the trunk* may already have been made in other segments of the examination. It includes

- Flexion, extension, and lateral bending of the spine (see Chapter 19)

- Thoracic expansion and diaphragmatic excursion during respiration (see Chapter 14)

Test flexion at the hip (L2, L3, L4—iliopsoas), place your hand on each client thigh in turn and ask the client to raise the leg against your hand. Expect equal effort bilaterally.

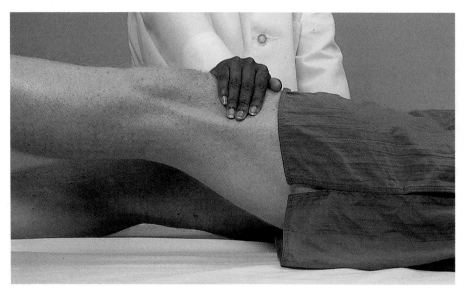

FLEXION OF THE THIGH

Test adduction at the hips (L2, L3, L4—adductors). Place both fists together and firmly on the bed between the client's knees. Ask the client to bring both legs together. Expect uniform and strong (5/5) adduction.

Test abduction at the hips (L4, L5, S1—gluteus medius and minimus). Place your fists firmly on the bed outside the client's knees. Ask the client to spread both legs against your hands. Expect strong (5/5) abduction bilaterally

Test extension at the hips (S1—gluteus maximus). Place your hand, palm down, under each of the client's thighs in turn. Ask the client to push the posterior thigh firmly down against your hand.

Test extension at the knee (L2, L3, L4—quadriceps). Support the knee in flexion and ask the client to straighten the leg against your hand placed firmly on the ankle. The quadriceps is the strongest muscle in the body, so expect a forceful response.

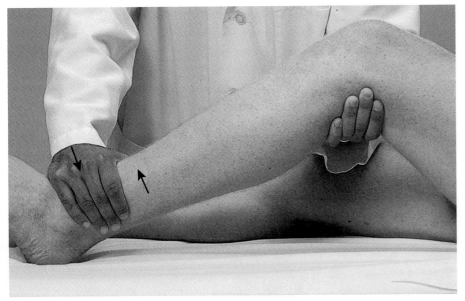

EXTENSION AT THE KNEE

Test flexion at the knee (L4, L5, S1, S2—hamstrings). Place the client's leg so that the knee is flexed with the foot resting on the bed. Tell the client to keep the foot on the bed as you try to straighten the leg by pulling up at the client's ankle. Expect a strong and equal effort bilaterally.

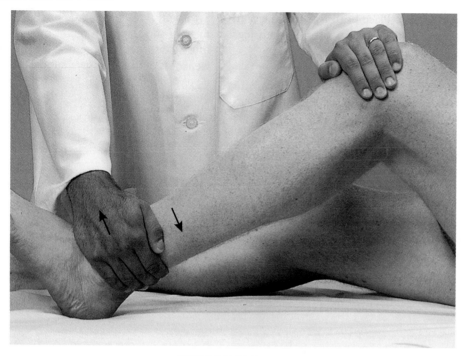

FLEXION AT THE KNEE

Test dorsiflexion (mainly L4, L5) and *plantar flexion* (mainly S1) at the ankle. Ask the client to pull up (dorsiflexion) and push down (plantar flexion) against your hand. Testing both legs at the same time facilitates comparison of the expected strong and equal effort

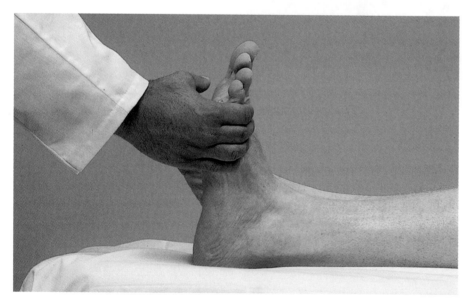

DORSIFLEXION

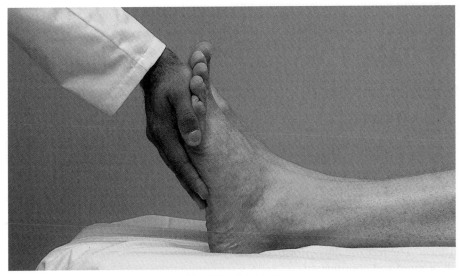

PLANTAR FLEXION

Coordination. Coordination of muscle movement requires that four areas of the nervous system function in an integrated way:

- The motor system, for muscle strength

- The cerebellar system (also part of the motor system), for rhythmic movement and steady posture

- The vestibular system, for balance and for coordinating eye, head, and body movements

- The sensory system, for position sense

To assess coordination, observe the client's performance in:

- Rapid alternating movements

- Point-to-point movements

- Gait and other related body movements

- Standing in specified ways

Rapid Alternating Movements

ARMS. Show the client how to strike one hand on the thigh, raise the hand, turn it over, and then strike the back of the hand down on the same place. Urge the client to repeat these alternating movements as rapidly as possible. Test each hand separately.

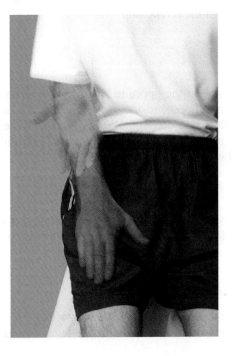

Observe the speed, rhythm, and smoothness of the movements. The nondominant hand often performs somewhat less well.

In cerebellar disease, one movement cannot be followed quickly by its opposite and movements are slow, irregular, and clumsy. This disorder is called *dysdiadochokinesis*. Upper motor neuron weakness and basal ganglia disease may also impair rapid alternating movements, but not in the same manner.

Show the client how to tap the distal joint of the thumb with the tip of the index finger, again as rapidly as possible. Again, observe the speed, rhythm, and smoothness of the movements. The nondominant side often performs less well.

Movements in both these tests should be rhythmic and coordinated.

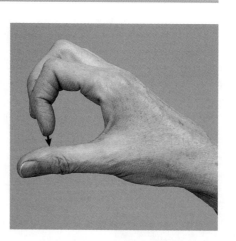

LEGS.   Ask the client to tap your hand as quickly as possible with the ball of each foot in turn. Note any slowness or awkwardness. The feet usually perform less well than the hands, but movements should still be rapid and coordinated.

Dysdiadochokinesis in cerebellar disease

Point-to-Point Movements

ARMS.   Ask the client to touch your index finger and then his or her nose alternately several times. Move your finger about so that the client has to alter directions and extend the arm fully to reach it. Observe the accuracy and smoothness of movements and watch for any tremor. Expect the client's movements to be smooth and accurate.

In cerebellar disease, movements are clumsy, unsteady, and inappropriately varying in their speed, force, and direction. The finger may initially overshoot its mark, but finally reaches it fairly well. Such movements are termed *dysmetria*. An *intention tremor* may appear toward the end of the movement (see p. 752).

Now hold your finger in one place so that the client can touch it with one outstretched arm and finger. Ask the client to raise the arm overhead and lower it again to touch your finger. After several repeats, ask the client to close both eyes and try several more times. Repeat on the other side. Expect the person to touch your finger successfully with eyes open or closed. These manoeuvres test position sense and the functions of both the labyrinth and the cerebellum.

Cerebellar disease causes incoordination that may get worse with eyes closed. If present, this suggests loss of position sense. Repetitive and consistent deviation to one side, referred to as *past pointing*, worse with the eyes closed, suggests cerebellar or vestibular disease.

LEGS.   Ask the client to place one heel on the opposite knee, and then run it down the shin to the big toe. Note the smoothness and accuracy of the movements. Repeat the tests, with the client's eyes closed, to determine position sense. Repeat on the other side. Expect the client to perform this test accurately and smoothly with either leg and equally coordinated with eyes open or closed.

In cerebellar disease, the heel may overshoot the knee and then oscillate from side to side down the shin. When position sense is lost, the heel is lifted too high and the client tries to look. With eyes closed, performance is poor.

Gait and Related Movements.   The following tests assess aspects of muscle strength, balance, and coordination. As the risk of a fall is ever present, it is advisable to stand close enough to offer assistance.

Physical irregularities in gait increase risk of falls.

Gait: Ask the client to:

- *Walk across the room* or down the hall, then turn, and come back. Observe posture, balance, swinging of the arms, and movements of the legs. The gait

A gait that lacks coordination, with reeling and instability, is called *ataxic*. Ataxia may be due to cerebellar disease, loss of position

should be performed with an easy balance, the arms swinging at the sides, and the turns accomplished smoothly.

sense, or intoxication. See Table 20-8, Deviations in Gait and Posture, pp. 754–755.

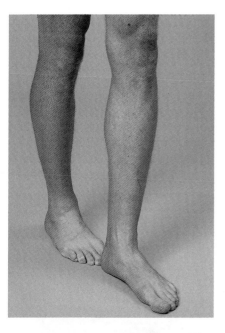

■ *Walk heel to toe—(tandem walking)*: Ask the client to walk heel to toe in a straight line with eyes open. This action should be accomplished accurately and without loss of balance.

Tandem walking may reveal an ataxia not previously obvious.

■ *Walk on the toes*, then *on the heels*: Ask the client to walk on heels, then toes. These movements test strength of plantar flexion (heel walking) and dorsiflexion (for walking) at the ankle as well as balance. Both movements should be strong and accomplished without loss of balance.

Walking on toes and heels may reveal distal muscular weakness in the legs. Inability to heel walk is a sensitive test for corticospinal tract weakness.

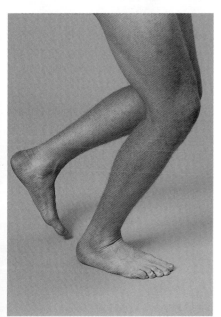

■ *Hop in place on* each foot in turn. Hopping involves the proximal muscles of the legs as well as the distal ones and requires both good position sense and intact cerebellar function.

Difficulty with hopping may be due to weakness, lack of position sense, or cerebellar dysfunction.

■ *Shallow knee bends* first on one leg, then on the other. Support the client's elbow if you think he or she is in danger of falling.

Difficulty here suggests proximal weakness (extensors of the hip), weakness of the quadriceps (the extensor of the knee), or both.

Both the hop and shallow knee bend should be performed easily and without loss of balance or need for assistance.

■ *Rising from a sitting position* without arm support and *stepping up* on a sturdy stool are more suitable tests than hopping or knee bends when clients are elderly or less robust.

Proximal muscle weakness involving the pelvic girdle and legs causes difficulty with both of these activities.

Stance. The following two tests can often be performed concurrently. They differ only in the client's arm position and in what you are looking for. In each case, stand close enough to the client to prevent a fall.

THE ROMBERG TEST. This is mainly a test of position sense. The client should first stand with feet together and eyes open and then close both eyes for 20 to 30

In ataxia due to loss of position sense, vision compensates for the

seconds without support. Note the client's ability to maintain an upright posture. Expect only minimal swaying with eyes either open or closed.

TEST FOR PRONATOR DRIFT. The client should stand for 20 to 30 seconds with both arms straight forward, palms up, and with eyes closed. A person who cannot stand may be tested for a pronator drift in the sitting position. In either case, a healthy person can hold this arm position well.

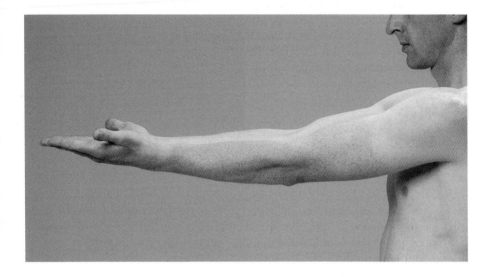

Now, instructing the client to keep the arms up and eyes shut, as shown above, *tap the arms briskly downward.* Expect the arms to return smoothly to the horizontal position. This response requires muscular strength, coordination, and a good sense of position.

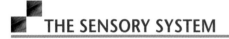

THE SENSORY SYSTEM

To evaluate the sensory system, you will test several kinds of sensation:

■ Pain and temperature (spinothalamic tracts)

■ Position and vibration (posterior columns)

■ Light touch (spinothalamic tracts and posterior columns)

■ Discriminative sensations, which depend on some of the above sensations, but also involve the cortex

Familiarize yourself with each kind of test so that you can use it as indicated. When you detect unexpected findings, correlate them with motor and reflex activity. Is the underlying lesion central or peripheral?

Patterns of Testing. Because sensory testing quickly fatigues many clients and then produces unreliable results, conduct the examination as efficiently as

sensory loss. The client stands fairly well with eyes open, but loses balance when they are closed, a *positive Romberg sign.* In *cerebellar ataxia,* the client has difficulty standing with feet together whether the eyes are open or closed.

The pronation of one forearm suggests a contralateral lesion in the corticospinal tract; downward drift of the arm with flexion of fingers and elbow may also occur. These movements are called *pronator drift,* shown on the next page.

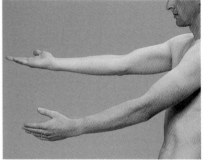

A sideward or upward drift, sometimes with searching, writhing movements of the hands, suggests loss of position sense.

A weak arm is easily displaced and often remains so. A client lacking position sense may not recognize the displacement and, if told to correct it, does so poorly. In cerebellar incoordination, the arm returns to its original position, but overshoots and bounces.

See Table 20-7, Disorders of the Central and Peripheral Nervous Systems, pp. 751–753.

Meticulous sensory mapping helps to establish the level of a spinal cord

possible. Pay special attention to those areas where there are (1) symptoms such as numbness or pain; (2) motor or reflex irregularities that suggest a lesion of the spinal cord or PNS; and (3) trophic changes, such as absent or excessive sweating, atrophic skin, or cutaneous ulceration. Repeated testing at another time is often required to confirm findings.

lesion and to determine whether a more peripheral lesion is in a nerve root, in a major peripheral nerve, or in one of its branches.

The following patterns of testing help you to identify sensory deficits accurately and efficiently:

- *Compare symmetric areas* on the two sides of the body, including the arms, legs, and trunk.

Hemisensory loss due to a lesion in the spinal cord or higher pathways

- When testing pain, temperature, and touch sensation, *compare symmetrical areas and also distal with the proximal areas* of the extremities. Further, scatter the stimuli so as to sample most of the dermatomes and major peripheral nerves (see p. 694). One suggested pattern includes both shoulders (C4), the inner and outer aspects of the forearms (C6 and T1), the thumbs and little fingers (C6 and C8), the fronts of both thighs (L2), the medial and lateral aspects of both calves (L4 and L5), the little toes (S1), and the medial aspect of each buttock (S3).

Symmetric distal sensory loss suggests a *polyneuropathy*, as described in the example on the next page. You may miss this finding unless you compare distal and proximal areas.

- When testing vibration and position sensation, first test the fingers and toes. If these are intact, you may safely assume that more proximal areas will also be intact.

- *Vary the pace of your testing.* This is important so that the client does not merely respond to your repetitive rhythm.

- When you detect an area of sensory loss or hypersensitivity, *map out its boundaries* in detail. Stimulate first at a point of reduced sensation, and move by progressive steps until the client detects the change. An example is shown at right.

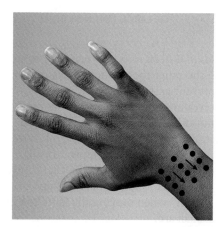

Here all sensation in the hand is lost. Repetitive testing in a proximal direction reveals a gradual change to intact sensation at the wrist. This pattern fits neither a peripheral nerve nor a dermatome (see pp. 694–695). If bilateral, it suggests the "glove and stocking" sensory loss of a polyneuropathy, often seen in *alcoholism* and *diabetes*.

By identifying the distribution of sensory deviations and the kinds of sensations affected, you can infer where the causative lesion might be. Any motor deficit or reflex irregularity also helps in this localizing process.

Before each of the following tests, show the client what you plan to do and what responses you want. Unless otherwise specified, the client's eyes should be closed during actual testing.

Pain. Use a sharp object, such as a broken cotton-tipped applicator or wooden tongue blade. Occasionally, substitute the blunt end for the point. "Retest" these areas with the point to ensure you are testing pain not pressure. Ask the client, "Is this sharp or dull?" or, when making comparisons, "Does this feel the same as this?" Apply the lightest pressure needed for the stimulus to feel sharp, and do not draw blood (see pattern of testing explained previously). Responses should be consistently accurate.

To prevent transmitting a blood-borne infection, *discard the sharp object safely. Do not reuse it on another person.*

Temperature.
(Testing is often omitted if pain sensation is intact, but include it if there is any question.) Use two test tubes, filled with hot and cold water, or a tuning fork heated or cooled by water. Touch the skin and ask the client to identify "hot" or "cold."

Light Touch.
With a fine wisp of cotton, touch the skin lightly, avoiding pressure. Ask the client to respond whenever a touch is felt, and to compare one area with another. Calloused skin is usually relatively insensitive and should be avoided. Test the dermatomes in a similar pattern as for pain. Responses should be consistently accurate.

Vibration.
Use a relatively low-pitched tuning fork of 128 Hz. Tap it on the heel of your hand and place it firmly over a distal interphalangeal joint of the client's finger, then over the interphalangeal joint of the big toe. Ask what the client feels. If you are uncertain whether it is pressure or vibration, ask the client to tell you when the vibration stops, and then touch the fork to stop it. If vibration sense is impaired, proceed to more proximal bony prominences (e.g., wrist, elbow, clavicles, medial malleolus, patella, anterior superior iliac spine, and spinous processes).

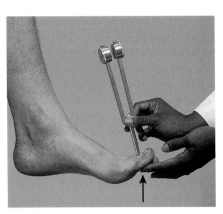

TUNING FORK ON PAD OF LARGE TOE, NOT BONE

Position.
Grasp the client's big toe, *holding it by its sides* between your thumb and index finger, and then pull it away from the other toes. (These precautions prevent extraneous tactile stimuli from revealing position changes that might not otherwise be detected.) Demonstrate "up" and "down" as you move the client's toe clearly upward and downward. Then, with the client's eyes closed, ask for a response of "up" or "down" when moving the large toe in a small arc.

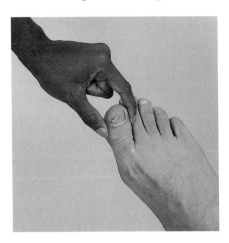

Discriminative Sensations.
Several additional techniques test the ability of the sensory cortex to correlate, analyze, and interpret sensations. Because discriminative sensations are dependent on touch and position sense, they are useful only when these sensations are either intact or only slightly impaired.

Screen a client with *stereognosis*, and proceed to other methods if indicated. The client's eyes should be closed during all these tests.

Analgesia refers to absence of pain sensation, *hypalgesia* to decreased sensitivity to pain, and *hyperalgesia* to increased sensitivity.

Anaesthesia is absence of touch sensation, *hypaesthesia* is decreased sensitivity, and *hyperesthesia* is increased sensitivity.

Vibration sense is often the first sensation to be lost in a peripheral neuropathy. Common causes include *diabetes* and *alcoholism.* Vibration sense is also lost in posterior column disease, as in *tertiary syphilis* or *vitamin B$_{12}$* deficiency.

Testing vibration sense in the trunk may be useful in estimating the level of a cord lesion.

Loss of position sense, like loss of vibration sense, suggests either posterior column disease or a lesion of the peripheral nerve or root.

Repeat several times on each side, avoiding simple alternation of the stimuli. If position sense is impaired, move proximally to test it at the ankle joint. In a similar fashion, test position sense in the metacarpophalangeal joints of the fingers, moving proximally if indicated to the wrist and elbow.

When touch and position sense are intact or only slightly impaired, a disproportionate decrease in or loss of discriminative sensations suggests disease of the sensory cortex. Stereognosis, number identification, and two-point discrimination are also impaired by posterior column disease.

■ *Stereognosis.* Stereognosis refers to the ability to identify an object by feeling it. Place in the client's hand a familiar object such as a coin, paper clip, key, pencil, or cotton ball, and ask the client to tell you what it is. Expect the client to skilfully manipulate the object in one hand and identify it correctly. Asking the client to distinguish "heads" from "tails" on a coin is a sensitive test of stereognosis.

Astereognosis refers to the inability to recognize objects placed in the hand.

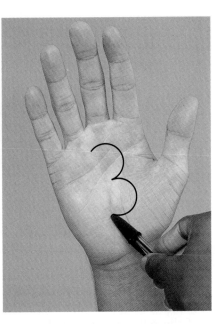

■ *Number identification (graphesthesia).* When motor impairment, arthritis, or other conditions prevent the client from manipulating an object well enough to identify it, test the ability to identify numbers. With the blunt end of a pen or pencil, draw a large number in the client's palm. Ensure the number is drawn in one fluid motion and correctly oriented for reading. A healthy person can identify most such numbers.

The inability to recognize numbers, like astereognosis, suggests a lesion in the sensory cortex.

■ *Two-point discrimination.* Using the two ends of an opened paper clip, touch a finger pad in two places simultaneously. Alternate the double stimulus irregularly with a one-point touch. Do not cause pain.

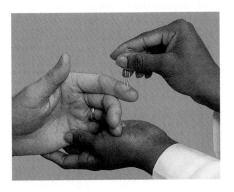

Find the minimal distance at which the client can discriminate one from two points (expect less than 5 mm on the finger pads). This test may be used on other parts of the body, but accurate perception of distances varies widely from one body region to another.

Lesions of the sensory cortex increase the distance between two recognizable points.

■ *Point localization.* Briefly touch a point on the client's skin. Then ask the client to open both eyes and point to the place touched. Expect a person to do so accurately. This test, together with the test for extinction, is especially useful on the trunk and the legs.

Lesions of the sensory cortex impair the ability to localize points accurately.

■ *Extinction.* Simultaneously stimulate corresponding areas on both sides of the body. Ask where the client feels your touch. Both stimuli should be felt.

DEEP TENDON REFLEXES

Eliciting the *deep tendon reflexes* involves a series of examiner skills. Be sure to select a properly weighted reflex hammer. Learn when to use either the pointed or the flat end of the hammer. For example, the pointed end is useful for striking small areas, such as your finger as it overlies the biceps tendon; the flat end causes less discomfort when you test the brachioradialis reflex. Now test the reflexes as follows:

■ Encourage the client to relax, then position the limbs properly and symmetrically.

■ Hold the reflex hammer loosely between your thumb and index finger so that it swings freely in an arc within the limits set by your palm and other fingers.

■ With your wrist relaxed, strike the tendon briskly using a rapid wrist movement. Your strike should be quick and direct, not glancing.

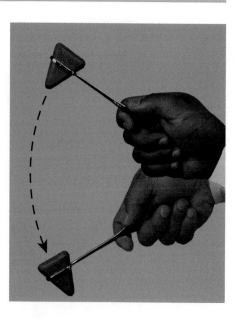

■ Note the speed, force, and amplitude of the reflex response and grade the response using the following scale. Always compare the response of one side with the other. Reflexes are usually graded on a 0 to 4+ scale.

SCALE FOR GRADING REFLEXES

4+ Very brisk, hyperactive, with *clonus* (rhythmic oscillations between flexion and extension)
3+ Brisker than average; possibly but not necessarily indicative of disease
2+ Average; expected
1+ Somewhat diminished; low average
0   No response

Hyperactive reflexes suggest central nervous system disease. Sustained clonus confirms it. Reflexes may be diminished or absent when sensation is lost, when the relevant spinal segments or the peripheral nerves are damaged. Diseases of muscles and neuromuscular junctions may also decrease reflexes.

Reflex response depends partly on the force of your stimulus. Use no more force than you need to provoke a definite response: Strike reflexes on symmetrical sides of the body with similar force. Differences between sides are usually easier to assess than symmetric changes. Symmetrically diminished or even absent reflexes may be found in healthy people.

If the client's reflexes are symmetrically diminished or absent, use *reinforcement*, a technique involving isometric contraction of other muscles that may enhance reflex activity. In testing arm reflexes, for example, ask the client to clench his or her teeth or to squeeze one thigh with the opposite hand. If leg reflexes are diminished or absent, reinforce them by asking the client to lock fingers and pull one hand against the other. Tell the client to pull just before you strike the tendon.

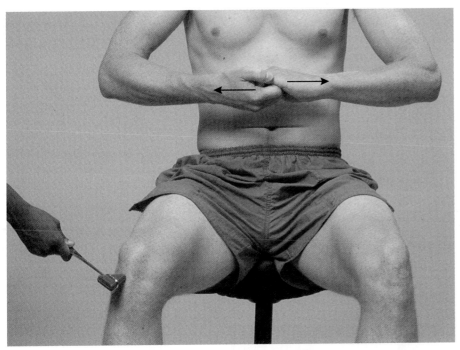

REINFORCEMENT OF KNEE REFLEX

The Biceps Reflex (C5, C6). The client's arm should be partially flexed at the elbow with palm down resting on the thigh (Sitting) or across the abdomen (Supine). Place your thumb or finger firmly on the biceps tendon. Strike with the reflex hammer so that the blow is aimed directly through your digit toward the biceps tendon.

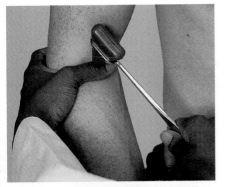

CLIENT SITTING

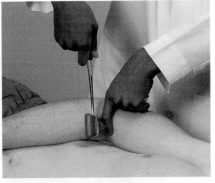

CLIENT LYING DOWN

Observe for flexion at the elbow, and watch for and feel the contraction of the biceps muscle.

The Triceps Reflex (C6, C7). The client may be sitting or supine. Flex the client's arm at the elbow, with palm toward the body, and pull it slightly across the chest. Strike the triceps tendon above the elbow. Use a direct blow from directly behind it. Watch for contraction of the triceps muscle and extension at the elbow.

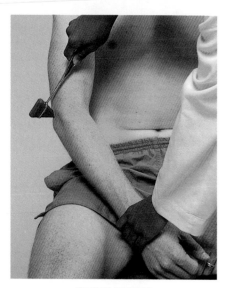

CLIENT SITTING

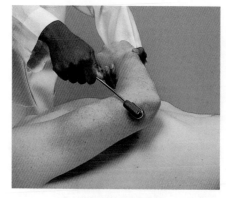

CLIENT SUPINE

If you have difficulty getting the client to relax, try supporting the upper arm as illustrated on the right. Ask the client to let the arm go limp, as if it were "hung up to dry." Then strike the triceps tendon.

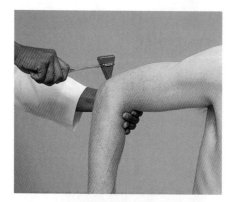

The Supinator or Brachioradialis Reflex (C5, C6). The client's hand should rest on the abdomen or the lap, with the forearm partly pronated. Strike the radius with the flat edge of the reflex hammer, about 2.5 to 5.0 cm above the wrist. Watch for flexion and supination of the forearm.

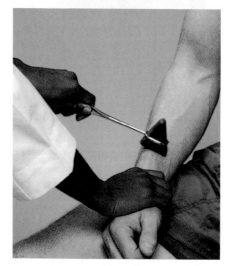

The Knee (Patellar) Reflex (L2, L3, L4). The client may be either sitting or supine as long as the knee is flexed. Briskly tap the patellar tendon just below the patella. Expect contraction of the quadriceps with extension at the knee. A hand on the client's anterior thigh lets you feel this reflex.

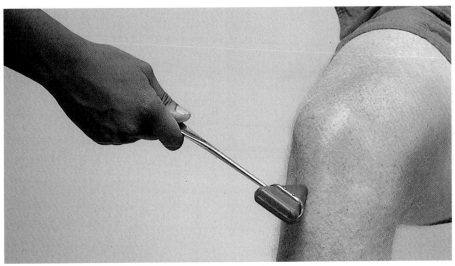

CLIENT SITTING

Two methods are useful when examining the supine client. Supporting both knees at once, as shown below on the left, allows you to assess small differences between knee reflexes by repeatedly testing one reflex and then the other. Sometimes, however, supporting both legs is uncomfortable for both the examiner and the client. You may wish to rest your supporting arm under the client's leg, as shown below on the right. Some clients find it easier to relax with this method.

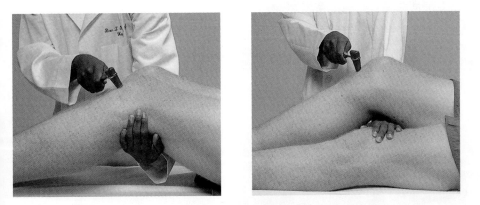

The Ankle (Achilles) Reflex (primarily S1). If the client is sitting, slightly dorsiflex the foot at the ankle. Persuade the client to relax. Strike the Achilles tendon. Watch and feel for plantar flexion at the ankle. Note also the speed of relaxation after muscular contraction.

The slowed relaxation phase of reflexes in *hypothyroidism* is often easily seen and felt in the ankle reflex.

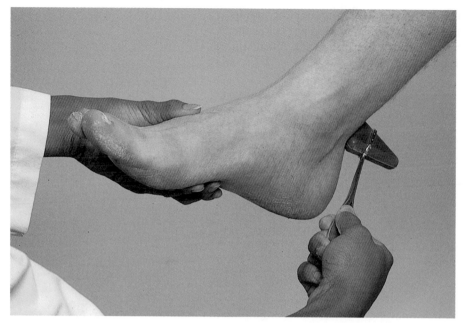

CLIENT SITTING

If the client is lying down, flex one leg at both hip and knee and rotate it externally so that the lower leg rests across the opposite shin. Then slightly dorsiflex the foot at the ankle and strike the Achilles tendon.

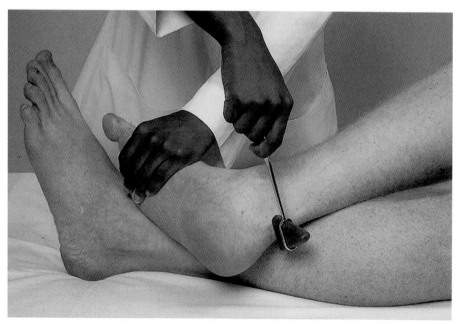

CLIENT LYING DOWN

Clonus. If the reflexes seem hyperactive, test for *ankle clonus.* Support the knee in a partly flexed position. With your other hand, dorsiflex and plantar flex the foot a few times while encouraging the client to relax, and then sharply dorsiflex the foot and maintain it in dorsiflexion. Look and feel for rhythmic oscillations between dorsiflexion and plantar flexion. In most healthy people, the ankle does not react to

Sustained clonus indicates central nervous system disease. The ankle plantar flexes and dorsiflexes repetitively and rhythmically.

this stimulus. A few clonic beats may be seen and felt, especially when the client is tense or has exercised.

Clonus may also be elicited at other joints. A sharp downward displacement of the patella, for example, may elicit patellar clonus in the extended knee.

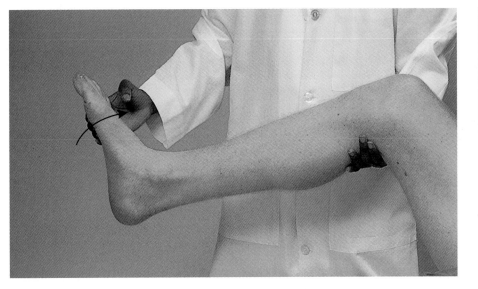

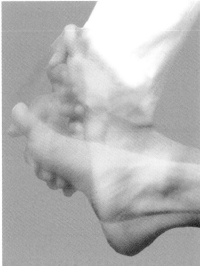

■ SUPERFICIAL (CUTANEOUS) REFLEXES

The Abdominal Reflexes. Test the abdominal reflexes by lightly but briskly stroking each side of the abdomen, above (T8, T9, T10) and below (T10, T11, T12) the umbilicus, in the directions illustrated. Use a key, the wooden end of a cotton-tipped applicator, or a tongue blade, twisted and split longitudinally. Note the contraction of the abdominal muscles and deviation of the umbilicus toward the stimulus. Obesity may mask an abdominal reflex. In this situation, use your finger to retract the client's

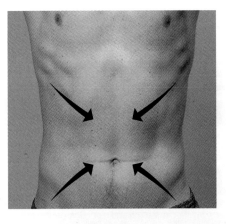

umbilicus away from the side to be stimulated. Feel with your retracting finger for the muscular contraction.

Abdominal reflexes may be absent in both central and peripheral nervous system disorders.

■ SPECIAL TECHNIQUES

ASTERIXIS

Asterixis helps identify a metabolic encephalopathy in clients whose mental functions are impaired. Ask the client to "stop traffic" by extending both arms, with hands cocked up and fingers spread. Watch for 1 to 2 minutes, coaxing the client as necessary to maintain this position.

Sudden, brief, nonrhythmic flexion of the hands and fingers indicates asterixis.

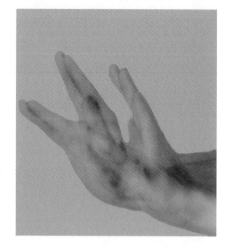

WINGING OF THE SCAPULA

When the shoulder muscles seem weak or atrophic, look for winging. Ask the client to extend both arms and push against your hand or against a wall. Observe the scapulae. Usually they lie close to the thorax.

In winging, shown below, the medial border of the scapula juts backward (posteriorly). It suggests weakness of the serratus anterior muscle, as in muscular dystrophy or injury to the long thoracic nerve.

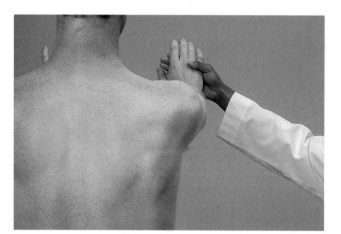

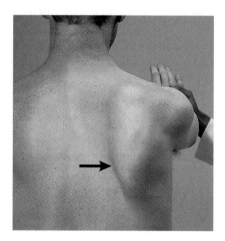

In very thin but healthy people, the scapulae may appear "winged" even when the musculature is intact.

MENINGEAL SIGNS

Testing for these signs is important if you suspect meningeal inflammation from infection or subarachnoid hemorrhage.

Neck Mobility. First make sure there is no injury to the cervical vertebrae or cervical cord. (In settings of trauma, this may require evaluation by x-ray.) Then, with the client supine, place your hands behind the client's head and flex the neck forward, until the chin touches the chest if possible. Generally the neck is supple, and the client can easily bend the head and neck forward.

Pain in the neck and resistance to flexion (nuchal rigidity) can arise from meningeal inflammation, arthritis, or neck injury.

Brudzinski's Sign. As you flex the neck, watch the hips and knees in reaction to your manoeuvre. Usually they remain relaxed and motionless.

Flexion of the hips and knees is a *positive Brudzinski's sign* and suggests meningeal inflammation.

Kernig's Sign. Flex the client's leg at both the hip and the knee, and then straighten the knee. Discomfort behind the knee during full extension occurs in many healthy people, but this manoeuvre should not produce pain.

Pain and increased resistance to extending the knee are a *positive Kernig's sign.* When bilateral, it suggests meningeal irritation.

Compression of a lumbosacral nerve root may also cause resistance, together with pain in the low back and the posterior thigh. Only one leg is usually involved. (Unilateral finding).

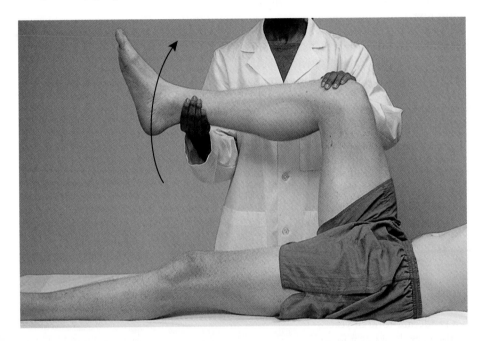

THE STUPOROUS OR COMATOSE CLIENT

Coma signals a potentially life-threatening event affecting the two hemispheres, the brainstem, or both. The usual sequence of history, physical examination, and laboratory evaluation does not apply. Instead, you must:

See Table 20-9, Metabolic and Structural Coma, p. 756.

- First assess the ABCs (airway, breathing, and circulation)

- Establish the client's level of consciousness

- Examine the client neurologically. Look for focal or asymmetric findings, and determine whether impaired consciousness arises from a metabolic or a structural cause.

Interview relatives, friends, or witnesses to establish the speed of onset and duration of unconsciousness, any warning symptoms, precipitating factors, or previous episodes, and the prior appearance and behaviour of the client. Any history of past medical and psychiatric illnesses is also useful.

As you proceed to the examination, remember two cardinal don'ts:

1. *Do not* dilate the pupils, the single most important clue to the underlying cause of coma (structural vs. metabolic)

2. *Do not* flex the neck if there is any question of trauma to the head or neck. Immobilize the cervical spine and get an x-ray first to rule out fractures of the cervical vertebrae that could compress and damage the spinal cord.

Airway, Breathing, and Circulation.

Quickly check the client's colour and pattern of breathing. Inspect the posterior pharynx and listen over the trachea for stridor to make sure the airway is clear. If respirations are slowed or shallow, or if the airway is obstructed by secretions, intubation may be considered as the spine is stabilized.

Assess the remaining vital signs: pulse, blood pressure, *rectal* temperature, and indicators of pain. If hypotension or haemorrhage is present, establish intravenous access and begin intravenous fluids. (Further emergency management and laboratory studies are beyond the scope of this text.)

Level of Consciousness.

Level of consciousness primarily reflects the client's capacity for arousal, or wakefulness. It is determined by the level of activity that the client can be aroused to perform in response to escalating stimuli from the examiner.

Five clinical levels of consciousness are described in the following table, together with related techniques for examination. Increase your stimuli in a stepwise manner, depending on the client's response.

When you examine clients with an altered level of consciousness, describe and record exactly what you see and hear. Imprecise use of terms such as lethargy, obtundation, stupor, or coma may mislead other examiners.

■ Level of Consciousness (Arousal): Techniques and Client Response

Level	Technique	Unexpected Response
Alertness	Speak to the client in a moderate tone of voice. An alert client opens the eyes, looks at you, and responds fully and appropriately to stimuli (arousal intact).	
Lethargy	Speak to the client in a loud voice. For example, call the client's name or ask "How are you?"	A lethargic client appears drowsy but opens the eyes and looks at you, responds to questions, and then falls asleep.
Obtundation	Shake the client gently as if awakening a sleeper.	An obtunded client opens the eyes and looks at you, but responds slowly and is somewhat confused. Alertness and interest in the environment are decreased.
Stupor	Apply a painful stimulus. For example, pinch a tendon, rub the sternum, or roll a pencil across a nail bed. (No stronger stimuli needed!)	A stuporous client arouses from sleep only after painful stimuli. Verbal responses are slow or even absent. The client lapses into an unresponsive state when the stimulus ceases. There is minimal awareness of self or the environment.
Coma	Apply repeated painful stimuli.	A comatose client remains unarousable with eyes closed. There is no evident response to inner need or external stimuli.

Neurologic Evaluation

Respirations. Observe the rate, rhythm, and pattern of respirations. Because neural structures that govern breathing in the cortex and brainstem overlap those that govern consciousness, irregularities in respiration often occur in coma.

See Table 20-9, Metabolic and Structural Coma, p. 756.

Pupils. Observe the size and equality of the pupils and test their reaction to light. The presence or absence of the light reaction is one of the most important signs distinguishing structural from metabolic causes of coma. The light reaction often remains intact in metabolic coma.

See Table 20-10, Pupils in Comatose Clients, p. 757.

Structural lesions such as stroke may lead to asymmetrical pupils and loss of light reaction.

Ocular Movement. Observe the position of the eyes and eyelids at rest. Check for horizontal deviation of the eyes to one side (gaze preference). When the oculomotor pathways are intact, the eyes look straight ahead.

In structural hemispheric lesions, the eyes "look at the lesion" in the affected hemisphere.

In irritative lesions due to epilepsy or early cerebral hemorrhage, the eyes "look away" from the affected hemisphere.

Posture and Muscle Tone. Observe the client's posture. If there is no spontaneous movement, you may need to apply a painful stimulus (see above). Classify the resulting pattern of movement as:

See Table 20-11, Irregular Posture in the Comatose Client, p. 758.

- *Expected avoidant*—the client pushes the stimulus away or withdraws.

- *Stereotypic*—the stimulus evokes irregular postural responses of the trunk and extremities.

Two stereotypic responses predominate: *decorticate rigidity* and *decerebrate rigidity* (see Table 20-11, Irregular Postures in the Comatose Client, p. 758.

- *Flaccid paralysis or no response.*

No response on one side suggests a corticospinal tract lesion.

The Arm:

Test muscle tone by grasping each forearm near the wrist and raising it to a vertical position. Note the position of the hand, which is usually only slightly flexed at the wrist.

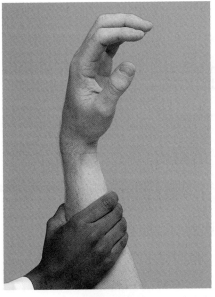

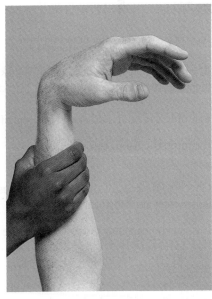

EXPECTED   **UNEXPECTED**

The hemiplegia of sudden cerebral accidents is usually flaccid at first. The limp hand drops to form a right angle with the wrist.

Then raise the arm to about 12 or 18 inches off the bed and drop it. Watch how it falls. With intact muscle tone, the arm drops somewhat slowly.

A flaccid arm drops rapidly, like a flail.

The Leg:

Support the client's flexed knees. Then extend one leg at a time at the knee and let it fall (see next page). Compare the speed with which each leg falls.

In *acute hemiplegia*, the flaccid leg falls more rapidly.

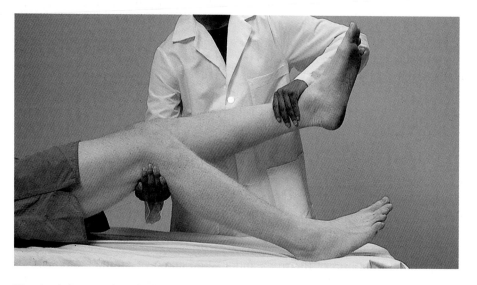

Flex both legs so that the heels rest on the bed and then release them. The leg with intact muscle tone returns slowly to its original extended position.

In acute hemiplegia, the flaccid leg falls rapidly into extension, with external rotation at the hip.

Further Examination.   As you complete the neurologic examination, check for facial asymmetry and asymmetries in motor, sensory, and reflex function. Test for meningeal signs if indicated using the neck mobility and Kernig's sign tests (p. 731).

Meningitis, subarachnoid hemorrhage

As you proceed to the general physical examination, check for unusual odours.

Alcohol, liver failure, uremia

Look for unexpected findings of the skin, including colour, moisture, evidence of bleeding disorders, needle marks, and other lesions.

Jaundice, cyanosis, cherry red colour of carbon monoxide poisoning

Examine the scalp and skull for signs of trauma.

Bruises, lacerations, swelling

Examine the fundi carefully.

Papilledema, hypertensive retinopathy

Check to make sure the corneal reflexes are intact. (Remember that use of contact lenses may abolish these reflexes.)

Reflex loss in coma and lesions affecting CN V or CN VII

Inspect the ears and nose, and examine the mouth and throat.

Blood or cerebrospinal fluid in the nose or the ears suggests a skull fracture; otitis media suggests a possible brain abscess.

Be sure to evaluate the heart, lungs, and abdomen.

Tongue injury suggests a seizure.

RECORDING AND ANALYZING FINDINGS

Nurses must describe findings from the physical examination of the nervous system precisely and clearly in their documentation. They analyze this information, in conjunction with relevant findings from the health history, to provide members of the interdisciplinary health care team with an integrated picture of the client's neurological functioning.

■ *Examples of Documentation for the Nervous System*

Area of Assessment	Expected Findings	Unexpected Findings
Cranial Nerves		
Olfactory, CN I	Sensation of smell intact bilaterally. See Chapter 12.	Detects pungent odour on right side, not on left side. See Chapter 12.
Optic, Oculomotor, Trochlear, Abducens, CNs II, III, IV, & VI		
Trigeminal, CN V	Sensations of pain and light touch intact over ophthalmic, maxillary, and mandibular branches bilaterally.	Sensations of pain and light touch intact over ophthalmic branch bilaterally and maxillary and mandibular branches on right side, absent on left side.
Sensory	Brisk bilateral blink.	Sluggish bilateral blink (wears contact lenses).
Motor	Temporal and masseter muscle strength 5/5 on palpation bilaterally.	Temporal and masseter muscle strength 3/5 on left, 5/5 on right.
Facial nerve, CN VII	Raises both eyebrows, frowns, shows teeth, smiles and puffs out cheeks symmetrically. Strongly resists eyelid opening bilaterally 5/5.	Unable to raise eyebrow, frown, resist eye opening, or show teeth, smile, puff out cheek on right side. Intact on left side.
Acoustic nerve, CN VIII	See Chapter 13.	See Chapter 13.
Glossopharyngeal and Vagus, CN IX and X	Gag reflex intact bilaterally.	Gag reflex depressed on right side, absent on left.
	Soft palate rises equally, uvula midline when client says, "ah."	Soft palate fails to rise on right side, uvula deviates to left when client says, "ah."
Spinal Accessory, CN XI	Shoulder shrug and sternomastoid muscle strength (5/5) bilaterally.	Shoulder shrug on right = 3/5, and left side = 5/5. Sternomastoid muscle strength right = 3/5, left = 5/5.
Hypoglossal, CN XII	Protrudes tongue midline, tongue movements to both sides equally strong. Words articulated clearly.	Tongue deviates to right side when protruded. Words often slurred.
Upper Extremities		
Muscle Tone	Slight tension felt during passive stretch bilaterally.	Left arm resists passive stretch. Slight tension felt in right arm.
Muscle Strength	Muscle strength 5/5 in hands, wrists, elbows, and shoulders bilaterally.	Muscle strength 2/5 in left wrist, elbow, and shoulder; 5/5 on right side.
Coordination	Bilaterally, performs rapid alternating movements smoothly. Point-to-point testing smooth and accurate with eyes open and closed, bilaterally.	Rapid alternating movements with right hand slow and awkward, rapid and smooth on left side. Point-to-point testing on right side slow but accurate with eyes open, inaccurate with eyes closed.

(continued)

■ *Examples of Documentation for the Nervous System (Continued)*

Area of Assessment	Expected Findings	Unexpected Findings
Sensation	Sensation of pain and light touch intact bilaterally over dermatomes C4-T1. Vibration and position sense intact bilaterally at fingers. Extinction, stereognosis, and graphesthesia intact bilaterally.	Pain and light touch absent over C5-C8 to 1 cm above the wrist bilaterally. Intact proximally. Vibration sense absent in finger joints and wrist, intact at elbows bilaterally. Stereognosis and graphesthesia absent on right, intact on left. Extinction absent on right at forearms.
Reflexes	Biceps 2+, triceps and brachioradialis reflexes 1+ bilaterally. Abdominal reflexes brisk bilaterally.	Bicep, tricep, and brachioradialis reflexes 3+ on right, 1+ on left. Abdominal reflexes sluggish bilaterally.
Lower Extremities		
Muscle Tone	Slight muscle tension noted during passive stretch bilaterally.	Left leg becomes spastic when passive movement attempted; slight muscle tension on right.
Muscle Strength	Muscle strength 5/5 over feet, ankles, knees, and hips bilaterally.	Muscle strength 2/5 over entire left leg (gravity eliminated); 5/5 on right side.
Coordination	Rapid alternating movements at toes rapid and moderately smooth bilaterally. Point-to-point testing smooth and accurate with eyes open and closed bilaterally.	Rapid alternating movements on right side slow and erratic, moderately smooth on left. Point-to-point slow and awkward on right side with eyes open, inaccurate with eyes closed, smooth and accurate on left.
Sensation	Pain and light touch intact over dermatomes L2 to S1 bilaterally. Vibration sense at great toes and position sense at toes intact bilaterally.	Pain and light touch absent over dermatomes L4-S1 to 2 cm superior to malleoli, intact proximally bilaterally. Vibration sense absent at toes and ankle on right leg, intact on left side. Position sense absent on right, intact on left.
Reflexes	Patellar and ankle reflexes 2+ without reinforcement bilaterally. Plantar reflex down-going bilaterally.	Patellar reflex 4+ on right, ankle reflex triggers clonus on right. Plantar reflex—dorsiflexion of right great toe. Patellar reflex in left leg 2+, Plantar reflex down-going.
Posture, gait, balance	Posture upright, gait coordinated with arm swing opposite to leg, heel strike with push-off at toe, head leads when turning.	Gait assisted with cane held in right hand, drags left toe slightly, left arm in sling.
Cerebellar/muscle strength	Romberg: Steady posture with eyes open, slight sway with eyes closed. Tandem walking smooth and coordinated; coordinated walking on heels and toes, strength and coordinated movement with shallow knee bend, and hop on one foot bilaterally.	Romberg: Steady stance with eyes open, moderate sway with eyes closed. Lost balance when tandem walking attempted. Unable to walk on toes or heels. Required assistance with slight knee bend, unable to hop on one foot bilaterally.

The reflexes may also be documented as follows:

	Biceps	Triceps	Brach	Knee	Ankle	Plantar
RT	4+	4+	4+	4+	4+	1
LT	2+	2+	2+	2+	1+	1

OR

ANALYZING FINDINGS FROM PHYSICAL EXAMINATION AND HEALTH HISTORY

After completing the history and physical examination and documenting findings related to the client concern, the nurse determines one or more nursing diagnoses in consultation with the client. For example:

Ms. Adams, a 53-year-old school teacher, presents with sensations of numbness and tingling in both lower extremities. She also reports a slow weight gain over the past 6 months. On examination, the area of numbness to both light touch and pain extends to 2 cm above the ankles bilaterally. The dorsalis pedis and posterior tibial pulses are 1+, and the ankle (Achilles) reflex is absent bilaterally. Both plantar reflexes are slightly down-going. The feet are cool to palpation, but no lesions are present. She denies any exposure to neurotoxins. The following nursing diagnoses are established:

- *Sensory perception, disturbed (kinaesthetic)*

- *Nutrition, imbalanced: more than body requirements*

An interdisciplinary approach ensures that Ms. Adams receives the needed interventions. Following consultation, the physician orders the appropriate diagnostic tests, including urinalysis, serum electrolytes and glucose levels, and thyroid tests. The nurse's baseline assessment includes vital signs, visual acuity (Snellen chart), height and weight, and blood glucose. Ms. Adams does not have hypertension, but her BMI is 30. Depending on the medical diagnoses, consultation with a diabetic, endocrine, or medical specialist may be appropriate. In addition to consultation with a dietician for weight and diet control, Ms. Adams might require the services of a diabetic teaching nurse. She may require medication for her condition and instruction on management by the nurse, physician, and pharmacist.

Critical Thinking Exercises

Answer the following questions about Ms. Adams.

- What is the expected response to the plantar reflex? (*Knowledge*)
- When testing pain, what is the rationale for testing all dermatomes with the sharp end of the splintered tongue blade and some with the blunt end? (*Comprehension*)
- How does the nurse test muscle strength at the knee? (*Application*)

- What specific information would you gather if Ms. Adams could maintain a steady stance during the Romberg test with her eyes open, but not with her eyes closed? (*Analysis*)
- What recommendations would you make for screening and follow-up, including client teaching, for Ms. Adams? (*Synthesis*)
- How would you evaluate the success of your client teaching, including the effects it might have on her lifestyle? (*Evaluation*)

BIBLIOGRAPHY

Canadian Research

Dryden, D. M., Saunders, L. D., Rowe, B. H., May, L. A., Yiannakoulias, N., Svenson, L., et al. (2003). The epidemiology of traumatic spinal cord injury in Alberta, Canada. *Canadian Journal of Neurological Sciences, 30*(2), 113–121.

Duff, D. (2002). Family concerns and responses following a severe traumatic brain injury: A grounded theory study. *AXON, 24*(2), 14–22.

Guttman, M., Kish, S. J., & Furukawa, Y. (2003). Current concepts in the diagnosis and management of Parkinson' disease. *CMAJ Canadian Medical Association Journal, 168*(3), 293–301.

Mirsattari, S. M., Johnston, J. B., McKenna, R., Del Bigio, M. R., Orr, P., Ross, R. T., et al. (2001). Aboriginals with multiple sclerosis: HLA types and predominance of neuromyelitis optica. *Neurology, 56*(3), 317–323.

Mouradian, M. S., Hussain, M. S., Lari, H., Salam, A., Senthilselvan, A., Dean, N., et al. (2005). The impact of a stroke prevention clinic in diagnosing modifiable risk factors for stroke. *Canadian Journal of Neurological Sciences, 32*(4), 496–500.

Pickett, G. E., Campos-Benitez, M., Keller, J. L., & Duggal, N. (2006) Epidemiology of traumatic spinal cord injury in Canada. *Spine, 31*(7), 799–805.

Stewart, T. C., Girotti, M. J., Nikore, V., & Williamson, J. (2003). Effect of airbag deployment on head injuries in severe passenger motor vehicle crashes in Ontario, Canada. *Journal of Trauma; Injury Infection & Critical Care, 54*(2), 266–272.

Van Neste-Kenny, J. (2003). Finding meaning after a head injury: The experience of clients' mothers and wives during the early phase of recovery. Unpublished doctoral dissertation, McGill University, Montreal, Canada. *CINAHL AN:* 2005090257.

Young, T. K., & Hachinski, V. (2003). The population approach to stroke prevention: A Canadian perspective. *Clinical & Investigative Medicine–Medecine Clinique et Experimentale, 26*(2), 78–86.

Test Questions

1. Characteristics of the 12 cranial nerves include all of the following **except** that
   a. they are paired.
   b. they emerge from within the cranium.
   c. each has motor and sensory functions.
   d. they include general or specialized functions.

2. The spinothalamic tracts transmit which of the following sensory impulses from the contralateral side of the body?
   a. Proprioception, pain, position
   b. Crude touch, pain, temperature
   c. Vibration, temperature, light touch
   d. Crude touch, temperature, vibration

3. The level of the spinal cord associated with the knee (patellar) deep tendon reflex is
   a. L1 and L2
   b. L3 and L4
   c. T9 and T10
   d. T11 and T12

4. When testing sensory function of the trigeminal nerve (CNV), which of the following sensations would the nurse assess?
   a. Pain and light touch
   b. Dull touch and vibration
   c. Vibration and stereognosis
   d. Proprioception and extinction

5. When conducting a Romberg test, the nurse asks the client to stand feet together with eyes open, then closed because
   a. position sense is affected with repetition.
   b. clients feel safer after testing with eyes open.
   c. vision can compensate for loss of position sense.
   d. vestibular defects become evident with eyes closed.

Bibliography

CITATIONS

Adams, S. M., & Standridge, J. B. (2006). What should we eat? Evidence from observational studies. *Southern Medical Journal, 99*(7), 744–748.

Agyeman, O., Nedeltchev, K., Arnold, M., Fischer, U., Remonda, L., Isenegger, J., et al. (2006). Time to admission in acute ischemic stroke and transient ischemic attack. *Stroke, 37*(4), 963–966.

BCHealthGuide. (2007). *Lead poisoning.* Retrieved October 1, 2007, from http://www.bchealthguide.org/kbase/major/hw119895/descrip.htm

Campbell, N. R., Petrella, R., & Kaczorowski, J. (2006). Public education on hypertension: A new initiative to improve the prevention, treatment and control of hypertension in Canada. *Canadian Journal of Cardiology, 22*(7), 599–603.

Canadian Immunization Guide. (2006). 7th ed. Retrieved March 24, 2009, from http://www.phac-aspc.gc.ca/publicat/cig.gci/index-eng.php

Canadian Institute of Health Information. (2006). *Head injuries in Canada: A decade of change (1994–1995 to 2003–2004).* Retrieved March 24, 2009, from http://secure.cihi.ca/cihiweb/en/downloads/analysis_ntr_2006_e.pdf (p.2)

Canadian Paraplegic Association. (2008). *Overview on spinal cord injuries (SCI) and its consequences.* Retrieved May 27,

2008, from http://canparaplegic.org/en/sci_Facts_67/items/6.html

Dryden, D. M., Saunders, L. D., Rowe, B. H., May, L. A., Yiannakoulias, N., Svenson, L. W., et al. (2003). The epidemiology of traumatic spinal cord injury in Alberta, Canada. *Canadian Journal of Neurological Sciences, 30*(2), 113–121.

Duff, D. (2002). Family concerns and responses following a severe traumatic brain injury: A grounded theory study. *AXON, 24*(2), 14–22.

Dworkin, M. S., Shoemaker, P. C., Fritz, D. L., Dowell, M. E., & Anderson D. E., Jr. (2002). The epidemiology of tick-borne relapsing fever in the United States. *American Journal of Tropical Medicine & Hygiene, 66*(6), 743–758.

Epilepsy Canada. (2005). *Epidemiology and basic information.* Retrieved October 1, 2005, from http://www.epilepsy.ca/eng/mainSet.html

Erstad, S., & Henley, C. (2007). *Avoiding mercury in fish.* Retrieved October 1, 2007, from http://www.bchealthguide.org/kbase/special/tn6745spec/sec1.htm

Giles, M. F., Flossman, E., & Rothwell, P. M. (2006). Client behaviour immediately after transient ischemic attack according to clinical characteristics, perception of the event, and predicted risk of stroke. *Stroke, 37*(5), 1254–1260.

Gillette Guyonnet, S., Abellan Van Kan, G., Andreiu, S., Barberger Gateau, P., Berr, C., Bonnefoy, M., et al. (2007). IANA task force on nutrition and cognitive decline with aging. *Journal of Nutrition, Health & Aging, 11*(2), 132–152.

Guttman, M., Kish, S. J., & Furukawa, Y. (2003). Current concepts in the diagnosis and management of Parkinson's Disease. *CMAJ Canadian Medical Association Journal, 168*(3), 293–301, 203.

He, R. J., Nowson, C. A., & MacGregor, G. A. (2006). Fruit and vegetable consumption and stroke: Meta-analysis of cohort studies. *Lancet, 367*(9507), 320–326.

Health Canada and Public Health Agency of Canada. (2007). *Lyme disease: It's your health.* Retrieved March 24, 2009 from http://www.hc-sc.gc.ca/hl-vs/iyh-vsv/diseases-maladies/lyme-eng.php

Health Canada and Public Health Agency of Canada. (2007). *West Nile virus.* Retrieved March 24, 2009 from http://www.hc-sc.gc.ca/dc-ma/wnv-vno/index-eng.php

Heart and Stroke Foundation of Canada. (2008). *Stroke.* Retrieved March 24, 2009 from http://www.heartandstroke.com/site/c.ikIQLcMWJtE/b.3483933/k.CD67/Stroke.htm?src

Hu, F. B. (2003). Plant-based foods and prevention of cardiovascular disease: An overview. *American Journal of Clinical Nutrition, 78*(3 Suppl.), 544S–551S.

Johnson, E. J., & Schaefer, E. J. (2006). Potential role of dietary n-3 fatty acids in the prevention of dementia and macular degeneration. *American Journal of Clinical Nutrition, 83*(6 Suppl), 1494S–1498S.

Kasper, D. L., & Harrison, T. R (Eds.). (2005). *Harrison's principles of internal medicine* (16th ed.). New York: McGraw Hill.

Kumar, A., Calne, S. M., Schulzer, M., Mak, E., Wszolek, Z., Van Netten, C., et al. (2004). Clustering of Parkinson's disease: Shared cause or coincidence? *Archives of Neurology, 61*(7), 1057–1060.

Larson, E. B., Wang, L., Bowen, J. D., McCormick, W. C., Teri, L., Crane, P., et al. (2006). Exercise is associated with reduced risk for incident dementia among persons 65 years of age and older. *Annals of Internal Medicine, 144*(2), 73–81.

Mirsattari, S. M., Johnston, J. B., McKenna, R., Del Bigio, M. R., Orr, P., Ross, R. T., et al. (2001). Aboriginals with multiple sclerosis: HLA types and predominance of neuromyelitis optica. *Neurology, 56*(3), 317–323.

Mouradian, M. S., Hussain, M. S., Lari, H., Salam, A., Senthilselvan, A., Dean, N., et al. (2005). The impact of a stroke prevention clinic in diagnosing modifiable risk factors for stroke. *Canadian Journal of Neurological Sciences, 32*(4), 496–500.

Multiple Sclerosis Society of Canada. (n.d.). *Frequently asked questions.* Retrieved May 27, 2008, from www.mssociety.ca/en/information/faq.htm

Noseworthy, J. H., Lucchinetti, C., Rodrigues, M., & Weinshenker, B. G. (2000). Multiple sclerosis. *New England Journal of Medicine, 343*(13), 938–952.

Parkinson Society of Canada. (2008). *Parkinson's awareness month.* Retrieved May 27, 2008, from http//www.parkinson.ca/en/home.htm

Pickett, G. E., Campos-Benitez, M., Keller, J. L., & Duggal, N. (2006). Epidemiology of traumatic spinal cord injury in Canada. *Spine, 31*(7), 799–805.

Qureshi, A. I., Suri, M. F., Guterman, L. R., & Hopkins, L. N. (2001). Ineffective secondary prevention in survivors of cardiovascular events in the US population: Report from the Third National Health and Nutrition Examination Survey. *Archives of Internal Medicine, 161*(13), 1621–1628.

Qureshi, A. I., Suri, M. F., Kirmani, J.F., Divani, A. A., & Mohammad, Y. (2005). Is prehypertension a risk factor for cardiovascular disease? *Stroke, 36*(9), 1859–1863.

Ridker, P. M., Cook, N. R., Lee, I. M., Gordon, D., Gaziano, J. M., Manson, J. E., et al. (2005). A randomized trial of low-dose aspirin in the primary prevention of cardiovascular disease in women. *New England Journal of Medicine, 352*(13), 1293–1304.

Schaefer, E. J., Bongard, V., Beiser, A. S., Lamon-Fava, S., Robins, S. J., Au, R., et al. (2006). Plasma phosphatidylcholine docosahexaenoic acid content and risk of dementia and Alzheimer's Disease: The Framingham Heart Study. *Archives of Neurology, 63*(11), 1545–1550.

Seshadri, S., Beiser, A., Kelly-Hayes, M., Kase, C. S., Au, R., Kannel, W. B., et al. (2006). The lifetime risk of stroke: Estimates from the Framingham Study. *Stroke, 37*(2), 345–350.

Spencer, C. (2005). *Alcohol and seniors.* Retrieved March 24, 2009, from www.agingincanada.ca/Seniors%20Alcohol/lg3ciii.htm

Statistics Canada. (2008). *Leading causes of deaths.* Retrieved March 24, 2009 from http://www.statcan.gc.ca/daily-quotidien/081204/dq081204c-eng.htm

Stewart, T. C., Girotti, M. J., Nikore, V., & Williamson, J. (2003). Effect of airbag deployment on head injuries in severe passenger motor vehicle crashes in Ontario, Canada. *Journal of Trauma: Injury Infection & Critical Care, 54*(2), 266–272.

Van Gelder, B. M., Tijhuis, M., Kalmijn, S., & Kromhout, D. (2007). Fish consumption, n-3 fatty acids, and subsequent 5-y cognitive decline in elderly men: The Zutphen Elderly Study. *American Journal of Clinical Nutrition, 85*(4), 1142–1147.

Van Neste-Kenny, J. (2003). Finding meaning after a head injury: The experience of clients' mothers and wives during the early phase of recovery. Unpublished doctoral dissertation, McGill University, Montreal, Canada. *CINAHL AN*: 2005090257.

Wieman, T. J. (2005). Principles of management: The diabetic foot. *American Journal of Surgery, 190*(2), 295–299.

BIBLIOGRAPHY

Willer, C. J., Dyment, D. A., Sadovnick, A. D., Rothwell, P. M., Murray, T. J., & Ebers, G. C. (2005). Canadian Collaborative Study Group. Timing of birth and risk of multiple sclerosis: Population based study. *British Medical Journal, 330*(7483), 120.

Willis, S. L., Tennstedt, S. L., Marsiske, M., Ball, K., Elias, J., Koepke, K. M., et al. (2006). Long-term effects of cognitive training on everyday functional outcomes in older adults. *Journal of the American Medical Association, 296*(23), 2805–2814.

Young, T. K., & Hachinski, V. (2003). The population approach to stroke prevention: A Canadian perspective. *Clinical & Investigative Medicine–Medecine Clinique et Experimentale, 26*(2), 78–86.

ADDITIONAL REFERENCES

Albers, G. W., Caplan, L. R., Easton, J. D., et al. (2002). Transient ischemic attack–Proposal for a new definition. *New England Journal of Medicine, 347*(21), 1713–1716.

Campbell, W. W., DeJong, R. N., & Haerer, A. F. (2005). *DeJong's the neurologic examination* (6th ed.). Philadelphia: Lippincott Williams & Wilkins.

Collins, R., Armitage, J., Parish, S., et al. (2004). Effects of cholesterol-lowering with simvastatin on stroke and other major vascular events in 20,536 people with cerebrovascular disease or other high-risk conditions. *Lancet, 363*(9411), 757–767.

Corvol, J. C., Bouzamondo, A., Sirol, M., et al. (2003). Differential effects of lipid lowering therapies on stroke prevention: A meta-analysis of randomized trails. *Archives of Internal Medicine, 163*(9411), 669–676.

Gilden, D. H. (2004). Bell's palsy. *New England Journal of Medicine, 351*(13), 1323–1331.

Gilman, S., Manter, J. T., Gatz, A. J., et al. (2003). *Manter and Gatz's essentials of clinical neuroanatomy and neurophysiology* (10th ed.). Philadelphia: F. A. Davis.

Goldstein, L. B., & Simel, D. L. (2005). Is this client having a stroke? *Journal of the American Medical Association, 293*(19), 2391–2402.

Griggs, R. C., & Joynt, R. J. (Eds.). (2003). *Baker and Joynt's clinical neurology on CD-ROM.* Philadelphia: Lippincott Williams & Wilkins.

Kaniecki, R. (2003). Headache assessment and management. *Journal of the American Medical Association, 289*(11), 1430–1433.

Katz, J. N., & Simmon, B. P. (2002). Carpal tunnel syndrome. *New England Journal of Medicine, 346*(23), 1807–1812.

Lavan, Z. P. (2005). Stroke prevention through community action. *Journal of Community Nursing, 19*(3), 4, 6, 8–10.

Louis, E. D. (2001). Essential tremor. *New England Journal of Medicine, 345*(12), 887–891.

McCance, K. L., & Huether, S. E. (2006). *Pathophysiology: The biologic basis for disease in adults and children* (5th ed.). Toronto, ON: Mosby.

Mendell, J. R., & Sahenk, Z. (2003). Painful sensory neuropathy. *New England Journal of Medicine, 348*(13), 1243–1294.

Merritt, H. H., & Rowland, L. P. (2005). *Merritt's neurology* (11th ed.). Philadelphia: Lippincott Williams & Wilkins.

Plum, F., & Posner, J. B. (1980). *Diagnosis of stupor and coma* (3rd ed.). Philadelphia: F. A. Davis.

Ropper, A. H., & Adams, R. D. (Eds.). (2005). *Adams and Victor's principles of neurology* (8th ed.). New York: McGraw-Hill.

Sherwood, L. (2007). *Human physiology: From cells to systems* (6th ed.). Belmont, CA: Thomson/Brooks/Cole.

Siderowf, A., & Stern, M. (2003). Update on Parkinson disease. *Annals of Internal Medicine, 138*(8), 651–658.

Soteriades, E. S., Evans, J. C., Larson, M. G., et al. (2002). Incidence and prognosis of syncope. *New England Journal of Medicine, 347*(12), 878–885.

Van de Beek, D., de Gans, J., Spanjaard, L., et al. (2004). Clinical features and prognostic factors in adults with bacterial meningitis. *New England Journal of Medicine, 351*(18), 1849–1859.

CANADIAN ASSOCIATIONS AND WEB SITES

Alcohol and Seniors: http://www.agingincanada.ca

BC Health Guide: http://www.bchealthguide.org

Brain Injury Association of Canada: http://www.biac-aclc.ca

Canadian Association of Neuroscience Nurses: http://www.cann.ca

Canadian Diabetic Association: http://www.diabetes.ca

Canadian Health Network: http://www.canadian-health-network.ca

Canadian Institute of Health Information: http://secure.cihi.ca/cihiweb/splash.html

Canadian Paraplegic Association: http://canparaplegic.org

Canadian Stroke Network: http://www.canadianstrokenetwork.ca

Epilepsy Canada: http://epilepsy.ca

Health Canada: http://www.hc-sc.gc.ca

Heart and Stroke Foundation of Canada: http://www.heartandstroke.ca

International Collaborators on Repair Discoveries (ICORD): http://www.icord.org

Multiple Sclerosis Society of Canada: http://mssociety.ca/en/information

Parkinson Society of Canada: http://www.parkinson.ca/

Public Health Agency of Canada: http://www.phac-aspc.gc.ca

Statistics Canada: http://www.statcan.ca

Spinal Cord Injury Rehabilitation Evidence (SCIRE): http://www.canparaplegic.org/en/Research_32/items/20.html

Think First Foundation: http://www.thinkfirst.ca

| TABLE 20-1 | Syncope and Similar Disorders |

Syncope

Syncope is defined as a brief loss of consciousness due to a sudden decrease in cerebral blood flow. Consciousness usually returns promptly but pallor, weakness, nausea, and/or slight confusion may persist for some time, dependent upon the underlying cause

Problem	Mechanism	Precipitating Factors
Vasodepressor or Vasovagal Syncope (*the common faint*)	Sudden peripheral vasodilatation, especially in the skeletal muscles, without a compensatory rise in cardiac output. Blood pressure falls. Often slow onset, slow offset. Associated with weakness, pallor, nausea, salivation, sweating, yawning.	A strong emotion such as fear or pain Fatigue, hunger, hot humid environment
Postural (*orthostatic*) **Hypotension**	■ *Inadequate vasoconstrictor reflexes* in both arterioles and veins, with resultant venous pooling, decreased cardiac output, and low blood pressure ■ *Hypovolemia,* a diminished blood volume insufficient to maintain cardiac output and blood pressure, especially in the upright position	■ Standing up usually from the supine position ■ Standing up after hemorrhage or dehydration
Micturition Syncope	Unclear	Emptying the bladder after getting out of bed to void
Cardiovascular Disorders		
Arrhythmias	Decreased cardiac output secondary to rhythms that are too fast (usually more than 180) or too slow (less than 35–40). Often sudden onset; sudden offset.	A sudden change in rhythm
Myocardial Infarction	Sudden arrhythmia or decreased cardiac output	Variable
Disorders Resembling Syncope		
Hypocapnia (decreased carbon dioxide) Due to Hyperventilation	Constriction of cerebral blood vessels secondary to hypocapnia that is induced by hyperventilation with the associated symptoms of dyspnea, palpitations, chest discomfort, numbness and tingling of the hands and around the mouth lasting for several minutes. Consciousness is often maintained.	Possibly a stressful situation Anxiety
Hypoglycemia	Insufficient glucose to maintain cerebral metabolism; secretion of epinephrine contributes to symptoms of sweating, tremor, palpitations, hunger, headache, confusion, abnormal behaviour, coma. True syncope is uncommon. Variable	Variable, including fasting insulin therapy and a variety of metabolic disorders.

TABLE 20-2 **Seizure Disorders**

Partial Seizures

Partial seizures start with focal manifestations. They are further divided into *simple partial seizures*, which do not impair consciousness, and *complex partial seizures*, which do. *Partial seizures may become generalized.* Partial seizures of all kinds usually indicate a structural lesion in the cerebral cortex, such as a scar, tumour, or infarction. The quality of such seizures helps the clinician to localize the causative lesion in the brain.

Problem	Clinical Manifestations	Postictal *(postseizure)* State
Partial Seizures		
Simple Partial Seizures		
■ With motor symptoms, Jacksonian	Tonic and then clonic movements that start unilaterally in the hand, foot, or face and spread to other body parts on the same side	Return to usual state of consciousness
Other motor	Turning of the head and eyes to one side, or tonic and clonic movements of an arm or leg without the Jacksonian spread	Return to usual state of consciousness
■ With sensory symptoms	Numbness, tingling; simple visual, auditory, or olfactory hallucinations such as flashing lights, buzzing, or odours	Return to usual state of consciousness
■ With autonomic symptoms	A "funny feeling" in the epigastrium, nausea, pallor, flushing, lightheadedness	Return to usual state of consciousness
■ With psychiatric symptoms	Anxiety or fear, feelings of familiarity (déjà vu) or unreality, dreamy states, fear or rage, flashback experiences, more complex hallucinations	Return to usual state of consciousness
Complex Partial Seizures	The seizure may or may not start with the autonomic or psychic symptoms outlined above. Consciousness is impaired, and the person appears confused. Automatisms include automatic motor behaviours such as chewing, smacking the lips, walking about, and unbuttoning clothes; also more complicated and skilled behaviours such as driving a car.	The client may remember initial autonomic or psychic symptoms (which are then termed an *aura*), but is amnesic for the rest of the seizure. Temporary confusion and headache may occur.
Partial Seizures That Become Generalized	Partial seizures that become generalized resemble tonic–clonic seizures (see next page). Unfortunately, the client may not recall the focal onset, and observers may overlook it.	As in a tonic–clonic seizure, described on the next page. Two attributes indicate a partial seizure that has become generalized: (1) the recollection of an *aura*, and (2) a *unilateral* neurologic deficit during the postictal period.

Source: Commission on Classification and Terminology of the International League Against Epilepsy. Proposal for revised classification of epilepsies and epileptic syndromes. Epilepsia 30:389–399, 1989. *See also* International League Against Epilepsy. A proposed diagnostic scheme for people with epileptic seizures and with epilepsy: report of the ILAE Task Force on Classification and Terminology. Available at: http://www.ilae-epilepsy.org/Visitors/Centre/ctf/index.cfm. Accessed October 4, 2007.

(table continues on next page)

TABLE 20-2   **Seizure Disorders** (*Continued*)

Generalized Seizures and Pseudoseizures

Generalized seizures begin with bilateral body movements, impairment of consciousness, or both. They suggest a widespread, bilateral cortical disturbance that may be either hereditary or acquired. When generalized seizures of the tonic–clonic (grand mal) variety start in childhood or young adulthood, they are often hereditary. When tonic–clonic seizures begin after the age of 30, suspect either a partial seizure that has become generalized or a general seizure caused by a toxic or metabolic disorder. Toxic and metabolic causes include withdrawal from alcohol or other sedative drugs, uremia, hypoglycemia, hyperglycemia, hyponatremia, and bacterial meningitis.

Problem	Clinical Manifestations	Postictal (*postseizure*) State
Generalized Seizures		
Tonic–Clonic Convulsion (grand mal)*	The person loses consciousness suddenly, sometimes with a cry, and the body stiffens into tonic extensor rigidity. Breathing stops, and the person becomes cyanotic. A clonic phase of rhythmic muscular contraction follows. Breathing resumes and is often noisy, with excessive salivation. Injury, tongue biting, and urinary incontinence may occur.	Confusion, drowsiness, fatigue, headache, muscular aching, and sometimes the temporary persistence of bilateral neurologic deficits such as hyperactive reflexes and Babinski responses. The person has amnesia for the seizure and recalls no aura.
Absence	A sudden brief lapse of consciousness, with momentary blinking, staring, or movements of the lips and hands but no falling. Two subtypes are recognized. *Petit mal absences* last less than 10 sec and stop abruptly. *Atypical absences* may last more than 10 sec.	No aura recalled. In petit mal absences, a prompt return to usual state; in atypical absences, some postictal confusion.
Atonic Seizure, or Drop Attack	Sudden loss of consciousness with falling but no movements. Injury may occur.	Either a prompt return to usual state or a brief period of confusion
Myoclonus	Sudden, brief, rapid jerks, involving the trunk or limbs. Associated with a variety of disorders	Variable
Pseudoseizures		
May mimic seizures, but are due to a conversion reaction (a psychological disorder)	The movements may have personally symbolic significance and often do not follow a neuroanatomic pattern. Injury is uncommon.	Variable

**Febrile convulsions* that resemble brief tonic–clonic seizures may occur in infants and young children. They are usually benign, but occasionally may be the first manifestation of a seizure disorder.

TABLE 20-3   Tremors and Involuntary Movements

Tremors

Tremors are relatively rhythmic oscillatory movements, which may be roughly subdivided into three groups: resting (or static) tremors, postural tremors, and intention tremors.

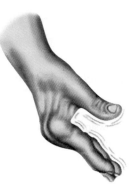

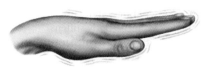

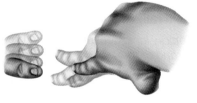

Resting (Static) Tremors

These tremors are most prominent at rest, and may decrease or disappear with voluntary movement. Illustrated is the common, relatively slow, fine, pill-rolling tremor of parkinsonism, about 5 per second.

Postural (Action) Tremors

These tremors appear when the affected part is actively maintaining a posture. Examples include the fine rapid tremor of hyperthyroidism, the tremors of anxiety and fatigue, and benign essential (and sometimes familial) tremor. Tremor may worsen somewhat with intention.

Intention Tremors

Intention tremors, absent at rest, appear with activity and often get worse as the target is neared. Causes include disorders of cerebellar pathways, as in multiple sclerosis.

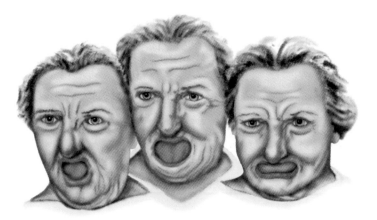

Oral–Facial Dyskinesias

Oral–facial dyskinesias are rhythmic, repetitive, bizarre movements that chiefly involve the face, mouth, jaw, and tongue: grimacing, pursing of the lips, protrusions of the tongue, opening and closing of the mouth, and deviations of the jaw. The limbs and trunk are involved less often. These movements may be a late complication of psychotropic drugs such as phenothiazines, termed *tardive* (late) dyskinesias. They also occur in long-standing psychoses, in some elderly individuals, and in some edentulous persons.

(table continues on next page)

TABLE 20-3   **Tremors and Involuntary Movements** (*Continued*)

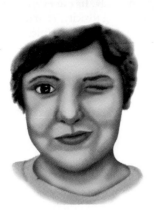

Tics

Tics are brief, repetitive, stereotyped, coordinated movements occurring at irregular intervals. Examples include repetitive winking, grimacing, and shoulder shrugging. Causes include Tourette's syndrome and drugs such as phenothiazines and amphetamines.

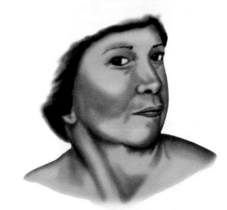

Dystonia

Dystonic movements are somewhat similar to athetoid movements, but often involve larger portions of the body, including the trunk. Grotesque, twisted postures may result. Causes include drugs such as phenothiazines, primary torsion dystonia, and as illustrated, spasmodic torticollis.

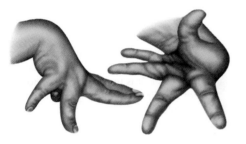

Athetosis

Athetoid movements are slower and more twisting and writhing than choreiform movements, and have a larger amplitude. They most commonly involve the face and the distal extremities. Athetosis is often associated with spasticity. Causes include cerebral palsy.

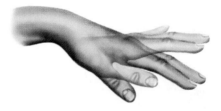

Chorea

Choreiform movements are brief, rapid, jerky, irregular, and unpredictable. They occur at rest or interrupt coordinated movements. Unlike tics, they seldom repeat themselves. The face, head, lower arms, and hands are often involved. Causes include Sydenham's chorea (with rheumatic fever) and Huntington's disease.

TABLE 20-4   **Nystagmus**

Nystagmus is a rhythmic oscillation of the eyes, analogous to a tremor in other parts of the body. Its causes are multiple, including impairment of vision in early life, disorders of the labyrinth and the cerebellar system, and drug toxicity. Nystagmus can occur when a healthy person watches a rapidly moving object (e.g., a passing train). Observe the three characteristics of nystagmus listed below and on the following page. Then refer to textbooks of neurology for differential diagnosis.

Direction of the Quick and Slow Components

Example: Left-Beating Nystagmus—A Quick Jerk to the Left in Each Eye, Then a Slow Drift to the Right

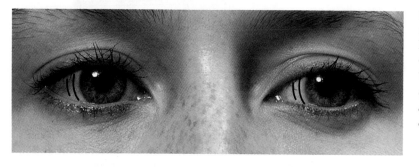

Nystagmus usually has both slow and fast movements, but is defined by its fast phase. For example, if the eyes jerk quickly to the client's left and drift back slowly to the right, the client is said to have nystagmus to the left.

Occasionally, nystagmus consists only of coarse oscillations without quick and slow components. It is then said to be *pendular*.

Plane of the Movements

Horizontal Nystagmus

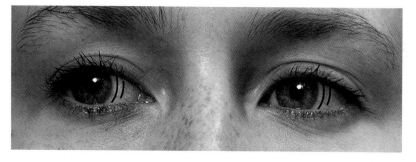

The movements of nystagmus may occur in one or more planes (i.e., horizontal, vertical, or rotary). It is the plane of the movements, not the direction of the gaze, that defines this variable.

Vertical Nystagmus

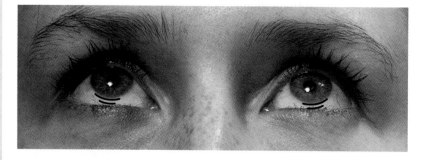

(table continues on next page)

TABLE 20-4   **Nystagmus** *(Continued)*

Rotary Nystagmus

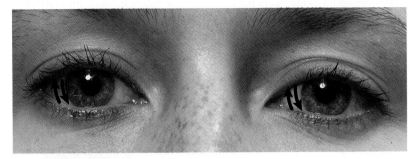

Direction of Gaze in Which Nystagmus Appears

Example: Nystagmus on Right Lateral Gaze

Nystagmus Present (Right Lateral Gaze)

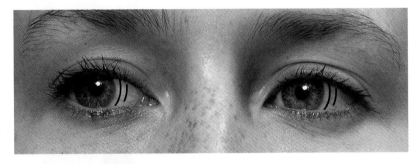

Although nystagmus may be present in all six directions of gaze, it may appear or become accentuated only on deviation of the eyes (e.g., to the side or upward). On extreme lateral gaze, the healthy person may show a few beats resembling nystagmus. Avoid making assessments in such extreme positions, and *observe for nystagmus only within the field of full binocular vision.*

Nystagmus not Present (Left Lateral Gaze)

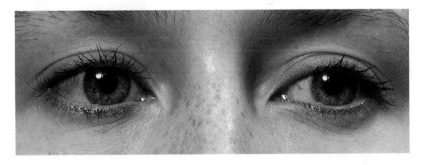

TABLE 20-5	Types of Facial Paralysis

Facial weakness or paralysis may result either (1) from a peripheral lesion of CN VII, the facial nerve, anywhere from its origin in the pons to its periphery in the face, or (2) from a central lesion involving the upper motor neuron system between the cortex and the pons. A peripheral lesion of CN VII, exemplified here by a Bell's palsy, is compared with a central lesion, exemplified by a left hemispheric cerebrovascular accident. These can be distinguished by their different effects on the upper part of the face.

CN VII—Peripheral Lesion

Peripheral nerve damage to CN VII paralyzes the entire right side of the face, including the forehead.

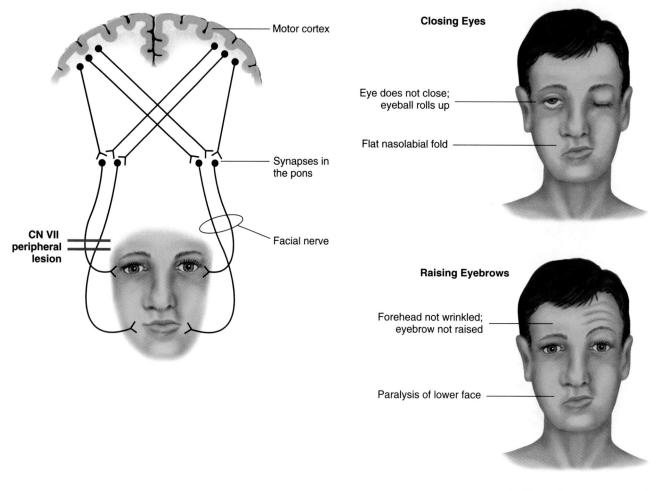

Motor cortex

Synapses in the pons

Facial nerve

CN VII peripheral lesion

Closing Eyes

Eye does not close; eyeball rolls up

Flat nasolabial fold

Raising Eyebrows

Forehead not wrinkled; eyebrow not raised

Paralysis of lower face

(table continues on next page)

TABLE 20-5   Types of Facial Paralysis (Continued)

CN VII—Central Lesion

The lower part of the face is controlled by upper motor neurons located on only one side of the cortex—the opposite side. *Left-sided damage to these pathways, as in a stroke, paralyzes the right lower face.* The upper face, however, is controlled by pathways from both sides of the cortex. Even though the upper motor neurons on the left are destroyed, others on the right remain, and the right upper face continues to function fairly well.

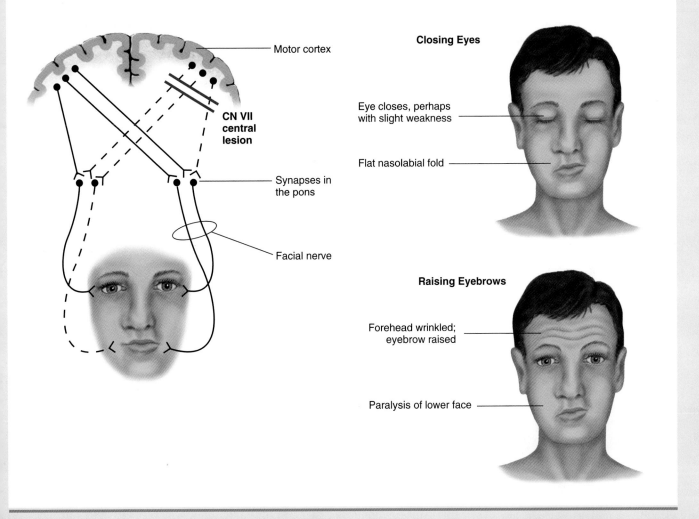

Motor cortex

CN VII central lesion

Synapses in the pons

Facial nerve

Closing Eyes

Eye closes, perhaps with slight weakness

Flat nasolabial fold

Raising Eyebrows

Forehead wrinkled; eyebrow raised

Paralysis of lower face

TABLE 20-6 Disorders of Muscle Tone

	Spasticity	Rigidity	Flaccidity
Location of Lesion	Upper motor neuron of the corticospinal tract at any point from the cortex to the spinal cord	Basal ganglia system	Lower motor neuron at any point from the anterior horn cell to the peripheral nerves
Description	Increased muscle tone (*hypertonia*) that is rate dependent. Tone is greater when passive movement is rapid, and less when passive movement is slow. Tone is also greater at the extremes of the movement arc. During rapid passive movement, initial hypertonia may give way suddenly as the limb relaxes. This spastic "catch" and relaxation is known as "clasp-knife" resistance.	Increased resistance that persists throughout the movement arc, independent of rate of movement, is called *lead-pipe rigidity*. With flexion and extension of the wrist or forearm, a superimposed rachetlike jerkiness is called *cogwheel rigidity*.	Loss of muscle tone (*hypotonia*), causing the limb to be loose or floppy. The affected limbs may be hyperextensible or even flail-like.
Common Cause	Stroke, especially late or chronic stage	Parkinsonism	Guillain-Barré syndrome; also initial phase of spinal cord injury (spinal shock) or stroke

TABLE 20-7   **Disorders of the Central and Peripheral Nervous Systems**

Central Nervous System Disorders

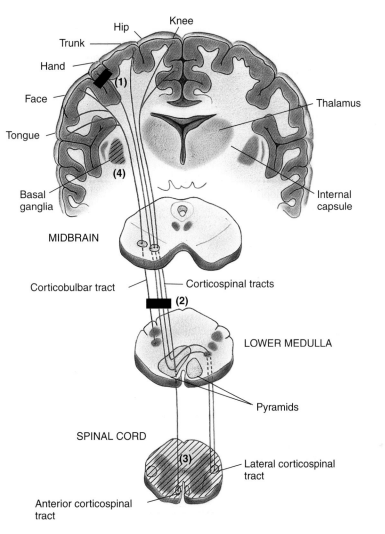

(table continues on next page)

Central Nervous System Disorders

	Typical Findings			
Location of Lesion	*Motor*	*Sensory*	*Deep Tendon Reflexes*	**Examples of Cause**
Cerebral Cortex (1)	Chronic contralateral upper motor neuron weakness and spasticity. Flexion is stronger than extension in the arm, plantar flexion is stronger than dorsiflexion in the foot, and the leg is externally rotated at the hip.	Contralateral sensory loss on the limbs and trunk on the same side as the motor deficits	↑	Cortical stroke
Brainstem (2)	Weakness and spasticity as above, plus cranial nerve deficits such as diplopia (from weakness of the extraocular muscles) and dysarthria	Variable. No typical sensory findings.	↑	Brainstem stroke, acoustic neuroma
Spinal Cord (3)	Weakness and spasticity as above, but often affecting both sides (when cord damage is bilateral), causing paraplegia or quadriplegia depending on the level of injury	Dermatomal sensory deficit on the trunk bilaterally at the level of the lesion, and sensory loss from tract damage below the level of the lesion	↑	Trauma, causing cord compression
Subcortical Grey Matter: Basal Ganglia (4)	Slowness of movement (bradykinesia), rigidity, and tremor	Sensation not affected	Average or ↓	Parkinsonism
Cerebellar (not illustrated)	Hypotonia, ataxia, and other abnormal movements, including nystagmus, dysdiadochokinesis, and dysmetria	Sensation not affected	Average or ↓	Cerebellar stroke, brain tumour

(table continues on next page)

Peripheral Nervous System Disorders

Posterior horn · Posterior root · Posterior root ganglion · Afferent sensory fibre · (1) · (2) · (3) · (4) · (5) · (6) · Efferent motor fiber · Anterior horn · Anterior horn cell · Anterior root · (1) · Muscle

Typical Findings

Location of Lesion	*Motor*	*Sensory*	*Deep Tendon Reflexes*	Examples of Cause
Anterior Horn Cell (1)	Weakness and atrophy in a segmental or focal pattern; fasciculations	Sensation intact	↓	Polio, amyotrophic lateral sclerosis
Spinal Roots and Nerves (2)	Weakness and atrophy in a root-innervated pattern; sometimes with fasciculations	Corresponding dermatomal sensory deficits	↓	Herniated cervical or lumbar disc
Peripheral Nerve— Mononeuropathy (3)	Weakness and atrophy in a peripheral nerve distribution; sometimes with fasciculations	Sensory loss in the pattern of that nerve	↓	Trauma
Peripheral Nerve— Polyneuropathy (4)	Weakness and atrophy more distal than proximal; sometimes with fasciculations	Sensory deficits, commonly in stocking-glove distribution	↓	Peripheral polyneuropathy of alcoholism, diabetes
Neuromuscular Junction (5)	Fatigability more than weakness	Sensation intact	Average	Myasthenia gravis
Muscle (6)	Weakness usually more proximal than distal; fasciculations rare	Sensation intact	Average or ↓	Muscular dystrophy

TABLE 20-8   Deviations in Gait and Posture

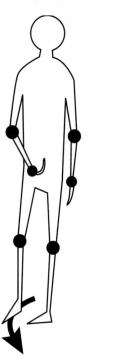

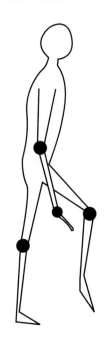

Underlying Defect	*Spastic Hemiparesis*	*Cerebellar Ataxia*	*Steppage Gait*
Description	Associated with lesion in corticospinal tract, as with stroke	Associated with bilateral spastic paresis of the legs	Associated with foot drop, usually secondary to lower motor neuron disease
	One arm is held immobile and close to the side, with elbow, wrist, and interphalangeal joints flexed. The leg is extended, with plantar flexion of the foot. On walking, the client either drags the foot, often scraping the toe, or circles it stiffly outward and forward (*circumduction*).	The gait is stiff. Each leg is advanced slowly, and the thighs tend to cross forward on each other at each step. The steps are short. The client appears to be walking through water.	These clients either drag their feet or lift them high, with knees flexed, and bring them down with a slap onto the floor, thus appearing to be walking up stairs. They are unable to walk on their heels. The steppage gait may involve one or both sides.

(table continues on next page)

TABLE 20-8 Deviations in Gait and Posture *(Continued)*

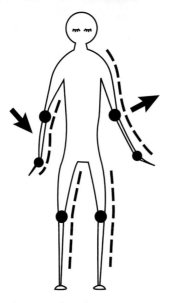
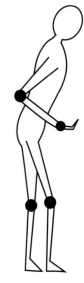

Underlying Defect	*Sensory Ataxia*	*Scissors Gait*	*Parkinsonian Gait*
	Associated with loss of position sense in the legs, as from polyneuropathy or posterior column damage	Associated with disease of the cerebellum or associated tracts	Associated with the basal ganglia defects of Parkinson's disease
Description	The gait is unsteady and wide-based (with feet wide apart). These clients throw their feet forward and outward and bring them down, first on the heels and then on the toes, with a double tapping sound. They watch the ground for guidance while walking. With eyes closed, they cannot stand steadily with feet together (a positive Romberg sign), and the staggering gait worsens.	The gait is staggering, unsteady, and wide-based, with exaggerated difficulty on the turns. These clients cannot stand steadily with feet together, whether their eyes are open or closed.	The posture is stooped, with head and neck forward and hips and knees slightly flexed. Arms are flexed at elbows and wrists. The client is slow in getting started. Steps are short and often shuffling. Arm swings are decreased, and the client turns around stiffly—"all in one piece."

TABLE 20-9   **Metabolic and Structural Coma**

Although there are many causes of coma, most can be classified as either structural or metabolic. Findings vary widely in individual clients; the features listed are general guidelines rather than strict diagnostic criteria. Remember that psychiatric disorders may mimic coma.

	Toxic–Metabolic	Structural
Pathophysiology	Arousal centres poisoned or critical substrates depleted	Lesion destroys or compresses brainstem arousal areas, either directly or secondary to more distant expanding mass lesions.
Clinical Features		
■ Respiratory pattern	If regular, may be regular in depth value rhythm or hyperventilation. If irregular, usually Cheyne-Stokes.	Irregular, especially Cheyne-Stokes or ataxic breathing
■ Pupillary size and reaction	Equal, reactive to light. If *pinpoint* from opiates or cholinergics, you may need a magnifying glass to see the reaction.	Unequal or unreactive to light (fixed) *Midposition, fixed*—suggests midbrain compression
	May be unreactive if *fixed and dilated* from anticholinergics or hypothermia	*Dilated, fixed*—suggests compression of CN III from herniation
■ Level of consciousness	Changes *after* pupils change	Changes *before* pupils change
Examples of Cause	Uremia, hyperglycemia	Epidural, subdural, or intracerebral hemorrhage
	Alcohol, drugs, liver failure	Cerebral infarct or embolus
	Hypothyroidism, hypoglycemia	Tumour, abscess
	Anoxia, ischemia	Brainstem infarct, tumour, or hemorrhage
	Meningitis, encephalitis	Cerebellar infarct, hemorrhage, tumour, or abscess
	Hyperthermia, hypothermia	

TABLE 20-10 | Pupils in Comatose Clients

Pupillary size, equality, and light reactions help in assessing the cause of coma and in determining the region of the brain that is impaired. Remember that unrelated pupillary abnormalities, including miotic drops for glaucoma or mydriatic drops for a better view of the ocular fundi, may have preceded the coma.

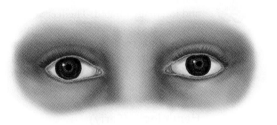

Small or Pinpoint Pupils

Bilaterally small pupils (1–2.5 mm) suggest (1) damage to the sympathetic pathways in the hypothalamus, or (2) metabolic encephalopathy (a diffuse failure of cerebral function that has many causes, including drugs). Light reactions are as expected usually.

Pinpoint pupils (<1 mm) suggest (1) a hemorrhage in the pons, or (2) the effects of morphine, heroin, or other narcotics. The light reactions may be seen with a magnifying glass.

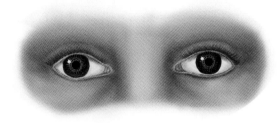

Midposition Fixed Pupils

Pupils that are in the *midposition or slightly dilated* (4–6 mm) and are *fixed to light* suggest structural damage in the midbrain.

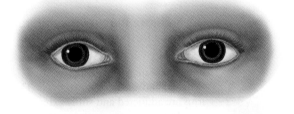

Large Pupils

Bilaterally fixed and dilated pupils may be due to severe anoxia and its sympathomimetic effects, as seen after cardiac arrest. They may also result from atropine-like agents, phenothiazines, or tricyclic antidepressants.

Bilaterally large reactive pupils may be due to cocaine, amphetamine, LSD, or other sympathetic nervous system agonists.

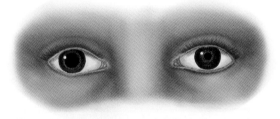

One Large Pupil

A pupil that is *fixed and dilated* warns of herniation of the temporal lobe, causing compression of the oculomotor nerve and midbrain.

TABLE 20-11	Irregular Postures in the Comatose Client

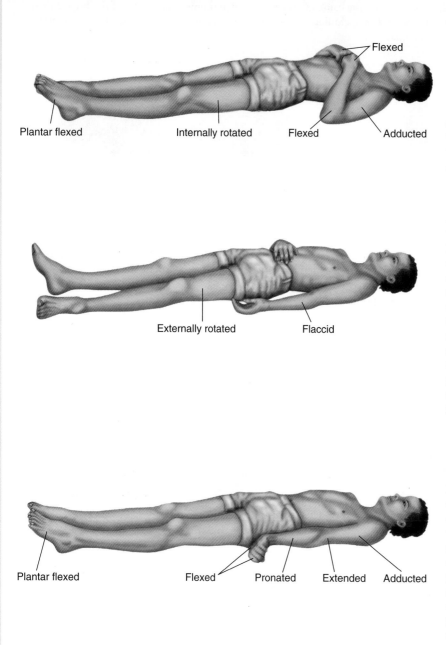

Decorticate Rigidity (Exaggerated Flexor Response)

In decorticate rigidity, the upper arms are held tight to the sides with elbows, wrists, and fingers flexed. The legs are extended and internally rotated. The feet are plantar flexed. This posture implies a destructive lesion of the corticospinal tracts within or very near the cerebral hemispheres. When unilateral, this is the posture of chronic spastic hemiplegia.

Hemiplegia (Early)

Sudden unilateral brain damage involving the corticospinal tract may produce a hemiplegia (one-sided paralysis), which early in its course is flaccid. Spasticity will develop later. The paralyzed arm and leg are slack. They fall loosely and without tone when raised and dropped to the bed. Spontaneous movements or responses to noxious stimuli are limited to the opposite side. The leg may lie externally rotated. One side of the lower face may be paralyzed, and that cheek puffs out on expiration. Both eyes may be turned away from the paralyzed side.

Decerebrate Rigidity (Exaggerated Extensor Response With Distal Flexion)

In decerebrate rigidity, the jaws are clenched and the neck is extended. The arms are adducted and stiffly extended at the elbows, with forearms pronated, wrists and fingers flexed. The legs are stiffly extended at the knees, with the feet plantar flexed. This posture may occur spontaneously or only in response to external stimuli such as light, noise, or pain. It is caused by a lesion in the diencephalon, midbrain, or pons, although severe metabolic disorders such as hypoxia or hypoglycemia may also produce it.

Male Genitalia and Hernias

William L. Diehl-Jones and Lynn S. Bickley

The male genitalia represent masculinity, sexuality, procreation, and elimination. When faced with disease of the genitalia, men may fear loss of sexual attractiveness and function, loss of reproductive function, or even loss of a significant other. Nurses have many opportunities to discuss with clients reproductive health, testicular self-examination, and risk factors for sexually transmitted infections (STIs) and cancer. In settings where male clients may be unable to practise self-hygiene or self-examination (e.g., continuing care), nurses ensure that care includes these.

The functional significance of the male genital system is twofold: It is an excretory organ for urine and the means of producing and delivering ejaculate (sperm and secretions). External structures include the penis and scrotum. The internal, palpable structures of the scrotal sac include the testes, epididymis, and spermatic cord. Accessory structures of the male genitalia include the paired seminal vesicles, Cowper's gland, and prostate gland. These accessory organs are involved in the production of seminal fluids; their assessment is not part of the physical examination, although a change in or lack of seminal secretions may indicate dysfunction in one or more of the glands. The prostate gland is associated with the male genitourinary system, and its structure and assessment are discussed in Chapter 23.

ANATOMY AND PHYSIOLOGY

Review the anatomy of the male genitalia.

The *shaft of the penis* is formed by three columns of vascular erectile tissue: the *corpus spongiosum,* containing the urethra, and two *corpora cavernosa.* The corpus spongiosum forms the bulb of the penis, ending in the cone-shaped *glans* with its expanded base, or *corona.* In uncircumcised men, the glans is covered by a loose, hoodlike fold of skin called the *prepuce* or *foreskin* where *smegma,* or secretions of the glans, may collect. The urethra is located ventrally in the shaft of the penis; urethral abnormalities may sometimes be felt there. The urethra opens into the vertical, slitlike *urethral meatus,* located somewhat ventrally at the tip of the glans.

The testes serve two primary functions: spermatogenesis, or sperm formation, and production of the steroid hormone *testosterone.* The testes are located in the scrotal sac, which is a loose, wrinkled pouch covered by thin, pigmented skin. Beginning at puberty, the scrotal skin usually has sparsely distributed hair follicles. A septum in the scrotum divides the testicles into right and left compartments. Both testicles are positioned external to the body cavity to help promote spermatogenesis, which can occur only if the testes remain approximately 3°C lower than core body temperature. The dartos and cremaster smooth muscles can reflexively change the surface area of the scrotal sac; this property, in turn, helps regulate scrotal temperature. Each testicle is ovoid and somewhat rubbery. Testicle size in adults varies from 3.5 cm to 5.5 cm.

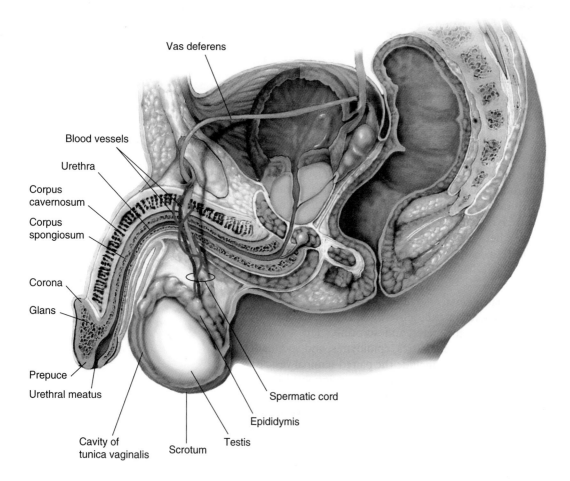

Except for the posterior surface, both testes are surrounded on all sides by a fibrous connective tissue sheath called the *tunica vaginalis*, which reflects posteriorly to form the *tunica albuginea*. This latter sheath of connective tissue further surrounds and divides the testes into separate lobules. Lying within each lobule are the actual sites of sperm formation, the *seminiferous tubules*. These uninterrupted, highly folded ducts are where sperm are continuously produced. Endocrine cells called *interstitial cells of Leydig* are located between loops of the seminiferous tubules. They are the principal site of testosterone production. Testosterone stimulates the development of male secondary sex characteristics, including facial and body hair, musculoskeletal growth, and enlargement of the larynx, which is associated with a low-pitched voice. Testosterone is also responsible for many of the physiological processes underlying sexual arousal.

The seminiferous tubules open into a network of channels called the *rete testis*, which is in turn connected to the epididymis. This firm, easily palpable, coiled, and tubular structure lies behind the testis and is nearly 6 m long when spread out. One of the main functions of the epididymis is fluid absorption; it may also contribute to the formation of seminal fluid. It is embedded in connective tissue, and gives rise to the vas deferens, which is a cordlike structure that begins at the tail of the epididymis, ascends within the scrotal sac, and passes through the external inguinal ring on its way to the abdomen and pelvis. Behind the bladder, it is joined by the duct from the seminal vesicle and enters the urethra within the prostate gland. Sperm thus pass from the testis and the epididymis through the vas deferens into the urethra. Secretions from the vasa deferentia, the seminal vesicles, and the prostate all contribute to the semen. Within the scrotum, each vas is closely associated with blood vessels, nerves, and muscle fibres. These structures make up the *spermatic cord*.

The blood supply to the testes and epididymis is via the *testicular artery,* which is a branch of the abdominal aorta. The testes are drained via the *pampiniform plexus,* a venous network that reduces to a single vein that ascends the inguinal canal.

A *vasectomy* is a procedure that involves tiny incisions through the scrotal sac and connective tissue sheath of the spermatic cord. The vas deferens is isolated from the accompanying artery, nerve, and vein, and is usually ligatured or clipped in two locations, between which the cord is cut. Therefore, vasectomies prevent spermatozoa from travelling up the vas deferens. The absence of sperm in semen makes no appreciable difference to the quality or quantity of semen ejaculated.

Male sexual function depends on expected levels of testosterone, adequate arterial blood flow to the inferior epigastric artery and its cremasteric and pubic branches, and intact neural innervation from α-adrenergic and cholinergic pathways. Erection from venous engorgement of the corpora cavernosa results from two types of stimuli. Visual, auditory, or erotic cues trigger sympathetic outflow from higher brain centres to the T11 through L2 levels of the spinal cord. Tactile stimulation initiates sensory impulses from the genitalia to S_2 to S_4 reflex arcs and parasympathetic pathways through the pudendal nerve. Both sets of stimuli appear to increase levels of nitric oxide and cyclic GMP, resulting in local vasodilation.

Lymphatics (lymph vessels) from the penile and scrotal surfaces ascend the spermatic cord and drain into the superficial inguinal nodes in the groin. The lymph drainage of the testes is into the deep lumbar lymph nodes on either side of the abdominal aorta. This arrangement is a consequence of early testicular development: The testes originate along the posterior abdominal wall and, during development, descend through the abdominal wall, dragging with them the blood and lymph vessels. This generates a natural weak point in the abdominal wall that can become patent when activities such as heavy lifting or straining increase abdominal pressure, resulting in a hernia (see p. 772).

Note that the lymphatics of the testes drain into the abdomen, where enlarged lymph nodes are clinically *undetectable* (see p. 566 for further discussion of the inguinal nodes).

ANATOMY OF THE GROIN

Because hernias are relatively common, it is important to understand the anatomy of the groin. The basic landmarks are the anterior superior iliac spine, the pubic tubercle, and the inguinal ligament that runs between them.

The *inguinal canal,* which lies above and approximately parallel to the inguinal ligament, forms a tunnel for the vas deferens as it passes through the abdominal muscles. The exterior opening of the tunnel—the *external inguinal ring*—is a triangular, slitlike structure palpable just above and lateral to the pubic tubercle. The internal opening of the canal—or *internal inguinal ring*—is approximately 1 cm above the midpoint of the inguinal ligament. Neither canal nor internal ring is palpable through the abdominal wall. When loops of bowel force their way through weak areas of the inguinal canal, they produce *inguinal hernias,* as illustrated on pp. 782–783.

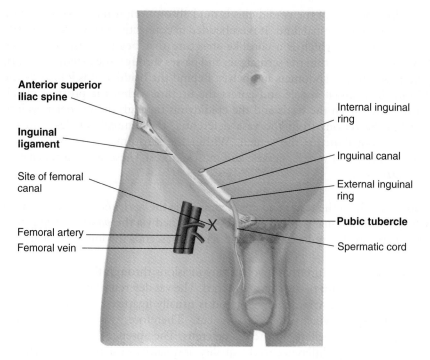

Another potential route for a herniating mass is the *femoral canal.* This lies below the inguinal ligament. Although you cannot see it, you can estimate its location by placing your right index finger, from below, on the right femoral artery. Your middle finger will then overlie the femoral vein and your ring finger will overlie the femoral canal. Femoral hernias protrude here.

THE HEALTH HISTORY: SUBJECTIVE DATA

Key Symptoms and Signs Reported by Client

- Change in sexual function (e.g., erectile dysfunction)
- Change in sexual desire (libido)
- Discharge from the penis
- Skin lesions on the penis or scrotum (e.g., chancroid)
- Scrotal heaviness, aching, or pain
- Scrotal swelling (e.g., varicocele)
- Bulge in the groin (e.g., hernia)

Begin the health history interview with broad opening questions, such as "What can I help you with today?" or "What concerns have you come about today?" Open-ended questions allow clients to express themselves freely. If a client reports a symptom or sign, start by completing a symptom/sign analysis before continuing with the health history that gathers more comprehensive information.

For men, questions about the genitalia follow naturally after those dealing with the urinary system. You will need to review sexual function and screen for symptoms of infection. Begin with general questions such as, "How is sexual function for you?" "Are you satisfied with your sexual life?" "What about your ability to perform sexually?" If the client reports a sexual problem, ask him to tell you about it. Ask whether there has been any change in desire or level of sexual activity recently. What does he think has caused it, what has he tried to do about it, and what are his hopes?

Identify the client's sexual preference as to partners (male, female, or both). Find out whether the client's partner has any concerns.

Direct questions help you to assess each phase of the sexual response. To assess *libido* or desire ask, "Have you maintained interest in sex?" For the *arousal phase* ask, "Can you achieve and maintain an erection?" Explore the timing, severity, setting, and any other factors that may be contributing to problems. Have any changes in his relationships or life circumstances coincided with onset of a problem? Are there circumstances when erection is as expected? On awakening in the early morning or during the night? With partners? With masturbation?

Erectile dysfunction may be from psychogenic causes, especially if early morning erection is preserved; also from decreased testosterone, decreased blood flow in the hypogastric arterial system, or impaired neural innervation.

Other questions relate to the phase of *orgasm* and *ejaculation* of semen. If ejaculation is premature, or early and out of control, ask, "About how long does intercourse last?" "Do you climax too soon?" "Do you feel as if you have any control over climaxing?" "Do you think your partner would like intercourse to last longer?" For reduced or absent ejaculation, "Do you find that you cannot have an orgasm even though you can have an erection?" Try to determine whether the problem involves the pleasurable sensation of orgasm, the ejaculation of seminal fluid, or both. Review the frequency and setting of the problem, medications, surgery, and neurologic symptoms.

Change in Sexual Function.   Assess any *change in sexual function* in a gentle, nonjudgemental manner. Sexual function usually changes during the lifespan, from puberty through older age. A client may feel confused or alarmed about the changes, and the nurse may be able to put these into perspective for him. Some examples include spontaneous erections and nocturnal ejaculation in prepubescent or pubescent males, and diminished erectile function in older clients.

Unexpected changes in sexual function may signal a pathophysiologic process or psychological disorder. For example, an inability to initiate or sustain an erection may be the consequence of psychosocial factors (e.g., stress, depression, confusion over gender identity/sexual orientation) or use of steroids, especially nonprescribed steroids. It may also signal a disorder such as hypertension, multiple sclerosis, Parkinson's disease, atherosclerosis, liver or kidney failure, or diabetes mellitus. Substances of abuse such as alcohol and tobacco can also cause changes in erectile function, as can medications, including antidepressants and certain heart medications (e.g., beta blockers, antihyperlipidemics).

Change in Sexual Desire (Libido).   Sexual desire (libido) is linked to, but not synonymous with, sexual function. The range of what clients consider desirable in terms of sexual frequency is wide and may change with age, whether or not the client is in a relationship. Change in libido ranges from low or nonexistent interest in sex to hypersexuality.

A common cause of decreased libido is stress and anxiety. The source of the stress may be relationship difficulties, work or financial problems, or other challenges. Alternatively, low libido may be drug-induced (e.g., antidepressants, marijuana) or the result of hypogonadism. Nurses know that illness and recovery states may also be associated with low libido and that it is important to have a full picture of the client's biopsychosocial state when addressing such an issue.

Hypersexuality is subjectively more difficult to assess. Again, there is a wide range of what is considered acceptable levels of sexuality. Cycles of mania and depression

Lack of libido may arise from psychogenic causes such as depression, endocrine dysfunction, or side effects of medications.

Premature ejaculation is common, especially in young men. Less common is reduced or absent ejaculation affecting middle-aged or older men. Possible causes are medications, surgery, neurologic deficits, or lack of androgen. Lack of orgasm with ejaculation is usually psychogenic.

Painful erections from *Peyronie's disease,* a bend in the erect penis. Curve not noticeable when penis flaccid, intercourse may be impossible. *Priapism* (sustained erection unrelated to sexual thoughts and lasting 1 hour or more), dysregulation of blood flow to the penis. Changes in viscosity, volume, and nature of penile secretions and ejaculate.

associated with bipolar disorder may be the cause, signalling the need for psychiatric evaluation. Endocrine disorders involving the adrenal glands or testes are another possible cause of hypersexuality. Nurses recall that the onset of puberty often coincides with heightened interest in sex.

Nurses pay attention to the discomfort that clients may feel in addressing sexual issues. They are sensitive to cultural differences because clients of some cultures may consider discussion of sexual function and libido improper.

Discharge from the Penis.
To assess the possibility of genital infection from STIs, ask about any *discharge from the penis*, dripping, or staining of underwear. If penile discharge is present, assess the amount, its colour and consistency, and any fever, chills, rash, or associated symptoms.

Penile discharge may accompany gonococcal (usually yellow) and nongonococcal urethritis (may be clear or white).

Penile, Testicular, or Scrotal Lesions or Skin Breakdown.
Inquire about *sores or growths on the penis*, and any *pain, aching or swelling in the scrotum*. Ask about previous genital symptoms or a past history of infections from herpes, gonorrhea, or syphilis. A client who has multiple partners, is homosexual, uses illicit drugs, or has a prior history of STIs is at increased risk for subsequent STIs.

See Table 21-1, Unexpected Findings of the Penis (p. 777); Table 21-2, Unexpected Findings of the Scrotal Sac (p. 778); and Table 21-3, Unexpected Findings of the Testes (p. 779). In addition to STIs, many skin conditions affect the genitalia; likewise, some STIs have minimal symptoms or signs.

Because STIs may involve other parts of the body, additional questions are often indicated. An introductory explanation may be useful. "Sexually transmitted infections can involve any body opening where you have sex. It's important for you to tell me which openings you use." And further, as needed, "Do you have oral sex? Anal sex?" If the client's answers are affirmative, ask about symptoms such as sore throat, diarrhea, rectal bleeding, and anal itching or pain.

Infections from oral–penile transmission include gonorrhea, Chlamydia, syphilis, and herpes. Symptomatic or asymptomatic proctitis may follow anal intercourse.

For the many clients without symptoms or known risk factors, it is wise to ask, "Do you have any concerns about HIV infection?" as an important screening question. Continue with the more general questions suggested on pp. 763–764.

Syphilitic chancroid lesions (painless, deep ulcerations), superficial abrasions secondary to physical trauma, and heat rashes.

Penile, testicular, or scrotal lesions or skin breakdown on the genitalia (either secondary to STIs or other pathologies) may not be present during examination. Questions such as, "Have you ever noticed any recurring rashes, irritations, sores, or bumps on your penis or scrotum?" may prompt the client to recall and disclose such symptoms and signs. If your client admits to any skin changes, conduct a complete symptom/sign analysis. Correlate responses to your questions with elements of the client's sexual history. Pay close attention to reports of other lesions that may not necessarily be present at the time of physical inspection. Rashes and trauma do not involve loss of skin beyond the epidermal layers.

Scrotal Heaviness, Aching, or Pain.
Heaviness, aching, or pain in the scrotum can have many causes, including testicular torsion, trauma, infection, testicular nodules, and inguinal hernias. *Prostatitis* may also cause pain and burning in the testicles. Testicular or scrotal pain may be *referred pain* from a different body part. For example, the client may experience a kidney stone passing through the urinary system as testicular pain.

Scrotal Swelling.
Scrotal swelling can occur at any age and may or may not be accompanied by pain or involve the testes. Inguinal hernias, hydroceles, and testicular torsion are a few causes of scrotal swelling that nurses should investigate

through questions such as, "Does the swelling affect one or both sides of the scrotum?" "Is it painful?" "How intense is the pain?" and "When did you notice the swelling?" In addition, the skin of the scrotal sac contains numerous hair follicles and associated sebaceous glands; these may become enlarged at puberty (from the influence of testosterone) or with an infection.

Bulge in the Groin. To assess the possibility of an *inguinal hernia* ask, "Do you have any pain in your groin when you cough or sneeze hard?" "Do you feel any tenderness or pressure in your groin above your testicle?" Increases in abdominal pressure, such as those caused by sneezing or coughing, can be sufficient to force a loop of small intestine into or through the inguinal canal. If your client answers "Yes" to any of these questions, follow up with a focused physical examination of the scrotum and inguinal canal, as noted under "Inspection" in Techniques (p. 772). An *inguinal* hernia may be detected by palpation, especially when the client coughs. Other signs and symptoms that can mimic a hernia, but are not detectable on physical examination, include a sports hernia or *osteitis pubis.* The former is a weakening of the internal inguinal canal. The latter is caused by micro-tears in the adductor muscles that originate on the pubic bone. Both are more common in young or middle-aged active men and are associated with sports (e.g., skating, running). A *femoral* hernia, although more common in women, may be confused with lymph nodes, and in men does not involve the scrotum or inguinal canal.

Example of Questions for Symptom Analysis: Genital Herpes

- Where have you noticed the lesions? (*Location*)
- Do they show up anywhere else? (*Radiation*)
- Describe the lesions. Are they raised? Painful? Blister-like? Red? Do they rupture? Are there any marks after they have healed? (*Quality*)
- How sore/painful are the lesions on a scale of 0 (*not painful*) to 10 (*the worst pain*)? How many lesions are there? Do they stop you from enjoying sexual intercourse? (*Intensity/severity*)
- When did you first notice the lesion(s)? (*Onset*)
- How long did they last? How long do they take to heal? (*Duration*)
- When did any blisters rupture? How often do you get them? (*Frequency*)

- What seems to trigger the lesions? Stress? Physical abrasion? Anything else? (*Aggravating factors*)
- What helps get rid of the lesions? (*Alleviating factors*)
- What else do you notice when you have these lesions? Fever? Flu symptoms? Tiredness? (*Associated symptoms*)
- What factors in your work, recreation, or home might be contributing to these lesions? (*Environmental factors*)
- How do these lesions affect your love life? Lifestyle? Work? Recreation? Relationships? (*Significance to client*)
- What do you think is the cause of these lesions? (*Client perspective*)

HEALTH PROMOTION

Important Topics for Health Promotion

- Sexual/reproductive health
- Risk factors and prevention of STIs and HIV
- Risk factors and prevention of hernias
- Risk factors and screening for testicular cancer

Sexual and Reproductive Health.   The key to promotion of sexual and reproductive health is education. Nurses can advise clients of best practices for both maintaining healthy lifestyles and avoiding risky behaviours. Hygiene, nutrition, and sleep are all essential elements of general health practices that can positively influence sexual and reproductive health.

Specific hygiene measures include retraction of the foreskin (if present) and cleaning of the glans penis. Parents need to teach their sons who have not been circumcised how to clean themselves, and to ensure that the foreskin retracts easily, thereby avoiding adhesions.

The effects of diet on male reproductive health have only recently been appreciated. Of particular interest is the B complex of vitamins, including folate, which is involved in metabolism of homocysteine. Folic acid supplementation appears to positively affect spermatogenesis and sperm parameters, either alone or in combination with other nutritional factors such as zinc (Forges et al., 2007). Information on other dietary supplements is more equivocal, although clients should be counselled that a nutritious diet is a component of reproductive health.

Exposures in the workplace can influence male reproductive health. With male clients who want to maintain fertility, nurses explore the potential for exposure to toxins (e.g., heavy metals, pesticides, styrene, acetone, solvents) and hazards in the physical environment (e.g., heat, welding processes, radiation).

Using condoms and limiting the number of sexual partners have long been recognized as important in preventing STIs and maintaining sexual and reproductive health. Nurses can reinforce these elements with clients. The benefits of regular physical examinations, including testicular examinations (particularly for those in the age group of 15-35 years) and prostate examinations (including digital rectal examinations), are well documented.

Incidence of testicular cancer in Canada is 4.2 per 100,000 (McLaughlin Centre, 2008), making it the most common malignancy in men 20 to 44 years (Cancer Care Ontario, PHAC, & Canadian Cancer Society, 2006); it constitutes the fastest growing malignancy in this population. These facts make it imperative that nurses be familiar with proper testicular screening techniques. Factors that increase the risk for developing testicular cancer include a history of an undescended testicle, age (especially 15–49 years), positive family history, and unusual development of a testicle (Canadian Cancer Society, 2008). Although *testicular self-examination (TSE)* has not been formally endorsed as a method of screening for testicular carcinoma, nurses may choose to teach clients the TSE to enhance health awareness and self-care. They would encourage men, especially those 15 to 35 years, to perform monthly TSE and to seek physician evaluation promptly for the following findings: any painless lump, swelling, or enlargement in either testicle; pain or discomfort in a testicle or the scrotum; a feeling of heaviness or a sudden fluid collection in the scrotum; or a dull ache in the lower abdomen or groin. Nurses always include questions in the health history pertaining to these issues.

The Testicular Self-Examination.   Incidence of testicular cancer in Canada is 4.2 per 100,000 (McLaughlin Centre, 2008), but it is the most common cancer of young men in the age group of 15 to 35 years. When detected early, testicular carcinoma has an excellent prognosis. Risk factors include *cryptorchidism*, which confers a high risk for testicular carcinoma in the undescended testicle; a history of carcinoma in the contralateral testicle; *mumps orchitis*, an inguinal hernia; and a hydrocele in childhood.

CLIENT INSTRUCTIONS FOR THE TESTICULAR SELF-EXAMINATION

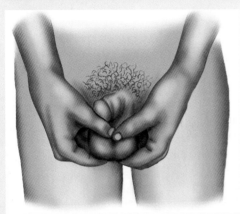

This examination is best performed after a warm bath or shower. The heat relaxes the scrotum and makes it easier to find anything unusual, such as tenderness or lumps. By being familiar with how the scrotum feels, you will detect changes more easily.

- Standing in front of a mirror, check for any swelling on the skin of the scrotum.

- Holding the scrotum, feel for the size and weight of the testicles (one may be slightly heavier and hang lower).
- Examine each testicle with both hands. Place thumbs on top and cup the index and middle fingers under the testicle.
- Rolling the testicle gently between the thumbs and fingers helps you check for smoothness. At the back of each testicle you will feel the epididymis, a soft tender tubelike structure. It carries the sperm.
- If you find any lump, see your doctor very soon. The lump may just be an infection, but if it is cancer, it will spread unless stopped by treatment.

Source: Modified from Canadian Cancer Society. (2006). *Early detection of testicular cancer.* Retrieved February 29, 2008, from http://www.cancer.ca/ccs/internet/standard/0,3182,3172_10175_74554325_langIden,00.html

Risk Factors and Prevention of STIs and HIV. Rates of bacterial STIs are increasing in Canada. These infections include genital chlamydia, gonorrhoea, and infectious syphilis, which are all reportable STIs. Unlike viral STIs, if any one of these diseases is diagnosed, the physician or care provider must report it to the Public Health Agency of Canada (PHAC). The PHAC's Canadian Sexually Transmitted Infections Surveillance Report (2007a) provides the trends.

The rate of chlamydia in 2000 was 89.1 per 100,000, or a 53.4% increase from 1997. The highest incidence and fastest rate of increase has been among men in their 20s. Also in 2000, males had a rate of gonorrhea infection of 25.3 per 100,000. This rate had been declining, but increased by 42.9% from 1997 to 2000. The highest reported incidence among males has been in the 20-to-29-year age group, and the rate of increase has been fastest in men in their 20s and 30s. Similarly, the rate of infectious syphilis had been declining until 1997, but increased significantly (62.2%) among males from 1997 to 2000. This translates to a rate of 0.73 per 100,000 among males. The highest incidence and fastest increase among males have occurred in the 25-to-29-year age group.

Marked geographic differences accompany the incidence of these STIs. Rates of infection with genital chlamydia and gonorrhea are highest in the North, followed by Manitoba and Saskatchewan. Rates of infectious syphilis are highest in British Columbia. Ontario, not surprisingly given its large population, reports the greatest number of cases for all three notifiable STIs (PHAC, 2007a).

Genital chlamydia is the most frequently reported STI nationally. Infectious syphilis is the STI with the fastest growing rate of incidence; men account for most cases. The incidence and prevalence of viral STIs in Canadian men are more difficult to ascertain; with the exception of human immunodeficiency virus (HIV), these are not reportable infections. As of 2005, 48,000 to 68,000 people in Canada were living with HIV, an increase of 16% from 2002 (PHAC, 2007b). Of these cases, approximately 80% are male. Aboriginal people are overrepresented in the Canadian HIV epidemic, comprising 7.5% of those with HIV infection, but 3.3% of the population.

Health promotion and counselling should address client education about STIs and HIV, early detection of infection during history taking and physical examination, and identification and treatment of infected partners. Discussion of risk factors for STIs and HIV is especially important for adolescents and younger clients, the age groups most adversely affected. Clinicians must be comfortable with eliciting the sexual history and with asking frank but tactful questions about sexual practices. A minimal history includes identifying the client's sexual orientation, the number of sexual partners in the past month, and any history of STIs (see Chapter 3). Questions should be clear and nonjudgemental. Identify use of alcohol and drugs, particularly injection drugs. Counsel clients at risk about limiting the number of partners, using condoms, and establishing regular medical care for treatment of STIs and HIV. It is important for men to seek prompt attention for any genital lesions or penile discharge.

Specific Prevention of Specific Diseases.
Risk of STIs and HIV is directly proportional to the number of sexual partners and frequency of unprotected sex. Clients should be encouraged to use latex condoms, although they must also be informed that condoms do not provide 100% protection from STIs. Female condoms are synthetic barriers worn by women, and which protect more of the surface area of the female genitalia. Clients should also be counselled that personal hygiene (e.g., washing before or after intercourse) does not confer adequate protection against STIs. Furthermore, sexual practices that cause excessive abrasion and increase the possibility of blood transfer pose an increased risk of HIV infection. Oral sex also transfers STIs from either partner.

As of May 1, 2003, HIV infection became legally notifiable in all provinces and territories, although each province/territory has a different system for reporting. At least one of three forms of testing is available in Canada: (1) nominal, or name based; (2) nonnominal, or nonidentifying; and (3) anonymous. Nonnominal testing relies on a code or initials, not the client's full or partial name. Anonymous testing involves using a unique, nonidentifying code that only the person being tested for HIV knows. Anonymous testing is available in only eight provinces. By facilitating access to testing and different test formats, it is hoped that more people will feel comfortable seeking out testing and counselling services for HIV infection.

Health promotion may also be directed at prevention of hernias. Two factors contribute to inguinal hernias: (1) activities that increase intra-abdominal pressure and (2) a possible genetic predisposition to weakness of the abdominal wall at the inguinal canal. Activities that increase intra-abdominal pressure include excessive straining during bowel movements, which is more likely in older men, and lifting heavy objects. Men involved in heavy construction work or manual labour are at increased risk of inguinal hernias; client teaching about these risks is required. Also, body builders and weight lifters are at increased risk, and should be encouraged to obtain proper coaching on technique and supportive equipment. Nurses and orderlies are also at risk of hernias, given that they are frequently called upon to lift clients. Again, proper techniques and the use of assistive devices can help ameliorate risk. Clients may be advised to use stool softeners if they are constipated, although the possibility of a bowel obstruction should be considered. Clients should be advised to avoid heavy lifting where possible, and if they are at risk of an inguinal hernia, they may be advised to have themselves fitted for an appropriate truss or abdominal support.

Emergency Concerns.   Certain findings are considered medical emergencies and require immediate follow-up and referral to a physician. *Torsion of the spermatic cord* is of particular concern because it can restrict blood flow to the testicle. If left untreated, torsion can result in ischemia and tissue death. *Priapism*, a sustained erection, is also an emergency, given that blood stasis in the penis may also result in poor tissue perfusion and damage. Another condition that may reduce blood flow and cause considerable pain is a *strangulated inguinal hernia*, in which a loop of the ileum descends through the inguinal canal, usually producing pain, and often restricting blood flow to the entrapped intestinal loop and the testicle itself. The intestinal loop may sometimes be gently pushed back through the inguinal canal, although prompt medical attention is invariably required to prevent ischemia.

In clients with an intact foreskin, the tissue may only partly retract. If it remains fixed in this position, the glans penis can become strangulated, which reduces blood flow and may prevent the voiding of urine.

The penis has a tough, connective tissue sheath. Particularly when erect, or even when not erect, trauma can actually cause this limiting membrane to break. An audible "snapping" sound accompanies asymmetric swelling of the penis. This form of *fracture* requires immediate medical attention.

Encourage men, especially those between the ages of 15 and 35, to perform monthly *testicular self-examinations* and to seek physician evaluation for the following findings: any painless lump, swelling, or enlargement in either testicle; pain or discomfort in a testicle or the scrotum; a feeling of heaviness or a sudden fluid collection in the scrotum; or a dull ache in the lower abdomen or the groin.

For younger clients, review the sexual maturity ratings, as shown in Table 21-4, Sexual Maturity Ratings in Boys, p. 780.

TECHNIQUES OF EXAMINATION: OBJECTIVE DATA

■ PROMOTING CLIENT COMFORT, DIGNITY, AND SAFETY

Nurses always safeguard the client's privacy, particularly in genitourinary examinations. Before proceeding with this type of assessment, inform each client about the process and purpose of the examination.

Factors that influence a client's comfort level with a genitourinary assessment include age, prior experience with physical examinations, the nature of the presenting complaint, gender identity, sexual preference, and ethnicity. In Canada's multicultural population, nurses are likely to encounter male clients with different cultural norms and differing comfort levels for genitourinary assessments. If it is unacceptable to the client that a female nurse perform a genital examination, the nurse requests that a male colleague carry out the procedure. Familiarity with influential factors and sensitivity to client preferences can facilitate completion of the health history and subsequent physical assessment.

When performing a genitourinary examination, nurses attend to client dignity. They ask in private questions relating to the client's health history and sexual practices, making sure to obtain prior consent from the client and before initiating the physical examination. Nurses avoid any statements with implied judgment. They always vacate the examination room while the client is changing, indicating that they will return, and then knock before reentering. During the physical examination, hospital gowns or towels are used to reveal only the area being examined.

As 96% of nurses in Canada are women, performing a physical assessment of male genitalia may present some awkwardness for both client and nurse. The examination may be performed with the client either standing or supine, but female nurses usually ask clients to lie in the left lateral position and drape them to minimize exposure but permit examination. It is acceptable for a nurse to request that an additional person be present in the examination room. Occasionally, a male client may have an erection during the examination. The nurse refrains from showing surprise, explains that this can be an expected physiological reaction, proceeds as expeditiously as possible, and is prepared to stop if the client declines to be examined further.

To check for hernias or varicoceles, the client stands to allow for the effects of gravity, and the examiner sits. The examiner asks the client to cough if a hernia is not immediately evident on palpation. The nurse should not encourage the client to cough if there is evidence of an entrapped (incarcerated) or strangulated hernia. The nurse wears nonlatex gloves throughout the examination and practices glove disposal and hand-washing procedures after the examination. Any equipment that comes in direct contact with the client (e.g., flashlight for transillumination, stethoscope for listening for bowel sounds in a scrotal swelling) requires disinfection.

Equipment

- Clean (sterile or nonsterile) nonlatex gloves
- Penlight or flashlight
- Sterile Q-tip or swab
- Glass slide
- Tissue fixative (5% buggered formalin or other cytological-grade fixative)
- Biohazard disposal container
- Sterile saline

THE PENIS

To examine the penile glans, the nurse may need to retract the foreskin if the man is not circumcised. Optimally, however, the nurse encourages the client to do this himself. The foreskin usually retracts smoothly, although white-coloured adhesions may prevent retraction in prepubescent males. In these cases, the foreskin should not be forcibly retracted. If males older than 3 years continue to have foreskin adhesions, the nurse encourages them to gently retract the foreskin during bathing to facilitate loosening of the adhesions and careful hygiene. Nurses note the presence and odour (if any) of smegma and ensure that a retracted foreskin is returned to its position covering the glans penis.

When the nurse finds an inflammatory or suspicious lesion on the penile shaft (or scrotal sac), he or she should assess the inguinal nodes very carefully for enlargement or tenderness.

Inspection. Inspect the penis, including:

■ The *skin*

See Table 21-1, Unexpected Findings of the Penis (p. 777).

■ The *prepuce* (foreskin). If it is present, retract it or ask the client to retract it. This step is essential for the detection of many chancres and carcinomas. Smegma, a cheesy, whitish material, commonly may accumulate under the foreskin.

Phimosis is a tight prepuce that cannot be retracted over the glans. *Paraphimosis* is a tight prepuce that, once retracted, cannot be returned. Edema ensues.

■ The *glans*. Look for any ulcers, scars, nodules, or signs of inflammation.

Balanitis (inflammation of the glans); *balanoposthitis* (inflammation of the glans and prepuce)

Check the skin around the base of the penis for excoriations or inflammation. Look for nits or lice at the bases of the pubic hairs.

Pubic or genital excoriations suggest the possibility of lice (crabs) or sometimes scabies.

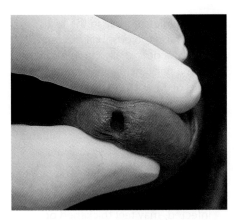

Note the location of the urethral meatus.

Compress the glans gently between your index finger above and your thumb below. This manoeuvre should open the urethral meatus and allow you to inspect it for discharge. Usually there is none.

Hypospedia is a congenital, ventral displacement of the meatus on the penis (p. 777).

Profuse yellow discharge in gonococcal urethritis; scanty white or clear discharge in nongonococcal urethritis. Definitive diagnosis requires Gram stain and culture.

If the client has reported a discharge that you are unable to see, ask him to strip, or milk, the shaft of the penis from its base to the glans. Alternatively, do it yourself. This manoeuvre may bring some discharge out of the urethral meatus for appropriate examination. Have a glass slide and culture materials ready.

Palpation. Palpate any abnormality of the penis, noting any tenderness or induration. Palpate the shaft of the penis between your thumb and first two fingers, noting any induration. Palpation of the shaft may be omitted in a young, asymptomatic male client.

Induration along the ventral surface of the penis suggests a urethral stricture or possibly a carcinoma. Tenderness of such an indurated area suggests periurethral inflammation secondary to a urethral stricture.

If you retract the foreskin, replace it before proceeding on to examine the scrotum.

THE SCROTUM AND ITS CONTENTS

Inspection. Inspect the scrotum, including:

See Table 21-2, Unexpected Findings of the Scrotal Sac (p. 778).

■ The *skin*; lift up the scrotum so that you can see its posterior surface.

Rashes, epidermoid cysts, rarely skin cancer

■ The *scrotal contours*. Note any swelling, lumps, or veins.

A poorly developed scrotum on one or both sides suggests *cryptorchidism* (an undescended testicle). Common scrotal swellings include indirect inguinal hernias, hydroceles, and scrotal oedema. Tender, painful

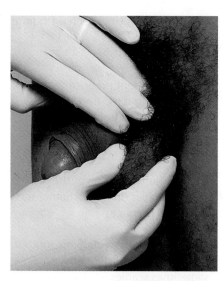

Palpation. *Palpate each testis and epididymis* between your thumb and first two fingers. Locate the epididymis on the superior posterior surface of each testicle. It feels nodular and cordlike and should not be confused with an unusual lump.

scrotal swelling in acute epididymitis, acute orchitis, torsion of the spermatic cord, or a strangulated inguinal hernia.

See Table 21-3, Unexpected Findings of the Testes (p. 779) and Table 21-5, Unexpected Findings of the Epididymis and Spermatic Cord (p. 781).

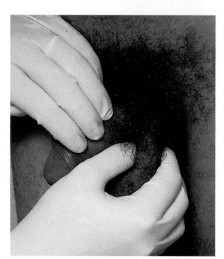

Note size, shape, consistency, and tenderness; feel for any nodules. Pressure on the testis usually produces a deep visceral pain.

Any painless nodule in the testis must raise the possibility of *testicular cancer,* a potentially curable cancer with a peak incidence between the ages of 15 and 35 years.

Palpate each spermatic cord, including the vas deferens, between your thumb and fingers from the epididymis to the superficial inguinal ring.

Multiple tortuous veins in this area, usually on the left, may be palpable and even visible. They indicate a *varicocele* (p. 781).

Note any nodules or swellings.

The vas deferens, if chronically infected, may feel thickened or beaded. A cystic structure in the spermatic cord suggests a hydrocele of the cord.

Swelling in the scrotum other than the testicles can be evaluated by transillumination. After darkening the room, shine the beam of a strong flashlight from behind the scrotum anteriorly through the mass. Look for transmission of the light as a red glow.

Swellings containing serous fluid, as in hydroceles, light up with a red glow, or transilluminate. Those containing blood or tissue, such as a normal testis, a tumour, or most hernias, do not.

◢ HERNIAS

Inspection. *Inspect the inguinal and femoral areas* carefully for bulges. While you continue your observation, ask the client to strain and bear down, as if having a bowel movement (the Valsalva manoeuvre) to enhance detection of hernias.

A bulge that appears on straining suggests a hernia.

Palpation. *Palpate for an inguinal hernia.* With the client still standing, and using in turn your right hand for the client's right side and your left hand for the client's left side, invaginate loose scrotal skin with your index finger. Start at a point low enough to be sure that your finger will have enough mobility to reach as far as the internal inguinal ring if this proves possible. Follow the spermatic cord upward to above the inguinal ligament and find the triangular, slitlike opening of the external inguinal ring. This is just above and lateral to the pubic tubercle. If the ring is somewhat enlarged, it may admit your index finger. If possible, gently follow the

See Table 21-6, Course and Presentation of Hernias in the Groin (p. 782).

inguinal canal laterally in its oblique course. With your finger located either at the external ring or within the canal, ask the client to strain down or cough. Note any palpable herniating mass as it touches your finger.

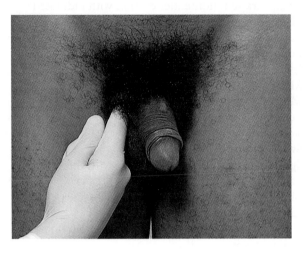
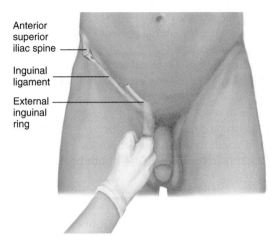

Anterior superior iliac spine

Inguinal ligament

External inguinal ring

See Table 21-7, Differentiation of Hernias in the Groin (p. 783).

Palpate for a femoral hernia by placing your fingers on the anterior thigh in the region of the femoral canal. Ask the client to strain down again or cough. Note any swelling or tenderness.

Evaluating a Possible Scrotal Hernia. If you find a large scrotal mass and suspect that it may be a hernia, ask the client to lie down. The mass may return to the abdomen by itself. If so, it is a hernia. If not:

■ Can you get your fingers above the mass in the scrotum?

If you can, suspect a hydrocele.

■ Listen to the mass with a stethoscope for bowel sounds.

Bowel sounds may be heard over a hernia, but not over a hydrocele.

If the findings suggest a hernia, gently try to reduce it (return it to the abdominal cavity) by sustained pressure with your fingers. Do not attempt this manoeuvre if the mass is tender or the client reports nausea and vomiting.

History may be helpful here. The client can usually tell you what happens to his swelling on lying down and may be able to demonstrate how he reduces it himself. Remember to ask him.

A hernia is *incarcerated* when its contents cannot be returned to the abdominal cavity. A hernia is *strangulated* when the blood supply to the entrapped contents is compromised. Suspect strangulation in the presence of tenderness, nausea, and vomiting, and consider surgical intervention.

RECORDING AND ANALYZING FINDINGS

Documentation of the information obtained from the health history and physical examination of the male genitalia and inguinal regions must be thorough, accurate, and clear for all members of the interdisciplinary team. Follow the principles of documentation to ensure the planning and implementation of comprehensive and appropriate care.

■ Examples of Documentation for Male Genitalia and Inguinal Regions

Area	Expected Findings	Unexpected Findings
Penis	Free of skin lesions and indurations	Oval, dark red, nontender erosion with indurated base, dorsal surface of glans penis
	Prepuce retracts easily	
	White, cheesy material present (smegma)	Prepuce not retractable
	Glans smooth	Foul-smelling smegma
	Urethral meatus at distal end of glans	Inflamed skin on glans penis dorsally
	Urethral meatus opens readily and is free of discharge	Meatus displaced to ventral surface of glans
		Meatus does not open
	Free of tenderness	Yellow discharge at meatus
	No lateral curvature or flexion	Tenderness on palpation of shaft
Scrotum	Wrinkled, loose, free of lesions	Swelling right scrotum
	Spermatic cord palpable, smooth bilaterally	Spermatic cord thicker on left side with thickenings along cord length
		Multiple, tortuous veins in left scrotal sac
Testes	Left testis lower than right	Right testicle unyielding
	Testes firm, smooth, slightly rubbery on palpation	Firm, fixed nontender nodule 1 cm × 1 cm on right lateral testis
	Free of nodules, tenderness	Right epididymis enlarged, tender
	Epididymis, palpable and nontender on posterior surface bilaterally	
Inguinal	Nonpalpable lymph nodes bilaterally	Tender lymph nodes left horizontal region >1 cm in size
	Bilaterally symmetrical and no inguinal or femoral bulges	Bulge right femoral canal
	Spermatic cord palpable into inguinal canal bilaterally	Mass touches palpating fingertip in left inguinal canal upon cough

■ ANALYZING FINDINGS FROM PHYSICAL EXAMINATION AND HEALTH HISTORY

After findings are documented, it is important to analyze the information from the health history and physical examination to determine one or more nursing diagnoses and plan an interdisciplinary approach. For example:

Robert, a 13-year-old boy, presents with his father and reports right scrotal pain that started suddenly, waking him from sleep 4 hours earlier. He denies any trauma and describes the pain as constant, throbbing, and not changing with position. He reports voiding as usual and no history of fever, chills, nausea, or vomiting.

During your assessment, you note that his temperature is 36.8°C and that he is in moderate distress secondary to right scrotal pain. His respiratory rate is rapid (30 breaths per minute). The right side of the scrotum appears edematous and red, with the testicle being markedly more tender on palpation than the left testicle. There is no cremasteric reflex on the right side and a partial cremasteric reflex on the left side. The uncircumcised penis is unremarkable in appearance; the foreskin retracts easily, and there are no signs of urethral discharge or rash. You note no testicular masses.

From this information, you develop the following nursing diagnosis:

Pain, acute*—potentially related to torsion of spermatic cord*

An interdisciplinary approach ensures immediate comprehensive care for Robert. The registered nurse monitors vital signs, fluid balance, and urinary elimination; manages pain; assesses psychosocial issues appropriate to age; establishes an intravenous line; ensures the client takes nothing by mouth; and provides facts and reassurance to Robert and his father. The urologist conducts a complete genital examination and refers Robert for emergency surgery. The anesthetist takes a history and explains the process of undergoing anesthesia to Robert and his father. The operating-room nurse explains the preparation for his emergency surgery and the procedures that will be followed in the operating and recovery rooms.

Critical Thinking Questions

- What are potential causes of scrotal swelling? (*Knowledge*)

- What might transillumination of the scrotum reveal? (*Comprehension*)

- How does the nurse assist the client to relax during inspection and palpation of the genitalia? (*Application*)

- What factors might contribute to client discomfort during the examination? (*Analysis*)

- What topics for health promotion are indicated with this client? (*Synthesis*)

- How would you evaluate the effectiveness of your postoperative teaching about testicular self-examination with this client? (*Evaluation*)

Canadian Research

Oliffe, J. L. (2005). Constructions of masculinity following prostatectomy-induced impotence. *Social Science and Medicine, 60*(10), 2240–2259.

Oliffe, J., & Mroz, L. (2005). Men interviewing men about health and illness: Ten lessons learned. *Journal of Men's Health and Gender, 2*, 257–260.

Oliffe, J. L. (2002). In search of a social model of prostate cancer: Finding out about Bronch. In S. Pearce & V. Muller (Eds.), *Manning the next millennium: Studies in masculinities.*Western Australia: Black Swan Press.

Shoveller, J. A., & Johnson, J. L. (2006). Risky groups, risky behaviour, and risky persons: Dominating discourses on youth sexual health. *Critical Public Health, 16*, (1), 47–60.

Shoveller, J. A., Johnson, J. L., Savoy, D., & Pietersma, W. A. W. (2006). Preventing sexually transmitted infections among adolescents: An assessment of ecological approaches and study methods. *Sex Education, 6*(2), 163–183.

Test Questions

1. All of the following are potential indicators of testicular disorders **except**
   a. scrotal discomfort.
   b. heaviness in the groin.
   c. painless testicular swelling.
   d. dull ache in the lower abdomen.

2. During assessment of the inguinal regions for herniating masses, the nurse instructs the standing male client to
   a. bear down.
   b. exhale fully.
   c. bend over and bear down.
   d. hold breath to count of ten.

3. When assessing for an inguinal hernia, the nurse asks the client to assume which of the following positions?
   a. Supine on examining table
   b. Standing, facing the examiner
   c. Lying on the left side, with right leg flexed
   d. Standing, upper body supported by examining table

4. During palpation of the male genitalia, an expected finding is
   a. palpable spermatic cord.
   b. beading of the vas deferens.
   c. painless testicular nodules.
   d. tortuous veins in the scrotum.

5. When invaginating the skin of the scrotum to assess the inguinal regions, an expected finding is
   a. intestinal contents in the inguinal canal.
   b. inability to introduce the index finger into the inguinal ring.
   c. movement of the examiner's index finger anteriorly when the client coughs.
   d. inability to follow the spermatic cord from the client's scrotum to inguinal ligament.

Bibliography

CITATIONS

Cancer Care Ontario, Public Health Agency of Canada, & Canadian Cancer Society. (2006). *Cancer in young adults in Canada*. Retrieved April 15, 2008, from http://www.phac-aspc.gc.ca/publicat/cyac-cjac06/index.html

Canadian Cancer Society. (2008). *Causes of testicular cancer.* Retrieved February 28, 2008, from http://www.cancer.ca/ccs/internet/standard/0,3182,3172_10175_272773_langId-en,00.html

Canadian Cancer Society. (2006). *Early detection of testicular cancer.* Retrieved February 29, 2008, from http://www.cancer.ca/ccs/internet/standard/0,3182,3172_10175_74554325_langId-en,00.html

Forges, T., Monnier-Barbarino, P., Alberto, J. M., Guéant-Rodríguez, R. M., Daval, J. L., & Guéant, J. L. (2007). Impact of folate and homocysteine metabolism on human reproductive health. *Human Reproduction Update, 13*(3), 225–238.

Goldman, B. D. (2000). Common dermatoses of the male genitalia: Recognition of differences in genital rashes and lesions is essential and attainable. *Postgraduate Medicine, 108*(4), 89, 95–96.

Gregory, D., Evans, J., Frank, B., & Kellett, P. (2008). Men's health: The need for change. *WellSpring, 19*(1), 1–4. Retrieved February 21, 2008, from http://www.centre4activeliving.ca/publications/wellspring/2008/febindex.html

Levy, B. S., & Wegman, D. H. (Eds.). (2006). *Occupational health: Recognizing and preventing work-related disease and injury* (5th ed). Philadelphia: Lippincott Williams & Wilkins.

McLaughlin Centre. (2008). *Testicular cancer.* Retrieved February 28, 2008, from http://www.emcom.ca/health/testicular.shtml

Public Health Agency of Canada. (2007a). *2004 Canadian sexually transmitted infections surveillance report.* CCDR 2007: 33S1; 1-69. Retrieved March 25, 2009, from http://www.phac-aspc.gc.ca/publicat/ccdr-rmte/07vol33/33s1/index_eng.php

Public Health Agency of Canada. (2007b). *HIV/AIDS—Epi updates.* Retrieved March 25, 2009, from http://www.phac-aspc.gc.ca/aids-sida/publication/epi-epi2007-eng.php

ADDITIONAL REFERENCES

Campbell, M. F., Walsh, P. C., Patrick, C., & Retik, A. B. (Eds.). (2002). *Campbell's urology* (8th ed.). Philadelphia: W. B. Saunders.

DeBusk, R. F. (2003). Sexual activity in clients with angina. *Journal of the American Medical Association, 290*(23), 3129–3132.

Eubanks, S. (2004). Hernias. In C. M. Townsend & D. C. Sabiston (Eds.), *Sabiston textbook of surgery: The biological basis of modern surgical practice* (17th ed.). Philadelphia: Elsevier Saunders.

Fitzgibbons, R. J., Filipi, C. J., and Quinn, T. H. (2005). Inguinal hernias. In F. C. Brunicardi, D. K. Andersen, T. R. Billiar, et al. (Eds.), *Schwartz's principles of surgery* (8th ed.) New York: McGraw-Hill.

Handsfield, H. H. (2001). *Colour atlas and synopsis of sexually transmitted diseases* (2nd ed.). New York: McGraw-Hill.

Tanagho, E. A., & McAninch, J. W. (Eds.). (2004). *Smith's general urology* (16th ed.). New York: Lange Medical Books, McGraw-Hill.

CANADIAN ASSOCIATIONS AND WEB SITES

Canadian Men's Health Network: http://www.mensnet.ca

Canadian HIV/AIDS Information Centre: http://www.aidssida.cpha.ca/

Public Health Agency of Canada (Men's Health): http://www.canadian-health-network.ca/

Public Health Agency of Canada (STI Link): http://www.phac-aspc.gc.ca/publicat/ccdr-rmtc/07vol33/33s1/index_e.html

R. Samuel McLaughlin Centre for Population Health Risk Assessment: http://www.mclaughlincentre.ca

TABLE 21-1   Unexpected Findings of the Penis

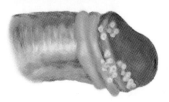

Venereal Wart
(Condyloma acuminatum)

Venereal warts are rapidly growing excrescences that are moist and often malodorous. They result from infection by human papillomavirus.

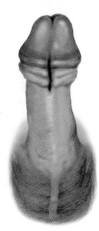

Hypospedia

Hypospedia is a congenital displacement of the urethral meatus to the inferior surface of the penis. A groove extends from the actual urethral meatus to its usual location on the tip of the glans.

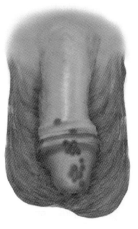

Genital Herpes

A cluster of small vesicles, followed by shallow, painful, nonindurated ulcers on red bases, suggests a herpes simplex infection. The lesions may occur anywhere on the penis. Usually there are fewer lesions when the infection recurs.

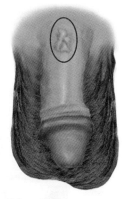

Peyronie's Disease

In Peyronie's disease, palpable nontender hard plaques are found just beneath the skin, usually along the dorsum of the penis. The client complains of crooked, painful erections.

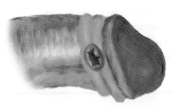

Syphilitic Chancre

A syphilitic chancre usually appears as an oval or round, dark red, painless erosion or ulcer with an indurated base. Nontender enlarged inguinal lymph nodes are typically associated. Chancres may be multiple and, when secondarily infected, may be painful. They may then be mistaken for the lesions of herpes. Chancres are infectious.

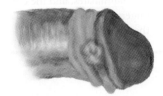

Carcinoma of the Penis

Carcinoma may appear as an indurated nodule or ulcer that is usually nontender. Limited almost completely to men who are not circumcised in childhood, it may be masked by the prepuce. Any persistent penile sore must be considered suspicious.

TABLE 21-2   **Unexpected Findings of the Scrotal Sac**

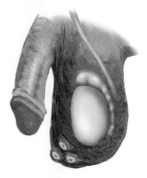

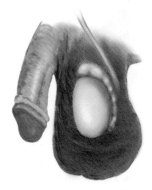

Epidermoid Cysts

These are firm, yellowish, nontender, cutaneous cysts up to about 1 cm in diameter. They are common and frequently multiple.

Scrotal Edema

Pitting edema may make the scrotal skin taut. This may accompany the generalized edema of congestive heart failure or nephrotic syndrome.

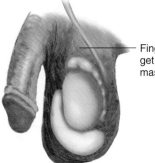

Fingers can get above mass

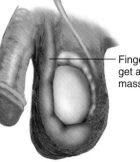

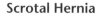

Fingers cannot get above mass

Hydrocele

A hydrocele is a nontender, fluid-filled mass within the tunica vaginalis. It transilluminates, and the examining fingers can get above the mass within the scrotum.

Scrotal Hernia

A hernia within the scrotum is usually an *indirect inguinal hernia*. It comes through the external inguinal ring, so the examining fingers cannot get above it within the scrotum.

TABLE 21-3   **Unexpected Findings of the Testes**

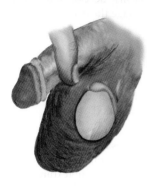

Cryptorchidism

In cryptorchidism, the testes are atrophied and may lie in the inguinal canal or the abdomen, resulting in an undeveloped scrotum, as shown. There is no palpable left testis or epididymis. Cryptorchidism markedly raises the risk for testicular cancer.

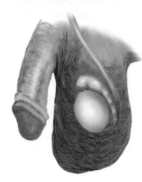

Small Testes

(In adult males, the length is usually ≤3.5 cm.) Small firm testes in *Klinefelter's syndrome*, usually ≤2 cm. Small soft testes suggesting atrophy seen in cirrhosis, myotonic dystrophy, use of estrogens, and hypopituitarism; may also follow orchitis.

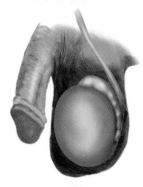

Acute Orchitis

The testis is acutely inflamed, painful, tender, and swollen. It may be difficult to distinguish from the epididymis. The scrotum may be reddened. Seen in mumps and other viral infections; usually unilateral.

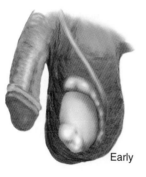

Early

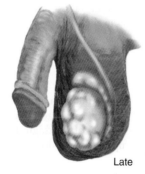

Late

Tumour of the Testes

Usually appears as a painless nodule. Any nodule within the testes warrants investigation for malignancy.

As a testicular neoplasm grows and spreads, it may seem to replace the entire organ. The testicle characteristically feels heavier than usual.

TABLE 21-4   Sex Maturity Ratings in Boys

In assigning sex maturity ratings in boys, observe each of the three characteristics separately because they may develop at different rates. Record two separate ratings: pubic hair and genital. If the penis and testes differ in their stages, average the two into a single figure for the genital rating.

	Pubic Hair	Penis	Testes and Scrotum
Stage 1	Preadolescent—no pubic hair except for the fine body hair (vellus hair) similar to that on the abdomen	Preadolescent—same size and proportions as in childhood	Preadolescent—same size and proportions as in childhood
Stage 2	Sparse growth of long, slightly pigmented, downy hair, straight or only slightly curled, chiefly at the base of the penis	Slight or no enlargement	Testes larger; scrotum larger, somewhat reddened, and altered in texture
Stage 3	Darker, coarser, curlier hair spreading sparsely over the pubic symphysis	Larger, especially in length	Further enlarged
Stage 4	Coarse and curly hair, as in the adult; area covered greater than in stage 3 but not as great as in the adult and not yet including the thighs	Further enlarged in length and breadth, with development of the glans	Further enlarged; scrotal skin darkened
Stage 5	Hair adult in quantity and quality, spread to the medial surfaces of the thighs but not up over the abdomen	Adult in size and shape	Adult in size and shape

Photos reprinted from *Pediatric Endocrinology and Growth*, 2nd ed., Wales & Wit, 2003, with permission from Elsevier.

| TABLE 21-5 | Unexpected Findings of the Epididymis and Spermatic Cord |

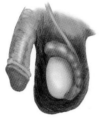

Acute Epididymitis

An acutely inflamed epididymis is tender and swollen and may be difficult to distinguish from the testes. The scrotum may be reddened and the vas deferens inflamed. It occurs chiefly in adults. Coexisting urinary tract infection or prostatitis supports the diagnosis.

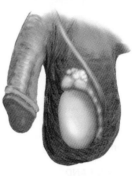

Spermatocele and Cyst of the Epididymis

A painless, movable cystic mass just above the testes suggests a spermatocele or an epididymal cyst. Both transilluminate. The former contains sperm, and the latter does not, but they are clinically indistinguishable.

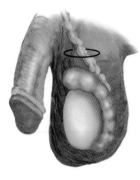

Tuberculous Epididymitis

The chronic inflammation of tuberculosis produces a firm enlargement of the epididymis, which is sometimes tender, with thickening or beading of the vas deferens.

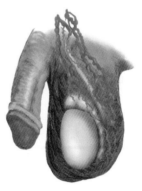

Varicocele

Varicocele refers to varicose veins of the spermatic cord, usually found on the left. It feels like a soft "bag of worms" separate from the testes, and slowly collapses when the scrotum is elevated in the supine client. Infertility may be associated.

Torsion of the Spermatic Cord

Torsion, or twisting of the testicle on its spermatic cord produces an acutely painful, tender, and swollen organ that is retracted upward in the scrotum. The scrotum becomes red and edematous. There is no associated urinary infection. Torsion, most common in adolescents, is a surgical emergency because of obstructed circulation.

TABLE 21-6   Course and Presentation of Hernias in the Groin

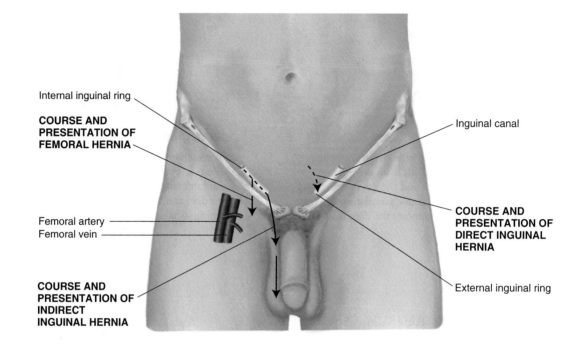

Internal inguinal ring

**COURSE AND
PRESENTATION OF
FEMORAL HERNIA**

Femoral artery

Femoral vein

**COURSE AND
PRESENTATION OF
INDIRECT
INGUINAL HERNIA**

Inguinal canal

**COURSE AND
PRESENTATION OF
DIRECT INGUINAL
HERNIA**

External inguinal ring

TABLE 21-7   **Differentiation of Hernias in the Groin**

Differentiation among these hernias is not always clinically possible. Understanding their features, however, improves your observation.

	Inguinal		Femoral
	Indirect	*Direct*	*Femoral*
Frequency	Most common, all ages, both sexes	Less common	Least common
Age and Sex	Often in children, may be in adults	Usually in men older than 40, rare in women	More common in women than in men
Point of Origin	Above inguinal ligament, near its midpoint (the internal inguinal ring)	Above inguinal ligament, close to the pubic tubercle (near the external inguinal ring)	Below the inguinal ligament; appears more lateral than an inguinal hernia and may be hard to differentiate from lymph nodes
Course	Often into the scrotum	Rarely into the scrotum	Never into the scrotum
With the examining finger in the inguinal canal during straining or cough	The hernia comes down the inguinal canal and touches the fingertip.	The hernia bulges anteriorly and pushes the side of the finger forward.	The inguinal canal is empty.

Female Genitalia

SARLA SETHI AND LYNN S. BICKLEY

The female genitalia represent femininity, sexuality, reproduction, and elimination. Unexpected signs and symptoms related to the female genitalia cause women to worry about how the changes may affect their health, sexual practices, and ability to conceive and bear children. They may delay seeing health professionals because of embarrassment, the probability of needing a pelvic examination, and fears about outcomes.

During history taking and physical examination, nurses engage in a focused conversation with female clients about questions and feelings regarding functioning of the female genitalia. Thorough examination is essential for early detection of health concerns. It is also an opportune time to provide accurate information about sexual health and self-care practices.

ANATOMY AND PHYSIOLOGY

The female genitourinary system consists of internal and external structures. The external genital area is known as the *vulva*, which includes the *mons pubis*, a hair-covered fat pad overlying the symphysis pubis; the *labia majora*, rounded folds of adipose tissue; the *labia minora*, thinner pinkish red folds that extend anteriorly to form the *prepuce*; and the *clitoris*. The *vestibule* is the boat-shaped fossa between the labia minora. In its posterior portion lies the vaginal opening, the *introitus*, which in virgins may be hidden by the *hymen*. The term *perineum*, as commonly used clinically, refers to the tissue between the introitus and the anus.

The *urethral meatus* opens into the vestibule between the clitoris and the vagina. Just posterior to it on either side lie the openings of the *paraurethral* (Skene's) *glands*.

The internal reproductive genitalia consist of the vagina, Skene's and Bartholin glands, cervix, uterus, fallopian tubes, and ovaries. The *vagina* is a musculomembranous tube extending upward and posteriorly between urethra and rectum. Its upper third takes a horizontal plane and terminates in the cup-shaped *fornix*. The vaginal mucosa lies in transverse folds, or rugae. The openings of *Bartholin's glands* are located posteriorly on either side of the vaginal opening, but are not usually visible. The glands are situated deeply.

Mons pubis

Prepuce

Clitoris

Urethral meatus

Opening of
paraurethral
(Skene's) gland

Vestibule

Introitus

Perineum

Labium majus

Labium minus

Hymen

Vagina

Opening of
Bartholin's gland

Anus

At almost right angles to the vagina lies the *uterus,* a flattened fibromuscular structure shaped like an inverted pear. The uterus has two parts: the body (corpus) and the cervix, which the isthmus joins together. The convex upper surface of the body is called the *fundus.* The lower part of the uterus, the *cervix,* protrudes into the vagina, dividing the fornix into anterior, posterior, and lateral fornices.

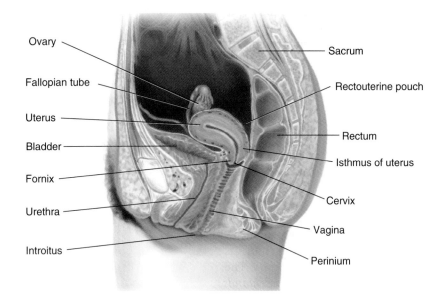

Ovary

Fallopian tube

Uterus

Bladder

Fornix

Urethra

Introitus

Sacrum

Rectouterine pouch

Rectum

Isthmus of uterus

Cervix

Vagina

Perinium

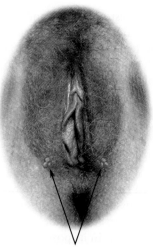

Location of
Bartholin's glands

The vaginal surface of the cervix, the *ectocervix,* is seen easily with a speculum. At its centre is a round, oval, or slitlike depression, the *external os,* which marks the opening into the endocervical canal. Epithelium of two possible types covers the ectocervix: a plushy, red columnar epithelium surrounding the os, which resembles the lining of the endocervical canal, and a shiny pink squamous epithelium continuous with the vaginal lining. The *squamocolumnar junction* forms the boundary between these two types of epithelium. At puberty, columnar epithelium gradually replaces the broad band of columnar epithelium encircling the os, called *ectropion*. The squamocolumnar junction migrates toward the os, creating the *transformation zone*. This is the area at risk for dysplasia, which is sampled by the Papanicolaou or Pap smear.

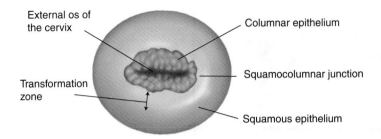

A *fallopian tube* with a fanlike tip extends from each side of the uterus toward the ovary. The two ovaries are almond-shaped structures that vary considerably in size but average about 3.5 × 2 × 1.5 cm from adulthood through menopause. The ovaries are palpable on pelvic examination in roughly half of women during the reproductive years. Usually, fallopian tubes cannot be felt. The term *adnexa*, a plural Latin word meaning appendages, refers to the ovaries, tubes, and supporting tissues.

The ovaries have two primary functions: the production of ova and the secretion of hormones, including estrogen, progesterone, and testosterone. Increased hormonal secretions during puberty stimulate the growth of the uterus and its endometrial lining. They stimulate enlargement of the vagina and thicken its epithelium. They also stimulate the development of secondary sex characteristics, including the breasts and pubic hair.

The parietal peritoneum extends downward behind the uterus into a cul de sac called the *rectouterine pouch* (pouch of Douglas). You can just reach this area on rectovaginal examination.

The pelvic organs are supported by a sling of tissues composed of muscle, ligaments, and fascia, through which the urethra, vagina, and rectum all pass.

Assessment of sexual maturity in girls, as classified by Tanner, depends not on internal examination, but on the growth of pubic hair and the development of breasts.

Physical changes in a young girl's breasts are one of the first signs of puberty. As in most developmental changes, there is a systematic progression of maturational changes. Generally, over a 4-year period, the breasts progress through five stages, called Tanner stages or Tanner sex maturity rating (SMR) stages, as shown on the next page. These progress from a preadolescent stage, to the appearance of breast buds, to subsequent enlargement and change in the contour of the breasts and areola. These stages are accompanied by the development of pubic hair and other secondary sexual characteristics, as shown on page 789. Menarche usually occurs when a girl is in breast stage 3 or 4, and by then she has passed her peak growth spurt (see the figure on p. 790).

For years the established expected age range for onset of breast development was 8 to 13 years of age (average age of 11 years), with breast development occurring before 8 years being unusual. Some recent studies suggest that the lower age cutoff should be 7 years for White females and 6 years for African American (and probably Hispanic) females, though there remains some controversy about the exact age.

Masses or nodules in the breasts of adolescent girls should be examined carefully. They are usually *benign fibroadenomas* or *cysts;* less likely etiologies include *abscesses* or *lipomas.* Breast carcinoma is extremely rare in adolescence, and nearly always occurs in families with a strong family history of the disease.

SEX MATURITY RATINGS IN GIRLS: BREASTS

Stage 1
Preadolescent. Elevation of nipple only

Stage 2

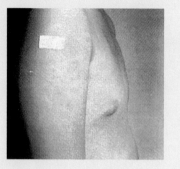

Breast bud stage. Elevation of breast and nipple as a small mound; enlargement of areolar diameter

Stage 3

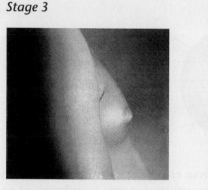

Further enlargement of elevation of breast and areola, with no separation of their contours

Stage 4

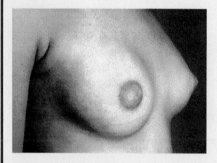

Projection of areola and nipple to form a secondary mound above the level of breast

Stage 5

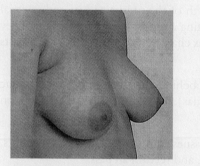

Mature stage; projection of nipple only. Areola has receded to general contour of the breast (although in some individuals, the areola continues to form a secondary mound).

(Photos used with permission of the American Academy of Pediatrics, *Assessment of Sexual Maturity Stages in Girls*, 1995.)

In approximately 10% of girls, the breasts develop at different rates, and considerable asymmetry may result in either size or Tanner stage. This generally resolves, and reassurance to the client is most helpful.

In older adolescent girls, a comprehensive breast examination should be accompanied by information about the Know Your Breasts approach (see Chapter 16).

It is helpful to counsel girls about this sequence and their current maturational stage. A girl's initial signs of puberty are hymeneal changes secondary to estrogen, widening of the hips, and beginning of a height spurt, although these changes are difficult to detect. The first easily detectable sign of puberty is usually the appearance

SEX MATURITY RATINGS IN GIRLS: PUBIC HAIR

Stage 1

Preadolescent—no pubic hair except for the fine body hair (vellus hair) similar to that on the abdomen

Stage 2

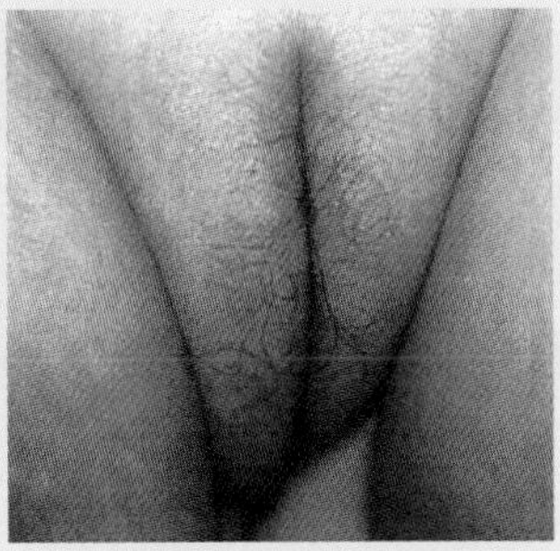

Sparse growth of long, slightly pigmented, downy hair, straight or only slightly curled, chiefly along the labia

Stage 3

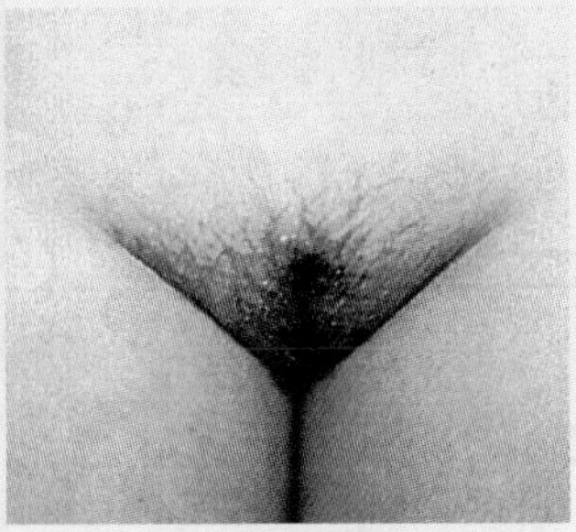

Darker, coarser, curlier hair, spreading sparsely over the pubic symphysis

Stage 4

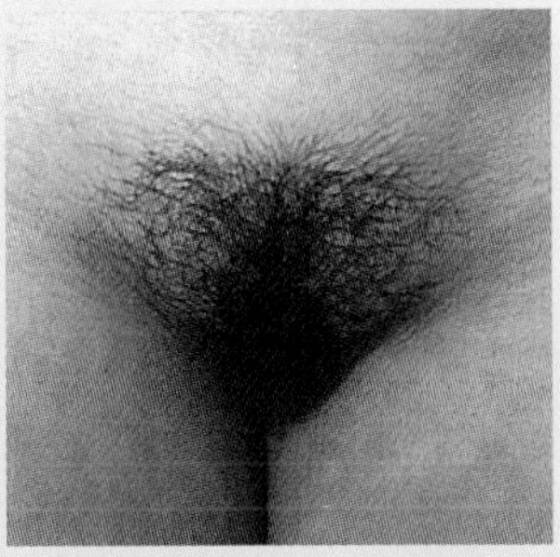

Coarse and curly hair as in adults; area covered greater than in stage 3 but not as great as in the adult and not yet including the thighs

Stage 5

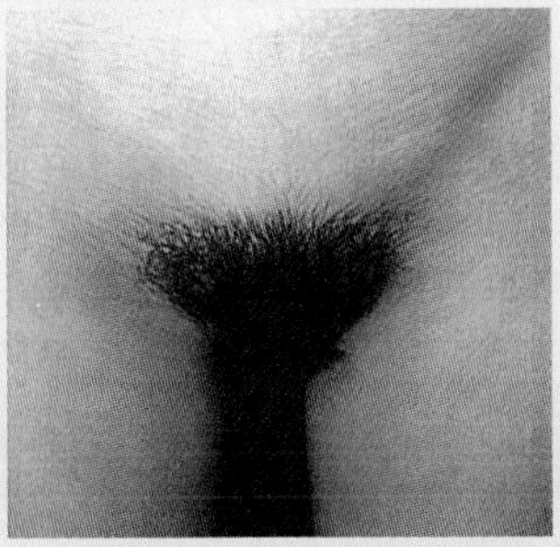

Hair adult in quantity and quality, spread on the medial surfaces of the thighs but not up over the abdomen

Photos used with permission of the American Academy of Pediatrics, *Assessment of Sexual Maturity Stages in Girls*, 1995.

of breast buds, although pubic hair sometimes appears earlier. The average age of the appearance of pubic hair has decreased in recent years, and current consensus is that the appearance of pubic hair as early as 7 years can be expected, particularly in dark-skinned girls who develop secondary sexual characteristics at an earlier age.

In most women, pubic hair spreads downward in a triangular pattern, pointing toward the vagina. In 10% of women, it may form an inverted triangle, pointing toward the umbilicus. Pubic hair growth is usually not completed until the mid-20s or later.

Just before menarche, there is a physiologic increase in vaginal secretions—a usual change that sometimes worries a girl or her mother. As menses become established, increased secretions (*leukorrhea*) coincide with ovulation. They also accompany

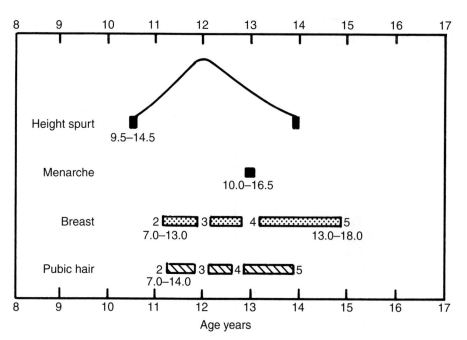

Numbers below the bars indicate the ranges in age within which certain changes occur. (Redrawn from Marshall WA, Tanner JM. Variations in the pattern of pubertal changes in girls. Arch Dis Child 45:22, 1970.)

sexual arousal. These usual kinds of discharges must be differentiated from those of infectious processes.

Lymphatics. Lymph from the vulva and the lower vagina drains into the inguinal nodes. Lymph from the internal genitalia, including the upper vagina, flows into the pelvic and abdominal lymph nodes, which are not palpable.

THE HEALTH HISTORY: SUBJECTIVE DATA

Key Symptoms and Signs Reported by the Client

- Changes related to menstrual periods
- Pregnancy
- Concerns related to sexual activity
- Discharge from the vagina

Inquiry about the genitalia and reproductive system requires nurses to be sensitive to the client's age and genetic background. Begin by explaining the purpose for taking a sexual history; for example, "I ask all my clients about their sexual health. May I ask you some questions about this?" (Chow & Day, 2007, p. 1380). Asking about a partner, or current meaningful relationship, may be a way to begin the sexual history. Ask about the client's present sexual activities, sexual orientation, and sexual concerns. Ask open-ended questions related to the symptoms, signs, and concerns reported by the client. Invite the client to fully participate in the discussion and dialogue regarding her concerns. Ensuring her comfort and privacy during history taking yields information that reflects the client's interpretation of the concerns being discussed. In addition, the nurse finds out from the client the effects the concern has on the quality of her life.

It may be appropriate to also screen for abuse. Three questions to use are as follows (Chow & Day, 2007, p. 1383):

- "In the past year, have you been hit, slapped, kicked, or otherwise physically hurt by someone?"

- "If pregnant, have you been hit, slapped, kicked, or otherwise physically hurt by someone?"

- "Have you ever been forced into sexual activity?"

Changes Related to Menstrual Periods.

For the menstrual history, ask the client how old she was when her monthly, or menstrual, periods began (age at *menarche*). When did her last period start and, if possible, the one before that? How often does she have periods, as measured by the interval between the first days of successive periods? How regular or irregular are they? How long do they last? How heavy is the flow? What colour is it? Flow can be assessed roughly by the number of pads or tampons used daily. Because women vary in their practices for sanitary measures; however, ask the client whether she usually soaks a pad or tampon, spots it lightly, and so on. Furthermore, does she use more than one at a time? Does she have any bleeding between periods? If sexually active, does she have any bleeding after intercourse?

Does the client have any discomfort or pain before or during her periods? If so, what is it like? How long does it last? Does it interfere with her usual activities? Are there other associated symptoms? What measures does she take to alleviate discomfort or pain? Ask a middle-aged or older woman if she has stopped menstruating. When? Did any symptoms accompany her change? Has she had any bleeding since?

Questions about *menarche, menstruation,* and *menopause* often provide an opportunity to explore the client's need for information and her attitude toward her body. When talking with an adolescent, for example, opening questions might include, "How did you first learn about monthly periods? How did you feel when they started? Many girls worry when their periods are not regular or come late. Has anything like that concerned you?" You can explain that girls in Canada usually begin to menstruate between the ages of 9 and 16 years (Estes & Buck, 2008), and often take 1 year or more before they settle into a regular pattern. Age at menarche is variable, depending on genetic endowment, socioeconomic status, and nutrition. The interval between periods ranges roughly between 24 and 32 days; the flow lasts between 3 and 7 days.

Menopause, the absence of menses for 12 consecutive months, usually occurs between the ages of 48 and 55 years (Van Noord et al., 1997). Associated symptoms include hot flashes, flushing, sweating, and disturbances of sleep. Often you will ask, "How do (did) you feel about not having your periods anymore? Has it affected your life in any way?" *Postmenopausal bleeding* is defined as bleeding that occurs after 6 months without periods and warrants further investigation.

Amenorrhea refers to the absence of periods. Failure to initiate periods is called *primary amenorrhea,* whereas the cessation of periods after they have been established is termed *secondary amenorrhea.* Pregnancy, lactation, and menopause are physiologic forms of the secondary type. *Oligomenorrhea* refers to infrequent periods, which may also be irregular. This pattern is common for as long as 2 years after menarche, and it also occurs before menopause.

The dates of previous periods signal possible pregnancy or menstrual irregularities.

Unlike the usual dark red menstrual discharge, excessive flow tends to be bright red and may include "clots" (not true fibrin clots).

Postmenopausal bleeding raises the question of endometrial cancer, although it also has other causes.

Other causes of *secondary amenorrhea* include low body weight from any cause, including malnutrition and anorexia nervosa, stress, chronic illness, and hypothalamic–pituitary–ovarian dysfunction.

Dysmenorrhea is pain with menstruation and is usually felt as a bearing down, aching, or cramping sensation in the lower abdomen and pelvis. Women may report *premenstrual syndrome (PMS)*, a complex of symptoms occurring 4 to 10 days before a period. PMS symptoms include tension, nervousness, irritability, depression, and mood swings; weight gain, abdominal bloating, edema, and tenderness of the breasts; and headaches. Though usually mild, PMS symptoms may be severe and disabling.

Chronic pelvic pain is described in relation to the menstrual cycle, to determine whether it is cyclic or acyclic. Common cyclic conditions are mittelschmerz (midcycle pain), primary and secondary dysmenorrhea, imperforate hymen, and pelvic congestion. Generally, women younger than 30 years experience mittelschmerz, and the pain may last from minutes to days. Usually, clients report it as aching, but on occasion it may be severe (Porth & Matfin, 2008).

Acyclic chronic pain may result from pelvic inflammatory disease, cysts or tumours, endometriosis, or uterine displacement. Young women most often notice it, describing a heavy feeling of discomfort in the lower abdomen, which is usually relieved when menstruation begins (Porth & Matfin, 2008).

Endometriosis primarily occurs in women of childbearing age, affecting 3% to 10% of them and 25% to 35% of infertile women (Memarzadeh et al., 2003). In this condition, some endometrial cells implant outside the uterine lining. During each menstrual cycle, these endometrial cells respond to hormonal fluctuations through physiologic changes and the formation of new lesions (McCance & Huether, 2006). The result is extensive adhesions and secondary dysmenorrhea. Women with endometriosis have a higher rate of infertility.

Polymenorrhea means unusually frequent periods, and *menorrhagia* refers to an increased amount or duration of flow. Bleeding may also occur between periods, termed *metrorrhagia* or *intermenstrual bleeding*, after intercourse (*postcoital bleeding*), or after other vaginal contact from practices such as douching.

Increased frequency, increased flow, or bleeding between periods may have systemic causes or may be dysfunctional. *Postcoital bleeding* suggests cervical disease (e.g., polyps, cancer) or, in an older woman, atrophic vaginitis.

Pregnancy. Questions relating to pregnancy include, "Have you ever been pregnant? How many times? How many living children do you have? Have you ever had a miscarriage? Or an abortion? How many times?" Ask about any difficulties during pregnancy and the timing and circumstances of any abortion, whether spontaneous or induced. How did the woman experience these losses? Record the pregnancy history using the "gravida-para" system, with the following abbreviations:

- G = gravida, or total number of pregnancies

- P = para, or outcomes of pregnancies. In addition, any pregnancy of 20 weeks or longer, regardless of delivery of a live or deceased infant, will be included in the para count. After P, you will often see the notations F (full-term), P (premature), A (abortion), and L (living child).

Inquire about methods of contraception used by the client and her partner. Is the client satisfied with the method chosen? Are there any questions about the options available?

If amenorrhea suggests a *current pregnancy*, inquire about the history of intercourse and *common early symptoms*: tenderness, tingling, or increased size of the breasts; urinary frequency; nausea and vomiting; easy fatigability; and feelings that the baby is moving, usually noted at about 20 weeks. Be considerate of the client's

Amenorrhea followed by heavy bleeding suggests a *threatened abortion* or *dysfunctional uterine bleeding* related to lack of ovulation.

feelings in discussing all these topics and explore them as seems indicated (see also Chapter 24, Assessing the Woman Who Is Pregnant).

Concerns Related to Sexual Activity.

Start with general questions such as, "Are you sexually active?" "Have you ever been sexually active?" If the client is sexually active ask, "How is sex for you?" Or "Are you having any concerns with sex?" You can also ask, "Are you satisfied with your sex life as it is now? Has there been any significant change in the last few years? Are you satisfied with your ability to perform sexually? How satisfied do you think your partner is? Do you feel that your partner is satisfied with the frequency of sexual activity?"

If the client has concerns about sexual activity, ask her to tell you about it. Direct questions help you assess each phase of the sexual response: desire, arousal, and orgasm. "Do you have an interest in sex?" inquires about the desire phase. For the orgasmic phase, "Are you able to reach climax (reach an orgasm or 'come')?" "Is it important for you to reach climax?" For arousal, "Do you get sexually aroused? Do you lubricate easily (get wet or slippery)? Do you stay too dry?"

Sexual dysfunctions are classified by the phase of sexual response. A woman may lack desire; she may fail to become aroused and to attain adequate vaginal lubrication; or, despite adequate arousal, she may be unable to reach orgasm much or all of the time. Causes include lack of estrogen, medical illness, psychosocial, and psychiatric conditions.

If appropriate, ask about *dyspareunia*, or discomfort or pain during intercourse. If present, try to localize the symptom. Is it near the outside, occurring at the start of intercourse, or does she feel it farther in, when her partner is pushing deeper? *Vaginismus* refers to an involuntary spasm of the muscles surrounding the vaginal orifice that makes penetration during intercourse painful or impossible. The cause of *vaginismus* may be physical or psychological.

Superficial pain suggests local inflammation, atrophic vaginitis, or inadequate lubrication; deeper pain may be from pelvic disorders or pressure on an ovary.

In addition to ascertaining the nature of a sexual concern, ask about its onset, severity (persistent or sporadic), setting, and factors, if any, which make it better or worse. What does the client think is the cause of the problem? What has she tried to do about it? What does she hope for? Sexual dysfunction is an important but complicated topic, involving the client's general health; medications and drugs, including use of alcohol; her partner's and her own knowledge of sexual practices and techniques; her attitudes, values, and fears; the relationship and communication between partners; and the setting in which sexual activity takes place.

More commonly, however, a sexual problem is related to situational or psychosocial factors.

Discharge from the Vagina.

The most common vulvovaginal symptoms are *vaginal discharge* and local *itching*. Follow your usual approach. If the client reports a discharge, inquire about its amount, colour, consistency, and odour. Ask about any local *sores* or *lumps* in the vulvar area. Are they painful or not? Because clients vary in their understanding of anatomic terms, be prepared to try alternative phrasing such as, "Any itching (or other symptoms) near your vagina? . . . Between your legs? . . . Where you urinate?"

See Table 22-1, Lesions of the Vulva, p. 821; also Table 22-6, Vaginal Discharge, p. 825.

Local symptoms or findings on physical examination may raise the possibility of *sexually transmitted infections* (STIs). Identify the sexual preference as to partners (male, female, or both). Inquire about sexual contacts and establish the number of sexual partners in the prior month and total number in client's lifetime. Ask whether the client has concerns about HIV disease, desires HIV testing, or has current or past partners at risk. Also ask about oral and anal sex and, if indicated, about symptoms involving the mouth, throat, anus, and rectum. If the client reports vaginal bleeding, use a symptom analyses approach to collect all relevant data.

Examples of Questions for Symptom Analysis—Vaginal Bleeding

- "Where is the bleeding coming from?" (*Location*)
- "Describe the bleeding—colour, odour, consistency, any clots?" (*Quality*)
- "Describe the amount of bleeding in 24 hours, as to number and size of pads/tampons used." "How often do you have to change?" "Are pads and tampons soaked when you change?" "Do you need to use more than one pad or tampon at a time?" "Is there a reason for seeking help today regarding your condition?" (*Severity*)
- "When did you first notice the bleeding?" "Did it start suddenly or gradually?" (*Onset*)
- "How long have you had the bleeding?" "Have you had it like this before?" (*Duration*)
- "When did the bleeding start?" "How long does it last?" "What is the interval between bleedings?" "When is it at its worst?" "Daytime or night time?" (*Time of day/month/year*)
- "What do you do to make the bleeding better?" Explore: "Medications?" "Dietary practices (eating or restricting certain foods)?" "Mental activities?" "Physical activities?" "Applying heat or cold to abdomen?" "What has worked in the past?" (*Alleviating factors*)
- "What makes the bleeding worse?" "Any activity?" "Sexual intercourse?" (*Aggravating factors*)
- "What other symptoms have you noticed with the bleeding?" Explore with the client: "Cramping?" "Bloating?" "Heavy feeling below?" "Abdominal pain?" "Constipation?" "Diarrhea?" "Fatigue?" (*Associated symptoms*)
- "What type of work do you do?" "Does anything in the work environment affect the bleeding?" "Anything in the home?" "Any recreational activities that affect the bleeding?" (*Environmental factors*)
- "How is this condition affecting your life?" (*Significance to client*)
- "What do you think is causing the bleeding?" (*Client's perspective*)

HEALTH PROMOTION

Important Topics for Health Promotion

- Options for family planning
- Menopause changes
- Risk factors and prevention of HPV and cancer
- Risk factors and prevention of other sexually transmitted infections (STIs), including HIV
- Genital self-examination and health practices

REPRODUCTIVE AND SEXUAL HEALTH

Options for Family Planning. It is important to counsel women, particularly teens, about the timing of ovulation in the menstrual cycle and how to plan or prevent pregnancy. Data indicate that more than half of pregnancies are unintended. Clinicians should be familiar with the numerous contraceptive methods and their effectiveness. These include natural (periodic abstinence, withdrawal, lactation), barrier (condom, diaphragm, cervical cap), implantable (intrauterine device, subdermal implant), pharmacologic (spermicide, birth-control pill, subdermal implant of levonorgestrel, estrogen/progesterone injectables and patch, vaginal ring), and surgical (tubal ligation) methods. Clinicians need to understand the concerns of the client or couple and respect their preferences when possible. Continued use of a preferred method is superior to a more effective method that is abandoned. For teens, a confidential setting eases discussion of topics that may seem private and difficult to them.

Menopause Changes. Be familiar with the psychological and physiologic changes of menopause—mood shifts; changes in self-concept; vasomotor changes ("hot flashes"); accelerated bone loss; increases in total and LDL cholesterol levels; and vulvovaginal atrophy leading to vaginal drying, dysuria, and, sometimes, dyspareunia.

Decisions about using hormone therapy (HT; formerly hormone replacement therapy [HRT]) in menopause are more challenging since the Women's Health Initiative (WHI) study. This randomized controlled trial of 16,000 women was stopped 3 years early when findings demonstrated that risks of HT outweighed benefits (those using HT had more risk of invasive breast cancer, heart attack, and blood clots than the control group (Writing Group for Women's Health Initiative Investigators [WGWHII], 2002). HT was effective in preventing hot flashes and decreasing osteoporotic fractures and colorectal cancer (WGWHII, 2002). Guidelines for managing menopausal symptoms are to use the lowest dose of HT (Canadian Institute for Health Information [CIHI], 2008) for as short as possible, preferably fewer than 5 years (Chow & Day, 2007). From 2000 to 2007, the number of women 65 years or older in Alberta, Saskatchewan, Manitoba, New Brunswick, and Nova Scotia taking estrogen-only HT decreased by 14.7% each year, while those taking combined HT dropped by 24.9% per year (CIHI, 2008).

RISK FACTOR ASSESSMENT

Risks for cervical cancer are both viral and behavioural. The most important is contracting the high-risk strains of human papillomavirus (HPV) 16 and 18, found in 95% to 100% of squamous cell cancers. There are more than 120 HPV genotypes (zur Haussen, 1996), and about 40 cause the following (de Villiers, 2001):

- Cancer of the cervix (95%)

- Nonmelanoma skin/cutaneous squamous cell cancer (90%)

- Anal cancer (more than 70%)

- Cancer of the vagina and vulva (50% for each)

- Oropharyngeal cancer (20%) (from oral sex; in newborns from vaginal birth)

Younger women have high rates of HPV. In a research study, more than 600 female college students received information before first intercourse on how to prevent HPV. Two years after first intercourse, 39% had HPV; 4 years after, 50% had it (Winer et al., 2003). While genital HPV appears particularly persistent in young sexually active women, 70% to 90% of cases clear over a 2-year period (Pinto & Crum, 2000). Thus, HPV DNA is no longer detectable on the mucosal or epithelial surface. In addition, clearance time varies with different HPV genotypes, from 5 to 6 months (HPV 6 and 11) to 8 to 14 months (HPV 16 and 18). It is unclear whether the virus is eliminated or remains latent in basal cells and can be reactivated under certain circumstances (Money & Provencher, 2007). In the remaining 10% to 30% of women, HPV continues to age of 15 to 25 years, becomes precancerous from 25 to 35 years, and moves to cancer of the cervix at 35 to 45 years. From 10 to 30 years can elapse between contracting HPV and cervical cancer (Lowy & Schiller, 2006).

Other risk factors include early sexual activity, multiple sexual partners, preference of partners (male, female, or both), history of STIs, failure to undergo screening, age, nutrition, smoking, immune status, and genetic polymorphism affecting the entry of HPV DNA into cervical cells. Having 10 or more lifetime sexual partners increases risk for HPV to 69%, compared with 21% for those with one partner (Ley et al., 1991). Each person brings to a sexual encounter possible exposure to HPV from all previous partners, thus the concern about number of partners of each sexual partner. Consistent use of condoms reduces risk of HPV by 70% but does not provide total protection (Winer et al., 2006). Women who use oral contraceptives may be less likely to use condoms, and thus have more possibilities of becoming infected with HPV.

Pap Smear. The Canadian Cancer Society/National Cancer Institute of Canada (2008) predicted that 1350 Canadian women would be diagnosed with and 385 would die from cervical cancer in 2008. Thus, on average, one Canadian woman dies from cervical cancer each day! While invasive cervical cancer is preventable and treatable, it is the second most common cancer in women worldwide (Parkin et al., 2001) as well as in Canadian women aged between 20 and 44 years (Society of Obstetricians and Gynaecologists of Canada, 2007).

Two primary types of cervical cancer are known: 80% to 90% are squamous cell carcinomas, and the remaining 10% to 20% are adenocarcinomas in glandular cells. Pap smear screening is not highly successful in isolating adenocarcinoma or its precursors. However, the actual proportion of adenocarcinomas appears to be increasing with the use of Pap screening in many Western countries (Money & Provencher, 2007): 1.83 out of 100,000 women in Canada may be diagnosed annually with adenocarcinomas (Liu et al., 2001).

Since the 1950s, Pap smear cervical cytology has contributed to a significant decline in incidence of and mortality from cervical cancer. Because screening practices differ among provinces/territories, health care professionals must be fully aware of the status of screening programs in their jurisdiction (Murphy, 2007). Also, the capacity of the provincial/territorial program influences the recommendations concerning initiation, intervals, and cessation of screening. This reinforces the need for regional recommendations in addressing issues pertaining to screening for cervical cancer (Murphy, 2007).

Cervical Screening in Canada

Conventional Cytology. The goal of screening is to determine who does and does not have a particular disease. How often the test correctly identifies those with a disease is called its *sensitivity*. How often it correctly identifies those without the disease is *specificity*. If early forms of disease precursors can be detected, interventions can be used to improve outcome (Murphy, 2007).

"The goal of cytologic screening is to sample the transformation zone, the area where physiologic transformation from columnar endocervical epithelium to squamous (ectocervical) epithelium takes place and where dysplasia and cancer arise" (U.S. Preventive Services Task Force, 2003). In Canada, the conventional glass slide is an accepted screening test for cervical cancer. But, "conventional Pap testing is less efficient at discriminating between women who have the disease and those who do not than is generally believed" (Nanda et al., 2000, p. 810). This means that Pap smear sensitivity estimates of women with cervical cancer were much lower than commonly understood. However, the specificity results (women without cervical cancer) were high. Thus, caution is necessary in placing full trust in the results obtained from one or occasional Pap smear(s) (Murphy, 2007). Ideally, women should initially have two Pap smears, 1 year apart. If both results are negative, then Pap smears every 2 to 3 years is recommended. This schedule provides a chronological picture of results, increasing the likelihood of an accurate diagnosis and effectiveness in reducing mortality (Murphy, 2007).

In Canada, two new tests have been introduced to screen for cervical cancer: liquid-based cytology (LBC) and HPV DNA testing. Their effectiveness is currently being evaluated.

LBC effectually reduces cervical cancer mortality (Murphy, 2007). Data are collected in the same way as for conventional cytology; however, specimens are placed in a vial containing cell-preserving fluid, not on slides. This ensures that almost all cellular material is preserved and available for analysis. Thus, LBC has greater sensitivity and specificity than the Pap smear, with a subsequent decreased need for repeat Pap screening. LBC is considered a highly promising technology for cervical screening programs (Murphy, 2007). At present, Ontario and Nunavat have incorporated LBC technology in a cervical screening program. In the near future, Newfoundland and British Columbia are planning to introduce LBC in their jurisdictions (Murphy, 2007).

HPV DNA testing is more sensitive than cytology and can be used for triage, primary screening, or posttherapeutic follow-up (Provencher & Murphy, 2007). Compared with cytology, it has higher sensitivity (95% vs. 84%), but slightly lower specificity (60% vs. 85%). While sensitivity of cytology varies from 19% to 76%, HPV DNA testing is consistently higher (85–100%) (Provencher & Murphy, 2007). Integrating HPV DNA testing will likely decrease the need for repeat cytology tests, thus lowering total costs of HPV screening. If LBC results are inconclusive, HPV DNA testing can be done automatically on the same sample. This eliminates the need to wait 3 to 6 months to repeat the cytology test. Clients with positive HPV DNA results can immediately undergo colposcopy (high-magnification microscope examination of the cervix) (Chow & Day, 2007) biopsy, if needed, and treatment. HPV DNA development for testing high-risk populations is promising (Provencher & Murphy, 2007). Newfoundland, Ontario, and Labrador have introduced HPV DNA testing (Murphy, 2007).

Brown et al. (2007) interviewed 22 Ontario women in the age group of 24 to 63 years about current knowledge of cervical screening practices, HPV, and HPV testing. Only 5 of the women had heard of HPV, while 15 knew some (mainly incorrect) information about genital warts. They were shocked at the prevalence of HPV and its link to cancer and questioned why they had not heard of it. When the women realized that HPV was transmitted sexually, they linked it to "infidelity, immorality and degenerate behaviour" (Brown et al., 2007, p. 792). They commented that "it would be totally embarrassing" to be positive, but "when it comes to your health, nothing is too embarrassing" (p. 792). They welcomed that the HPV DNA test could be done immediately, thereby reducing anxious waiting between cytology tests (usually 3–6 months) and having repeated pelvic examinations. Also, having more definitive results sooner meant that right treatment could start earlier. "Because if I have something, I want it looked after immediately, I don't want it to linger on any longer than it has to" (p. 793).

Recording Findings. The standardized Bethesda System of cytologic interpretation and terminology is highly valuable in presenting results to clients and health care providers, and in comparing results across Canada (Murphy, 2007). Since its development in 1988, it has been revised in 1991, 2001, and 2006 (report pending; Murphy, 2007). Most Canadian provinces use the 1991 version, while Ontario and Nova Scotia use 2001 terminology (Murphy, 2007).

The principal categories are as follows:

- *Negative for intraepithelial lesion or malignancy:* No cellular evidence of neoplasia is present, although organisms like *Trichomonas*, *Candida*, or *Actinomyces* may be reported. Shifts in flora consistent with bacterial vaginosis or cell changes from herpes simplex may also be reported.

■ *Epithelial cell abnormalities:* These include precancerous or cancerous lesions:

■ *Squamous cells,* including *atypical squamous cells* (ASC), which may be of undetermined significance (ASC-US); *low-grade squamous intraepithelial lesions* (LSIL), including mild dysplasia; *high-grade squamous intraepithelial lesions* (HSIL), including moderate and severe dysplasia with features suspicious for invasion; and invasive *squamous cell carcinoma.*

■ *Glandular cells,* including *atypical endocervical cells* or *atypical endometrial cells,* specified or not otherwise specified (NOS); *atypical endocervical cells* or *atypical glandular cells, favour neoplastic; endocervical adenocarcinoma in situ;* and *adenocarcinoma*

■ *Other malignant neoplasms* (e.g., sarcomas, lymphomas), both rare

Screening and Maintenance. While objectives for screening practices vary among provinces/territories, recommendations across Canada are similar and relate to the target population, initiation of Pap smear, intervals between Pap smears, and cessation of Pap smears (Murphy, 2007):

■ Annual screening is recommended after initiation of sexual intercourse regardless of age, or by age 18 to 20 years.

■ Interval between screenings is determined by the findings of the most recent Pap test. For example, after two negative results, the recommended interval is every 2 to 3 years.

■ More frequent Pap smears are recommended for women with unexpected cytology results and who engaged in intercourse before 18 years, have had multiple sexual partners, are HIV positive, and are immunocompromised.

■ In most of Canada, cessation of Pap screening is at age 69 or 70 years.

■ For women who have had a hysterectomy, screening is discontinued if the cervix was removed for benign reasons and there is no history of abnormal or cancerous cell growth. Women with a history of abnormal cell growth should be screened annually; screening is discontinued for such clients if three consecutive vaginal cytology tests are negative.

Challenges with Having Pap Smears. Several research teams have explored why women do or do not have initial Pap smears and then do not return for future tests. Having a Pap test is related to:

■ Age and level of education (Coe et al., 2007)

■ Age, having a clinical breast examination or a medical checkup within the past year, or having a physician recommend the test (Wallace et al., 2007)

■ Being examined by female health care providers (Buetow et al., 2007; Coe et al., 2007; Wallace et al., 2007; Van Til, 2003).

Not having a Pap test is related to:

■ Fear of the results

■ Poor access to the test (no doctor, waiting 6 months for appointment)

- "No time to look after themselves" but encouraging daughters to have the test (Van Til, 2003, p. 1122)

- Embarrassment over asking for the test

- Being examined by a male physician (Buetow et al., 2007; Coe et al., 2007; Wallace et al., 2007; Van Til, 2003)

- Feeling that the physician might be "too cavalier—routine thing for the doctor but to us it is very traumatic" (Van Til, 2003, p. 1123)

- Distress over disrobing because of age-related changes in appearance

- Failure of physicians to recommend the test (while 85% of participants in Van Til's earlier study in Prince Edward Island [1999] had seen doctors in the previous year, no physician had suggested the need for a Pap test)

Van Til et al. (2003) held focus groups with 60 women in Prince Edward Island. Three themes emerged. *Personal experiences* (value of self and relationship with the physician) interacted with *system issues* (accessibility, request for the Pap test, and valuing prevention), leading to *recommendations for improvement* (more female physicians, more pleasant environment, appointments, and knowledge). The women during their reproductive years generally saw obstetricians for pregnancies and birth control and were comfortable with them because they were considered "experts." As the women aged and if these physicians retired, women were often left with their family physician as the only option. For some, especially in small rural communities, the physician might be their neighbour or friend.

Comments such as "I don't have to have a Pap because I am no longer sexually active" (Van Til et al., 2003, p. 1126) and "I figured that I'm old, not old but 65— so I don't need a Pap anymore" (p. 1127) speak to the need for education and services for women older than 40 years. Pap screening may be "least accessible and least perceived as needed, however, among women over 40 years who are at the highest risk" for cervical cancer (Wallace et al., 2007, pp. 800–801). All Canadian provinces report fewer Pap smears for women older than 50 years (Snider et al., 1997). Nurses have a role to play in encouraging older women to have regular Pap tests.

Two other groups of women have fewer Pap tests. In a Canadian study of 38,000 women aged 20 to 69 years, those who were obese (BMI ≥ 30) were 30% to 40% less likely to have Pap smears than those with BMIs of 18.5 to 24.9. The main reason the women who were obese gave for not having Pap smears was fear—of embarrassment, pain, or finding something wrong (Mitchell et al., 2008). Women with disabilities, chronic disabling conditions, or both may also have fewer Pap smears. Issues relate to reduced mobility and dexterity (transportation to the health provider's office, getting undressed and dressed, getting on the examining table, and being able to assume an appropriate position for the pelvic examination; see p. 807 for alternate positions). For example, in a study of 220 women with multiple sclerosis, 25% did not have regular pelvic examinations and 11% had not had a Pap smear in 3 to 5 years (Shabas & Weinreb, 2000). There is rarely justification for omitting the pelvic examination (Chow & Day, 2007).

Regular gynecology examinations (including swabs and Pap tests) are necessary to detect infections, cancer, and other gynecologic conditions. The Canadian Cancer Society/National Cancer Institute of Canada (2008) predicted the following numbers of cancer cases and deaths for women in 2008:

Location of Cancer	Number of Cases	Number of Deaths
Body of Uterus	4287	805
Ovary	2461	1715
Bladder	1667	525
Cervix	1349	385

The high rate of deaths from ovarian cancer is of note because it is equal to the total number of deaths from cancer of the body of the uterus, bladder, and cervix. While currently no test is available for early detection of cancer of the ovary (other than regular pelvic examinations), a blood test is in development.

RISK FACTORS AND PREVENTION OF STIs AND HIV

The Canadian Guidelines on Sexually Transmitted Infections (2006) reflect the change in terminology from sexually transmitted diseases (STDs) to the more inclusive term of STIs (Public Health Agency of Canada [PHAC], 2006, 2008). In Canada, chlamydia, gonorrhoea, infectious syphilis, and HIV/AIDS are reportable STIs. While HPV is the most common STI, it is not reportable. Rates of genital chlamydia, gonorrhea, infectious syphilis, and HIV/AIDS continue to increase (PHAC, 2007a, 2007b).

Infection	Cases	Rates	Increases by Provinces
Genital chlamydia	72,390	219.5/100,00	British Columbia, Alberta, Manitoba, Ontario, Quebec, Nova Scotia, Northern Territory, Nunavut
Gonorrhea	11,515	34.9/100,000	British Columbia, Ontario, New Brunswick, Prince Edward Island, Newfoundland, Northern Territory
Infectious Syphilis	1168	3.5/100,000	Alberta, Manitoba, New Brunswick, Nova Scotia, Prince Edward Island, Newfoundland

For infectious syphilis, overall cases fell in 2005; however, from 2005 to 2007, nine Alberta women (15–40 years) gave birth to babies with congenital syphilis (Singh et al., 2007). Total cases of syphilis in pregnant women in the rest of Canada were only 3 in 2005 and 4 in 2006 (PHAC, 2006). Since July 2007, five more Alberta babies have been born with syphilis, and a total of five newborns have died from congenital syphilis (Simons, 2008; Zabjek, 2008). Factors that contribute to continual increases in rates of chlamydia, gonorrhea, and infectious syphilis are early age of sexual intercourse, lack of knowledge about risk-decreasing behaviours, and continuation of sex in later years.

In 2005, 10,000 to 13,500 Canadian women were living with HIV/AIDS. Women account for 20% of the total cases of HIV/AIDS (PHAC, 2007b).

 Cultural Consideration

Aboriginal Canadians are overrepresented in the number of cases of HIV/AIDS, with a rate 2.8 times higher than for non-Aboriginal people (PHAC, 2007b).

Prevention and control of STIs require implementation of primary and secondary prevention measures. Primary prevention focuses on identifying at-risk people and giving necessary information and education such as use of latex condoms (for male partners), female condoms (which cover more of the female genital area), and dental dams for oral sex (for both sexes). Researchers report that increased parent communication with adolescents led to delayed onset of initiating sexual intercourse (Hutchinson, 2002), less sexual activity (Hutchinson et al., 2003), increased condom use (Hutchinson & Cooney, 1998), more consistent condom use (Hutchinson et al., 2003), and more comfort with sexual risk-related discussions with partners (Hutchinson & Cooney, 1998). They also found that such communication influenced adolescents' behavioural, narrative, and control beliefs related to engaging in sexual risk behaviour (Hutchinson & Wood, 2007). When mothers talked with their adolescent daughters about high-risk sexual behaviours, there were fewer sexual episodes and unprotected sexual episodes, but no change in number of sexual partners (Hutchinson et al., 2003).

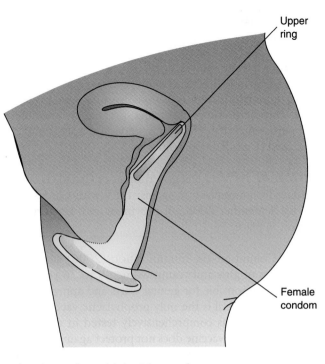

Secondary prevention centres attention on detection of infection in at-risk populations and treating infected people using available remedies and counseling. Also, acting to prevent further spread of infection, by partner notification and treating infected persons, is important (World Health Organization, 2006). Nurses working with people with STIs need:

- Awareness of their own beliefs and attitudes and values

- Respectful and open-minded views of different lifestyles and sexual preferences

- Comfortable with clients of all ages

- Awareness of the importance of nonverbal communication (e.g., eye contact, tone of voice, body language)

- Comfortable with topics such as anal sex, oral sex, past sex, and future sex

The five *Rs* for counselling clients with an STI are as follows (Parker, 2007):

- Be *Real* with clients—help them explore the psychosocial effects of their diagnosis. Clients may report disgust, embarrassment, anger, fear, self-blame, betrayal, low self-esteem, and diminished sexual desirability. They may ask, "How did I get this?" "Who did I get it from?" "How long have I had it?" and "Will I ever be able to have sex without a condom?"

- *Review* what clients know and what Internet sources they have used.

- Be a *Resource*—help clients build on current knowledge (transmission and characteristics of the infection, treatment options, and prevention).

- **Reassure** clients that they have a commonly occurring infection and that they will have help to manage it.

- **Reiterate** the plan and what was discussed.

Untreated chlamydia, gonorrhea, and infectious syphilis can result in pelvic inflammatory disease, chronic pelvic pain, ectopic pregnancy, and infertility. In addition, the role of persistent HPV infection in cervical dysplasia and carcinoma has already been discussed (Canadian Guidelines on STIs, 2006).

Specific Prevention of HPV.   The government of Canada is committed to ensuring federal funding for immunization against HPV with Gardasil vaccine for girls 9 to 10 years. By September 2008, all provinces and territories had HPV immunization programs in place.

The National Advisory Committee on Immunization (2006) supports research findings that immunization of girls and young women 9 to 26 years will protect them from strains of HPV responsible for genital warts and approximately 70% of cervical cancers. Currently, Gardasil is the only prophylactic vaccine against HPV available in North America. It was comprehensively tested in clinical trials with 25,000 women over a decade. The vaccine does not protect against all types of HPV that cause cervical cancers. Nevertheless, Gardasil is considered an important prophylactic measure to stem the increase of cervical cancer in young women (HPV Awareness, 2006).

Ideally, the vaccine is given before the sexual debut. Also, it is important for females to receive it at the right times for full benefits: in three doses at 1 month, 3 months, and 6 months. Women who have already acquired a type of HPV may not get full advantage of the vaccine (Shier & Bryson, 2007).

SPECIFIC PREVENTION OF SPECIFIC DISEASES

Pap Smears for Cervical Cancer.   Health professionals know that regular gynecologic examinations and Pap smears throughout a woman's life will result in early detection of cervical and other cancers. Attention is needed on how to make the Pap smear/pelvic examination more tolerable. Part of this includes a more pleasant environment, female health care providers for the examination, ways for providers rather than clients to make appointments automatically, and having a women's health clinic where both Pap smears and mammograms could be done at the same time (Buetow et al., 2007; Coe et al., 2007; Wallace et al., 2007; Van Til, 2003).

Female Genital Self-Examination.   A self genital examination is a systematic approach for detecting changes such as lesions, warts, and discharge. The following are instructions:

- Do the examination *sitting* on the edge of a chair or *standing*.

- Have a good light source and use a hand mirror to see the structures.

- Check pubic hair for nits (pubic lice) and at base of hairs for skin rashes.

- Gently spread apart the outer folds (labia majora), one side at a time. Look for swelling, redness, bumps, sores, blisters, lacerations, or warts (cauliflower-like sores).

- Gently spread apart the inner folds (labia minora), one side at a time. Look for swelling, redness, bumps, sores, blisters, lacerations, or warts.

- Look near the top of the inner folds for the clitoris—check colour and look for any sores.

- Look at the vaginal opening. (It appears as a slit if you have not had sexual intercourse. It is larger if you have had sexual intercourse and more so if you had a baby by vaginal birth.) Look for vaginal discharge, if you find any note its amount, colour, and appearance.

- Examine the anal area for rashes, sores, or warts.

Self-Care Practices. Review these self-care practices with female clients:

WAYS TO PREVENT STIs:

- Delay first sexual intercourse.
- Restrict the number of sexual partners.
- Avoid sex with people who have multiple partners.
- Use condoms regardless of whether you use other birth-control methods (e.g., oral contraceptives).
- Obtain the HPV vaccine. Ideally you should have the vaccine before you are sexually active. It protects against cancer of the cervix; some skin cancers; cancer of the vulva, vagina, and anus; and genital warts.

Use of Oral Contraceptives (Chow & Day, 2007):

- Use a condom.
- Take birth-control pill at same time each day.
- Stop smoking, or cut down.
- Report the following symptoms immediately: ACHES
  A – abdominal pain
  C – chest pain
  H – headaches
  E – eye problems (blurred vision, seeing spots)
  S – severe leg pain.

Plan B to Prevent Pregnancy

- If you have intercourse without birth control or the birth-control method fails (e.g., the condom breaks), see a pharmacist right away about Plan B to prevent pregnancy. The drug is available without a prescription.

Know the Warning Signs/Symptoms of STIs:

- Pain in pelvic area
- Itchy rash around the vagina
- Changes in vaginal discharge (colour, amount, appearance)
- Bleeding between menstrual periods
- Pain or burning on urination (passing urine)

Practice Genital Hygiene

- Wash external genitals with water and a very mild (nonperfumed) soap.
- The vagina is self-cleaning, so there is no need to put solutions into it (e.g., douching). Douching solutions may cause irritation or an allergic reaction in the vagina and nearby tissue.
- Reduce a moist genital environment by wearing cotton panties (or at least ones with a cotton crotch) and not wearing jeans in hot weather.

Reduce Risk of Bladder Infections:

- Increase intake of fluids (avoid fluids containing caffeine).
- Pass urine every 2–3 hours during the day and evening.
- Pass urine before and after sexual intercourse.
- Avoid bubble baths.

Source: Adapted from Potter, P. A., Perry, A. G., Ross-Kerr, J. C., & Wood, M. J. (Eds.) (2006). *Canadian fundamentals of nursing* (3rd ed.). Toronto, ON: Elsevier Canada.

EMERGENCY CONCERNS

Excessive Vaginal Bleeding. Abnormal bleeding is not uncommon during the childbearing years and around menopause. During the childbearing years, causes of bleeding are attributed to clinical types of abortion (threatened, missed, inevitable, incomplete, and septic). Bleeding also may occur with ectopic pregnancy. In this case, pain prior to the bleeding is a telling sign.

In contrast, excessive vaginal bleeding does not always accompany many gynecologic conditions. Nurses must be aware that there is always a possibility of concealed excessive bleeding. It is highly important to obtain a focused health history and to conduct a physical examination germane to the presenting problem to reach an accurate diagnosis before intervening. Some important signs to monitor are pulse rate, breathing, skin colour, and blood pressure.

Excess bleeding is associated with interstitial tumours and subendometrial fibromyomata. Bleeding after menopause is highly significant, and malignancy of the endometrium must be ruled out (Porth & Matfin, 2008).

Abdominal Pain. Abdominal pain, acute or chronic, can be of gynecologic origin. Causes include infection related to acute salpingo-oophoritis, septic abortion, or ruptured abscess; irritation from blood in the peritoneal cavity following a ruptured ectopic pregnancy, retrograde menstruation, an intrauterine device (IUD), dilatation and curettage (D & C), or uterine perforation; vascular complications from torsion of an adnexal or a paraovarian cyst; and carcinoma of the body of the uterus or cervix (Porth & Matfin, 2008).

Bartholin's Gland Infection. Bartholin glands play a significant role in keeping the internal labial surfaces continuously lubricated. Inflammation of them usually results from infection with streptococci, staphylococci, chlamydia, or *Escherichia coli*. Affected glands are typically inflamed and painful, and the client may be febrile. In addition, the ducts leading to the gland are susceptible to obstruction, which may result in Bartholin cysts (Porth & Matfin, 2008).

Route of entry of these organisms is through infection of the lower part of the female external genitalia. Nurses can help reduce Bartholin's glands infections by teaching clients to follow appropriate hygiene practices, have protected sex, and engage in a monogamous sexual relationship.

Pelvic Inflammatory Disease (PID). PID is most often the result of an STI of the fallopian tubes (salpingitis) or tubes plus ovaries (salpingo-oophoritis). It is caused by *Neisseria gonorrhoeae*, *Chalmydia trachomatis*, and other organisms. Clients with PID experience lower abdominal pain. *Acute* disease is associated with very tender, bilateral adnexal masses, although pain and muscle spasm usually make it impossible to delineate them. Movement of the cervix produces pain. If not treated, a tubo-ovarian abscess or infertility may ensue (Porth & Matfin, 2008). Clients with multiple sexual partners have a greater occurrence of PID than those who are monogamous.

Ruptured Tubal Pregnancy. Ruptured tubal pregnancy spills blood into the peritoneal cavity, causing severe abdominal pain and tenderness. Guarding and rebound tenderness are sometimes associated. A unilateral adnexal mass may be palpable, but tenderness often prevents its detection. Faintness, syncope, nausea, vomiting, tachycardia, and shock may occur, reflecting the hemorrhage (Porth & Matfin, 2008). The client may have a prior history of amenorrhea or other symptoms of pregnancy.

Important Areas of Examination

External Examination	Internal Examination
■ Mons pubis	■ Vagina, vaginal walls
■ Labia majora and minora	■ Cervix
■ Urethral meatus, clitoris	■ Uterus, ovaries
■ Vaginal introitus	■ Pelvic muscles
■ Perineum	■ Rectovaginal wall

◤ PROMOTING CLIENT COMFORT, DIGNITY, AND SAFETY

Of all the physical assessment examinations, the pelvic examination causes the most concerns for women. Canadian women expressed negative reactions about the following aspects of the environment and pelvic examination (Van Til, 2003): the cold and uncomfortable room, being exposed, lack of dignity, discomfort and embarrassment, and feeling vulnerable because they didn't know what to expect. One subject described the pelvic examination this way:

"Well, just there with my feet stuck up in the air. *Did you know what the doctor was doing? (Researcher)* Well no, the sheet was up and you couldn't see him. But I could feel him probing around. But it was embarrassing, And I never went back" (p. 1120). Another subject commented: "I just gave up going (*for a Pap smear*) because I'm uncomfortable and I'm shivering and I'm uptight when they're doing it and he's there hollering at me, 'Relax! Relax!'. Well I couldn't relax and it's cold and it's hard" (p. 1126). Some women had the feeling they were "being molested" during the exam and some reported having flashbacks (p. 1120).

It is significant to note that not one of the 60 women in the PEI study shared any positive comments about the Pap smear test (Van Til et al., 2003).

Many students feel anxious or uncomfortable when first examining the genitalia of another person. At the same time, clients have their own concerns. Some women have had painful, embarrassing, or even demeaning experiences during previous pelvic examinations, whereas others may be facing their first examination. Clients may fear what the clinician will find and how these findings may affect their lives.

The woman's reactions and behaviour give important clues to her feelings and to attitudes toward sexuality. If she adducts her thighs, pulls away, or expresses negative feelings during the examination, you can gently talk with her as you would during the interview. "I notice you are having some trouble relaxing. Is it just being here? Or are you troubled by the examination? Is anything worrying you?" Behaviours that seem to present an obstacle to your examination may become the key to understanding your client's concerns. Adverse reactions may be a sign of prior abuse, and these issues should be explored.

A client who has never had a pelvic examination is often unsure of what to expect. Try to shape the experience so that she learns about her body and the steps of the pelvic examination, and becomes more comfortable with them. Before she undresses, explain the relevant anatomy with the help of 3D models. Show her the speculum and other equipment and encourage her to handle them during the examination so that she can better understand your explanations and procedures. It is especially important to inform the client fully regarding the procedure to reduce discomfort. Ideally, have a warm examining room and a bath blanket for the client. Allow the client time to get undressed and to sit on the examining table. Knock and ask permission before re-entering the room. Assist the client into an appropriate position on the examining table. Also, this is an opportune time for the client to learn more about her body—the examiner can use the mirror to show the client the areas being examined. Discussion following the examination (with the client dressed) could include what measures the client can institute to enhance and maintain the health of her reproductive system.

TIPS FOR THE SUCCESSFUL PELVIC EXAMINATION

The Client

- Avoids intercourse, douching, or use of vaginal suppositories for 24–48 hours before examination
- Empties bladder before examination
- Lies supine, with head and shoulders elevated, arms at sides or folded across chest to enhance eye contact and reduce tightening of abdominal muscles

The Examiner

- Explains each step of the examination in advance
- Drapes client from mid-abdomen to knees; depresses drape between knees to provide eye contact with client
- Avoids unexpected or sudden movements
- Warms speculum with tap water
- Monitors comfort of the examination by watching the client's face
- Uses excellent but gentle technique, especially when inserting the speculum

---

Indications for a pelvic examination during adolescence include menstrual abnormalities such as amenorrhea, excessive bleeding, or dysmenorrhea, unexplained abdominal pain; vaginal discharge; the prescription of contraceptives; bacteriologic and cytologic studies in a sexually active client, and the client's own desire for assessment.

All female clients who have been raped require specific support and assessment. Specially prepared nurses (Sexual Assault Nurse Examiners [SANEs]) work in emergency departments and provide comprehensive care to women who have been sexually assaulted. Their role includes providing the support needed before, during, and after the general and gynecologic examinations so that the client does not feel that she is being violated again. Collection of specimens (using a special rape kit) and photographs requires meticulous attention to detail in terms of the quality and identification (name, date, time) to maintain the chain of custody for evidence. SANEs are also prepared to testify in legal proceedings.

Equipment

- Bath blanket
- Gloves
- Good light
- Mirror
- Vaginal specula—several types and sizes
- Water-soluble lubricant
- Equipment for taking Pap smears, bacteriologic cultures, or other diagnostic equipment

Be sure always to wear gloves, both during the examination and when handling equipment and specimens. Plan ahead, so that any needed equipment and culture media are readily at hand.

Helping the client to relax is essential for an adequate examination. Adopting the tips above will help ensure the client's comfort.

Note that male examiners should be accompanied by female assistants. Female examiners should also be assisted if the client is physically or emotionally challenged. Also be aware of the cultural requirements for being with female clients during the examination.

Choosing Equipment.   You should have within reach a good light, a vaginal speculum of appropriate size, water-soluble lubricant, and equipment for taking Pap smears, bacteriologic cultures, or other diagnostic tests. Review the supplies and procedures of your own facility before taking cultures and other samples.

Specula are made of metal or plastic and come in two basic shapes, named for Pedersen and Graves. Both are available in small, medium, and large sizes. The medium Pedersen speculum is usually most comfortable for sexually active women. The narrow-bladed Pedersen speculum is best for the client with a relatively small introitus, such as a virgin or an elderly woman. The Graves specula are best suited for parous women with vaginal prolapse.

Before using a speculum, become thoroughly familiar with how to open and close its blades, lock the blades in an open position, and release them again. Although the instructions in this chapter refer to a metal speculum, you can easily adapt them to a plastic one by handling the speculum before using it.

Plastic specula typically make a loud click or may pinch when locked or released. Forewarning the client helps to avoid unnecessary surprise.

Positioning the Client.   Drape the client appropriately and then assist her into the lithotomy position. Help her to place first one heel and then the other into the stirrups. She may be more comfortable with shoes on than with bare feet. Then ask her to slide all the way down the examining table until her buttocks extend slightly beyond the edge. Her thighs should be flexed, abducted, and externally rotated at the hips. A pillow should support her head.

Alternate, more comfortable, positions are available for the pelvic examination. Their use depends on the physical limitations of the client and the personal preferences of the client and nurse. Three examples include the following (Seidel et al., 1995):

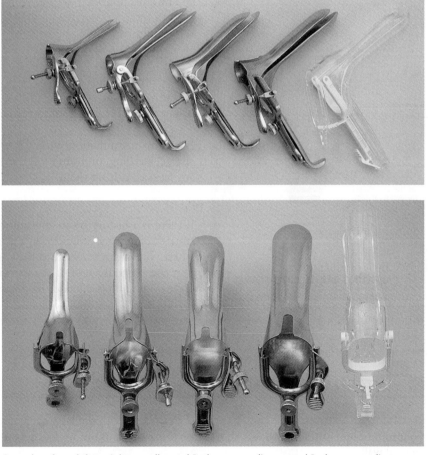

Speculae, from left to right: small metal Pedersen, medium metal Pedersen, medium metal Graves, large metal Graves, and large plastic Pedersen

- Side-lying position with the bottom leg bent or straight and the top leg bent and pulled up close to the chest

- Diamond-shaped position: The client lies on her back, with heels together and knees spread apart

- M-shaped position: The client lies on her back, with knees bent and apart, and feet flat on the examining table, close to her buttocks

In some of these positions, it may be necessary to insert the vaginal speculum with the handle up.

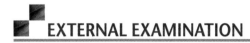

EXTERNAL EXAMINATION

Assess the Sexual Maturity of an Adolescent Client. You can assess pubic hair during either the abdominal or the pelvic examination. Note its character and distribution, and rate it according to Tanner's stages described on p. 787.

Delayed puberty is often familial or related to chronic illness. It may also be from abnormalities in the hypothalamus, anterior pituitary gland, or ovaries.

Examine the External Genitalia. Seat yourself comfortably and warn the client that you will be touching her genital area. Inspect the mons pubis, labia, and perineum. Separate the labia and inspect

Excoriations or itchy, small, red maculopapules suggest *pediculosis pubis* (lice or "crabs"). Look for nits or lice at the bases of the pubic hairs.

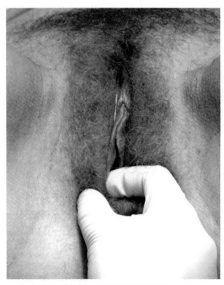

PALPATING BARTHOLIN'S GLAND

- The labia minora

- The clitoris

Enlarged clitoris in masculinizing conditions

- The urethral meatus

Urethral caruncle, prolapse of the urethral mucosa (p. 822)

- The vaginal opening, or introitus

Note any inflammation, ulceration, discharge, swelling, or nodules. If there are any lesions, palpate them.

Herpes simplex, Behcet's disease, syphilitic chancre, epidermoid cyst. See Table 22-1, Lesions of the Vulva (p. 821).

If there is a history or an appearance of labial swelling, check Bartholin's glands. Insert your index finger into the vagina near the posterior end of the introitus. Place your thumb outside the posterior part of the labium majus. On each side in turn, palpate between your finger and thumb for swelling or tenderness. Note any discharge exuding from the duct opening of the gland. If any is present, culture it.

A *Bartholin's gland* may become acutely or chronically infected and then produce a swelling. See Table 22-2, Bulges and Swelling of the Vulva, Vagina, and Urethra (p. 822).

INTERNAL EXAMINATION

Assess the Support of the Vaginal Walls. With the labia separated by your middle and index fingers, ask the client to bear down. Note any bulging of the vaginal walls.

Bulging from a *cystocele or rectocele.* See Table 22-2, Bulges and Swelling of the Vulva, Vagina, and Urethra (p. 822).

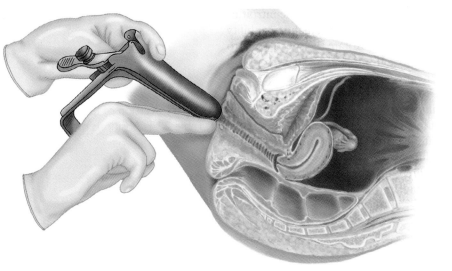

Insert the Speculum. Select a speculum of appropriate size and shape, and lubricate it with warm, but not hot, water. (Other lubricants may interfere with cytologic studies and bacterial or viral cultures.) You can enlarge the vaginal introitus by lubricating one finger with water and applying downward pressure at its lower margin. Check the location of the cervix to help angle the speculum more accurately. Enlarging the introitus greatly eases insertion of the speculum and the client's comfort. With your other hand (usually the left), introduce the closed speculum past your fingers at a somewhat downward slope. Be careful not to pull on the pubic hair or pinch the labia with the speculum. Separating the labia majora with your other hand can help to avoid this.

THE SMALL INTROITUS

Many virginal vaginal orifices admit a single examining finger. Modify your technique so as to use your index finger only. A small Pedersen speculum may make inspection possible. When the vaginal orifice is even smaller, a fairly good bimanual examination can be performed by placing one finger in the rectum rather than in the vagina, but warn the client first!
Similar techniques may be indicated in elderly women if the introitus has become atrophied and tight.

An *imperforate hymen* occasionally delays menarche. Be sure to check for this possibility when menarche seems unduly late in relation to the development of a girl's breasts and pubic hair.

Two methods help you to avoid placing pressure on the sensitive urethra. (1) When inserting the speculum, hold it at an angle (shown below on the left), and then (2) slide the speculum inward along the posterior wall of the vagina, applying downward pressure to keep the vaginal introitus relaxed.

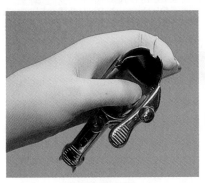

ENTRY ANGLE

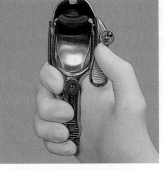

ANGLE AT FULL INSERTION

After the speculum has entered the vagina, remove your fingers from the introitus. You may wish to switch the speculum to the right hand to enhance manoeuvrability of the speculum and subsequent collection of specimens. Rotate the speculum into a horizontal position, maintaining the pressure posteriorly, and insert it to its full length. Be careful not to open the blades of the speculum prematurely.

Inspect the Cervix.

Open the speculum carefully. Rotate and adjust the speculum until it cups the cervix and brings it into full view. Position the light until you can visualize the cervix well. When the uterus is retroverted, the cervix points more anteriorly than illustrated. If you have difficulty finding the cervix, withdraw the speculum slightly and reposition it on a different slope. If discharge obscures your view, wipe it away gently with a large cotton swab.

See retroversion of the uterus, Table 22-7, Positions of the Uterus.

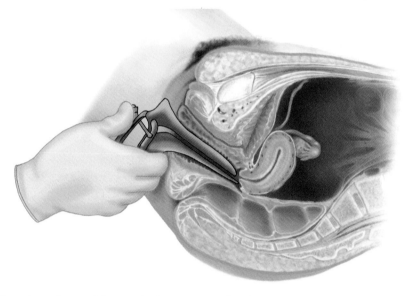

Note the colour of the cervix, its position, the characteristics of its surface, and any ulcerations, nodules, masses, bleeding, or discharge. Inspect the cervical os for discharge.

See Table 22-3, Variations in the Cervical Surface (p. 823), Table 22-4, Shapes of the Cervical Os (p. 824), and Table 22-5, Unexpected Changes in the Cervix (p. 824).

Maintain the open position of the speculum by tightening the thumb screw.

A yellowish discharge on the endocervical swab suggests a mucopurulent cervicitis, commonly caused by *Chlamydia trachomatis, Neisseria gonorrhoeae,* or herpes simplex (Table 22-6, Vaginal Discharge). Raised, friable, or lobed wartlike lesions in *condylomata* or *cervical cancer.*

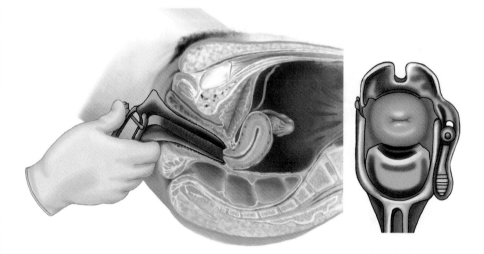

Obtain Specimens for Cervical Cytology (Papanicolaou Smears).
Obtain one specimen from the endocervix and another from the ectocervix, or a combination specimen using the cervical brush ("broom"). For best results the client should not be menstruating. She should avoid intercourse and use of douches, tampons, contraceptive foams or creams, or vaginal suppositories for 48 hours before the examination. In addition to obtaining the Pap smear, for sexually active women aged 25 or younger, and for other asymptomatic women at increased risk for infection, plan to culture the cervix routinely for *Chlamydia trachomatis*.

Chlamydial infection is linked to urethritis, cervicitis, pelvic inflammatory disease, ectopic pregnancy, infertility, and chronic pelvic pain. Risk factors include age younger than 25, multiple partners, and prior history of STIs.

OBTAINING THE PAP SMEAR: OPTIONS FOR SPECIMEN COLLECTION

Cervical Scrape and Endocervical Brush

Cervical Scrape. Place the longer end of the scraper in the cervical os. Press, turn, and scrape in a full circle, making sure to include the *transformation zone* and the *squamocolumnar junction.* Smear the specimen on a glass slide. Set the slide in a safe spot that is easy to reach. Note that doing the cervical scrape first reduces obscuring cells with blood, which sometimes appears with use of the endocervical brush.

Endocervical Brush. Take the endocervical brush and place it in the cervical os. Roll it between your thumb and index finger, clockwise and counterclockwise. Remove the brush and pick up the slide you have set aside. Smear the slide with the brush, using a gentle painting motion to avoid destroying any cells. Place the slide into an ether–alcohol solution at once, or spray it promptly with a special fixative.

Note that for women who are pregnant, a cotton-tip applicator, moistened with saline, is advised in place of the endocervical brush.

Cervical Broom

Many clinicians now use a plastic brush tipped with a broomlike fringe for collection of a single specimen containing both squamous and columnar epithelial cells. Rotate the tip of the brush in the cervical os, in a full clockwise direction, then stroke each side of the brush on the glass slide. Promptly place the slide in solution or spray with a fixative as described previously.

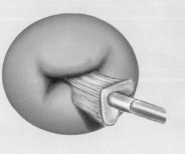

Alternatively, place the sample directly into preservative so that the laboratory can prepare the slide (liquid-based cytology).

Inspect the Vagina. Withdraw the speculum slowly while observing the vagina. As the speculum clears the cervix, release the thumb screw and maintain the open position of the speculum with your thumb. Close the speculum as it emerges from the introitus, avoiding both excessive stretching and pinching of the mucosa. During withdrawal, inspect the vaginal mucosa, noting its colour and any inflammation, discharge, ulcers, or masses.

See Table 22-6, Vaginal Discharge (p. 825).

Cancer of the vagina

Perform a Bimanual Examination. Lubricate the index and middle fingers of one of your gloved hands, and *from a standing position,* insert them into the vagina, again exerting pressure primarily posteriorly. Your thumb should be abducted, your ring and little fingers flexed into your palm. Pressing inward on the perineum with your flexed fingers causes little if any discomfort and allows you to position your palpating fingers correctly. Note any nodularity or tenderness in the vaginal wall, including the region of the urethra and the bladder anteriorly.

Stool in the rectum may simulate a rectovaginal mass, but, unlike a tumour mass, can usually be dented by digital pressure. Rectovaginal examination confirms the distinction.

Palpate the cervix, noting its position, shape, consistency, regularity, mobility, and tenderness. Usually the cervix can be moved somewhat without pain. Feel the fornices around the cervix.

Pain on movement of the cervix, together with adnexal tenderness, suggests *pelvic inflammatory disease.*

Palpate the uterus. Place your other hand on the abdomen about midway between the umbilicus and the symphysis pubis. While you elevate the cervix and uterus with your pelvic hand, press your abdominal hand in and down, trying to grasp the uterus between your two hands. Note its size, shape, consistency, and mobility, and identify any tenderness or masses.

See Table 22-7, Positions of the Uterus (p. 826) and Table 22-8, Disorders of the Uterus (p. 827).

Uterine enlargement suggests pregnancy or benign or malignant tumours.

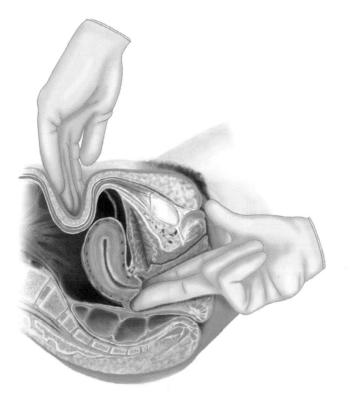

Now slide the fingers of your pelvic hand into the anterior fornix and palpate the body of the uterus between your hands. In this position your pelvic fingers can feel the anterior surface of the uterus, and your abdominal hand can feel part of the posterior surface.

Nodules on the uterine surfaces suggest *myomas* (Table 22-8, Disorders of the Uterus).

If you cannot feel the uterus with either of these manoeuvres, it may be tipped posteriorly (retrodisplaced). Slide your pelvic fingers into the posterior fornix and feel for the uterus butting against your fingertips. An abdominal wall that is obese or poorly relaxed may also prevent you from feeling the uterus even when it is located anteriorly.

See *retroversion* and *retroflexion of the uterus* (p. 826).

Palpate each ovary. Place your abdominal hand on the right lower quadrant, your pelvic hand in the right lateral fornix. Press your abdominal hand in and down, trying to push the adnexal structures toward your pelvic hand. Try to identify the right ovary or any adjacent adnexal masses. By moving your hands slightly, slide the adnexal structures between your fingers, if possible, and note their size, shape, consistency, mobility, and tenderness. Repeat the procedure on the left side.

Three to five years after menopause, the ovaries have usually atrophied and are no longer palpable. If you can feel an ovary in a postmenopausal woman, consider an abnormality such as a cyst or a tumour.

Ovaries are usually somewhat tender. They are usually palpable in slender, relaxed women but are difficult or impossible to feel in others who are obese or poorly relaxed.

Adnexal masses include ovarian cysts, tumours, and abscesses, also the swollen fallopian tube(s) of pelvic inflammatory disease, and a tubal pregnancy. A uterine myoma may simulate an adnexal mass. See Table 22-9, Adnexal Masses (p. 828).

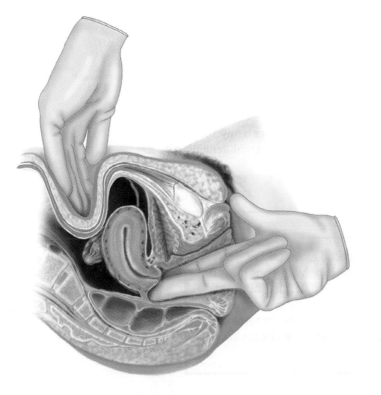

Assess the Strength of the Pelvic Muscles.
Withdraw your two fingers slightly, just clear of the cervix, and spread them to touch the sides of the vaginal walls. Ask the client to squeeze her muscles around them as hard and long as she can. A squeeze that compresses your fingers snugly, moves them upward and inward, and lasts 3 seconds or more is full strength.

Impaired strength may be due to age, vaginal deliveries, or neurologic deficits. Weakness may be associated with urinary stress incontinence.

Do a Rectovaginal Examination.
Withdraw your fingers. Lubricate and change your gloves again if necessary (see note on using lubricant). Then slowly reintroduce your index finger into the vagina, your middle finger into the rectum. Ask the client to strain down as you do this so that her anal sphincter will relax. Tell her that this examination may make her feel as if she has to move her bowels but

that she will not do so. Repeat the manoeuvres of the bimanual examination, giving special attention to the region behind the cervix that may be accessible only to the rectal finger.

Rectovaginal palpation is especially valuable in assessing a retrodisplaced uterus, as illustrated. It also allows palpation of the uterosacral ligaments, the cul-de-sac, and the adnexa.

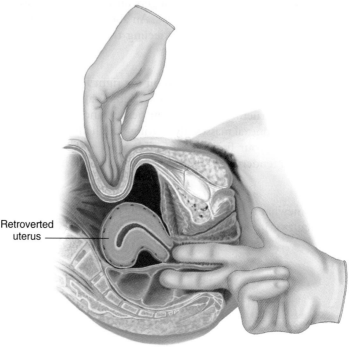

Retroverted uterus

Proceed to the rectal examination (see Chapter 23). If a hemoccult test is planned, you should change gloves to avoid contaminating fecal material with any blood provoked by the Pap smear. After the examination, wipe off the external genitalia and rectum, or offer the client some tissue so she can do it herself.

USING LUBRICANTS

If you use a tube of lubricant during a pelvic or rectal examination, you may inadvertently contaminate it by touching the tube with your gloved fingers after touching the client. To avoid this problem, let the lubricant drop onto your gloved fingers without allowing contact between the tube and the gloves. If you or your assistant should inadvertently contaminate the tube, discard it. Small disposable tubes for use with one client circumvent this problem.

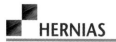 **HERNIAS**

Hernias of the groin occur in women as well as in men, but they are much less common. The examination techniques (see Chapter 23) are basically the same as for men. A woman too should stand up to be examined. To feel an indirect inguinal hernia, however, palpate in the labia majora and upward to just lateral to the pubic tubercles.

An indirect inguinal hernia is the most common hernia that occurs in the female groin. A femoral hernia ranks next in frequency.

SPECIAL TECHNIQUES

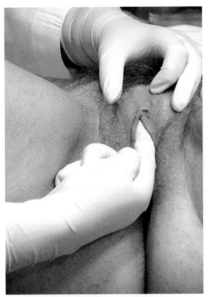

MILKING THE URETHRA

If you suspect urethritis or inflammation of the paraurethral glands, insert your index finger into the vagina and milk the urethra gently from inside outward. Note any discharge from or about the urethral meatus. If present, culture it.

Urethritis may arise from infection with *Chlamydia trachomatis* or *Neisseria gonorrhoeae*.

RECORDING AND ANALYZING FINDINGS

Recording and analysis of data must be accurate, comprehensive, and organized, and use terminology that all interprofessional team members understand to maintain continuity of care. The following is an example:

Examples of Documentation: Female Genitalia		
Areas of Assessment	**Expected Findings**	**Unexpected Findings**
External Genitalia	■ Mons Pubis: Skin colour consistent; labia majora and minora symmetrical. No ecchymosis, excoriation, rashes, swelling, or inflammation. Even hair distribution in shape of inverted triangle. No nits or lice. No tenderness elicited on light and deep palpation. ■ Clitoris: Not enlarged ■ Urethral opening slitlike, midline, and not prolapsed ■ No discharge or odour ■ No evidence of female circumcision ■ Vaginal opening: no lesions or discharge noted ■ Anal area pigmented and clear	■ Mons Pubis: Pubic hair sparse. Asymmetry of labia majora and minora. ■ Rash over mons pubis ■ Hypertrophy of clitoris ■ Urethral opening slightly reddish and indurated ■ Vaginal opening ulcerated, and a large amount of thick yellow, foul-smelling discharge noted ■ External genitalia tender to touch ■ Evidence of female circumcision ■ Evidence of trauma to vaginal region

(continued)

■ *Examples of Documentation: Female Genitalia (Continued)*

Areas of Assessment	Expected Findings	Unexpected Findings
Internal Genitalia	**Inspection and Palpation** ■ Cervix midline, smooth, evenly pink. Projects 3 cm into the vagina ■ No lacerations or ulceration noticed ■ Vaginal wall pink, moist, smooth, and totally rugated ■ Vaginal discharge clear and odourless ■ Vaginal walls strong without bulging of anterior or posterior walls ■ Vaginal muscle strong; tone intact	**Inspection and Palpation** ■ Cervical surface asymmetrical, reddened; ulceration and lacerations noted. ■ During Pap smear, cervical area bleeding noted ■ Tenderness on palpation of cervix ■ Lacerations all over vaginal mucosa ■ Thick, copious, green, foul-smelling discharge ■ Vaginal area tender to touch ■ Weak vaginal muscle strength/tone
	Bimanual Examination ■ Cervix smooth and firm ■ No pain while cervix moved from side to side ■ No tenderness elicited ■ Uterus not enlarged ■ Fundus round and firm ■ Uterus moves freely ■ No tenderness elicited on palpation	**Bimanual Examination** ■ Cervix firm but not smooth, contour irregular, mobility intact, tenderness to palpation ■ Uterus enlarged, irregular in shape ■ Does not move freely ■ Tenderness elicited during palpation
	Rectovaginal Examination ■ On palpation posterior wall of uterus firm, smooth, moves freely ■ No tenderness elicited ■ No nodules felt	**Rectovaginal Examination** ■ On palpation tenderness elicited ■ A mass and/or small nodules felt

ANALYZING FINDINGS FROM HISTORY AND PHYSICAL EXAMINATION

Nurses analyze findings from a client's history (subjective data) and physical examination (objective data) to arrive at nursing diagnoses. The following case study provides an example of the plan of care for Mrs. B. Huck:

Mrs. Huck, 45 years old, G2, P2 (children 17 and 15 years) has come to the clinic concerned that "for the last 3 months I have been experiencing pain during sex with my husband. Hence, I'm not enjoying sex with him." She states that before the presenting condition, she always enjoyed sex with her husband. She also mentions that she is very apprehensive before sex because of the vaginal odour and discharge that she has been experiencing, particularly during intercourse. Mrs. Huck states that she and her husband have sex 4 to 6 times a week. She is amazed that her husband does not notice that she is uncomfortable and carries on as usual. She states, "I am worried something is wrong with me, and if I continue having sex, am I harming myself or him?"

Provision of comprehensive care means that the nurse refers Mrs. Huck to her family physician for complete physical and pelvic examinations, including vaginal swabs, Pap smear, and laboratory tests. Mrs. Huck requires medical treatment to resolve her presenting problem. Also, it is necessary to examine Mr. Huck to determine whether he is infected. If so, he requires relevant medical and nursing interventions to resolve his condition. If swabs from either or both Mr. and Mrs. Huck come back positive for an STI, additional team members (e.g., nurse from an STI clinic, possibly a psychologist) may become involved. Based on collected subjective and objective data, the team constructs and implements appropriate interventions in a timely manner. This is crucial to stop the chances for recurrence of the present condition affecting Mr. and Mrs. Huck.

Two nursing diagnoses are:

■ ***Sexual dysfunction*** *related to altered body function (vaginal discharge and pain)*

■ ***Alteration in relationship with spouse*** *related to altered body function (vaginal discharge and pain)*

Critical Thinking Exercise

Answer the following questions about Mrs. Huck's presenting condition:

■ What are some causes of vaginal discharge? (*Knowledge*)
■ What are the implications of Mrs. Huck's presenting condition for her, her marriage, and her children? (*Comprehension*)

■ Describe your approach with rationale that will help Mrs. Huck in the resolution of her presenting concern. (*Application*)
■ What factors related to Mrs. Huck's present condition do you consider to fully illuminate her situation? (*Analysis*)
■ What will be your recommendations for maintaining continuity of care for Mrs. Huck? (*Synthesis*)
■ How would you evaluate the effectiveness of your implemented interventions for Mrs. Huck? (*Evaluation*)

Research

*Ahlberg, K., Ekman, T., Wallgren, A., & Gaston-Johansson, F. (2004). Fatigue, psychological distress, coping, and quality of life in clients with uterine cancer. *Journal of Advanced Nursing, 45*(2), 205–213.

Cockell, S. J., Oates-Johnson, T., Gilmour, D. T., Vallis, T. M., & Turnbull, G. K. (2003). Postpartum flatal and fecal incontinence quality-of-life scale: A disease-and population-specific measure. *Qualitative Health Research, 13*(8), 1132–1144.

Daly, M. B., & Ozols, R. F. (2004). Symptoms of ovarian cancer—where to set the bar. *Journal of the American Medical Association, 291*(22), 2755–2756.

*Denny, E. (2004). Women's experiences of endometriosis. *Journal of Advances in Nursing, 46*(6), 641–648.

Hutchinson, M. K. (2002). Sexual risk communication with mothers and fathers: Influence on sexual risk behaviours of adolescent daughters. *Family Relations, 51*, 238–245.

*Hutchinson, M. K., & Cooney, T. M. (1998). Patterns of parent-teen sexual risk communication: Implications for intervention. *Family Relations, 47*, 185–194.

Hutchinson, M. K., Jemmott, J. B., Jemmott, L. S., Braverman, P., & Fong, G. T. (2003). The role of mother-daughter sexual risk communication in reducing sexual risk behaviours among urban adolescent females: A prospective study. *Journal of Adolescent Health, 33*, 98–107.

*Hutchinson, M. I., & Wood, E. B. (2007). Reconceptualizing adolescent sexual risk in a parent-based expansion of the theory of planned behaviour. *Journal of Nursing Scholarship, 39*(2), 141–146.

*Lemaire, G. S. (2004). More than just menstrual cramps: Symptoms and uncertainty among women with endometriosis. *Journal of Obstetrical, Gynecologic and Neonatal Nurses, 33*(1), 71–79.

Mitchell, H. (2004). Vaginal discharge – Causes, diagnosis, and treatment. *British Medical Journal, 328*(7451), 1306–1308.

*Van Til, L., MacQuarrie, C., & Herbert, R. (2003). Understanding the barriers to cervical screening among older women. *Qualitative Health Research, 13*(8), 1116–1131.

------

*Indicates nursing research.

Test Questions

1. The most important risk factor for cervical cancer is
   a. immunosuppressive illnesses.
   b. failure to seek Pap smear screening.
   c. persistent human papillomaviral infections.
   d. poor nutrition and smoking during adolescence.

2. Menopausal women experience which of the following symptoms?
   a. Polyuria, weight loss, increased sweating
   b. Vasomotor changes, increased cholesterol levels, bone loss
   c. Increased self-concept, decreased cholesterol levels, polyuria
   d. Decreased cholesterol levels, vaginal atrophy, mood instability

3. When palpating the internal female genitalia, the nurse separates the client's labia and asks her to strain down to assess
   a. vaginal mucosa lesions.
   b. edematous labia majora.
   c. support of vaginal walls.
   d. Bartholin's gland inflammation.

4. When collecting a specimen for cytology from the cervix, the nurse
   a. presses firmly on a glass slide with the applicator end.
   b. labels glass slides and treats immediately with fixative.
   c. uses water-soluble lubricant to ease insertion of the speculum.
   d. collects specimens from endocervix, ectocervix, and lateral fornices.

5. When inserting the vaginal speculum, the nurse angles the blades obliquely and presses along the posterior vaginal wall to
   a. promote relaxation.
   b. facilitate identification of the cervix.
   c. prevent pressure on the urethra.
   d. avoid sensitive posterior structures.

Bibilography

CITATIONS

Brown, L., Ritvo, P., Howlett, R., Cotterchio, M., Matthew, A., Rosen, B., et al. (2007). Attitudes toward HPV testing: Interview findings from a random sample of women in Ontario, Canada. *Health Care for Women International, 28,* 728–798.

Buetow, S., Janes, R., Steed, R., Ihimaera, L., & Elley, C. R. (2007). Why don't some women return for cervical smears? A hermeneutic phenomenological investigation. *Health Care for Women International, 28,* 843–852.

Canadian Cancer Society/National Cancer Institute of Canada. (2008). *Canadian cancer statistics 2008.* Toronto, ON: Author.

Canadian Institute for Health Information (CIHI). (2008). Analysis in brief. *Hormone replacement therapy: An analysis focusing on drug claims by female seniors, 2000 to 2007.* Retrieved October 30, 2008, from http://secure.cihi.ca/cihiweb/displ Page.jsp?cw_page=AR_2130_E

Chow, J., & Day, R. A. (2007). Assessment and management of female physiologic processes. In R. A. Day, P. Paul, B. Williams, S. C. Smeltzer, & B. Bare (Eds.), *Brunner & Suddarth's textbook of medical-surgical nursing* (1st Canadian ed., pp. 1374–1415). Philadelphia: Lippincott Williams & Wilkins.

Coe, K., Martin, L., Nuvayestewa, L., Attaki, A., Papenfull, M., Guernsey De Zapien, J., et al. (2007). Predictors of Pap test use among women living on the Hopi reservation. *Health Care for Women International, 28*(9), 764–781.

Cox, J. T. (2006). Epidemiology and natural history of HPV. *Journal of Family Practice, 55*(Suppl.), 3–9.

de Villiers, E.-M. (2001). Taxonomic classification of papillomaviruses. *Papillomavirus Report, 12*(3), 57–63.

Harris, M. M. B. (2004). *Medical statistics made easy.* London: Martin Dunitz.

Health Canada. (2007). *Summary of basis of decision: Gardasil.* Retrieved October 19, 2008, from http://www.hc-sc.gc.ca/dhp-mps/prodpharma/sbd-smd/phase1-decision/drug-med/sbd_smd_2007_gardasil_102682-eng.php

Hutchinson, M. K. (2002). Sexual risk communication with mothers and fathers: Influence on sexual risk behaviours of adolescent daughters. *Family Relations, 51,* 238–245.

Hutchinson, M. K., & Cooney, T. M. (1998). Patterns of parent-teen sexual risk communication: Implications for intervention. *Family Relations, 47,* 185–194.

Hutchinson, M. K., Jemmott, J. B., Jemmott, L. S., Braverman, P., & Fong, G. T. (2003). The role of mother-daughter sexual risk communication in reducing sexual risk behaviours among urban adolescent females: A prospective study. *Journal of Adolescent Health, 33.* 98–107.

Hutchinson, M. I., & Wood, E. B. (2007). Reconceptualizing adolescent sexual risk in a parent-based expansion of the theory of planned behaviour. *Journal of Nursing Scholarship, 39*(2), 141–146.

Ley, C., Bauer, H. M., Reingold, A., Schiffman, M. H., Chambers, J. C., Tashiro, C. J., et al. (1991). Determinants of genital human papillomavirus infection in young women. *Journal of the National Cancer Institute, 83*(14), 997–1003.

Liu, S, Semenciw, R., & Mao, Y. (2001). Cervical cancer: The increasing incidence of adenocarcinoma and adenosquamous carcinoma in younger women. *Canadian Medical Association Journal, 164,* 1151–1152.

Lowy, D. R., & Schiller, J. T. (2006). Prophylactic human papillomavirus vaccines. *The Journal of Clinical Investigation, 116*(5), 1167–1173.

McCance, K. L., & Huether, S. E. (Eds.). (2006). *Pathophysiology: The biologic basis for disease in adults and children* (5th ed.). St. Louis, MO: Elsevier Mosby.

Memarzadeh, S., Muse, K. N., Jr., & Fox, M. D. (2003). Endometriosis. In A. H. Miller, B. A., Kolonel, L. N., Bernstein, L., Young, J. L., Swanson, G. M., West, D. W., et al. (Eds.), *Racial/ethnic patterns of cancer in the United States 1988—1992.* Bethesda, MD: National Cancer Institute.

Mitchell, R. S., Padwal, R. S., Chuck, A. W., & Klarenbach, S. W. (2008). Cancer screening among the overweight and obese in Canada. *American Journal of Preventive Medicine, 35*(2), 127–132.

Morgan, K., McCance, K. L., & Robinson. (2004). Alterations of the reproductive systems. In S. E. Huether & K. L. McCance (Eds.), *Understanding pathophysiology* (4th ed., pp. 861–916). St. Louis, MO: Mosby.

Murphy, K. J. (2007). Screening for cervical cancer. *Journal of the Society of Obstetrics and Gynaecology Canada, 29*(8, Suppl. 3), S27–S36.

Nanda, K., McCrory, D. C., Myers, E. R., Bastian, L. A. Hasselblad, V., Hickey, J. D., et al. (2000). Accuracy of Papanicolaon test in screening for and follow up to the cervical cytologic abnormalities: A systematic review. *Annals of Internal Medicine, 132,* 810–819.

National Advisory Committee on Immunization. (2006). *Statement on human papillomavirus vaccine.* Retrieved November 3, 2008, from http://www.phac-aspc.gc.ca/publicat/cig-gci/index-eng.php

Parker, P. (2007). Approaches for counseling clients with sexually transmitted infections. Sexually Transmitted Disease (STD) Centre, Alberta Health Services — M Capital Health, Edmonton, AB. (STD/HIV Information Line: 1-800-772-2437).

Parkin, D. M., Bray, F., Ferlay, J., & Pisani, P. (2001). Estimating the world cancer burden: Globocan 2000. *International Journal of Cancer, 94*(2), 153–156.

Pinto, A. P., & Crum, C. P. Natural history of cervical neoplasia: Defining progression and its consequence. *Clinical Obstetrics & Gynecology, 43*(2), 352–362.

Porth, C. M., & Matfin, G. (2008). *Pathophysiology: Concepts of altered health states* (8th ed., North American Ed.). Philadelphia: Lippincott Williams & Wilkins.

Potter, P. A., Perry, A. G., Ross-Kerr, J. C., & Wood, M. J. (Eds.). (2006). *Canadian fundamentals of nursing* (3rd ed.). Toronto, ON: Elsevier Canada.

Provencher, D. M., & Murphy, K. J. (2007). The role of HPV testing. *Journal of the Society of Obstetrics and Gynaecology Canada, 29*(8, Suppl. 3), S15–S21.

Public Health Agency of Canada. (2006). *Canadian guidelines on sexually transmitted infections, 2006 edition.* Ottawa, ON: Author. Retrieved October 29, 2008, from http://www.phac-aspc.gc.ca/std-mts/sti_2006/pdf/sti2006_e.pdf

Public Health Agency of Canada, Centre for Communicable Diseases and Infection Control. (2007a). *Reported cases of notifiable STI from January 1 to December 31, 2006 and January 1 to December 31, 2007 and corresponding rates for January 1 to December 31, 2006 and 2007.* Retrieved October 16, 2008, from http://www.phac-aspc.gc.ca/std-mts/stdcases-casmts/cases-cas-08-eng.php

Public Health Agency of Canada. (2007b). National HIV prevalence and incidence estimates for 2005. *HIV/AIDS Epi Update,* November 2007. Retrieved October 16, 2008, from http://www.phac-aspc.gc.ca/aids-sida/publication/epi-epi2007-eng.html

Public Health Agency of Canada. (2007c). *Recommendations on a human papillomavirus immunization program.* Retrieved October 16, 2008, from http://www.phac-aspc.gc.ca/publicat/2008/papillomavirus-papillome/papillomavirus-papillome-index-eng.php

Public Health Agency of Canada. (2008). *Updates to the Canadian guidelines on sexually transmitted infections.* Retrieved September 15, 2008, from http://www.phac-aspc.gc.ca/std-mts/sti_2006/pdf/Guidelines_Eng_complete_06-26-08.pdf

Seidel, H. M., Ball, J. W., Dains, J. E., & Benedict, G. W. (1995). *Mosby's guide to physical examination* (3rd ed.). St. Louis, MO: Mosby.

Shabas, D., & Weinreb, H. (2000). Preventive healthcare in women with multiple sclerosis. *Journal of Women's Health & Gender-Based Medicine, 9*(4), 389–395.

Shier, M., & Bryson, P. (2007). Vaccines. *Journal of Obstetrics and Gynaecology Canada, 29*(8, Suppl. 3), S51–S54.

Simons, P. (2008, November 11). Province hushes up syphilis outbreak. *The Edmonton Journal,* pp. A1, A2.

Singh, A. E., Sutherland, K., Lee, B., Robinson, J. L., & Wong, T. (2007). Resurgence of early congenital syphilis in Alberta. *Canadian Medical Association Journal, 177*(1), 33–36.

Snider, J., Beauvais, J., Levy, I., Villeneuve, P., & Pennock, J. (1997). Trends in mammography and Pap smear utilization in Canada. *Chronic Diseases in Canada, 17*(3). Retrieved November 17, 2008, from http://www.phac-aspc.gc.ca/publicat/cdic-mcc/17-3/c_e.html

Society of Obstetricians and Gynaecologists of Canada. (2007). *SOGC Position Statement on CMAJ Commentary, "Human papillomavirus, vaccines Women's health questions and cautions."* Retrieved May 9, 2008, from http://sogc.medical.org/media/guidelines-hpv-commentary_e.asp

van Noord, P. A., Dubas, J. A., & Dorland, M. (1997). Age at natural menopause in a population-based screening cohort: The role of menarche, fecundity, and life style factors. *Fertility and Sterility, 68*(1), 95–102.

Van Til, L. D. (1999). *An evaluation of PEI Well Women Clinics as a recruitment stategy for cervical cancer screening.* Charlottetown, PEI: Department of Health and Social Services.

Van Til, L. D., MacQuarrie, C., & Herbert, R. (2003). Understanding the barriers to cervical cancer screening among older women. *Qualitative Health Research, 13*(8), 1116–1131.

Wallace, D., Hunter, J., Papenfuss, M., Guernsey De Zapien, J., Denman, C., & Giuliano, A. R. (2007). Pap smear screening among women ≥ 40 years residing at the United States-Mexico border. *Health Care for Women International, 28,* 799–816.

Winer, R. L., Lee, S. K., & Hughes, J. P. (2003). Human papillomavirus infection incidence and risk factors in a cohort of female university students. *American Journal of Epidemiology, 157,* 218–226.

Winer, R. L., Lee, S. K., Hughes, J. P., Feng, Q., O'Reilly, S., Kiviat N. B., et al. (2006). Condom use and the risk of genital human papillomavirus infection in young women. *New England Journal of Medicine, 354*(25), 2645–2654.

World Health Organization. (2006). *Preventing and treating sexually transmitted and reproductive tract infections.* Geneva, Switzerland: Author. Retrieved May 10, 2008, from www.who.int/hiv/topics/sti/prev/en/print.html

Writing Group for Women's Health Initiative Investigators (WGWHII). (2002). Risks and benefits of estrogen plus progestin in healthy postmenopausal women: Principal results from the Women's Health Initiative randomized controlled trial. *Journal of the American Medical Association, 288*(3), 321–333.

Zabjek, A. (2008, August 9), Syphilis cases broken down. *The Edmonton Journal*, pp. B1, B4.

zur Haussen, H. (1996). Roots and perspectives of contemporary papillomavirus research. *Journal of Cancer Research and Clinical Oncology, 122*(1), 3–13.

ADDITIONAL REFERENCES

Brisson, M., Van De Velde, N., De Wais, P., & Boily, M. C. (2007). Estimating the number needed to vaccinate to prevent diseases and death related to human papillomavirus infection. *Canadian Medical Association Journal, 177*(5), 464–468.

Dawar, M., Deeks, S., & Dobson, S. (2007). Human papillomavirus vaccines launch a new era in cervical cancer prevention. *Canadian Medical Association Journal, 177*(5), 456–461.

Franco, E. L., & Harper, D. M. (2005). Vaccination against human papillomavirus infection: A new paradigm in cervical cancer control. *Vaccine, 23*(17-18), 2388–2394.

Monga, A. (Ed.). (2006). *Gynaecology by ten teachers* (18th ed.). London: Arnold.

U.S. Preventive Services Task Force. (2003). *Screening for cervical cancer: Clinical considerations.* Retrieved October 18, 2008, from http://www.ahrq.gov/clinic/3rduspstf/cervcan/cervcanrr.htm#clinical

CANADIAN ASSOCIATIONS AND WEB SITES

Canadian Women's Health Network: http://www.cwhn.ca/indexeng.html

Female Genital Mutilation: http://www.cirp.org/pages/female

Health Canada and Society of Gynecologic Oncologists of Canada. Programmatic Guidelines for Screening of Cancer of Cervix: http://www.phac-aspc.gc.ca/ccdpc-cpcmc/cc-ccu/pdf/screening.pdf

Human Papillomavirus (HPV) Society of Obstetricians and Gynaecologists of Canada (SOGC): http://www.sexualityandu.ca

Ontario Human Rights Commission. Policy on Female Genital Mutilation: http://www.ohrc.on.ca/en/resources/Policies/PolicyFGM2/view

Public Health Agency of Canada: http://www.phac-aspc.gc.ca

Society of Obstetricians and Gynaecologists of Canada (SOGC). Human Papillomavirus (HPV) Awareness: http://www.sogc.org/projects/hpv_e.asp

INTERNATIONAL

The North American Menopause Society (NAMS): http://www.menopause.org/

TABLE 22-1 **Lesions of the Vulva**

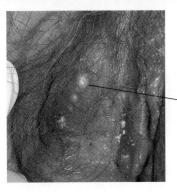

Cystic
nodule
in skin

Epidermoid Cyst

A small, firm, round cystic nodule in the labia suggests an epidermoid cyst. These are yellowish in colour. Look for the dark punctum marking the blocked opening of the gland.

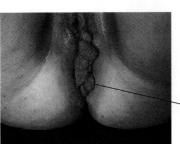

Warts

Genital (Venereal) Wart

(Condyloma Acuminatum)

Warty lesions on the labia and within the vestibule suggest condyloma acuminatum. They result from infection with human papillomavirus.

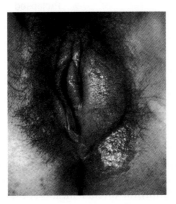

Syphilitic Chancre

A firm, painless ulcer suggests the chancre of primary syphilis. Because most chancres in women develop internally, they often go undetected.

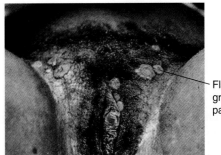

Flat,
gray
papules

Secondary Syphilis

(Condyloma Latum)

Slightly raised, round or oval, flat-topped papules covered by a grey exudate suggest condylomata lata. These constitute one manifestation of secondary syphilis and are contagious.

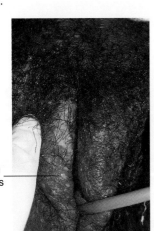

Shallow
ulcers on
red bases

Genital Herpes

Shallow, small, painful ulcers on red bases suggest a herpes infection. Initial infection may be extensive, as shown. Recurrent infections usually are confined to a small local patch.

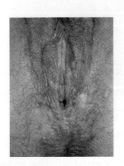

Carcinoma of the Vulva

An ulcerated or raised red vulvar lesion in an elderly woman may indicate vulvar carcinoma.

TABLE 22-2   Bulges and Swelling of the Vulva, Vagina, and Urethra

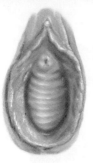

Cystocele

A cystocele is a bulge of the upper two thirds of the anterior vaginal wall, together with the bladder above it. It results from weakened supporting tissues.

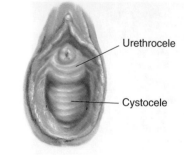

Cystourethrocele

When the entire anterior vaginal wall, together with the bladder and urethra, is involved in the bulge, a cystourethrocele is present. A groove sometimes defines the border between urethrocele and cystocele, but is not always present.

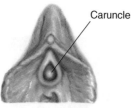

Urethral Caruncle

A urethral caruncle is a small, red, benign tumour visible at the posterior part of the urethral meatus. It occurs chiefly in postmenopausal women and usually causes no symptoms. Occasionally, a carcinoma of the urethra is mistaken for a caruncle. To check, palpate the urethra through the vagina for thickening, nodularity, or tenderness, and feel for inguinal lymphadenopathy.

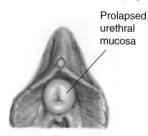

Prolapse of the Urethral Mucosa

Prolapsed urethral mucosa forms a swollen red ring around the urethral meatus. It usually occurs before menarche or after menopause. Identify the urethral meatus at the centre of the swelling to make this diagnosis.

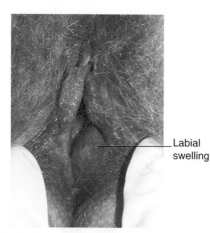

Bartholin's Gland Infection

Causes of a Bartholin's gland infection include trauma, gonococci anaerobes like bacteroides and peptostreptococci, and *Chlamydia trachomatis*. Acutely, it appears as a tense, hot, very tender abscess. Look for pus coming out of the duct or erythema around the duct opening. Chronically, a nontender cyst is felt. It may be large or small.

Rectocele

A rectocele is a herniation of the rectum into the posterior wall of the vagina, resulting from a weakness or defect in the endopelvic fascia.

TABLE 22-3   **Variations in the Cervical Surface**

Two kinds of epithelia may cover the cervix: (1) shiny pink *squamous epithelium*, which resembles the vaginal epithelium, and (2) deep red, plushy *columnar epithelium*, which is continuous with the endocervical lining. These two meet at the *squamocolumnar junction*. When this junction is at or inside the cervical os, only squamous epithelium is seen. A ring of columnar epithelium is often visible to a varying extent around the os—the result of an expected process that accompanies fetal development, menarche, and the first pregnancy.*

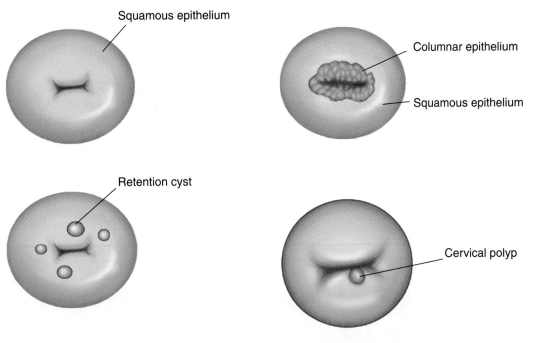

With increasing estrogen stimulation during adolescence, all or part of this columnar epithelium is transformed into squamous epithelium by a process termed *metaplasia*. This change may block the secretions of columnar epithelium and cause *retention cysts* (sometimes called *nabothian cysts*). These appear as one or more translucent nodules on the cervical surface and have no pathologic significance.

A cervical polyp usually arises from the endocervical canal, becoming visible when it protrudes through the cervical os. It is bright red, soft, and rather fragile. When only the tip is seen, it cannot be differentiated clinically from a polyp originating in the endometrium. Polyps are benign but may bleed.

*Terminology is in flux. Other terms for the columnar epithelium that is visible on the ectocervix are *ectropion, ectopy,* and *eversion.*

| TABLE 22-4 | Shapes of the Cervical Os |

Expected

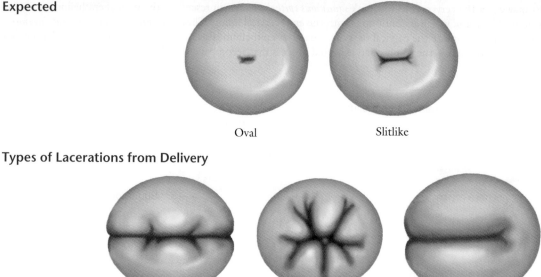

Oval   Slitlike

Types of Lacerations from Delivery

Unilateral transverse   Bilateral transverse   Stellate

| TABLE 22-5 | Unexpected Changes of the Cervix |

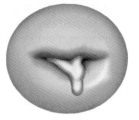

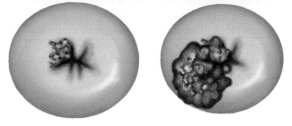

Mucopurulent Cervicitis

Mucopurulent cervicitis produces purulent yellow drainage from the cervical os, usually as a result of infection from *Chlamydia trachomatis, Neisseria gonorrhoeae,* or herpes. These infections are sexually transmitted and may occur without symptoms or signs.

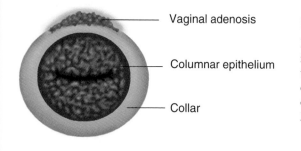

— Vaginal adenosis

— Columnar epithelium

— Collar

Carcinoma of the Cervix

Carcinoma of the cervix begins in an area of metaplasia. In its earliest stages, it cannot be distinguished from the usual appearance of the cervix. In a late stage, an extensive, irregular, cauliflower-like growth may develop. Early frequent intercourse, multiple partners, smoking, and infection with human papillomavirus increase the risk for cervical cancer.

Fetal Exposure to Diethylstilbestrol (DES)

Daughters of women who took DES during pregnancy are at greatly increased risk for several disorders, including (1) columnar epithelium that covers most or all of the cervix, (2) vaginal adenosis, that is, extension of this epithelium to the vaginal wall, and (3) a circular collar or ridge of tissue, of varying shapes, between the cervix and vagina. Much less common is an otherwise rare carcinoma of the upper vagina.

TABLE 22-6 Vaginal Discharge

The vaginal discharge that often accompanies vaginitis must be distinguished from a physiologic discharge. The latter is clear or white and may contain white clumps of epithelial cells; it is not malodorous. It is also important to distinguish vaginal from cervical discharges. Use a large cotton swab to wipe off the cervix. If no cervical discharge is present in the os, suspect a vaginal origin and consider the causes below. Remember that diagnosis of cervicitis or vaginitis hinges on careful collection and analysis of the appropriate laboratory specimens.

	Trichomonal Vaginitis	**Candidal Vaginitis**	**Bacterial Vaginosis**
			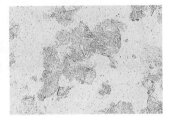
Cause	*Trichomonas vaginalis*, a protozoa; often but not always acquired sexually	*Candida albicans*, a yeast (overgrowth of vaginal flora); many factors predispose, including antibiotic therapy.	Bacterial overgrowth probably from anaerobic bacteria; may be transmitted sexually
Discharge	Yellowish green or grey, possibly frothy; often profuse and pooled in the vaginal fornix; may be malodorous	White and curdy; may be thin but typically thick; not as profuse as in trichomonal infection; not malodorous	Grey or white, thin, homogeneous, malodorous; coats the vaginal walls; usually not profuse, may be minimal
Other Symptoms	Pruritus (though not usually as severe as with *Candida* infection); pain on urination (from skin inflammation or possibly urethritis); dyspareunia	Pruritus; vaginal soreness; pain on urination (from skin inflammation); dyspareunia	Unpleasant fishy or musty genital odour
Vulva and Vaginal Mucosa	Vestibule and labia minora may be reddened. Vaginal mucosa may be diffusively reddened, with small red granular spots or petechiae in the posterior fornix. In mild cases, the mucosa looks as expected.	The vulva and even the surrounding skin are often inflamed and sometimes swollen to a variable extent. Vaginal mucosa often reddened, with white, often tenacious patches of discharge. The mucosa may bleed when these patches are scraped off. In mild cases, the mucosa looks as expected.	Vulva usually unchanged. Vaginal mucosa usually as expected.
Laboratory Evaluation	Scan saline wet mount for trichomonads	Scan potassium hydroxide (KOH) preparation for branching hyphae of *Candida*	Scan saline wet mount for *clue cells* (epithelial cells with stippled borders); sniff for fishy odour after applying KOH ("whiff test"); vaginal secretions with pH >4.5

TABLE 22-7	Positions of the Uterus

Both retroversion and retroflexion are common variants.

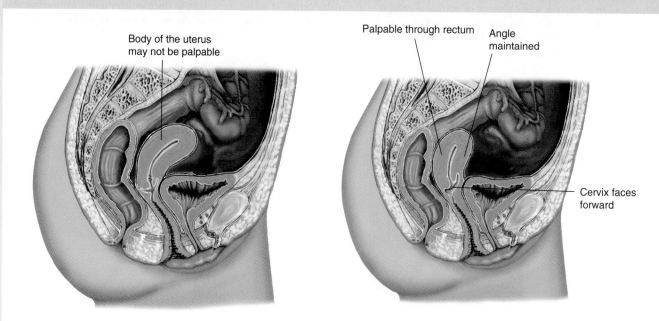

Body of the uterus
may not be palpable

Palpable through rectum

Angle
maintained

Cervix faces
forward

Retroversion of the Uterus

Retroversion of the uterus refers to a tilting backward of the entire uterus, including both body and cervix. It is a common variant occurring in approximately 20% of women. Early clues on pelvic examination are a cervix that faces forward and a uterine body that cannot be felt by the abdominal hand. In *moderate retroversion*, the body may not be palpable with either hand. In *marked retroversion*, the body can be felt posteriorly, either through the posterior fornix or through the rectum. A retroverted uterus is usually both mobile and asymptomatic. Occasionally, such a uterus is fixed and immobile, held in place by conditions such as endometriosis or pelvic inflammatory disease.

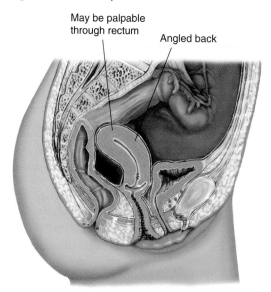

May be palpable
through rectum

Angled back

Retroflexion of the Uterus

Retroflexion of the uterus refers to a backward angulation of the body of the uterus in relation to the cervix. The cervix maintains its usual position. The body of the uterus is often palpable through the posterior fornix or through the rectum.

TABLE 22-8   Disorders of the Uterus

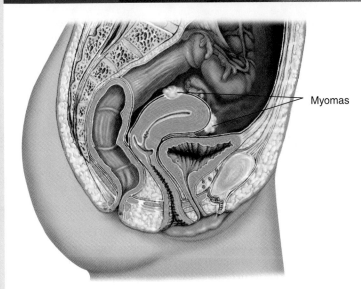

Myomas of the Uterus (Fibroids)

Myomas are very common benign uterine tumours. They may be single or multiple and vary greatly in size, occasionally reaching massive proportions. They feel like firm, irregular nodules in continuity with the uterine surface. Occasionally, a myoma projecting laterally can be confused with an ovarian mass; a nodule projecting posteriorly can be mistaken for a retroflexed uterus. Submucous myomas project toward the endometrial cavity and are not themselves palpable, although they may be suspected because of an enlarged uterus.

Myomas

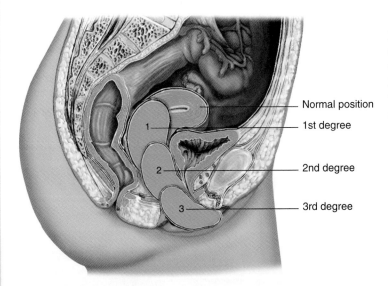

Normal position

1st degree

2nd degree

3rd degree

Prolapse of the Uterus

Prolapse of the uterus results from weakness of the supporting structures of the pelvic floor and is often associated with a cystocele and rectocele. In progressive stages, the uterus becomes retroverted and descends down the vaginal canal to the outside:

- In first-degree prolapse, the cervix is still well within the vagina.
- In second-degree prolapse, it is at the introitus.
- In third-degree prolapse (procidentia), the cervix and vagina are outside the introitus.

TABLE 22-9   Adnexal Masses

Adnexal masses most commonly result from disorders of the fallopian tubes or ovaries. Three examples, often hard to differentiate, are described. In addition, inflammatory disease of the bowel (such as diverticulitis), carcinoma of the colon, and a pedunculated myoma of the uterus may simulate an adnexal mass.

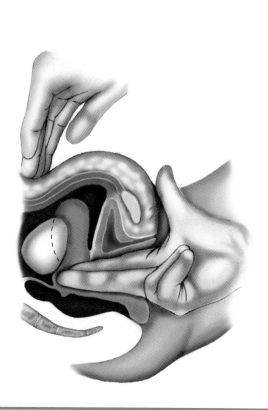

Ovarian Cysts and Tumours

Ovarian cysts and tumours may be detected as adnexal masses on one or both sides. Later, they may extend out of the pelvis. Cysts tend to be smooth and compressible, tumours more solid and often nodular. Uncomplicated cysts and tumours are not usually tender.

Small (≤6 cm in diameter), mobile, cystic masses in a young woman are usually benign and often disappear after the next menstrual period.

Ruptured Tubal Pregnancy

A ruptured tubal pregnancy spills blood into the peritoneal cavity, causing severe abdominal pain and tenderness. Guarding and rebound tenderness are sometimes associated. A unilateral adnexal mass may be palpable, but tenderness often prevents its detection. Faintness, syncope, nausea, vomiting, tachycardia, and shock may be present, reflecting the haemorrhage. There may be a prior history of amenorrhea or other symptoms of a pregnancy.

Pelvic Inflammatory Disease

Pelvic inflammatory disease (PID) is most often a result of sexually transmitted infection of the fallopian tubes (salpingitis) or of the tubes and ovaries (salpingo-oophoritis). It is caused by *Neisseria gonorrhoeae, Chlamydia trachomatis,* and other organisms. *Acute* disease is associated with very tender, bilateral adnexal masses, although pain and muscle spasm usually make it impossible to delineate them. Movement of the cervix produces pain. If not treated, a *tubo-ovarian abscess* or infertility may ensue.

Infection of the fallopian tubes and ovaries may also follow delivery of a baby or gynecologic surgery.

CHAPTER

23

The Anus, Rectum, and Prostate

Judy A. Bornais and Lynn S. Bickley

Often, one of the last components of the comprehensive physical examination for all clients is assessment of the anus and rectum, with the addition of the prostate in males. Examiners usually save these areas for the end of the examination because of the uncomfortable nature of such assessment. Nurses must be cognizant of the potential embarrassment and uneasiness of the client when answering related personal questions and experiencing the invasive portion of the assessment. Despite the potential for discomfort for both clients and nurses, examination of the anus, rectum, and prostate is a vitally important part of overall health assessment. The significant role of the nurse in screening and health promotion during this portion of the assessment cannot be underestimated.

ANATOMY AND PHYSIOLOGY

The gastrointestinal tract terminates in a short segment, the *anal canal*. The entire anal canal is approximately 3 cm to 4 cm in length, ending posteriorly with the anal orifice. Its external margin is poorly demarcated, but the skin of the anal canal can usually be distinguished from the surrounding perianal skin by its moist, hairless appearance. The anal canal is usually held in a closed position by the muscle action of the voluntary *external anal sphincter* skeletal muscle, which the client can control. Along with the external anal sphincter, the involuntary *internal anal sphincter*, which is an extension of the muscular coat of the rectal wall, also plays a role in keeping the anal canal closed.

Note carefully the direction of the anal canal on a line roughly between the anus and umbilicus. Unlike the rectum above it, which contains only autonomic nerves, the canal is liberally supplied by somatic sensory nerves, and as a result, a poorly directed finger, instrument, or any trauma will produce pain in the client.

A serrated line marks the change from the skin of the anal canal to the mucous membrane of the rectum. This anorectal junction also denotes the boundary between somatic and visceral nerve supplies. The junction is not palpable, but is visible on proctoscopic examination.

Above the anorectal junction, the rectum balloons out and turns posteriorly into the hollow of the coccyx and the sacrum. The prostate gland lies on the anterior surface of the male rectal wall and inferior to the bladder. The three lobes of the *prostate gland* surround the urethra. The prostate gland is small during childhood,

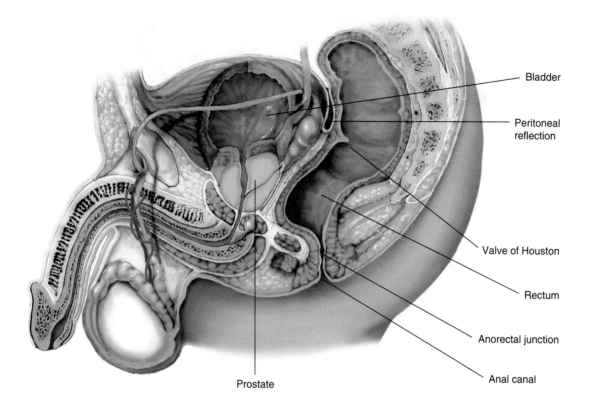

Bladder

Peritoneal reflection

Valve of Houston

Rectum

Anorectal junction

Anal canal

Prostate

but between puberty and the age of about 20 years, it increases roughly five-fold in size. Prostate volume further expands as the gland becomes hyperplastic (see p. 845). The two lateral lobes lie against the anterior rectal wall, where they are palpable as a rounded, heart-shaped structure approximately 2.5 to 3 cm long and 4 cm in diameter. They are separated by a shallow median sulcus or groove, also palpable. The third, or median, lobe is anterior to the urethra and cannot be examined by palpation. The *seminal vesicles,* shaped like rabbit ears above the prostate, are also not usually palpable.

The prostate gland produces fluid that makes up part of the semen. The semen plays an important role in carrying sperm and also alters the acidic pH of the vagina during intercourse. Prostate glands produce prostate-specific antigen (PSA), which is mostly found in the semen but can also be present in small amounts in the blood. The PSA is a glycoprotein produced by prostate epithelial cells. It can be elevated in benign conditions such as hyperplasia and prostatitis, and transiently elevated by ejaculation, prostate biopsy, and urinary retention. It can also be low in aggressive prostate cancers.

In the female, the uterine *cervix* can usually be felt through the anterior wall of the rectum.

The rectal wall contains three inward foldings, called *valves of Houston.* These valves retain feces so that air may pass (flatus) without feces. The lowest of these can sometimes be felt, usually on the client's left. Most of the rectum that is accessible to digital examination does not have a peritoneal surface. The anterior rectum usually does, and may be reached with the tip of the examining finger. This may allow the examiner to verify the tenderness of peritoneal inflammation or the nodularity of peritoneal metastases.

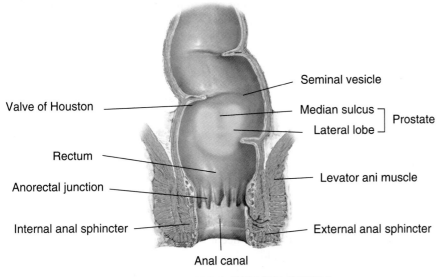

**CORONAL SECTION OF THE ANUS AND RECTUM.
VIEW FROM BEHIND, SHOWING THE ANTERIOR WALL**

Note that the estimated length of the anal canal and rectum in the adult client is approximately 16 cm. The examination finger of most nurses is 6 to 10 cm in length, allowing for a significant portion of the anal/rectal canal to be palpated.

THE HEALTH HISTORY: SUBJECTIVE DATA

Key Symptoms and Signs Reported by the Client

- Rectal bleeding
- Anal pain
- Itching and burning at the anal opening
- Inability to pass stool (impaction)
- Inability to pass urine (obstruction)
- Flatulence
- "Thin" stools
- Hemorrhoids
- Fecal incontinence
- Difficulty sitting for long periods

Start your inquiry with open-ended questions concerning symptoms related to the anorectal area and prostate. Other chapters have already addressed many of the relevant questions, for example, what medications the client takes, both over-the-counter (e.g., iron supplements) and prescription. You will want to ask your client about current bowel movements. Are they regular? How often do they occur? Are there any changes in the pattern of bowel function or the size or calibre of the stools? What about diarrhea, constipation, or fecal incontinence?

See Table 17-3, Constipation, p. 549, and Table 17-5, Black and Bloody Stools, p. 552.

Ask the client to describe the colour of the stools. Are they clay-coloured? Is there blood in the stool, ranging from black stools, suggesting melena, to the red blood of hematochezia, to bright-red blood from the rectum? Turn to p. 832 to review the health history regarding these symptoms. Does the client have excessive fat, pus, or mucus in the stools, or a need to pass gas (flatus) often?

Change in bowel pattern, especially stools of thin pencil-like calibre, may warn of cancer. Blood in the stool may be from polyps or cancer, also from gastrointestinal bleeding or local hemorrhoids; mucus may appear in villous adenoma and in bacillary or amoebic dysentery.

Is there any pain on defecation? Any itching? Any extreme tenderness in the anus or rectum? Is there any mucopurulent discharge or bleeding? Any ulcerations? Does the client have anal intercourse?

Proctitis with anorectal pain, pruritus, tenesmus, discharge or bleeding in anorectal infection from gonorrhea, *Chlamydia*, lymphogranuloma venereum, receptive anal intercourse, ulcerations in *herpes simplex*, chancre in *primary syphilis*. Itching in younger clients from pinworms.

Is there any history of anal warts or anal fissures?

Genital warts from *human papillomavirus, condylomata lata* in secondary syphilis. Anal fissures in *proctitis, Crohn's disease*

In men, review the pattern of urination (see p. 518). Does the client feel the need to void often? Does he have any difficulty starting the urine stream or holding back urine? Is the flow weak? What about urination at night? Or pain or burning as urine is passed? Any blood in the urine or semen, or pain with ejaculation? Any sense of not emptying the bladder completely? Any increased urgency to void? Is there frequent pain or stiffness in the lower back, hips, or upper thighs?

These symptoms suggest urethral obstruction as in *benign prostatic hyperplasia* or *prostate cancer*, especially in men older than age 70.

Also in men, is there any feeling of discomfort or heaviness in the prostate area at the base of the penis? Any associated malaise, fever, or chills?

Suggests possible *prostatitis*

Is there any family history of colorectal or prostate cancer, or inflammatory bowel disease?

Has the client recently travelled? Could excess stress have preceded the change in bowel habits?

When was the client's last digital rectal examination? Has a stool sample been sent for occult blood? Has a PSA test or colonoscopy ever been done?

Does the client follow Canada's Food Guide for healthy eating? How many servings of fruit, vegetables, and grain products does the client consume per day? How much water or noncaffeinated fluid does he or she consume daily? (See Chapter 8). Does the client exercise? How active is the client's lifestyle?

Examples of Questions for Symptom Analysis—Rectal Bleeding

- When you notice the bleeding, is it coming from the anal canal? Where does it stain on your underwear? (*Location, radiation*)
- What colour are your stools (e.g., black/tarry/clay/ grey/brown)? (*Quality*)
- How much blood is there? Scant amount? Spotty intermittent amount? Moderate amount? Copious? (*Quantity*)
- When did the bleeding first start? Did it start suddenly or gradually? (*Onset*)
- How long has the bleeding been occurring? (*Duration*)
- Is the bleeding continuous? Or is it only during/ immediately after a bowel movement? (*Timing*)

- What makes it (the bleeding) better? Sitz baths? Increased fluids? Increased fibre intake? (*Alleviating factors*)
- What makes it (the bleeding) worse? Constipation? Large bowel movements? Hard stools? Straining at stool? (*Aggravating factors*)
- Do you have any other symptoms with the bleeding? (*Associated symptoms*)
- Have you had any trauma to the pelvic area? Do you sit for long periods at work? At home? (*Environmental factors*)
- Tell me how this is affecting your life. (*Significance to client*)
- What do you think is happening? (*Client perspective*)

HEALTH PROMOTION

Important Topics for Health Promotion

- Pattern of bowel function
- Voiding pattern and ability
- Screening for prostate cancer
- Screening for polyps and colorectal cancer

RISK FACTOR ASSESSMENT

Over the last few decades, significant evidence has accumulated regarding the causes of cancer. Researchers have identified several factors, such as tobacco use, unhealthy diet, and environmental and workplace carcinogens. Inquiring about these risk factors during the health history provides essential information. Nurses also should assess family history, demographics, and workplace/lifestyle issues, which can increase the risk of prostate and colon cancer. Other risks include a diet high in fat, particularly animal and saturated fat, and certain genetic backgrounds (Canadian Cancer Society [CCS], 2007a, b). Many health care providers believe that reducing the number of people exposed to substances that increase risk, improving cancer-protective behaviours, or both may prevent cancer or diminish its risk (Public Health Agency of Canada [PHAC], 2004). Promoting healthy bowel and prostate function includes the following:

- A diet of fibre-rich foods, with 25 to 38 g/day of fibre from fruits, vegetables, beans, and whole-wheat breads and cereals (Dieticians of Canada, 2007)

- A low-fat diet

- Limited alcohol intake

- Smoking cessation

- A healthy weight

- Regular physical activity

SPECIFIC PREVENTION FOR SPECIFIC DISEASES

Health promotion is an important role of nurses. Its significance in the prevention and screening for prostate and colorectal cancers cannot be overemphasized.

In Canadian men, *prostate cancer* is the leading type of cancer diagnosed and the third leading type resulting in death, following lung and colorectal cancer (CCS, 2009c). An estimated 24,700 new cases of prostate cancer were diagnosed in 2008. While no single cause is linked to prostate cancer, increasing age, family history of prostate cancer, high-fat (particularly animal and saturated fat) diet, and certain ethnicities or genetic backgrounds all appear to increase risk (CCS, 2007b). During his lifetime, one out of seven men will develop prostate cancer, most of whom are older than 60 years (CCS, 2009a). Men of African ancestry have the highest incidence of prostate cancer and also present most often with advanced disease, while men of Asian and Aboriginal genetic background have the lowest incidence (Hoffman et al., 2001). Obesity, physical inactivity, and working with metal cadmium are currently being investigated as other possible links to the development of prostate cancer (CCS, 2007b). Investigations of nonsteroidal anti-inflammatory drugs, vasectomy, and testosterone supplements as possible risk factors have been inconclusive.

Early androgen suppression therapy has been shown to significantly improve the overall survival of men with prostate cancer (Wilt et al., 2007). In 2007, a new "therapeutic vaccine" was shown to mobilize the immune system of clients already diagnosed with prostate cancer (Peres, 2007). Studies of the vaccine demonstrated that the immune system can recognize and respond to fight prostate cancer. This breakthrough in active cellular immunotherapy was sufficiently promising to lead to permission for U.S. researchers to conduct further investigations.

Early detection (secondary prevention) is the best approach for prostate cancer, but to date there is no consensus among health care professionals regarding screening for it (PHAC, 2004). One method used to detect prostate cancer is the PSA blood test, which measures the level of free and bound PSA in the blood. The PSA is an enzyme produced in the ducts of the prostate and absorbed into the bloodstream, where it may become bound to two proteins. With benign prostate conditions such as infection and urinary retention, there is more free PSA, while cancer produces more of the bound form. For the average male, an expected PSA level ranges from 0 to 4 nanograms per millilitre (ng/mL). A PSA level of 4 to 10 ng/mL is considered slightly elevated, levels between 10 and 20 ng/mL are considered moderately elevated, and anything greater is considered highly elevated. Various factors can cause levels to fluctuate, and approximately 40% of clients with organ-confined prostate cancer show no elevation of serum PSA (European Randomized Control Study for Prostate Cancer, 2007).

The PSA test, although controversial in preventing cancer death, is used to detect and follow the progress of prostate cancer (Kopec et al., 2005). Although evidence shows that PSA testing helps to identify early prostate cancer, and randomized control trials have found that prostate cancer screening decreases the risk of being diagnosed with metastatic prostate cancer, evidence that early identification improves mortality is insufficient (Aus et al., 2007; Thompson et al., 2007).

Health care providers also have used the digital rectal examination (DRE) to detect prostate cancer. The DRE reaches only the lateral and posterior surfaces of the prostate, missing 25% to 35% of tumours that are nonpalpable or in other areas (U.S. Preventive Services Task Force, 1996). With DRE there is a tendency to detect larger tumours. Small multifocal lesions with an aggressive biologic potential are not detectable with DRE alone. The general opinion is that DRE is highly subjective and variable between examiners.

Currently, no recommended screening tests for prostate cancer are available (CCS, 2009b). Despite the numerous studies on screening with PSA tests, the Canadian Task Force on Preventive Health Care recommends against PSA screening (Canadian Task Force on Preventive Health Care Guidelines as cited in PHAC, 2004). Until very large combined screening efforts from the European Randomized Study of Screening for Prostate Cancer (ERSPC) and the U.S. Prostate, Lung, Colorectal, and Ovarian Cancer Study (PLCO) are analyzed, decisions on large-scale screening efforts are being deferred (Aus et al., 2007; Thompson et al., 2007), and a shared approach to decision making between health care providers and their clients is encouraged (Ilic et al., 2007). The Canadian Task Force on Preventive

Health Care recommendations for screening for prostate cancer (1998) state that poor evidence exists to include or exclude DRE from the periodic health examination for men older than 50 years, and, therefore, does not recommend that health care providers who currently include DRE in their examinations change their behaviour. Further changes to the recommendations await the results of the large studies in progress.

Colorectal cancer (CRC) is the second leading cause of death from cancer when numbers for men and women are combined (CCS, 2009c). An estimated 21,500 new cases were diagnosed in 2008, and 8,900 were expected to die from it. Colorectal cancer is believed to begin as benign tumours or polyps in the large intestine or rectum, which develop over time, often 7 to 10 years, and later invade the wall and other organs. One third of CRC is found in the rectum (PHAC, 2004). Among the many risk factors for CRC described in Chapter 17 (see pp. 523–524) related to age, chronic disease, other cancers, family history, and lifestyle factors, is the additional factor of certain ethnic and genetic backgrounds (Health Canada, 2007; CCS, 2009d). Increasing physical activity, limiting alcohol consumption, using nonsteroidal anti-inflammatory drugs, and eliminating tobacco use have been found to reduce the risk of colorectal cancer (Asano & McLeod, 2007a; Health Canada, 2007). It has been suggested that a diet of fibre-rich foods from fruit and vegetables and low in red meat consumption helps prevent colorectal cancer (Dieticians of Canada, 2007; Health Canada, 2007), but to date no evidence from randomized control trials suggests that increased dietary fibre reduces the incidence or recurrence of adenomatous polyps and carcinomas in a 2- to 4-year intervention period (Asano & McLeod, 2007b).

Screening for CRC has reduced both the incidence and mortality of colorectal cancer (CCS/National Cancer Institute of Canada, 2006). Use of hemoccult or fecal occult blood tests (FOBTs) has been shown to reduce mortality from CRC (Hewitson et al., 2007). As bowel cancers often bleed, FOBTs are used to detect small amounts of blood in the stool. Clients collect stool samples over a period of 3 days. Certain raw fruits and vegetables and specific medications (e.g., nonsteroidal anti-inflammatory drugs, more than 1 aspirin a day) can affect the results of the test; therefore, clients must observe precautions for 7 days prior to and during stool collection. Three days prior and during collection, clients are required to limit alcohol to one drink daily; avoid red meats, citrus fruits, and juices; and not take more than 250 mg of vitamin C. They must also avoid specified raw fruits and vegetables. Results from FOBT are not diagnostic, but they provide information that helps health care personnel to determine the need for further investigations. Health Canada recommends that screening for CRC using unrehydrated Hemoccult II or its equivalent as the entry test be offered to adults aged between 50 and 74 years. Clients are to be screened at least every 2 years, and those with positive test results should undergo follow-up colonoscopy, with the option of barium enema and flexible sigmoidoscopy where appropriate (PHAC, 2002).

Barium enemas and scoping procedures that allow direct visualization of the colon (colonoscopy and sigmoidoscopy) have been used in early detection of CRC (National Cancer Institute of Canada, 2003). People who are at increased risk for CRC should discuss an individual plan of surveillance with their health care provider, including the possibility of screening with colonoscopy or sigmoidoscopy (National Cancer Institute of Canada, 2003; PHAC, 2002). Increased risk includes those who have had CRC, inflammatory bowel disease, familial adenomatous polyposis or hereditary nonpolyposis colon cancer, benign polyps, or a first-degree relative with CRC.

◼ EMERGENCY CONCERNS

Clients who report difficulty voiding or inability to void within a 24-hour period require immediate attention from a primary health care provider. Clients who have experienced trauma to the anus or rectum, or who report frank rectal bleeding, tarry stools, rectal pain (e.g., abscess of anal glands), or symptoms of a fecal impaction also require prompt attention.

TECHNIQUES OF EXAMINATION: OBJECTIVE DATA

◼ PROMOTING CLIENT COMFORT, DIGNITY, AND SAFETY

For many clients, the rectal examination is the least popular segment of the physical examination. It may cause discomfort and even embarrassment for the client, but if the examination is skilfully done, it should not be truly painful. You may choose to omit the rectal examination in adolescents who have no relevant complaints, but in middle-aged or older adults, omission risks missing an asymptomatic carcinoma. A successful examination requires a calm demeanour, an explanation to the client of what he or she may feel, gentleness, and slow movement of your finger. Remember to provide your client with draping to provide as much privacy as possible.

Equipment
◼ Gloves
◼ Lubricant

◼ INSPECTION OF THE ANUS

Choose one of several suitable client positions for conducting the examination. Often, the male clinician asks the male client to stand and lean forward with his upper body resting across the examining table and hips flexed. While asking the male client to lie bent over is an option for the examination, 96% of nurses in Canada are female, and, therefore, a more appropriate examination position for the male client is the side-lying position. For most purposes, the side-lying position, depicted in the following illustration, is satisfactory and allows good visualization of the perianal and sacrococcygeal areas. If you need to examine only the rectum of the female client, the lateral position is satisfactory and affords a good view of the perianal and sacrococcygeal areas. Do not mistake a retroverted uterus or vaginal tampon for a tumour.

Ask the client to lie on the left side with the buttocks close to the edge of the examining table near you. Flexing the client's hips and knees, especially the top leg, stabilizes the client's position and improves visibility. Drape the client appropriately and adjust the light for the best view. Glove your hands and spread the buttocks apart.

No matter how you position the client, your examining finger cannot reach the full length of the rectum. If a rectosigmoid cancer is suspected or screening is warranted, turn to the interdisciplinary team for sigmoidoscopy or colonoscopy.

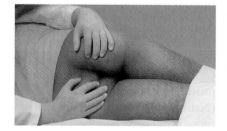

The anus is usually hairless with rough wrinkles and often more darkly pigmented than the surrounding skin. It should appear symmetrical, and the anal opening should remain closed. The area is expected to be moist and free of inflammation. Ask the client to hold his breath and bear down while you examine the anus; expect it to be free of lesions, protrusions, and fissures.

Inspect the sacrococcygeal and perianal areas for lumps, ulcers, inflammation, rashes, or excoriations. Adult perianal skin is usually more pigmented and somewhat coarser than the skin over the buttocks.

Anal and perianal lesions include hemorrhoids, venereal warts, herpes, syphilitic chancre, and carcinoma. A *perianal abscess* produces a painful, tender, indurated, and reddened mass. Pruritus ani causes swollen, thickened, fissured skin with excoriations.

◼ PALPATION OF THE ANUS, RECTUM, AND PROSTATE

Palpate any unusual areas, noting lumps or tenderness. Lubricate your gloved index finger, explain what you are going to do, and tell the client that the examination may make him or her feel that the bowels will move, but that will not happen. Ask the client to strain down. Inspect the anus again as it relaxes, noting any lesions.

As the client strains, place the pad of your gloved and lubricated index finger over the anus. Inform the client that you are about to begin the internal examination.

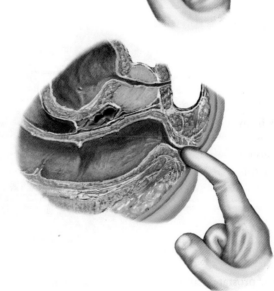

Soft, pliable tags of redundant skin at the anal margin are common. Though sometimes caused by past anal surgery or previously thrombosed hemorrhoids, they are often unexplained.

See Table 23-1, Unexpected Findings of the Anus, Surrounding Skin, and Rectum (pp. 843–844).

Sphincter tightness in anxiety, inflammation, or scarring; laxity in some neurologic diseases or sexual practices

As the sphincter relaxes, gently insert your fingertip into the anal canal in the direction pointing toward the umbilicus. If you feel the sphincter tighten, pause and reassure the client. When in a moment the sphincter relaxes, proceed.

Occasionally, severe tenderness prevents entry and internal examination. Do not try to force it. Instead, place your fingers on both sides of the anus, gently spread the orifice, and ask the client to strain down. Look for a lesion, such as an anal fissure, that might explain the tenderness.

If you can proceed without undue discomfort, note:

- The sphincter tone of the anus. Usually, the muscles of the anal sphincter close snugly around your finger.

- Tenderness, if any

- Induration

Induration may be caused by inflammation, scarring, or malignancy.

- Irregularities or nodules

The irregular border of a rectal cancer is shown below.

Insert your finger into the rectum as far as possible. Rotate your hand clockwise to palpate as much of the rectal surface as possible on the client's right side, then counterclockwise to palpate the surface posteriorly and on the client's left side.

Note any nodules, irregularities, or induration. To bring a possible lesion into reach, take your finger off the rectal surface, ask the client to bear down, and palpate again.

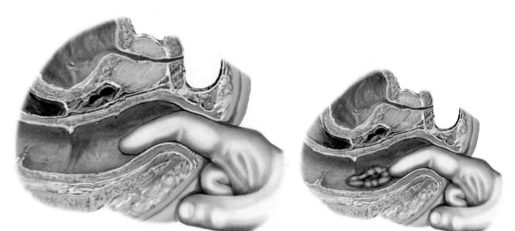

Palpation of the Prostate.

With the male client bearing down and your palpating finger in the rectum, rotate your hand further counterclockwise so that your finger can examine the *posterior surface of the prostate gland*. By turning your body somewhat away from the client, you can feel this area more easily. Tell the client that you are going to feel his prostate gland, and that this may prompt an urge to urinate.

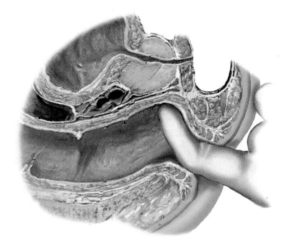

Sweep your finger carefully over the prostate gland, identifying its lateral lobes and the median sulcus between them. Note the size, shape, and consistency of the prostate, and identify any nodules or tenderness. The prostate is expected to be rubbery and nontender.

See Table 23-2, Unexpected Findings of the Prostate (p. 845).

If possible, *extend your finger above the prostate* to the region of the seminal vesicles and the peritoneal cavity. Note any nodules or tenderness.

Gently withdraw your finger and wipe the anus or give the client tissues. Note the colour of any fecal matter on your glove, and test it for occult blood.

A rectal "shelf" of peritoneal metastases (see p. 844) or the tenderness of peritoneal inflammation

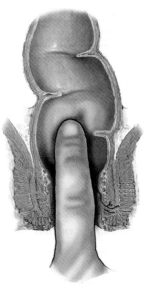

**PALPATING THE PROSTATE—
VIEW FROM BELOW**

Alternate Palpation of the Female Client. If a woman is in the lithotomy position for examination of the genitalia, you may decide to examine the rectum at this time. It allows you to conduct the bimanual examination (see Chapter 22) and delineate a possible adnexal or pelvic mass. It is suitable for testing the integrity of the rectovaginal wall and may also help you to palpate a cancer high in the rectum. Note that the cervix is readily palpated through the anterior wall.

RECORDING AND ANALYZING FINDINGS

Documentation of the information obtained through the client history and physical examination of the anus, rectum, and prostate needs to be thorough, accurate, and clear for all members of the interdisciplinary team. Such documentation optimizes the planning and implementation of comprehensive and appropriate care for the client.

■ *Examples of Documentation for the Anus, Rectum, and Prostate*

Area of Assessment	Expected Findings	Unexpected Findings
Sacrococcygeal and perianal areas	Skin intact, coarse, colour of surrounding skin	Red, tender, ulcerated skin perianal area
Anus	Anal opening darkly pigmented, hairless, moist, closed; external sphincter tone intact	Tender swollen bluish mass .5 cm × .5 cm protruding from anal margin at 7 o'clock position
Rectum	Smooth, nontender rectal walls	Nonintact mucous membrane and tenderness posterior rectal wall
Prostate gland	Smooth, rubbery heart-shaped gland; slightly moveable and nontender; defined median sulcus	1.0 cm × 1.0 cm firm hard nodule, left lateral prostate lobe; obscured median sulcus
Rectovaginal wall	Smooth, regular, symmetrical wall	Fixed, immobile uterus palpated

ANALYZING FINDINGS FROM PHYSICAL EXAMINATION AND HEALTH HISTORY

After documenting the findings, nurses complete an analysis of the health history information and physical examination findings to develop a nursing diagnosis and plan an interdisciplinary approach. For example:

Mr David Bondy, 63 years old, presents to the clinic with concerns about the difficulty he is experiencing when voiding. He states that he often wakens in the middle of the night to void and has difficulty initiating a stream. He has been experiencing this difficulty for more than 1 month, sometimes has blood in his urine, and is concerned that something is wrong. He reports a nonsignificant health history. Upon examination Mr. Bondy is overweight (BMI of 30) and states that he is a "real meat and potatoes guy." During the DRE, you palpate an enlarged, firm smooth prostate gland lacking a central groove.

*Nursing Diagnosis: **Difficulty voiding** related to possible benign prostatic hypertrophy (BPH)*

To ensure comprehensive care for Mr. Bondy, his primary health care physician or nurse practitioner orders a few additional tests. A fasting plasma glucose test is performed to rule out the possibility that diabetes mellitus is causing the increased voiding, particularly at night. Mr. Bondy is at risk for developing diabetes mellitus because of his age and weight. Urinalysis is completed to rule out a urinary tract infection. A PSA test is discussed with Mr. Bondy in light of ruling out cancer as the cause of the urinary symptoms. A urologist performs a complete urologic assessment to determine the indicated steps in treatment. Mr. Bondy requires counselling by the nurse about the importance of a healthy weight and regular physical activity. He may also benefit from a referral to a dietician, who can further discuss healthy eating and reduction of the client's high-fat, red-meat intake.

Critical Thinking Exercise

- What are the differences in findings between palpating a healthy prostate and a prostate enlarged from benign prostatic hypertrophy (BPH) or prostate cancer? (*Knowledge*)
- How can you distinguish between the finding for BPH and prostate cancer? (*Comprehension*)
- How does the nurse assist clients to relax during inspection and palpation of the anus and rectum? (*Application*)
- What lifestyle factors might be contributing to the symptoms of BPH? (*Analysis*)
- What recommendations for screening and follow-up would you make to a client who reports frequent difficulty with voiding? (*Synthesis*)
- How would you evaluate the success of your client teaching with Mr. Bondy? (*Evaluation*)

Canadian Research

Canadian researchers have found that screening men with the prostate-specific antigen (PSA) test before any symptoms of cancer are evident may reduce their risk of getting metastatic prostate cancer by 35%. The research was funded in part by the CCS (2005).

Kopec et al. (2005). Screening with prostate-specific antigen and metastatic prostate cancer risk: A population based case-control study. *Journal of Urology, 174*, 495-499.

Test Questions

1. Symptoms of prostate disorder include which of the following?
   a. Nocturia, daytime polyuria, strong urinary stream
   b. Incomplete emptying, nocturia, weak urinary stream
   c. Elevated PSA level, daytime polyuria, low back pain
   d. Decreased urination, painful urination, elevated PSA level

2. To assess the rectal mucosa when palpating the rectum, the nurse rotates the examining hand
   a. from the left to the right.
   b. anteriorly, then posteriorly.
   c. counterclockwise, then clockwise.
   d. clockwise, then counterclockwise.

3. If the anal sphincter tightens as the nurse palpates it, he or she
   a. instructs the client to mouth-breathe.
   b. pauses, reassures the client, and proceeds.
   c. proceeds only if the client's internal sphincter muscle relaxes.
   d. puts two fingers on the client's anus and instructs the client to relax.

4. The prostate gland is characterized by a
   a. coronal groove.
   b. rounded heart shape.
   c. palpable median lobe.
   d. palpable anterior surface.

5. Specific characteristics the nurse assesses when palpating the anal canal include all of the following **except**
   a. scarring.
   b. alignment.
   c. ulceration.
   d. induration.

Bibliography

CITATIONS

Asano, T. K., & McLeod, R. S. (2007a). Nonsteroidal anti-inflammatory drugs (NSAID) and aspirin for preventing colorectal adenomas and carcinomas (Review). *Cochrane Library* 3.

Asano, T. K., & McLeod, R. S. (2007b). Dietary fibre for the prevention of colorectal adenomas and carcinomas (Review). *Cochrane Library* 3.

Aus, G., Bergdahl, S., Lodding, P., Lilja, H., & Hugosson, J. (2007). Prostate cancer screening decreases the absolute risk of being diagnosed with advanced prostate cancer–Results from a prospective, population-based randomized controlled trial. *European Urology, 51,* 659–664.

Canadian Cancer Society. (2007a). *Detailed guide: Prostate cancer.* Retrieved October 17, 2007, from http://www.cancer.ca/ccs/internet/standard/0,3182,3172_10175_74550606_langId-en,00.html

Canadian Cancer Society. (2007b). *Causes of prostate cancer.* Retrieved September 10, 2007, from http://www.cancer.ca/ccs/internet/standard/0,3182,3172_10175_272747_langId-en,00.html

Canadian Cancer Society. (2009a). *Prostate cancer statistics.* Retrieved March 26, 2009, from http://www.cancer.ca/Canada-wide/About%20cancer/Cancer%20statistics/Stats%20at%20a%20glance/Prostate%20cancer.aspx?sc_lang=en

Canadian Cancer Society. (2009b). *Research into prostate cancer screening.* Retrieved March 26, 2009, from http://www.cancer.ca/Canada-wide/Prevention/Get%20screened/Research%20into%20prostate%20cancer%20screening.aspx?sc_lang=en

Canadian Cancer Society. (2009c). *Colorectal cancer stats.* Retrieved March 26, 2009, from http://www.cancer.ca/Canada-wide/About%20cancer/Cancer%20statistics/Stats%20at%20

Canadian Cancer Society. (2009d). *Causes of colorectal cancer.* Retrieved March 26, 2009, from http://www.cancer.ca/Canada-wide/About%20cancer?Types%20of%20cancer/Caues%20of%20colorectal%20cancer.aspx?sc_lang=en

Canadian Cancer Society/National Cancer Institute of Canada. (2006). *Canadian cancer statistics 2006* (Special Topic). Toronto, ON: Authors.

Canadian Cancer Society. (2005). *Funded study adds important information to early PSA screening issue.* Retrieved August, 27, 2007, from http://www.cancer.ca/ccs/internet/mediareleaselist/0,3208,3172_343093094_468761888_langId-en,00.html

Canadian Task Force on Preventive Health Care. (1998). *Summary table of recommendations: Screening for prostate cancer.* Retrieved October 15, 2007, from http://www.ctfphc.org/Tables/Ch67tab.htm

Dieticians of Canada. (2007). *Fibre-up factsheet.* Retrieved September 10, 2007, from http://www.dietitians.ca/public/content/eat_well_live_well/english/faqs_tips_facts/fact_sheets/index.asp?fn=view&id=8370&idstring=6040%7C8370%7C986%7C2540%7C2518%7C1035%7C2359%7C1267%7C1151%7C2526%7C2520%7C1288%7C987%7C2525%7C2546%7C1070

European Randomized Study of Screening for Prostate Cancer. (2007). Retrieved September 14, 2007, from http://www.erspc.org/ERSPC_FAQ.pdf

Health Canada. (2007). *Screening for colorectal cancer.* Retrieved September 10, 2007, from http://www.hc-sc.gc.ca/iyh-vsv/diseases-maladies/colorectal_e.html#ri

Hewitson, P., Glasziou, P., Irwig, L., Towler, B., & Watson, E. (2007). *Screening for colorectal cancer using the faecal occult blood test, Hemoccult* (Review). *The Cochrane Library* 3.

Hoffman, R. M., Gilliland, F. D., Eley, J. W., Harlan, L. C., Stephenson, R. A., & Stanford, J. L. et al. (2001). Racial and ethnic differences in advanced-stage prostate cancer: The prostate cancer outcomes study. *Journal of the National Cancer Institute, 93*(5), 388–395.

Ilic, D., O'Connor, D., Green, S., & Wilt, T. (2007). Screening for prostate cancer (Review). *The Cochrane Library, 3.*

BIBLIOGRAPHY

Kopec, J. A., Goel, V., Bunting, P. S., Neuman, J., Sayre, E. C., Warde, P., et al. (2005). Screening with prostate specific antigen and metastatic prostate cancer risk: A population based case-control study. *Journal of Urology, 174,* 495–499.

National Cancer Institute of Canada. (2003). *Review of trends in colorectal cancer.* Retrieved August 30, 2007, from http://www.ncic.cancer.ca/ncic/internet/standard/0,3621,84658243_857 87780_91035926_langId-en,00.html

Peres, J. (2007, March 31). Prostate cancer breakthrough: Vaccine-like drug closer to approval. *The Edmonton Journal,* p. A 16.

Public Health Agency of Canada. (2004). *Progress report on cancer control in Canada.* Retrieved August 16, 2007, from http://www.phac-aspc.gc.ca/publicat/prccc-relccc/index.html

Public Health Agency of Canada. (2002). *Technical report for the National Committee on Colorectal Cancer Screening.* Retrieved September 10, 2007, from http://www.phac-aspc.gc.ca/publicat/ncccs-cndcc/techrep_e.html

Thompson, I., Thrasher, J. B., Aus, G., Burnett, A. L., Canby-Hagino, E. D., Cookson, M. S., et al. (2007). Guidelines for the management of clinically localized prostate cancer: 2007 update. *Journal of Urology, 177,* 2106–2131.

U.S. Preventive Task Force. (1996). *Guide to clinical preventive services* (2nd ed.). Baltimore: Williams & Wilkins.

Wilt, T., Nair, B., MacDonald, R., & Rutks, I. (2007). Early versus deferred androgen suppression in the treatment of advanced prostatic cancer (Review). *The Cochrane Library,* 3.

ADDITIONAL REFERENCES

Schrock, T. R. (2000). Examination and diseases of the anorectum. In M. Feldmen, M. Friedman, & M. H. Sleisinger (Eds.), *Sleisinger's and Fortran's gastrointestinal and liver disease: Pathophysiology/diagnosis/management* (7th ed.). Philadelphia: Elsevier Saunders.

CANADIAN ASSOCIATIONS AND WEB SITES

Canadian Cancer Society: http://www.ccs.ca

Canadian Library Association: http://www.cla.ca

Canadian Prostate Health Network: http://www.canadian-prostate.com

Canadian Prostate Cancer Network: http://www.cpcn.org

Canadian Prostate Cancer Research Initiative: http://www.prostateresearch.ca/

Colorectal Cancer Association of Canada: http://www.ccac-accc.ca/

Prostate Cancer Research Foundation of Canada: http://www.prostatecancer.ca/

Prostate Centre at Princess Margaret Hospital, Toronto: http://www.prostatecentre.ca/

Prostate Centre at Vancouver General Hospital: http://www.prostatecentre.com

Pilonidal Cyst and Sinus

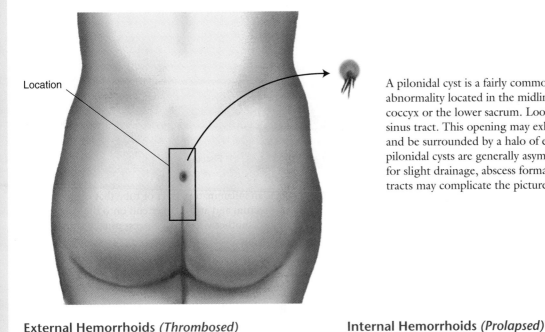

Location

A pilonidal cyst is a fairly common, probably congenital, abnormality located in the midline superficial to the coccyx or the lower sacrum. Look for the opening of a sinus tract. This opening may exhibit a small tuft of hair and be surrounded by a halo of erythema. Although pilonidal cysts are generally asymptomatic, except perhaps for slight drainage, abscess formation and secondary sinus tracts may complicate the picture.

External Hemorrhoids (*Thrombosed*)

External hemorrhoids are dilated hemorrhoidal veins that originate below the pectinate line and are covered with skin. They seldom produce symptoms unless thrombosis occurs. This causes acute local pain that increases with defecation and sitting. A tender, swollen, bluish, ovoid mass is visible at the anal margin.

Internal Hemorrhoids (*Prolapsed*)

Anterior

Posterior

Internal hemorrhoids are enlargements of the usual vascular cushions located above the pectinate line. Here, they are not usually palpable. Sometimes, especially during defecation, internal hemorrhoids may cause bright-red bleeding. They may also prolapse through the anal canal and appear as reddish, moist, protruding masses, typically located in one or more of the positions illustrated.

Prolapse of the Rectum

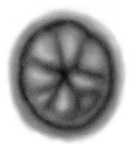

On straining for a bowel movement, the rectal mucosa, with or without its muscular wall, may prolapse through the anus, appearing as a doughnut or rosette of red tissue. A prolapse involving only mucosa is relatively small and shows radiating folds, as illustrated. When the entire bowel wall is involved, the prolapse is larger and covered by concentrically circular folds.

(table continues on next page)

Anal Fissure

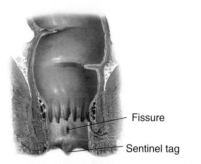

Fissure

Sentinel tag

An anal fissure is a very painful oval ulceration of the anal canal, found most commonly in the midline posteriorly, less commonly in the midline anteriorly. Its long axis lies longitudinally. There may be a swollen "sentinel" skin tag just below it, and gentle separation of the anal margins may reveal the lower edge of the fissure. The sphincter is spastic; the examination is painful. Local anesthesia may be required.

Anorectal Fistula

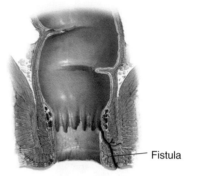

Fistula

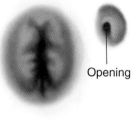

Opening

An anorectal fistula is an inflammatory tract or tube that opens at one end into the anus or rectum and at the other end onto the skin surface (as shown here) or into another viscus. An abscess usually antedates such a fistula. Look for the fistulous opening or openings anywhere in the skin around the anus.

Polyps of the Rectum

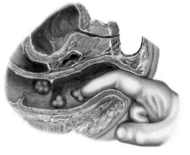

Polyps of the rectum are fairly common. Variable in size and number, they can develop on a stalk (*pedunculated*) or lie on the mucosal surface (*sessile*). They are soft and may be difficult or impossible to feel even when in reach of the examining finger. Proctoscopy and biopsy are needed for differentiation of benign from malignant lesions.

Cancer of the Rectum

Asymptomatic carcinoma of the rectum makes routine rectal examination important for adults. Illustrated here is the firm, nodular, rolled edge of an ulcerated cancer.

Rectal Shelf

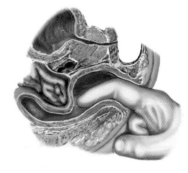

Widespread peritoneal metastases from any source may develop in the area of the peritoneal reflection anterior to the rectum. The sensation of external compression on the rectum or a rectal shelf—a firm, hard nodular area—is associated with malignancy. In a woman, this shelf of metastatic tissue develops in the rectouterine pouch, behind the cervix and the uterus.

Expected Prostate Gland

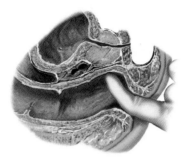

As palpated through the anterior rectal wall, the prostate is a rounded, heart-shaped structure about 2.5 cm long. The median sulcus can be felt between the two lateral lobes. Only the posterior surface of the prostate is palpable. Anterior lesions, including those that may obstruct the urethra, are not detectable by physical examination.

Prostatitis

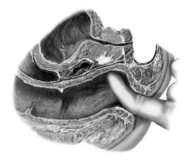

Acute prostatitis (illustrated here) is an acute, febrile condition caused by bacterial infection. The gland is very tender, swollen, firm, and warm. Examine it gently.

Chronic prostatitis does not produce consistent physical findings and must be evaluated by other methods.

Benign Prostatic Hyperplasia

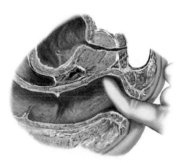

Starting in the third decade of life, benign prostatic hyperplasia (BPH) becomes increasingly prevalent. The affected gland usually feels symmetrically enlarged, smooth, and firm though slightly elastic. It seems to protrude more into the rectal lumen. The median sulcus may be obliterated. Finding an expected-sized gland by palpation, however, does not rule out BPH. Prostatic hyperplasia may obstruct urinary flow, causing symptoms, yet not be palpable.

Cancer of the Prostate

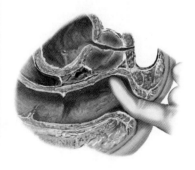

Cancer of the prostate is suggested by an area of hardness in the gland. A distinct hard nodule that alters the contour of the gland may or may not be palpable. As the cancer enlarges, it feels irregular and may extend beyond the confines of the gland. The median sulcus may be obscured. Hard areas in the prostate are not always malignant. They may also result from prostatic stones, chronic inflammation, and other conditions.

Special Populations

24

Assessing the Woman Who Is Pregnant

ANGELA BOWEN AND LYNN S. BICKLEY

During pregnancy, significant changes in a woman's body help nourish and accommodate the developing fetus, prepare for the process of childbirth, and enable the mother to potentially breastfeed her baby. It can be a period of excitement and fear, happiness or despair, with major implications for the woman's health and well-being. A thorough assessment of all aspects of pregnancy is essential to ensure effective care for mother, baby, and family. Nurses have opportunities to interact with women during the preconception phase, pregnancy, and postnatal phase. One specific community example includes prenatal classes. The focus of this chapter is history taking and assessment of the healthy adult woman during preconception and pregnancy.

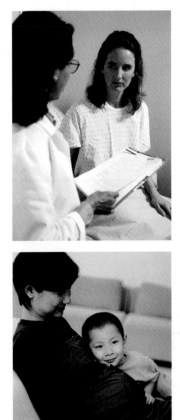

PRECONCEPTION

This period usually refers to the 3 months immediately before a pregnancy; however, because 50% of pregnancies are unplanned (Society of Obstetricians and Gynaecologists of Canada [SOGC], 2007a), sexually active women of childbearing age are potentially in the preconception phase at all times unless they have been sterilized or are in menopause. When a pregnancy is planned, preconception is a time for preparing the woman's body to promote a healthy pregnancy and fetus. During this phase, health care providers may work with women to address several factors.

ASSESSMENT OF RISK FACTORS

Risks include all factors that may affect fertility, pregnancy, or childbirth and existing conditions that pregnancy may worsen. Awareness of and appropriate planning to address such factors help minimize their effects on pregnancy and childbirth. During preconception, the woman also may eliminate some risk factors, such as smoking and drinking alcohol.

Medical Conditions. Those that can affect maternal and fetal health during pregnancy include hypertension, diabetes, obesity, anemia, and bowel disorders. Preconception interventions to increase the chances for successful pregnancy include changing antihypertensive drugs that are unsafe during pregnancy to those that are safe, losing weight, and stabilizing blood glucose levels.

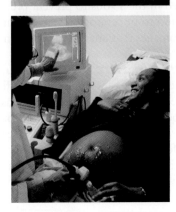

Medications. Several prescription and over-the-counter medications are *teratogenic* (have adverse effects on the fetus and pregnancy). Identifying potential teratogenic medications before pregnancy begins helps decrease these effects. Some medications can be substituted with drugs that have been proven safe during pregnancy.

Maternal Age. Increased maternal age is linked with decreased fertility and other conditions affecting pregnancy. Although nothing can be done to change a client's age, planning and careful monitoring may help minimize some associated risks.

Genetic Concerns. Identifying genetic concerns related to the client's age or to the family or individual history of conditions in either partner helps during pregnancy planning. Genetic counselling is offered to couples at risk for conceiving a baby with genetic disorders.

 Cultural Considerations

In some cultures, a woman may undergo female genital mutilation (FGM). FGM can contribute to chronic pelvic inflammatory disease, infertility, fear of intimacy, and challenges with labour and birth (Hacker, Moore, & Gambone, 2004).

■ *Risks for Genetic Disorders and Maternal Age*		
Maternal Age (years)	Risk for Down Syndrome	Total Risk for Chromosomal Abnormalities
20	1/1667	1/526
30	1/952	1/384
35	1/385	1/192
40	1/106	1/66
45	1/30	1/21
48	1/14	1/10

Adapted from the SOGC, 2006.

Exposure to Diethylstilbestrol (DES) as a Fetus. The drug DES was used in the 1960s to prevent premature labour and spontaneous abortion. It was found to be teratogenic, and women exposed to DES as fetuses may have cervical anomalies that affect their pregnancy and childbirth.

Rubella Titre, Blood Group, and Type. Maternal exposure to rubella (German measles) can seriously affect the fetus if the pregnant client has not had or been immunized against the disease. Rubella causes birth defects and miscarriage, especially in the first trimester. Routine immunization programs to prevent rubella are standard in Canada (Public Health Agency, 2005). Checking the titre of a client before she is pregnant is necessary to determine whether her immunity to rubella is active. If the client has not been immunized or the titre is not at an expected level, the rubella vaccination can be administered before the pregnancy begins.

Checking blood group and type also assists with comprehensive planning. Women who are Rh negative require an injection of Rho (D) Immune Globulin (Human) to prevent hemolytic disease in the newborn. It is important to identify this as early as possible in a pregnancy. Other blood tests include antibody serum, CBC, VDRL, and hepatitis B and C.

Sexually Transmitted Infections (STIs).   Many STIs affect the pregnant woman and fetus. Some, such as syphilis and HIV, can be transmitted from mother to fetus. Testing both female and male partners for STIs is beneficial for possible treatment of them before pregnancy begins or for effective management of pregnancy and delivery. Include testing for chlamydia, gonorrhea, and human papillomavirus (HPV).

Workplace Exposures.   Numerous workplace substances have been identified as potentially harmful to the fetus. Exposure of either parent to various chemicals, metals, vinyl monomers, anaesthetic gases, or radiation needs to be assessed to determine potential fetal effects.

Risk Behaviours.   These include high-risk activities that may affect pregnancy or the growing fetus. Examples are having multiple sexual partners and engaging in extreme sports (e.g., skydiving, race car driving).

Use of tobacco, alcohol, or recreational drugs and exposure to secondhand smoke have been proven to have several negative effects on pregnancy, the developing fetus, childbirth, and breastfeeding (Health Canada, 2005; Lander et al., 2005). Encouraging women to stop smoking, avoid recreational drugs, and limit alcohol and exposure to secondhand smoke in the preconception phase helps improve the potential for a healthy pregnancy, mother, and baby.

PROMOTING WELLNESS IN PREPARATION FOR PREGNANCY

Nutrition.   Recommendations are for the woman planning to become pregnant to eat a well-balanced daily diet (see accompanying table) that includes a folic acid supplement. The correct value is 400 mcg/day (0.4 mg) for all women, particularly during the 3 months before conception. Once pregnancy occurs, 600 mcg (0.6 mg) of folic acid is required daily (Health Canada, 2007d). Up to 1000 mcg/day (1.0 mg) is recommended for women with increased risk of neural tube defects (e.g., those taking anticonvulsants or with a history of delivering a baby with neural tube defects) (Wilson et al., 2007).

■ *Recommended Daily Servings for Females*	
	All Women Aged 19–50 Years
Vegetables and fruit	7–8
Grain products	6–7
Milk and alternatives	2
Meat and alternatives	2

Source: Health Canada, 2007a,d.

Exercise. Exercise before and during pregnancy promotes overall maternal and fetal health (Public Health Agency of Canada [PHAC], 2008b). Guidelines for exercise during pregnancy are available at http://www.healthycanadians.gc.ca/hp-gs/pdf/hpguide-eng.pdf.

Dental and Gum Health. Healthy teeth and gums are essential to a healthy pregnancy. Any dental procedures should be done prior to pregnancy to minimize exposure to x-rays and anesthetics (Bulechek, Butcher, & Dochterman, 2008; PHAC, 2008a).

Social Support. Assessing the client's available support systems helps with planning and assistance during and after the pregnancy. Partner, family, friends, and spiritual support systems can benefit the client during these periods.

CONTRACEPTION

Stopping contraception methods is necessary before pregnancy can occur. It is recommended to discontinue hormonal contraception (e.g., birth-control pill) at least 2 to 3 usual periods before and to remove uterine contraceptive devices at least one usual period before planned conception.

PREGNANCY

The techniques of assessment and examination are similar to those of the nonpregnant woman; however, nurses need to understand and be able to distinguish the unique physiologic changes associated with pregnancy, which are amplified with twin and other multiple pregnancies. Pregnancy is divided into three trimesters: first trimester, 1 to 12 weeks; second trimester, 13 to 27 weeks; third trimester, 28 to 40+ weeks.

ANATOMY AND PHYSIOLOGY

HORMONAL CHANGES

During pregnancy, hormonal changes lead to extensive anatomical and physiologic changes in every major organ system. Increased levels of estradiol, progesterone, and placental hormones, especially human chorionic gonadotropin (HCG), drive many of the endocrine and metabolic changes of pregnancy, which are briefly summarized here:

- Estradiol appears to stimulate lactotrophs in the *anterior lobe of the pituitary gland*. These cells may triple in size as increasing prolactin output readies the breast tissue for lactation (Petraglia et al., 2004).

- The *posterior pituitary gland* stores oxytocin and antidiuretic hormone (ADH)—HCG appears to reset the receptors for thirst and ADH release, leading to decreased serum sodium concentration and, in some women, polyuria.

- The *thyroid gland* remains normal size; however, estrogen effects on thyroxine-binding globulin and HCG stimulation of the thyrotropin (TSH) receptor lead to fluctuations in free T4 and T3 levels and in TSH, usually within the normal range (Berghout & Wiersinga, 1998).

■ *Placental hormones* contribute to increased *insulin resistance* in later pregnancy and a shift from carbohydrate to fat metabolism. Insulin resistance is linked to transient hyperglycemia after meals, but between meals, fasting glucose levels fall, partly because of the demands of fetal growth and increased peripheral use of glucose (Boden, 1996).

■ At the end of pregnancy, increases in placental corticotrophin-releasing factor and adrenal adrenocorticotropic hormone produce "a state of *relative hypercortisolism*" that may be a trigger for labour (Mazjoub et al., 1999; Petraglia et al., 2004).

■ Rising *progesterone* levels have several effects. Although respiratory rate does not change, tidal volume and minute ventilation increase, sometimes leading to complaints of dyspnea. Progesterone and estradiol lower esophageal sphincter tone, contributing to symptoms of reflux and heartburn. Progesterone also relaxes tone and contraction in the ureters, causing hydronephrosis, and in the bladder, increasing risk for bacteriuria.

■ *Cardiovascular changes* in pregnancy are significant. Plasma volume increases up to 50% by the end of pregnancy, causing a dilutional but physiologic anemia. Cardiac output increases, and systemic vascular resistance and blood pressure fall.

■ Finally, *musculoskeletal changes* ensue from weight gain and *relaxin*, a hormone secreted in the corpus luteum and placenta: lumbar lordosis as the gravid uterus enlarges, contributing to mechanical low back discomfort, and ligamentous laxity in the sacroiliac joints and the pubic symphysis, to ease passage of the baby through the birth canal.

RESPIRATORY SYSTEM

Relaxin may be responsible for laxity of the chest-wall ligaments, a 20% increase in oxygen consumption, increased pliability of connective tissue with decreased pulmonary resistance, and increased levels of sensitivity to CO_2 by progesterone (Hacker et al., 2004). The enlarging uterus can also affect respiratory status by placing pressure on the diaphragm.

The diaphragm rises as the uterus grows, which causes the rib cage to flare, vertical diameter to decrease, and anterior–posterior and transverse diameters to increase. Chest circumference increases by up to 6 cm. These compensatory changes prevent loss of intrathoracic volume (Nichols & Zwelling, 1997). Thoracic breathing occurs as the uterus grows.

Because total oxygen consumption increases by 15% to 20% and tidal volume increases by 40%, the respiratory rate does not increase in pregnancy (Hacker et al., 2004; London et al., 2007).

Airway resistance is unchanged or decreased; however, many women experience dyspnea. The costal angle increases from 68° to 103° (Hacker et al., 2004). Increased vascularity may cause nasal stuffiness and epistaxis.

CARDIOVASCULAR SYSTEM

Systolic Murmur. As the uterus grows, the diaphragm is elevated. The heart shifts upward, forward, and to the left, which can lead to a systolic murmur in up to

90% of pregnant women. About 20% of women may have a diastolic murmur and 10% a continuous murmur. No expected changes in ECG occur (Nichols & Zwelling, 1997).

Total Blood Volume, Cardiac Output, and Anemia. Blood flow increases in early pregnancy, with ongoing increases to the uterus, kidneys, breasts, and skin. Two areas of major increase are the kidneys (for elimination of waste) and skin (for elimination of heat). Total blood volume and cardiac output increase by approximately 40%. A disproportionate increase in plasma compared to red blood cells causes hemodilution and decreased hematocrit values, often referred to as "physiologic anemia of pregnancy"(London et al., 2007; Nichols & Zwelling, 1997).

Syncope. Feelings of lightheadedness and syncope (temporary loss of consciousness) occur in early pregnancy as a combination of postural hypotension, vasomotor instability, and hypoglycemia (Nichols & Zwelling, 1997).

Venous Compression. Pressure from the growing fetus and gravid uterus compresses the iliac veins and inferior vena cava. Decreased venous return in the supine position can lead to supine hypotension and bradycardia in 10% of pregnant women. Venous compression elevates pressure in the veins that drain the pelvic organs and legs, which increases edema and varicosities in the legs, vulva, and rectum (hemorrhoids). It also predisposes the woman to thrombosis. In the third trimester, compression of the uterus by the aorta, the "Poseiro effect," can decrease blood flow to the fetus. This is suspected when the femoral pulse cannot be felt (Hacker et al., 2004).

Changes in Blood Values. Platelet levels remain stable. There is a 40% increase in fibrin levels; however, bleeding time and clotting time are unchanged. Overall, pregnancy is a hypercoagulable state (increases in clotting factors I, II, V, VII, VIII, X, XII), which along with decreased protein S (anticoagulant) and venous stasis, increases the risk of thromboembolism and subsequent pulmonary embolism (Simpson & Creehan, 2008).

VITAL SIGNS

Changes in vital signs are described in this section.

■ *Changes in Vital Signs*		
Parameter	**Change**	**Gestation**
Arterial blood pressure		
Systolic	↓ 4–6 mm Hg	Lowest at 20–24 weeks, gradually increases to term
Diastolic	↓ 8–15 mm Hg	
Mean	↓ 6–10 mm Hg	
Pulse	↑ 10–18 beats/min	Early 2nd trimester, then stable
Respirations	No change	
Temperature	May be slightly elevated	As pregnancy progresses

Adapted from Hacker et al., 2004, and London et al., 2007.

GASTROINTESTINAL SYSTEM

Progesterone relaxes the smooth muscle, which can decrease peristalsis and delay gastric emptying. Estrogen decreases gastric secretion of hydrochloric acid and pepsin, and the growing uterus exerts abdominal pressure, which can result in bloating and constipation.

The gums are softer, spongier, and more prone to bleeding. This is a result of the effect of estrogen on the collagenous tissue (Nichols & Zwelling, 1997). Increased hCG and carbohydrate metabolism can promote nausea and vomiting, and alterations in taste. *Ptylism* is the increased sensation of saliva, but there is no evidence of saliva increase in pregnancy (Nichols & Zwelling, 1997). Relaxation of the cardiac sphincter causes gastroaesophageal reflux disease (GERD) in 40% to 80% of women who are pregnant (Winbery & Blaho, 2001). Estrogen decreases bile flow, which along with smooth muscle relaxation leads to biliary stasis with prolonged emptying of the gallbladder. Higher levels of cholesterol predispose to cholelithiasis (Hacker et al., 2004).

RENAL AND URINARY TRACTS

Increased vascularity results in the kidneys enlarging by 1.5 cm. Progesterone causes smooth muscle relaxation and dilatation of the ureters. Dextrorotation of the uterus causes further dilatation of the right ureter. As the uterus enlarges it can obstruct the ureters. The changes begin early in pregnancy and can remain until the 16th week postpartum (Hacker et al., 2004; Sanders & Lucas, 2001) and predispose the woman to bladder and kidney infections.

Urinary Frequency.   Pressure on the bladder increases in the first and third trimesters, which results in the need to urinate frequently.

Increased Renal Blood Flow.   Renal plasma flow and glomerular filtration rate (GFR) increase by up to 50% by 20 weeks, then remain at a plateau until term. The increased GFR is reflected in a 25% decrease in serum creatinine and urea nitrogen (Hacker et al., 2004).

Glycosuria/Glucosuria.   Increased renal blood flow decreases the renal threshold for glucose; however, glycosuria is not to be ignored, because it may indicate gestational diabetes and can promote vaginal infections.

INTEGUMENTARY SYSTEM

Stretching of the skin and hormones lead to changes in the integumentary system of the pregnant client.

Increased Pigmentation.   Pigmentation of the areola, nipples, vulva, and perineum increases. In some women, a darkened line up the abdomen appears, which is called linea nigra. Chloasma, or "mask of pregnancy," is a blotchy brown discoloration on the face, caused by stimulation of the anterior pituitary hormone melanotropin. It increases with sun exposure (Nichols & Zwelling, 1997).

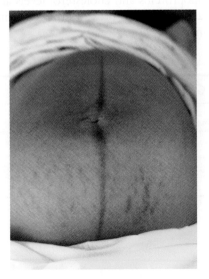

Increased Secretions. Sweat and sebaceous glands are hyperactive during pregnancy, resulting in increased production of sweat and sebum (an oily, colourless, odourless fluid). Increased sebum leads to an increase in acne (London et al., 2005).

Hair. Women may experience *hirsutism* (increased hair growth). Nail growth may also be affected, with nails being longer but thinner and softer (Nichols & Zwelling, 1997; Hacker et al., 2004).

Striae. Separation of underlying connective tissue causes striae on the abdomen, thighs, buttocks, and breasts. These appear as purplish lines on affected areas of skin, and then change to whitish, gray lines over time.

Vascular Changes in Skin. Spider angioma, vascular spiders, or spider nevi may appear. Also, small red lines from ruptured capillaries caused by increased blood volume and estrogen may appear on the chest, neck, face, arms, and legs. Palmar erythema, or redness of the palms, results from increased subcutaneous blood flow.

Itchiness. Itching, or "cholestasis of pregnancy," may result from the reduced flow of bile into the intestines, which causes bile salts to accumulate in the bloodstream. It usually begins on the palms of the hands and the soles of feet and can become generalized. Jaundice can develop.

MUSCULOSKELETAL SYSTEM

Increased progesterone and estrogen levels affect the musculoskeletal system and result in several changes. Joints and ligaments relax from increased relaxin levels during pregnancy, which can result in injury. Lordosis increases with the increasing size of the uterus; low backache is common. The pelvis relaxes and the ligaments elongate from increased estrogen and progesterone levels, resulting in an unstable, waddling gait. The anterior–posterior diameter ratio increases as well. The rectus abdominus muscle may separate with diminished muscle tone (diastasis recti). In severe cases, an examiner may be able to palpate the fetus.

METABOLIC CHANGES

During pregnancy, metabolic needs increase and the basal metabolic rate (BMR) can increase by 20% to 25%. Increased water retention, increased need for protein and carbohydrates, and increased lipoproteins and cholesterol levels also occur during pregnancy. Health Canada (2007a, 2007b) provides the following guidelines for ranges in weight gain in pregnancy.

■ *Guidelines for Gestational Weight Gain Ranges*	
BMI Category*	**Recommended Gain (kg)**
BMI <20	12.5–18.0
BMI 20–27	11.5–16.0
BMI >27	7.0–11.5

*Does not apply to multiple gestation pregnancies.
Source: Health Canada, 2007a,b.

ENDOCRINE SYSTEM

Several changes in the endocrine system result from increased hormone levels.

Thyroid. Thyroid function increases by 50%. Thyroxine increases; however, there is no increase in TSH. Parathyroids enlarge, especially if a woman is not getting enough calcium. Parathyroid levels decrease in the first trimester and then increase throughout pregnancy. Hyperparathyroidism of pregnancy causes an increase in the availability of calcium and vitamin D for the fetus.

Adrenals. There is no structural change in the adrenal glands, but cortisol and aldosterone levels increase.

Pancreas. Insulin decreases as the fetus uses the woman's glucose stores, while insulin needs increase with rising levels of estrogen, progesterone, HCG, HPL, and cortisol. The placenta produces insulinase, which counteracts maternal insulin. This is called the diabetogenic effect of pregnancy (Nichols & Zwelling, 1997). Compromised pancreatic function leads to an increased risk of gestational diabetes.

BREASTS

Breasts are very sensitive to higher levels of estrogen and progesterone, resulting in several changes during pregnancy. Sensations of tingling, tenderness, or fullness are common. The nipples become more erectile and darken, the areolae darken, venous patterns become more visible, and Montgomery's tubercles (small bumps around the areolae) enlarge. The greater number and size of mammary glands result in breast enlargement. The woman may produce colostrum as early as the second trimester.

REPRODUCTIVE SYSTEM

A bluish discoloration of the vagina, cervix, uterus, and vulva (Chadwick's sign) may occur. The mucosa thickens as a result of hormonal and vascular changes.

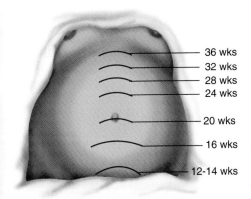

EXPECTED HEIGHT OF THE UTERINE FUNDUS BY MONTH OF PREGNANCY

36 wks
32 wks
28 wks
24 wks
20 wks
16 wks
12-14 wks

Vaginal Changes. Increased estrogen levels and vascularity affect the vagina. Leukorrhea (white, thick, acidic secretions) occurs, and vaginal pH becomes more acidic from the action of *Lactobacillus acidophilus* on increased levels of glycogen in the vaginal epithelium. Also, clients are at an increased risk for monilial (yeast) infections.

Uterus. There is hypertrophy of existing cells and increased fibrous tissue in the uterus. The weight of the uterus increases from 60 g to 1100 g, and volume increases from 10 mL to 5000 mL (London et al., 2007). The uterus softens (Hegar's sign). The abdomen becomes increasingly prominent to accommodate the growing uterus and fetus. Early distention from fluid retention and relaxation of abdominal muscles can be detected even before the uterus expands into the abdominal cavity at 12 to 14 weeks' gestation. Expected growth patterns of the gravid uterus are illustrated to the left, and the standing contours of the primigravid abdomen in each trimester of pregnancy are shown to the right.

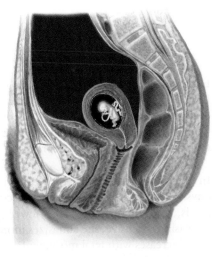

FIRST TRIMESTER

As the uterus grows, it changes shape and position. The nongravid uterus may be anteverted, retroverted, or retroflexed. Until up to 12 weeks of gestation, the gravid uterus is still a pelvic organ. Regardless of its initial positioning, the enlarging uterus becomes anteverted and quickly fills space usually occupied by the bladder, triggering frequent voiding. By 12 weeks' gestation, the uterus straightens and rises out of the pelvis and can be felt when palpating the abdomen.

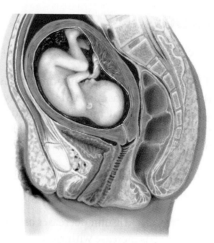

SECOND TRIMESTER

The enlarging uterus pushes the intestinal contents laterally and superiorly and stretches its supporting ligaments, sometimes causing "round ligament pain" in the lower quadrants, more typically on the right. The uterus adapts to fetal growth and positions, and tends to rotate to the right to accommodate the rectosigmoid structures on the left side of the pelvis.

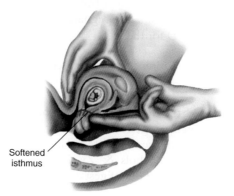

Softened isthmus

HEGAR'S SIGN

Cervix. The vaginal portion of the cervix softens (Goodell's sign), and a mucous plug forms and blocks the cervix to prevent bacteria from entering the uterus. Red velvety mucosa, termed *cervical erosion* or *eversion*, also commonly appears on the cervix and is an expected finding.

Ovaries and Fallopian Tubes. Changes are less noticeable on physical examination. Corpus luteum, the ovarian follicle that discharged the ovum, may be felt as a small nodule on the affected ovary. This nodule disappears by mid-pregnancy.

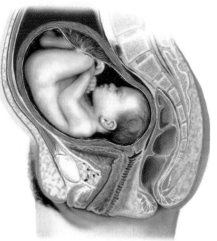

THIRD TRIMESTER

Placenta. The placenta develops by the third week and continues to grow until it covers 50% of the uterine wall at 20 weeks. By delivery it is 3 cm thick and weighs 400 to 600 g.

PSYCHOLOGICAL CHANGES OF PREGNANCY

Each trimester poses unique psychological challenges for the woman and her family. In the first trimester, she may experience many uncomfortable physical symptoms (e.g., fatigue, nausea, vomiting). She may be ambivalent about the pregnancy. The woman can be more introspective and forgetful. She may have emotional lability with increased anxiety and depression.

In the second trimester, the woman is likely to be more psychologically and physically robust. The pregnancy becomes obvious as the uterus rises out of the pelvis, and there are usually fewer physical concerns. The woman becomes increasingly pensive; she fantasizes more about the baby, and her attachment to the fetus increases with fetal movement.

The third trimester can bring increased reports of fatigue and insomnia because of increased fetal activity and physical discomforts such as backache and urinary frequency. The woman may be very self-absorbed and may experience increasing anxiety about the birth and impending motherhood. She may be more susceptible to depression at this time than at any other time in the pregnancy (Kendell et al., 1976; Spinelli, 2001).

THE HEALTH HISTORY: SUBJECTIVE DATA

The pregnant woman may experience several signs and symptoms. Not all women experience the same signs or symptoms and may experience differing severity of the symptoms or signs.

Begin the health history with a general open-ended question such as, "Describe how you have been feeling during this pregnancy" or "Tell me about any concerns you have." From this, follow the information that the client gives you to gather more data.

■ *Key Symptoms and Signs of Pregnancy Reported by Clients*

Sign and Symptom	Time in Pregnancy	Explanation
Amenorrhea—no menses	Throughout	High levels of estrogen, progesterone, and HCG support the developing pregnancy and avert menses and shedding of the endometrial lining.
Nausea and/or vomiting	Usually first trimester	Hormones slow peristalsis and causes changes in taste or smell.
Breast tenderness, tingling	Usually first trimester	Increased estrogen and progesterone stimulate growth of breast tissue and mammary glands. Vascularity increases. The woman may complain of pain between the shoulder blades from the increased weight.
Weight loss	Usually first trimester	Woman may lose 1–2 kg from nausea and vomiting or change in food preferences.
Groin/lower abdominal pain	Second trimester	Growing uterus causes tension, spasms, and stretching of round ligaments.
Urinary frequency, incontinence	First and third trimesters	Increased blood volume and glomerular filtration increase urine production, leaving less room for the bladder until the uterus rises out of the pelvis at approximately 13 weeks and when the head descends (third trimester). Uterine pressure and smooth muscle relaxation may cause stress incontinence.
Fatigue	First and third trimesters	The woman may be tired from rapid changes in energy requirements, progesterone (sedative effect), physical discomforts, sleep disturbances, fetal movement, depression.
Edema	Third trimester	Increased venous pressure in the legs, obstruction of lymph flow, and reduced plasma colloid osmotic pressure.
Heartburn	Throughout	Relaxation of lower esophageal sphincter allows stomach contents to back up into lower esophagus.
Constipation	Throughout	Relaxed smooth muscle slows peristalsis. Iron supplements may also cause constipation.
Backache, shooting pain down right leg	Throughout	Relaxation of joints and ligaments and lordosis is required to balance the growing uterus. The increased pressure of uterus aggravates the sciatic nerve.
Leukorrhea-white vaginal discharge	Throughout	Increased blood flow and high estrogen levels. Change in colour, itchiness, or odour may indicate infection.
Headaches	Throughout	Estrogen and progesterone contribute to migraine and other headaches.
Leg cramps	As pregnancy progresses	Pressure of the growing uterus and/or excessive intake of phosphorus and a shortage of calcium.
Bleeding gums or "pregnancy gingivitis"	Second and third trimesters	Rising progesterone levels—gums react to the bacteria in plaque, increased vascularity of mouth, hypertrophy of gums.

KEY DATA REQUIRED BY HEALTH PROFESSIONALS

Confirmation of Pregnancy. This can be done by detection of HCG in the woman's urine. Many home pregnancy urine tests can detect a pregnancy a few days before the first missed period and are up to 99% accurate. Ultrasound can be used as early as 5 weeks; blood levels of HCG are also used to confirm pregnancy.

Expected Date of Confinement (EDC) or Delivery (EDD) or Birth (EDB). This can be calculated from the date of the last menstrual period, blood levels of beta HCG, and ultrasound. A modified Nagele's rule is often used to determine the expected delivery date by counting ahead 7 days and 9 months from the first day of the last menstrual period.

Current Health Status and Medical History. Data such as current age, health status, previous medical history, and medications are essential for assessment. Women who are older than 35 years or younger than 15 years are at increased risk for maternal and fetal complications during pregnancy. Hypertension, diabetes, thyroid disorders, peripheral vascular disorders, obesity, and allergies are some examples of conditions that may affect pregnancy and childbirth. Other important data include previous hospitalizations and surgeries, current medications, supplements and alternative therapies, blood transfusions, vital signs, urinalysis, psychiatric disorders (depression, anxiety, anorexia, bipolar disorder, schizophrenia, addictions) and hemoglobin levels.

Obstetrical and Gynecological History. Review the following:

- Fertility concerns or interventions

- Number, duration, and outcome of pregnancies

- Type of delivery, anesthesia, complications

- Birth weight and health

- Present health of children. Are they alive and well? Do they live with the client?

- Unexpected vaginal bleeding

- Sexually transmitted infections

- Gynaecologic surgeries or other procedures

- Date of last Pap smear and results

- Contraceptive history including type and duration used

Lifestyle and Work Factors. Review information that pertains to the client's work and lifestyle behaviours that may affect the pregnancy and fetal development.

Tobacco, Alcohol, Caffeine, or Recreational Drug Use/Abuse. Ask the client about amounts used, type, motivation to quit, and client's knowledge of the risks associated with the use of these substances.

Risk Behaviours. Multiple sexual partners, competitive or extreme sports, and use of safety measures such as seatbelts and helmets are important data to gather.

Exercise. Collect information about the type and amount of exercise, and safety measures the woman uses during exercise.

Nutrition.   Gather information about the client's understanding of Canada's Food Guide and nutritional needs during pregnancy. Ask her to give an overview of the foods and beverages she consumes in a typical day.

Work History.   Review the client's past and current employment to determine any potential workplace exposures that may affect the pregnancy. Also consider potential for injury related to the client's type of work.

Family History.   Information about the client's biological family helps assess the potential for some conditions that may affect the pregnancy and development of the fetus.

Genetically Transmitted Diseases.   Key concerns include history of muscular dystrophy, hemophilia, cystic fibrosis, fragile X syndrome, congenital heart disease, phenylketonuria, sickle cell anemia, and Tay-Sach's disease.

Congenital Anomalies.   Kye concerns include history of congenital anomalies such as spina bifida, anencephaly, cleft palate and lip, hypospadias, and congenital heart disease.

Obstetrical History of Mother and/or Sisters.   Obtain information about family members relative to their pregnancies and outcomes.

Chronic Diseases.   Ask about conditions such as diabetes mellitus, asthma, hypertension, psychosis, epileptic disorders, rheumatoid arthritis, and deafness.

Psychosocial Stressors.   This includes any information regarding the psychological adjustment of the client to the pregnancy, delivery, and parental role. Identify positive coping mechanisms, stress management techniques, and support systems (father, partner, friends, family, spiritual, and other) that can help the client. Assess whether the client plans to continue with the pregnancy, raise the baby, or give the child to an adoptive couple. Inquire about financial concerns, because low income is associated with poor pregnancy outcomes (Joseph et al., 2007). Ask about current stressors in the woman's life or work, and whether there is any risk to her or the baby for family violence.

Begin with a symptom or sign reported by the client. Always start with an open-ended question. Health professionals use a symptom analysis approach to collect data related to all aspects of a symptom. The symptom of "fatigue" is used as the topic for symptom analysis that follows:

Example of Questions for Symptom Analysis—Fatigue

- "Where in your body are you most aware of your fatigue?" (*Location*)
- "Describe your fatigue." (*Quality*)
- "To what degree does the fatigue affect your ability to perform your usual daily activities?" (*Severity*)
- "When did you notice your energy levels change?" (*Onset*)
- "Have your energy levels stayed low? Or do they change?" (*Constancy*)
- "Is there a time of day that you feel more fatigued?" (*Timing*)
- "What makes the fatigue worse?" (*Aggravating factors*)
- "What helps reduce the fatigue?" "Can you put your feet up during the day?" "Can you take a nap?"

"Do you get any help with household chores?" "Or help with other children?" (*Alleviating factors*)
- "Are you noticing any other symptoms?" "Are you feeling sad?" "Depressed?" "How are you sleeping?" "Have you had your blood checked for anemia?" (*Associated symptoms*)
- "What is going on in your work/school/home/recreational environment that might be affecting your fatigue?" "How much stress is in your life right now?" (*Environmental factors*)
- "Tell me how the fatigue is affecting your life." (*Significance to client*)
- "What do you think is contributing to the fatigue you feel?" (*Client perspective*)

HEALTH PROMOTION AND RISK FACTOR ASSESSMENT

Pregnancy is a time of increased contact with health care professionals. This provides an excellent opportunity to introduce and support lifestyle changes that will promote health throughout life.

Important Topics for Health Promotion

- Prevention of gestational diabetes
- Promotion of mental health and safety
- Promotion of healthy lifestyle
- Promotion of good nutrition and oral health
- Prenatal and breastfeeding classes
- Follow-up visits and prenatal monitoring

PREVENTION OF GESTATIONAL DIABETES

A pregnant woman who exercises and eats a balanced diet is less likely to gain excessive weight or develop gestational diabetes. Women with gestational diabetes have increased risks for gestational hypertension, infection, and operative delivery or giving birth to a baby with macrosomia, other anomalies, or health problems. A woman without or with well-managed gestational diabetes has a decreased risk for developing type 1 or type 2 diabetes later in life (London et al., 2007). For a woman with multiple risk factors, diabetes testing should be done during the first trimester, then again during the second and third trimesters, even if results from the first test are negative (Canadian Diabetes Association, 2007).

Risk factors include previous diagnosis of gestational diabetes, past delivery of a high-birthweight infant; Aboriginal, Hispanic, South Asian, Asian, or African heritage; age ≥35 years; obesity; history of polycystic ovary syndrome or aconthosis nigricans; and use of corticosteroids.

PROMOTION OF MENTAL HEALTH AND SAFETY

Pregnancy is a time of change and increased stress, which can trigger anxiety and depression. Depression can affect up to 20% of pregnant women (Marcus et al., 2003). Untreated, these illnesses have deleterious effects on the fetus, the pregnancy and the mother. The Edinburgh Postnatal Depression scale is a 10-item screen validated for use in pregnancy and post partum (Cox, Holden, & Sagovsky, 1987).

Cultural Considerations

For women considered at high risk during pregnancy, as many as 29% have depression and anxiety (Bowen & Muhajarine, 2006).

Intimate partner violence (IPV) is reported in 6% to 8% of pregnancies, which is considered conservative due to underreporting. The SOGC (2005) suggests health care providers assess IPV as part of prenatal care and in response to symptoms or conditions associated with abuse such as bruises on abdomen. IPV can have serious effects on the woman who is pregnant, the pregnancy, and the fetus (SOGC, 2005). Ask the client in a nonjudgmental manner about potential exposure to violence. Ensure that you are in a private setting to foster the client's feeling of safety to promote reporting of violence.

■ Potential Effects of Intimate Partner Violence

Maternal	Pregnancy	Fetal
■ Delayed prenatal care ■ Insufficient weight gain ■ Maternal infections (vaginal, cervical, kidney, uterine) ■ Exacerbation of chronic illness ■ Maternal stress ■ Maternal depression	■ Abdominal trauma ■ Miscarriage ■ Antepartum hemorrhage ■ Premature rupture of membranes ■ Premature labour and birth ■ Abruptio placenta ■ Complications during labour	■ Low birth weight ■ Fetal injury ■ Fetal death

National Domestic Violence Hotline (bilingual): 1-800-363-9010.
National Clearinghouse on Family Violence, Public Health Agency of Canada: 1-800-267-1291.
Source: PHAC, 2006.

■ PROMOTION OF HEALTHY LIFESTYLE HABITS

Encourage the client to quit smoking, stop drinking alcohol, decrease caffeine intake, avoid over-the-counter medications, and reduce risk behaviours, Smoking has been linked to (1) increased rates of spontaneous abortion and perinatal mortality (Health Canada, 2005; London et al., 2005); (2) complications of labour such as placental abruption, placenta previa, and preterm delivery (Health Canada, 2005); and (3) increased incidence of low-birth weight newborns, babies with cleft lip and palate, and sudden infant death syndrome (SIDS; London et al., 2005). The woman should stop all alcohol intake to prevent the risk of (1) mental retardation, (2) cardiac anomalies, (3) interuterine growth restriction, and (4) fetal alcohol spectrum disorder (London et al., 2005). Drugs such as narcotics (heroin and methadone), barbituates, tranquilizers, stimulants (amphetamines and cocaine), psychotropics (PCP "angel dust," LSD, marijuana) and "club drugs" (MDMA—"Ecstasy," Rohypnol—"date rape drug") can cause various congenital abnormalities as well as challenges for the newborn such as withdrawal symptoms (London et al., 2005).

Sexually Transmitted Infections (STIs). Unprotected or risky sexual activity may increase the chance of acquiring STIs; however, all women should be assessed for STIs. Considerations related specifically to pregnancy are bolded in the following table.

■ Sexually Transmitted Infections

Infection	Signs and Symptoms	Considerations
Chlamydia	Vaginal discharge, painful urination, lower abdominal pain, bleeding, pain during intercourse, eye/rectal infection (rare)	Pelvic inflammatory disease (PID), **ectopic pregnancy, infertility,** chronic pelvic pain, rashes, sores, joint pain
Gonorrhea	Increased vaginal discharge; painful urination; lower abdominal pain; bleeding, pain during intercourse; rectal pain, discharge, or itching	PID, chronic pelvic pain, **infertility, ectopic pregnancy,** systemic gonococcal infection

(continued)

■ *Sexually Transmitted Infections (Continued)*

Infection	Signs and Symptoms	Considerations
Syphilis	*Primary*: small painless chancre where bacteria entered the body. This will heal on its own. *Secondary*: general feeling of being unwell; rash, particularly on the palms of the hands or soles of the feet; patchy hair loss; flat smooth condylomata acuminate-genital warts *Early latent*: generally asymptomatic, but lesions or rashes may reappear for the first year of infection *Tertiary*: damage to cardiovascular and neurological systems and other major organs; may lead to death.	■ Increased risk of contracting or transmitting HIV; **during the pregnancy syphilis can be transmitted to the fetus. In Alberta from 2005 to 2007, 14 babies were born with congenital syphilis and 5 died (Simons, 2008).** ■ Treatment must be monitored to ensure effectiveness. ■ Longer course of treatment and closer follow-up may be necessary for people with HIV co-infection.
Genital herpes	Not all infected people are symptomatic. Tingling, burning sensations where infection first entered; outbreaks may include painful sores, inflammation and redness, fever, muscular pain, tender lymph nodes. Atypical symptoms are genital pain, urethritis, aseptic meningitis, cervicitis.	■ Avoid sexual activity from the start of the tingling until after all lesions have healed. ■ Condoms and medications can reduce but not eliminate the risk of transmission. ■ **Precautions can be taken during pregnancy and delivery to reduce the risk of transmission to the baby.**
Hepatitis B	Tiredness, nausea, and vomiting, decreased appetite, rash, joint pain, yellowing of the eyes and skin	■ Sexual partners and household contacts should be advised to be vaccinated. ■ Can lead to cirrhosis and cancer of the liver ■ May require liver-functioning monitoring ■ **Babies born to mothers with hepatitis B are at high risk of becoming carriers. Injections of antibodies and the vaccine should be administered immediately after birth.**
Human immunodeficiency virus (HIV)	Frequent fever or sweats; joint or muscle pain; persistent skin rashes; swollen glands, sore throat; fatigue or lack of energy; headaches; rapid, unexplained weight loss; nausea, vomiting, diarrhea	**HIV can be transmitted during pregnancy, childbirth, and breastfeeding.**
Human papillomavirus (HPV) can cause condylomata acuminate, venereal/genital warts, cancer	■ May be asymptomatic ■ Anogenital warts may develop on the vulva, cervix, anus, or urethra ■ Itchiness ■ Discomfort during intercourse ■ Bleeding with intercourse	■ **During pregnancy, genital warts may increase in size and number and then resolve after delivery.** ■ **Rarely transmitted to infant during delivery** ■ Cervical, vulvar, vaginal, anal, and other cancers ■ Obstruction of the urethra or vaginal opening ■ Depression and sexual dysfunction in chronic cases ■ Vaccination is available to prevent certain types of HPV (See Chapter 22, p. 802)

(continued)

- *Sexually Transmitted Infections (Continued)*

Infection	Signs and Symptoms	Considerations
Candidiasis	Vaginal itching; swollen or red vulva and vagina; thick, white clumpy discharge resembling cottage cheese; burning of the external genitalia with urination; pain with intercourse from vaginal dryness and irritation of the vulva	**Yeast overgrowth can be caused by glucosuria of pregnancy.**
Trichomoniasis	Off-white or yellowish-green frothy discharge; sore or itchy vagina; pain during intercourse or urination	**May increase the risk of preterm delivery and low birth weight**

Source: Adapted from SOGC, 2007a.

Exercise.   Exercise increases demands for oxygen on the cardiovascular system, which is already altered by the pregnancy. Maternal cardiac reserves are lower, which may cause shunting of blood from the fetus during or after exercise (Hacker et al., 2004). Ideally, the woman will begin an exercise program at least 3 months before conception. The SOGC (2003b) recommends all pregnant women, without contraindications, participate in aerobic exercise and strength conditioning. Exercise should not lead to any loss of balance or fetal trauma. Walking, prenatal swimming, or yoga classes are beneficial. Contraindications to exercise in pregnancy are included below. The SOGC (2003b) heart rate target zones for the woman who is pregnant are also listed.

- *Contraindications for Exercise in Pregnancy*

Absolute Contraindications	Relative Contraindications
- Ruptured membranes - Preterm labour - Hypertensive disorders of pregnancy - Incompetent cervix - Growth-restricted fetus - High order multiple gestation - Placenta previa after 28th week - Persistent second or third trimester bleeding - Uncontrolled type 1 diabetes - Thyroid, cardiovascular, or other chronic disease	- Previous spontaneous abortion - Previous preterm birth - Mild/moderate cardiovascular disorder - Mild/moderate respiratory disorder - Anemia (Hb < 100 g/L) - Malnutrition or eating disorder - Twin pregnancy >28 weeks - Other significant medical conditions

Source: Adapted from SOGC, 2003b.

- *Heart Rate Target Zones for Aerobic Exercise in Pregnancy*

Maternal Age	Heart Rate Target Zone (beats/min)	Heart Rate Target Zone (beats/10 sec)
<20	140–155	23–26
20–29	135–150	22–25
30–39	130–145	21–24
≥40	125–140	20–23

■ PROMOTION OF GOOD NUTRITION AND ORAL HEALTH

A woman who eats a balanced diet during pregnancy is less likely to gain excessive weight or develop gestational diabetes, while being more likely to have less heartburn and give birth to a healthier baby (Beck, 2004).

Food Requirements. Health Canada recommends that women who are pregnant eat two to three additional servings per food group per day. Adolescents who are pregnant need more calcium, so milk and milk products are encouraged, while sodas and high-sugar, high-fat snack foods are discouraged.

■ Recommended Daily Servings for Women Who Are Pregnant	
	Pregnant Women
Vegetables and fruit	5–11
Grain products	8–10
Milk and alternatives	4–5
Meat and alternatives	4–5

Source: Health Canada, 2007a,d.

Health Canada (2002) provides "The Healthy Eating Checklist":

■ How many food groups did I eat from? What groups are missing? (Grain products and vegetables/fruit should be included in most meals/snacks if the number of daily servings is to fall within the recommended range.)

■ How many servings from each food group did I get?

■ Of the grain products chosen, were most whole grain or enriched foods?

■ Have I included dark green or orange vegetables or orange fruit?

■ Are my meals/snacks low or high in fat? What makes it so?

■ How many caffeine-containing foods or beverages did I have today?

■ How many alcoholic drinks have I had today?

■ Did I enjoy eating today?

■ Was I active today?

■ Lastly, what should my meals/snacks look like over the next day or next several days to balance what I have recently eaten?

Nutritional Supplementation. Encourage women to take a daily prenatal supplement. Caution them to take no more than 10,000 IU of vitamin A (retinol) per day (Health Canada, 2007d). Daily intake should provide the following:

■ Calcium: 1000 mg/day can decrease blood pressure and leg cramps (Beck, 2004)

■ Magnesium: 350 to 400 mg/day (Health Canada, 2007c)

■ Iron: 27 mg/day, and up to 48 mg/day for vegetarians (Beck, 2004)

■ Folic acid: usually 600 mcg/day during pregnancy and up to 1000 mcg/day for women with increased risk of neural tube defects or who are taking anticonvulsant medication

■ Protein: Necessary for placental function and fetal growth. Protein-rich foods supply vitamin B_6, iron, and zinc. Protein requirements increase with activity from 48 g per day in the least active to 81 g in the most active woman per day (Beck, 2004).

Women with uncontrolled or newly diagnosed diabetes or those experiencing difficulty maintaining appropriate dietary intake and weight gain may need referral to a registered dietician.

Oral Health. Maintaining good oral health is important in pregnancy. Women with poor oral health and gingivitis are more likely to deliver preterm and have problems such as preeclampsia (Boggess et al., 2003).

Cultural Considerations

Aboriginal and other high-risk pregnant women can access prenatal and postpartum information and support through the Canada Prenatal Nutrition Program (PHAC, 2008a).

PRENATAL AND BREASTFEEDING CLASSES

Women and their families can benefit from various classes to help with adaptation to pregnancy and impending parenthood.

Prenatal Classes. These are available in most communities. In larger centres, the classes may be specialized for single women, adolescents, or those with certain cultural backgrounds. Prenatal classes help the client and her partner or support person understand the birth process, potential complications and interventions, coping techniques to help the woman feel less pain during labour, and hospital procedures and policies. Some prenatal classes also include preparation for the postpartum period, and parenting strategies.

Breastfeeding Classes. The Breastfeeding Committee for Canada (2007) recommends exclusive breastfeeding of infants to age 6 months, with safe and appropriate foods along with complementary breastfeeding from 6 months to 2 years of age and beyond. Information about breastfeeding through individual counselling and classes during pregnancy increases success. Referral to a lactation consultant may be indicated if the woman has:

■ Inverted nipples

■ Unusual breast shape or breasts that differ greatly from each other

■ Breast reduction or augmentation surgery, particularly when there has been a circumareolar incision

■ Previous difficulties with breastfeeding

■ Medical indications such as breast cancer, or undergoing chemotherapy, having diagnostic/treatment procedures using radioactive compounds, HIV antibody positive, herpes simplex infection (involving the breast), continued street drug use (PHAC, 2002)

■ FOLLOW-UP VISITS AND MONITORING

Follow-up Visits. Careful monitoring of the client is essential. The frequency of follow-up visits varies depending on risk factors. Check urinary protein and glucose at each visit.

In an uncomplicated pregnancy, see the client:

■ Every 4 weeks until 28 weeks

■ Every 2 to 3 weeks until 36 weeks

■ Weekly until delivery (Hacker et al., 2004)

Assess blood pressure. Reassess any unexpected findings.

Gestational hypertension is systolic blood pressure (SBP) ≥140 and diastolic blood pressure (DBP) ≥ 90, first occurring after week 20 and *without proteinuria.*

Chronic hypertension is SBP ≥ 140 and DBP ≥ 90 before pregnancy, before week 20, and after 12 weeks postpartum.

Preeclampsia is SBP ≥ 140 and DBP ≥ 90 after week 20 and *with proteinuria* (American College of Obstetrics and Gynecology, 2001).

Blurred vision, nausea/vomiting, epigastric pain may indicate HELLP syndrome (H = hemolysis, EL = elevated liver enzymes, LP = low platelet count) (London et al., 2007).

Monitor fetal well-being through a nonstress test; note fetal movements.

Assess edema (see Chapter 18) and reflexes (see Chapter 20).

Evaluate amount and colour of urine. Use a dipstick for protein 1+ to 4+ and glucose.

Premature rupture of membranes (PROM)—membranes rupture prior to 37 weeks:

Malodorous, yellow, green, brown, or bloody amniotic fluid

■ Assess vital signs, fetal well-being nonstress test; note fetal movements.

■ Screen for GBS, prophylactic antibiotics as necessary (SOGC, 2007b).

Preterm labour (PTL)—labour that begins before 37 weeks' gestation:

■ Assess vital signs, particularly temperature and pulse.

■ Monitor fetal well-being with a nonstress test; note fetal movements.

■ Assess quality and frequency of contractions.

■ Avoid vaginal examinations.

■ Assess for amount, colour of vaginal secretions for amniotic fluid, blood, meconium.

Changes in Medical Conditions. Conditions may intensify, reappear, or appear in pregnancy:

- Preexisting rheumatic or congenital heart disease, which increases maternal and fetal mortality (Hacker et al., 2004)

- Chronic renal failure—hypertension and proteinuria

- Chronic inflammatory bowel disease, which pregnancy is unlikely to alter (Hacker et al., 2004)

- Thromboembolic disorders (e.g., thrombophlebitis, deep vein thrombosis, pulmonary embolus) occur in 1.4% of pregnancies (Hacker et al., 2004) and require immediate medical attention.

- Lung disease (Hacker et al., 2004)

  - Asthma, which affects 1% of pregnant women. The effect of pregnancy on asthma is unknown, but severe asthma is linked to fetal demise and growth restriction.

  - Cystic fibrosis, which does not pose any expected problems in pregnancy, may cause problems in women with pulmonary hypertension and malabsorption.

- Seizures, which may increase, decrease, or remain the same

  - Epilepsy, which increases risk for preeclampsia, bleeding, hyperemesis, and preterm or prolonged labour. Anticonvulsant medications can be teratogenic (Hacker et al., 2004).

- Infection

- Human immunodeficiency virus (HIV)—there is no apparent effect from pregnancy, but women may be at risk for opportunistic and other infections.

- Rubella, which can cause congenital rubella syndrome in the first trimester

- Hepatitis B and C, which pregnancy does not affect but are associated with poorer fetal outcomes (Hacker et al., 2004)

- Genital herpes, which increases risks for abortion, growth restriction, and preterm labour. Women with active lesions should have a caesarean section.

- Urinary tract infections—symptomatic or asymptomatic; incidence of asymptomatic is up to 10% (Hacker et al., 2004)

- Group B Streptococcus (GBS), which is found in the vagina, rectum, or bladder of up to 40% of pregnant women. Serious infection for newborns of untreated women can occur (SOGC, 2007b).

- Toxoplasmosis, which occurs in 0.01% of women and passes to the fetus (Hacker et al., 2004)

- "Thyroid storm," which may be triggered by hyperthyroidism (0.05% of pregnancies), infection, or other complications (Hacker et al., 2004).

Tests and Procedures. Different tests or procedures may be done throughout the pregnancy. See the accompanying table.

■ *Tests Done in Pregnancy*

Test	Gestation and Frequency	Purpose	Comments
Ultrasound	5–12 weeks 16–20 weeks 35+ weeks	Confirm pregnancy and rule out threatened abortion Gestation, anomalies, position of placenta and fetus	SOGC (2003a) recommends ultrasound to rule out threatened abortion, but some practitioners do use it to confirm pregnancy. Transvaginal if <12 weeks gestation, otherwise abdominal.
Chorionic Villus Sampling (CVS)	Weeks 10–12	Detects chromosomal abnormalities, e.g., Down's syndrome	CVS is performed earlier than amniocentesis, same criteria for testing (SOGC, 2006)
Maternal Serum Screening (MSS)	11–13 weeks (Down's syndrome) 6 days (Trisomy 18) and 16–18 weeks (neural tube defects)	Screen risk for Down's syndrome, Trisomy 18, neural tube defects	Guidelines for the type and gestation timing of MSS vary between provinces/territories
Amniocentesis	Weeks 15 and 18	Screen for genetic conditions, for example, Down's syndrome, cystic fibrosis	Needle inserted through the abdomen into the uterus to collect a small sample of amniotic fluid. Test offered to woman if: ■ ≥35 years old ■ maternal serum screening test shows increased risk ■ individual or family history of baby with a genetic disorder
Asymptomatic Bacteriuria	12–16 weeks	Decrease acute pyleonephritis and intrauterine growth restriction (Ontario Guidelines Advisory Committee [OGAC], 2005).	Varies between centres. The Ontario Guidelines Advisory Committee advises to screen once in pregnancy (OGAC, 2005).
Glucose Tolerance Test (GTT)	24–28 weeks	Screen gestational diabetes	The Clinical Practice Guidelines for the Prevention and Management of Diabetes in Canada recommends universal screening (Canadian Diabetes Association, 2007).
Group B Streptococcus (GBS)	Weeks 35 to 37	GBS can cause neonatal pneumonia or meningitis	GBS commonly found in the vagina or rectum of healthy women. Antibiotics can be administered during labour to prevent infection in the infant (SOGC, 2007b).

(continued)

■ Tests Done in Pregnancy (Continued)

Test	Gestation and Frequency	Purpose	Comments
Nonstress Test (NST)	32–36 weeks depends on circumstances—may be weekly or more frequently	Fetal distress, reduced fetal movement, intrauterine growth restriction, oligo or polyhydramnios, postdates, complications such as bleeding, diabetes, hypertension	NST determines fetal heart rate reactivity to fetus with movement
Biophysical Profile (BPP)	32–36 weeks, may be done frequently	Fetal distress, ↓ fetal movement, intrauterine growth restriction, oligo or polyhydramnios, postdates, complications such as bleeding, diabetes, hypertension	BPP consists of a nonstress test and an ultrasound

EMERGENCY CONCERNS

The following are conditions for which the client needs to seek immediate attention for assessment and possible intervention.

■ In **ectopic pregnancy**, which occurs in 2% of pregnancies, the pregnancy implants in the fallopian tubes or abdominal cavity. Ectopic pregnancy accounts for 6% to 16% of cases of pain and bleeding in the first trimester (Murray et al., 2005). An undetected, untreated ruptured ectopic pregnancy can result in maternal hemorrhage and death.

■ **Vaginal bleeding** is unexpected and may indicate threatened or missed abortion, ectopic or molar pregnancy, or trophoblastic disease.

■ **Absence of fetal movement** requires emergency attention.

■ **Pain in the calf** may be accompanied by edema and redness. It may indicate a deep vein thrombosis, which requires immediate attention to ensure prompt treatment and prevention of pulmonary embolism (see Chapter 18).

■ **Dyspnea and/or chest pain** may indicate a cardiovascular emergency or potential pulmonary embolism. Emergency attention is critical.

Abdominal Conditions During Pregnancy. Common examples include the following:

■ Appendicitis occurs in 0.05% to 0.13% of pregnant women. Pregnancy may mask symptoms, leading to increased rate of perforation (Guttman, Goldman, & Gideon, 2004).

■ Cholecystitis (1%) and cholelithiasis (4%) may develop from biliary stasis and increased serum cholesterol and lipid levels (Hacker et al., 2004).

- Pancreatitis, which occurs in 0.1% to 0.4% of pregnancies, usually in the third trimester, is confirmed by elevated serum amylase (> 200 U/dL; Hacker et al., 2004).

- Bowel obstruction is most common in third trimester.

- Adnexal torsion is common, probably as a result of ligament elongation (Hacker et al., 2004).

- Abdominal trauma may cause abruptio placenta.

- Ovarian tumours happen in 0.05% of pregnancies (Hacker et al., 2004).

The second trimester is considered the safest time for surgery (Varner, 1994).

Obstetrical Complications. The most common examples are as follows:

- **Placenta previa** is when the placenta is over or near the cervical os. Symptoms include painless bleeding at around 34 weeks' gestation. Assess vital signs for shock; do a fetal well-being nonstress test and note fetal movements. **Do not perform a vaginal examination.** Refer the client for ultrasound.

- In **abruptio placenta**, the placenta separates from the uterine wall.

- Painful, bright red bleeding (disseminated intravascular coagulation [DIC])— excessive clotting and bleeding—is an urgent situation. It may follow trauma. Assess the client's vital signs for shock; monitor fetal well-being with a nonstress test and note fetal movements. Refer for ultrasound.

- Gestational hypertension, pre-eclampsia/eclampsia involves blood pressure > 140/90 with or without edema and/or proteinuria (Magee et al., 2008). It is an emergency.

TECHNIQUES OF EXAMINATION: OBJECTIVE DATA

PROMOTING CLIENT COMFORT, DIGNITY, AND SAFETY

- Provide a warm, private, draft-free room.

- Start the health history while the woman is fully dressed.

- Ask the client whether she has had a complete physical, including a pelvic examination. If not, take time to explain what will happen and why, as it relates to the pregnancy. Use this opportunity to explain any pregnancy changes in her body (e.g., linea nigra, urinary frequency, leukorrhea).

- Women may be embarrassed by the examination; a woman who has been sexually abused may resist a pelvic examination (see Chapter 22).

- Not all women are comfortable with a casual approach.

- Always knock on the door and ask if you may enter once the woman has started disrobing for the examination.

- Provide adequate draping.

- Have all equipment at hand.

- Avoid interruptions.

Equipment

- Stethoscope
- Fetoscope or doptone
- Sphygmomanometer
- Weigh scale with height measure
- Nasal speculum
- Penlight
- Tongue blades
- Cup of water (for the thyroid examination)

- Reflex hammer
- Tape measure
- Gynecological speculum—different types and sizes
- Equipment for Pap smear, cytology, and bacteriology specimens
- Clean gloves
- Water-soluble lubricant

THE EXAMINATION

GENERAL INSPECTION

Observe the woman's overall emotional state, nutritional status, and neuromuscular coordination as she walks into the room and climbs on the table. Discuss her priorities for the examination, responses to pregnancy, and perception of overall health. This helps to develop rapport and trust.

VITAL SIGNS

Assess pulses, respirations, blood pressure, and heart sounds to establish baseline measurements.

Measure height and weight. Calculate BMI using standard tables; consider 19 to 25 as usual BMI for pre-pregnant state.

Weight loss of more than 5% during the first trimester may be from excessive vomiting, or *hyperemesis*.

HEENT AND NECK

Stand facing the seated woman and observe the following:

- **Face.** Check for chloasma, dryness, edema, or oiliness.

Facial edema after 24 weeks of gestation may suggest gestational hypertension.

- **Hair.** Look for any hirsutism or thinness.

Localized patches of hair loss should not be attributed to pregnancy (though hair loss is common postpartum).

- **Eyes.** Note conjunctival colour and whether the woman wears glasses or contacts.

- **Ears.** There should be no change during pregnancy.

- **Nose.** Assess mucous membrane and the septum; bleeding and congestion are common.

Nosebleeds are more common during pregnancy. The nasal septum can show signs of cocaine use.

- **Mouth.** Check for the condition of the gums and teeth and halitosis. Ask about dental pain or impending procedures.

Gingival enlargement with bleeding is common during pregnancy.

- **Thyroid.** Inspect and palpate the gland. Modest symmetric enlargement is expected.

- **Lymph nodes.** Palpate.

THORAX AND LUNGS

Inspect the thorax for symmetry. Auscultate the lungs, and listen to the breath sounds and air entry.

HEART

Palpate the apical impulse. In advanced pregnancy, it may be slightly higher than usual in the 4th intercostal space because of transverse and leftward rotation of the heart from the higher diaphragm.

Auscultate the heart. A venous hum and systolic or continuous mammary souffle are common in pregnancy, reflecting increased blood flow in healthy vessels. Listen for a mammary souffle (pronounced *soo-fl*), late in pregnancy and during lactation. It is most easily heard in the second or third interspace in the parasternal areas and is typically both systolic and diastolic. Only the systolic component may be audible.

Murmurs may also accompany anemia. New diastolic murmurs should be investigated.

BREASTS AND AXILLAE

Inspect breasts and nipples for symmetry and color. The venous pattern may be marked, the nipples and areolae dark, and Montgomery's glands prominent.

An inverted nipple needs attention if breast-feeding is planned.

Palpate for masses. During pregnancy, breasts are tender and nodular.

A pathologic mass may be difficult to isolate.

Compress each nipple between your index finger and thumb. This manoeuvre may express colostrum.

A bloody or purulent discharge should not be attributed to pregnancy.

Refer client to lactation consultant as necessary. Offer to discuss the Canadian Cancer Society's Know Your Breasts approach (2007).

SKIN

Check colour and temperature. Observe for any pregnancy-related changes, such as striae, linea nigra, and itchiness. Inspect injection sites throughout body for signs of illicit drug use.

Anemia of pregnancy may cause pallor.

ABDOMEN

Position the client for physical examination:

■ The woman should not be flat on her back after 20 weeks' gestation because this position may cause supine hypotension.

Supine hypotensive syndrome after 20 weeks is a form of diminished circulation and may lead the woman to feel dizzy and faint, especially when lying down.

■ Keep the client's head slightly elevated; you may put a pillow under her knees or a wedge under the right hip.

■ Ask how she is feeling.

■ Let her sit up as needed, especially before doing the pelvic examination.

Inspect the abdomen for scars from previous caesarean section or other surgeries and from injuries. Look for rashes, tattoos, piercings, or striae. Check the symmetry of the abdomen.

Palpate the abdomen. Your hands should be warm and firm, yet gentle. Keep your fingers together and flat against the abdomen or pelvic tissue to prevent discomfort. Use the finger pads; make smooth, continuous contact rather than kneading or sharp, abrupt motions. Palpate for masses, pain, or guarding.

Leopold's Manoeuvres.

These manoeuvres are important adjuncts to palpation of the pregnant abdomen beginning at 28 weeks' gestation. They help determine where the fetus is lying in relation to the woman's back (longitudinal or transverse), what end of the fetus is presenting at the pelvic inlet (head or buttocks), where the fetal back is located, how far the fetal presenting part has descended into the maternal pelvis, and the estimated fetal weight. This information is necessary to assess the adequacy of fetal growth and probability of successful vaginal birth.

Common deviations include *breech presentation* (fetal buttocks present at the outlet of the maternal pelvis) and absence of the presenting part well down into the maternal pelvis at term. Neither situation necessarily precludes vaginal birth. The most serious findings are a *transverse lie* close to term and slowed fetal growth that may indicate *intrauterine growth retardation (IUGR)*.

First Manoeuvre (Upper Pole).

Stand at the woman's side facing her head. Keeping the fingers of both examining hands together, palpate gently with the fingertips to determine what fetal part is in the upper pole of the uterine fundus.

The fetal buttocks are usually at the upper pole. They feel firm but irregular, and less globular than the head. The fetal head feels firm, round, and smooth.

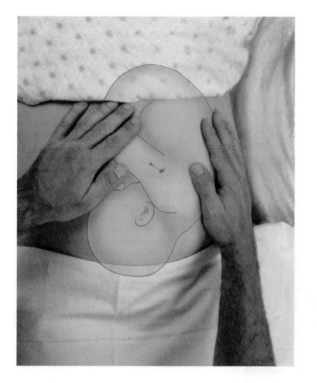

Second Manoeuvre (Sides of Maternal Abdomen).

Place one hand on each side of the woman's abdomen, aiming to capture the fetal body between them. Use one hand to steady the uterus and the other to palpate the fetus.

The hand on the fetal back feels a smooth, firm surface the length of the hand (or more) by 32 weeks' gestation. The hand on the fetal arms and legs feels irregular bumps and perhaps kicking if the fetus is awake and active.

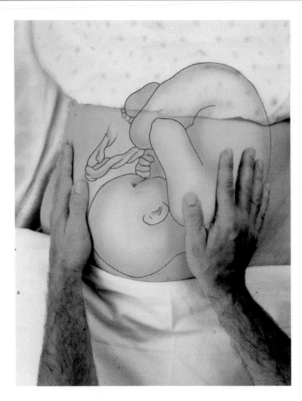

Third Manoeuvre (Lower Pole).   Turn and face the woman's feet. Using the flat palmar surfaces of the fingers of both hands and, at the start, touching the fingertips together, palpate just above the symphysis pubis. Note whether the hands diverge with downward pressure or stay together. This tells you whether the presenting fetal part, head or buttocks, is descending into the pelvic inlet.

If the fetal head is presenting, the fingers feel a smooth, firm, rounded surface on both sides. If the hands diverge, the presenting part is descending into the pelvic inlet (as shown). If the hands stay together and you can gently depress the tissue over the bladder without touching the fetus, the presenting part is above your hands.

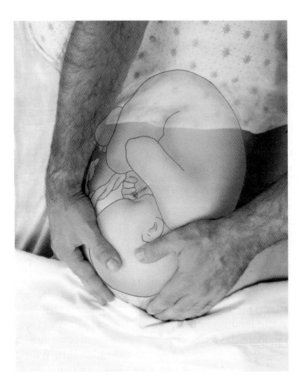

If the presenting fetal part is descending, palpate its texture and firmness. If not, gently move your hands up the lower abdomen and capture the presenting part between your hands.

The fetal head feels smooth, firm, and rounded; the buttocks, firm but irregular.

Fourth Manoeuvre (Confirmation of Presenting Part). With your dominant hand, grasp the fetal part in the lower pole; with your nondominant hand, the fetal part in the upper pole. This manoeuvre may help you distinguish between the head and buttocks.

The head is usually in the lower pole, and the buttocks in the upper pole. If the head is above the pelvic inlet, it moves somewhat independently of the rest of the fetal body.

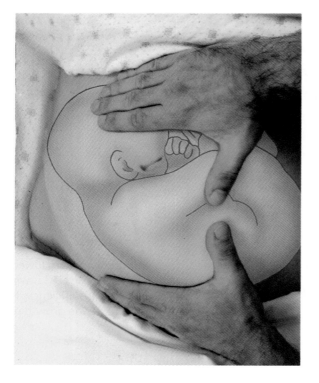

Fetal Movements ("Quickening"). The woman usually feels these by 18 to 20 weeks; others can feel them after 24 weeks. Advise the woman that if she has fewer than 10 movements over 2 hours to seek assessment by a health care provider (London et al., 2007).

If movements cannot be felt after 24 weeks, consider error in calculating gestation, fetal death or morbidity, or false pregnancy.

Uterine Contractility. Uterine contractions may occur as early as 6 weeks' gestation. Braxton–Hicks are painless contractions that the woman may or may not be aware of. The uterus often contracts (feels tense) during palpation in the third trimester. Allow contraction to subside before continuing. Painful, regular contractions of increasing intensity may indicate labour.

SYMPHYSEAL-FUNDAL HEIGHT

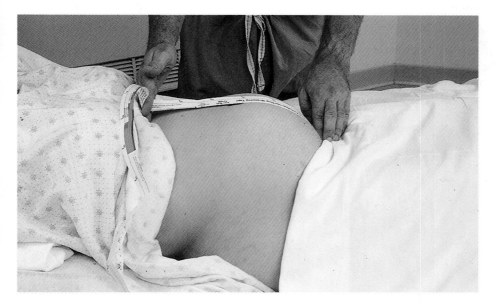

If more than 4 cm higher than expected, consider inaccurate dates, multiple pregnancy, macrosomia, uterine leiomyoma, or polyhydramnios.

- Perform after 13 weeks' gestation.

- Use a tape measure.

- Start from the top of symphysis to the top of the fundus in the midline.

- Follow MacDonald's rule: length in cm × 8/7 = week's gestation.

- 20 to 32 weeks, SFH = gestation in weeks ±2 cm.

If more than 4 cm lower than expected, the EDC is wrong, there is placental insufficiency, transverse lie, or intrauterine growth restriction.

AUSCULTATION OF FETAL HEART

The fetal heart is audible after 10 weeks' gestation with doptone, and after 18 weeks with a fetoscope.

Lack of an audible fetal heart may mean false pregnancy, pregnancy of fewer weeks than expected, or fetal demise.

DOPTONE (LEFT) AND FETOSCOPE (RIGHT)

- From 12 to 18 weeks, listen at midline of the woman's lower abdomen.

- After 28 weeks, listen over the fetal back or through the chest (doing Leopold's manoeuvres).

- Encourage woman and partner to listen.

Fetal Heart Rate. The usual range is 120 to 160 bpm, with higher values earlier in the pregnancy. Rhythm is a regular galloping sound, and variability can range from 10 to 15 bpm over 60 seconds. After 34 weeks, accelerations of 15 beats for 15 seconds with movement indicates reactive FHR.

EXTREMITIES (LEGS AND ARMS)

Look for varicosities, spider nevi, and thrombophlebitis (redness and edema) in the legs.

Measure circumference of each lower leg at intervals and compare measurements. Palpate for increased temperature and pain.

Patellar Reflex. Obtain baseline rating (0 to 4+).

- 1+ is a diminished response.

- 2+ is the expected response.

- 3+ is brisker than expected.

- 4+ is hyperactive (very brisk, jerky, or clonic).

Circulation. Check colour and temperature of skin and nail beds (expect pink colour).

Edema. Assess hands, feet, legs, and face.

GENITALIA

Pelvic Examination. Begin by telling the client when you are going to touch her body, especially before you insert your fingers into her vagina or rectum.

After 24 weeks, auscultation of more than one FHR with varying rates in different locations suggests more than one fetus.

FHR that drops noticeably near term with fetal movement could indicate poor placental circulation or decreased amniotic fluid volume. Lack of beat-to-beat variability late in pregnancy warrants investigation with an FHR monitor.

Varicose veins may begin or worsen during pregnancy.

Look for pitting edema (Dillon, 2007):

- 1+ depresses 2 mm, depression ends quickly—expected in late pregnancy

- 2+ depresses 4 mm, depression remains for 10 to 15 seconds—mild edema

- 3+ depresses 6 mm, depression remains more than 1 minute—moderate edema

- 4+ depresses 8 mm, depression remains 2 to 3 minutes—severe edema

Assess the vulva for appropriate hair distribution, location of urinary and vaginal orifices, varicosities, discharge *other* than leukorrhea (unexpected), or odour (unexpected).

Some women have labial varicosities that become tortuous and painful.

Assess the vagina for pregnancy-related changes; episiotomy or other scars; any discharge or odour; warts, lesions, or tender spots (unexpected).

Review Chapter 22 for instruments and techniques used to take cervical smears (see pp. 811–812).

Speculum Examination.

The examination is easier in pregnancy because of relaxation of the vaginal walls. However, structures may be soft and difficult to distinguish at first. Lubricate a warm speculum with water. Tell the woman that it may be uncomfortable. Encourage her to bear down slightly. Insert the speculum carefully because of relaxation of the pelvis and increased vascularity. Visualize the cervix and vaginal walls. Note any lesions and any discharge.

A pink vagina suggests a nonpregnant state. Vaginal irritation and itching with discharge suggest infection.

Collection of Specimens.

Perform a Papanicolaou test (Pap smear) at first visit if the woman has not had one in the past year. Collect cultures of discharge and lesions for STI or vaginal infection.

Vaginal Examination.

Insert two lubricated fingers into the woman's introitus, palmar side down, with slight pressure downward on the perineum. Slide the fingers into the posterior vaginal vault. Maintaining downward pressure, gently turn the fingers palmar side up. Avoid the sensitive urethral structures at all times.

Palpate Bartholin's and Skene's glands.

Tenderness or discharge is unexpected.

Bimanual Examination.

For the bimanual examination, place one hand on the woman's abdomen and the lubricated fingers of the other hand in the vagina.

The cervix is closed in primipara women (first pregnancy), but the examiner can insert one finger in a multiparous external os (a woman who has had a vaginal delivery) but should not be able to go beyond to the internal os. The multiparous cervix may feel irregular. At less than 34 weeks the cervix should be 1.5–2 cm long.

Check for cystocele (prolapse of bladder into vagina) or rectocele (prolapse of rectum into vagina). This may be pronounced from relaxation of the muscles.

A shortened cervix before 32 weeks may indicate preterm labour.

Uterus. Assess size. With internal fingers placed on either side of cervix, palmar surface upward, gently lift the uterus toward your abdominal hand. Capture the fundal portion of the uterus between your two hands to estimate size. Assess shape. It is an inverted pear at 8 weeks, and then becomes globular. Check consistency and position. Early softening of the isthmus is called Hegar's sign.

An irregularly shaped uterus suggests uterine myomata or a *bicornuate uterus*, which has two distinct uterine cavities separated by a septum.

Adnexa. Check both sides. Ovaries should be small and walnut shaped, with no masses. Expect the client to have pain when you palpate over the ovaries.

Early in pregnancy, it is important to rule out a tubal (*ectopic*) pregnancy (see Table 22-9, Adnexal Masses, p. 828).

ANUS AND RECTUM

Inspect for rashes, lesions, hemorrhoids, inflammation, or prolapses.

Prepare the client for the bimanual recto-vaginal examination. Lubricate the index and middle fingers of one hand. Conduct the bimanual recto-vaginal examination. Place one hand on the client's abdomen and the index finger of your other hand in her vagina and your middle finger in her rectum. Feel the rectum for lumps and masses. Assess the cervix as described previously.

Hemorrhoids often engorge later in pregnancy. They may be painful and bleed.

Perform a rectal examination if necessary.

CONCLUDING THE VISIT

Once you have finished the examination and the woman is dressed, review findings with her. If further data are necessary to confirm pregnancy, blood type, or any other matter, discuss steps to obtain them. Reinforce the importance of the client attending her follow-up visits and performing health promotion actions.

RECORDING AND ANALYZING FINDINGS

Most nurses will use the provincial/territorial prenatal record to document the health history as well as the initial and follow-up assessments. It will be updated at each subsequent visit. A copy of this prenatal record is usually given to the woman at 36 to 37 weeks' gestation, and the woman will be encouraged to take it to the hospital when she presents for delivery or in case of emergency.

■ Examples of Documentation for Examination of the Woman Who Is Pregnant

Area of Assessment	Expected Findings	Unexpected Findings
Psychosocial	States "getting excited about meeting the baby"; discusses preparations for the upcoming birth, accompanied by husband	Crying, reports "crying all the time" and "scared." Unaccompanied.
General inspection	Upright posture, appears relaxed, smiles readily, walks with widened gait, sits and rises from chair easily	Limping favouring right leg, difficulty sitting in chair and mobilizing, looking down, teary
Vital signs	T 37.2 P 76 R 18 BP sitting right arm 120/70	T 38.2 P 84 R 22 BP sitting right arm 135/85
Weight gain at 26 weeks	4 kg	10 kg total weight gain, 4 kg in last 4 weeks
Head and neck	Chloasma present, hair dry, sclera white, slightly reddened gums	Facial edema bilaterally, patches of hair loss distributed over scalp, swollen gums
Thorax and lungs	Thoracic breathing, vesicular sounds throughout lung fields	Use of accessory muscles, fine crackles in both lower lobes
Heart	S1, S2, systolic murmur present, heart rate 80	Heart rate 135, radial pulse, and apical beat unequal
Breasts	Venous patterns present bilaterally, darkened areola, symmetrical, Montgomery glands visible	Venous pattern more prominent on right breast. Bloody discharge from right nipple
Abdomen	Fundal height 27 cm at 26 weeks gestation. Striae present bilaterally. Fetal heart rate (FHR) 155.	Fundal height 32 cm at 26 weeks. Singleton. FHR 105.
Genitalia, anus, rectum	Hemorrhoids present, milky white vaginal discharge	Dark yellowish vaginal discharge, labial varicosities present bilaterally
Extremities	Pink, edema to ankles and feet 1+ bilaterally, all reflexes 1+	Edema in left ankle and foot 4+, all reflexes 3+

ANALYZING FINDINGS FROM HEALTH HISTORY AND PHYSICAL EXAMINATION

Analyzing subjective and objective data from the health history and physical examination leads to the formulation of nursing diagnoses and a plan for interprofessional care. The particular aspects of the client and her input into the proposed plan are key. For example:

Anita Perez, 37 years old, recently got married and wishes to become pregnant. She comes to see the nurse for preconception care. The nurse discusses potential risks for genetic disorders and other complications in women older than 35 years. Findings of the health history and physical examination are as follows:

- *Psychiatric/psychological—history of anxiety and depression, states is worried about her age and the health of a baby*

- *BP 142/90, weight 79 kg height 160 cm, BMI 27.3*

- *Pelvic examination—no unexpected findings*

- *Menstrual history—periods regular every 28 days for 3 days, becoming lighter in last 2 years*

- *Contraception—has used birth-control pill for 17 years*

- *Pap smear taken*

- *Breast examination—does self-examinations every few months*

- *Smoker—one-half package per day*

- *Alcohol—occasional glass of wine*

- *Drug use—denies recreational or prescription drugs, no supplements*

- *Exercise—rarely*

- *Employment—works as a teacher in primary school; two students recently had rubella*

- *Husband—45 years old, car salesman, no health concerns, had two children with previous wife, both healthy*

- *Family history—mother died of stroke at 60 years, father is hypertensive, sister had two miscarriages and a set of healthy twins at age 35 after two sessions of in vitro fertilization*

From this information the nurse identifies the following nursing diagnosis:

***Anxiety** related to advanced maternal age for pregnancy*

The nurse asks about specific questions or concerns the client has related to pregnancy and presents accurate information about risks. Comprehensive care for Ms. Perez includes seeing an obstetrician and possibly a geneticist to discuss options for genetic testing. A laboratory technologist will take blood samples to determine group and type, rubella titre, and HIV and STI status. Pap smear and vaginal swabs will also be assessed. Blood pressure needs to be re-evaluated; if it remains high, the client will need to see a primary care physician or nurse practitioner regarding treatment options before and during pregnancy. A dietitian can give helpful instruction about a healthy diet for conception and pregnancy, and will encourage reduced caffeine and elimination of alcohol. Referral to a smoking cessation program could be helpful. The nurse encourages activities such as walking, prenatal swimming, and yoga to promote cardiovascular health and relaxation.

Critical Thinking Exercise

- What may be the cause of heartburn in a woman at 32 weeks of pregnancy? (*Knowledge*)
- What is the expected date of delivery for a woman with a last menstrual period of May 10, 2009? (*Comprehension*)
- How do you position the woman who is pregnant for a physical examination? (*Application*)

- What factors might contribute to edema during pregnancy? (*Analysis*)
- What recommendations for screening and follow-up would you make for a 15-year-old girl who is pregnant? (*Synthesis*)
- How would you evaluate the effectiveness of your teaching related to the risks of alcohol use during pregnancy? (*Evaluation*)

Canadian Research

Brennand, E. A., Dannenbaum, D., & Willows, N. D. (2005). Pregnancy outcomes of First Nations women in relation to pregravid weight and pregnancy weight gain. *Journal of Obstetrics and Gynaecology of Canada, 27*, 936–944.

Heaman, M. I., & Chalmers, K. (2005). Prevalence and correlates of smoking during pregnancy: A comparison of aboriginal and non-aboriginal women in Manitoba. *Birth, 32*, 299–305.

Heaman, M., Sprague, A. E., & Stewart, P. J. (2006). Reducing the preterm birth rate: A population health strategy. *Journal of Obstetric, Gynecologic, & Neonatal Nursing, 30*, 20–29.

Joseph, K. S., Liston, R. M., Dodds, L., Dahlgren, L., & Allen, A. C. (2007). Socioeconomic status and perinatal outcomes in a setting with universal access to essential health care services. *Canadian Medical Association Journal, 177*, 583–590.

Porteous, J. (2008). Oh, by the way, the patient is pregnant! *Canadian Operating Room Nursing Journal, 26*(2), 35, 37–39, 41–42.

Smylie, J. (2001). A guide for health professionals working with Aboriginal peoples. *Journal of the Society of Obstetricians and Gynaecologists of Canada, 100*, 1–15.

Strass, P., & Billay, E. (2008). A public health nursing initiative to promote antenatal health. *The Canadian Nurse, 104*(2), 29–35.

Tough, S. C., Siever, J. E., & Johnston, D. W. (2007). Retaining women in a prenatal care randomized controlled trial in Canada: Implications for program planning. *BMC Public Health, 7*, 148.

International Nursing Research

Brooten, D., Youngblut, J. M., Donahue, D., Hamilton, M., Hannan, J., & Neff, D. F. (2007). Women with high-risk pregnancies, problems, and APN interventions. *Journal of Nursing Scholarship, 39*(4), 349–357.

Drake, E. E., Humenick, S. S., Amankwaa, L., Younger, J., & Roux, G. (2007). Predictors of maternal responsiveness. *Journal of Nursing Scholarship, 39*(2), 119–125.

Gaffney, K. F. (2006). Postpartum smoking relapse and becoming a mother. *Journal of Nursing Scholarship, 38*(1), 26–30.

Gaffney, K. F., & Henry, L. L. (2007). Identifying risk factors for postpartum tobacco use. *Journal of Nursing Scholarship, 39*(2), 126–132.

Sauls, D. J. (2006). Dimensions of professional labor support for intrapartum practice. *Journal of Nursing Scholarship, 38*(1), 36–41.

Wilson, B. L. (2007). Assessing the effects of age, gestation, socioeconomic status, and ethnicity on labor inductions. *Journal of Nursing Scholarship, 39*(3), 208–213.

Test Questions

1. The risk for chromosomal abnormalities in babies born to women who are 40 years of age is
   a. 1/98.
   b. 1/66.
   c. 1/10.
   d. 1/148.

2. Which of the following changes in vital signs occurs in the female client who is pregnant:

   a. Pulse decreases
   b. Respirations increase
   c. Blood pressure decreases
   d. Temperature decreases

3. Nausea and vomiting in pregnancy is primarily caused by
   a. gastroesophageal reflux disease (GERD).
   b. increased HCG and carbohydrate metabolism.
   c. ptylism.
   d. decreased bile flow due to increased estrogen.

4. The increased pigmentation that occurs on the face of some pregnant women is called
   a. nigra.
   b. melanotropin.
   c. striae.
   d. cholasma.

5. When positioning the client for assessment after the 20th week of pregnancy, you should position the client
   a. supine to facilitate accurate measurements of the level of the uterus.
   b. on left side to increase circulation to the fetus.
   c. on right side to increase circulation to the fetus.
   d. supine with head slightly elevated to ensure comfort.

Bibliography

CITATIONS

Beck, L. (2004). *Leslie Beck's nutrition guide to a healthy pregnancy.* Toronto, ON: Penguin.

Boggess, K. M., Lieff, S., Murtha, A. P., Moss, K., Beck, J., & Offenbacher, S. (2003). Maternal periodontal disease is associated with an increased risk for preeclampsia. *Obstetrics & Gynecology, 101,* 227–231.

Bowen, A. N., & Muhajarine, N. (2006). Prevalence of depressive symptoms in an antenatal outreach program in Canada. *Journal of Obstetrical, Gynecological, and Neonatal Nursing, 35*(4), 492–498.

Breastfeeding Committee for Canada. (2007). *Breastfeeding statement for the Breastfeeding Committee for Canada.* Retrieved September 10, 2008, from http://breastfeedingcanada.ca/html/webdoc5.html

Bulechek, G. M., Butcher, H. K., & Dochterman, J. M. (Eds.). (2008). *Nursing interventions classification (NIC)* (5th ed., pp. 576–578, 580). St Louis, MI: Mosby Elsevier.

Canadian Cancer Society. (2009). *Know your breasts.* Retrieved March 22, 2009, from http://www.cancer.ca/canada-wide/prevention/get%20screened/know%20your%20breasts.aspx?sc_lang=en

Canadian Diabetes Association. (2007). *Gestational diabetes: Preventing complications in pregnancy.* Retrieved September 10, 2008, from http://www.diabetes.ca/about-diabetes/what/gestational/

Cox, J. L., Holden, J. M., & Sagovsky, R. (1987). Detection of postnatal depression: Development of the 10-item Edinburgh Postnatal Depression Scale. *British Journal of Psychiatry, 150,* 782–786.

Dillon, P. M. (2007). *Nursing health assessment. Clinical pocket guide* (2nd ed.). Philadelphia: F. A. Davis.

Guttman, R., Goldman, R. D., & Gideon, K. (2004). Appendicitis during pregnancy. *Canadian Family Physician, 50,* 355–357.

Hacker, N. F., Moore J. G., & Gambone, J. C. (2004). *Essentials of obstetrics and gynecology* (4th ed.). Philadelphia: Elsevier Saunders.

Health Canada. (2002). *Canada's food guide to healthy eating—healthy eating checklist.* Retrieved September 10, 2008, from http://www.hc-sc.gc.ca/fn-an/nutrition/prenatal/national_guidelines-lignes_directrices_nationales-07_eng.php

Health Canada. (2005). *Smoking and your body.* Retrieved September 10, 2008, from http://www.hc-sc.gc.ca/hl-vs/tobac-tabac/body-corps/index-eng.php

Health Canada. (2007a). *Eating well with Canada's food guide.* Retrieved September 10, 2008, from http://www.hc-sc.gc.ca/fn-an/food-guide-aliment/index-eng.php

Health Canada. (2007b). *Guidelines for gestational weight gain ranges.* Retrieved September 10, 2008, from http://www.hc-sc.gc.ca/fn-an/nutrition/prenatal/national_guidelines-lignes_directrices_nationales-06_e.html

Health Canada. (2007c). *Magnesium monograph.* Retrieved September 10, 2008, from http://www.hc-sc.gc.ca/dhp-mps/prodnatur/applications/licen-prod/monograph/mono_magnesium_e.html

Health Canada. (2007d). *Nutrition for a healthy pregnancy: National guidelines for the childbearing years.* Retrieved September 10, 2008, from http://www.hc-sc.gc.ca/fn-an/nutrition/prenatal/national_guidelines-lignes_directrices_nationales-06_e.html

Joseph, K. S., Liston, R. M., Dodds, L., Dahlgren, L., & Allen, A. C. (2007). Socioeconomic status and perinatal outcomes in a setting with universal access to essential health care services. *Canadian Medical Association Journal, 177,* 583–590.

Kendell, R. E., Wainright, S., Hailey, A., & Shannon, B. (1976). The influence of childbirth on psychiatric morbidity. *Psychological Medicine, 6,* 297–302.

London, M. L., Ladewig, P. W., Ball, J. W., & Bindler, R. C. (2007). *Maternal and child nursing care* (2nd ed.). Upper Saddle River, NJ: Pearson Prentice Hall.

Magee, L. A., Helewa, M., Moutquin, J.-M., & Dadelszen, P. von. (2008). Diagnosis, evaluation, and management of the hypertensive disorders of pregnancy. *Journal of Obstetrics and Gynaecology Canada, 30*(3), S9–S15.

Marcus, S. M., Flynn, H. A., Blow, F. C., & Barry, K. L. (2003). Depressive symptoms among pregnant women screened in obstetrics settings. *Journal of Women's Health, 12,* 373–380.

Murray, H., Baakdah, H., Bardell, V., & Tulandi, T. (2005). Diagnosis and treatment of ectopic pregnancy. *Canadian Medical Association Journal, 173,* 905–912.

Nichols, F. H., & Zwelling, E. (1997). *Maternal-newborn nursing: Theory and practice.* Philadelphia: W. B. Saunders Company.

Ontario Guidelines Advisory Committee. (2005). *UTI screening: Pregnancy.* Retrieved September 10, 2008, from http://www.gacguidelines.ca/index.cfm?ACT=topics&Summary_ID=112&Topic_ID=60

Public Health Agency of Canada. (2002). *Family-centred maternity and newborn care: National guidelines.* Retrieved September 10, 2008, from http://www.phac-aspc.gc.ca/dca-dea/publications/fcmc07_e.html

Public Health Agency of Canada. (2005). *Public health advisory on rubella (German measles).* Retrieved October 22, 2008, from http://www.phac-aspc.gc.ca/media/advisories_avis/rubella-eng.php

Public Health Agency of Canada. (2006). *National clearinghouse on family violence.* Retrieved September 10, 2008, from http://www.phac-aspc.gc.ca/ncfv-cnivf/familyviolence/index. html

Public Health Agency of Canada. (2008a). *Canada prenatal nutrition program.* Retrieved September 10, 2008, from http://www.phac-aspc.gc.ca/dca-dea/programs-mes/cpnp_main_e.html

Public Health Agency of Canada. (2008b). *The sensible guide to a healthy pregnancy.* Retrieved October 22, 2008, from http://www.healthycanadians.gc.ca/hp-gs/pdf/hpguide-eng.pdf

Sanders, C. L., & Lucas, M. J. (2001). Medical complications of pregnancy: Renal disease in pregnancy. *Obstetrics and Gynecology Clinics of North America, 28,* 593–600.

Saskatchewan Prevention Institute. (2007). *Routine and special tests during pregnancy.* Retrieved September 10, 2008, from http://www.preventioninstitute.sk.ca/home/Program_Areas/Maternal__Infant_Health/Prenatal_Health/Routine_and_Special_Tests_During_Pregnancy/

Simons, P. (2008, November 11). Province hushes up syphilis outbreak. *The Edmonton Journal,* pp. A1, A2.

Simpson, K. R., & Creehan, P. A. (2008). *Perinatal nursing* (3rd ed.). Philadelphia: AWHONN, Lippincott Williams & Wilkins.

Society of Obstetricians and Gynaecologists of Canada. (2001). *A guide for health professionals working with Aboriginal peoples. Health issues affecting Aboriginal people.* Retrieved October 28, 2008, from http://www.sogc.org/guidelines/public/100E-PS3-January2001.pdf

Society of Obstetricians and Gynaecologists of Canada. (2003a). *The use of first trimester ultrasound.* Retrieved September 14, 2008, from http://www.sogc.org/guidelines/public/135E-CPG-October2003.pdf

Society of Obstetricians and Gynaecologists of Canada. (2003b). *Exercise in pregnancy and the postpartum period.* Retrieved September 10, 2008, from http://www.sogc.org/guidelines/public/129E-JCPG-June2003.pdf

Society of Obstetricians and Gynaecologists of Canada. (2005). Intimate partner violence consensus statement. *Journal of Obstetrics and Gynecology Canada, 27,* 365–388.

Society of Obstetricians and Gynaecologists of Canada. (2006). *Prenatal diagnosis.* Retrieved September 10, 2008, from http://www.sogc.org/health/pregnancy-prenatal_e.asp

Society of Obstetricians and Gynaecologists of Canada. (2007a). *Understanding sexually transmitted infections.* Ottawa, ON: Author.

Society of Obstetricians and Gynaecologists of Canada. (2007b). *Group B Streptococcus infection in pregnancy.* Retrieved September 10, 2008, from http://www.sogc.org/health/pregnancy-groupb_e.asp

Spinelli, M. G. (2001). Interpersonal psychotherapy for antepartum depressed women. In B. L. K. A. Yonkers (Ed.), *Management of psychiatric disorders in pregnancy* (pp. 105–121). London: Arnold.

Varner, C. M. W. (1994). Physiologic changes in pregnancy: Surgical implications. *Clinical Obstetrics and Gynecology, 37,* 241.

Wilson, R. D., Désilets, V., Wyatt, P., Langlois, S., Gagnon, A., Allen, V., et al. (2007). *Pre-conceptional vitamin/folic acid supplementation 2007: The use of folic acid in combination with a multivitamin supplement for the prevention of neural tube defects and other congenital anomalies.* Retrieved September 10, 2008, from http://www.sogc.org/guidelines/documents/guiJOGC201JCPG0712.pdf

Winbery, S. L., & Blaho, K. E. (2001). Dyspepsia in pregnancy. *Obstettrics and Gynecology Clinics of North America, 28,* 333–350.

ADDITIONAL RESOURCES

Cockell, S. J., Oates-Johnson, T., Gilmour, D. T., Vallis, T. M., & Turnbull, G. K. (2003). Postpartum flatal and fecal incontinence quality- of- life scale: A disease-and population-specific measure. *Qualitative Health Research, 13*(8), 1132–1144.

Hacker, N. F., Moore J. G., & Gambone, J. C. (2004). *Essentials of obstetrics and gynecology* (4th ed.). Philadelphia: Elsevier Saunders.

London, M. L., Laewig, P. W., Ball, J. W., & Bindler, R. C. (2007). *Maternal and child nursing care* (2nd ed.). Upper Saddle River, NJ: Pearson Prentice Hall.

CANADIAN ASSOCIATIONS AND WEB SITES

Association of Women's Health, Obstetric, and Neonatal Nurses (AWHONN): http://www.awhonncanada.org/site/awhonn/

Best Start: http://www.beststart.org/

Breastfeeding Committee of Canada: http://breastfeedingcanada.ca

British Columbia Reproductive Care Program (BCRCP): http://www.bcphp.ca

Canada Prenatal Nutrition Program: http://www.phac-aspc.gc.ca/dca-dea/programs-mes/cpnp_main_eng.php

Canadian Perinatal Web site: http://www.preinet.org/perinet/Directory.htm

Canadian Perinatal Surveillance System (CPSS): http://www.phac-aspc.gc.ca/rhs-ssg/index.html

Childbirth and Postpartum Professional Association of Canada: http://www.cappacanada.ca

Health Canada and the Public Health Agency of Canada: http://www.hc-sc.gc.ca/hl-vs/preg-gros/index-eng.php

Motherisk: http://www.motherisk.org/prof/index.jsp

Perinatal Education Program: http://www.usak.ca/nursing/cne/perinatal/guidelines.htm

Perinatal Partnership Program of Eastern and Southern Ontario (PPPESO): http://www.pppeso.on.ca/site/pppeso/

Perinatal Research Centre, University of Alberta: http://www.ualberta.ca/PERINATAL/

Public Health Agency of Canada. The sensible guide to a healthy pregnancy: http://www.healthycanadians.gc.ca/hp-gs/pdf/hpguide-eng.pdf.'

Regional Perinatal Outreach Program of Southwestern Ontario: http://www.sjkc.london.ca/sjh/profess/periout/index.htm

Reproductive Care Program of Nova Scotia: http://rcp.nshealth.ca

Saskatchewan Prevention Institute: http://www.preventioninstitute.sk.ca/

Society of Obstetricians and Gynaecologists of Canada (SOGC): http://www.sogc.org

The Older Adult

MARJORIE C. ANDERSON, KATHLEEN HUNTER, AND LYNN S. BICKLEY

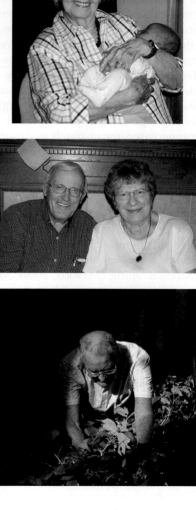

Canadian seniors are a heterogeneous population in terms of health status, cultural origins, functional ability, financial status, and living arrangements. Because of this heterogeneity, seniors often are subcategorized into three age groups: 65 to 74 years, 75 to 84 years, and 85 years or older. Overall, people 65 years or older currently make up 13.1% of Canada's population. By 2036, almost 9.8 million Canadians will be older than 65 years, comprising approximately 25% of the total population. In the past two decades, the number of seniors 85 years or older has grown rapidly, increasing from 200,000 to 500,000. By 2021, almost 800,000 Canadians will belong to this age group. Canadians now live longer, with life expectancy in 2003 at approximately 80 years and further increases projected (Turcotte & Schellenberg, 2006).

Although chronic disease increases with age, leaving older people at risk for changes in function and overall health, most Canadian seniors report themselves in good health (Shields & Martin, 2006). In fact, older Canadians now live longer with fewer disabilities than in previous generations. The vast majority of older Canadians (93%) live independently in the community; only 7% reside in collective dwellings (e.g., continuing-care facilities). Institutional living is age associated, with 2% of those aged 65 to 74 years living in institutions, a rate that rises to 32% among those 85 years or older (Turcotte & Schellenberg, 2006). In response to the growing proportion of seniors in the population, public awareness has increased of the need for the Canadian health care system to promote healthy aging and to support the continued independence of as many seniors as possible (Healthy Aging and Wellness Working Group of the Federal/Provincial/Territorial Committee of Officials–Seniors, 2006).

Assessing the older adult presents special opportunities and challenges. Much of the focus for assessing older adults is different from the disease-oriented approach of history taking and physical examination for younger clients: the focus on healthy or successful aging; the need to understand and mobilize family, social, and community supports; the importance of skills directed to functional assessment, the sixth vital sign; and the opportunities for promoting the older adult's long-term health and safety.

In this chapter, we review the physiologic changes of aging in *Anatomy and Physiology,* as well as the heterogeneity of the aging process and the challenges of distinguishing expected from unexpected physical findings. Then follows *The Health History,* which begins with the Approach to the Client. This section presents how to adjust the office environment and adapt the content and pace of the interview to the older client; the varying meanings and significance of symptoms in older adults, especially when linked to one of the geriatric syndromes; and the cultural dimensions of aging. The next section explores the importance of assessing activities of daily living, medications, nutrition, acute and chronic pain, lifestyle behaviours such as alcohol use and smoking, and advance directives and palliative care. *Health Promotion* provides guidelines for health screening in older adults, including recommendations for topics such as vision and hearing, exercise, immunizations, household safety, cancer, depression, dementia, and elder mistreatment. *Techniques of Examination* presents Functional Assessment: The "Sixth Vital Sign," and provides an efficient tool for office evaluation, the 10-Minute Geriatric Screener. Then follows the Physical Examination of the Older Adult, which builds on the techniques you already have learned for physical examinations in general, but highlights special aspects for older clients when surveying general appearance, measuring vital signs, and completing each regional examination. *Recording and Analyzing Your Findings* contains a sample of the written history and physical examination of the older adult.

ANATOMY AND PHYSIOLOGY

Primary aging reflects physiological changes over time that are independent of and not induced by disease or environmental influences (Masoro, 2006). Over time, these changes decrease physiologic reserves, with consequences that may not become apparent except during periods of stress, such as exposure to fluctuating temperature, dehydration, or hypovolemic shock. For example, decreased cutaneous vasoconstriction and sweat production can impair responses to heat; declines in thirst sensation may delay recovery from dehydration; and the physiological decrease in maximum cardiac output, left ventricular filling, and maximum heart rate seen with aging may impair the response to hypovolemic shock. Age-related physiological changes cannot be reversed and must be compensated for as much as possible. In contrast, environmental influences and lifestyle choices (e.g., not smoking, exercising regularly, eating a nutritious diet) can slow some age-related changes and enhance the possibility of healthy aging (Miller, 2009).

Coincident with primary aging, the aging population displays marked heterogeneity. Investigators have identified vast differences in how people age and have distinguished *secondary aging*—changes involving interactions of primary aging processes with environmental influences and disease processes—from successful aging (Masoro, 2006; Miller, 2009). Successful (healthy) aging occurs in people who escape debilitating disease entirely and maintain healthy lives late into their 80s and 90s. Studies of centenarians show that genes account for approximately 20% of the probability of living to 100, and healthy lifestyles account for approximately 20% to 30% (Perls, 2003; Perls et al., 2002; Rowe & Kahn, 1997). This evidence is compelling for nurses to promote optimal nutrition, smoke-free environments, strength training and aerobic exercise, and social and intellectual engagement for older adults to delay unnecessary depletion of physiologic and cognitive reserves (Bradshaw & Klein, 2007).

VITAL SIGNS

Blood Pressure. In Western societies, beginning at approximately 40 years for women and 50 years for men, systolic blood pressure rises 5 to 8 mm Hg per decade. Diastolic blood pressure rises at a rate of 1 m Hg per decade in both sexes, plateaus at 60 years for women, but continues to rise slowly in men. As a result, pulse pressure (systolic blood pressure minus diastolic blood pressure) widens. The gradual increase in systolic blood pressure and widening pulse pressure largely result from the gradual stiffening of the large arteries and blunting of the baroreceptor mechanism with age. The stiffened noncompliant aorta is less able to buffer pulsatile cardiac outflow (Taffet & Lakatta, 2003). Furthermore, increased weight, high sodium intake, cigarette smoking, and physical inactivity contribute to increases in blood pressure. Recall that blood pressures between 120/80 and 139/89 mm Hg are considered prehypertensive and increase the client's risk for hypertension (see Chapter 15).

Older adults are at risk for postural (orthostatic) hypotension—a sudden drop in systolic or diastolic blood pressures of more than 20 mm Hg or 10 mm Hg, respectively, within 1 minute of standing from a lying or sitting position. In addition, older adults are at risk for postprandial hypotension—a fall in blood pressure of 20 mm Hg within 75 minutes of eating a meal. Both forms of hypotension increase risk for falls and hip fractures (Miller, 2009).

When assessing blood pressure, nurses should be aware that older adults can exhibit *pseudohypertension*—an artificially elevated systolic blood pressure. This phenomenon can occur when arteriosclerosis so stiffens the arteries that the external cuff cannot compress them. Clues to this condition are radial and/or brachial arteries that resist compression when palpated and the absence of end-organ damage (e.g., in the kidneys) that usually accompanies severe hypertension (Duthie, 2007; Miller, 2009).

Heart Rate and Rhythm. Resting heart rate remains unchanged in healthy older adults. The quality of the peripheral pulse, because of the arteriosclerotic changes that stiffen the arteries, may seem full and bounding (Duthie, 2007; Taffet & Lakatta, 2003). Pacemaker cells in the sinoatrial node, atrioventricular node, and His bundle decrease with age. As a result, generally benign ventricular and supraventricualar ectopic beats increase (Taffet & Lakatta, 2003). By contrast, if atrial fibrillation, a common arryhthmia in this age group, is detected, it is pathological with more serious sequelae.

Respiratory Rate and Temperature. Respiratory rate in older adults can be expected to increase to 16 to 24 breaths per minute; however, respiratory pattern should not change. Many eccrine sweat glands become fibrotic, while others function poorly, reducing the effectiveness of sweating. Older adults also lose subcutaneous fat. These factors combine to make older adults more susceptible to hyperthermia and hypothermia. In addition, core temperature tends to decrease to an average of 36°C (Fetzer & McQueen, 2006).

HEIGHT AND WEIGHT

Over the years, height tends to decrease because of compression of intervertebral discs and changes in posture (see Chapter 19). With aging, lean body mass decreases, in women more than men. Some clients gain body fat. A lower percentage of body water accompanies these changes (Duthie, 2007; Miller, 2009).

SKIN, NAILS, AND HAIR

With age, because collagen and elastin fibres in the dermis lose their elasticity, the skin wrinkles, becomes lax, and loses turgor. Thickness of the dermal layer decreases, and the junction between the epidermis and dermis flattens, which increases the susceptibility of the skin to shearing forces (Gilchrest, 2007). Vascularity of the dermis decreases, causing lighter skin to look pale and more opaque. Eccrine, apocrine, and sebaceous glands atrophy and decrease in number and function. Decreased production of eccrine sweat, loss of subcutaneous fat, and impaired dermal vascular responsiveness to changes in ambient temperature increase the risk of older adults to hypothermia and hyperthermia. Slowed maturation of the epidermal layer contributes to skin dryness (*xerosis*), which is often accompanied by itching (*pruritus*). The ability of the epidermis to produce pre-vitamin D in response to sun exposure decreases, contributing to vitamin D deficiency and osteomalacia. Subcutaneous tissue is lost, especially over the dorsum of the hands, feet, lower legs, and sun-exposed areas of the face. The skin on the back of the hands, forearms, and lower legs becomes thin, fragile, loose, transparent, and more susceptible to tears. Regeneration of healthy skin slows, which is particularly noticeable in delayed healing of superficial, surgical, and traumatic wounds (Gilchrest, 2007, 2009). With loss of subcutaneous fat, dermal capillaries become poorly supported and more easily damaged. Blood leaks and spreads within the dermis, resulting in purple patches or macules, termed *actinic purpura*, which fade over time. In addition, as the repair function of skin cells becomes slower and less accurate with age, incidence of skin cancers increases.

Nail growth slows, and nails lose lustre. Fingernails tend to become increasingly soft, brittle, and prone to splitting. They lose the half-moon lunula and develop longitudinal striations. Toenails tend to yellow, thicken, and become longitudinally striated (Kenney, 1987).

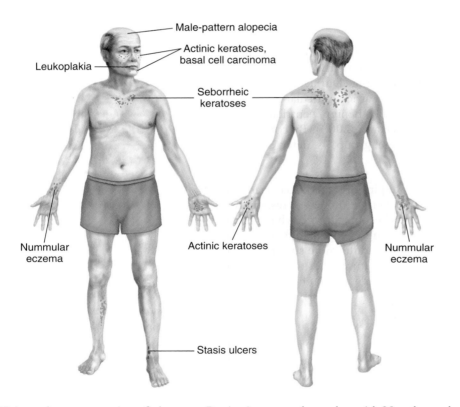

Hair undergoes a series of changes. Beginning as early as the mid-30s, the scalp hair of Caucasians loses its pigment and becomes gray from a decline in melanin. Hair loss on the scalp is genetically determined. As early as 20 years, a man's hairline may start to recede at the temples; hair loss at the vertex follows. In women, hair loss follows a similar but less severe pattern. With aging, most adults can expect gradual hair loss elsewhere on the body, first on the trunk and limbs, then in the pubic areas and axillae. As women approach 55 years, coarse terminal facial hairs may appear on the chin and upper lip, but do not increase after that. Older men may experience coarse terminal hair growth in the nares, ears, and eyebrows (Kenney, 1987, 2009).

Cultural Considerations

In the Japanese population and in African Canadians, greying of terminal hair does not appear until the mid-40s at the earliest.

HEAD AND NECK

The eyes, ears, and mouth bear the brunt of age-related change.

Vision. The fat that surrounds and cushions the eye within the bony orbit tends to atrophy, and the eyeball recedes somewhat. This, and the loss of elasticity in the eyelid muscles and accumulation of dark pigment around the eyes contribute to the appearance of sunken eyes (*enophthalmos*) (Miller, 2009). The skin of the eyelids becomes wrinkled, and eyelid muscles weaken. Fat may accumulate in the inner third of the upper eyelid, creating a fold that can impair vision (*blepharochalasis*). A combination of weakened muscle and fat accumulation may push the lower lid forward, creating soft bulges. An *ectropion* is created if the lower lid falls away from the conjunctiva, while an *entropion* develops if the lower lid inverts. The ectropion may block the flow of tears through the punctum. The eyelashes in an entropion may irritate the cornea, causing infection. The lacrimal gland produces fewer secretions, often precipitating the condition of dry eyes.

The cornea becomes increasingly opaque and yellowed, which interferes with the passage of light. Ongoing changes in the lens gradually increase its size and density. These changes result in impaired passage of light to the retina, requiring older adults to use more light for reading and fine work. The increased density and opacity of the lens contribute to the formation of cataracts with 20% of Canadian seniors reporting this vision problem (Millar, 2004). The increased size of the lens may push the iris outward, narrowing the angle between iris and cornea and increasing the risk of *narrow-angle glaucoma* (see Chapter 12, p. 314; Watson, 2003).

The iris (a sphincter muscle) becomes more rigid and less responsive to changes in light, resulting in reduced pupillary size and less light getting to the retina, especially in environments with subdued lighting. The ciliary body atrophies with age. It produces less aqueous humor and no longer acts effectively on an already stiffened lens to control accommodation—the ability to focus on near objects. Ensuing *presbyopia* usually becomes noticeable during the fifth decade, leading adults to require corrective reading glasses (Millar, 2004; Watson, 2003). With aging, the vitreous body begins to shrink, which may lead to the formation of floaters and scatter light, resulting in less light reaching the retina. Retinal arteries become thinner and increasingly sclerotic, resulting in A-V nicking (Table 12-10, p. 335). Changes in the retina increase the risk for *macular degeneration* (see Chapter 12).

Visual acuity remains fairly constant between 20 and 50 years, diminishing gradually until approximately 70 years, and then more rapidly. Nevertheless, most elderly people retain good to adequate vision (20/20 to 20/70 as measured by standard charts) with the aid of corrective lenses. Colour discrimination, especially for dark colours (black, brown, navy) and pastels, declines with age, and dark adaptation becomes slower. Finally, a decline in the quantity and quality of the retinal–neural pathways in the brain adversely affects the speed of processing visual information (Miller, 2009; Watson, 2003).

Hearing. Acuity of hearing usually diminishes. Age-related changes in the inner ear include gradual loss of sensory hair cells in the cochlea and neurons in the cochlear nuclei. Loss of hearing sounds beyond the range of human speech begins in young adulthood and, with prolonged exposure to loud noise and aging, gradually extends to sounds in the middle and lower ranges (Medwetsky, 2007, 2009). When a person fails to catch the upper tones of words while hearing the lower tones, words sound distorted and are difficult to understand, especially in noisy environments. This age-related inner-ear hearing impairment is termed *presbycusis* and affects more than 50% of Canadians older than 65 years (Public Health Agency of Canada [PHAC], 2006). In addition, the ossicles in the middle ear can become calcified, which impedes transfer of sound vibrations from the tympanic membrane to the oval window. Also, sweat gland secretion in the external ear canal decreases, making cerumen dryer and more difficult to remove. Eventually, the external canal can become impacted with cerumen, impeding the movement of sound waves to the tympanic membrane.

Taste and Smell. As a result of changes in the central nervous system, the ability to smell declines gradually after age 30 years. Factors such as cigarette smoking, medications, and periodontal disease also contribute to this decline. The ability of healthy older adults to perceive the intensity of sour, salty, and bitter tastes declines with age, but they retain the perception for sweet taste.

Oral Cavity. Although humans continue to produce salivary secretions across the lifespan, many older adults experience a dry mouth (*xerostomia*), most likely as a result of medications and chronic diseases. Even healthy, well-maintained teeth show signs of aging. The chewing cusps of the teeth wear down; as tooth enamel becomes harder and more brittle, the teeth are more susceptible to fractures. Poor hygiene and maintenance may lead to dental caries or periodontal disease, and subsequent tooth loss (see Chapter 13). Alveolar bone matrix that once surrounded tooth sockets is gradually resorbed over time, a process accelerated when teeth are lost. If a person has no teeth, the lower portion of the face looks small and sunken with accentuated "purse-string" wrinkles radiating from the mouth. Overclosure of the mouth may lead to maceration of the skin at the corners, a condition known as *angular cheilitis* (see Chapter 13).

Cervical Lymph Nodes and Thyroid Gland. Aging of the immune system is reflected in the loss of lymphoid tissue in lymph nodes, thymus gland, and spleen (Kenney, 1989). Therefore, the frequency of palpable cervical nodes gradually diminishes with age and, according to one study, falls below 50% between 50 and 60 years. The submandibular glands may become easier to feel. The thyroid gland decreases in size and becomes more nodular to palpation, but it retains function and responds appropriately to stressors (Hassani & Hershman, 2003; Kenney, 1989).

THORAX AND LUNGS

Although the respiratory system does undergo age-related changes, healthy, nonsmoking seniors can compensate for this decline in functional capacity. In the upper respiratory tract, the mucous secreted by goblet cells is more viscous and difficult to expectorate. Older adults experience blunting of the cough reflex and a less effective gag reflex, likely from reduced laryngeal nerve endings. With age, the costal cartilage becomes calcified and respiratory muscles weaken, necessitating the use of more energy to move the chest wall. Accentuation of the dorsal curvature of the thoracic spine with age may produce a kyphosis. This increases the anteroposterior diameter of the chest; however, the resulting barrel chest has little effect on function. Age-related changes in lung tissue include an overall decrease in lung mass, alveolar surface area, and pulmonary capillary blood flow, and a thickening of the alveolar–capillary diffusion interface. These changes result in increased residual volume and decreased effective diffusion capacity between the pulmonary capillaries and alveoli. In addition, decreased natural elastic recoil of lung tissue along with weakened muscles of respiration leads to a lower forced expiratory volume. Also, arterial oxygen partial pressure (PaO^2) declines, stabilizing by age 75 years to approximately 80 mm Hg (Enright, 2003, 2009).

CARDIOVASCULAR SYSTEM

Lifestyle choices significantly influence cardiovascular performance, making it difficult to distinguish age-related from disease-related changes. Factors such as tobacco smoking, hypercholesterolemia, physical deconditioning, and hypertension adversely affect the cardiovascular system. Maximal heart rate and oxygen consumption achieved during maximal effort does decline with age, but continued regular physical activity may moderate the rate of decline (Kenney, 1989; O'Brien Cousins & Horne, 1998; Taffet, 2003; Taffet & Lakatta, 2003). Because of the patchy fibrosis of connective tissue in the myocardium, the ventricular walls become stiffer, especially on the left side. Age-related changes in the large arteries, specifically stiffening of the smooth muscle layer, cause increased peripheral resistance. Consequently, the left ventricle must work harder against resistance of less compliant arteries, resulting in left ventricle hypertrophy and enlargement of the left atrium (Taffet & Kakatta, 2003).

Neck Vessels. The aorta enlarges, lengthens, and becomes tortuous and less compliant. Arterial stiffening is uniform in all the larger arteries, not patchy and increased at points of stress as is found with atherosclerosis (Taffet & Lakatta, 2003). The right carotid artery may buckle, resulting in a pulsatile palpable mass low in the neck. This mass appears chiefly in women with hypertension and may be mistaken for an aneurysm—a true dilatation of the artery. In older adults, systolic bruits heard in the middle or upper portions of the carotid arteries suggest, but do not prove, partial arterial obstruction from atherosclerosis. By contrast, cervical bruits in younger people are usually innocent (Kenny, 1989; Miller, 2009; Taffet & Lakatta, 2003). A tortuous aorta occasionally raises pressure in the jugular veins on the left side of the neck by impairing drainage within the thorax.

Extra Heart Sounds—S3 and S4. A physiologic *third heart sound*, commonly heard in children and young adults, may persist as late as age 40 years, especially in women. After 40 years, however, an S3 strongly suggests congestive heart failure from volume overload of the left ventricle, as found with coronary artery disease or valvular heart disease (e.g., mitral regurgitation). In contrast, a *fourth heart sound* is seldom heard in young adults other than well-conditioned athletes. An S4 can be heard in otherwise healthy older people, suggesting decreased ventricular compliance and impaired ventricular filling. Reliance on atrial contraction to complete ventricular filling becomes increasingly necessary and contributes to the S4 commonly heard in older adults (Taffet & Lakatta, 2003). See Table 15-7, Extra Heart Sounds in Diastole, p. 473.

Cardiac Murmurs. Middle-aged and older adults commonly have a short *systolic aortic ejection murmur* detected in approximately one-third of people close to age 60 years, and in more than half of those reaching 85 years. With age, the bases of the aortic cusps thicken with fibrous tissue and calcification follows. Turbulence produced by blood flow into a dilated aorta may further augment this murmur. In most people, the process of fibrosis and calcification (*aortic sclerosis*) does not impede blood flow. In some people, the aortic valve leaflets become calcified and immobile, resulting in *aortic stenosis* and outflow obstruction. A brisk carotid upstroke may help distinguish aortic sclerosis from aortic stenosis with its delayed upstroke, but clinical differentiation between aortic sclerosis and aortic stenosis may be difficult. Both carry increased risk for cardiovascular morbidity and mortality (Kenney, 1989; Miller, 2009). See Table 15-10, Midsystolic Murmurs, pp. 476–477.

Similar changes alter the mitral valve, usually approximately one decade later than aortic sclerosis. Calcification of the mitral valve annulus (valve ring) impedes valve closure during systole, causing the systolic murmur of *mitral regurgitation*. This murmur may become pathologic as volume overload increases in the left ventricle. See Table 15-8. Pansystolic (Holosystolic) Murmurs, p. 474.

BREASTS AND AXILLAE

The female adult breast may be soft, but also granular, nodular, or lumpy. This uneven texture represents physiologic nodularity. It may be bilateral and palpable throughout the breast or only in parts of it. With menopause and decline in endogenous estrogen, mammary glandular tissue atrophies and is replaced by fat. Although the proportion of fat increases, its total amount may decrease. Change in connective tissue with age causes breasts to become flaccid and more pendulous. The ducts surrounding the nipple may become more easily palpable as firm, stringy strands. As the incidence of breast cancer increases with age, any breast lump found is more likely to be cancerous than a cyst or fibroadenoma. Axillary hair diminishes, as do secretions from axillary apocrine glands (Kimmick & Muss, 2003; Miller, 2009).

ABDOMEN

During the middle and later years, as lean body mass decreases, body fat increases and tends to accumulate in the lower abdomen, around the hips, and intra-abdominally. Total body weight may remain stable or even decline with this change in body composition, but waist circumference often increases (Harris, 2003). The accumulation of abdominal fat together with weakening of the abdominal muscles can result in a potbelly. Occasionally a person notes this change with alarm and interprets it as fluid or evidence of disease.

Aging may blunt the manifestations of acute abdominal disease. Pain may be less severe, fever is often less pronounced, and signs of peritoneal inflammation (e.g., muscular guarding and rebound tenderness [p. 530]) may be diminished or even absent.

Because of decreased strength of the abdominal muscles and conditions contributing to increased intra-abdominal pressure (e.g., straining to void or defecate), hernias are often seen in the elderly population (Sinanan et al., 2003).

MALE AND FEMALE GENITALIA; ANUS, RECTUM, AND PROSTATE

As *men* age, sexual interest appears to remain intact, although frequency of intercourse declines. Several physiologic changes accompany decreasing testosterone levels. The penis decreases in size, and the testicles drop lower in the scrotum. Erections take longer and require more tactile stimulation to achieve, and respond less to erotic cues. The volume of seminal fluid decreases, and ejaculation is less forceful; nevertheless, men sustain their fertility well into the 70s. Pubic hair decreases and becomes gray. Erectile dysfunction (inability to have an erection) affects approximately 50% of older men, often influencing quality of life (Mulligan & Saddiqi, 2003). Usual causes include hypogastric-cavernous arterial insufficiency or venous leakage through the subtunical venules. Other contributing factors include several groups of medications (e.g., antihypertensives, cardiovascular agents, antidepressants, benzodiazepines, anticholinergics, histamine H2 antagonists, alcohol) and chronic diseases (e.g., diabetes mellitus, vascular disease; Butler & Lewis, 2003, 2009; Mulligan & Saddiqi, 2003).

In men, proliferation of prostate epithelial and stromal tissue, termed *benign prostatic hyperplasia* (BPH), begins in the third decade. The rate of growth is slow with prostate gland enlargement detectable in about half of men by midlife and accompanied by symptoms of trouble urinating observed in half of these men (DuBeau, 2003). Symptoms of urinary hesitancy, dribbling, and incomplete emptying can often be traced to causes other than BPH, such as coexisting disease, use of medication, and lower urinary tract abnormalities (Miller, 2009). Hyperplasia continues to increase prostate volume until the seventh decade, then appears to plateau. These changes are androgen dependent.

In women, ovarian function usually starts to diminish during the fifth decade; on average, menopause typically occurs between 49 and 51 years. As endogenous estrogen levels fall, many women experience hot flashes, some for 5 years or longer. Symptoms include flushing, profuse sweating, palpitations, chills, mood changes, and sleep disturbances. Vulvovaginal changes include the following: pubic hair becomes sparse and grey, the labia and clitoris become smaller as subcutaneous fat decreases, Bartholin's glands atrophy and secrete less fluid, the length and width of the vagina decreases, and the vaginal wall becomes thin, pale, and dry, with loss of lubrication. The latter problem contributes to dyspareunia (painful intercourse). The cervix, uterus, ovaries, and fallopian tubes diminish in size; within 10 years after menopause, the ovaries are no longer palpable. The suspensory ligaments of the adnexa, uterus, and bladder may also relax, resulting in stress incontinence, cystocele, and vaginal prolapse. As with men, the level of sexual activity declines with age, but sexuality and sexual interest remain unchanged, particularly in the absence of partner issues, partner loss, or unusual life stress. Women also experience medication-induced sexual dysfunction (Kaiser, 2003, 2009).

PERIPHERAL VASCULAR SYSTEM

Changes in the tunica intima (endothelial layer) and tunica media (smooth muscle layer) include thickening and increased collagen. Calcification of elastin fibres results in stiffening of the larger arteries, increased peripheral vascular resistance, and less responsive baroreflex mechanism (regulates blood pressure) (Miller, 2009). Peripheral arteries tend to lengthen and to feel harder and less resilient. The aorta is particularly affected because its lumen increases in diameter and becomes more tortuous to compensate for increased peripheral vascular resistance. Atherosclerosis, the major cause of arterial disorders, affects older adults more frequently, and peripheral vascular disease is a leading cause of morbidity in the elderly. Its disease pattern, as noted, is quite distinct from age-related change (Taffet & Lakatta, 2003). Age-related changes do not necessarily indicate atherosclerosis or pathologic changes in the coronary or cerebral vessels.

The common changes in skin, nails, and hair discussed earlier are not specific for arterial insufficiency, even though they are classically associated with it. Loss of peripheral arterial pulsations is not typical and demands careful evaluation. Temporal arteritis can occur in some older adults, with symptoms that include headache, facial pain, and possible loss of vision in 15% of those affected (Gonzales & Goodwin, 2007).

Aging of the tunica media in the larger veins results in their elongation, thickening, dilatation, and loss of elasticity. Also, valves in the saphenous and femoral leg veins become increasingly incompetent, resulting in compromised venous return and venous stasis (Miller, 2009).

MUSCULOSKELETAL SYSTEM

Musculoskeletal changes continue throughout the adult years. Decreased mobility including subtle changes in gait and posture may be expected but not profound. Maximal bone mass density is achieved in early adulthood. Bone remodelling continues but changes as bone resorption increases, calcium absorption decreases, and other aspects of bone metabolism change. Decreased estrogen secretion in women and testosterone in men accelerates the rate of bone loss, resulting in osteopenia in both sexes, but earlier in women. If unchecked, osteoporosis with all its problems ensues.

Soon after maturity, subtle losses in height begin; significant shortening is obvious by old age. Most loss of height occurs in the trunk as intervertebral discs thin and vertebral bodies collapse because of weakened trabecular bone from osteoporosis. Flexion at the knees and hips may also contribute to shortened stature. Vertebral compression fracture and intervertebral disc compression contribute to the kyphosis of aging and increased anteroposterior diameter of the chest, especially in women. For these reasons, the limbs of an elderly person tend to look long in proportion to the trunk.

With aging, there is a net loss of skeletal muscle fibres, a decrease in muscle mass and a subsequent loss of muscle strength, particularly in the legs. The hands of an aged person often look thin and bony as a result of atrophy of the interosseous muscles that leaves concavities or grooves in the back of the hands. As illustrated on page 631, this change may first appear between the thumb and the hand (1st and 2nd metacarpals) but may also be seen between the other metacarpals. Small muscle wasting may also flatten thenar and hypothenar eminences of the palms. Loss of muscle mass in the arms and legs may exaggerate the apparent size of adjacent joints.

Endurance and coordination also diminish as a result of age-related changes in muscle fibres and the central nervous system. Even in the highly trained older athlete, the rate of decline in level of performance is similar to the untrained older athlete, suggesting age-related deficits will occur regardless. Exercise is still the most effective way to slow this inevitable decline in muscle strength (Loeser & Delbono, 2003).

Joint function, including flexibility and range of motion in the extremities and back, declines with age. This decline is partly from osteoarthritis but also from age-related changes in joint cartilage, such as decreased hydration and roughening of the cartilage surfaces from wear. Likely age-related changes in cartilage contribute to the prevalence of osteoarthritis, which increases with age. Tendons and ligaments decline in strength and flexibility with age. The degree of loss in range of motion is directly related to use (Loeser & Delbono, 2003).

Older women walk and stand using a narrower base, whereas men shorten their stride, decrease their step height when walking, and stand using a wider base. Overall, both walk slower and in a more flexed posture, contributing to an increased risk for falls. Exercise and an active lifestyle can significantly improve gait (Duthie, 2007; Miller, 2009).

NERVOUS SYSTEM

Aging may affect all aspects of the nervous system, from mental status to motor and sensory function and reflexes. Brain weight and volume decline with age from shrinkage of larger neurons and loss of white matter and some neurons, primarily in the frontal and temporal lobes. Function of neurotransmitters such as dopamine decreases. Nevertheless, most adults adapt well to getting old. They maintain self-esteem. They adapt to their changing mental and physical capacities and social and financial circumstances, and eventually prepare themselves for death.

Most elderly people do well on mental status examinations, but selective impairments may become evident, especially at advanced ages. Successfully aging older adults typically retain memory functions adequate for the societal demands of independent living. Short-term and remote memory remains largely intact, as does memory for vocabulary and general information. Language comprehension also remains intact. Many older people voice concern about their memories. *Benign senescent forgetfulness* or *age-associated memory impairment* is the usual explanation. This term refers to difficulty recalling names of people or objects or certain details of specific events. Identifying this common phenomenon, when appropriate, may calm worries about Alzheimer's disease. As people age, slowed psychomotor and cognitive processing can affect how quickly people retrieve and process data, learn new material, complete visuospatial tasks, and negotiate tasks (e.g., driving) that require rapid perceptual speed, attention, and working memory (Craft et al., 2003).

Frequently, the examiner must distinguish age-related changes in the nervous system from manifestations of specific mental disorders (e.g., depression, dementia), the prevalence of which increases with age. Sorting out psychological ailments from medical conditions may be difficult, particularly because both mood disturbances and cognitive changes can alter clients' ability to recognize or report symptoms. Older adults are significantly more susceptible to delirium, a reversible state of sudden onset of confusion that frequently follows surgery or is the first clue to infection or problems with medication. The examiner must recognize and successfully reverse this condition promptly (see Table 25-1, p. 932).

Occasionally, an older person develops a benign essential tremor that gradually progresses from the hands and arms to involve the jaw, head, voice, and trunk. It may be confused with a parkinsonism tremor (p. 744; Marshall, 2007). Unlike parkinsonian tremors, benign tremors are slightly faster, disappear at rest, and have no associated muscle rigidity.

Aging may also affect the sensory system, balance, and reflexes. Older adults frequently lose some or all vibration sense in the feet and ankles bilaterally, but not in the fingers or knees. Sensations of light touch and pain may also be mildly impaired. Less commonly, position sense may diminish or disappear. Expect increased sway in the Romberg test from diminished vibratory and position sense in the lower extremities. The gag reflex and abdominal reflexes may be diminished or absent (Miller, 2009). Ankle reflexes may be symmetrically decreased or absent, even when reinforced, but patellar reflexes persist (Pakkar & Cummings, 2003). Partly because of musculoskeletal changes in the feet, the plantar response becomes less obvious and more difficult to interpret, but the Babinski sign is a pathological finding. If reflex changes are asymmetric, search for an explanation other than age alone. Except for the age-related changes documented for hearing, vision, taste, and the gag reflex, function of the remaining cranial nerves remains intact (CVI, VII, XI, XII) with aging.

THE HEALTH HISTORY: SUBJECTIVE DATA

APPROACH TO THE CLIENT

As you talk with older adults, begin to refine your usual techniques for obtaining the health history. Your demeanour should convey respect, patience, and cultural awareness. Be sure to address clients by their last name.

> ### APPROACH TO THE OLDER ADULT CLIENT
> - Adjusting the office environment
> - Shaping the content and pace of the visit
> - Eliciting symptoms.
> - Addressing the cultural dimensions of aging

Adjusting the Office Environment. When you expect to interview elderly clients, take the time to adapt the environment of the office, hospital room, or continuing-care facility to facilitate the client's ease in responding to your questions, and later to the physical examination. In the hospital or continuing-care environment, with permission from the client, lower side rails or move a walker to remove barriers between you and the client. Face the client directly, sitting at eye level. Use your understanding of cultural differences to assist you in determining the appropriate distance to sit from the client (see Chapter 2). Ensure as much privacy as possible during the interview. Drawing the curtain around the bed or examination table enhances the perception of privacy. Equip the office setting with chairs with higher seating to aid clients with quadriceps weakness to sit and rise from a chair, and a wide stool with handrails leading up to the examining table to facilitate safe movement to the examination table. Do not leave the elderly client alone if there is any concern about safety with mobility or cognitive decline.

Recall the older client's physiologic changes in temperature regulation. Make sure the office is neither too cool nor too warm and that the bed- or wheelchair-bound client is comfortably warm. The examining gown should be of appropriate length, preferably to mid-thigh. Brighter natural lighting helps compensate for changes in vision—a well-lit room allows the older adult to see your facial expressions and gestures.

> Avoid sitting with your back to a window because this will put your face in shadow, making it difficult for the client to read your facial expressions.

More than 50% of older Canadian adults have hearing deficits, especially loss of high-tone discrimination (PHAC, 2006). Keeping the interview environment free of distractions or noise is more conducive to accurate reactions and responses. In the hospital or continuing-care setting, ask the client to turn off the radio or television before starting the interview. If appropriate, consider using an assistive listening device, a microphone that amplifies your voice and connects to an earpiece inserted by the client. Try to adopt low speaking tones, which are best perceived by older adults with hearing impairment. Ensure the client is appropriately using glasses, hearing aids, and dentures to assist with communication (Tangarorang et al., 2003, 2009). Allow for additional time to undress and for transfers from a seated to lying position and vice versa. You and the client may benefit from the presence of a relative or aide to assist with undressing, dressing, transfers, and validation of interview data.

Shaping the Content and Pace of the Visit. With older adults, you will often need to alter the traditional format of the initial or follow-up visit.

From middle age on, people begin to measure their lives in terms of years left rather than years lived. Older people often reminisce about the past and reflect on previous experiences. Listening to this process of life review provides important insights and helps you support clients as they work through painful feelings or recapture joys and accomplishments.

At the same time, it is important to balance the need to assess complex problems with the client's endurance and possible fatigue. To provide enough time to fully listen to the client but prevent him or her from becoming exhausted, make ample use of brief screening tools (see p. 911); information from home visits and the medical record; and reports from family members, caretakers, and allied health disciplines. Consider dividing the initial assessment into two visits. Two or more shorter visits may be less fatiguing and more productive because older clients frequently need more time to respond to questions, and their explanations may be slow and lengthy. Balance this against the physical and mental challenges of getting to an appointment.

Eliciting Symptoms in the Older Adult.   Eliciting the history from older adults calls for the clinician to be careful and astute: Clients may accidentally or purposefully underreport symptoms, the presentation of acute illnesses may be different, common symptoms may mask a geriatric syndrome, and clients may have cognitive impairment.

Older clients tend to overestimate healthiness even when increasing disease and disability are obvious (Tangarorang et al., 2003). It is best to start the visit with open-ended questions like, "How can I help you today?" Older clients may be reluctant to report their symptoms. Some are afraid or embarrassed; others try to avoid medical expenses or the discomforts of diagnosis and treatment. Still others overlook their symptoms, thinking them to be merely part of aging, and simply forget about them. To reduce the risk for late recognition and delayed intervention, you may need to adopt more directed questions or health screening tools, as well as consult with family members and caretakers.

Acute illnesses present differently in older adults than in younger age groups. Older clients with infections are less likely to have fever. In those with myocardial infarction, reports of chest pain fall with increasing age, and complaints of shortness of breath, syncope, stroke, and acute confusion become more common (Tullman et al., 2007). Older clients with hyperthyroidism and hypothyroidism present with fewer symptoms and signs. In hyperthyroidism, fatigue, weight loss, and cardiac findings are the most common symptoms in older clients (ACCE Task Force, 2002/2006). In hypothyroidism, older clients present with fewer symptoms and signs. Fatigue and weakness are common but notably nonspecific; the usual chilliness, paresthesias, weight gain, and cramps found in younger clients are uncommon.

Managing an increasing number of chronic conditions calls for recognizing the symptom clusters typical of different *geriatric syndromes.* Geriatric syndromes are health conditions that share risk factors, including advancing age and cognitive, functional, and mobility impairments stemming from factors associated with multiple organ systems. They include delirium, falls, functional decline, incontinence, and pressure ulcers (Inouye et al., 2007). Student examiners need to learn about these syndromes because one symptom may relate to several others in a pattern of which the client is unaware.

Finally, nurses need to be knowledgeable about how cognitive impairment affects the client's history. Information can be obtained from the client or a proxy if there are communication limitations (McClane, 2006), although nurses are aware that the closeness of the relationship between the older client and the proxy can affect the accuracy of information given by that proxy (Dewey & Parker, 2000). Whenever possible, direct questions to the client. Use simple sentences with prompts about necessary information. For clients with more severe impairments, confirm key symptoms with family members or caretakers in the client's presence and with his or her consent.

Learn to recognize and avoid stereotypes that keep you from viewing each client as a unique person with a treasure of life experiences. When listening to them, discover how these clients see themselves and their situations, as well as their priorities, goals, and coping skills. Such knowledge strengthens your alliance with older clients as you collaborate on plans for care and treatment.

TIPS FOR COMMUNICATING EFFECTIVELY WITH OLDER ADULTS

- Provide a well-lit, moderately warm setting with minimal background noise and safe chairs and access to the examining table.
- Face the client and speak in low tones; make sure the client is using glasses, hearing devices, and dentures if needed.
- Adjust the pace and content of the interview to the stamina of the client; consider two visits for initial evaluations when indicated.
- Allow time for open-ended questions and reminiscing; include family and caretakers when needed, especially if the client has cognitive impairment.
- Make use of brief screening instruments, the medical record, and reports from interdisciplinary team members.
- Carefully assess symptoms, especially fatigue, loss of appetite, dizziness, and pain, for clues to underlying disorders.
- Make sure written instructions are in large print and easy to read.

Key Symptoms and Signs Reported by the Older Adult

- Falls
- Leaking (urinary or fecal incontinence)
- Inability to get around (mobility impairment)
- Pain (acute, chronic)
- Vision or hearing changes (sensory impairments—visual, auditory, taste, tactile, olfactory)
- Skin lesions
- Symptoms of vascular disorders (cerebrovascular, peripheral vascular)

Falls are a major concern of older adults and may result from a single cause (e.g., a cardiac condition) or from multiples causes (e.g., visual impairment and gait impairment combined with poor lighting in the environment). Clients who report falls require a falls assessment (see p. 909 and the algorithm on p. 910 of this chapter for further information on falls).

The client may be reluctant to bring up the potentially embarrassing symptom of urinary or fecal *incontinence*. The nurse should tactfully ask whether the client has experienced any loss. Overactive bladder syndrome is the presence of urgency, frequency, and nocturia, with or without incontinence (Abrams et al., 2002). It can be bothersome and may increase risk of falls for some people. The nurse should also inquire about these and any other lower urinary tract symptoms, such as hesitancy or a sensation of not emptying the bladder, as a part of the review of symptoms.

Mobility impairment and reduced physical endurance can arise from various acute or chronic conditions such as arthritis, joint inflammation, stroke, or respiratory or cardiovascular disease. It is important to have the client describe the change and any associated symptoms. Functional assessment and the physical examination are also important components in assessing mobility changes and their effects on a client's ability to carry out activities of daily living.

Acute and chronic pain can be problematic for older people. Pain and associated complaints account for 80% of clinician visits (Ferrell, 2003). Prevalence of pain may reach 25% to 50% in community-dwelling adults and 40% to 80% in continuing-care residents. Pain usually arises from musculoskeletal concerns such as back and joint pain (Ferrell, 2003).

Headache, neuralgias from diabetes and herpes zoster, nighttime leg pain, and cancer pain are also common. Older clients are less likely to report pain, leading to undue suffering, depression, social isolation, physical disability, and loss of function. Inquire about pain, now considered the "fifth vital sign," each time you meet with the older client. Ask specifically, "Are you having any pain right now?" and "How about during the past week?" If the client reports pain, analyze the symptom in detail. Also, learn to distinguish acute pain from chronic pain and thoroughly investigate the causes of each.

Assessment of pain in clients with cognitive impairment is a challenge. Look for behavioural cues such as facial grimaces, groaning with movement, increased restlessness, and change in personal interaction. These signs may indicate pain.

The management of acute pain is usually quite straightforward, but chronic pain is more difficult, at times requiring a multidimensional approach including the concurrent use of analgesia and nondrug interventions. Perhaps a more positive term for this type of pain is *persistent pain* because the pain is persistent and long-term (Ferrel & Chodosh, 2003). Nurses are responsible for assessing the effectiveness of pain management and make use of unidimensional scales such as the Visual Analog scale, graphic pictures, and the Verbal 0-10 scale; all have been validated and are easy to use. It is important for nurses to become familiar with the many modalities of pain relief and the analgesics most appropriate for older adults.

Concerns about *sensory impairments* such as visual or auditory changes are frequent symptoms described by older people. It is important to assess these concerns as a part of the physical examination and determine whether corrective devices (glasses, hearing aids) are effective. In addition, older people reporting a loss of taste or smell, affecting food intake, may benefit from diet counselling to improve the appeal of food.

Benign *skin lesions* such as actinic or seborrheic keratoses are common in older adults. Skin lesions require careful evaluation to differentiate between benign lesions and the malignant lesion of basal or squamous cell carcinoma or malignant melanoma (see Tables in Chapter 10, for colour plates on skin lesions).

Symptoms of vascular disorders can be variable. The five warning signs of *cerebrovascular* disease (stroke) include weakness, trouble speaking, vision problems, headache, and dizziness (Heart and Stroke Foundation of Canada, 2008). Stroke is a medical emergency, and nurses should teach clients to seek immediate medical help should they experience symptoms such as dizziness, visual changes, hemiparesis, or hemiplegia. *Peripheral vascular disease* may have symptoms that include numbness, coldness of the limbs, or pain on walking (intermittent claudication) in arterial disease or lower limb edema and discoloration (brown or reddish purple) in venous stasis. These symptoms should be further assessed through physical examination.

Examples of Questions for Symptom Analysis—Falls

- "Where have you fallen?" (*Location*)
- "What does it feel like when you fall?" "Do you lose consciousness (black out)?" "Does it feel as if your legs give out?" (*Quality*)
- "How many falls have you had in the past year?" (*Quantity*)
- "When did the falls start?" (*Onset*)
- "How often do they occur?" (*Frequency*)
- "What makes the falls worse/more frequent for you?" (*Aggravating factors*)
- "What do you do to try to avoid falling?" (*Alleviating factors*)

- "What else do you notice about yourself when you fall?" (*Associated symptoms*)
- "What are you doing at the time of your fall?" "What is going on in your life?" "What things in your home might contribute to falls?" (*Environmental factors*)
- "How do these falls affect your day-to-day living?" (*Significance to client*)
- "What do you think is the cause of your falls?" (*Client perspective*)

Addressing Cultural Dimensions. As Canada is a multicultural society, senior First Nations, Métis, Inuit, and immigrants contribute to our ethnic and linguistic diversity. Only 1% of Canadian seniors are First Nations. While the First Nations population tends to be younger than the Canadian population in general, it is expected that the proportion of seniors will increase in the future. Slightly more than half of First Nations seniors live on reserves, which has implications for planning of health care services (Turcotte & Schellenberg, 2006).

Many seniors in Canada are immigrants: 28.6% of people 65 to 74 years and 28% of those 75 to 84 years compared to only 21.3% of those 25 to 54 years. Most seniors who immigrated to Canada came when they were young and have lived here for many decades. The small proportion who immigrate after 65 years usually come with family (Turcotte & Schellenberg, 2006). Although 54% of immigrant seniors are currently originally from Western Europe, patterns of immigration have been changing. Between 1981 and 2002, the immigrant seniors from Asia increased from 5.6% to 19.1%. This led to an increase in the number of immigrant seniors who do not speak either official language, creating a communication challenge for health professionals (Turcotte & Schellenberg, 2006).

Cultural differences affect the epidemiology of illness and mental health, the process of acculturation, the specific concerns of the elderly, the potential for misdiagnosis, and disparities in health outcomes (Xakellis et al., 2004). Learn culturally specific ways to show respect to elders and use appropriate nonverbal communication styles. Direct eye contact or handshaking, for example, may not be culturally appropriate. Identify critical experiences that affect the client's outlook and psyche arising from the country of origin or migration history. Ask about spiritual advisors and native healers.

Cultural values particularly affect decisions about the end of life. Elders, family, and even an extended community group may make these decisions with or for the older client. Such group decision making is in contrast to the client autonomy and informed consent that many contemporary health care providers value, expect, and automatically assume to be desired by all (Nunez, 2003). Being sensitive to the stresses of migration and acculturation, using translators effectively, enlisting "client navigators" from the family and community, and accessing culturally validated assessment tools like the Geriatric Depression scale are important for empathetic care of older adults.

SPECIAL AREAS OF CONCERN WHEN ASSESSING COMMON OR CONCERNING SYMPTOMS

TOPICS TO ASSESS IN THE OLDER ADULT

- Physical activities of daily living (ADL)
- Instrumental activities of daily living (IADL)
- Medications
- Nutrition
- Intimacy and sexuality
- Smoking and alcohol
- Advanced directives and palliative care

Certain signs and symptoms in older adults can greatly affect the person's ability to function safely and independently in the community. For example, geriatric syndromes such as urinary incontinence, hearing and vision loss, and instability and falls can adversely affect older adults' ability and desire to socialize and sustain independent living. Explore the meaning of these symptoms for the older client as you would for all clients, and review the **Topics to Assess** section in previous chapters. Be sure to place signs and symptoms in the context of your overall functional assessment. Several areas warrant special attention as you gather the health history. Approach the following areas with extra thoroughness and sensitivity, always focusing on helping the older adult maintain optimal well-being and level of functioning.

Physical and Instrumental Activities of Daily Living.
Learning how older adults, especially those with chronic illness, function in terms of daily activities is essential and provides an important baseline for the future. First, assess the client's ability for self-care. Ask about his or her capacity to perform the *activities of daily living (ADLs)*—these consist of basic self-care abilities—then move on to inquiries about capacity for higher level functions of the *instrumental activities of daily living (IADLs)* listed in the following table. Can the client perform these activities independently? Does he or she need some help? Is the client entirely dependent on others?

You may wish to start with an open-ended request, "Tell me about your typical day," or "Tell me about your day yesterday." Then move to a greater level of detail … You got up at 8 a.m.? How is it getting out of bed? … "What did you do

---

ACTIVITIES OF DAILY LIVING AND INSTRUMENTAL ACTIVITIES OF DAILY LIVING

Physical Activities of Daily Living (ADLs)	Instrumental Activities of Daily Living (IADLs)
Bathing	Using the telephone
Dressing	Shopping
Toileting	Preparing food
Transferring	Housekeeping
Continence	Laundry
Feeding	Transportation
Managing money	Taking medicine

---

next?" Ask how things have changed, who is available for help, and what the helpers actually do. Ask whether there is anything the client would like to do but no longer can. Remember that assessing the client's safety is one of your priorities.

Medications. Older Canadians are becoming healthier and living longer. Nonetheless, among community-dwelling Canadian seniors, 81% have at least one chronic condition, while 33% report three or more chronic conditions (Gilmour & Park, 2006). The increased prevalence of chronic conditions is associated with increased use of medications. On average, community-based seniors take three different types of medications, the most common of which are non-narcotic pain relievers, blood pressure and heart medications, diuretics, and stomach remedies (Rotermann, 2006). On a more encouraging note, the Canadian Institute of Health Information (CIHI, 2007) issued a report in fall 2007 stating that seniors on public drug programs in Alberta, Saskatchewan, Manitoba, and New Brunswick (information from other provinces and territories was unavailable) were prescribed fewer potentially harmful drugs between 2005 and 2007 than between 2000 and 2001. The most commonly prescribed drugs from the Beers list (Fick et al., 2003) were oral, conjugated estrogens (hormone replacement, use declining), amitriptyline (antidepressant, use increasing), digoxin, oxybutynin (for incontinence), and temazepam (a benzodiazepine; CIHI, 2007). With aging, both the pharmacokinetics (how the body absorbs, distributes, metabolizes, and excretes a drug) and pharmacodynamics (how the drug affects the body at a cellular level) change. These changes, along with the fact that many seniors take several medications daily, increase the risk for adverse drug interactions and reactions often necessitating hospitalization (Miller, 2009). In a recent study of medical inpatients in a large Canadian hospital, 24% of hospitalizations were drug related, and 98% of these were considered preventable (Samoy et al., 2006).

It is vital to document accurately a thorough medication history. Record the indication for each drug, its name, dose, and frequency. Be sure to explore all components of potential polypharmacy, including the use of multiple medications for the same disease often from multiple sources. Inquire about all prescription drugs, over-the-counter drugs, vitamin and nutrition supplements, herbal and homeopathic remedies, folk medicines, narcotics, benzodiazepines, and recreational substances. Also, explore inappropriate use, under use, and nonadherence to medications; assess the medication regimen for possible drug interactions and drugs contraindicated for older adults and polypharmacy (Fick et al., 2003; Reuben et al., 2004). Be particularly careful when assessing sleep disturbances (e.g., insomnia), which are common in older adults. Increased exercise may be the best remedy. Recall that medications are a common modifiable risk factor associated with falls Miller (2009).

Nutrition. Another option for screening is the Mini Nutritional Assessment (MNA; from Nestle Nutrition Services. ® Nestle, 1994, available at http://www. mna-elderly.com). The latter assessment tool provides a malnutrition indicator score. Prevalence of undernutrition increases with age, affecting 5% to 10% of elderly outpatients and 30% to 50% of hospitalized clients (Takahashi et al., 2004). Those with chronic disease are particularly at risk, especially those with poor dentition, oral, or gastrointestinal disorders; depression or other psychiatric illness; and drug regimens that affect appetite and oral secretions. In January 2001, the Food and Nutrition Board, the Institute of Medicine, the National Academy of Science, and Health Canada jointly revised the Dietary Reference Intakes (DRIs) to include the 51- to 75-year-olds and those aged 76 years and older (Health Canada, 2004).

Energy and nutritional requirements for healthy men and women decline with age but may need to be adjusted in the presence of disease and nutritional deficiencies (see the following table for insights into requirements; Mirie, 2001).

■ Energy and Nutritional Requirements for Older Adults

	51–75 Years	76 Years and Older
Energy in kcal/day	Men: 2000–2800[a] Women: 1400–2000	Men: 1650–2450 Women: 1200–2000
Protein	0.8 g/kg/d[a,b]; or possibly— 1.0–1.25 g/kg/day[d] 10–35% of total kcal[a,b]	Same
Carbohydrate	Men: 100 g/day[a] Women: 100 g/day 45–65% of total kcal/day[a,b]	Same
Fats Saturated fats	Men and Women: g/day not determined[a] 20–30% total kcal/day[a,b] 10% of total fat intake	Same
Fibre	Men: 30 g/day[a] Women: 21 g/day 20–35 g/day[d]	Same
Vitamin D	Men: 400–2000 IU/day[a] Women: 400–2000 IU/day	Men: 600–2000 IU/day Women: 600–2000 IU/day
Calcium	Men: 1200 mg/day[a] Women: 1200 mg/day, 1500 mg/day if osteoporotic[c]	Same 1500 mg /day in osteoporotic
Water	30 ml/kg body weight[d]	Same

[a]Health Canada, 2004; [b]Mirie, 2001; [c]Hansen & Binkley, 2007; [d]Sullivan & Johnson, 2003.

Being aware of nutritional requirements for older adults assists nurses to analyze the dietary intake of their clients. As protein–energy malnutrition can become a concern for older adults, especially those who are frail, it is important for nurses to assess dietary intake for calories and protein to determine whether they are under body requirements. The consequences of protein–energy malnutrition include loss of muscle mass (sarcopenia), poor wound healing, and decline in cognition and energy. Monitoring serum albumin provides laboratory data to support concern that visceral body protein stores are less than body requirements. In addition, there is value in assessing water intake. The sensation of thirst diminisheds in the older adult and dehydration can increase the possibility of delirium. Finally, adequate fibre intake is important as this will decrease the incidence of constipation and improve the management of diverticulosis if present (Miller, 2009; Mirie, 2001).

Obesity, as for any age group, is a concern for older adults. About 25% of older Canadians are obese (BMI >30; Tjepkema, 2005). Of those obese seniors, 19% were male and 27% female (Turcotte & Schellengerg, 2006). Obesity is highly correlated with hypertension and arthritis, and visceral body fat contributes to type 2 diabetes mellitus, decreases ventilatory capacity, and affects overall activity level (Miller, 2009; Wilcox & King, 2003). Nurses and dieticians have an important role in recommending nutritional and exercise programs for overweight seniors and monitoring results.

Intimacy and Sexuality. Lifelong patterns of intimacy and sexuality remain stable into old age. Of 1000 Canadians aged 40 to 80 years who were polled, 73% reported being sexually active in the past 12 months, and 90% expressed strong emotional and physical satisfaction in their relationships (Pfizer, 2002). In a recently reported Canadian study (Robinson & Molzahn, 2007), intimacy and sexual activity contributed significantly to overall quality of life. The frequency of sexual activity does decline with age and is greatly influenced by the availability of desirable partners, especially for women. Older adults sustain their ability to respond to sexual stimulation, but responses are slower and less intense. Unfortunately, medications needed to manage heart disease, hypertension, and depression contribute to erectile dysfunction in men and related sexual dysfunction in women. In both men and women, these medications cause decreased or absent libido and inability to achieve orgasm. Also, men experience difficulty achieving and sustaining an erection, and women experience decreased vaginal lubrication. All older adults may have difficulty engaging in sexual intercourse because of the pain and decreased flexibility caused by arthritis; breathlessness caused by chronic obstructive pulmonary disease, penile neuropathy, or delayed vaginal lubrication caused by diabetes mellitus; neurological impairments resulting from strokes; and urinary incontinence from prostatic hyperplasia or changes in pelvic floor support (Calgary Health Region, n.d.; Capital Health, 2004; Miller, 2009).

It is evident that older adults have the potential to remain sexually active. Although many North Americans continue to view older adults as no longer needing or desiring sexual activity, this attitude is changing. Increasingly, seniors are acknowledging the importance of sexual activity to their psychosocial well-being. Nurses understand that sexual dysfunction is often amenable to intervention, and they listen intelligently to concerns about sexual activity that older adults express. Counselling regarding age-related changes in sexuality may reduce fears that sexual performance is inadequate. For example, nurses advise that sexual arousal requires a longer period of foreplay (touching and manual stimulation) to achieve an erection and orgasm. They suggest that women use a water-based lubricant or an estrogen cream to alleviate painful intercourse and that they practise Kegel exercises regularly to enhance pelvic-floor muscle tone, which may help maintain an erection in a partner. Women should void before and after sexual intercourse to decrease the risk of urinary tract infections related to age-related thinning of the vaginal wall. Both men and women may benefit from a medication review if medication-induced sexual dysfunction is a possible problem. Nurses should discuss the possible satisfaction for both partners from the simple acts of intimacy such as hugging, kissing, and hearing loving words. Open and honest communication between partners about sexual relationships and between clients and health care providers remains important throughout life (Calgary Health Region, n.d.; Capital Health, 2004; Miller, 2009).

Smoking and Alcohol. Smoking and exposure to environmental tobacco smoke is harmful at all ages. In 2005, almost 9% of Canadians aged 65 years and older admitted to smoking, down from 11% in 2003 (Statistics Canada, 2007b, Turcotte & Schellenberg, 2006). These data are encouraging, because smoking contributes significantly to the risk for lung diseases, coronary heart disease, and allergies (Miller, 2009). Smoking also contributes to skin wrinkling, increases the risk of osteoporosis, and interferes with the smell and taste of food. At each visit, nurses should advise elderly smokers to quit. The commitment to stop smoking may take time, but the longer the interval following the cessation of smoking, the greater the reduction in risk for heart and lung disease.

Although seniors are less likely to drink (as little as one drink per month) than are other age groups, 48% of surveyed seniors indicated they drink regularly (men more often than women; Turcotte & Schellenberg, 2006). An estimated 22% of Canadians older than 65 years drink four times per week. Two-thirds of these people began drinking at an earlier age, while the remaining one third started drinking as seniors, often in response to losses in their lives (Health Canada, 2007). Older adults are more vulnerable to the effects of alcohol because of their lower body mass, which results in higher peak blood alcohol for a given dose of alcohol. As well, blood flow through the liver and the capacity of the liver to metabolize alcohol decreases with age. Alcohol is a source of empty calories, interferes with absorption of B-complex vitamins and vitamin C, and can lead to malnutrition. Admission to hospital can result in alcohol-induced delirium (Miller, 2009).

Use the CAGE questions to uncover problem drinking. Although symptoms and signs are subtle in older adults, making early detection more difficult, the four CAGE questions (see p. 74) remain sensitive and specific in this age group using the conventional cutoff score of 2 or more (Jones et al., 1993).

Advanced Directives and Palliative Care.

Many older clients want to express their wishes about end-of-life decisions and would like care providers to initiate these discussions before any serious illness develops (Miller, 2009; Tulsky, 2003). Advanced care planning involves discussing and documenting advanced directives that include a living will and durable power of attorney. Both should be completed when the person is competent and preferably in the presence of a lawyer, perhaps at a time when the person's will is updated. The living will describes the client's preferences for initiating, continuing, and terminating certain forms of treatment including "Do Not Resuscitate" orders specifying life support measures should respiratory and/or cardiac arrest occur. Durable power of attorney designates a health care proxy or agent to make decisions on the client's behalf that will reflect the client's wishes in case of cognitive confusion or an emergency. Increasingly, acute care hospitals and continuing care centres in Canada are creating policies addressing end-of-life decisions. Nurses in both active treatment and continuing care centres will need to assist with and carry out end-of-life directives. On admission of older adults to a care facility, nurses should address clients' preferences regarding the end-of-life phase and enter the appropriate documents into the record. Advanced directives are legally binding and provide important guidelines for family and staff. These conversations, although difficult at first, convey your respect and concern for clients and help them and their families prepare openly and in advance for a peaceful death (Callahan, 2004).

For clients with advanced or terminal illnesses, advanced care planning must be part of an overall plan for palliative care. When curative or restorative treatments are no longer an option, quality of life rather than quantity becomes the focus (Miller, 2009). The goal of palliative care is "to relieve suffering and improve the quality of life for clients with advanced illnesses and their families through specific knowledge and skills, including communication with clients and family members; management of pain and other symptoms; psychosocial, spiritual, and bereavement support; and coordination of an array of medical and social services" (Morrison & Meier, 2004, p. 2582). With this goal in mind, the nurse in palliative care uses assessment skills to guide and evaluate interventions.

HEALTH PROMOTION

Important Topics for Health Promotion in the Older Adult

- Risk factors
- Screening
- Exercise and physical activity
- Immunizations

As the life span for older adults extends into the 80s, new issues for health promotion emerge. Given the heterogeneity of the aging population, guiding principles for deciding who might benefit from screening and when it might be stopped are not always helpful, especially because evidence for making screening decisions is not always available. In general, nurses should base screening decisions on each older person's particular circumstances, rather than on his or her age alone. Studies have shown that health screening among older adults is effective in preventing disability and decreasing placement in nursing homes (Struck et al., 2004).

RISK FACTOR ASSESSMENT

Demographics. A decline in mortality rates among older people has contributed to the increased life expectancy of Canadians. Between 1991 and 2002 mortality rates for all age groups decreased, except those 90 years or older (Turcotte & Schellenberg, 2006).

Several factors have contributed to the overall improvement of health of Canadians and the decline in mortality rates. Examples include advances in medical knowledge, improved public health measures, and income support programs for older adults. Nevertheless, chronic diseases such as diabetes, stroke, and dementia become more prevalent as the population ages. Chronic disease can lead to decline in function and potentially limit quality of life. Leading causes of death among seniors in Canada are cancer and heart disease. "Cancer is primarily a disease of older Canadians" (Canadian Cancer Society, 2008, p. 43). Lung, colorectal, prostate, and breast cancers are responsible for the most deaths. Influenza and pneumonia are of concern as well, but the death rate from these diseases, particularly among very old people, has declined in Canada (Turcotte & Schellenberg, 2006).

Family History. Neurodegenerative disorders and mood disorders are important to include when gathering the history of the older client. As well, information on the health of the clients' children and grandchildren may provide insight into family health issues (Duthie, 2007).

Lifestyle/Workplace Issues. Past as well as present behaviours can affect quality of life and influence the likelihood of healthy aging (Martel et al., 2005). Physical inactivity, obesity, smoking, and alcohol consumption can influence the development or exacerbation of chronic disease and concomitant functional decline. Although seniors are less likely to smoke and use alcohol than younger adults (Turcotte & Schellenberg, 2006), nurses should include questions related to lifestyle in the history. Also, information on occupation prior to retirement may alert the nurse to the potential of previous exposure to occupational risks and development of latent diseases such as asbestosis. Older farmers who remain actively working have increased risk of injury associated with use of equipment as well as falls (Golonka et al., 2007). From 1996 to 2004, men 65 to 69 years increased their participation in the labour force by 5%, while women in the same age group increased it by 11%. Among seniors 70 years or older, up to 8% of men and 2% of women are in the labour force (Turcotte & Schellenberg, 2006). The percentage of seniors who work postretirement is higher among those with a university degree.

Household/Environmental Safety. Many injuries among older adults occur at home, and most of these result from falls (further discussed in the following section). Home safety review for seniors should include ensuring the adequacy of lighting, decreasing clutter, ensuring that surfaces are nonskid, and keeping the hot-water temperature set to the recommended 49°C (120°F; Public Health Agency of Canada [PHAC], 2005a). Discussion should include the importance of outside lighting and avoidance of hazards such as cracked sidewalks. Driving can also pose safety risks for older people, so nurses should inquire whether clients are still driving. Specialized driving assessments for older drivers are available in some provinces if there is a concern regarding cognitive or motor skills.

Falls. Falls are a significant risk for older adults. They can lead to serious injuries and may result in hospitalization, admission to long-term care, or even death (Lockett et al., 2004). Between 1998 and 2003, almost 85,000 Canadian seniors sustained injury to the femur, pelvis, hip, or thigh, accounting for 56% of all fall-related injuries for seniors treated in hospital. Another 24% of fall-related hospitalizations among this group included injuries to an upper limb, lower limb, or spine. Among community-dwelling seniors, home is the most frequently reported location of falls. Although only 7.4% of Canadian seniors live in residential care, they tend to have more chronic diseases and functional impairments than those in the community; in addition, fall rates are much higher in residential settings (PHAC, 2005b). Loss of confidence from fear of falling and postfall anxiety syndrome further impair functional status, even after recovery. Hip fracture from falling is associated with excess mortality in older adults. Women who suffer a hip fracture are more than twice as likely to die compared to those who do not have a fracture, a risk that is more pronounced in the first 6 months after fracture (Empana et al., 2004). In a recent prospective cohort study, the mortality risk was highest in the first 6 months after the fracture, with gender differences. For men, the risk of death after hip fracture approximated that of men without fracture after the 6-month interval. For women, a moderately greater risk of death persisted through to the fourth year after fracture (Robbins et al., 2006). Hip fractures have also been associated with increased dependency as measured through admission to a nursing home. Among community-living older adults, the incidence of nursing home admission was 60% for those who experienced a hip fracture compared with 3% who did not, when measured at 3 months after baseline (Leibson et al., 2002).

A brief risk assessment is the initial step in assessment of fall risk among seniors, both in the community and in residential care, and can be undertaken by nurses, family physicians, and other health professionals. Health care providers can identify those

---

COMPREHENSIVE CLINICAL RISK ASSESSMENT FOR FALLS

- Review of falls (history and circumstances)
- History of urinary incontinence
- Risk for osteoporosis
- Client perception of functional ability
- Client fear of falling
- Review of medications
- Identification of home hazards
- Assessment for gait/balance/mobility and visual impairment
- Assessment of muscle strength
- Neurological assessment
- Cardiovascular examination

Source: National Institute for Clinical Excellence, 2004.

who may benefit from a more comprehensive falls assessment (PHAC, 2005b). International evidence-based guidelines on falls in older people suggest a more comprehensive assessment for the following seniors: those who present for medical attention with one or more falls, those who report recurrent falls, and those with gait and/or balance abnormalities (American Geriatric Society, British Geriatric Society & American Academy of Orthopedic Surgeons, 2001). After assessing for multifocal risk factors associated with falls, nurses can implement general prevention strategies including a review of environmental hazards (e.g., obstacles between the bed and bathroom) or education for clients who use assistive devices. They can teach strategies such as prevention of postural hypotension by sitting at the end of the bed for a few minutes before rising slowly (Registered Nurses Association of Ontario, 2007).

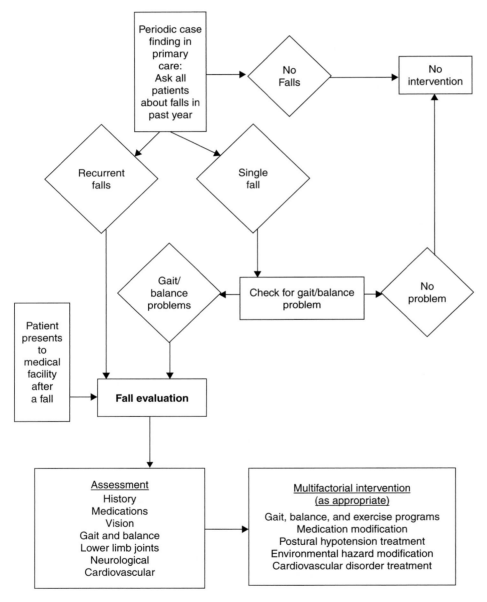

PREVENTION OF FALLS IN OLDER ADULTS

Source: American Geriatric Society, British Geriatrics Society, American Academy of Orthopaedic Surgeons. Guideline for the prevention of falls in older persons. J Am Geriatr Soc. 49(5):664–672, 2001.

Specific fall risk assessment tools have been developed for community, hospital, and residential care. Nurses use a tool appropriate for the specific population they are assessing (RNAO, 2005). As members of multidisciplinary teams, nurses participate in the design and implementation of multifactorial fall prevention plans based on the client's fall risk assessment. Evidence-based interventions can include strength training, exercise such as Tai Chi, medication reviews, avoidance of high-risk medications (e.g., benzodiazepines, antipsychotics), hip protectors, environmental modification, and client education (RNAO, 2005).

Elder Abuse.   Nurses give consideration to screening older clients for elder mistreatment. This encompasses psychological, financial, or physical abuse (including neglect or overuse of medications). Older clients may not report abuse because of cognitive impairment, shame, or dependence on the abuser. Signs that may indicate abuse include unexplained physical injury, dehydration/malnutrition, poor hygiene, oversedation, depression, fear, and anxiety. Although several screening instruments are available, no single instrument has emerged for rapid, accurate assessment and diagnosis of elder mistreatment (Fulmer & Hernandez, 2003; Fulmer et al., 2004). In Canada, several jurisdictions have legislation to protect older adults and those in residential care (Department of Justice, 2007). Nurses are informed about relevant legislation in their area of practice and the reporting mechanism for suspected abuse.

SCREENING

▪ Common Screening Instruments for Use with Older Adults		
Instrument	**Focus of Instrument**	**Comments**
10-Minute Geriatric Screener (p. 915)	Vision Hearing Memory Affect/depression Leg mobility Urinary incontinence Nutrition/weight loss Physical disability	▪ A focused assessment ▪ Includes a variation of the Timed Up and Go test (Podsiadlo & Richardson, 1991)
Geriatric Depression Scale	Depression	
Mini Mental State Examination (MMSE)	Cognitive impairment	▪ A gross assessment ▪ Level of education and cultural variables such as language may affect scores ▪ May miss depression, delirium, and type of dementia
Montreal Cognitive Assessment (MoCA)	Mild cognitive impairment	▪ More recent than MMSE ▪ Has high sensitivity and specificity for identifying mild cognitive impairment ▪ Dementia has slow insidious onset (Nasreddine et al., 2005)
Confusion Assessment Method (CAM) (Inouye et al., 1990)	Delirium	▪ A medical emergency ▪ CAM is one of the most widely used assessment instruments for delirium

Vision and Hearing.   Screening for age-related changes in vision and hearing is important for helping older adults to maintain optimal function (Bogardus et al., 2003). Test vision objectively using an eye chart. Asking the client about any hearing loss may be adequate, followed by the whisper test and more formal testing if indicated (see Chapter 13, p. 357).

Cancer. In Canada, 44% of new cases of cancer and 60% of cancer-related deaths are among people 70 years or older (Canadian Cancer Society/National Cancer Institute of Canada, 2008). As the increased number of new cancers is partly due to the aging population, cancer screening for seniors is important. Interestingly, while prostate cancer (males) and breast cancer (females) are not among the main causes of cancer deaths, they are the most likely cancers to be diagnosed among seniors (Turcotte & Schellenberg, 2006).

SCREENING RECOMMENDATIONS OF THE CANADIAN CANCER SOCIETY (2007)

- *Prostate cancer:* Digital rectal examination (DRE) during annual check-up for men after age 50 years
- *Breast cancer:* Mammogram every 2 years up to age 69 years for women. After age 70 years, the client and physician determine the frequency of mammography.
- *Cervical cancer:* Pap smear every 1 to 3 years for sexually active women (no age-related recommendations)
- *Colorectal cancer:* Fecal occult blood test (FOBT) at least every 2 years (both men and women) after age 50 years

---

Depression. Depression commonly affects older adults but is both under-diagnosed and undertreated. A positive response to asking, "Do you often feel sad? Depressed?" is approximately 80% sensitive and specific and should prompt further investigation. Depressed men older than 65 years are at increased risk for suicide and require particularly careful evaluation.

Dementia. Dementia is global impairment of cognitive function that interferes with day-to-day activities and affects 8% of Canadians older than 65 years. Prevalence increases dramatically with age, with dementia affecting 34.5% of people 85 years and older (Lindsay et al., 2004). Prominent features include short- and long-term memory deficits, impaired judgement, and difficulty carrying out tasks. Thought processes are impoverished; speech may be hesitant as a result of difficulty finding words. Loss of orientation to place may make navigating by foot or car problematic or even dangerous. In Canada, Alzheimer's disease accounts for 64% of dementias, with vascular (19%) or Lewy body dementia (15% to 20%) being the next most common forms. Alzheimer's disease and vascular dementia that occur together are referred to as mixed dementia (Alzheimer Society of Canada, 2007).

Dementia often has a slow insidious onset and may escape detection by both families and clinicians, especially in the early stages of mild cognitive impairment. Look for problems with memory, then later for changes in cognitive function or ADLs. Watch for family concerns about new or unusual behaviours. If you identify cognitive changes, investigate contributing factors such as medications, depression, metabolic abnormalities, or other medical and psychiatric conditions. If clients have dementia, counsel families about the potential for disruptive behaviour, accidents, falls, and termination of driving privileges. Foster discussion of legal arrangements such as power of attorney and advanced directives while the client can still contribute to decision making.

Sundowning appears in mid-stage dementia and slowly worsens to the point where the person can no longer be cared for at home. Nurses are alert to reports by caregivers of physical aggression (e.g., biting), resistiveness (e.g., refusing to eat or take medications), disconcerted verbalizing (e.g., very loud singing or cursing), night-time sleeplessness (e.g., up all night), wandering (e.g., relentless motion), and daytime sleepiness (in late morning or early afternoon). Such behaviours peak between 2.00 p.m. and 9.00 p.m. and 12.00 a.m. to 6.00 a.m. (Nowak & Davis, 2007).

Delirium.   Delirium, a common condition among older people, results from a medical condition, substance intoxication or withdrawal, or other multiple etiologies. In older adults, modifiable factors such as medications, dehydration, and sensory impairment can potentially contribute to delirium (Canadian Coalition for Seniors' Mental Health, 2006). Key features of delirium are a disturbed level of consciousness (hypo- or hyperactivity or alertness) and changes in cognition that evolve over a short period (days). Delirium is associated with high rates of morbidity and mortality in older people and should be considered a medical emergency.

EXERCISE

Regular aerobic exercise can be recommended for almost any adult and is one of the most widely advocated health promotion interventions. In 2005, Canadian seniors reported 40.2% of their household population were at least moderately physically active, up from 34.5% in 2001 (Statistics Canada, 2007a). This finding is encouraging because a regular program of aerobic exercise improves cardiovascular function, decreases blood pressure, decreases risk of diabetes, reduces obesity, and has a positive effect on cognition (Larson et al., 2006). Resistance training improves balance and muscle strength and decreases risk of osteoporosis. Stretching and Tai Chi improve balance, coordination, and flexibility. All these forms of exercise combat the negative effects of inactivity, decrease the risk of falls, promote socialization, and counteract depression (Miller, 2009). Exercise programs can begin with 30 minutes of brisk walking most days in a week. Indoor mall walking is popular in winter months when sidewalks may be slippery. Wheelchair exercises assist seniors with limited mobility. Physical therapists can provide more tailored recommendations.

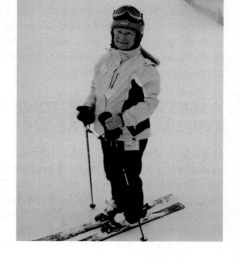

IMMUNIZATIONS

In Canada, the National Advisory Committee on Immunization (2006) has outlined immunization recommendations for all adults. All adults should be immunized against diphtheria, tetanus, pertussis, measles, mumps, rubella, and varicella. Schedules exist for those with a completed primary series, who do not have a record of prior immunization, or with an unclear history. When the primary series is complete, clients can maintain immunity to tetanus and diphtheria by receiving a combined toxoid every 10 years and a single dose of acellular pertussis vaccine once in adulthood. Adults older than 65 years should have one lifetime dose of pneumococcal vaccine as well as yearly influenza vaccine. Health care providers, including those working in continuing care facilities, require annual influenza vaccination. People who live with seniors also require influenza vaccine.

EMERGENCY CONCERNS

An acute onset of any of the geriatric syndromes (delirium, falls, incontinence, vascular disorders) or change in functional ability should alert the clinician to further assess the older person. As older adults often have an altered presentation of illness, nurses should never attribute changes in a client to "old age."

TECHNIQUES OF EXAMINATION: OBJECTIVE DATA

As you have gathered, assessment of the older adult does not follow the traditional format of the history and physical examination. It calls for enhanced techniques of interviewing, special emphasis on daily function and key topics related to elder health, and a focus on functional assessment during the physical examination. Because of its importance to the health of older adults and the order of your assessment, this section begins with Assessing Functional Status: The "Sixth Vital Sign." This segment includes how to evaluate risk for falls, one of the greatest threats to health and well-being in elders. Next follows features of the traditional head-to-toe examination tailored to the older adult.

PROMOTING CLIENT COMFORT, DIGNITY, AND SAFETY

Age-related changes to the immune system leave older adults with a declining ability to fight infection (Htwe et al., 2007). Handwashing, the use of routine practices, and additional precautions during the examination are required. Pressure ulcers are one of the geriatric syndromes (Inouye et al., 2007), and many older clients may have decreased mobility. Ensure that clients do not lie in one position on a bony prominence for long periods and provide assistance for getting on and off the examination table. Pain from osteoarthritis or other conditions may limit the physical examination, either because clients cannot assume a needed position or have a limited range of motion. Be alert for signs of discomfort such as facial grimacing. Strive to promote dignity. When working with older clients, ask clients how they would prefer to be addressed. Never use potentially disrespectful terms such as "grandma," "grandpa," or "dear." Such terminology assumes a familiarity that clients may not appreciate. Ensure clients are adequately draped to minimize exposure and avoid chilling.

ASSESSING FUNCTIONAL STATUS: THE "SIXTH VITAL SIGN"

During assessment of older adults, the examiner places a special premium on maintaining the client's health and well-being. In a sense, all visits are opportunities for health promotion and counselling directed to sustaining the client's independence and optimal level of function. Although the specific goals of care may vary, a primary focus is preserving the client's functional status, the sixth vital sign. Functional status specifically means the ability to perform tasks and fulfill social roles associated with daily living across a wide range of complexity (Kortez & Reuben, 2003; Reuben, 2003). As noted in the General Survey section on p. 129, your assessment of functional status begins when the client enters the room. Several well-validated and time-efficient assessment tools can help maintain focus on these observations and assist with this approach.

Assessing Functional Ability. The goal associated with assessing functional ability of older clients is to determine the therapy, assistance, or aids they require to maximize independence and compensate for any deficits (Duthie, 2007). The 10-minute Geriatric Screener (p. 915) incorporates some functional issues. More in-depth assessment of function includes assessment of ADLs and IADLs, and use of specific problem-focused instruments such as the Tinetti Gait and Balance Tool (Tinetti, 1986) or the Berg Balance scale (Berg et al., 1992).

Assessing Cognitive Ability. Screening instruments, including the Mini Mental State Examination and Montreal Cognitive Assessment, can help to identify cognitive impairment, but may not be diagnostic for depression, delirium, or type of dementia. The Geriatric Depression scale and CAM are helpful when clinicians suspect depression or delirium. Dementia-specific instruments and neuropsychological testing in complex cases usually require referral to an occupational therapist or neuropsychologist.

■ Modified 10-Minute Geriatric Screener

Problem	Screening Measure	Positive Screen
Vision	2 Parts: Ask: "Do you have difficulty driving, or watching television, or reading, or doing any of your daily activities because of your eyesight?" If yes, then: Test each eye with Snellen chart while patient wears corrective lenses (if applicable).	Yes to question and inability to read greater than 20/40 on Snellen chart
Hearing	Use audioscope set at 40 dB. Test hearing using 1,000 and 2,000 Hz.	Inability to hear 1,000 or 2,000 Hz in both ears or either of these frequencies in one ear
Leg mobility	Time the patient after asking: "Rise from the chair. Walk 20 feet briskly, turn, walk back to the chair and sit down."	Unable to complete task in 15 seconds
Urinary incontinence	2 Parts: Ask: "In the last year, have you ever lost your urine and gotten wet?" If yes, then ask: "Have you lost urine on at least 6 separate dates?"	Yes to both questions
Nutrition/ weight loss	2 Parts: Ask: "Have you lost 10 lbs over the past 6 months without trying to do so?" Weigh the patient.	Yes to the question or weight <100 lbs
Memory	Three-item recall	Unable to remember all three items after 1 minute
Depression	Ask: "Do you often feel sad or depressed?"	Yes to the question
Physical disability	Six questions: "Are you able to … : do strenuous activities like fast walking or bicycling? do heavy work around the house like washing windows, walls, or floors? go shopping for groceries or clothes? get to places out of walking distance? bathe, whether a sponge bath, tub bath, or shower? dress, like putting on a shirt, buttoning and zipping, or putting on shoes?	Yes to any of the questions

Source: Moore AA, Siu AL. Screening for common problems in ambulatory elderly: clinical confirmation of a screening instrument. Am J Med 100:438-440, 1996.

PHYSICAL EXAMINATION OF THE OLDER ADULT

UNEXPECTED FINDINGS

General Survey. From your first contact with the client, you have begun to compile an objective database from the client's appearance and behaviours. You likely made an observation about grip strength when shaking hands and noted skin colour, an obvious tremor or physical deformity, and disturbances in speech (Duthie, 2007). What is the client's apparent state of health and degree of vitality?

Flat or impoverished affect may be seen in *depression, Parkinson's disease,* or *Alzheimer's disease.*

Does the client look his or her stated age? What about mood and affect? Note the client's personal grooming, hygiene, and the fit, appropriateness, and cleanliness of clothing. How does the client walk and transfer onto the examining table? Can the client follow directions? Is speech coherent and appropriate? Are thought processes unusually slowed? At all times be conscious of differences between expected age-related change and pathology.

Undernutrition, slowed motor performance, loss of muscle mass, or weakness suggests frailty or caregiver neglect.
Kyphosis or disturbances in gait can impair balance and increase risk for falling.

Vital Signs. Weight should be taken yearly because it can change for various reasons. Height decreases with age and should be taken periodically. Determine the BMI. Although BMI tables may not be appropriate for some adults older than 65 years, current guidelines in these tables are likely appropriate for healthy older adults. Expect a weight appropriate for height, and know that being overweight in old age increases the morbidity risks for osteoarthritis in the hips and knees, heart disease, diabetes, and breast and colon cancers (Harris, 2004).

A marked change in weight should be investigated. Overweight is commonly seen and underweight to a lesser extent (Harris, 2004).

Measure the blood pressure in both arms using recommended techniques, including palpation to detect an auscultatory gap. Measure blood pressure in two positions: supine after resting for up to 10 minutes, then within 3 minutes of standing. Check for increased systolic blood pressure (SBP) and widened pulse pressure (PP). With aging, SBP and diastolic blood pressure (DBP) increase, but SBP does to a greater degree. A blood pressure between 120/80 and 139/89 is considered prehypertensive, even in the elderly population. Review the categories of prehypertension from the Joint National Committee on Prevention, Detection, Evaluation, and Treatment of High Blood Pressure (2003) for help with the detection and management of hypertension (p. 109). Assess the client for orthostatic hypotension and if possible postprandial hypotension.

Isolated systolic hypertension (SBP ≥ 140) after age 50 triples the risk for coronary heart disease in men. PP ≥ 60 is a risk factor for cardiovascular and renal disease and stroke (Bobrie et al., 2001; Chaudry et al., 2004; Papademetriou, 2003; Vaccarino et al., 2001).
Orthostatic hypotension occurs in 10% to 20% of older adults and in up to 30% of frail continuing care residents, especially when they first arise in the morning. It can present with lightheadedness, weakness, unsteadiness, visual blurring, and, in 20% to 30% of clients, syncope. Causes include medications, autonomic disorders, diabetes, prolonged bed rest, blood loss, and cardiovascular disorders (Bobrie et al., 2001).

Measure heart rate with the client lying and standing, respiratory rate, and temperature. The apical heart rate may yield more information about arrhythmias in older clients. Expect occasional premature ventricular ectopic beats but not an irregular rhythm. As peripheral vascular resistance increases with age, the radial or brachial artery may resist compression. If the pulse is still palpable when the blood pressure cuff is inflated above SBP, pseudohypertension may be present. Expect a respiratory rate between 16 to 24 breaths per minute and a regular pattern. Take the temperature in the usual way, but use a thermometer that records lower temperatures.

Respiratory rate ≥ 25 breaths per minute indicates lower respiratory infection (e.g., pneumonia). Absence of fever (temperature > 38°C) does not exclude infection. Hypothermia is more common in elderly clients (Tangarorang et al., 2003).

Weight and height are especially important in the elderly and needed for calculation of the BMI. Weight should be measured at every visit.

Skin. Note physiologic changes of aging, such as thinning, loss of elastic tissue and turgor, and wrinkling. Skin may be dry, flaky, rough, and often itchy *(asteatosis)*, with a latticework of shallow fissures that creates a mosaic of small polygons, especially on the legs. Observe any patchy changes in colour. Check the extensor

Low weight is a key indicator of poor nutrition.
Undernutrition is seen with depression, alcoholism, cognitive impairment, malignancy, chronic organ failure (cardiac, renal, pulmonary), medication use, social

surface of the hands and forearms for white depigmented patches (*pseudoscars*) and for well-demarcated vividly purple macules or patches that may fade after several weeks (*actinic purpura*).

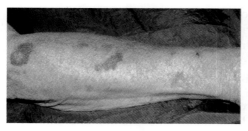

ACTINIC PURPURA

isolation, poverty, and caregiver neglect.

Look for changes from sun exposure. Areas of skin may appear weatherbeaten, thickened, yellowed, and deeply furrowed; there may be *actinic lentigines*, or "liver spots," and *actinic keratoses*, superficial flattened papules covered by a dry scale (p. 249).

Inspect for the benign lesions of aging, namely *comedones*, or blackheads, on the cheeks or around the eyes; *cherry angiomas* (p. 268), which often appear early in adulthood; and *seborrheic keratoses*, raised yellowish lesions that feel greasy and velvety or warty (p. 269).

Distinguish such lesions from a *basal cell carcinoma*, initially a translucent nodule that spreads and leaves a depressed center with a firm elevated border, and from a *squamous cell carcinoma*, a firm reddish-appearing lesion often emerging in a sun-exposed area (p. 269). A dark, raised, asymmetric lesion with irregular borders may be a *melanoma*.

Watch for any painful vesicular lesions in a dermatomal distribution.

Suspect *herpes zoster* from reactivation of latent varicella-zoster virus in the dorsal root ganglia. Risk increases with age and impaired cell-mediated immunity (Gnann & Whitely, 2002).

In older bed-bound clients, especially when emaciated or neurologically impaired, inspect the skin thoroughly for damage or ulceration.

Pressure sores may develop from obliteration of arteriolar and capillary blood flow to the skin or from shear forces during movement across sheets or when lifted upright incorrectly. See Table 10-11, Pressure Ulcers.

HEENT. Conduct a careful and thorough evaluation of the head and neck, as detailed in Chapters 11 to 13.

Inspect the head as detailed in Chapter 11. Expect the hair to be greying (or coloured), somewhat thinner, and perhaps coarser than when the client was younger. Note the expected receding hairline in most men and to a lesser extent in women. Men's eyebrows may become quite bushy, and you may notice coarse hairs protruding from the nares and ears. You can expect to find a few coarse hairs on the face of many women. Facial skin in many older adults will often appear wrinkled and lack turgor. Carefully inspect the face and neck for benign and malignant skin lesions such as *actinic keratoses* and *squamous cell carcinomas,* often found on exposed areas. Make the appropriate referral if you find any suspicious lesions. Palpate the temporomandibular joint to detect degenerative changes resulting from osteoarthrosis within the joint secondary to excessive compression on the joint because of the lost teeth; record the presence of crepitations and pain with movement.

Test visual acuity using a wall-mounted or pocket Snellen chart. Note the need for corrective lenses for uncorrected myopia and presbyopia.

Refractive errors are common in Canadians (see Chapter 12).

Pupillary reaction to light (direct and consensual) should be brisk. Observe for pupillary dilation for distance and constriction with near effort. Except for possible impairment in upward gaze, extraocular movements remain intact. Observe for the eyes to converge as they focus on a near object. A greying ring (arcus senilis) at the edge of the cornea is an expected finding.

Using your ophthalmoscope, carefully examine the lenses and fundi.

Cataracts, glaucoma, and macular degeneration all increase with aging (Congdon et al., 2003).

Inspect each lens carefully for any opacities. Do not depend on the flashlight alone because the lens may look clear superficially. The formation of cataracts is expected but warrants further evaluation.

Cataracts are the world's leading cause of blindness. Risk factors include cigarette smoking, exposure to UVB light, high alcohol intake, diabetes, medications (including steroids), and trauma. See Table 12-5, Opacities of the Cornea and Lens

In older adults, the fundi lose their youthful shine and light reflections, and the arteries look narrowed, paler, straighter, and less brilliant. Assess the cup-to-disc ratio, usually ≤ 1:2.

An increased cup-to-disc ratio suggests open-angle *glaucoma,* caused by irreversible optic neuropathy and leading to loss of peripheral and central vision and blindness. Prevalence is three to four times higher in Afro Canadians than in the general population.

Inspect the fundi for colloid bodies called *drusen,* causing alterations in pigmentation of the retina.

Macular degeneration causes poor central vision and blindness. Types include *dry atrophic* (more common but less severe) and *wet exudative,* or neovascular. Drusen may be hard and sharply defined, or soft and confluent with altered pigmentation, shown below and on p. 339.

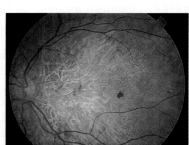

Test hearing by occluding one ear and using the techniques for whispered voice (see p. 357). If appropriate, the Weber–Rinne tests and audioscope can be used for more formal screening. Be sure to inspect the ear canals for cerumen impaction.

Removing cerumen often quickly improves hearing.

Examine the oral cavity for odour, gingival mucosa for colour and edema, teeth for dental caries and mobility, buccal surfaces for moisture and lesions, tonsillar cavities for tonsils (expect tonsillar tissue to have receded), and salivary glands for quantity

Malodour may occur with poor oral hygiene, *periodontitis,* and dental caries. *Gingivitis* may arise from

of saliva. Dilated veins under the tongue are often found. Ask the client to remove dentures so you can examine the gums for denture sores.

periodontal disease. Dental plaque, dry mouth, poor oral hygiene, and neglected dental care contribute to *dental caries*. Increased tooth mobility from abscesses or advanced caries warrants removal of the tooth to prevent aspiration. Decreased salivation may develop from dehydration, medications, radiation, and possibly *Sjogren's syndrome*. Leukoplakia may arise on the lateral borders of the tongue and floor of the mouth (Shay, 2007).

Continue by examining the thyroid gland and lymph nodes. Enlarged submandibular salivary glands are sometimes easily felt. Expect the thyroid gland to be difficult to palpate.

Any enlarged cervical lymph node or nodule in the thyroid must be fully investigated.

Inspect range of motion of the neck including active flexion, extension, lateral flexion, and rotation. Expect limitations in range of motion from degeneration of the intervertebral discs and facet joints that contribute to osteoarthritic changes in the spine (Loeser & Delbono, 2003).

Thorax and Lungs.

Complete the usual examination, making note of subtle signs of changes in pulmonary function. Inspect the thorax for evidence of kyphosis. Expect auscultation to reveal full air entry and vesicular breath sounds over anterior and posterior lung fields.

Increased anteroposterior diameter, purse-lipped breathing, and dyspnea with talking or minimal exertion suggest *chronic obstructive pulmonary disease.*

Cardiovascular System.

Review your findings from measurement of the blood pressure and heart rate. The occasional premature ventricular or supraventricular arrhythmia is expected. The apical beat may provide more information about rate and rhythm than the radial pulse.

Isolated systolic hypertension and a widened pulse pressure are cardiac risk factors, prompting a search for *left ventricular hypertrophy (LVH).*

As with younger adults, begin by inspecting the JVP, palpating the carotid upstrokes, and listening for any overlying carotid bruits. Pressure in the right jugular vein is often more reliable because a tortuous aorta can impede venous return into the right atrium.

A *tortuous atherosclerotic aorta* can raise pressure in the left jugular veins by impairing their drainage into the right atrium. It may also cause kinking of the carotid artery low in the neck on the right, chiefly in women with hypertension, which can be mistaken for a carotid aneurysm (Tuffet & Lukatta, 2003). Carotid bruits in the elderly warrant further investigation for possible carotid stenosis due to risk for ipsilateral stroke.

Assess the apical impulse, then auscultate S_1 and S_2. Listen also for the extra sounds of S_3 and S_4. Physiological splitting of the S_2 may be difficult to hear.

Sustained apical impulse in LVH; diffuse apical impulse in congestive heart failure (see p. 451).

In older adults an S_3 suggests dilatation of the left ventricle from congestive heart failure or cardiomyopathy; an S_4 often accompanies hypertension and stiff left ventricular wall (Duthie, 2007).

Beginning in the second right interspace, listen for cardiac murmurs in all areas of auscultation (see p. 454). Describe the timing, shape, location of maximal intensity, radiation, intensity, pitch, and quality of each murmur you detect. The murmur of aortic stenosis peaks early and is rarely heard in the carotid arteries (Miller, 2009).

A systolic crescendo–decrescendo murmur in the second right interspace suggests aortic sclerosis or aortic stenosis, seen in approximately 30% and 2% of community-dwelling elders, respectively.
A harsh holosystolic murmur at the apex suggests mitral regurgitation, also common in the elderly.

Breasts and Axillae. Inspect the breasts for puckering or asymmetry, and the axillae for rashes. Palpate the breasts carefully for lumps or masses. Include palpation of the tail of Spence that extends into the axilla. Examine the axillae for lymphadenopathy, an unexpected finding.

Lumps or masses in older women, and rarely in older men, mandate further investigation for possible malignancy.

Abdomen. Conduct your usual examination of the abdomen. Check for any bruits over the aorta, renal arteries, and femoral arteries. Inspect the upper abdomen; palpate to the left of the midline for any aortic pulsations. Try to assess the width of the aorta by pressing more deeply with one hand on each of its lateral margins (see p. 536).

Bruits may be noted in atherosclerotic vascular disease. Widened aorta and pulsatile mass may be found in *abdominal aortic aneurysm.*

Inspect for surgical scars and inquire about their origin if the history is incomplete. Inspect for symmetry, ventral hernias, and inguinal hernias. Expect weaker abdominal muscles. Palpate for masses, abdominal tenderness, and evidence of urinary retention. Auscultate for frequency and quality of bowel sounds.

Masses, abdominal tenderness require further investigation.
An acute abdomen resulting from peritonitis from any cause may present with a soft abdomen and minimal tenderness.

Female Genitalia and Pelvic Examination. Take special care to explain the steps of the examination and allow time for careful positioning. Ask an assistant to help the older woman move onto the examining table, then into the lithotomy position. Raising the head of the table may make her more comfortable. For the woman with arthritis or spinal deformities who cannot flex her hips or knees, an assistant can gently raise and support the legs, or help the woman into the left lateral position.

Inspect the vulva for changes related to menopause such as thinning of the skin, loss of pubic hair, and decreased distensibility of the introitus. Identify any labial masses. Note that bluish swellings may be varicosities. Bulging of the anterior vaginal wall below the urethra may indicate an urethrocele or urethral diverticulum.

Benign masses include condylomata, fibromas, leiomyomas, and sebaceous cysts. See Table 22-2, Bulges and Swellings of the Vulva, Vagina, and Urethra, p. 822.
A cough may trigger stress incontinence.

Look for any vulvar erythema.

Erythema with satellite lesions results from infection with *Candida;* erythema with ulceration or necrotic center is associated with *carcinoma.* Multifocal reddened lesions with white scaling plaques are consistent with *Paget's disease.*

Inspect the urethra for *caruncles*, or prolapse of fleshy erythematous mucosal tissue at the urethral meatus. Note any enlargement of the clitoris.

Clitoral enlargement may accompany *androgen-producing tumours* or use of androgen creams.

Spread the labia, press downward on the introitus to relax the levator muscles, and gently insert the speculum after moistening it with warm water or a water-soluble lubricant. If you find severe vaginal atrophy, a gaping introitus, or an introital stricture from estrogen loss, you will need to vary the size of the speculum.

Inspect the vaginal walls, which may be atrophic, dry, and lacking rugal folds, and the cervix. Note any thin cervical mucus or vaginal or cervical discharge.

Estrogen-stimulated cervical mucus with ferning is seen with use of hormone replacement therapy, *endometrial hyperplasia,* and *estrogen-producing tumours.* Discharge may accompany vaginitis or cervicitis. See Table 22-6, Vaginal Discharge, p. 825.

Use a wooden spatula or endocervical brush to obtain endocervical cells for the Pap smear. A blind swab may be indicated if the atrophic vagina is too small.

See Table 22-7, Positions of the Uterus, p. 826, and Table 22-8, Disorders of the Uterus, p. 827.

After removing the speculum, ask the client to bear down to detect uterine prolapse, cystocele, urethrocele, or rectocele.

Perform the bimanual examination. Check for motion of the cervix and for any uterine or adnexal masses. Expect the uterus to be small and the ovaries nonpalpable.

Mobility of the cervix is restricted with inflammation, malignancy, or surgical adhesion. Enlarging uterine fibroids, or leiomyomas, are found in *malignant leiomyosarcoma.* The ovaries are palpable with *ovarian cancer.*

Perform the rectovaginal examination. Assess for uterine and adnexal irregularities through the anterior rectal wall and for rectal masses. Change gloves first if blood from the bimanual examination is on the vaginal examining glove to obtain an accurate stool sample.

A uterus that is enlarged, fixed, or irregular may indicate adhesions or possible malignancy. Rectal masses are found in *colon cancer.*

Male Genitalia and Prostate.
Examine the penis, retracting the foreskin if present. Examine the scrotum, testes, and epididymis.

Findings include smegma, penile cancer, and scrotal hydroceles.

Proceed with the rectal examination, paying special attention to any rectal masses and any nodularity or masses of the prostate. Note that the anterior and median lobes of the prostate are inaccessible to rectal palpation, limiting the utility of the digital rectal examination for detecting prostate enlargement or possible malignancy.

Rectal masses are found in *colon cancer. Prostate hyperplasia* may be linked with enlargement; *prostate cancer* is possible with nodules or masses.

Peripheral Vascular System.
Auscultate the abdomen for aortic, renal, or femoral artery bruits.

Bruits over these vessels are found in *atherosclerotic disease.*

Assess the width of the abdominal aorta in the epigastric area and examine for a pulsatile mass.

Consider *abdominal aortic aneurysm* if aortic width is ≥ 3 cm or with a pulsatile mass, especially in older male smokers with coronary disease.

Palpate pulses carefully, comparing sides.

Diminished or absent pulses may indicate *arterial occlusion.* Consider confirmation with an office ankle–brachial index. Note that ≤33% of clients with peripheral vascular disease have symptoms of claudication (McDermott et al., 2002).

Inspect the lower legs for brownish discolouration around and superior to the malleoli. Note condition and colour of the skin and presence of hair over the lower legs, feet, and toes. Palpate all peripheral pulses carefully. Compare sides and proximal to distal pulses in the extremities. Observe for symmetry and amplitude. Compress the radial and brachial arteries to determine their rigidity. With the client standing, inspect the saphenous veins for distention and tortuosity. Assess for edema (see Chapter 18).

Shiny skin and brownish discolouration around the malleoli are indicative of venous stasis. Look for stasis ulcers. Radial and brachial arteries that resist compression suggest arteriosclerosis and the possibility of pseudohypertension. Absent or markedly diminished peripheral pulses and absence of hair suggests arterial insufficiency.

Musculoskeletal System. You began the assessment of the musculoskeletal system as the client entered the room, sat down, was positioned on the examination table, and was asked the last question on the 10-Minute Geriatric Screener (p. 915). Inspect active range of motion (ROM) in all the joints, evaluating for limitations in range. Inspect the extremities for loss of muscle mass, expecting losses appropriate to level of activity. Expect atrophy of interosseous muscles and thenar eminences of the hand. Palpate all joints for tenderness, swelling, warmth, redness, and crepitations. Review the techniques for examining individual joints in Chapter 19.

Inability to perform active ROM in any joint following a stroke. Heberden's and Bouchard's nodes in the fingers. Fallen arches and hammer toes.
Degenerative joint changes in *osteoarthritis;* joint inflammation in *rheumatoid* or *gouty arthritis.* See Tables 19-1 to 19-10.

Nervous System. For a complete examination of the neurological system, assess cranial nerves, motor function, sensory function, and mental status. Any evidence of lateralizing (asymmetrical) motor and/or sensory signs warrants a detailed neurological examination. The 10-Minute Geriatric Screener will direct your efforts to a more focused assessment, for example, a focus on memory and affect. Expect an elderly person to process and retrieve information and memories more slowly. An alteration in level of consciousness, orientation, judgement, calculations, speech, and language cannot be attributed solely to age.

Learn to distinguish delirium from depression and dementia (see Table 25-1, Delirium, Depression, and Dementia). Nonetheless, careful search for underlying causes is warranted.

For detailed examination of the cranial nerves, see Chapters 11, 12, 13, and 20, and for mental status, see Chapter 9.

Assess the *motor functions* of strength, coordination, gait, and reflexes. Expect strength to be congruent with muscle mass, sustained, and symmetrical. Muscle tone may be slightly increased. Deep tendon reflexes generally remain intact, but the ankle reflex may be absent (an acceptable variant with aging). The *sensations* of pain, light touch, and position should remain intact. Vibratory sensation is frequently absent in the toes and ankles. A Babinski reflex is an unexpected finding. Observe the client walk across the room. Expect a diminished arm swing, a shorter step length, and a foot lift less than seen in young people. To assess leg strength and balance, ask the client to rise from a chair without using the arms, walk on heels and toes, then sit down. The client should perform these actions without assistance. To assess fine motor ability, determine whether the client can dress and undress without assistance. If tremor is present, evaluate it for amplitude, rhythm, distribution, frequency, and time of occurrence; note if it occurs at rest, with motion, or with intention.

Muscle atrophy and loss of motor and sensory function are seen following a stroke. Jerky movements and cogwheel rigidity are observed in *Parkinson's disease.* The tremor of Parkinson's disease is of slow frequency and occurs at rest, with a "pill-rolling" quality. It is aggravated by stress and inhibited during sleep or movement. Essential tremor is bilateral and symmetric, diminished by alcohol, and associated with a positive family history (Marshall, 2007).

RECORDING AND ANALYZING FINDINGS

Documentation of findings from the physical examination of the older adult could include data from every system of the body, including the mental status examination. Nurses analyze this information, in conjunction with relevant findings from the health history, to provide members of the geriatric team with an integrated picture of this older client.

Abnormalities of gait and balance, especially widening of base, slowing and lengthening of stride, and difficulty turning, are correlated with risk for falls (Baloh, 2003).

■ Examples of Documentation—The Older Adult

Area of Assessment	Expected Findings	Unexpected Findings
General survey	Dressed in a clean, pressed pant suit; neatly groomed 70-year-old *female*. Responds articulately to questions. Walks with assurance. Hand grip firm. Skin colour light pink.	Frail-looking 70-year-old *male*. Clothes rumpled, tie soiled. Walks slowly using a cane. Requires assistance to mount examining table. Colour pale. Responds slowly and hesitantly to questions.
Vital signs	TPR: 36.5°C; 80; regular with occasional extra beat; 24 and regular. BP 130/82 sitting, right arm; 132/84, left arm. Height: 165 cm, Weight: 55 kg, BMI: 20	TPR: 36.4°C; 88, irregular irregularity; 26 regular, increases with effort. BP 146/96 sitting, right arm, 148/94 left arm. Height: 180 cm, Weight: 85 kg, BMI: >27
Skin	Face: light pink. Forearm skin thin, warm and dry; small purpura lesion on right forearm. Skin over lower legs pale and dry, states uses lotions twice daily. Few coarse hairs under chin.	Face: skin pale, reddish patch on right cheek, purpura lesions on left forearm; brown, shiny skin over lower shins and malleoli bilaterally, without ulceration.
HEENT	Hair grey, full, carefully groomed. Vision 20/20 bilaterally with corrective glasses. Pupils equal (3 mm), react briskly—direct and consensual. Extraocular movements intact bilaterally. Conjunctivae clear. Disc margins soft, no foveal light reflex, arterial light reflex increased bilaterally. Tympanic membrane with intact cone of light bilaterally. AC>BC bilaterally. Nasal mucosa pink. No sinus tenderness bilaterally. Oral mucosa pink, moist, without lesions. Dentition—molars capped, several fillings, no obvious caries, gums moist and pink. Tongue midline, bilaterally strong. Pharynx without exudates. Uvula rises midline with phonation. Neck ROM intact bilaterally, slight restriction to lateral flexion, especially to right. Thyroid not palpable. No cervical lymph nodes palpable.	Marked receded hairline at temples. Vision 20/30 in right eye, 20/40 in left. Conjunctivae reddened. Ectropion bilaterally. Disc margins dull, drusen patches within macular area and frequent A-V nicking bilaterally. Tympanic membrane with intact cone of light on right, obscured with dry, dark brown cerumen on left. Right ear -AC>BC, left ear AC = BC. Oral mucosa pink, less moist, breath slightly malodorous, no lesions. Dentition—partial dental plates upper and lower, possible caries, gums moist, dark pink, slightly edematous. Tongue deviates to right. Uvula deviates to left. Neck ROM restricted in lateral flexion and rotation, forward flexion and extension intact bilaterally. Palpable tender tonsillar lymph node, 1 cm × 1.5 cm on right.
Thorax and lungs	Chest excursion upward, outward, equal bilaterally. Slight kyphosis. Lungs resonant throughout. Vesicular breath sounds over anterior and posterior lung fields bilaterally.	Chest excursion equally decreased. Lungs resonant and breath sounds vesicular over upper lung fields, dull with late inspiratory coarse crackles in bases bilaterally.

(continued)

■ *Examples of Documentation—The Older Adult (Continued)*

Area of Assessment	Expected Findings	Unexpected Findings
Cardiovascular system	Carotid pulses strong and equal bilaterally, without bruits. Apical impulse in left 5th ICS, MCL, 2 cm in diameter. No splitting of S2, no S3, S4, or murmurs.	Carotid bruit on right, none on left. Apical impulse 3.5 cm in diameter, 6th ICS, left of MCL. S3 and S4 present. Harsh midsystolic murmur in 2nd right interspace, radiates down left sternal border.
Breasts and axillae	Left breast slightly larger than right breast, nipples erect without discharge, areola round, colour pinkish brown, no dimpling or retractions, soft, slightly stringy to palpation, no nodules felt. Minimal greying hair in axillae, no rashes bilaterally.	Small mobile lump, 1.5 cm × 1.5 cm in right axilla, left clear, both without hair.
Abdomen	Flat, without lateral bulges, soft, nontender, without masses. Active bowel sounds all 4 quadrants. Liver span 7 cm in right mid-clavicular line; edges smooth.	Protuberant, lateral bulging, left> right, soft mass 3 cm × 2 cm left lower quadrant. Hyperactive bowel sounds all 4 quadrants. Liver span 11 cm in right mid-clavicular line, edges firm.
Female genitalia and pelvic examination	Pubic hair greying and thinned. Labia and clitoris small without lesions. Introitus tight, vaginal walls pink, moist, slightly rugated. No lesions, or bulges noted. Cervix pink, tight, without lesions. Pap smear taken. Uterus small, ovaries nonpalpable. Anorectal area without lesions, no masses felt with rectal exam. Stool negative for occult blood.	Shiny, red vaginal mucosa Right ovary palpable
Male genitalia and prostate	Sparse gray pubic hair Small noncircumcized penis Prostate walnut-sized, rubbery, with identifiable median sulcus	Enlarged left scrotal sac. Enlarged nontender prostate; median sulcus not defined.
Peripheral vascular system	Aorta, renal, iliac, and femoral arteries without bruits. Brachial and radial pulses 2+ bilaterally. Popliteal, dorsalis pedis, posterior tibial pulses 1+ bilaterally. ROM over arms and legs intact bilaterally.	Bruits over aortic and iliac arteries. Aorta 4 cm in diameter. Brachial and radial pulses 2+, firm to palpation. Popliteal, posterior tibial and dorsalis pedis pulses nonpalpable bilaterally.
Musculoskeletal system	ROM in thoracic and lumbar spine intact, decreases slightly with lateral flexion. Most joints nontender. Mild tenderness at left acromioclavicular joint.	Flexion at knees and hips very limited bilaterally. Knee joints enlarged and tender, hip joints tender bilaterally.
Nervous system	Oriented to person, place, and time. Mini Mental State: score 29. Cranial nerves II–XII intact bilaterally. Decreased muscle mass over all extremities. Tone intact. Strength 4/5 throughout. Rapid alternating movements and point-to-point testing intact over arms and legs bilaterally with eyes open and closed. Gait: slightly	Mini Mental State score = 26, unable to recall three items on 10-minute Geriatric Screener. Muscle mass markedly decreased over legs, used arms of chair to rise. Gait shuffling, leans on cane. Rapid alternating movements slow in hands. Point to point slow but intact with eyes open, inaccurate with eyes closed, upper and lower

(continued)

■ Examples of Documentation—The Older Adult (Continued)

Area of Assessment	Expected Findings	Unexpected Findings
	wide base. Sensations of pain, light touch, and position sense intact throughout. Vibration sense absent in toes, intact at ankle bilaterally. Romberg: slight sway, increased with eyes closed. Reflexes 2+, symmetric over arms, patella, 1+ at ankles. Plantar flexion bilaterally to stimulus.	extremities. Vibration sense absent at toes and ankles. Romberg: slight sway with eyes open, marked sway with eyes closed. Reflexes 1+ over arms and patella, none responsive at ankles.

■ ANALYZING FINDINGS FROM HEALTH HISTORY AND PHYSICAL EXAMINATION

Mr. Irving, a 75-year-old retired accountant, presents with a history of moderate cognitive impairment and current concerns about increasing pain in his right hip. The pain has necessitated use of a cane for walking and two tablets of Tylenol four times a day. He has had the hip pain for at least 5 years. He is accompanied by his eldest daughter, who does his grocery shopping. He lives alone in a seniors' self-contained apartment. His wife died 3 years ago. He employs a cleaning agency for his apartment biweekly. He reports increasing difficulty in preparing his own meals. Driving is becoming increasingly difficult because of hip pain. On examination, he scores 25/30 on the Mini Mental, and 20 on the Mini Nutritional Assessment. His BMI is 20; he reports a gradual weight loss. Any movement at the right hip causes considerable pain (7/10), even with analgesia. The joint is tender to palpation. Both knees show evidence of osteoarthritis. Quadriceps strength is decreased, requiring assistance from arms of chair to sit and rise from chair.

The above information gives rise to the following nursing diagnoses:

- ■ *Mobility impaired, physical, related to inflammatory and joint-degenerative changes in right hip*

- ■ *Ineffective coping with independent community living related to impaired mobility and moderate dementia*

An interdisciplinary team of health care professionals specializing in care of the elderly ensures the assessment and evaluation of all aspects of Mr. Irving's physical and psychosocial health, as well as the development of a plan of action. The client would benefit from consultation with a geriatrician, geriatric nurse practitioner, physical and occupational therapists, orthopedic surgeon, and social worker. Further assessment of his mental status, hip pain, and limited mobility are needed. Given his age, and if other aspects of his physical condition are adequate, he may benefit from a total hip replacement. He should not drive given his deteriorating mental and physical status. He might benefit from relocation to a facility where meal preparation and opportunities for socialization are available.

Critical Thinking Exercise

- Define *primary* and *secondary* aging. (*Knowledge*)
- What is your rationale for applying the Mini Mental State Examination and the Mini Nutritional Assessment? (*Comprehension*)
- What screening tests would you recommend for this 75-year-old male client? (*Application*)

- What factors might contribute to the accuracy of information given by a proxy (Mr. Irving's daughter) providing the history for her father? (*Analysis*)
- What recommendations for immunization would you make to this older client? How often should immunization be reviewed on his behalf? (*Synthesis*)
- How would you evaluate your counselling regarding nutritional intake with Mr. Irving and his daughter? (*Evaluation*)

Canadian Research

Hirdes, J. P. (2006). Predictors of influenza immunization among home care clients in Ontario. *Canadian Journal of Public Health, 97*, 335–339.

King, K. M., LeBlanc, P., Sanguins, J., & Mather, C. (2006). Gender-based challenges faced by older Sikh women as immigrants: Recognizing and acting on the risk of coronary artery disease. *Canadian Journal of Nursing Research, 38*, 16–40.

Low, G., & Molzahn, A. (2007). A replication study of predictors of quality of life in older age. *Research in Nursing & Health, 30*(2), 141–150.

Low, G., & Gutman, G. (2006). Does gender play a role in health-related quality of life? *Journal of Gerontological Nursing, 32*(11), 42–49.

Martel, L., Bélanger, A., Berthelot, J-M., & Carrière, Y. (2005). *Healthy aging: Healthy today, healthy tomorrow? Findings from the National Population Health Survey.* Catalogue No. 82-618. Ottawa: Statistics Canada.

Robinson, J. G., & Molzahn, A. E. (2007). Sexuality and quality of life. *Journal of Gerontological Nursing, 33*(3), 19–29.

Wilson, D. M., & Palha, P. (2007). A systematic review of published research articles on health promotion at retirement. *Journal of Nursing Scholarship, 39*(4), 330–337.

Test Questions

1. During inspection of the abdomen, all of the following signs are expected age-related changes except for the following:
   a. Pink-purple striae
   b. Aortic pulsations in the epigastrium
   c. Weakening of the abdominal muscles
   d. Fat accumulation in the hypogastrium.

2. When auscultating the heart of an older client, the nurse recognizes that the diameter of the anteroposterior diameter of the thorax with age contributes to decreased audibility of the following:
   a. Aortic closure at the base
   b. The first heart sound at the apex
   c. Pulmonic closure during splitting
   d. The first heart sound during expiration

3. When testing cerebellar function of an older client using the Romberg test, which of the following findings is expected?
   a. Slight sway with eyes closed
   b. Moderate sway with eyes open
   c. Inability to sustain balance with eyes open
   d. Inability to sustain balance with eyes closed.

4. The nurse observes the gait and stature of an elderly client entering the room. Which of the following findings is an age-related change?
   a. Gait is wide based
   b. Arms appear long in proportion to the trunk
   c. Shoulder of dominant hand is higher than the shoulder of the nondominant hand
   d. Knees are flexed throughout the stance phase

5. When palpating the prostate gland of a 75-year-old man, which of the following is an expected finding?
   a. Dribbling of urine
   b. Firm, enlarged, warm prostate gland
   c. Firm, smooth, enlarged lateral lobes of the prostate gland
   d. Areas of hardness in the lateral lobes of the prostate gland.

6. When inspecting the toenails of an elderly client, an expected finding is
   a. Painless separated nail plate
   b. Yellowed, thickened lustreless nails
   c. Thinned, slightly curved free nail edge
   d. Whitish nail plate with reddish band near free edge

7. In relation to the peripheral vascular system, all the following are considered to be age-related changes except for the following:
   a. Thickened toe nails bilaterally
   b. Diminished left dorsalis pedis pulse
   c. Thinned hair distribution over lower legs and feet
   d. Loss of subcutaneous tissue in skin over lower legs

8. When inspecting the breast of an elderly female client, which of the following is considered unexpected?
   a. Peau d'orange skin
   b. Slight breast asymmetry
   c. Flaccid, pendulous breasts
   d. Long-standing nipple inversion

9. When inspecting the pharynx of an older client, which of the following is an age-related finding?
   a. Tonsils are not visualized
   b. Uvula deviates to the right
   c. Soft palate moves upward
   d. Small reddish spots on anterior pillars

10. With a client suspected of suffering from presbycusis, the nurse would expect difficulty hearing:
    a. full range of tones.
    b. low-pitched sounds.
    c. high-pitched sounds.
    d. medium-frequency sounds.

Bibliography

CITATIONS

AACE Task Force. (2002/2006). American Association of Clinical Endocrinologists and the American College of Endocrinology: Medical guidelines for clinical practice for the evaluation and treatment of hyperthyroidism and hypothyroidism. *Endocrine Practice, 8*(6), 457–469.

Abrams, P., Cardozo, L., Fall, M., Griffiths, D., Rosier, P., Ulstem, U., et al. (2002). The standardisation of terminology of lower urinary tract function: Report from the standardisation sub-committee of the International Continence Society. *Neurourology and Urodynamics, 21,* 167–178.

Alzheimer Society of Canada. (2007). *What is Alzheimer's disease and related dementias?* Retrieved January 18, 2008, from http://www.alzheimer.ca/

American Geriatric Society, British Geriatric Society and American Academy of Orthopedic Surgeons. (2001). Guideline for prevention of falls in older person. *Journal of the American Geriatrics Society, 49,* 664–672.

Apfeldorf, W. J., & Alexopoulos, G. S. (2003). Late-life mood disorders. In W. R. Hazzard, J. P. Blass, J. B. Halter, J. G. Ouslander, & M. E. Tinetti (Eds.), *Principles of geriatric medicine & gerontology* (5th ed., pp. 1443–1458). New York: McGraw-Hill.

Baloh, R. W., Ying, S. H., & Jacobson, K. M. (2003). A longitudinal study of gait and balance dysfunction in normal older people. *Archives of Neurology, 60,* 835–839.

Berg, K. O., Wood-Dauphinee, S. L., Williams, J. I., & Maki, B. (1992). Measuring balance in the elderly: Validation of an instrument. *Canadian Journal of Public Health, 83*(Suppl. 2), S7–S11.

Bobrie, G., Genes, N., Vaur, L., Clerson, P., Vaisse, B., Mallion, J. M., et al. (2001). Is "isolated home" hypertension as opposed to "isolated office" hypertension a sign of greater cardiovascular risk? *Archives of Internal Medicine, 161*(18), 2205–2211.

Bogardus, S. T., Yeuh, B., & Shekelle, P. G. (2003). Screening and management of hearing loss in primary care: Clinical applications. *Journal of the American Medical Association, 289,* 1986–1990.

Bradshaw, J., & Klein, W. C. (2007). Health promotion. In J. A. Blackburn & C. N. Dulmus (Eds.), *Handbook of gerontology.* *Evidence-based approaches to theory, practice, and policy* (pp. 171–200). Hoboken, NJ: John Wiley & Sons.

Butler, R. N., & Lewis, M. I. (2003). Sexuality and aging. In W. R. Hazzard, J. P. Blass, J. B. Halter, J. G. Ouslander, & M. E. Tinetti (Eds.), *Principles of geriatric medicine & gerontology* (5th ed., pp. 1277–1282). New York: McGraw-Hill.

Calgary Health Region. (2004). *Sexual and reproductive health.* Retrieved January 11, 2008, from http://www.calgaryhealthregion.ca/hecomm/sexual/sexandsexualityasyouage.htm

Callahan, D. (2003). The value of achieving a peaceful death. In C. K. Cassel, R. M. Leipzig, H. J. Cohen, et al. (Eds.), *Geriatric medicine* (4th ed., pp. 351–360). New York: Springer.

Canadian Cancer Society/National Cancer Institute of Canada. (2007). *Canadian cancer statistics 2007.* Toronto, ON: Author.

Canadian Cancer Society/National Cancer Institute of Canada. (2008). *Canadian cancer statistics 2008.* Toronto, ON: Author.

Canadian Coalition for Seniors' Mental Health. (2006). *National guidelines for seniors' mental health: The assessment and treatment of delirium.* Toronto, ON: Author.

Capital Health. (2004). Sexuality and the older adult. Retrieved January 11, 2008, from http://www.capitalhealth.ca/YourHealth/BrowsebyAlpha/content.asp?L=&NavType=Alpha&guid=D2197006-1F9E-48FE-94E

Canadian Institute for Health Information. (2007). *Study shows decrease in seniors taking potentially harmful drugs between 2000 and 2006.* Retrieved January 17, 2008, from http://www.icis.ca/cihiweb/dispPage.jsp?cw_page=media_13sep2007_e

Chaudhry, S. I., Krumholz, H. M., & Foody, J. M. (2004). Systolic hypertension in older persons. *Journal of the American Medical Association, 292*(9), 1074–1080.

Congdon, N. G., Friedman, D. S., & Lietman, T. (2003). Important causes of visual impairment in the world today. *Journal of the American Medical Association, 290*(15), 2057–2060.

Consensus Committee of the American Autonomic Society and the American Academy of Neurology. (1996). Consensus statement on the definition of orthostatic hypotension, pure autonomic failure, and multiple system atrophy. *Neurology, 46,* 1470.

Craft, S., Cholerton, B., & Reger, M. (2003). Aging and cognition: What is normal? In W. R. Hazzard, J. P. Blass, J. B. Halter, J. G. Ouslander, & M. E. Tinetti (Eds.), *Principles of geriatric medicine & gerontology* (5th ed., pp. 1355–1372). New York: McGraw-Hill.

Department of Justice. (2007). *Abuse of older adults: A fact sheet from the Department of Justice Canada.* Ottawa, ON: Department of Justice.

Dewey, M. E., & Parker, C. J. (2000). Survey into the health problems of elderly people: A comparison of self-report with proxy information. *International Journal of Epidemiology, 29,* 684–698.

DuBeau, C. E. (2003). Benign prostatic hyperplasia. In C. K. Cassel, R. M. Leipzig, H. J. Cohen, et al. (Eds.), *Geriatric medicine* (4th ed., pp. 755–768). New York: Springer.

Duthie, E. H. (2007). History and physical examination. In E. H. Duthie, P. R. Katz, & M. L. Malone (Eds.), *Practice of geriatrics* (4th ed., pp. 3–15). Philadelphia: Saunders Elsevier.

Empana, J. P., Dargent-Molina, P., & Breart, G. (2004). Effect of hip fracture on mortality in elderly women: The EPIDOS prospective study. *Journal of the American Geriatrics Society, 52,* 685–690.

Enright, P. L. (2003). Aging of the respiratory system. In W. R. Hazzard, J. P. Blass, J. B. Halter, J. G. Ouslander, & M. E. Tinetti (Eds.), *Principles of geriatric medicine & gerontology* (5th ed., pp. 511–515). New York: McGraw-Hill.

Ferrell, B. A. (2003). Acute and chronic pain. In C. K. Cassel, R. M. Leipzig, H. J. Cohen, et al. (Eds.), *Geriatric medicine* (4th ed., pp. 323–342). New York: Springer.

Ferrell, B. A., & Chodosh, J. (2003). Pain management. In W. R. Hazzard, J. P. Blass, J. B. Halter, J. G. Ouslander, & M. E. Tinetti (Eds.), *Principles of geriatric medicine & gerontology* (5th ed., pp. 303–321). New York: McGraw-Hill.

Fetzer, S. J., & McQueen, M. (2006). Vital signs. In P. A. Potter, A. G. Perry, J. C. Ross-Kerr, & M. J. Wood (Eds.), *Canadian fundamentals of nursing* (3rd ed., pp. 561–615). Toronto, ON: Elsevier Canada.

Fick, D. M., Cooper, J. W., Wade, W. E., Waller, J. L., Maclean, J. R., Beers, M. H., et al. (2003). Updating the Beers criteria for potentially inappropriate medication use in older adults: Results of a US consensus panel of experts. *Archives of Internal Medicine, 163,* 2716–2724.

Fulmer, T., Guadagno, L., Bitondo Dyer, C., & Connolly, M. T. (2004). Progress in elder abuse screening and assessment instruments. *Journal of the American Geriatrics Society, 52,* 297–304.

Gilchrest, B. A. (2007). Skin disorders. In E. H. Duthie, P. R. Katz, & M. L. Malone (Eds.), *Practice of geriatrics* (4th ed., pp. 531–546). Philadelphia: Saunders Elsevier.

Gilmour, H., & Park, J. (2006). Dependency, chronic conditions and pain in seniors. *Health Reports Supplement, 16,* 21–31.

Gnann, J. W., & Whitely, R. J. (2002). Herpes zoster. *New England Journal of Medicine, 347*(5), 340–346.

Golonka, R., Belton, K., Strain, L., Hunter, K. & Voaklander, D. (2007). *Agricultural fatalities in Canada 1990–2000: Focus on older farmers and workers.* Ottawa, ON: Canadian Agricultural Safety Association.

Gonzales, E. B., & Goodwin, J. S. (2007). Musculoskeletal disorders. In E. H. Duthie, P. R. Katz, & M. L. Malone (Eds.), *Practice of geriatrics* (4th ed., pp. 495–509). Philadelphia: Saunders Elsevier.

Harris, T. B. (2003). Weight and age: Paradoxes and conundrums. In W. R. Hazzard, J. P. Blass, J. B. Halter, J. G. Ouslander, & M. E. Tinetti (Eds.), *Principles of geriatric medicine & gerontology* (5th ed., pp. 1171–1177). New York: McGraw-Hill.

Hassani, S., & Hershman, J. M. (2003). Thyroid diseases. In W. R. Hazzard, J. P. Blass, J. B. Halter, J. G. Ouslander, & M. E. Tinetti (Eds.), *Principles of geriatric medicine & gerontology* (5th ed., pp. 837–853). New York: McGraw-Hill.

Healthy Aging and Wellness Working Group of the Federal/Provincial/Territorial Committee of Officials (Seniors). (2006). *Healthy aging in Canada: A new vision, a vital investment from evidence to action.* Ottawa, ON: Public Health Agency of Canada.

Health Canada. (2007). *Best practices: Treatment and rehabilitation for seniors with substance use problems.* Retrieved January 11, 2008, from http://www.hc-sc.gc.ca/hl-vs/pubs/apd/treat_senior-trait_ainee/review-3-recension_e.html#1

Health Canada. (2004). *Dietary reference intakes.* Retrieved January 11, 2008, from http://www.hc-sc.gc.ca/fn-an/nutrition/reference/index_e.html

Heart and Stroke Foundation of Canada. (2008). *Stroke warning signs.* Retrieved January 11, 2008, from http://www.heartandstroke.com/site/c.ikIQLcMWJtE/b.3483937/k.8989/Warning_Signs.htm

Htwe, T. H., Mushtaq, A., Tobinson, S. B., Rosher, R. B., & Khardori, N. (2007). Infection in the elderly. *Infectious Diseases Clinics of North America, 21,* 711–743.

Inouye, S. K., van Dyck, C., Alessi, C., Balkin, S., Seigal, A., & Horowitz, R. (1990). Clarifying confusion: The confusion assessment method. *Annals of Internal Medicine, 113,* 941–948.

Inouye, S. K., Studenski, S., Tinetti, M. E., & Kuchel, G. A. (2007). Geriatric syndromes: Clinical, research, and policy implications of a core geriatric concept. *Journal of the American Geriatrics Society, 55,* 780–791.

Jones, T. V., Lindsey, B. A., Yount, P., Soltys, R., Farani-Enayat, B. (1993). Alcoholism screening questionnaires: Are they valid in elderly medical outpatients? *Journal of General Internal Medicine, 8*(12), 674–678.

Kaiser, F. E. (2003). Sexual function and the older woman. In C. K. Cassel, R. M. Leipzig, H. J. Cohen, et al. (Eds.), *Geriatric medicine* (4th ed., pp. 727–736). New York: Springer.

Kenney, R. A. (1987). *Physiology of aging* (2nd ed.). Chicago: Year Book Medical Publishers.

Kimmick, G. G., & Muss, H. B. (2003). Breast disease. In W. R. Hazzard, J. P. Blass, J. B. Halter, J. G. Ouslander, & M. E. Tinetti (Eds.), *Principles of geriatric medicine & gerontology* (5th ed., pp. 685–694). New York: McGraw-Hill.

Koretz, B., & Reuben, D. B. (2003). Instruments to assess functional status. In C. K. Cassel, R. M. Leipzig, H. J. Cohen, et al. (Eds.), *Geriatric Medicine* (4th ed., pp. 195–204). New York: Springer.

Larson, E. B., Wang, L., Bowen, J. D., McCormick, W. C., Teri, L., Crane, P., et al. (2006). Exercise is associated with reduced risk for incident dementia among persons 65 years of age and older. *Annals of Internal Medicine, 144*(2), 73–81.

Leibson, C. L., Tosteson, A. N., Gabriel, S. L., Ransom, J. E., & Melton, L. J. (2002). Mortality, disability, and nursing home use for persons with and without hip fracture: A population-based study. *Journal of the American Geriatrics Society, 50,* 1644–1650.

Lindsay, J., Sykes, E., McDowell, I., Verreault, R., & Laurin, D. (2004). More than the epidemiology of Alzheimer's disease: Contributions of the Canadian Study of Health and Aging. *Canadian Journal of Psychiatry—Revue Canadienne de Psychiatrie, 49,* 83–91.

Lockett, D., Bonnefant, D., Asselin, G., Kuhn, M., & Edwards, N. (2004). *Active independent aging: A community guide for falls prevention and active living.* Ottawa, ON: University of Ottawa and City of Ottawa, Public Health and Long-Term Care Branch.

Lorser, T. F., & Delbono, O. (2003). Aging of the muscles and joints. In W. R. Hazzard, J. P. Blass, J. B. Halter, J. G. Ouslander, & M. E. Tinetti (Eds.), *Principles of geriatric medicine & gerontology* (5th ed., pp. 903–918). New York: McGraw-Hill.

Marshall, F. J. (2007). Movement disorders. In E. H. Duthie, P. R. Katz, & M. L. Malone (Eds.), *Practice of geriatrics* (4th ed., pp. 381–395). Philadelphia: Saunders Elsevier.

Martel, L., Bélanger, A., Berthelot, J-M., & Carrière, Y. (2005). *Healthy aging: Healthy today, healthy tomorrow? Findings from the National Population Health Survey.* Catalogue No. 82-618. Ottawa, ON: Statistics Canada.

Masoro, E. J. (2006). Are age-associated diseases an integral part of aging? In E. J. Masoro & S. N. Austad (Eds.), *Handbook of the biology of aging* (6th ed., pp. 43–62). Boston: Elsevier.

McClane, K. S. (2006). Screening instruments for use in a complete geriatric assessment. *Clinical Nurse Specialist, 20,* 201–207.

McDermott, M. M., Greenland, P., Liu, K., Guralnik, J. M., Celic, L., Criqui, M. H., et al. (2002). The ankle brachial index is associated with leg function and physical activity: The walking and leg circulation study. *Annals of Internal Medicine, 136*(12), 873–883.

Medwetsky, L. (2007). Hearing loss. In E. H. Duthie, P. R. Katz, & M. L. Malone (Eds.), *Practice of geriatrics* (4th ed., pp. 285–300). Philadelphia: Saunders Elsevier.

Millar, W. J. (2004). Vision problems among seniors. *Health Reports, 16*(1), 1–5. Statistics Canada Catalogue 82-003. Retrieved May 30, 2008, from www.statcan.ca/english/studies/82-003/archieve/2004/16-1-d.pdf

Miller, C. A. (2009). *Nursing for wellness in older adults. Theory and practice* (5th ed.). Philadelphia: Lippincott.

Mirie, W. (2001). Aging and nutritional needs. In R. R. Watson, *Handbook of nutrition in the aged* (3rd ed., pp. 43–48). Boca Raton, FL: CRC Press.

Morrison, R. S., & Meier, D. E. (2004). Palliative care. *New England Journal of Medicine, 350,* 2582–2590.

Mulligan, T., & Saddiqi, W. (2003). Changes in male sexuality. In C. K. Cassel, R. M. Leipzig, H. J. Cohen, et al. (Eds.), *Geriatric medicine* (4th ed., pp. 719–726). New York: Springer.

Nasreddine, Z. S., Phillips, N. A., Bedirian, V., Charbonneau, S., Whitehead, V., Collin, I., et al. (2005). The Montreal cognitive assessment, MoCA: A brief screening tool for mild cognitive impairment. *Journal of the American Geriatrics Society, 53,* 695–699.

National Advisory Committee on Immunization. (2006). *Canadian immunization guide* (7th ed.). Ottawa, ON: Public Health Agency of Canada Infectious Disease and Emergency Preparedness Branch, Minister of Public Works and Government Services Canada.

National Institute for Clinical Excellence. (2004). *Clinical guideline 21: The assessment and prevention of falls in older people.* Retrieved June 1, 2008, from http://www.nice.org.uk/nicemedia/pdf/CG021fullguideline.pdf

Nowak, L., & Davis, J. (2007). A qualitative examination of the phenomenon of sundowning. *Journal of Nursing Scholarship, 39*(3), 256–258.

Nunez, G. R. (2003). Culture, demographics, and critical care issues: An overview. *Critical Care Clinics, 19,* 619–639.

O'Brien Cousins, S., & Horne, T. (Eds.). (1991). *Active living among older adults: Health benefits and outcomes.* Ann Arbor, MI: Edward Brothers.

Pakkar, A., & Cummings, J. (2003). Mental status and neurologic examination in the elderly. In W. R. Hazzard, J. P. Blass, J. B. Halter, J. G. Ouslander, M. E. Tinetti (Eds.), *Principles of geriatric medicine & gerontology* (5th ed., pp. 111–119). New York: McGraw-Hill.

Papademetriou, V. (2003). Comparative prognostic value of systolic, diastolic, and pulse pressure. *American Journal of Cardiology, 91*(4), 433–435.

Perls, T. T. (2003). Understanding the determinants of exceptional longevity. *Annals of Internal Medicine, 139*(5 Suppl.), 445.

Perls, T. T., Kunkel, L. M., & Puca, A. A. (2002). The genetics of exceptional human longevity. *Journal of the American Geriatric Society, 50,* 359–368.

Pfizer (2002). *First global sexual health survey finds older adults aged 40-80 enjoy sex regularly.* Retrieved January 11, 2008, from http://www.Pfizer.ca/English/newsroom/press%20releases/default.asp?s=1&year=2002releaseID=70

Podsiadlo, D., & Richardson, S. (1991). The timed "Up & Go": A test of basic functional mobility for frail elderly persons. *Journal of the American Geriatrics Society, 39,* 142–148.

Public Health Agency of Canada. (2006). *Hearing loss info-sheet for seniors.* Retrieved May 27, 2008 from http://www.phac-aspc.gc.ca/seniors-aims/pubs/info_sheets/hearing_loss/pdf/hearing_e.pdf

Public Health Agency of Canada. (2005a). *The safe living guide: A guide to home safety for seniors.* Ottawa, ON: Minister of Public Works and Government Services Canada.

Public Health Agency of Canada. (2005b). *Report on seniors' falls in Canada.* Ottawa, ON: Minister of Public Works and Government Services Canada.

Registered Nurses Association of Ontario. (2007). *Falls prevention: Building the foundations for patient safety: A self learning package.* Toronto, ON: Author.

Registered Nurses Association of Ontario. (2005). *Prevention of falls and fall injuries in the older adult* (Revised). Toronto, ON: Author.

Reuben, D. B., Herr, K. A., Pacala, J. T., et al. (2004). *Geriatrics at your fingertips: 2008–2009,* 10th edition. NY: The American Geriatrics Society.

Reuben, D. B. (2003). Comprehensive geriatric assessment and system approaches to geriatric care. In C. K. Cassel, R. M. Leipzig, H. J. Cohen, et al. (Eds.), *Geriatric medicine* (4th ed., pp. 195–204). New York: Springer.

Robbins, J. A., Biggs, M. L., & Cauley, J. (2006). Adjusted mortality after hip fracture: From the cardiovascular health study. *Journal of the American Geriatrics Society, 54,* 1885–1891.

Robinson, J. G., & Molzahn, A. E. (2007). Sexuality and quality of life. Journal of Gerontological Nursing, 33(3), 19–29.

Rotermann, M. (2006). Seniors' healthcare use. Health Reports Supplement, 16, 33–45. Statistics Canada, Catalogue 82-003-XPE. http://www.statcan.ca/english/freepub/82-003-SIE/2004000/pdf/82-003-SIE2005000.pdf

Rowe, J. W., & Kahn, R. L. (1997). Successful aging. *The Gerontologist, 37,* 433–440.

Samoy, L. J., Zed, P. J., Wilbur, K., Balen, R. M., Abu-Laban, R. B., & Roberts, M. (2006). Drug-related hospitalizations in a tertiary care internal medicine service of a Canadian hospital: A prospective study. *Pharmacotherapy, 26,* 1578–1586.

Shay, K. (2007). Dental and oral disorders. In E. H. Duthie, P. R. Katz, & M. L. Malone (Eds.), *Practice of geriatrics* (4th ed., pp. 547–561). Philadelphia: Saunders Elsevier.

Shields, M., & Martin, L. (2006). Healthy living among seniors. Health at older ages. *Health Reports, 16*(Suppl.). Ottawa, ON: Statistics Canada.

Sinanan, M., Kao, L., & Vedovatti, P. A. (2003). Surgery in the elderly population. In W. R. Hazzard, J. P. Blass, J. B. Halter, J. G. Ouslander, & E. Tinetti (Eds.), *Principles of geriatric medicine & gerontology* (5th ed., pp. 385–399). New York: McGraw-Hill.

Statistics Canada. (2007a). *Leisure-time physical activity, by age group.* Retrieved March 26, 2009, from http://www41. statcan.ca.2007/2966/grafx/htm/ceb2966_000_2_eng.htm

Statistics Canada. (2007b). *Smokers, by province and territory.* Retrieved January 11, 2008, from http://www40.statcan.ca/101/cst01/health07a.htm

Stuck, A. E., Beck, J. C., & Egger, M. (2004). Preventing disability in elderly people. *Lancet, 364*(9446), 1641–1643.

Taffet, G. E. (2003). Physiology of aging. In C. K. Cassel, R. M. Leipzig, H. J. Cohen, et al. (Eds.), *Geriatric medicine* (4th ed., pp. 27–36). New York: Springer.

Taffet, G. E., & Lakatta, E. G. (2003). Aging of the cardiovascular system. In W. R. Hazzard, J. P. Blass, J. B. Halter, J. G. Ouslander, & M. E. Tinetti (Eds.), *Principles of geriatric medicine & gerontology* (5th ed., pp. 403–421). New York: McGraw-Hill.

Takahashi, P. Y., Okhravi, H. R., Lim, L. S., Kasten, M. J. (2004). Preventive health care in the elderly population: A guide for practicing physicians. *Mayo Clinic Proceedings, 79*, 416–427.

Tangarorang, G. L., Kerins, G. J., & Besdine, R. W. (2003). Clinical approach to the older patient: An overview. In C. K. Cassel, R. M. Leipzig, H. J. Cohen, et al. (Eds.), *Geriatric medicine* (4th ed., pp. 149–162). New York: Springer.

Tinetti, M. E. (1986). Performance-oriented assessment of mobility problems in elderly patients. *Journal of the American Geriatrics Society, 34*, 119–126.

Tjepkema, M. (2005). *Adult obesity in Canada: Measured weight and height.* Statistics Canada, Cat. No. 82-620-MWE. Retrieved May 27, 2008, from http://www.statcan.ca/english/research/82-620-MIE/2005001/pdf/aobesity.pdf

Tulsky, J. A. (2003). Doctor-patient communication issues. In C. K. Cassel, R. M. Leipzig, H. J. Cohen, et al. (Eds.), *Geriatric medicine* (4th ed., pp. 287–298). New York: Springer.

Turcotte, M., & Schellenberg, G. (2006). *A portrait of seniors in Canada 2006.* Ottawa, ON: Statistics Canada.

Vaccarino, V., Berger, A. K., Abramson, J., Black, H. R., Setaro, J. F., Davey, J. A., et al. (2001). Pulse pressure and risk of cardiovascular events in the systolic hypertension in the elderly program. *American Journal of Cardiology, 88*(9), 980–986.

Watson, G. R. (2003). Assessment and rehabilitation of older adults with low vision. In W. R. Hazzard, J. P. Blass, J. B. Halter, J. G. Ouslander, & M. E. Tinetti (Eds.), *Principles of geriatric medicine & gerontology* (5th ed., pp. 1223–1237). New York: McGraw-Hill.

Wilcox, S., & King, A. C. (2003). Health behaviours & adherence. In W. R. Hazzard, J. P. Blass, J. B. Halter, J. G. Ouslander, & M. E. Tinetti (Eds.), *Principles of geriatric medicine & gerontology* (5th ed., pp. 1223–1237). New York: McGraw-Hill.

Xakellis, G., Brangman, S. A., Hinton, W. L., Jones, V. Y., Masterman, D., Pan, C. X., et al. (2004). Curricular framework: Core competencies in multicultural geriatric care. *Journal of the American Geriatric Society, 52*, 137–142.

ADDITIONAL RESOURCES

Amin, S. H., Kuhle, C. L., & Fitzpatrick, L. A. (2003). Comprehensive evaluation of the older woman. *Mayo Clinic Proceedings, 78*(9), 1157–1185.

Cassel, C. K. (2003). *Geriatric medicine: An evidence-based approach* (4th ed.). New York: Springer.

Duthie, E. H., Katz, P. R., & Malone, M. L. (Eds.). (2007). *Practice of geriatrics* (4th ed.). Philadelphia: Saunders Elsevier.

Hazzard, W. R., Blass, J. P., Halter, J. B., Ouslander, J. G., & Tinetti, M. E. (Eds.). (2003). *Principles of geriatric medicine and gerontology* (5th ed.). New York: McGraw-Hill.

Kane, R. L., Ouslander, J. G., & Abrass, I. B. (2004). *Essentials of clinical geriatrics* (5th ed.). New York: McGraw-Hill.

Kennedy-Malone, L., Fletcher, K. R., & Plank, L. R. (2004). *Management guidelines for gerontological nurse practitioners* (2nd ed.). Philadelphia: F. A. Davis.

Public Health Agency of Canada. (1999). *No. 36 – Seniors taking medication.* Retrieved January 14, 2008, from http://www.phac-aspc.gc.ca/seniors-aines/pubs/factoids/2001/no36_e.htm

Public Health Agency of Canada. (1996). *Working together on seniors' medication use: A federal/provincial/territorial strategy for action.* Retrieved January 11, 2008, from http://www.hc-sc.ca/seniors-aines/pubs/working_together/index_e.htm

Tullman, D. F., Haugh, K. H., Dracup, K. A., & Bourguignon, C. (2007). A randomized controlled trial to reduce delay in older adults seeking help for symptoms of acute myocardial infarction. *Research in Nursing and Health, 30*(5), 485–497.

CANADIAN ASSOCIATIONS AND WEB SITES

Alzheimer Society of Canada: http://www.alzheimer.ca/

Canadian Association on Gerontology: http://www.cagacg.ca/

Canadian Coalition for Seniors' Mental Health: http://www.ccsmh.ca/en/natlGuidelines/natlGuidelinesInit.cfm

Canadian Gerontological Nursing Association: http://www.cgna.net/

Canadian Health Network: http://www.canadian-health-network.ca

The Canadian Continence Foundation: http://www.continence-fdn.ca/

TABLE 25-1   Delirium, Depression, and Dementia

	Delirium	Dementia	Depression
Clinical Features			
Onset	Acute	Insidious	Gradual with symptoms that persist for at least 2 weeks
Course	Fluctuating, with lucid intervals; worse at night	Slowly progressive	Relapse (symptoms return within 6 months of remission), Recurrence (symptoms return after more than 6 months of remission)
Duration	Hours to weeks	Months to years	Months, if responsive to medication. Chronic, if comorbidities and personal losses preclude favourable response to medication.
Sleep/Wake Cycle	Always disrupted	Sleep fragmented	Insomnia or hypersomnia, frequent awakening
General Medical Illness or Drug Toxicity	Either or both present	Often absent, especially in Alzheimer's disease	Often occurs in conjunction with bereavement and medical illnesses (e.g., major surgery, central nervous system disorders, nutritional deficiencies, cardiovascular disturbances, metabolic and endocrine disorders)
Mental Status			
Level of Consciousness	Disturbed. Person less clearly aware of the environment and less able to focus, sustain, or shift attention	Usually autoresponsive until late in the course of the illness	Usually responsive to surroundings
Behaviour	Activity often abnormally decreased (somnolence) or increased (agitation, hypervigilance)	Normal to slow; may become inappropriate	Socially appropriate, may avoid social interaction, may be somnolent or agitated
Speech	May be hesitant, slow or rapid, incoherent	Difficulty in finding words, aphasia	May be slowed, in a monotone
Mood	Fluctuating, labile, from fearful or irritable to normal or depressed	Often flat, depressed	Sad, downcast, frequent tearfulness, loss of pleasure in life
Thought Processes	Disorganized, may be incoherent	Impoverished. Speech gives little information.	Slowed, difficulty in making decisions
Thought Content	Delusions common, often transient	Delusions may occur.	Feelings of hopelessness, worthlessness, thoughts of death or suicide
Perceptions	Illusions, hallucinations, most often visual	Hallucinations may occur.	Delusions of guilt, persecution
Judgement	Impaired, often to a varying degree	Increasingly impaired over the course of the illness	Difficulty in planning ahead, initiating new projects
Orientation	Usually disoriented, especially for time. A known place may seem unfamiliar.	Fairly well maintained, but becomes impaired in the later stages of illness	Well maintained

(table continues on next page)

	Delirium	**Dementia**	**Depression**
Attention	Fluctuates. Person easily distracted, unable to concentrate on selected tasks.	Usually unaffected until late in the illness	Problems concentrating
Memory	Immediate and recent memory impaired	Recent memory and new learning especially impaired	May have problems concentrating sufficiently to remember
Examples of Cause	Delirium tremens (due to withdrawal from alcohol) Uremia Acute hepatic failure Acute cerebral vasculitis Atropine poisoning	*Reversible:* Vitamin B_{12} deficiency, thyroid disorders *Irreversible:* Alzheimer's disease, vascular dementia (from multiple infarcts), dementia due to head trauma	Etiology not fully understood. Risk factors for late-onset depression include grief, persistent insomnia, and many chronic medical conditions, including pain, central nervous system disorders (stroke, dementia, Parkinson's disease), metabolic and endocrine disorders (hypothyroidism, diabetes), arthritis, and cancers.

Index

right ventricle of, 424, 425
during pregnancy, 874
surface projections of, 424–425
valves of, 425–426
Heartburn, 388, 512
during pregnancy, 859b
Heart failure
left-sided
cough and hemoptysis in, 416t
dyspnea in, 412t–413t
physical findings in, 420t
left ventricular, 436–437
Heart murmurs, 429–430
attributes of, 457–459, 459b
diastolic, 457, 475t
in older adults, 893, 919
pansystolic (holosystolic), 474t
systolic, 457–458
Heart rate, 141, 432, 445, 467t
fetal, auscultation of, 879
measurement of, 445
in older adults, 889
Heart rhythms, 141, 467t
irregular, 468t
in older adults, 889
Heart sounds, 429, 454
auscultation of, 456, 456b–457b
diastolic, in systole, 473t
extra, in systole, 472t
in older adults, 893
splitting of, 429, 471t
variations in, 470t–471t
Heart valves, 425–426. *See also specific valves*
auscultation of sounds from, 430, 454
semilunar, 426
stenotic, 473t
Heaviness, 764
Heberden's nodes, 632, 634, 677t
Hegar's sign, 857, 858
Height, 174
in general survey, 131
measurement of
in older adults, 916
during pregnancy, 873
Height and weight, in older adults, 889
Heliotrope, 260t
Helix, 341, 342
Hematemesis, 513
Hematochezia, 831
Hematuria, 519
Hemianopsia, 306
Hemiparesis, 711
spastic, 754t
Hemiplegia, 711, 734
in comatose patients, 758t
Hemoccult blood tests, for colorectal cancer, 835
Hemochromatosis, skin in, 273t
Hemolytic anemia, 517
Hemoptysis, 389, 416t
Hemorrhage, subconjunctival, 329t
Hemorrhagic telangiectasia, hereditary, 373t
Hemorrhoids, 517, 843b
during pregnancy, 880
Hepatitis, 531
fulminant, 531
infectious, prevention of, 522–523

Hepatitis A, 522
Hepatitis B, 522, 864b
Hepatitis C, 522–523
Hepatocellular jaundice, 518
Hepatomegaly, 561t
Hereditary hemorrhagic telangiectasia, 373t
Hernias
epigastric, 556t
examination techniques for, 772–773
inspection as, 772
palpation as, 772–773
in females, 814
femoral, female, 814
incisional, 556t
inguinal, 648
female, 814
in males, 772–773
course and presentation of, 782t
differentiation of, 783t
femoral, 783t
incarcerated, 773
inguinal, 783t
inspection or, 772
palpation of, 772–773
scrotal, evaluating, 773
strangulated, 773
scrotal, 778t
umbilical, 556t
ventral, assessment techniques for, 541
Herniated intervertebral discs, 642
Herpes simplex infections
genital, 810
female, 821t
in males, 777t
of lips, 372t
of skin, 262t, 264t
Herpes zoster infections
in older adults, 917
of skin, 254, 274t
Hidradenitis suppurativa, 498
Higher cognitive functions, in mental status examination, 218b, 230–231
Hinge joints, 603b, 604
Hip(s), 645–650
abduction at, testing, 715
adduction at, testing, 715
bony structures and joints of, 645
examination techniques for, 646–650
inspection as, 646–647
palpation as, 647–648
range of motion and manoeuvers as, 648–650
extension at, testing, 715
flexion at, testing, 714
flexion deformity of, 649
fracture of, 647
muscle groups of, 646
Hip fracture, due to fall
in older adults, 909
Hirsutism, 287
during pregnancy, 856
History. *See* Health history
HIV, 800–802
prevention of, 767–768
risk factors of, 800
Hives, 264t

Hoarseness, 351
Holosystolic murmurs, 457, 474t
Horizontal inguinal lymph nodes, 567
Horizontal nystagmus, 746
Hormonal changes, during pregnancy, 852–853
Hormone replacement therapy, 444
Horner's syndrome, 314, 331t
Hot tub folliculitis, 271t
Household/environmental safety, of older adults, 909
Housemaid's knee, 653, 655
Houston, valves of, 830
HPV (human papillomavirus), 832
cervical cancer and, 795–796, 797
prevention of, 802
HPV DNA testing, 797
Human immunodeficiency virus (HIV), 864b
Human papillomavirus (HPV), 832
cervical cancer and, 795–796, 797
prevention of, 802
Humeroulnar joint, 628
Humerus, greater tubercle of, 621
Huntington's disease, 745t
Hutchinson's teeth, 378t
Hydroceles, 772, 773, 778t
Hydrocephalus, 287
Hydrostatic pressure, 568
Hymen, 785, 786
imperforate, 809
Hyoid bone, 281
Hypaesthesia, 722
Hypalgesia, 722
Hyperalgesia, 722
Hypercortisolism, relative, during pregnancy, 853
Hyperemesis, during pregnancy, 873
Hyperesthesia, 722
cutaneous, 539
Hyperkinetic ventricular impulse, 469t
Hyperopia, 306
Hyperplasia, 830
Hyperpyrexia, 141
Hyperresonance, as percussion note, 399b, 404
Hypertension
control of, 699
in older adults, 889
prevention of, 438b, 439–440
pulmonary, 453, 454
systemic, 454
with unequal blood pressure in arms and legs, 140
"White Coat," 140
Hypertensive retinopathy, 337t
Hyperthyroidism, 283, 285, 286, 315–316
apical impulse in, 452
signs and symptoms of, 298t
skin in, 253, 273t
Hypertrophic cardiomyopathy, 477t
Hypertrophic osteoarthropathy, 607
Hypertrophy, 709
Hyperventilation, 120t, 388
anxiety with, dyspnea in, 412t–413t
hypercapnia due to, 741t
Hypervolemia, jugular venous pressure and, 446

Swelling. *See also* Edema
  musculoskeletal, 618
Swinging flashlight test, 321
Swing phase of gait cycle, 647
Sydenham's chorea, 745t
Symphyseal-fundal height (SFH), during
    pregnancy, 878
Symphysis pubis, 645
Symptoms
  eliciting from older adults, 899–902, 900b
  principal, ten key attributes of, 7, 57–59,
    58b–59b
Syncope, 697
  micturition, 741t
  during pregnancy, 854
Synovial cavity, 603
Synovial fluid, 603
Synovial joints, 602b, 603
  structure of, 603–604, 603b
Synovial membrane, 603
  of shoulder, examination techniques for,
    627b
Syphilis, 864b
  congenital, facies in, 803t
  mucous patch of, 380t
  secondary, female, 821t
  skin in, 274t
Syphilitic chancre, 267t, 373t
  female, 821t
  in males, 777t
Systemic lupus erythematosus (SLE), 606
  skin in, 274t
Systole, 427, 426
Systolic aortic murmur, in older adults, 893
Systolic blood pressure, 428
Systolic clicks, 472t
Systolic hypertension, in older adults, 889
Systolic murmurs, 457–458
  aids to identify, 460, 460b
  during pregnancy, 853–854
Systolic pressure, 445

T

Talkative clients, interviewing, 68
Talocalcaneal joint, 659, 661
Talofibular ligament
  anterior, 659
  posterior, 659
Talus, 659
Tandem walking, 719
Tanner stages, 787–788
Tardive dyskinesia, 744t
Tarsal joint, transverse, 661
Tarsal plates, 299, 300
Taste and smell senses, in older adults, 892
Teeth
  abrasion of, with notching, 378t
  anatomy and physiology of, 347
  attrition of, 378t
  caries of
    in older adults, 918
  erosion of, 378t
    in children, 806t
  examination techniques for, 361
  findings in, 377t–378t
  health promotion and, 354–355
  Hutchinson's, 378t

Telangiectasia, 271t
  hemorrhagic, hereditary, 373t
Temperature, body
  of feet and legs, 585
  measurement of, 141–142
  in older adults, 889
Temperature intolerance, with goiter, 283
Temperature sensation, 693
  assessment of, 706, 722
Temporal arteritis, headache and, 296t–297t
Temporal artery, superficial, 279, 280
Temporal bone, 279, 299
  mastoid portion of, 279
Temporal muscles, 619, 620
  palpation of, 706
Temporomandibular joint, 618–620
Tenderness
  abdominal, 559t–560t
  in chest, 396
  of kidneys, 536
  musculoskeletal, 618
  of nonpalpable liver, 540
  rebound, 539
  spine and, 640
Tendonitis, 605
  bicipital, 675t
  calcific, of shoulder, 674t
  rotator cuff, 674t
Tenesmus, 517
Tenosynovitis, 606, 634, 635
  acute, 679t
  de Quervain's, 633, 634, 635
  gonococcal, 633
Tension headache, 282, 294t
Teres minor muscle, 622, 628
Terminal hair, 246
Terry's nails, 277t
Testes, 772
  painless nodules in, 772
  small, 779t
  tumours of, 779t
  undescended, 725, 813t
  unexpected findings of, 779t
Testicular, 764
Testicular artery, 761
Testicular cancer, 772
Testicular self-examination, 766–767
Testosterone, 759
Tetralogy of Fallot, in infants, 809t
Thalamus, 685, 693
Thenar atrophy, 678t
Thenar space infection, 679t
Therapeutic relationship, 61–66, 62b
  active listening for, 62
  building, 61
  empathic responses and, 64
  empowering client and, 65–66, 66b
  guided questioning and, 62–63, 62b
  nonverbal communication and, 63–64
  partnering and, 65
  reassurance and, 65
  sexuality and, 79–80
  transitions and, 65
  validation and, 64
Thin patients, blood pressure measurement in,
    140
Third heart sound, in older adults, 893

Thoracic kyphosis, 641
Thoracohumeral muscle group, 628
Thorax. *See also* Chest *entries; specific organs*
  anatomic terms for locations on, 386
  anatomy and physiology of, 382–387
  anterior, examination of, 403–405
    auscultation in, 405
    inspection in, 403
    palpation in, 403–404
    percussion in, 404–405
  anterioposterior diameter of, 396
  deviations of, 417t
  documentation for, 406b
  examination techniques for, 395–405
    in older adults, 918
    during pregnancy, 874
  expansion of, testing, 397, 403
  in health history, 387–390, 387b
  initial survey of, 395–396
  locating findings on, 382–386
  in older adults, 892–893
  posterior, examination of, 396–403
    auscultation in, 400–403
    inspection in, 396
    palpation in, 396–397
    percussion in, 397–400
  during pregnancy, 874
  recording and analyzing findings for,
    405–407, 406b
Thought content, in mental status examina-
    tion, 218b
Thought processes
  content of, in mental status examination,
    225, 226b
  in general survey, 131
  in mental status examination, 218b, 225,
    226b
Thrills, 448–449
Throat. *See also* Pharynx
  documentation for, 362b–363b
  examination techniques for
    in older adults, 917–919
  strep (streptococcal pharyngitis), 351
Thromboangiitis obliterans, 586, 594t–595t
Thrombocytopenic purpura, skin in, 274t
Thrombophlebitis, superficial, 570, 585,
    594t–595t
Thrombosis, 575
  iliofemoral, 585
Thrush, 711
  palatal, 375t
Thumbs
  abduction of, carpal tunnel syndrome and,
    662
  opposition of, testing, 713
  range of motion and manoeuvers for, 636
Thyroid
  enlargement of, 298t
  during pregnancy, 857–873
  signs and symptoms of dysfunction of, 298t
  single nodules of, 298t
Thyroid cartilage, 281
Thyroid gland, 281
  examination techniques for, 288–290
  in older adults, 892
  during pregnancy, 852, 873
Thyroid health, 284–285

Valgus stress test, 657b
Validation, in interview, 64
Valsalva manoeuver
    to identify systolic murmurs, 460
Values, 78
Valves
    cardiac. *See* Heart valves
    venous, evaluating competency of, 588
Valves of Houston, 830
Varicella
    skin in, 274t
Varicocele, 781t
Varicose veins, 585
    mapping, 588
    during pregnancy, 879
    prevention, 574
    risk factor assessment, 574
    screening and maintenance, 574
    of tongue, 380t
Varus stress test, 657b–658b
Vascular changes in skin, during pregnancy, 856
Vascular disorders, in older adults, 901
Vascular lesions, of skin, 268t
Vas deferens, 760, 761
    infection of, 772
Vasectomy, 761
Vasodepressor syncope, 697, 741t
Vasomotor rhinitis, 350
Vasovagal syncope, 697
Veins. *See also specific veins*
    anatomy and physiology of, 565–566
    communicating (perforating), 565
    deep, 565, 566
    spider, 268t
    superficial, 565
    varicose, 585
        mapping, 588
        during pregnancy, 879
        of tongue, 380t
Vellus hair, 246
Venae cavae, 424, 425
Venereal warts, 832
    female, 821t
Venous compression, during pregnancy, 854
Venous hum, 478t
    abdominal, 558t
Venous insufficiency
    chronic, 585, 594t–595t, 596t, 597t, 599t
    stasis ulcer of, 267t
Venous peripheral vascular disease, 570
Venous stasis ulcers, 570
Venous valves, evaluating competency of, 588
Ventricular gallop, 473t
Ventricular impulses, variations and unexpected findings of, 469t
Ventricular premature contractions, 468t
Ventricular septal defect, 450, 474t
Vertebrae. *See also* Spine
    spinous processes of, 383, 638, 640
Vertebral arch, 638
Vertebral bodies, 638
Vertebral foramen, 638
Vertebral line, 384
Vertical inguinal lymph nodes, 567

Vertical nystagmus, 746t
Vertigo, 367t, 696
Vesicles, 264t, 271t, 272t
Vesicular breath sounds, 400, 401b
Vestibular function, assessment of, 707
Vestibular dysfunction, 354
Vestibular neuronitis, 367t
Vestibule, 342, 344, 358, 359, 785, 786
Vibration sense, 693
    assessment of, 722
    in older adults, 897
Viral exanthems, 274t
Viral meningitis, 702
Viral pneumonia, cough and hemoptysis in, 416t
Viral rhinitis, 359
Visceral pain, 514
Visceral tenderness, 559t, 560t
Visible minority, 33–35
Vision, in older adults, 891
    screening in older adults, 911
Visual acuity, 310
    assessment of, 705
    in older adults, 911
    of older adults, 891
Visual aura, with migraine, 282
Visual fields, 302–303
    assessment of, 705
    defects of, 326t
    testing, 311–312
Visual loss, 307–308
    emergency concerns, 309
    interviewing and, 71
    risk factor assessment, 308
    screening and maintenance, 309
    specific prevention for specific diseases, 308–309
Visual pathways, 303
Vital signs, 12, 129, 133. *See also* Blood pressure; Heart rate; Heart rhythms; Respiratory rate; Temperature, body
    blood pressure
        classification of, 139–140
        cuff, 135–136
        preparation for measuring, 136b–137b
        technique for measuring, 136, 137–139
    client, promotion of, 134
    comfort, 134
    dignity, 134
    documentation, 143
    equipment for, 134b
    examination techniques for, in older adults, 916
    in older adults, 888–889
    during pregnancy, 854, 854b, 873
    safety, 134
    sequence, 135
Vitamin B$_{12}$, 190
Vitamin D, 179, 185, 190, 610
Vitiligo, 259t
Vitreous body, 301, 302
Vitreous detachment, 306
Vitreous floaters, 306, 320
Vitreous hemorrhage, 306
Vocabulary, in mental status examination, 230

Voice
    assessment of, 705, 708
Voice sounds, transmitted, 402–403, 405, 418t
Volume overload, 432
Vomiting, 513
    during pregnancy, 859b, 873
von Recklinghausen's syndrome, skin in, 273t
Vulva, 785
    carcinoma of, 821t
    lesions of, 821t
Vulvovaginal symptoms, 793

W

Waist circumference, 176
Warmth, musculoskeletal, 618
Warts
    genital, 832
        female, 821t
        in males, 777t
    plantar, 681t
Weakness, 696–697
Weaver's bottom, 648
Weber test, 358
Weight, 174–175
    in general survey, 132
    measurement of, in older adults, 916
    during pregnancy, 873
Weight gain, 513
    during pregnancy, 177–178
    symptom analysis and, 172
Weight loss, 513
    after pregnancy, 178
    during pregnancy, 859b
    symptoms and signs of pregnancy, 859b
Wharton's ducts, 347
Wheals, 264t, 272t
Wheezes, 402, 402b, 419t
Wheezing, 390, 396
Whispered pectoriloquy, 403
White lines, transverse, on nails, 278t
White matter, 685
White spots, on nails, 278t
Workplace substances, effect on pregnancy and fetus, 851
Wrists, 630–637
    bony structures of, 631
    examination techniques for, 632–636
        inspection and, 632–633
        palpation as, 633–634
        range of motion and manoeuvers as, 634–636
    extension at, testing, 712
    joints of, 631
    muscle groups of, 631–632

X

Xanthelasma, 328t
Xerostomia, 892
Xiphoid process, 511

Z

Zinc, 190
Zygomatic bone, 279, 299